PRINCIPLES of EXERCISE TESTING & INTERPRETATION
INCLUDING PATHOPHYSIOLOGY AND CLINICAL APPLICATIONS   Third Edition

PRINCIPLES of EXERCISE TESTING & INTERPRETATION

INCLUDING PATHOPHYSIOLOGY AND CLINICAL APPLICATIONS

Third Edition

KARLMAN WASSERMAN, MD, PhD
Professor of Medicine, UCLA School of Medicine
Division of Respiratory and Critical Care Physiology and Medicine
Department of Medicine
Harbor-UCLA Medical Center
Torrance, California

JAMES E. HANSEN, MD
Professor of Medicine, UCLA School of Medicine
Division of Respiratory and Critical Care Physiology and Medicine
Department of Medicine
Harbor-UCLA Medical Center
Torrance, California

DARRYL Y. SUE, MD
Professor of Medicine, UCLA School of Medicine
Division of Respiratory and Critical Care
Physiology of Medicine
Department of Medicine
Harbor-UCLA Medical Center
Torrance, California

RICHARD CASABURI, PhD, MD
Professor of Medicine, UCLA School of Medicine
Chief, Division of Respiratory and Critical Care Physiology and Medicine
Department of Medicine
Harbor-UCLA Medical Center
Torrance, California

BRIAN J. WHIPP, PhD, DSc
Professor, Department of Physiology
St. George's Hospital Medical School
London, England

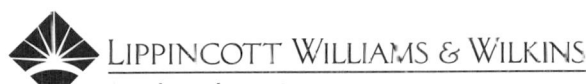
LIPPINCOTT WILLIAMS & WILKINS
A **Wolters Kluwer** Company

Philadelphia • Baltimore • New York • London
Buenos Aires • Hong Kong • Sydney • Tokyo

Editor: Ruth Weinberg
Development Editor: Raymond E. Reter
Marketing Manager: Melissa Harris

Copyright © 1999 Lippincott Williams & Wilkins

351 West Camden Street
Baltimore, Maryland 21201–2436 USA

Printed in the United States of America
First Edition, 1987
Second Edition, 1994

Library of Congress Cataloging-in-Publication Data

Principles of exercise testing and interpretation/Karlman Wasserman...[et al.].—3rd ed.
    p.   cm.
  Includes bibliographical references and index.
  ISBN 0-683-30646-4
  1. Exercise tests.   2. Heart function tests.   3. Pulmonary function tests. I. Wasserman, Karlman. II. Wasserman, Karlman.
    [DNLM: 1. Exercise Test. 2. Exertion—physiology. 3. Exercise Test. 4. Exertion—physiology. WG 141.5.F9 P957 1999]
  RC683.5.E94P75   1999
  616.07′5—dc21
  DNLM/DLC
  for Library of Congress   98-43362
                                                                             CIP

To purchase additional copies of this book, call our customer service department at **(800) 638–0672** or fax orders to **(800) 447–8438.** For other book services, including chapter reprints and large quantity sales, ask for the Special Sales department.

Canadian customers should call **(800) 665–1148**, or fax **(800) 665–0103.** For all other calls originating outside of the United States, please call **(410) 528–4223** or fax us at **(410) 528–8550.**

99 00 01 02 03
2 3 4 5 6 7 8 9 10

Dedicated to our families

Preface

The third edition of *Principles of Exercise Testing and Interpretation* was prepared to update the monograph on important advances, made since the preparation of the second edition, on the physiology and pathophysiology of exercise performance. It was also stimulated by an increased appreciation of the wide application of cardiopulmonary exercise testing in the diagnosis of disease and also its contribution to decision making in the management of patients. A new chapter has been added to the monograph to describe the latter applications.

The most important requirement for exercise performance is transport of oxygen to support the bioenergetic processes in the muscle cells (including, of course, the heart) and elimination of the carbon dioxide formed as a by-product of exercise metabolism. Thus, an appropriate cardiovascular and respiratory response is required to match the muscle energy requirement. Appropriate treatment requires that patient symptoms be thought of in terms of a defect in the gas exchange between the cell and the environment. The defect may be in the lungs, heart, peripheral or pulmonary circulations, the muscles themselves, or there may be a combination of defects. This book describes the pathophysiology in gas transport resulting from diseases affecting each site in the cardiorespiratory coupling mechanism, and illustrates how the functional competency of each component can be evaluated by cardiopulmonary exercise testing.

Often, the treatment of patients with exercise intolerance induced by fatigue or dyspnea is not focused because indirect diagnostic approaches are used. However these symptoms occurring at unusually low levels of exercise can usually be traced to abnormal gas exchange between the atmosphere and the mitochondria in response to exercise. By measuring gas exchange during cardiopulmonary exercise tests, not only can the exercise limitation be quantified, but also the functional adequacy of the heart, circulatory systems and lungs can be assessed simultaneously. Fortunately, this assessment can usually be non-invasive.

The gas exchange responses to exercise are likely to indicate to the physician which organ(s) are functioning poorly and which are functioning well. The pattern of the gas exchange response has been found in most instances to be characteristic of the disease process. For instance, cardiopulmonary exercise testing might not only detect cardiovascular limitation but could be used to distinguish which cardiovascular disease is restricting the patient's exercise performance, e.g., coronary artery disease, chronic heart failure or peripheral vascular disease. In addition, it is likely that no test in medicine can quantify improvement in organ function leading to increased exercise tolerance better than cardiopulmonary exercise testing. As a referral center for problematic cases, we are often impressed with the revelations of pathophysiology provided by cardiopulmonary exercise testing.

This book describes how to evaluate the patient with exercise intolerance using the physiology and pathophysiology of exercise gas exchange as frames of reference. The absence of detailed electrocardiographic displays in this book should not be interpreted to mean that the authors do not regard the electrocardiogram as an essential component of exercise tests. On the contrary, we routinely record and analyze a 12 lead ECG throughout the exercise. Because many other sources are available for interpreting the exercise electrocardiogram, we provide only the interpretation of the records rather than presenting the ECG records themselves.

As important background chapters to the interpretation of exercise tests, we again devote the first two chapters to bioenergetic and physiological principles underpinning exercise performance. In the third chapter, we apply this knowledge to specific variables that detect abnormalities in function during exercise. The fourth chapter describes the pathophysiology of exercise limitation caused by diseases of the cardiovascular, respiratory, musculoskeletal and other systems. The next chapter proceeds to describe how to prepare the patient for and perform a cardiopulmonary exercise test. Chapter six provides an analysis of normal values. Next is a chapter that presents an interpretive method using flow charts with which the large amount of data derived from a cardiopulmonary exercise test can be used for making specific diagnoses. Chapter eight describes many applications of cardiopulmonary exercise testing that have largely become apparent since the preparation of the second edition. Importantly it describes certain clinical diagnoses that can only be made by cardiopulmonary exercise testing. The final chapter consists of studies performed on 84 patients. Each case, illustrating common and not so common disorders, was selected to make a teaching point in pathophysiology. In this respect, this chapter serves as an atlas of disorders that result in exercise limitation.

Detailed practical information is provided in the Appendix to assist the reader in setting up a laboratory, testing the subject, and making necessary calculations. Although this is of special importance to anyone wishing to establish a laboratory, we believe that this information is very helpful to the interpreter's understanding of the technical aspects of the measurements and calculations.

This book is therefore designed to help cardiologists, pulmonologists and exercise physiologists keep pace with the expanding knowledge gained from computerized measurements of gas exchange during exercise. It serves as a guide for those who wish to use exercise testing to: 1) diagnose the pathophysiology of exercise limitation; 2) evaluate the severity of a patient's pathophysiology; 3) evaluate the effect of medical or surgical therapy; and 4) provide a physiological basis for training strategies for patient rehabilitation or athletic performance. This book spans the field of "exercise," from basic concepts in exercise physiology to a meaningful report. In summary, our goal was to write a comprehensive and practical book for physiologists, physicians, cardiologists, pulmonologists, and technicians interested in exercise physiology, pathophysiology, and testing.

KARLMAN WASSERMAN
JAMES E. HANSEN
DARRYL Y. SUE
RICHARD CASABURI
BRIAN J. WHIPP

Torrance, California

Acknowledgments

We are indebted to our colleagues, our former fellows, and the many physicians and scientists who have participated in our semi-annual postgraduate course (practicum) in Exercise Testing and Interpretation, for which the two prior editions served as a syllabus. This third edition, like the second, was stimulated by the many useful discussions we have had with our students, as well as knowledge gained from recent research. We hope that continuing discussions of these kinds will not only benefit our search for a better understanding of exercise physiology and pathophysiology, but also help to close the gap between physiologic knowledge and the application of cardiopulmonary exercise testing.

K.W. is especially indebted to his wife, Gail, for tolerating his diversions during innumerable evenings and weekends in his effort to see this book reach fruition.

K. W.
J.E.H.
D.Y.S.
R.C.
B.J.W.

Contents

4. Pathophysiology of Disorders Limiting Exercise 95

5. Clinical Exercise Testing 115

6. Normal Values 143

7. Principles of Interpretation: A Flow Chart Approach 165

8. Clinical Applications of Cardiopulmonary Exercise Testing 178

9. Case Presentations 215

CHAPTER 1

Exercise Testing and Interpretation: An Overview

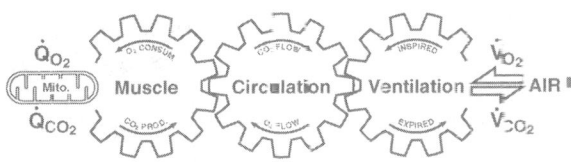

PHYSICAL EXERCISE requires the interaction of physiological mechanisms that enable the cardiovascular and respiratory systems to support the increased energy demands of contracting muscles. The responses of each system must be coupled to cell respiration and to each other (Fig. 1.1) to preserve the state of the internal environment, i.e., maintain homeostasis. Both systems are consequently stressed during exercise. Their abilities to respond adequately to this stress is a measure of their functional competence or "health."

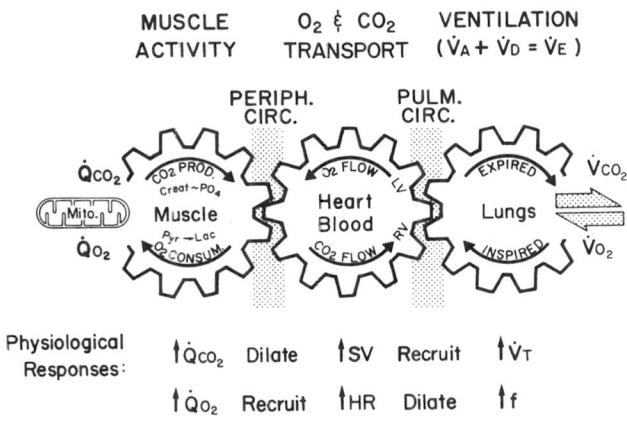

FIGURE 1.1.   Gas transport mechanisms for coupling cellular (internal) to pulmonary (external) respiration. The gears represent the functional interdependence of the physiological components of the system. The large increase in O_2 utilization by the muscles ($\dot{Q}O_2$) is achieved by increased extraction of O_2 from the blood perfusing the muscles, the dilatation of selected peripheral vascular beds, an increase in cardiac output (stroke volume and heart rate), an increase in pulmonary blood flow by recruitment and vasodilatation of pulmonary blood vessels, and finally, an increase in ventilation. O_2 is taken up ($\dot{V}O_2$) from the alveoli in proportion to the pulmonary blood flow and degree of O_2 desaturation of hemoglobin in the pulmonary capillary blood. In the steady-state, $\dot{V}O_2 = \dot{Q}O_2$. Ventilation (tidal volume (V_T) × breathing frequency (f)) increases in relation to the newly produced CO_2 ($\dot{Q}CO_2$) arriving at the lungs and the drive to achieve arterial CO_2 and hydrogen ion homeostasis. These variables are related in the following way:

$$\dot{V}CO_2 = \dot{V}_A \times P_{ACO_2}/P_B$$

where: $\dot{V}CO_2$ = minute CO_2 output, $\dot{V}_A$ = minute alveolar ventilation, P_{ACO_2} = arterial CO_2 tension, and P_B = barometric pressure.

The representation of gears uniformly sized is not intended to imply equal changes in each of the components of the coupling. For instance, the increase in cardiac output is relatively small for the increase in metabolic rate. This implies an increased extraction of O_2 from and CO_2 loading into the blood by the muscles. In contrast, at moderate work intensities, minute ventilation increases in approximate proportion to the new CO_2 brought to the lungs by the venous return. The development of metabolic acidosis at heavy and very heavy work intensities accelerates the increase in ventilation to provide respiratory compensation for the metabolic acidosis.

WHY MEASURE GAS EXCHANGE TO EVALUATE CARDIOVASCULAR FUNCTION AND CELLULAR RESPIRATION?

Exercise testing offers the investigator the unique opportunity to study simultaneously the cellular, cardiovascular, and ventilatory systems' responses under conditions of precisely controlled metabolic stress. Exercise tests in which gas exchange is not determined cannot realistically evaluate the ability of the cardiovascular and ventilatory systems to perform their common major function, i.e., gas exchange with cells. But, in addition, exercise testing with appropriate gas exchange measurements can also serve to grade the adequacy of cardiorespiratory function. This is of significant practical importance because cardiopulmonary exercise testing, in which gas exchange is measured, provides what is probably the most sensitive assessment of the effect of new therapy on function of any diseased organ system whose major function is to couple pulmonary gas exchange to cellular respiration. For example, it is important to determine whether new medical, surgical, and rehabilitative procedures can effectively intervene to improve the gas transport capability of a diseased organ system.

Making the correct diagnosis is essential to rational treatment of exercise limitation. Cardiopulmonary exercise testing is actually one of the most inexpensive ways of diagnosing the pathophysiology of the cardiovascular and ventilatory systems because, in contrast to other diagnostic tests that evaluate one organ system, cardiopulmonary exercise testing evaluates all of the organ systems essential for exercise, simultaneously. An exercise test that restricts its measurements to the electrocardiogram can only support a diagnosis of myocardial ischemia. However, an individual patient may have mixed defects (e.g., cardiac and pulmonary). Consequently it is often necessary to determine the relative contribution of each to the patient's symptoms before embarking on major therapeutic procedures directed at either one (1).

CARDIAC STRESS TEST AND PULMONARY STRESS TEST: NOMENCLATURE FALLACIES

The authors would like to dispel a concept that has developed in medicine, i.e., that there is *cardiac stress testing* and *pulmonary stress testing*. It is impossible to stress only the heart or only the lungs. Exercise requires the coordinated function of the heart, the lungs, and the peripheral and the pulmonary circulations to match the increased cellular respiration required to live and work. The major function of the cardiovascular as well as the ventilatory system is to support cellular respiration. Diseases of the heart cause both abnormal breathing and gas exchange responses to exercise as do many disorders of the lungs.

Abnormalities of the heart might cause "pulmonary symptoms" with abnormalities in lung gas exchange during exercise (2–5). Similarly, pulmonary disorders might result primarily in abnormalities in cardiovascular responses to exercise (6, 7). Although the cardiovascular and pulmonary gas exchange responses to exercise tend to be relatively uniform and predictable in normal subjects, different diseases affect the responses in specific ways depending on the disease pathophysiology. Thus the knowledgeable examiner can not only detect abnormality but can often define the disease process. Therefore, gas exchange measurements are important components of an exercise test designed to diagnose specific pathophysiology involving the cardiovascular or ventilatory systems. Because cardiopulmonary exercise testing is quantitative, it allows the severity of dysfunction to be graded.

CELL RESPIRATION AND BIOENERGETICS

The most immediate requirement of exercise is the release of the energy of the terminal phosphate bond of adenosine triphosphate (ATP) to fuel the contractile and related demands of the muscle at a rate commensurate with that required to perform the task. The bioenergetic process for the ATP generation in the muscle is achieved by three mechanisms (Fig. 1.2): the aerobic oxidation of substrates (primarily glycogen and fatty acids), the anaerobic

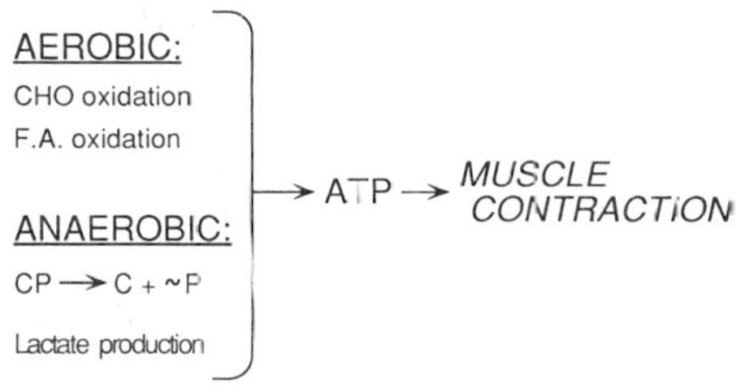

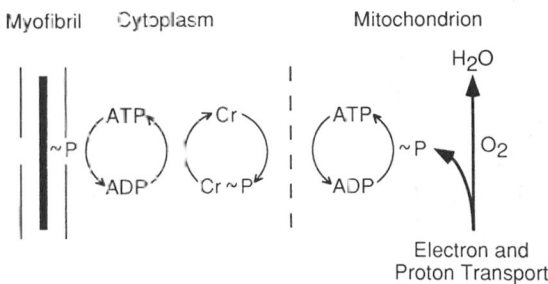

FIGURE 1.3.   Scheme by which phosphocreatine (creatine phosphate, $Cr \sim P$) supplies high energy phosphate ($\sim P$) to adenosine diphosphate (ADP) at the myofibril. Because of its quantity in muscle, $Cr \sim P$ serves as a reservoir of readily available $\sim P$ as well as a shuttle mechanism to translocate $\sim P$ from mitochondria to the myofibril contractile sites.

hydrolysis of phosphocreatine (PCr), and the breakdown of glycogen or glucose to lactic acid. Each is critically important for a normal exercise response, and each plays a different role in the total bioenergetic response. For instance, the aerobic oxidation of carbohydrate and fatty acids provides the major source of ATP production, and becomes the only source during sustained exercise of moderate intensity. This mechanism is naturally dependent on an adequate response of the cardiorespiratory system so that the O_2 supply to the cells is adequate to regenerate, aerobically, all the ATP needed for the activity. On the other hand, local stores of PCr provide most of the high energy phosphate needed in the early phase of exercise. PCr is quickly hydrolyzed by creatine kinase to creatine and inorganic phosphate (Pi). The energy released in this reaction can be used to regenerate ATP from adenosine diphosphate (ADP) and Pi at the myofibril (Fig. 1.3). This reaction is essential because the O_2 reserves in the muscle, and blood in the immediate vicinity of the muscle at the start of exercise, are relatively small. Thus PCr serves as an immediate source of ATP regeneration. But in addition, it is also intimately linked to the control of O_2 utilization so the profile of change of PCr is often considered to be a proxy variable for that of muscle O_2 consumption (8–10).

If the exercise is too heavy for the energy needs of the cell to be met entirely by O_2 and PCr-linked energy generation, then another source of ATP contributes. Anaerobic glycolysis produces ATP from glucose or glycogen without the need for O_2, but with the production of lactic acid. The lactic acid is produced by reduction of pyruvate, the latter taking place to replenish the oxidized form of the cytosolic co-enzyme, nicotinamide adenine dinucleotide (NAD^+), when the coenzyme shifts to a more re-

FIGURE 1.2.   Sources of adenosine triphosphate (ATP) regeneration.

duced state ($NADH+H^+$). Thus pyruvate serves as the oxidant to regenerate NAD^+ when the cell becomes critically O_2–poor. This reaction is required for glycolysis to proceed. The energy produced by anaerobic glycolysis is relatively small for the amount of glycogen and glucose consumed, and the consequence of lactate accumulation has important implications with respect to gas exchange which will be described in the next chapter.

Gas exchange (O_2 consumption and CO_2 production) is affected in a different way by each of the three sources of ATP. For instance, when the regeneration of ATP is aerobic, O_2 is consumed and CO_2 is produced in proportion to the ratio of carbohydrate to fatty acid in the substrate being oxidized in the muscle cells. On the other hand, when PCr is split, it is converted to creatine (Cr) and Pi. Because Cr is neutral in water while PCr reacts like a relatively strong acid, the hydrolysis of PCr decreases cell acidity. This reaction therefore retains CO_2 in the tissues as HCO_3^- and reduces net CO_2 output produced by aerobic metabolism. Finally when high energy phosphate is generated from anaerobic glycolysis, the H^+ produced with lactate is buffered primarily by HCO_3^-, thereby adding CO_2 to that produced by aerobic processes.

Because these different mechanisms of ATP regeneration have different effects on gas exchange, study of the gas exchange responses to exercise can reveal information on the relative contributions of aerobic respiration, PCr hydrolysis, and anaerobic glycolysis to the total bioenergetic response.

The purpose of this monograph is to present recent advances in our understanding of normal gas transport and related mechanisms that support the increased muscle respiration needed to perform exercise. It also describes the abnormal gas exchange responses that characterize the many pathophysiological states that cause patients to suffer from exercise intolerance.

NORMAL COUPLING OF EXTERNAL TO CELLULAR RESPIRATION

Figure 1.1 schematizes the coupling of pulmonary to cellular respiration by the circulation. Obviously, the circulation must increase at a rate which is adequate for O_2 supply to the cells. In fact, cardiac output increases in proportion to the metabolic rate in normal subjects, approximately 6 liters per minute of cardiac output per liter per minute of O_2 consumption (11). Since 5 liters of blood contain slightly less than 1 liter of O_2, the normal circulatory re-

sponse seems to be sufficient to provide enough O_2 to the contractile units to meet their requirement and a little more. In other words, O_2 is not completely extracted from the muscle blood flow, and an O_2 diffusion gradient is maintained between the end-capillary blood and myocyte. Disease of the cardiovascular system is often characterized by the failure of O_2 uptake to increase at a rate appropriate for the work rate increase (13, 14). This phenomenon is accompanied by a lactic acidosis.

Because the total H^+ in the body is only on the order of 3.4 micromoles, and the total H^+ equivalent produced per minute from metabolism in the form of CO_2, even for moderate speed walking, is about 40,000 micromoles per minute, elimination of the increased CO_2 must be accomplished quickly and precisely. Therefore, to regulate arterial pH closely, ventilation must be closely linked to CO_2 production during exercise. Even a small failure of the ventilatory system to keep pace with the rate of CO_2 generated from aerobic metabolism will cause a respiratory acidosis. Ventilation must increase more when a lactic acidosis is superimposed on the respiratory acid (CO_2) load. Thus, exercise work rates producing a lactic acidosis cause a marked increase in the ventilatory response (15). Furthermore, failure to accelerate ventilation to achieve ventilatory compensation for the exercise-induced lactic acidosis will cause a pronounced reduction in arterial pH (16).

QUANTIFYING STATE AND TIME COURSE OF CELLULAR RESPIRATION FROM MEASUREMENTS OF EXTERNAL RESPIRATION

Physical activity is a major challenge to homeostasis of the cellular environment. Walking at a pace of 3 MPH requires a 16- to 20-fold increase in O_2 consumption of the muscles of locomotion. The rate of acid production, in the form of CO_2, increases by a like amount. Despite these major rapid changes in cellular respiration, external respiration is normally able to increase with almost equal rapidity and with such precision that the blood is rearterialized with no, or only minor, changes in PO_2, PCO_2, and pH. Thus, blood recirculates to the highly metabolic muscle in virtually the same aerated and acid-base state as existed at rest (17–20). The normal subject is able to perform level walking, at typical rates of ambulation, without developing a metabolic acidosis (17, 19). This is because the response of the transport systems (Fig. 1.1) can increase the rate of O_2 delivery to meet all of the energy requirements of the muscles aerobically within 3 minutes of starting exercise. Thus, by 3 minutes, the $\dot{V}O_2$ achieves a constant or steady-state value. It is during this early exercise period, while $\dot{V}O_2$ is increasing (i.e., the period of the O_2 deficit), that ATP derived from PCr hydrolysis and aerobic oxidation of substrate from O_2 stores (evidenced by venous hemoglobin and possibly local myoglobin desaturation) make their contribution to the exercise bioenergetics.

The patterns of $\dot{V}O_2$ and $\dot{V}CO_2$ kinetics are characteristic, but different, for work rates without or with a lactic acidosis (i.e., below and above the subject's anaerobic threshold, AT) as shown on the right side of Figure 1.4. At the start of upright exercise, there is an immediate increase in both $\dot{V}O_2$ and $\dot{V}CO_2$, the increases last about 15 seconds (Fig. 1.4). These increases have been attributed to the rapid increase in pulmonary blood flow that accompanies the immediate increase in both stroke volume and heart rate at the start of exercise (21). The subsequent increases in $\dot{V}O_2$ and $\dot{V}CO_2$ depend on the rate of hydrolysis of PCr, the aerobic rephosphorylation of ADP to ATP (Fig. 1.2), and the change in O_2 stores, primarily in the venous circulation. In the steady state, the O_2 stores are reduced, but constant, and no longer contribute to ATP regeneration. PCr also decreases to a constant level within 2 to 3 minutes of exercise (8), indicating that it, too, no longer contributes to ATP regeneration. The level of ATP in muscle remains essentially constant until $\dot{V}O_2$ increases to levels approaching $\dot{V}O_2$max (22), reflecting the ability of these mechanisms to regenerate ATP at a sufficient rate to match the rate of ATP utilization.

Because of the precise quantitative relationship between the O_2 consumed in the muscle and high energy phosphate ($\sim$P) produced (23), and the features of the O_2 stores utilization, the time course of the changes in $\dot{V}O_2$ is thought to closely reflect the rate of aerobic $\sim$P regeneration (24). Although the initial changes in $\dot{V}CO_2$ are similar to those of $\dot{V}O_2$ in the first 15 sec of exercise, $\dot{V}CO_2$ subsequently rises more slowly than $\dot{V}O_2$ to steady state because of an increase in CO_2 stores during this early exercise period. The changes in intracellular pH associated with PCr hydrolysis and the Haldane effect (CO_2 stored as carbamate in proportion to the degree of oxyhemoglobin desaturation) as O_2 extraction increases during early exercise, in addition to the increasing tissue PCO_2, contribute to this early increase in CO_2 stores.

In the steady-state of exercise below the AT, $\dot{V}CO_2$ typically remains below $\dot{V}O_2$ because metabolism is

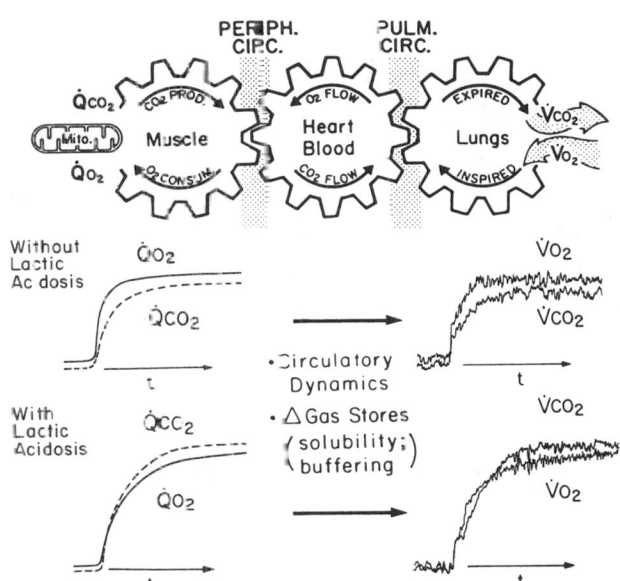

FIGURE 1.4.   Scheme of coupling of external to cellular respiration. Right side of figure shows breath-by-breath data for 6 minutes of constant work rate exercise for work with and without lactic acidosis. Each study is an overlay of four repetitions to reduce random noise in the data and enhance the physiological features. Measurements of external respiration (right) can be used as a basis for reconstructing the changes in muscle cellular respiration. The left side of the figure schematically shows the changes in muscle cellular respiration that would account for the observed changes in external respiration. The factors that modulate the relationship between cellular respiration and external respiration are shown in the center. At the start of exercise there is normally a step increase in both $\dot{V}O_2$ and $\dot{V}CO_2$ consequent to the abrupt increase in pulmonary blood flow due to an immediate increase in heart rate and stroke volume. After an approximate 15-second "delay," $\dot{V}O_2$ and $\dot{V}CO_2$ increase further, when venous blood formed after exercise started arrives at the lungs, albeit with $\dot{V}CO_2$ increasing more slowly than $\dot{V}O_2$. The slower rise in $\dot{V}CO_2$ than $\dot{V}O_2$, for exercise capable of being performed without a lactic acidosis, is accounted for by chemical reactions in the tissues which store some of the metabolic CO_2. For work rates without a lactic acidosis, $\dot{V}O_2$ reaches a steady-state by 3 minutes and $\dot{V}CO_2$ by 4 minutes. For work rates with a lactic acidosis, $\dot{V}O_2$ does not reach a steady-state by 3 minutes and may not reach a steady-state before the subject fatigues. In contrast, $\dot{V}CO_2$ kinetics remain relatively unchanged with the level of $\dot{V}CO_2$ exceeding $\dot{V}O_2$ after the first several minutes of heavy intensity exercise (see text for discussion of mechanisms).

solely aerobic. The ratio of increase in $\dot{V}CO_2$ relative to $\dot{V}O_2$ in the steady-state should define the respiratory quotient (RQ) of the muscle substrate. When $\dot{V}O_2$ does not achieve a steady state by 3 minutes, as illustrated by the measurements shown on the lower right of Figure 1.4, lactate increases in the body, i.e, the work rate is above the subject's AT, and a number of physiological and biochemical processes are not in a steady state including: arterial HCO_3^- and H^+ concentrations; ventilation; and heart rate. $\dot{V}CO_2$ increases relative to $\dot{V}O_2$ when lactate increases because HCO_3^- is the principal buffer of the newly formed lactic acid; 22.3 ml of CO_2 are released for each mmol of HCO_3^- buffering lactic acid (derived from Avogadro's number whereby 1 mole or 6.02×10^{23} molecules of CO_2 occupies 22.3L under standard conditions). Consequently, $\dot{V}CO_2$ rises to a level higher than $\dot{V}O_2$. In contrast to the slowing of $\dot{V}O_2$ kinetics for above AT exercise, the $\dot{V}CO_2$ kinetics are similar for work rates below and above the AT (25). The reason for this is that the total $\dot{V}CO_2$ is the sum of the CO_2 produced by aerobic metabolism plus that produced when HCO_3^- buffers an increasing lactic acid concentration and a relatively small amount of CO_2 exhaled depending on the degree of hyperventilation in response to the lactic acidosis. If the work rate is not too high above the AT, $\dot{V}O_2$ may reach a constant value before the subject fatigues. Otherwise, $\dot{V}O_2$ progressively increases until the subject is forced to stop from fatigue.

PATTERNS OF CHANGE IN EXTERNAL RESPIRATION (O_2 UPTAKE AND CO_2 OUTPUT) AS RELATED TO FUNCTION, FITNESS, AND DISEASE

This book is devoted largely to describing patterns of gas exchange that relate to function, fitness and disease states, and it should be acknowledged that the increases in external respiration ($\dot{V}O_2$ and $\dot{V}CO_2$) needed for exercise are intimately and predictably linked to the increases in cellular respiration. The linkage is through the circulation. The contribution of aerobic and anaerobic metabolism can often be inferred from measurements of external respiration. For example, gas exchange kinetics differ in response to exercise depending on whether work is performed above or below the AT (Fig. 1.4). For work rates at which a lactic acidosis develops, the O_2 supply is probably inadequate to meet the total O_2 need of all the contracting units. Therefore, $\dot{V}O_2$ increase is slow, with the slow component in $\dot{V}O_2$ being a marker of increased anaerobiosis. There is an accompanying increase in $\dot{V}CO_2$ in excess of $\dot{V}O_2$ due to the CO_2 release from bicarbonate as it buffers lactic acid. In contrast, when work is done in a true steady-state in which all the O_2 required by the muscle is provided to and utilized by the muscle, the $\dot{V}O_2$ increases rapidly and no lactic acidosis develops.

Individuals who are highly fit for endurance work do not develop a lactic acidosis until work rates become high. Their $\dot{V}O_2$ kinetics are relatively rapid compared with less fit subjects. However, patients with circulatory disorders usually have slow $\dot{V}O_2$ kinetics, even at relatively low work rates. Thus the difference between the steady-state $\dot{V}O_2$ requirement and the actual $\dot{V}O_2$ during the transition from rest to exercise, the O_2 deficit, varies depending on fitness for aerobic work. The O_2 deficit is made up of O_2 equivalents from the energy generated when phosphocreatine hydrolyzes, O_2 from the venous pool as O_2 extraction increases, a small amount of O_2 from myoglobin as muscle PO_2 decreases, and for work above the anaerobic threshold, anaerobic glycolysis. The amounts from each depend on the relative intensity of the exercise for the subject. The mechanisms and the components contributing to the O_2 deficit will be discussed in greater detail in Chapter 2.

FACTORS LIMITING EXERCISE

Symptoms that stop people from performing exercise are fatigue, dyspnea, or pain (angina or claudication). By observing external respiration during a quantitative exercise test in which large muscle groups are stressed (walking, running or cycling), it can be determined whether exercise tolerance is reduced and, if so, whether abnormal cardiovascular and/or ventilatory responses to exercise account for the reduction.

Fatigue

During large muscle group exercise, fatigue will occur relatively early when the O_2 requirement of the contracting muscles is not met by the O_2 transport system. A number of investigators (13, 14, 26) have measured $\dot{V}O_2$ during submaximal work rate exercise in both patients with heart failure and normal subjects. $\dot{V}O_2$, and therefore aerobic ATP production, was reduced below the expected value in heart failure patients at the symptom limiting work rate. The more severely impaired the patient, the greater was the reduction. Because aerobic ATP production is below that required, the muscles do not have the chemical energy to contract when anaerobic mechanisms become exhausted, i.e., muscle fatigue.

The exact mechanisms of muscle fatigue remain a topic of debate. Because lactic acidosis accompanies an increased rate of anaerobic ATP production, it is tempting to attribute the fatigue to the intracellular consequences of the exercise lactic acidosis. Low cellular pH, increased inorganic phosphate, impaired calcium release from the sarcoplasmic reticulum, and decreased levels of ATP have also been proposed as mediators of fatigue. However, regardless of the proximate mechanisms, the consistent physiological signal for impending fatigue during exercise is the failure for $\dot{V}O_2$ to reach a steady-state and thereby meet the cellular O_2 requirement.

Dyspnea

The symptom of dyspnea is a common abnormal consequence of exercise. It occurs in patients in whom the ventilation is relatively ineffective, such as in patients with a high fraction of the breath which is physiological dead space (low gas exchange efficiency), and in those with hypoxemia, metabolic acidosis or impaired ventilatory mechanics.

The ventilatory control system determines the exercise ventilation through its role in the regulation of arterial pH during exercise and as a compensating mechanism for hypoxemia—should it occur. If the CO_2 generated during aerobic ATP regeneration is not excreted by the lungs as quickly as it is added to the circulation, arterial H^+ increases due to the reaction of CO_2 with water to yield carbonic acid. An additional source of H^+ at work rates above the *AT* is that produced from lactic acid. Since HCO_3^- is the major buffer in acute acid-base disturbances, CO_2 production increases as HCO_3^- buffers lactic acid. The buffer CO_2 load, added to the aerobic CO_2 production, results in a disproportionate increase in H^+ with respect to the increase in $\dot{V}O_2$ or work rate. The resultant H^+ stimulus is a major cause of increased ventilation during exercise and is a contributor to dyspnea.

Normal sedentary subjects usually experience fatigue rather than dyspnea as their limiting symptom during exercise involving large muscle groups. Three types of normal subjects, however, seem to be prone to experience dyspnea, a limiting factor to exercise. Females may report dyspnea with exertion when performing the same work rate as a male who is asymptomatic. This is because they characteristically have about 2/3 of the ventilatory capacity of males of the same height; thus women use a larger proportion of their ventilatory capacity for the same level of exercise when compared to men of the same size. Also, because of the reduction in maximal ventilatory capacity with aging, normal elderly people may experience exertional dyspnea at maximum exercise rather than fatigue. Finally, some athletes with very high aerobic capacity may produce enough CO_2 combined with a high rate of accumu-

lation of lactic acid to become limited by their ventilatory capacity.

Pain

Pain in the chest or other related areas is the most common symptom of patients with coronary artery disease. This is a reflection of an inadequate O_2 supply to the myocardium relative to the myocardial O_2 demand. Reducing the O_2 demand by decreasing myocardial work or increasing myocardial O_2 supply can eliminate anginal pain. Reducing O_2 demand, however, may necessitate a reduced maximal work capacity. That is, the patient may be forced to trade a less active life style for relief of angina.

Claudication occurs because of an O_2 supply/demand imbalance in the muscles of the exercising extremity. Because walking at a normal pace requires an increase in O_2 utilization by the muscles of locomotion of approximately 20-fold, the ability to increase blood flow to the lower extremities is critically important to be able to walk without pain. If atherosclerotic changes in the conducting vessels to the lower extremity limit the increase in leg blood flow, an O_2 supply/demand imbalance will result. This will result in slowed O_2 uptake kinetics (27), and critically low levels of O_2 tension in the muscles (28) and leg pain.

EVIDENCE OF SYSTEMIC DYSFUNCTION UNIQUELY REVEALED BY INTEGRATIVE CARDIOPULMONARY EXERCISE TESTING

Obligatory changes in exercise gas exchange occur when diseases of the cardiovascular and/or ventilatory systems affect function. The gas exchange responses to exercise are likely to indicate to the physician which organ(s) is functioning poorly and which is functioning well.

Chapter 8 describes pathophysiological diagnoses uniquely made as a result of cardiopulmonary exercise testing. For example, cardiopulmonary exercise testing might not only distinguish between lung and cardiovascular disease, but it may be used to distinguish one cardiovascular disease from another as the cause of exercise limitation. For instance, coronary artery disease, chronic heart failure, and peripheral vascular disease may be distinguished by the pattern of abnormal gas exchange response to exercise (29). Measuring gas exchange during an exercise test may also increase the information that can be obtained from an ECG-positive test because the gas exchange measurements can confirm ischemia-induced left ventricular dysfunction during exercise and the precise metabolic rate at which the ischemia and dysfunction take place. Further, it is unlikely that there is any test in medicine, short of a lung biopsy, that will identify the pulmonary vasculopathy that might lead to primary pulmonary hypertension earlier than cardiopulmonary exercise testing.

Because about 25% of the population has a potentially patent foramen ovale, if these individuals develop primary or secondary pulmonary vascular disease, they might develop a transient right-to-left shunt during exercise. The development of a shunt depends on conditions in which right atrial pressure increases above left atrial pressure. This is more likely to take place during exercise than when the subject is at rest. Currently, vascular indicators are injected in the venous circulation and imaging is used to detect the test agent in the left side of the circulation. This is usually done at rest, when the right atrial pressure may not be great enough to shunt blood right to left. Thus, relatively expensive and invasive technology is being used under unfavorable conditions for making a diagnosis of pathophysiology that exists primarily under conditions of exercise. By measuring gas exchange during exercise, in addition to evaluating the functional capacity of the cardiovascular and ventilatory systems, a right-to-left shunt could be detected (without additional cost) because of the unique gas exchange response that takes place when part of the venous return bypasses the lungs. For greater sensitivity of detection, performing the exercise test while breathing 100% O_2 and measuring Pa_{O_2}, allows a right-to-left shunt of even less than 5% to be detected. These are just a few examples of diagnoses uniquely made by cardiopulmonary exercise testing. Others will be presented in the chapter on "Applications."

The cardiopulmonary exercise test, in which gas exchange is measured with the ECG, should be among the most sensitive tests to evaluate causes of exercise intolerance because it evaluates the function of all organs that couple lung to cellular respiration. In addition, no test in medicine can likely quantify improvement in organ function leading to increased exercise tolerance better than cardiopulmonary exercise testing. Thus, the addition of gas exchange measurements to the standard exercise test would greatly reduce the need to do additional tests. However, maximal benefit cannot be obtained from a cardiopulmonary exercise test unless the diagnosing physician is trained to recognize both the pathophysiological processes that limit exercise and their manifestations during the test.

For the diagnosing physician to interpret easily the large mass of data collected during a cardiopulmonary exercise study, the results should be displayed graphically so that the relationships between the functional variables can be seen. Chapter 9 shows the cardiopulmonary exercise test data from patients with a variety of diseases. A nine-panel graphic array was developed, after refinement with time and experience, to facilitate diagnosis of the pathophysiology of exercise. This nine-panel graphic array is shown on a single page to provide a picture of all of the critical data needed to determine the physiological state of each of the links in the coupling of external to cellular respiration.

Because of the important attributes of cardiopulmonary exercise testing and its relatively small expense and morbidity, it is surprising that cardiopulmonary exercise testing is not used more frequently by specialists who treat patients with heart and lung diseases. However, we anticipate that cardiopulmonary exercise tests will be used with greater frequency in the future because of its growing number of applications in medicine.

In summary, symptoms that limit exercise can usually be detected by an abnormality in the gas transport coupling of external to cellular respiration. Integrative exercise tests in which gas exchange is measured dynamically, rather than as a single steady-state measurement, can usually identify the pathophysiology of reduced exercise tolerance. This diagnosis of pathophysiology might even provide sufficient information for an anatomical diagnosis or, if not, may suggest other tests that would narrow the diagnostic choices. When the cause of the patient's exercise intolerance is not clinically obvious, we believe that often it is more cost-effective to do an integrative cardiopulmonary exercise test before proceeding with more invasive and expensive testing.

References

1. Weber KT. What can we learn from exercise testing beyond the detection of myocardial ischemia? Clin Cardiol 1997;20:684–696.
2. Wasserman K, Zhang Y-Y, Gitt A, Belardinelli R, Koike A, Lubarsky L, Agostoni PG. Lung function and exercise gas exchange in chronic heart failure. Circulation 1997; 96:2221–2227.

3. Sullivan MJ, Higginbotham MB, Cobb FR. Increased exercise ventilation in patients with chronic heart failure: intact ventilatory control despite hemodynamic and pulmonary abnormalities. Circulation 1988;77:552–559.
4. Kleber F, Reindl I, Wernecke K, Baumann G. Dyspnea in heart failure. In: Wasserman K (ed). Exercise Gas Exchange in Heart Disease. Arrmonk, NY: Futura Publishing Company, 1996;95–108.
5. Metra M, Raccagni D, Carini G, Orzan F, Papa A, Nodari S, Cody RJ, Dejours P. Ventilatory and arterial blood gas changes during exercise in heart failure. In: Wasserman K (ed). Exercise Gas Exchange in Heart Disease. Arrmonk, NY: Futura Publishing Co., 1996;125–143.
6. Hansen JE, Wasserman K. Pathophysiology of activity limitation in patients with interstitial lung disease. Chest 1996;109:1566–1576.
7. Butler J, Schrijen F, Henriguez A, Polu JM, Albert RK. Cause of the raised wedge pressure on exercise in chronic obstructive pulmonary disease. Am Rev Respir Dis 1988;138:350–354.
8. Mahler M. First-order kinetics of muscle oxygen consumption, and an equivalent proportionality between $\dot{Q}o_2$ and phosphorylcreatine level: Implications for the control of respiration. J Gen Physiol 1985;86:135–165.
9. Balaban R. Regulation of oxidative phosphorylation in mammalian cell. Am J Physiol 1990;258:C377–C389.
10. Chance B, Leigh J, Clark B, Maris J, Kent J, Nioka S, Smith D. Control of oxidative metabolism and oxygen delivery in human skelectal muscle: a steady-state analysis of the work/energy cost transfer function. Proc Natl Acad Sci USA 1985;82:8384–8388.
11. Weber KT, Janicki JS. Cardiopulmonary exercise (CPX) testing in heart and lung disease. In: Anonymous. Cardiopulmonary Exercise Testing Physiologic Principles and Clinical Applications. Philadelphia: W.B. Saunders, 1986;200.
12. Wasserman K. Coupling of external to cellular respiration during exercise: the wisdom of the body revisited. Am J Physiol 1994;266:E519–E539.
13. Wilson JR, Ferraro N, Weber KT. Respiratory gas analysis during exercise as a noninvasive measure of lactate concentration in chronic congestive heart failure. Am J Cardiol 1983;51:1639–1643.
14. Kitzman DW, Higginbotham MB, Cobb FR, Sheikh KH, Sullivan MJ. Exercise intolerance in patients with heart failure and preserved left ventricular systolic function: failure of the Frank-Starling mechanism. J Am Coll Cardiol 1991;17:1065–1072.
15. Wasserman K, VanKessel A, Burton GG. Interaction of physiological mechanisms during exercise. J Appl Physiol 1967;22:71–85.
16. Wasserman K, Whipp BJ, Koyal SN, Cleary M. Effect of carotid body resection on ventilatory and acid-base control during exercise. J Appl Physiol 1975;39:354–358.
17. Bouyhus A, Pool J, Binkhorst RA, VanLeeuwen P. Metabolic acidosis of exercise in healthy males. J Appl Physiol 1966;21(3):1040–1046.
18. Holmgren A, McIlroy MB. Effect of temperature on arterial blood gas tensions and pH during exercise. J Appl Physiol 1964;19:243–245.
19. Koyal SN, Whipp BJ, Huntsman D, Bray GA, Wasserman K. Ventilatory responses to the metabolic acidosis of treadmill and cycle ergometry. J Appl Physiol 1976; 40:864–867.
20. Barr DP, Himwich HE. Studies in the physiology of muscular exercise. II. Comparison of arterial and venous blood following vigorous exercise. J Biol Chem 1923;58: 525–537.
21. Sietsema KE, Daly JA, Wasserman K. Early dynamics of O_2 uptake and heart rate as affected by exercise work rate. J Appl Physiol 1989;67:2535–2541.
22. Meyer R, Foley J. Cellular processes integrating the metabolic response to exercise. In: Rowell LB, Shepherd JT, eds. Handbook of Physiology, Section 12: Exercise: Regulation and Integration of Multiple Systems. Bethesda, MD: American Physiological Society, 1996;841–869.
23. McGilvery RW. Biochemistry: A functional approach. In: McGilvery RW, ed. Biochemistry. Philadelphia: Saunders, 1983;390–497.
24. Barstow TJ, Lamarra N, Whipp BJ. Modulation of muscle and pulmonary O_2 uptakes by circulatory dynamics during exercise. J Appl Physiol 1990;68(3):979–989.
25. Casaburi R, Barstow TJ, Robinson T, Wasserman K. Influence of work rate on ventilatory and gas exchange kinetics. J Appl Physiol 1989;67:547–555.
26. Sullivan MJ, Knight D, Higginbotham MB, Cobb FR. Relation between central and peripheral hemodynamics during exercise in patients with chronic heart failure. Muscle blood flow is reduced with maintenance of arterial perfusion pressure. Circulation 1989;80:769–781.
27. Auchincloss JH, Ashutosh K, Rana S, Peppi D, Johnson LW, Gilbert R. Effect of cardiac, pulmonary, and vascular disease on one-minute oxygen uptake. Chest 1976;70: 486–493.
28. Bylund-Fellenius A-C, Walker PM, Elander A, Holm S, Holm J, Schersten T. Energy metabolism in relation to oxygen partial pressure in human skeletal muscle during exercise. Biochem J 1981;200:247–255.
29. Wasserman K. Diagnosing cardiovascular and lung pathophysiology from exercise gas exchange. Chest 1997; 112:1091–1101.

Physiology of Exercise

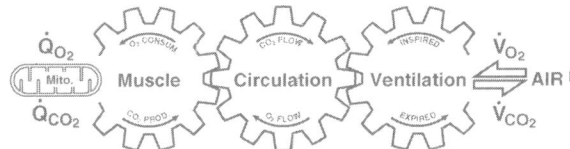

THE PERFORMANCE of muscular work requires the physiological responses of the cardiovascular and ventilatory systems to be coupled to the increase in metabolic rate. Efficient coupling minimizes the stress to the component mechanisms supporting energy production. In other words, cellular respiratory requirements (internal respiration) can only be met by the interaction of physiological mechanisms that link gas exchange between the muscle cells and the atmosphere (external respiration) (see Fig. 1.1). Inefficient coupling increases the stress to these systems, and, when sufficiently severe, can impair or limit work performance. Normal gas exchange between the cells and the environment requires:

1. Appropriate intracellular structure, energy substrate, and enzyme concentrations
2. A heart capable of pumping the quantity of oxygenated blood needed to sustain energy production
3. An effective system of blood vessels that can selectively distribute blood flow to match local tissue gas exchange requirements
4. Blood with normal hemoglobin of adequate concentration
5. An effective pulmonary circulation through which the regional blood flow is matched to the appropriate ventilation
6. Normal lung mechanics and chest bellows
7. Ventilatory control mechanisms capable of regulating arterial blood gas tensions and pH

The response of each of the coupling links in the gas exchange process is usually quite predictable and can be used as a frame of reference for evidence of impaired responses.

In this chapter, we will review the essentials of skeletal muscle physiology, including the relationship of structure and function, cellular respiration, substrate metabolism, and the effect of an inadequate O_2 supply. After considering internal respiration, we will examine the circulatory and ventilatory links between internal and external respiration. These will include the factors that determine the magnitude and time course of the cardiovascular and ventilatory responses and how they are coupled with the metabolic stress of exercise.

SKELETAL MUSCLE
Mechanical Properties and Fiber Types

Human skeletal muscles consist of two basic fiber types, Types I and II (Table 2.1). These fiber types are classified on the basis of both their contractile and biochemical properties (1). Type I (or "slow-twitch") fibers take a relatively long time to develop peak tension following their activation, i.e., some 80 msec, compared with the 30 msec average for Type II (or "fast-twitch") fibers. The slow contractile properties of Type I fibers appear to result largely from the relatively low activity of the myosin ATPase at the myofibril that catalyzes the splitting of the terminal high energy phosphate from ATP, the lower Ca^{++} activity of the regulatory protein, troponin, and the slower rate of Ca^{++} uptake by sarcoplasmic reticulum. These same properties appear to confer a relatively high resistance to fatigue on the Type I fibers.

Biochemical differences between the two basic fiber types center chiefly on their capacity for oxidative and glycolytic activities. The Type I fibers, being especially rich in myoglobin, are classified as red fibers, while the Type II fibers, which contain considerably less myoglobin, are classified as white fibers. The Type I slow-twitch fibers tend to have significantly higher levels of oxidative enzymes than the Type II fast-twitch fibers that typically have a high glycolytic activity and enzyme profile. The Type II fibers are further classified into Type IIa and Type IIb, based on the greater oxidative and lesser glycolytic potential of the Type IIa fibers compared with the Type IIb fibers (Table 2.1). With respect to substrate stores, muscle glycogen concentration is, in fact, similar in Type I and Type II fibers, but the triglyceride content is two to three times greater in the Type I slow-twitch fibers. Evidence suggests that the Type I slow-twitch fibers are more efficient than the Type II fast-twitch fibers, performing more work or developing more tension per unit of substrate energy utilized (2).

TABLE 2.1.   Characteristics of Muscle Fiber Types

	Slow Oxidative (Type I)	Fast Oxidative (Type IIa)	Fast Glycolytic (Type IIb)
Contraction	Slow twitch	Fast twitch	Fast twitch
Fiber Size	Small	Intermediate	Large
Color	Red	Red	White
Myoglobin Concentration	High	High	Low
Mitochondrial Content	High	High	Low

Considerable potential for change exists in the enzyme concentrations of a particular fiber by specific training. For example, a fast-twitch fiber in an endurance-trained athlete could have higher concentrations of oxidative enzymes than slow-twitch fibers in a chronically sedentary subject (3).

These structural and functional differences between fiber types depend to a large extent on the neural innervation of the fibers. A single motor neuron supplies numerous individual muscle fibers; this functional assembly is termed a "motor unit." These fibers are distributed throughout the muscle, rather than being spatially contiguous. Fibers comprising a motor unit are characteristically of the same "fiber type" and substrate depletion occurs rather uniformly within each fiber of the contracting unit.

Fiber type distribution within human skeletal muscle varies from muscle to muscle. For example, the soleus muscle typically has a much higher density of slow-twitch fibers (greater than 80%) than the gastrocnemius muscle (about 50%) or the triceps brachii (about 20 to 50%). The vastus lateralis muscle (on average, approximately 50% slow-twitch fibers) has been used widely for analysis of fiber type characteristics in humans. The basic fiber type pattern of this muscle varies in different subjects. Elite endurance-trained athletes typically have a high percentage of slow-twitch fibers in this muscle (greater than 90% not being uncommon) compared with untrained, control subjects (about 50%) or elite sprinters (20 to 30%).

Whereas basic fiber type pattern is genetically determined, it is greatly influenced by the neural characteristics of the efferent motor neuron. When the motor nerves innervating the fast flexor digitorum longus and the slow soleus muscles of the cat are cut and cross-spliced, the contractile and biochemical characteristics of the muscle begin to resemble the features of the muscle originally innervated by the nerve (4). Thus an important trophic influence on muscle function is conferred by its nerve supply. A program of exercise training, however, does not cause appreciable interchanges between Type I and Type II fibers, but can cause changes within Type II fibers (e.g., from Type IIb to Type IIa) (5). Evidence is accumulating, however, that long-term inactivity and/or chronic disease can result in a shift toward a greater percentage of Type II fibers.

The pattern of activation of fiber types depends on the form of exercise. For low-intensity exercise, the Type I slow-twitch fibers tend to be recruited predominantly, whereas the Type II fast-twitch fibers (which produce greater force) are recruited at higher work rates, especially at or above 70 to 80% of the maximal aerobic power (6).

Energetics

Skeletal muscle may be considered to be a machine that is fueled by the chemical energy of substrates derived from ingested food and stored as carbohydrates and lipids in the body. Although protein is a perfectly viable energy source, it is not used to fuel the energy needs of the body to any appreciable extent, except under conditions of starvation.

The free energy of the substrate (i.e., that fraction of the total chemical energy that is capable of doing work) is not used directly for muscle contraction. It must first be stored in the terminal phosphate bond of adenosine triphosphate (ATP). The terminal phosphate bond of this compound has a high free energy of hydrolysis (ΔG) and is designated as a "high energy" phosphate bond ($\sim P$). Current estimates of ΔG per $\sim P$, for physiological conditions such as those occurring in contracting muscle, are as high as 12 to 14 Kcal/mole. Muscle is ultimately, therefore, a digital device operating in discrete multiple units of $\sim P$ energy, with one $\sim P$ thought to be utilized per myosin cross-bridge linkage to and subsequent release from actin. The muscle uses this energy for the conformational changes externally manifested by shortening or increasing tension. Thus, muscular exercise depends on the intrinsic structural characteristics of muscle and on the body's systems, which maintain an appropriate physicochemical milieu for adequate ATP regeneration.

Sources of High Energy Phosphate and Cell Respiration

Energy for muscular contraction is obtained predominantly by the oxidation in the mitochondria of three (pyruvate) and two carbon (acetate) metabolic intermediaries from carbohydrate and fatty acid catabolism (Fig. 2.1). A small additional amount of energy comes from biochemical mechanisms in the cell cytoplasm which metabolize glucose and glycosyl units (from glycogen) to pyruvate (Fig. 2.1). Both the mitochondrial and cytosolic sources of energy are transformed into high-energy phosphate ($\sim P$) compounds, predominantly as creatine phosphate and ATP. During the splitting of $\sim P$ from these compounds, energy is made available for cellular reactions such as biosynthesis, active transport, and muscle contraction. Exercise entails an acceleration

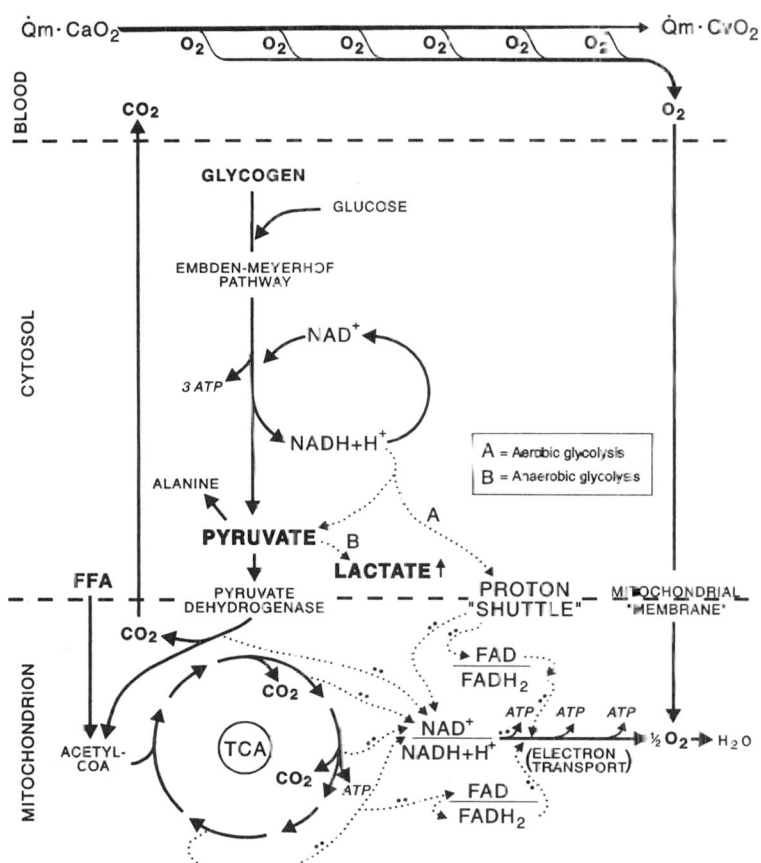

FIGURE 2.1. Scheme of the major biochemical pathways for production of ATP. The transfer of H^+ and electrons to O_2 by the electron transport chain in the mitochondrion and the "shuttle" of protons from the cytosol to the mitochondrion (Pathway A) are the essential components of aerobic glycolysis. This allows the efficient use of carbohydrate substrate in regenerating ATP to replace that consumed by muscle contraction. Also illustrated is the important O_2 flow from the blood to the mitochondrion, without which the aerobic energy generating mechanisms within the mitochondrion would come to a halt. At the sites of inadequate O_2 flow to mitochondria, Pathway B serves to reoxidize $NADH+H^+$ to NAD^+ with a net increase in lactic acid production (lactate accumulation). Lactate will increase relative to pyruvate as $NADH+H^+/NAD^+$ increases in the cytosol (see figure insert and text).

of the energy-yielding reactions in the muscles to regenerate ~P at the increased rate needed for the increased energy expenditure of physical work. Thus, the cellular consumption of O_2 is increased; this must be matched by an increased delivery of O_2 from the atmosphere to the mitochondria. Simultaneously, CO_2, the major catabolic end-product of exercise, is removed from the cell by muscle blood flow and excreted by the lungs.

Acetate, produced from the catabolism of carbohydrates, fatty acids, or (in nutritionally deficient states) amino acids reacts with oxaloacetate in the mitochondrion, after esterification with coenzyme-A (also known as acetyl-CoA), to form citrate in the Krebs or tricarboxylic acid (TCA) cycle (see Fig. 2.1). Here the catabolic reactions result in CO_2 release and the transfer of hydrogen ions (protons) and their associated electrons to the mitochondrial electron transport chain. These then flow down the energy gradient of the electron transport chain, transferring energy to resynthesize ATP from ADP and inorganic phosphate (Pi) (i.e., oxidative phosphorylation). At the end of the electron transport chain, cytochrome oxidase catalyzes the reaction of each pair of protons and electrons with an atom of

oxygen to form a molecule of water. For each transfer of a pair of protons and electrons, sufficient energy is released to form either two or three ATP: three if the electron transport process begins at nicotinamide adenine dinucleotide (NAD^+) but only two if it begins at flavin adenine dinucleotide (FAD) (see Fig. 2.1).

Six ATP molecules are gained during the catabolism of glucose to pyruvate if the reduced nicotinamide adenine dinucleotide ($NADH+H^+$) in the cytosol, formed during glycolysis, is reoxidized by the proton shuttle and FAD (Pathway A of Fig. 2.1) (7). Of the six ATP molecules regenerated from glucose (seven from glycogen) by this mechanism, two are formed in the cytosol by the Embden-Meyerhof (glycolytic) pathway and four in the mitochondrion during the coupled reoxidation of cytosolic $NADH+H^+$ by the mitochondrion, via the mitochondrial membrane proton shuttle and the cytochrome electron transport chain (7). The shuttle accepts hydrogen ions from the cytosolic $NADH-H^+$ and transfers them to mitochondrial coenzymes, NAD^+ or FAD as illustrated in Figure 2.1. This method of regenerating oxidized NAD^+ in the cytosol maintains the cytosolic redox state and enables glycolysis to continue. Because O_2 is the ultimate recipient of the protons which are generated by glycolysis and transported into the mitochondria, this glycolysis is aerobic (see Pathway A, Fig. 2.1).

The formation of acetyl-CoA from pyruvate and its subsequent entry into the TCA cycle yields a total of five reduced mitochondrial NAD molecules, i.e., $NADH+H^+$. Since the reoxidation of each $NADH+H^+$ by the electron transport chain yields 3 ATP molecules, there is a net gain of 15 ATP. However, two molecules of acetyl-CoA are formed from each glucose molecule so that the total gain is 30 ATP from these reactions. When added to the 2 ATP gained from glycolysis and the 4 others obtained from reoxidation of cytosolic $NADH+H^+$ by the proton shuttle with the subsequent transfer of its protons and electrons to oxygen (see Fig. 2.1), the total gain in ATP from the complete oxidation of glucose is 36. However, because glycogen is the major carbohydrate source in the normally nourished person, an additional $\sim$P is obtained because when a glycosyl unit combines with inorganic phosphate it becomes $\sim$P. Thus there is a net yield of 37 ATP from the aerobic oxidation of each glycosyl unit. Because 6 molecules of O_2 are used for glucose (glycosyl)oxidation and 36 high energy phosphate bonds are formed, the $\sim$P:$O_2 = 6$, for glucose (6.18 for glycogen). Six molecules of CO_2 and H_2O are catabolic end-products of these reactions.

Under conditions in which the mitochondrial proton shuttles fail to reoxidize the $NADH+H^+$, generated by glycolysis, at a rate sufficient to keep cytosolic $NADH+H^+/NAD^+$ normal (Fig. 2.1), the redox state of the cytosol is lowered. As $NADH+H^+$ accumulates in the cytosol at the expense of NAD^+, glycolysis would slow if it were not for an alternate pathway capable of reoxidizing cytosolic $NADH+H^+$. When $NADH+H^+$ accumulates, pyruvate can reoxidize the $NADH+H^+$ to NAD^+. However, pyruvate is reduced to lactate in this process (Pathway B, Fig. 2.1). This pyruvate oxidation of $NADH+H^+$ results in lactate accumulation. Because the breakdown of glucose or glycosyl to lactate occurs without use of oxygen, it is termed anaerobic glycolysis. The substrate price for the production of energy from this reaction is expensive compared with the complete oxidation of glycogen to CO_2 and H_2O. The net gain in *ATP* is only 3 from each glycosyl unit instead of 37. For the same work rate, therefore, this pathway causes glycogen (and glucose) to be used at a considerably faster rate than when the production of $\sim$P is totally aerobic (8, 9). Moreover,

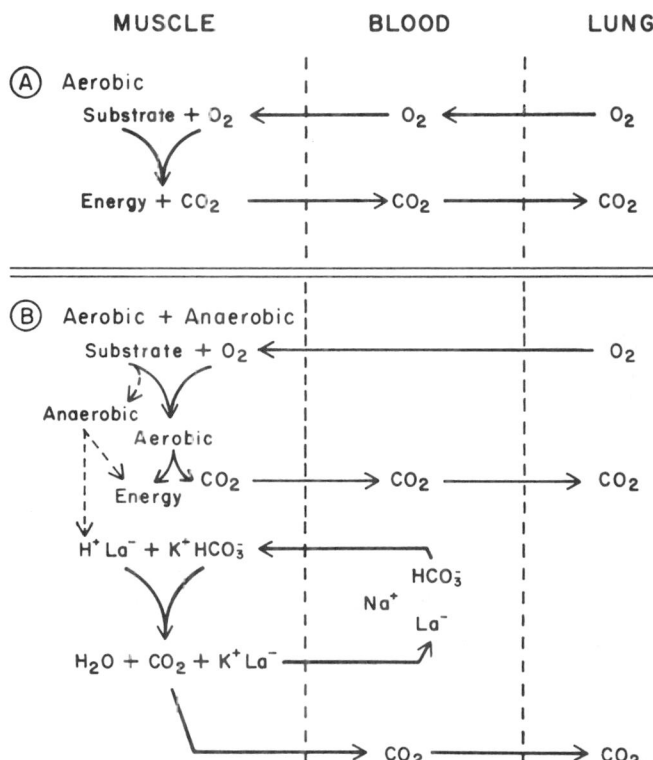

FIGURE 2.2. Gas exchange during aerobic (A) and aerobic plus-anaerobic (B) exercise. The acid-base consequence of the latter is a net increase in cell lactic acid production. The buffering of the accumulating lactic acid takes place in the cell at the site of formation, predominantly by bicarbonate. The latter mechanism will increase the CO_2 production of the cell by approximately 22 ml per mEq of bicarbonate buffering of lactic acid. The increase in cell lactate and decrease in cell bicarbonate will result in chemical concentration gradients causing lactate to be transported out of and bicarbonate to be transported into the cell.

the two lactic acid molecules which accumulate when each glucose molecule or glycosyl unit undergoes anaerobic metabolism cause a disturbance in acid-base balance in the cell and blood (Fig. 2.2). That the *turn-on* of anaerobic *ATP* production does not signal the *turn-off* of aerobic *ATP* production deserves emphasis. Both aerobic and anaerobic mechanisms share in energy generation at high work rates with the anaerobic mechanism providing an increasing proportion of energy as the work rate is increased.

Substrate Utilization and Regulation

At this point, several terms need to be clarified for precision and to avoid possible confusion (see Fig. 1.1). The symbol $\dot{V}O_2$ indicates O_2 uptake by the lungs. It is distinguished from O_2 consumption by the cells, which is symbolized by $\dot{Q}O_2$. The symbol

$\dot{V}_{CO_2}$ indicates CO_2 output by the lungs to distinguish it from CO_2 production by the cells, symbolized by $\dot{Q}_{CO_2}$. Thus the substrate mixture undergoing oxidation is characterized by the net rates of CO_2 yield or production ($\dot{Q}_{CO_2}$), and oxygen utilization or consumption ($\dot{Q}_{O_2}$). The ratio $\dot{V}_{CO_2}/\dot{V}_{O_2}$ as measured at the mouth (i.e., the gas exchange ratio, R) reflects $\dot{Q}_{CO_2}/\dot{Q}_{O_2}$, the metabolic respiratory quotient (RQ), only when there is a steady state, i.e., CO_2 is not being added to or being removed from the body CO_2 stores and the O_2 stores are constant, i.e., when $\dot{Q}_{CO_2} = \dot{V}_{CO_2}$ and $\dot{Q}_{O_2} = \dot{V}_{O_2}$.

During acute hyperventilation (resulting, for example, from acute hypoxia, pain or anxiety, or of volitional origin), considerably more CO_2 is unloaded from the body CO_2 stores than O_2 is loaded into the O_2 stores. This is because hemoglobin is almost completely saturated with O_2 at the end of the pulmonary capillaries at sea level and the physical solubility of O_2 in blood is low; on the other hand, appreciable amounts of CO_2 can be unloaded from blood and tissue stores as alveolar ventilation is increased and Pa_{CO_2} is reduced. Thus, the gas exchange ratio, R, will exceed the metabolic RQ until a steady state is again attained at the new level of ventilation. Similarly, during the acute metabolic acidosis of exercise, "extra" CO_2 is evolved when HCO_3^--buffers lactic acid (see Fig. 2.2). This, too, will result in R exceeding RQ until a new steady state in CO_2 stores is attained (i.e., the CO_2 pool size is again constant although depleted) at which time R again equals RQ. Differences between R and RQ will also occur during acute hypoventilation and recovery from metabolic acidosis, but in the opposite direction.

As seen in the following equations, carbohydrate (e.g., glycogen or glucose) is oxidized with RQ = 1.0 (i.e., 6 CO_2 produced and 6 O_2 consumed) and has a ~P:O_2 = 6.0 or 6.18 depending on whether glucose or glycogen is the substrate:

$$C_6H_{12}O_6 + 6\,O_2 \rightarrow 6\,CO_2 + 6\,H_2O + 36 \text{ or } 37 \text{ ATP}$$
$$(1)$$

Lipid (e.g., palmitate) is oxidized with RQ = 0.71 (i.e., 16 CO_2 produced/23 O_2 consumed) and has a ~P:O_2 = 5.65 (i.e., 130 ATP/23 O_2):

$$C_{16}H_{32}O_2 + 23\,O_2 \rightarrow 16\,CO_2 + 16\,H_2O + 130 \text{ ATP}$$
$$(2)$$

Intermediate steady state RQ values reflect different proportions of carbohydrate and fat being utilized in the metabolic process (Fig. 2.3). For storage economy, fat is more efficient energy but, for economy of O_2 utilization, carbohydrate is the more efficient substrate.

When a steady state of gas exchange exists, R provides an accurate reflection of RQ. During exercise, the muscle RQ can be estimated from the increase in $\dot{V}_{CO_2}$ relative to the increase in $\dot{V}_{O_2}$ over the range of moderate work rates. These gas exchange measurements (10–12) suggest that the muscle substrate RQ during exercise is approximately 0.95. This is in close agreement with the muscle substrate RQ in normal humans, found by Bergstrom et al. (13), based on the rate of muscle glycogen consumption during exercise determined from repeated muscle biopsies. Thus, a greater proportion of carbohydrate as compared to fatty acids is used for energy during muscular work as compared with the resting state.

Because muscle RQ is high relative to that of most other organs (nervous system excluded), the total body RQ increases from a resting value of approximately 0.8 (on an average "Western diet") toward approximately 0.95 during moderate exercise, depending on the exercise metabolic rate (Fig.

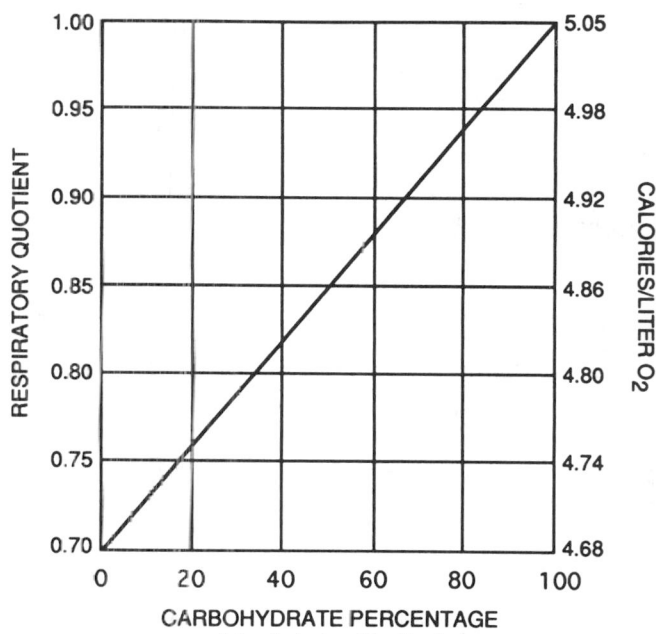

FIGURE 2.3. The percentage of carbohydrate substrate in the diet estimated from the respiratory quotient measurement. The calories of energy obtained per liter of oxygen consumed for each combination is given on the right ordinate. (Plot of data reprinted with permission from Lusk G. Science of Nutrition. Johnson Reprint Corp., New York, 1976;65.)

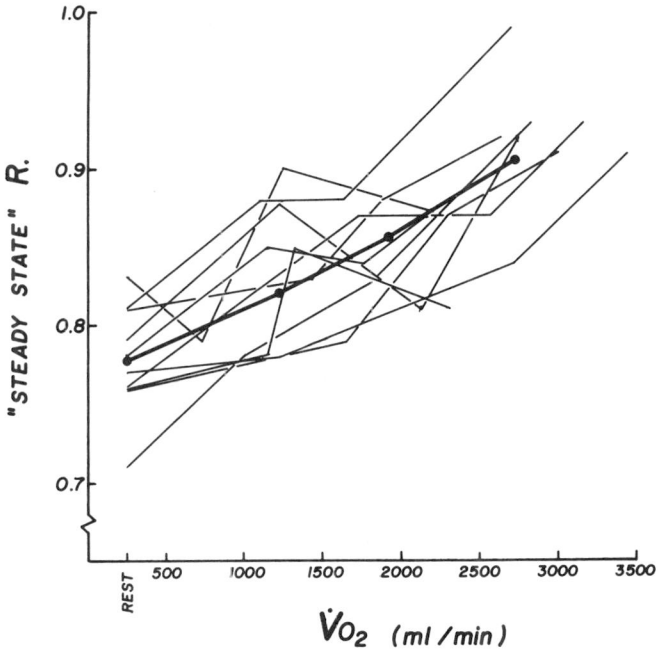

FIGURE 2.4.   The steady state R (RQ) at various levels of exercise for the whole body determined as the ratio of steady state $\dot{V}CO_2$ to $\dot{V}O_2$ for the levels of exercise indicated on the x-axis for 10 subjects. The heavy line is the average response.

2.4). An RQ of 0.95 indicates that about 84% of the substrate during exercise is derived from carbohydrate (Fig. 2.3). Although the fuel mixture for the total body derives proportionally more from carbohydrate than from lipid stores during exercise as work rate increases (Fig. 2.4), RQ decreases slowly over time during prolonged constant load exercise (Fig. 2.5), reflecting a reduction in muscle glycogen stores. When muscle glycogen becomes depleted, the exercising subject senses

exhaustion (14). Acute ingestion of glucose allows the work to continue (15).

The rate of decrease in muscle glycogen during exercise can be slowed by raising blood glucose levels with a continued infusion of glucose (16). The importance of muscle glycogen in work tolerance is well described by the experiments of Bergstrom et al. (13), who demonstrated a high positive correlation between the tolerable duration of high intensity work and the muscle glycogen content before exercise.

Physical fitness affects the substrate utilization pattern. A fitter subject uses a greater proportion of fatty acids for energy than an unfit one for submaximal work (17). This mechanism conserves glycogen allowing more work to be performed before glycogen depletion and consequent exhaustion. The specific regulation of different substrates is considered later.

Carbohydrates. Skeletal muscle in humans contains, on average, 80 to 100 mmols (15 to 18 g) glucose per kilogram of wet weight stored as glycogen. For the "standard" 70 kg man, this amounts to approximately 400 g of muscle glycogen. Note that this represents an estimate of the total skeletal muscle carbohydrate pool, whereas a contracting muscle can draw only on its own glycogen reserves and not on the pools in non-contracting muscles.

Normally, there are 5 to 6 g of glucose available in the blood (100 mg/100 ml). Although muscle uptake of blood glucose increases considerably during exercise, the blood concentration does not fall, except during prolonged work, due to an increased rate of glucose release from the liver.

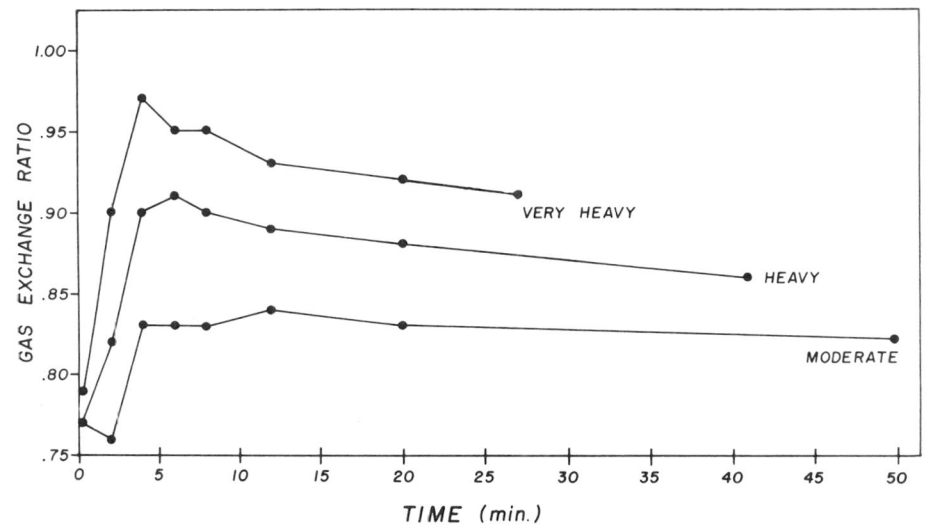

FIGURE 2.5.   Effect of exercise duration on the gas exchange ratio (R) for constant work rate exercise of moderate, heavy, and very heavy work intensity. Note that the gas exchange ratio is higher for the higher work intensities, but declines with time after the initial increase. Results are those for a single healthy subject.

The liver represents a highly labile glycogen reserve of some 50 to 90 g. This glycogen is broken down into glucose and released into the blood by glycogenolysis. Glucose can also be produced in the liver (gluconeogenesis) from lactate, pyruvate, glycerol, and alanine precursors. The rate of glucose release from the liver into the circulation depends on both the blood glucose concentration and a complex interaction of hormones such as insulin, glucagon, and the catecholamines, epinephrine and norepinephrine (18, 19). As exercise intensity and duration increase, the circulating levels of catecholamines and glucagon increase, thereby maintaining the level of blood glucose despite its increased utilization by the exercising muscles. These regulatory processes maintain physiologically adequate concentrations of glucose except when muscle and liver glycogen stores become greatly depleted.

Lipids. Skeletal muscles have access to their own intramuscular store of lipids, averaging 20 gm of triglycerides per kg wet weight. This source accounts for a considerable proportion of the total energy required by the muscles, depending on the duration of exercise and the rate of depletion of muscle glycogen.

Extramuscular lipid sources are also utilized during exercise. These derive from adipose tissue where triglycerides undergo hydrolysis to glycerol and free fatty acids (mainly palmitic, stearic, oleic, and linoleic acids). The fatty acids are transported in the blood, bound predominantly to albumin. The store of extramuscular lipid is large. In the "standard" 70 kg man, fat accounts for approximately 15 kg of triglycerides, equivalent to about 135,000 Kcal of energy.

The sympathetic nervous system, along with catecholamines from the adrenal medulla, regulate adipose tissue lipolysis. Epinephrine and norepinephrine increase the local concentration of cyclic 3',5'AMP through activation of adenyl cyclase. This leads to increased rates of hydrolysis of the stored adipose tissue triglycerides. Other factors reduce the rate of adipose tissue lipolysis during exercise, including increased blood lactate and exogenous glucose loads.

The free fatty acids account for only a small proportion (usually less than 5%) of the total plasma fatty acid pool; the remainder are triglycerides. Resting plasma free fatty acid concentrations are approximately 0.5 mmol/L, rising during exercise to approximately 2 mmol/L. The turnover rate of the plasma free fatty acid pool is high, with a half-time of 2 to 3 minutes at rest and less during exercise. As a consequence, the flux of free fatty acids to the exercising muscle (i.e., plasma flow × plasma FFA concentration) is an important determinant of skeletal muscle uptake.

The plasma concentration of free fatty acids does not increase, and may even decrease slightly, with physical training. Therefore, the increased proportional contribution of free fatty acid oxidation to exercise energetics, when measured at a specific work rate after training, may reflect increased utilization from intramuscular sources. Adipose tissue lipolysis does not appear to be enhanced by training and may even be depressed.

Amino Acids. During exercise, the rate of release of intramuscular alanine increases appreciably, but with little or no change in other amino acids (20). The arterial alanine concentration increases as much as twofold during severe exercise (21). The source of the alanine released from muscle is predominantly from the transamination of pyruvate (derived from increased rates of carbohydrate metabolism). The amino groups are derived from the deamination of inosine monophosphate during purine nucleotide metabolism and the branch-chain amino acids (valine, leucine, and isoleucine).

A highly linear relationship exists between the plasma concentrations of alanine and pyruvate at rest and during exercise. A decreased muscle release of alanine is observed in phosphorylase-deficient muscle (McArdle's syndrome) associated with the decreased output of pyruvate (22). The alanine formed by transamination in muscle is transported in the blood to the liver where it serves as a precursor for gluconeogenesis. Thus an alanine-glucose cycle is established between muscle and liver, with the carbon skeleton of alanine supporting hepatic glucose synthesis.

OXYGEN COST OF WORK

The oxygen cost of performing work depends on the work rate. Figure 2.6 shows the time course of oxygen uptake ($\dot{V}O_2$) from unloaded cycling for various levels of cycle ergometer exercise in a normal individual. Note that, in this individual, a steady state is reached by 3 minutes up to a work rate of 150 watts. At higher work rates, $\dot{V}O_2$ continues to increase above the 3-minute value. In this range of work rate, the rate at which $\dot{V}O_2$ increases is greater, the higher the work rate (23, 24). The maximum $\dot{V}O_2$ for each of the work rates above 200 watts is

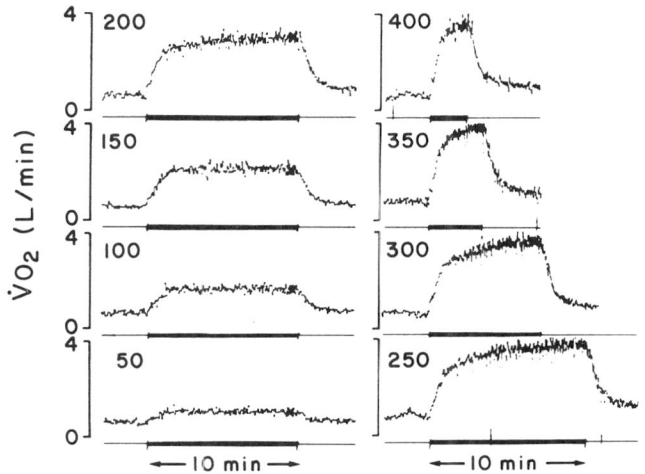

FIGURE 2.6. Breath-by-breath time course of oxygen uptake for eight levels of constant work rate cycle ergometer exercise, starting from unloaded cycling. The work rate (watts) for each study is shown in the respective panel. The bar on the X-axis indicates the period of the imposed work rate. The $\dot{V}_{O_2}$ asymptote (steady-state) is significantly delayed for work above the anaerobic threshold. (Reprinted with permission from Whipp BJ, Mahler M. Dynamics of pulmonary gas exchange during exercise. In: West JB, ed. Pulmonary Gas Exchange. New York: Academic Press, 1980;2:33–96.)

the same, thereby identifying the subject's $\dot{V}_{O_2}$max. However, the $\dot{V}_{O_2}$max is reached in a shorter time, forcing the subject to fatigue earlier, the higher the work rate.

When plotting the steady-state $\dot{V}_{O_2}$ values for those cycle ergometer work rates in which a steady state is achieved, such as shown for 50, 100, and 150 watts in Figure 2.6, a linear relationship between $\dot{V}_{O_2}$ and work rate is obtained (Fig. 2.7). The slope of this relationship is approximately the same for all normal people (approximately 10 ml/min/watt). This means that work efficiency in humans is relatively fixed for a given work task. However, while the slope of the $\dot{V}_{O_2}$-work rate relationship is not affected by training, age or gender, the position of the relationship depends on body weight.

On the cycle ergometer, obese subjects exhibit an upward displacement of approximately 5.8 ml/min/kg body weight (25). This reflects the added work rate generated as a result of moving the heavier lower extremities. The effect of body weight on $\dot{V}_{O_2}$ is more pronounced on the treadmill since an even greater work rate must be done to support the movement of the entire body through space.

Work Efficiency

Cycle ergometer work rate and the steady-state $\dot{V}_{O_2}$ measurement are commonly used interchangeably

when describing the level of exercise being performed because work efficiency or the increase in work rate (ΔWR) as related to the increase in $\dot{V}_{O_2}$ required to perform the work ($\Delta\dot{V}_{O_2}$) varies only slightly from one individual to another (26). Trained and untrained individuals, whether old or young, male or female, all have similar work efficiencies. This similarity reflects the basic biochemical energy-yielding reactions needed for muscle contraction. However it is important to recognize that the $\dot{V}_{O_2}$ of the "unloaded" ergometer can vary considerably from one subject to another because of differences in subject size and actual work rate of the "unloaded" cycle. Thus ΔWR/$\Delta\dot{V}_{O_2}$ is much more uniform among subjects than WR/$\dot{V}_{O_2}$.

Care must be taken not to confuse changes in skill or motor efficiency due to practice with the assessment of work efficiency. To measure work efficiency, relatively simple tasks must be employed which do not depend on technique and for which the work output can be measured, e.g., cycling. To calculate muscle work efficiency, the caloric equivalent of the steady-state $\dot{V}_{O_2}$ (4.96 Cal/L $\dot{V}_{O_2}$ at RQ = 0.95, see Fig. 2.3) and the external power (0.014 Cal/min/watt) for at least two measured work rates must be known. For lower extremity cycle ergometer

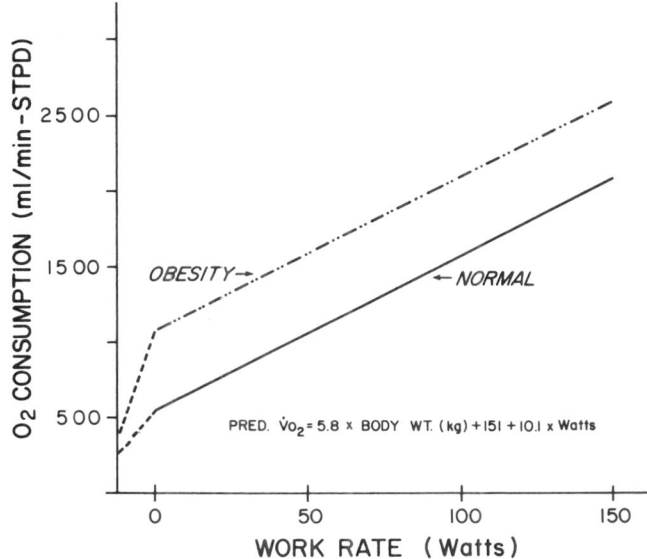

FIGURE 2.7. The effect of work rate on steady-state oxygen consumption during cycle ergometer exercise. The oxygen consumption response in normal subjects is quite predictable for cycle ergometer work regardless of age, gender, or training. The predicting equation is given in the figure. In obese subjects, the oxygen requirement to perform work is displaced upward, the displacement dependent on body weight. (Reprinted with permission from Wasserman K, Whipp BJ. Exercise physiology in health and disease. Am Rev Respir Dis 1975;112:219–249.)

work, normal subjects have an efficiency of approximately 28% (25, 27).

$\dot{V}_{O_2}$ Non-Steady-State

The continued slow increase in $\dot{V}_{O_2}$ observed after 3 minutes during constant work rate exercise is only seen for work rates that are accompanied by a lactic acidosis (23, 24, 28). The rate of increase in $\dot{V}_{O_2}$ in response to constant work rate exercise correlates well with the increase in blood lactate (24, 28–30), as discussed in the section entitled "Gas Exchange Kinetics" in this chapter. At least five mechanisms may contribute to the slow increase in $\dot{V}_{O_2}$ after 3 minutes of exercise:

1. Progressive vasodilation to the local muscle units by metabolic vasodilators produced in response to relative O_2 lack (e.g., $[H^+]$) thereby increasing O_2 flow and O_2 consumption at the O_2 deficient sites
2. Acidemia facilitating O_2 unloading from hemoglobin by shifting the oxyhemoglobin dissociation curve downward for a given P_{O_2}
3. O_2 cost of conversion of lactate to glycogen in the liver, as the lactate concentration rises
4. Increase in $\dot{V}_{O_2}$ needed to satisfy the increased work of the muscles of respiration and the heart at high ventilatory and cardiac output responses
5. Reduced muscular efficiency during heavy work either by recruiting more low efficiency "fast-twitch" muscle fibers or by calling into play additional groups of muscles (such as more forceful pulling on the handlebars)

Other mechanisms, such as increased catecholamine levels, and increased body temperature at high work rates could also add to the O_2 cost of heavy work.

LACTATE INCREASE

Lactate Increase as Related to Work Rate

Figure 2.8 shows the arterial blood lactate concentration as related to $\dot{V}_{O_2}$ in three groups of subjects performing progressively increasing cycle ergometer work: normal subjects who are relatively active, sedentary normal subjects and patients with heart disease. All show similar resting and low level exercise lactate concentrations. The pattern of lactate increase is the same for each group, but the $\dot{V}_{O_2}$ at which the lactate starts to increase differs. Lactate

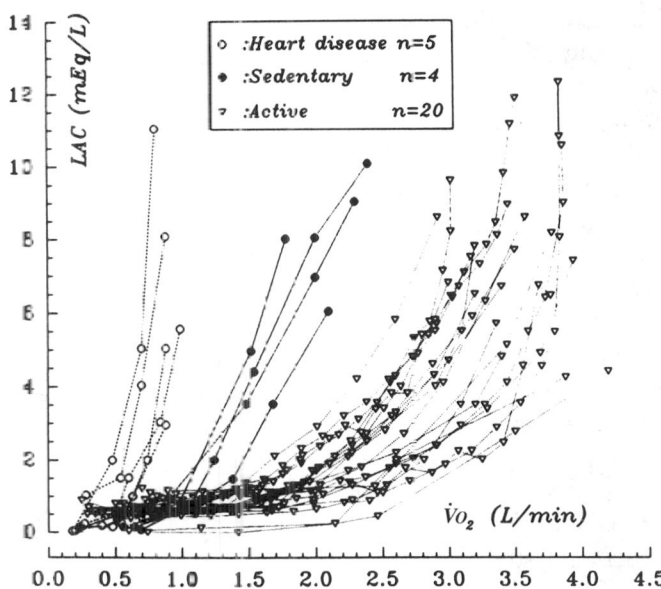

FIGURE 2.8. Pattern of increase in arterial lactate in active and sedentary healthy subjects and patients with heart disease as related to increasing exercise oxygen uptake ($\dot{V}_{O_2}$). Lactate (LAC) concentration rises from approximately the same resting value to approximately the same concentration at maximal exercise in each of the three groups. The fitter the subject for aerobic work, the higher the $\dot{V}_{O_2}$ before lactate starts to increase significantly above resting levels. (Modified from Wasserman K. Coupling of external to cellular respiration during exercise: the wisdom of the body revisited. Am J Physiol 1994;266:E519–E539.)

does not start to increase in subjects who are relatively physically active until $\dot{V}_{O_2}$ is increased to as much as 10 times the resting metabolic rate. In contrast, the $\dot{V}_{O_2}$ at which lactate starts to increase in sedentary subjects is about 4 times the resting level (equivalent to the $\dot{V}_{O_2}$ required for adults to walk at a normal pace). In cardiac patients with a low, symptom-limited maximum $\dot{V}_{O_2}$, arterial lactate increases at exceedingly low exercise levels. Activity that only doubles the resting metabolic rate can result in a marked increase in lactate. The $\dot{V}_{O_2}$ at which lactate starts to increase in normal subjects is, on average, about 50–60% of their $\dot{V}_{O_2}$max. However, it can be considerably higher in aerobically fit subjects. As we age, on average, the $\dot{V}_{O_2}$ at which lactate starts to increase, as a percent of $\dot{V}_{O_2}$max increases as a result of $\dot{V}_{O_2}$max declining at a proportionately greater rate; this ratio is also slightly higher for females than males.

Lactate Increase as Related to Time

Work rate or power output is an absolute quantity of work performed per unit of time. However, a given work rate may be stressful for one individual, limiting the duration that the work can be sustained, while not a significant physical stress for a more fit individual. Therefore, we use adjectives to describe the degree of physical stress, e.g., moderate, heavy, very heavy, based on the pattern of arterial lactate change, as suggested by Wells et al. (31), since the magnitude of arterial lactate increase for a given work rate closely reflects the fitness of an individual for endurance (aerobic) exercise (32).

For constant-load cycle ergometer exercise, three patterns of arterial blood lactate concentration are observed (Fig. 2.9) (33). The first pattern is one in which either no increase in lactate is observed or lactate rises slowly and then peaks early in exercise after which it returns to its resting value as $\dot{V}O_2$ reaches a steady state. This is defined as moderate work intensity and implies that the work is not uncomfortable and hence can be sustained in a true steady-state. Heavy intensity exercise is defined as a sustained but constant increase in arterial lactate resulting from a balance between increased rate of production and increased rate of utilization. This

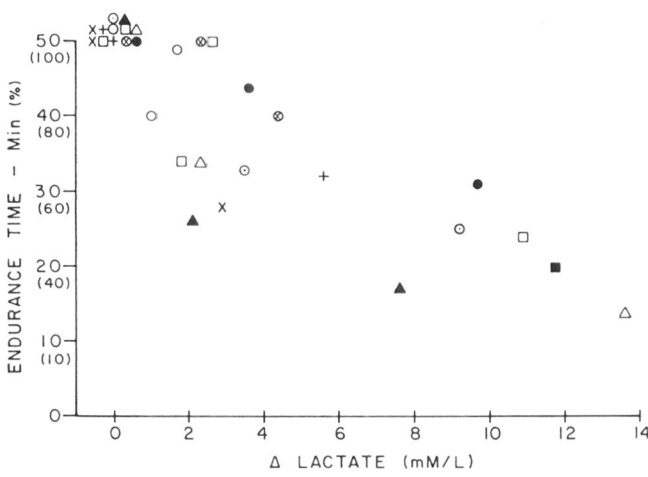

FIGURE 2.10. The endurance time as related to the increase in arterial lactate (above the preexercise resting value) during the last minute of constant work rate cycle ergometer exercise. Data are from thirty experiments on ten male subjects studied at three work rates, each for a target time of 50 minutes. Endurance time is reduced when lactate is increased. (Reprinted with permission from Wasserman K. The anaerobic threshold measurement to evaluate exercise performance. Am Rev Respir Dis (Suppl.) 1984;129:535–540.)

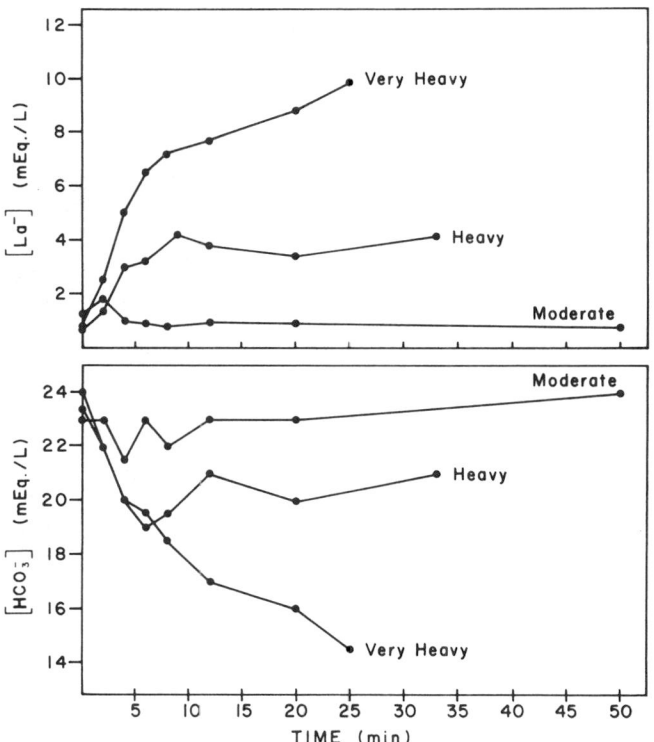

FIGURE 2.9. Arterial lactate increase and bicarbonate decrease with time for moderate, heavy, and very heavy exercise intensities for a normal subject. Bicarbonate changes in opposite direction to lactate and in a quantitatively similar manner. While the target exercise duration was 50 minutes for each work rate, the endurance time was reduced for the heavy and very heavy work rates.

work can only be sustained for a limited duration (Figs. 2.9, 2.10) and a true metabolic steady state does not exist. The latter is evident from a continuously increasing minute ventilation and development of a metabolic acidosis (34).

When arterial lactate continues to increase throughout the exercise to the point of fatigue (Fig. 2.9), this is termed very heavy work. At these work rates, arterial lactate typically continues to increase to levels >5 mmol/L. The higher the lactate, the earlier the fatigue, whether arterial lactate is in the heavy or very heavy work intensity range (Fig. 2.10).

Lactate Increase in Response to Increasing Work Rate

As illustrated in Figure 2.8, arterial lactate does not appreciably increase above resting values until a $\dot{V}O_2$ is reached above which lactate increases at a progressively steeper rate. To determine the best fit mathematical model describing the $\dot{V}O_2$ at which lactate starts to increase, we tested both continuous exponential and threshold models (35–37). The purpose of this model testing was to better understand the physiological events that accompany the development of the highly reproducible lactic acidosis engendered by heavy exercise. To obtain a better picture of the systematic pattern of the change in

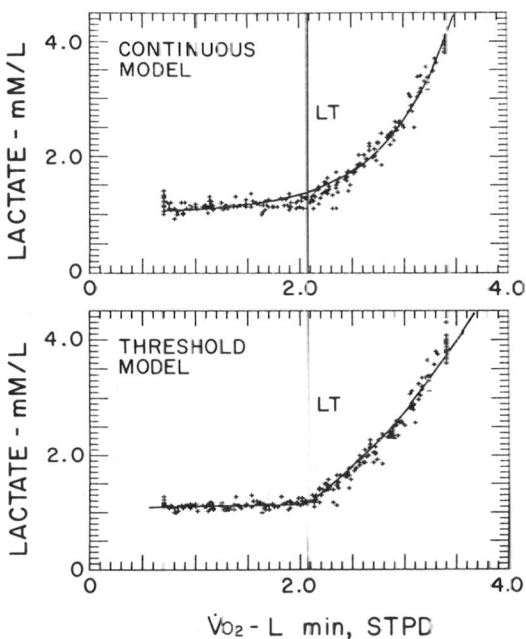

FIGURE 2.11. The threshold behavior of arterial lactate increase as related to $\dot{V}O_2$ in response to exercise. Data are arterial lactate measurements from 17 active healthy subjects shown in Figure 2.8. Points are plotted only up to a lactate level of 4.5 mmol/L, (the region of interest in evaluating threshold versus a continuous exponential model). The vertical solid line shows the average threshold for the 17 subjects. The points for the individual subjects are plotted in the same relation to the threshold $\dot{V}O_2$ as existed in their individual plot. In the upper panel, the solid line describes the continuous exponential model. Lactate values fall above the exponential model line at the lowest $\dot{V}O_2$ while the lactate values are below the model curve in the region of the threshold. In contrast, the threshold model (solid lines, lower panel) is a better fit to the actual lactate measurements. Details of the mathematical analysis for a smaller number of subjects are presented in reference 37.

arterial lactate with increasing $\dot{V}O_2$, we plotted the arterial blood lactate against the simultaneously measured $\dot{V}O_2$, after the $\dot{V}O_2$ scale was normalized to that demonstrating a significant increase in arterial lactate for the 17 physically active, healthy young male subjects shown in Figure 2.11. In this plot, the data points are distributed with the same deviation relative to the average curve as they were distributed in the individual curves for each subject. Because lactate increases steeply with little increase in $\dot{V}O_2$ as $\dot{V}O_2$max is approached, the data examined to address the question of model behavior for lactate increase are restricted to the region of interest, from resting lactate to that below an arterial lactate of 4.5 mmol/L. As illustrated in Figure 2.11 (upper panel), a mono-exponential model of lactate increase from rest as a function of $\dot{V}O_2$ does not describe the lactate data well. Lactate points fall above

the model curve at the low $\dot{V}O_2$ values, while in the region of $\dot{V}O_2$ just below that at which lactate starts to rise (identified as the threshold in the threshold model), the points fall below the model curve. In contrast, the points distribute evenly around the two components of the threshold model (Fig. 2.11, lower panel). This threshold is denoted as the lactate threshold (*LT*).

Neither the threshold nor the mono-exponential models are perfect fits for the lactate–$\dot{V}O_2$ relationship at all work levels. But the data in the region of interest, i.e., below 4.5 mmol/L, clearly fit the threshold model better than the exponential model. Supporting the threshold model are numerous muscle biopsy studies that show that muscle lactate does not increase at mild to moderate work rates (38–42). The $\dot{V}O_2$ at which lactate begins to increase in arterial blood coincides with that of the muscle (38).

Mechanisms of Lactate Increase

Several mechanisms have the potential to yield increases in lactate production as $\dot{V}O_2$ increases during exercise.

Overload of the Tricarboxylic Acid Cycle

Lactate can accumulate in the muscle and blood during exercise if glycolysis proceeds at a rate faster than pyruvate can be utilized by the mitochondrial tricarboxylic acid cycle (Fig. 2.1). This mechanism should cause lactate to increase *as a result of* and *in proportion to* pyruvate increase. i.e., a mass action effect. Alternatively, when cytosolic nicotinamide adenine dinucleotide ($NADH+H^+$), reduced in the process of glycolysis, cannot be reoxidized rapidly enough by the mitochondrial membrane proton shuttle—electron transport chain—cytochrome oxidase—O_2 pathway (Pathway A of Fig. 2.1), reoxidation of cytosolic $NADH+H^+$ can take place by the reaction: Pyruvate + $NADH+H^+$ → Lactate + NAD^+ (Pathway B of Fig. 2.1). This mechanism is operant when the oxygen required by the exercising muscles cannot be supplied at a sufficiently rapid rate to reoxidize $NADH+H^+$ by Pathway A. Thus, the cell redox state is lowered, forcing lactate to be increased *relative* to pyruvate.

Change in Cytosolic Redox State

Figure 2.12 shows a plot of the log-log transformation of arterial lactate, pyruvate and lactate/pyruvate (L/P) ratio as a function of $\dot{V}O_2$ in one normal subject

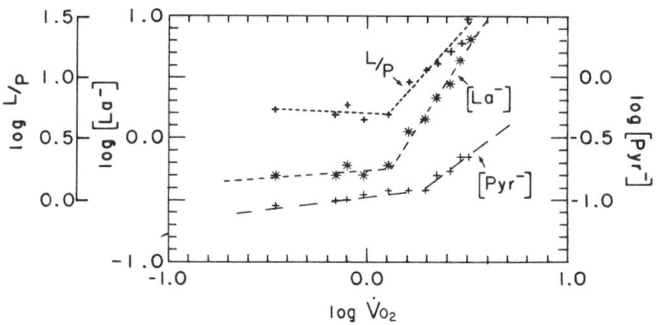

FIGURE 2.12. Log lactate [La⁻], log pyruvate [Pyr⁻], and log lactate/pyruvate (L/P) ratio plotted against log $\dot{V}O_2$. The loglog transform of the lactate-$\dot{V}O_2$ and pyruvate-$\dot{V}O_2$ relationships allows easy detection of the lactate and pyruvate inflection points. The pyruvate inflection point is at a higher $\dot{V}O_2$ than the lactate inflection point. Because the pre-threshold pyruvate slope is the same as the lactate slope, the L/P ratio does not increase until the lactate inflection point. (Reprinted with permission from Wasserman K, Beaver WL, Davis JA, et al. Lactate, pyruvate, and lactate to pyruvate ratio during exercise and recovery. J Appl Physiol 1985; 59:935–940.)

who was representative of the average response of 10 healthy subjects (43). Below the lactate threshold (*LT*), lactate increased by a few tenths of a mmol/L as pyruvate increased, but the L/P ratio did not increase until the *LT* was reached. Pyruvate also increased steeply, but not until a $\dot{V}O_2$ was reached which was well above that of the *LT*. Also, the rate of increase in pyruvate was always slower than lactate. Consequently the L/P ratio increased *at the LT* and continued to increase until $\dot{V}O_2$max. A similar phenomenon has been observed in the muscle cells of humans (44). The increase in muscle L/P was accompanied by a reduction in the muscle energy charge indicated by an increase in the ADP/ATP ratio (44).

The increase in lactate with an increase in L/P ratio indicates that the increase in lactate during exercise is not simply a mass action phenomenon resulting from increased glycolysis. Rather, the lactate increase results from a shift in equilibrium between lactate and pyruvate *as a result of* change in $NADH+H^+/NAD^+$ ratio (cytosolic redox state) (Fig. 2.1). The conversion of pyruvate to lactate results in the reoxidation of cytosolic $NADH+H^+$ providing NAD^+ for continued glycolysis even under anaerobic conditions. Since no O_2 is used in the reoxidation of Pathway B (Fig. 2.1), this glycolysis is *an*aerobic. Simultaneously, reoxidation of cytosolic $NADH+H^+$ can take place, aerobically, in better oxygenated contracting muscle cells by pathway A, i.e., aerobic glycolysis (Fig. 2.1). The reversal of the exercise-induced increase in arterial L/P is seen at

the start of recovery (Fig. 2.13) and provides an important clue to the mechanism(s) of the lactic acidosis of exercise. The exercise-induced rise in arterial lactate continues into the recovery phase, but at a slowed rate before it starts to decrease. Pyruvate concentration, on the other hand, actually increases more rapidly at the start of recovery. Thus, as soon as exercise stops (and the O_2 requirement decreases), the L/P ratio reverses, supporting the evidence obtained during exercise that the exercise-induced lactate increase is not simply a mass action effect consequent to pyruvate increase. The same reversal in L/P ratio, with lactate decreasing and pyruvate increasing, takes place in the muscle cell at the start of recovery (45).

Sequential Recruitment of Fiber Types

Another mechanism proposed for the increase in lactate during exercise is the increased contraction of Type IIb muscle fibers above the lactate threshold (46). These fibers contain high levels of glycogen. However, it has never been demonstrated that these fibers are activated at the lactate threshold. Furthermore, it would be necessary to demonstrate that Type IIb fibers have a redox state with a higher $NADH+H^+/NAD^+$ ratio and, therefore, higher L/P ratio than Types I or IIa fibers. Additionally, there is no evidence that suggests that activation of Type IIb fiber types is influenced by changes in oxygenation as is the case for arterial lactate concentration.

In summary, it is difficult to attribute the increase in lactate with an increase in L/P ratio, as seen with heavy exercise, to accelerated glycolysis, inadequate tricarboxylic acid cycle enzymes, or changes in contracting muscle fiber type. Rather, the experimental studies support the concept that the major mechanism accounting for the lactate increase at the lactate threshold is the lowering of cytosolic redox state induced by a net increase in anaerobic glycolysis.

O_2 Supply, Critical Capillary PO_2 and Lactate Increase

O_2 is extracted from the capillary blood as it flows past the actively contracting muscles because O_2 is required for the aerobic production of ATP (Fig. 2.1). While isolated mitochondria can respire and rephosphorylate ADP to ATP at a PO_2 of 1 mmHg or less (47), the capillary PO_2 must be appreciably greater than 1 mmHg to provide the pressure for O_2 to diffuse from the red cell to the sarcoplasm to sustain muscle mitochondrial respiration during

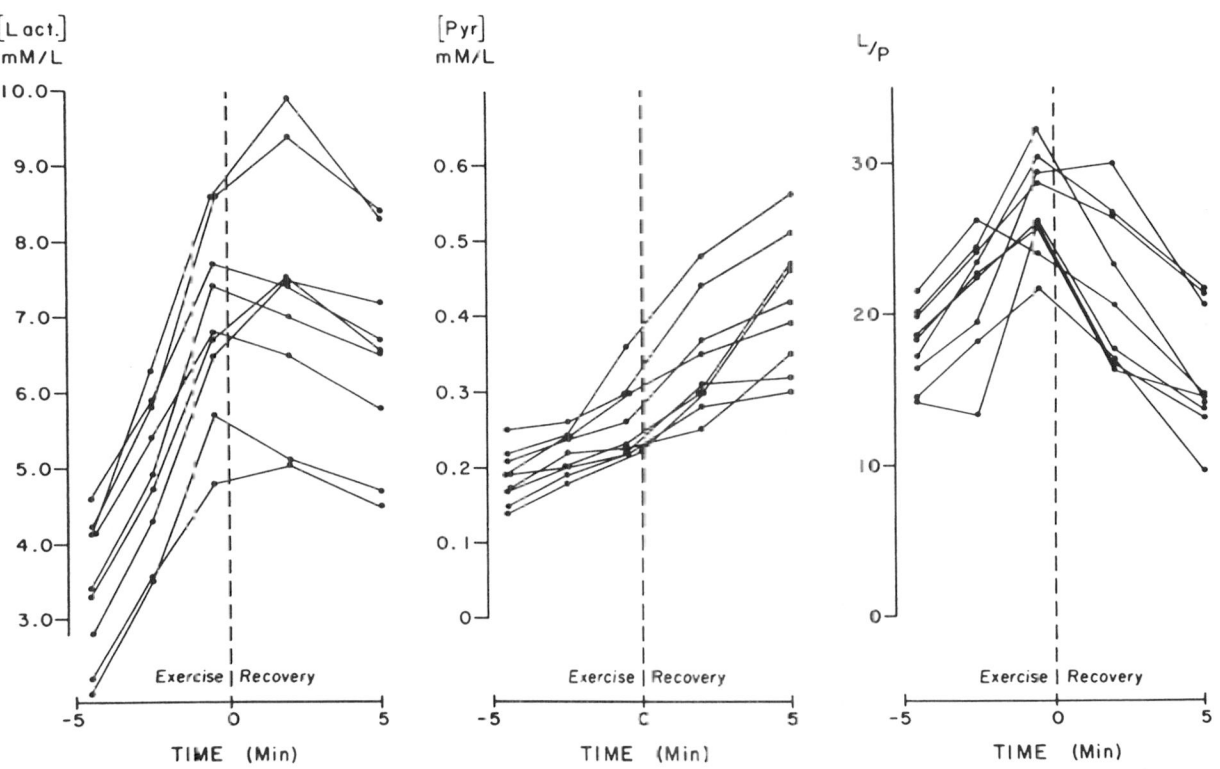

FIGURE 2.13.   Lactate (Lact), pyruvate (Pyr), and lactate-to-pyruvate (L/P) ratio during last 5 min (highest 3 work rates) of exercise and first 5 min of recovery. Studies show that lactate either increases or decreases slightly by 2 min of recovery. All subjects show a decrease by 5 min of recovery. In contrast, pyruvate continues to rise through first 5 min of recovery. As a consequence, L/P ratio decreases by 2 min and continues to decrease by 5 min of recovery toward control value. (Reprinted with permission from Wasserman K, Beaver WL, Davis JA, et al. Lactate, pyruvate, and lactate-to-pyruvate ratio during exercise and recovery. J Appl Physiol 1985;59:935–940.)

exercise. Wittenberg and Wittenberg estimated this pressure to be 15 to 20 mmHg (48). It was termed the "critical" capillary PO_2 because it represents the lowest capillary PO_2 that allows the muscle mitochondria to receive the O_2 required to perform exercise aerobically. The major factors determining the PO_2 difference between red cell and sarcoplasm are the resistances to O_2 diffusion by the red cell membrane, plasma, capillary endothelium, interstitial space and sarcolemma (48). By measuring oxymyoglobin saturation in the dog gracilis muscle during a moderate level of exercise, Gayeski and Honig (49) estimated the PO_2 in the sarcoplasm to be about 5 mmHg. The P_{50} for oxymyoglobin in humans is 6 mmHg (50). Because it would be less than 1/2 saturated, oxymyoglobin can serve as an O_2 store to support only very short bursts of heavy exercise. However, it may play a role in facilitating O_2 diffusion in muscle fibers containing myoglobin.

To obtain a PO_2 of 15 mmHg at the end-capillary, a muscle blood flow of at least 6 liters would be needed for a muscle O_2 consumption of 1 liter/minute, assuming a hemoglobin concentration of 15 gm/dl and an alveolar PO_2 adequate to saturate the arterial oxyhemoglobin to at least 95%. This would leave less than 1/6 of the O_2 inflow into the capillary bed remaining at the venous end of the capillary.

Figure 2.14 illustrates the change in PO_2 along the muscle capillary for various blood flow/metabolic rate ratios thought to be physiologic. This model allows for the Bohr effect resulting from aerobic metabolism (modeling decreasing pH in the capillary from aerobic CO_2 production) but not for anaerobic metabolism (lactic acidosis). A blood flow/O_2 consumption ratio of 5:1 would cause obligatory anaerobiosis and lactic acidosis since its PO_2 would fall below the critical level well before the blood has reached the venous end of the capillary bed.

A lactic acidosis secondary to cellular hypoxia would be expected only if the critical capillary PO_2 was reached at the metabolic rate required to perform the exercise. When reaching the critical capillary PO_2, capillary PO_2 would no longer decrease despite increasing work rate. However, as work rate increased, lactate would increase, because the criti-

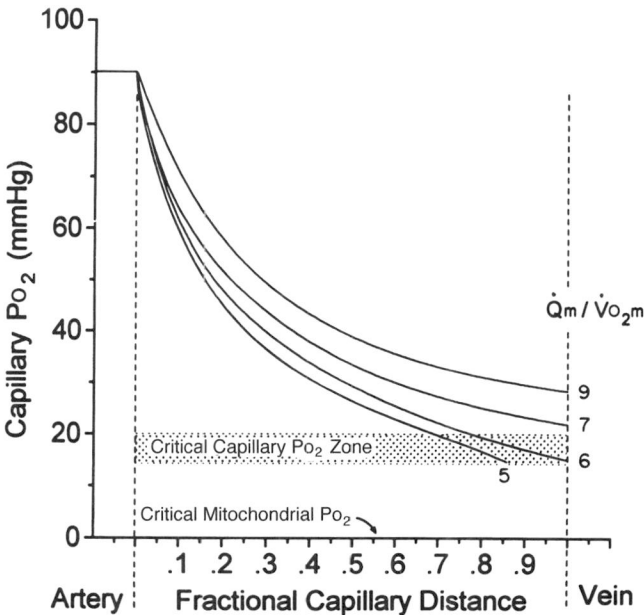

FIGURE 2.14.   Model of muscle capillary bed O_2 partial pressure (P_{O_2}) as blood travels from artery to vein. The model assumes hemoglobin concentration of 15 g/dl, arterial P_{O_2} of 90 mmHg and a linear O_2 consumption along the capillary. The rate of fall of capillary P_{O_2} depends on the muscle blood flow ($\dot{Q}m$)/muscle $\dot{V}_{O_2}$ ($\dot{V}_{O_2}m$) ratio. The curves include a Bohr effect due to a respiratory CO_2 production. The capillary P_{O_2} is heterogeneous along the capillary bed even with a homogenous $\dot{Q}m/\dot{V}_{O_2}m$. The end-capillary P_{O_2} cannot decrease below the critical capillary P_{O_2}. Any muscle unit with a theoretical $\dot{Q}m/\dot{V}_{O_2}$ less than 6 will have increased anaerobic metabolism and lactate production. See text for application of model. (Reprinted with permission from Wasserman K. Coupling of external to cellular respiration during exercise: the wisdom of the body revisited. Am J Physiol 1994;266:E519–E539.)

cal capillary P_{O_2} would occur earlier during the course of the blood flow through the capillary. In comparison to the metabolic rate increase of the exercising muscles (including respiratory muscles and heart), the metabolic rate of other tissues do not change their metabolic rate appreciably as work rate increases. Therefore, it might be assumed that the increase in $\dot{V}_{O_2}$ during leg cycling exercise is due primarily to the increase in lower extremity muscle metabolism. Further, it can be assumed that femoral vein P_{O_2} and lactate closely approximate the average end-capillary value.

The capillary P_{O_2} must be heterogeneous, even if there were a single "ideal" blood flow/metabolic rate ratio in the muscle, because the blood enters the muscle with a $P_{O_2} = 90$ mmHg (in a normal subject at sea level) and leaves the capillary bed at a P_{O_2} which is approximately equal to that of the femoral vein P_{O_2} (Fig. 2.14). The "critical" capillary P_{O_2} would be the lowest P_{O_2} to which the end-capillary P_{O_2} could fall. The capillary P_{O_2} cannot

decrease below the critical capillary P_{O_2} because the mitochondrial P_{O_2} would be too low to consume O_2. That the critical capillary P_{O_2} was reached should be evidenced by the failure of end capillary or femoral vein P_{O_2} to decrease further despite increasing work rate.

Critical Capillary P_{O_2}

The model shown in Figure 2.14 is instructive in several respects: 1) it illustrates that the capillary P_{O_2} is heterogeneous even when the muscle blood flow/metabolic rate ratios ($\dot{Q}m/\dot{V}_{O_2}m$) for individual capillary beds in the muscle are homogeneous, ranging from high values at the arterial to low values at the venous end of the capillary bed; and 2) it shows that estimates of "mean" muscle P_{O_2}, calculated from femoral vein P_{O_2}, are erroneous unless it is certain that there is no heterogeneity in $\dot{Q}m/\dot{V}_{O_2}m$ ratios and that the $\dot{Q}m/\dot{V}_{O_2}m$ ratio is at least 6, i.e., lactate is not increased. Rather than the "mean" capillary P_{O_2}, the question must be asked whether the muscle blood flow and therefore capillary P_{O_2} are sufficiently high to prevent a muscle lactic acidosis. When exercise is performed above the *LT*, aerobic and anaerobic metabolism take place simultaneously, because O_2 is consumed by the muscle supplied by the capillary on the arterial end while lactate is released by muscle on the venous end.

In an organ such as skeletal muscle, if the increase in ATP requirement increases beyond the increase in O_2 flow, the end-capillary P_{O_2} must decrease. At high metabolic rates, the capillary P_{O_2} must remain above the critical capillary P_{O_2} to allow continued aerobic energy transfer (53). This is the P_{O_2} needed to overcome the diffusive resistance between the capillary and mitochondria to achieve the O_2 flow required for aerobic regeneration of high energy phosphate in the myocyte. The diffusive resistance is determined by the medium for diffusion and the physical distance between the red cells in the muscle capillary (O_2 source) and the mitochondria or myoglobin (O_2 sink).

Experimental support for the critical capillary P_{O_2} concept is provided by the studies of Stringer et al. (51), and Koike et al. (52) in which femoral vein P_{O_2} and lactate were measured during leg cycling exercise in normal subjects and patients with chronic heart failure, respectively. During progressively increasing work rate studies, femoral vein blood P_{O_2} reached a "floor" or lowest value in the middle of the subjects' work capacities and before lactate concentration started to increase (Fig. 2.15).

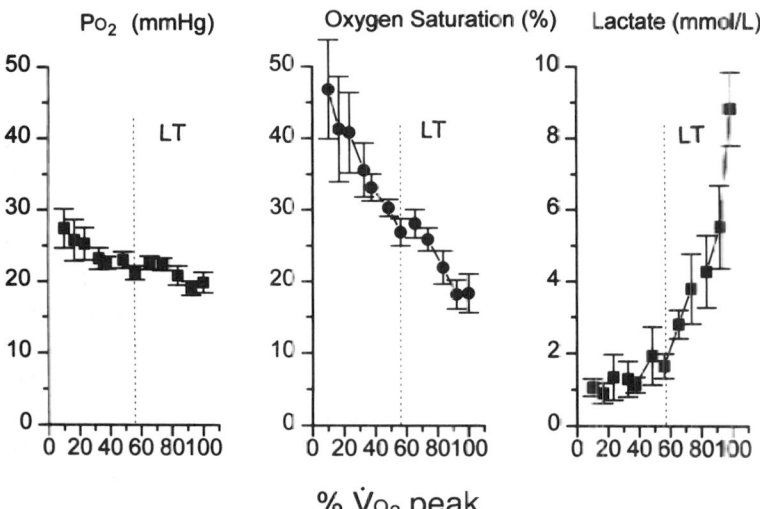

FIGURE 2.15.   Average (5 normal subjects) femoral vein oxygen tension (PO₂) (left panel), oxyhemoglobin saturation (middle panel) and lactate concentration (right panel) during increasing work rate exercise in ramp pattern to the maximal V̇O₂. Vertical dashed line indicates the average lactate threshold (*LT*) determined by gas exchange using the V-slope method (74). Vertical bars indicate standard error of mean. There is no significant difference between the PO₂ values from the *LT* to V̇O₂ max, but the oxyhemoglobin saturation decreased significantly above the *LT*. (Modified from data reported in Stringer WW, Wasserman K, Casaburi R, et al. Lactic acidosis as a facilitator of oxyhemoglobin dissociation during exercise. J Appl Physiol 1994;76:1462–1467.)

To determine the critical capillary PO₂ in normal subjects, 10 healthy adults were studied with femoral vein and arterial catheters, five during progressively increasing and five during two levels of constant work rate leg cycling exercise, one below and one above the *LT*. As would be predicted from the critical capillary PO₂ concept, femoral vein and therefore end-capillary PO₂ decreased to its lowest value before lactate started to increase (Fig. 2.16).

This was true of all subjects, whether performing incremental or heavy constant work rate exercise, consistent with the model shown in Figure 2.14. When end-capillary blood reaches a 'floor' or 'critical' value of 15 to 20 mmHg, anaerobic metabolism developed and lactate concentration increased. It is important to note that femoral vein lactate increased before arterial lactate increased and lactate remained higher in the femoral venous than the arterial blood (Fig. 2.17). This is in agreement with prior studies on lactate balance across the exercising extremity (54–56). To investigate further the hypothesis that femoral vein PO₂ reaches a 'floor' value by the time the *LT* is reached, normal subjects performed two constant work rate exercise tests for 6 minutes, one at a moderate work rate and one at a heavy work rate. The moderate work rate was

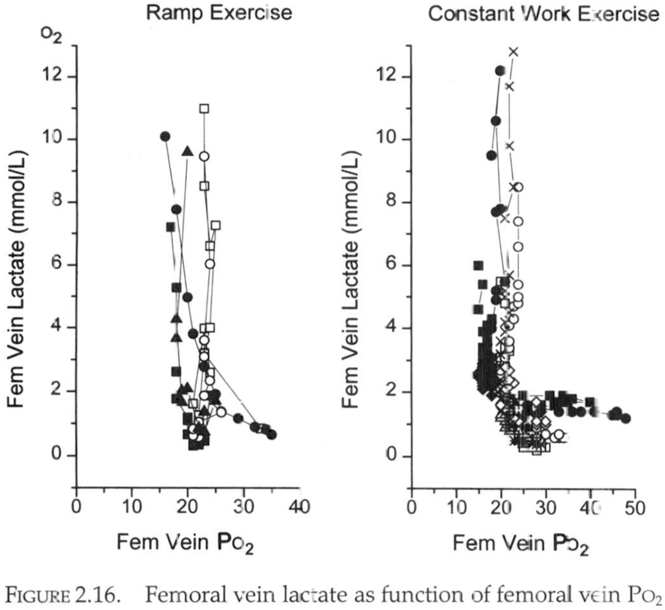

FIGURE 2.16.   Femoral vein lactate as function of femoral vein PO₂ for incremental (ramp) exercise in 5 normal subjects (left panel) and 10 constant work rate exercise tests (five below and five above the *LT*) in 5 normal subjects (right panel). The highest PO₂ values are where exercise starts. Different symbols represent different subjects. (Modified from Stringer WW, Wasserman K, Casaburi R, et al. Lactic acidosis as a facilitator of oxyhemoglobin dissociation during exercise. J Appl Physiol 1994;76:1462–1467.)

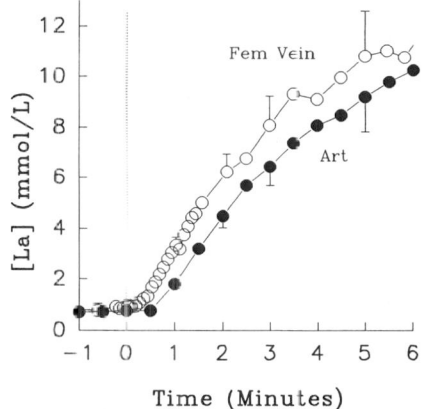

FIGURE 2.17.   Average (5 normal adult subjects) femoral vein and arterial lactate concentration during heavy constant work rate leg cycling exercise. By rapid blood sampling, it is clear that the increase in arterial lactate lags the increase in femoral vein lactate concentration.

calculated to be at 80% of the *LT* (avg = 113 W, $\dot{V}_{O_2}$ = 1.76 L/min). The heavy work rate studied was calculated to be at the *LT* plus 75% of the difference between the *LT* and $\dot{V}_{O_2}$max (avg = 265 W, $\dot{V}_{O_2}$ = 3.36 L/min). These tests were done with a high sampling density of femoral vein blood (every 5 sec during the first 2 minutes and then every 30 sec for 4 minutes) to accurately describe the changes. The results of these studies are shown in Figure 2.18. The femoral vein P_{O_2} decreased to the same 'floor' value at 30 to 60 sec after the start of exercise for both the moderate and heavy work intensities (Fig. 2.18, left panel). This value remained the same for the remainder of the exercise period, despite the large difference in work rate and $\dot{V}_{O_2}$. In contrast to P_{O_2}, oxyhemoglobin saturation continued to decrease past the time when the end-capillary P_{O_2} (as evidenced from the femoral vein measurements) became constant (middle panel of Fig. 2.18).

Oxyhemoglobin Dissociation above the Lactic Acidosis Threshold

As shown in Figure 2.18, for the work rates selected to be below the *LT*, oxyhemoglobin desaturation proceeds rapidly for the first minute and then more slowly for the next 1 to 2 minutes before reaching a constant value. The change after 1 minute followed the decrease in pH. For the work rate above the *LT*, the oxyhemoglobin desaturation was much more marked and continued for the entire 6 minutes of exercise. The femoral vein oxyhemoglobin desaturation, which was not accounted for by the P_{O_2} decrease, could be completely accounted for by the

pH decrease (Fig. 2.18, right panel). To illustrate this, the data shown in Figure 2.18 were replotted with femoral vein oxyhemoglobin saturation values plotted against the independently measured femoral vein P_{O_2} values (Fig. 2.19); pH isopleths are overlaid on these data. This plot, when compared with the pH changes shown in the right panel of Figure 2.18, shows that the decrease in oxyhemoglobin saturation that could not be accounted for by a decrease in P_{O_2} could be completely accounted for by the decrease in measured pH. Also, Figure 2.19 shows that the decrease in oxyhemoglobin saturation below 25% was completely accounted by the Bohr effect (acidification of the capillary blood). Thus blood acidification appears to account for oxyhemoglobin dissociation for work above the *LT*. However, although to a much lesser degree, acidification from increasing P_{CO_2} should also contribute to oxyhemoglobin dissociation below the *LT*, along with the much more important decrease in P_{O_2}.

Because the net increase in lactic acid production during exercise is buffered by intracellular HCO_3^-, additional CO_2 is produced in the muscle over that expected from aerobic metabolism as HCO_3^- dissociates. This results in an increase in end-capillary P_{CO_2} without a further fall in P_{O_2} (Fig. 2.20). Simultaneously, the decrease in intracellular HCO_3^- results in a decrease in extracellular and therefore femoral vein HCO_3^-. Both the decrease in femoral vein HCO_3^- and the increase in P_{CO_2} serve to acidify the capillary blood of the muscle cells producing lactate (53). The lactic acidosis of exercise thereby facilitates oxyhemoglobin dissociation. Consequently, it is an essential mechanism for achieving maximal O_2 extraction while simultaneously maintaining the par-

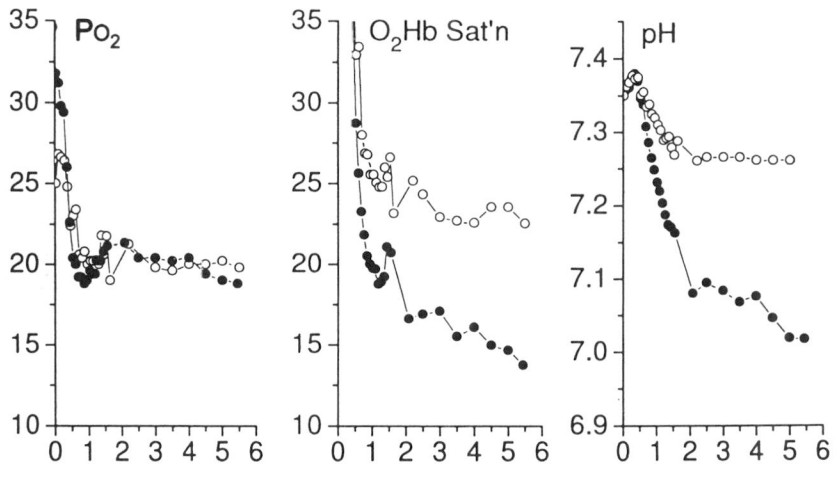

FIGURE 2.18.   Femoral venous P_{O_2}, oxyhemoglobin saturation (O_2Hb Sat'n) and pH as related to time of exercise for two constant work rate tests, one below (open circles) and one above (solid circles) the lactate threshold (*LT*). The data are the average of five subjects. The below and above *LT* work rates averaged 113 and 265 watts, respectively. Note that O_2Hb saturation is lower during the higher intensity exercise despite identical P_{O_2} values. This is related to the Bohr shift resulting from the decreasing pH in the high intensity test. (Modified from Stringer WW, Wasserman K, Casaburi R, et al. Lactic acidosis as a facilitator of oxyhemoglobin dissociation during exercise. J Appl Physiol 1994;76:1462–1467.)

Exercise Time (Minutes)

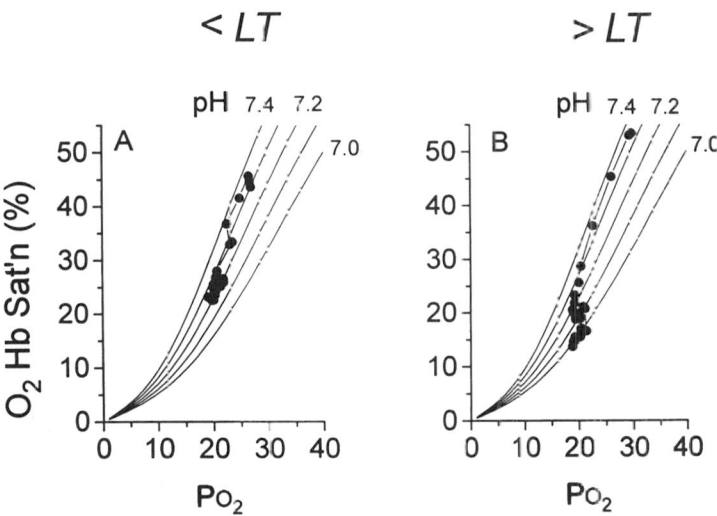

FIGURE 2.19.   Changing femoral vein oxyhemoglobin saturation (O_2Hb Sat'n; see Fig. 2.18, middle panel) as a function of femoral vein P_{O_2} (Fig. 2.18, left panel) for the 6-min constant work rate exercise tests shown in Figure 2.18. Superimposed are the lower part of oxyhemoglobin dissociation curves for pH values of 7.0–7.4, calculated from equations reported in reference 148. Left panel: data for below *LT*. Right panel: data for above *LT* exercise. Start of exercise is where O_2Hb saturation is highest. Femoral vein oxyhemoglobin saturation progressively decreased as exercise continued, as shown in Figure 2.18. Oxyhemoglobin saturations fell on pH isopleths in agreement with measured pH (Fig. 2.18, right panel). Thus the entire decrease in O_2Hb saturation that took place after P_{O_2} reached its lowest value could be accounted for by Bohr effect. (Reprinted with permission from Stringer WW, Wasserman K, Casaburi R, et al. Lactic acidosis as a facilitator of oxyhemoglobin dissociation during exercise. J Appl Physiol 1994;76:1462–1467.)

tial pressure gradient needed to allow O_2 to diffuse into the myocyte at an adequate rate to perform heavy exercise. Thus, for work rates demanding more O_2 than that at the *LT*, the further extraction of O_2 from oxyhemoglobin is H^+ concentration dependent.

BUFFERING THE EXERCISE-INDUCED LACTIC ACIDOSIS

Lactic acid is the predominant fixed acid produced during exercise. It has a pK of approximately 3.9 and therefore is essentially totally disassociated at the pH of the muscle cell (approximately 7.0). The H^+ produced in the cell, as lactate accumulates, must

be buffered immediately on its formation. Because HCO_3^- is a volatile buffer (the resulting acid does not remain in the cell but leaves on its formation), it is the primary buffer for the new H^+. Thus CO_2 production by the cell must increase at a rate commensurate with the *rate* of HCO_3^- buffering of lactic acid. Approximately 22.3 ml of CO_2 will be produced over that from aerobic metabolism for each mmol of lactic acid buffered by HCO_3^- (Fig. 2.2). The increase in cell lactate and decrease in cell HCO_3^- concentrations stimulate transmembrane exchange of these ions, with $[HCO_3^-]$ decreasing in the blood almost mmol for mmol with the increase in lactate concentration (Fig. 2.21) (33, 57–61).

The mechanism for lactate movement out of the cell is primarily carrier mediated. The studies of Trosper and Philipson, working with cardiac sarco-

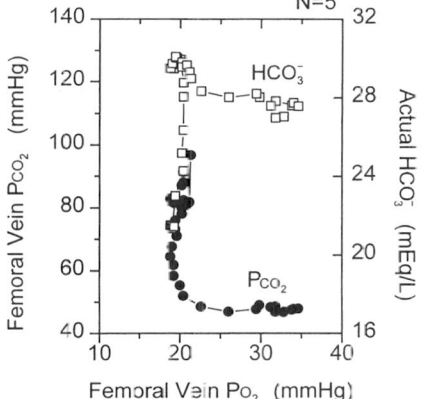

FIGURE 2.20.   Femoral vein (end-capillary) P_{CO_2} and HCO_3^- as a function of end-capillary P_{O_2} during constant work rate heavy exercise. Values are the average for the five normal subjects whose data are shown in Figure 2.18. Values at the start of exercise are at the right and move leftward as P_{O_2} decreases.

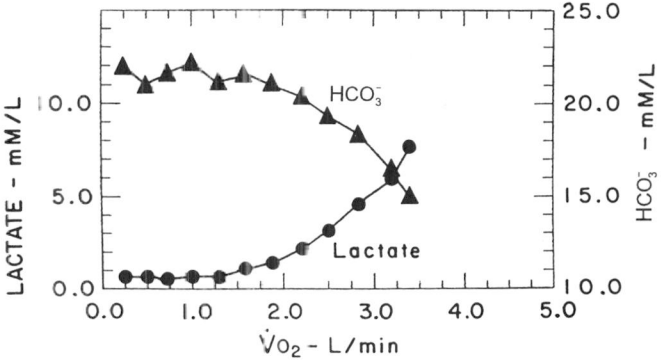

FIGURE 2.21.   The increase in arterial lactate and decrease in standard HCO_3^- as related to the increase in O_2 uptake ($\dot{V}_{O_2}$) during a progressively increasing work rate test on a cycle ergometer in a normal subject. (Modified from Wasserman K, Beaver WL, Davis JA, et al. Lactate, pyruvate, and lactate-to-pyruvate ratio during exercise and recovery. J Appl Physiol 1985;59:935–940.)

lemmal vesicles, suggest that transport is accelerated by the pH gradient across the sarcolemmal membrane (62). At the cellular level, this will be established primarily by the $[HCO_3^-]$ gradient since the intra- and extracellular fluid will have similar partial pressures of CO_2. Mainwood et al. (63) and Hirsche et al. (64) found that lactate efflux from muscle was highly influenced by the HCO_3^- concentration of the muscle perfusate. The reciprocal changes of lactate and HCO_3^- in the extracellular fluid during heavy exercise suggest that permeation of lactate across the sarcolemmal membrane is a coupled HCO_3^-—lactate antiport carrier mechanism. This is supported by the study of Korotzer et al. (65) which shows that intravenous injection of the carbonic anhydrase inhibitor, acetazolamide, during low levels of exercise about 1/2 hour before performing heavy exercise, significantly attenuates the increase in arterial lactate and decrease in bicarbonate. Replacing the intracellular HCO_3^-, which is consumed when it buffers newly produced lactic acid with HCO_3^- from the blood stream, minimizes the decrease in intracellular pH.

To better appreciate the dynamics of lactate and HCO_3^- movement between the cell and perfusing blood, arterial lactate and standard (Std) HCO_3^- were measured every 7.5 sec during the first 3 minutes and then every 30 sec during the remaining 3 minutes of a 6-minute moderate, heavy and very heavy constant load exercise (Fig. 2.22). For the latter two work intensities, lactate started to increase at about 40 sec and Std HCO_3^- started to decrease at about 50 seconds, on average. Thereafter, lactate and Std HCO_3^- changed reciprocally. The simultaneous decrease in Std HCO_3^- and lactate increase for all arterial samples for heavy and very heavy exercise intensities for the 8 subjects whose data contribute to the concentration-time plots shown in Figure 2.22, are shown in Figure 2.23. Std HCO_3^- and lactate changes were highly correlated after lactate increased by about 0.5 mmol/L and 1.0 mmol/L for heavy and very heavy intensity exercise,

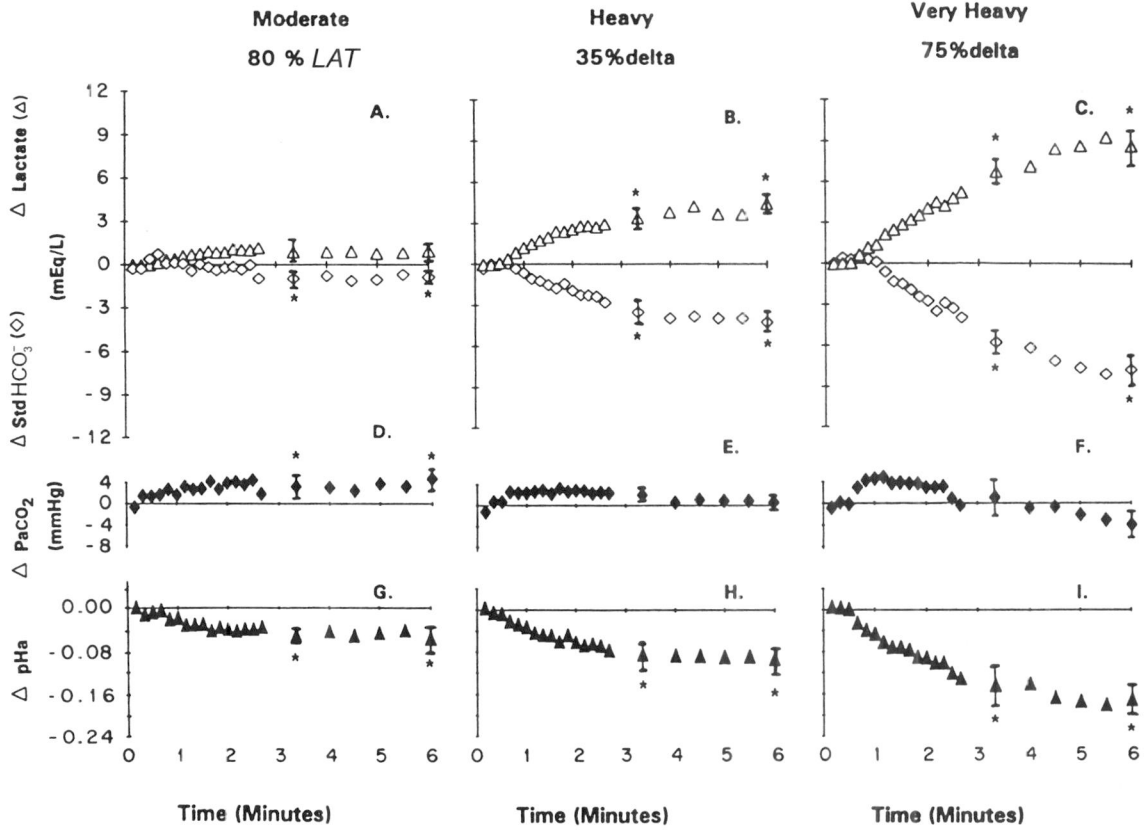

FIGURE 2.22.   Average responses to three exercise intensities displayed as change from resting measurements for arterial lactate, standard bicarbonate (Std HCO_3^-), P_{CO_2}, and pH (n = 8 subjects). Resting values for arterial pH, P_{CO_2}, Std HCO_3^-, lactate, and hemoglobin are 7.40 ± 0.03 (SD), 39.8 ± 3.1 torr, 24.5 ± 1.3 meq/l, 0.89 ± 0.47 meq/l, and 14.2 g/dl, respectively. At selected times during exercise (3 and 6 min), SEs (bars) and significant differences (*P < 0.05 from rest) are shown. (Reprinted with permission from Stringer W, Casaburi R, Wasserman K. Acid-base regulation during exercise and recovery in man. J Appl Physiol 1992;72:954–961.)

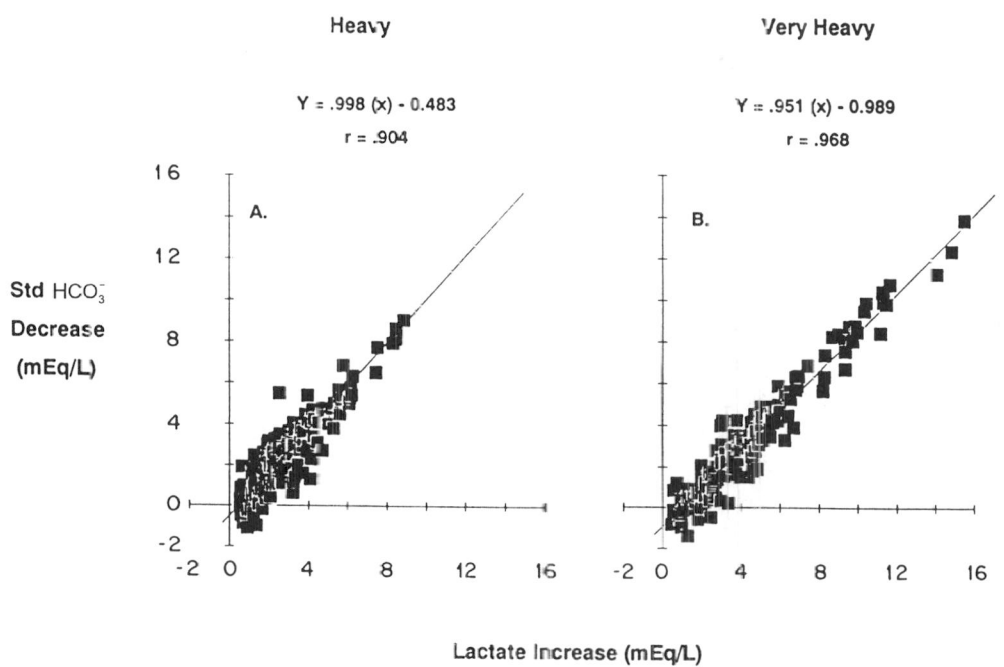

Heavy

$Y = .998 (x) - 0.483$

$r = .904$

Very Heavy

$Y = .951 (x) - 0.989$

$r = .968$

Std HCO_3^- Decrease (mEq/L)

Lactate Increase (mEq/L)

FIGURE 2.23.   Standard (Std) HCO_3^- decrease as function of lactate increase from resting values for the heavy and very heavy work intensities shown in Figure 2.22. Fall in Std HCO_3^- is delayed until after lactate starts to increase (see regression equations). Thereafter, changes are approximately equal and opposite [heavy, $n = 181$: slope = 0.998 (CI 0.92 to 1.06), intercept = -0.48 (CI -0.71 to -0.26; very heavy, $n = 141$: slope = 0.951 (CI 0.92 - 0.98), intercept = -0.99 (CI -1.12 to -0.78)]. (Reprinted with permission from Stringer W, Casaburi R, Wasserman K. Acid-base regulation during exercise and recovery in man. J Appl Physiol 1992;72:954-961.)

respectively (58). This suggests that the earliest H^+ produced with lactate is buffered by a mechanism other than HCO_3^- buffer, or new HCO_3^- buffer is produced at the start of exercise. Supporting the latter mechanism is the study of Wasserman et al. (66), showing the development of a femoral vein alkalemia during the first 30 s of exercise before the development of the expected acidemia. This alkalemia was due to the early release of K^+ from the muscle cell accompanied by a stoichiometric increase in HCO_3^-. This development of a metabolic alkalosis during the first 30 sec of exercise accounts for the failure of arterial HCO_3^- to decrease until lactate increased by approximately 0.5 to 1.0 mmol/L. The release of muscle K^+, and the development of muscle and femoral vein metabolic alkalosis, is thought to be due to the increase in intracellular pH caused by the hydrolysis of phosphocreatine (66). This early exercise-induced metabolic alkalosis masks the initial metabolic acidosis caused by the increase in lactate. Thus the lactate threshold, i.e., the $\dot{V}O_2$ above which there is a sustained lactate increase, slightly precedes the decrease in arterial Std HCO_3^- i.e., the $\dot{V}O_2$ above which metabolic acidosis develops, as previously shown by Beaver et al. (57) and Stringer et al. (58). Consequently, the lactic acidosis develops at a slightly higher $\dot{V}O_2$ as

compared with the LT. The lactic acidosis threshold (LAT) contrasts with the LT in methodology, only. The latter is determined from actual measurements of arterial lactate increase while the former is determined by the decrease in arterial standard HCO_3^- concentration or the gas exchange evidence of excess CO_2 produced over that from aerobic metabolism. This excess CO_2 derives from the dissociation of HCO_3^- as it buffers lactic acid. While the LT and LAT are systematically related and conceptually interchangeable, they are not identical, quantitatively.

THE ANAEROBIC THRESHOLD (AT) CONCEPT

The finding that the lactic acidosis of exercise does not take place until after the critical capillary PO_2 is reached supports the concept that lactate accumulation in the active muscle takes place when the muscle O_2 supply becomes critical. Thus the anaerobic threshold, measured by arterial lactate increase, arterial HCO_3^- decrease or the CO_2 generated from the HCO_3^- buffering of lactic acid (53) describes a $\dot{V}O_2$ at which the critical capillary PO_2 had been reached for a given work task. The decrease in PO_2 to its lowest or critical value before lactate concentration starts to increase in femoral vein blood lends support to the concept that the lactate increase during exercise is tissue O_2-supply dependent.

That the lactic acidosis of exercise results from tissue hypoxia is further supported by the observation that the muscle lactate/pyruvate ratio (L/P), a measure of the cell redox state, increases when the lactate threshold is reached (44, 67–68). Arterial blood lactate and pyruvate measurements in humans also show that the arterial L/P ratio increases at the lactate threshold (37). Because the cytosolic $NADH+H^+/NAD^+$ ratio is regulated by the mitochondrial redox state through the mitochondrial membrane shuttle (Fig. 2.1), failure to reoxidize mitochondrial coenzymes with molecular O_2 would also limit the reoxidation of cytosolic $NADH+H^+$ to NAD^+, thereby causing the cytosolic L/P ratio to increase.

Studies during exercise in which carboxyhemoglobin (COHb) was experimentally increased, provide further evidence that lactate concentration and $\dot{V}O_2$ above the LT are O_2 transport dependent, but work below the LT are O_2 transport independent (29, 69). Progressively increasing work rate exercise tests were done without increasing COHb in the blood and compared with the same work rate protocol in which COHb was increased to 10% and (on a separate day) to 20%. These levels do not affect cellular respiration and ventilation at rest and low work rates (70). The LT decreased, systematically, as COHb concentration increased (Fig. 2.24) (69). Lactate increased in response to increased COHb (10 and 20%) only for work rates above LT exercise (29, 71). Also, consistent with the concept that work above the LT is partially anaerobic, is the finding that $\dot{V}O_2$ above the LT, but not below the LT, was

reduced the higher the COHb level (Fig. 2.24). Thus, a commonly made statement used to argue that lactate increase is not mechanistically linked to anaerobiosis, that $\dot{V}O_2$ is not affected in the work rate range in which lactate is increased, is clearly untrue.

The rate of anaerobic glycolysis is affected by blood oxygenation. Experimental observations demonstrate that blood lactate concentration can be reduced or increased as a result of changes in blood oxygenation (8, 29, 71–73). For example, increasing blood O_2 content during exercise above the LT reduces arterial blood lactate, whereas reducing it increases blood lactate (32, 73). The diversion of pyruvate from the tricarboxylic acid cycle to the production of lactate results in accelerated use of carbohydrate stores (8, 9).

Identifying AT by Gas Exchange

Figure 2.25 shows the effect of an increasing work rate on ventilation and gas exchange for a cycle ergometer exercise test in which the work rate was increased at 1-minute intervals, after a 4-minute warm-up period of pedaling without load. As the work rate is increased, $\dot{V}O_2$, $\dot{V}CO_2$, and $\dot{V}E$ rapidly enter a region in which they increase linearly until the exercise lactic acidosis develops. At work rates above the LAT, CO_2 output increases more rapidly than O_2 uptake because CO_2 generated by the bicarbonate buffering of lactic acid is added to the metabolic CO_2 production. This is the basis of the V-slope plot for measuring the anaerobic threshold (74) (described below). Initially, $\dot{V}E$ increases in proportion to the increased CO_2 output (isocapnic buffering). Thus, $\dot{V}E$ retains a linear relationship with

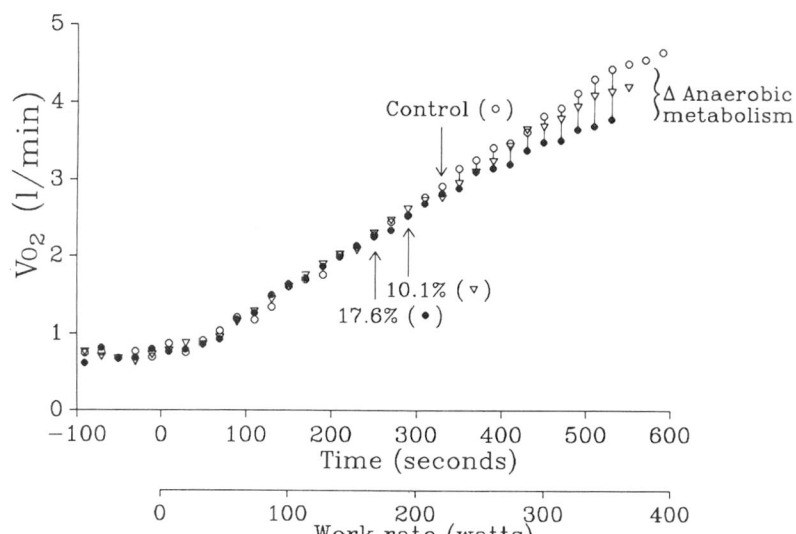

FIGURE 2.24. $\dot{V}O_2$ response to three ramp tests (work rate increased at 40 watt/min) during air breathing (control test) and air plus carbon monoxide breathing that resulted in COHb levels of 10.1% and 17.6% in 1 subject. Points to the left of 0 are measured during unloaded cycling. Each point is average of 20 sec of data. Arrows show time (and work rate) and $\dot{V}O_2$ of the anaerobic threshold for the three tests. Area enclosed in bracket is metabolic equivalent of increased anaerobic metabolism caused when COHb was increased to 17.6%. (Reprinted with permission from Koike A, Weiler-Ravell D, McKenzie DK, et al. Evidence that the metabolic acidosis threshold is the anaerobic threshold. J Appl Physiol 199;8:2521–2526.)

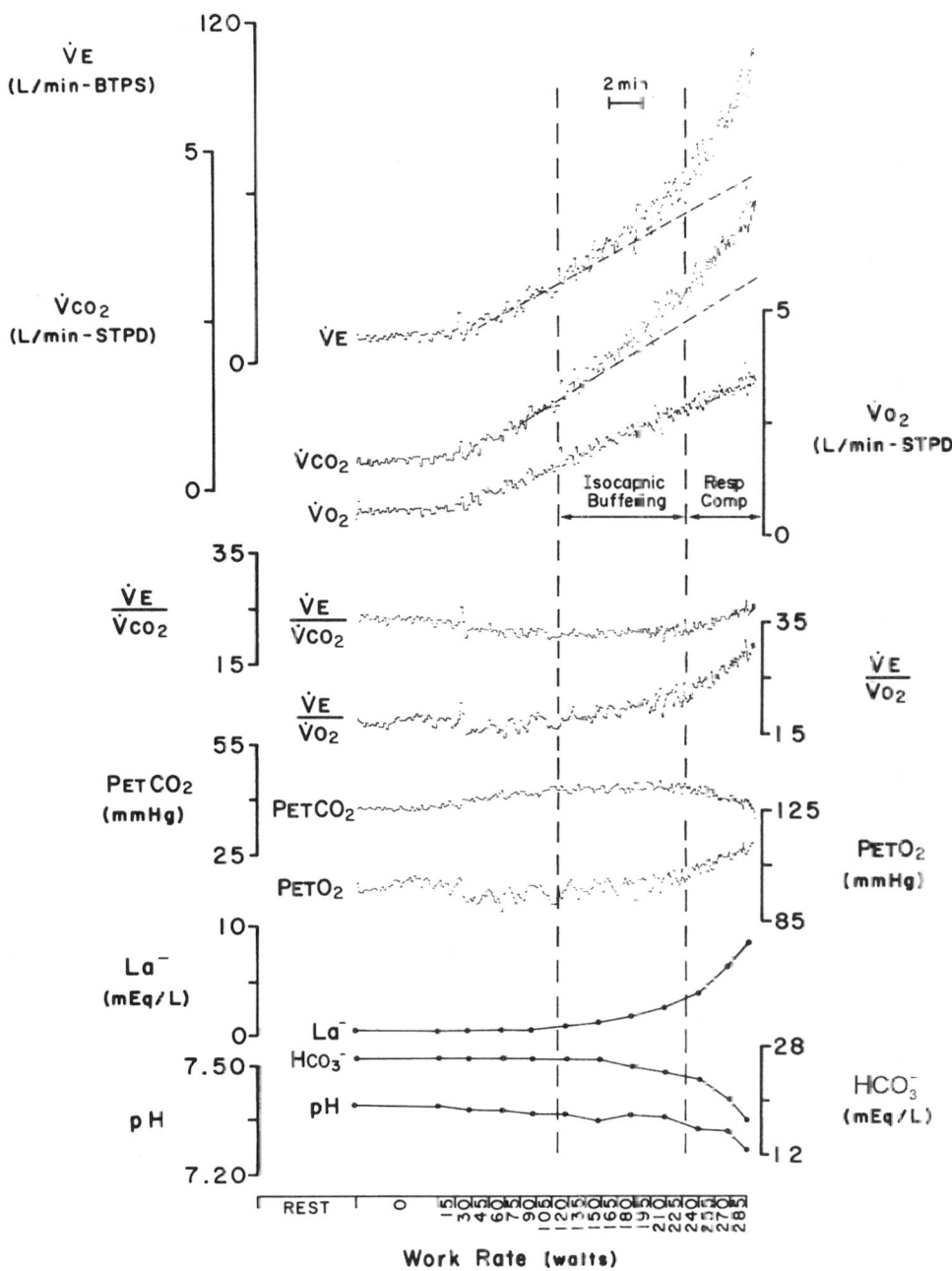

FIGURE 2.25. Breath-by-breath measurements of minute ventilation ($\dot{V}E$), CO_2 output ($\dot{V}CO_2$), O_2 uptake ($\dot{V}O_2$), $\dot{V}E/\dot{V}CO_2$ $\dot{V}E/\dot{V}O_2$, $PETCO_2$, $PETO_2$, arterial lactate and bicarbonate, and pH for a one-minute incremental exercise test on a cycle ergometer. The *LT* occurs when lactate increases (left vertical dashed line). This is accompanied by a fall in HCO_3^- (*LAT*) and generally an increase in $\dot{V}E/\dot{V}O_2$. "Isocapnic buffering" refers to the period when $\dot{V}E$ and $\dot{V}CO_2$ increase curvilinearly at the same rate without an increase in $\dot{V}E/\dot{V}CO_2$, thus retaining a constant $PETCO_2$. After the period of isocapnic buffering, $PETCO_2$ decreases and $\dot{V}E/\dot{V}CO_2$ increases, reflecting ventilatory compensation for the metabolic acidosis of exercise.

$\dot{V}CO_2$ ($\dot{V}E/\dot{V}CO_2$ appears constant or decreases slightly) while it increases relative to O_2 ($\dot{V}E/\dot{V}C_2$ increases) above the *LAT* (see Fig. 2.25). As the work rate is increased further, $\dot{V}E$ starts to increase even more rapidly than CO_2 output (increase in $\dot{V}E/\dot{V}CO_2$), causing $PaCO_2$ and $PETCO_2$ to decrease. This additional ventilatory response reflects the ventilatory compensation for the exercise-induced lactic acidosis. The increased H^+ concentration stimulates the carotid bodies to increase ventilatory drive (34). By increasing the ventilatory drive, arterial PCO_2 is reduced, providing a ventilatory constraint to the

lactic acid-induced fall in pH (75). Table 2.2 contrasts the exercise gas exchange responses for constant work rate exercise performed below and above the *AT*.

Figure 2.2 shows the effect of buffering the cellular lactic acidosis with HCO_3^- on $\dot{V}CO_2$ relative to $\dot{V}O_2$. The increases in $\dot{V}O_2$ and $\dot{V}CO_2$, as a function of progressively increasing work rate, are shown in Figure 2.26. Plotting $\dot{V}CO_2$ as a function of $\dot{V}O_2$ for a progressively increasing work rate test (V-slope plot) yields a progression of points which most commonly appear to be linear with a slope of approxi-

TABLE 2.2 Differences in Response to Exercise for Work Rates below and above the Anaerobic Threshold (*AT*)

Measurement	Below AT	Above AT
Exercise duration	Prolonged; limited by muscular and skeletal trauma or substrate, fluid balance, thermoregulation	Reduced; limited by inadequate O_2 transport, "fatigue" or dyspnea
$\dot{V}O_2$, time to steady-state	<3 min	>3 min; steady-state may not occur
$\dot{V}CO_2$, time to steady-state	<4 min	<4 min
$\dot{V}E$, time to steady-state	<4 min	>4 min; steady-state usually does not occur
$PaCO_2$	Constant	Decreasing
pHa	Approx. 7.4	Metabolic acidosis

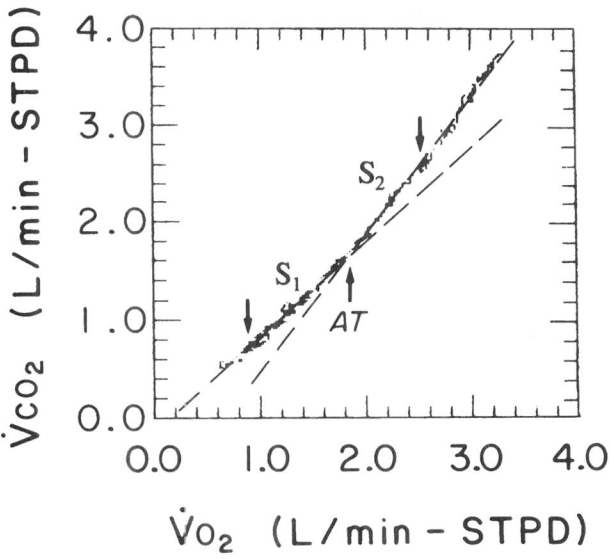

FIGURE 2.27. CO_2 output ($\dot{V}CO_2$) as a function of oxygen uptake ($\dot{V}O_2$) during a progressively increasing work rate test (v-slope plot). The transition from aerobic metabolism, in which $\dot{V}CO_2$ increases linearly with $\dot{V}O_2$ with a slope (S_1) slightly less than 1, to anaerobic plus aerobic metabolism, where the slope increases to a value greater than 1 (S_2), defines the lactic acidosis threshold (*LAT*) or anaerobic threshold (*AT*) by gas exchange. The steeper S_2 reflects the production of additional CO_2 from HCO_3^- buffering of lactic acid over that produced by aerobic metabolism. Hyperventilation does not occur at the *AT* during a progressively increasing work rate test and, therefore, does not contribute to the steepening of S_2. The lower downward directed arrow indicates where CO_2 stores are no longer increasing and calculation of S_1 starts. The upper downward directed arrow indicates the $\dot{V}O_2$ above which hyperventilation in response to metabolic acidosis starts. S_1 and S_2 are calculated from the data between these two arrows. (Modified from Beaver WL, Wasserman K, Whipp BJ. A new method for detecting the anaerobic threshold by gas exchange. J Appl Physiol 1986;60 2020–2027.)

mately 1, after the first minute of the progressively increasing work rate test. The curve then breaks with the $\dot{V}CO_2$ increasing faster than $\dot{V}O_2$ so that the slope is now clearly above 1. The break-point where the slopes coincide is the anaerobic or lactic acidosis threshold (Fig. 2.27). This slope transition coincides with the *LAT*, as confirmed with arterial standard HCO_3^- measurements. It is slightly higher than the *LT* for the reasons described in the section

entitled "Buffering the exercise-induced lactic acidosis (74)." The slope of the increase in $\dot{V}CO_2$ relative to $\dot{V}O_2$ below the threshold (S_1 in Fig. 2.27), has an average value of 0.95 with a small variation (10, 11). The transition to a slope greater than 1 (S_2 in Fig. 2.27) occurs, on average, in the mid-range of healthy subjects' aerobic capacities.

The intercept of S_1 and S_2 is the *LAT*, measured by gas exchange, and estimates the *AT*. The term *LAT* describes the biochemical event that causes the $\dot{V}CO_2$ vs $\dot{V}O_2$ slope to exceed 1, although the underlying mechanism is the lactic acidosis resulting from exercise above the *AT*. Hyperventilation (reduction in $PaCO_2$ and increase in $\dot{V}E/\dot{V}CO_2$) almost never occurs at the *LAT*. As shown in Figure 2.25, when hyperventilation does occur during a progressively increasing work rate test, it does so at a higher $\dot{V}O_2$ (at the upper, downward-directed arrow in Fig. 2.27) and represents the ventilatory

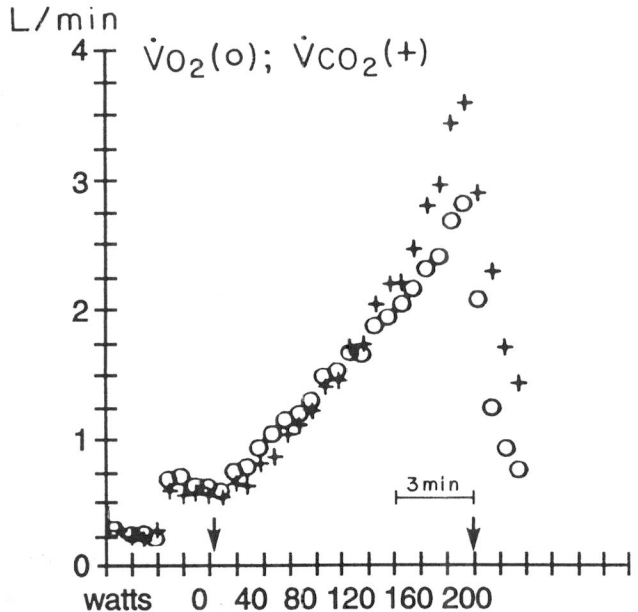

FIGURE 2.26. $\dot{V}CO_2$ and $\dot{V}O_2$ as related to work rate for 1-minute incremental (20 W/min) cycle ergometer exercise test. $\dot{V}CO_2$ starts to increase more steeply than $\dot{V}O_2$ in the middle work-rate range, reflecting buffering of lactic acid above the lactic acidosis threshold.

compensation for the lactic acidosis. S_2 being steeper than 1 during the progressively increasing work rate test signifies that CO_2 is being released from cell HCO_3^- as it dissociates during the buffering of lactic acid (Fig. 2.2).

Cooper et al. (10) reported that S_1 did not vary with different rates of increase in work rate. However, S_2 becomes steeper the faster the work rate increase (10, 76), presumably because of the faster rate of lactate formation relative to $\dot{V}_{O_2}$ increase. However, with glycogen depletion, S_1 becomes more shallow, consistent with the lower respiratory quotient of the metabolic substrate (10).

Altered Physiological Responses to Exercise Above the *AT*

Table 2.2 contrasts the gas exchange responses to constant load exercise performed below and above the *AT*. The *AT* appears to be an excellent discriminator of the highest work rate that can be endured for a prolonged period of exercise, such as a marathon (77, 78). $\dot{V}_{O_2}$ and $\dot{V}_E$ reach a steady-state early for exercise at or below the *AT*. However, a steady state in $\dot{V}_{O_2}$ and $\dot{V}_E$ is delayed or not achieved for exercise above the *AT*. Acid-base balance is essentially the same as at rest below the *AT* (acid-base homeostasis). In contrast, there is a metabolic acidosis above the *AT* with $P_{a CO_2}$ decreasing as arterial acidemia is sustained.

Table 2.3 lists the physiological changes that take place when performing exercise above the *AT*. These include important functional adaptations which affect ATP production and mitochondrial O_2 supply such as further vasodilatation in the vascular bed with high H^+ production (79), a shift in the

TABLE 2.3. Altered Physiological Responses to Exercise above the *AT*

1. Accelerated muscle glycogen utilization and anaerobic regeneration of ATP
2. Reduced exercise endurance
3. Metabolic acidosis
4. Bohr effect rather than decreasing capillary P_{O_2} increases O_2 extraction from blood
5. Increased plasma electrolyte concentration
6. Hemoconcentration
7. Increased production of metabolic intermediaries, e.g., glycerol phosphate and alanine
8. Delay in $\dot{V}_{O_2}$ steady state
9. Increased $\dot{V}_{CO_2}$ over that predicted from aerobic metabolism
10. Increased ventilatory drive
11. Increased catecholamine levels
12. Increased double product

oxyhemoglobin dissociation curve to the right allowing O_2 to unload more readily from hemoglobin (80) and increase in hemoglobin concentration (81). A description of the physiological responses to exercise which are altered above the *AT* follows.

Accelerated Glycolysis

A.V. Hill and associates (82) showed a correlation between blood lactate increase and the O_2 debt (the amount of O_2 consumed, over resting levels, during the recovery from exercise). When the mechanism for glycolysis was better understood, it was appreciated that three ATP molecules were generated during the anaerobic metabolism of one glycosyl unit of glycogen to two lactate molecules (83). By this mechanism, anaerobic glycolysis provided energy without molecular oxygen during exercise (Fig. 2.1), and, accordingly, O_2 consumption decreased slowly to resting values during recovery as lactate was metabolized.

Exercise Endurance

Exercise endurance is reduced for work rates above the *AT*, the reduction being greater the higher the blood lactate that the exercise engenders (Fig. 2.10). Reduced endurance may not be due to the increased lactate concentration or the associated increase in H^+, per se, but rather due to the inadequate rate of aerobic production of ATP, reflected by the rising lactate concentration as work rate approaches the subject's peak $\dot{V}_{O_2}$.

Oxyhemoglobin Dissociation

Perhaps the most important beneficial effect of net lactate accumulation during exercise is to cause H^+ to increase in the capillary bed where lactate is produced. This mechanism serves to facilitate the dissociation of oxyhemoglobin. As described, the rightward shift in the oxyhemoglobin dissociation curve caused by H^+ defends the capillary P_{O_2} and allows arterial-venous O_2 difference to increase maximally when performing heavy intensity exercise (53). Dissociation of oxyhemoglobin at work rates above the *AT* occurs because of the Bohr effect created by the increase in lactic acid. Thus in a disorder in which lactate can not increase, such as in McArdle's syndrome (84) or disorders of glycolysis in which lactate can not increase, it is not possible to extract O_2 to the extent seen in normal subjects during maximal exercise. This has been experimentally demonstrated by the finding that the maximum

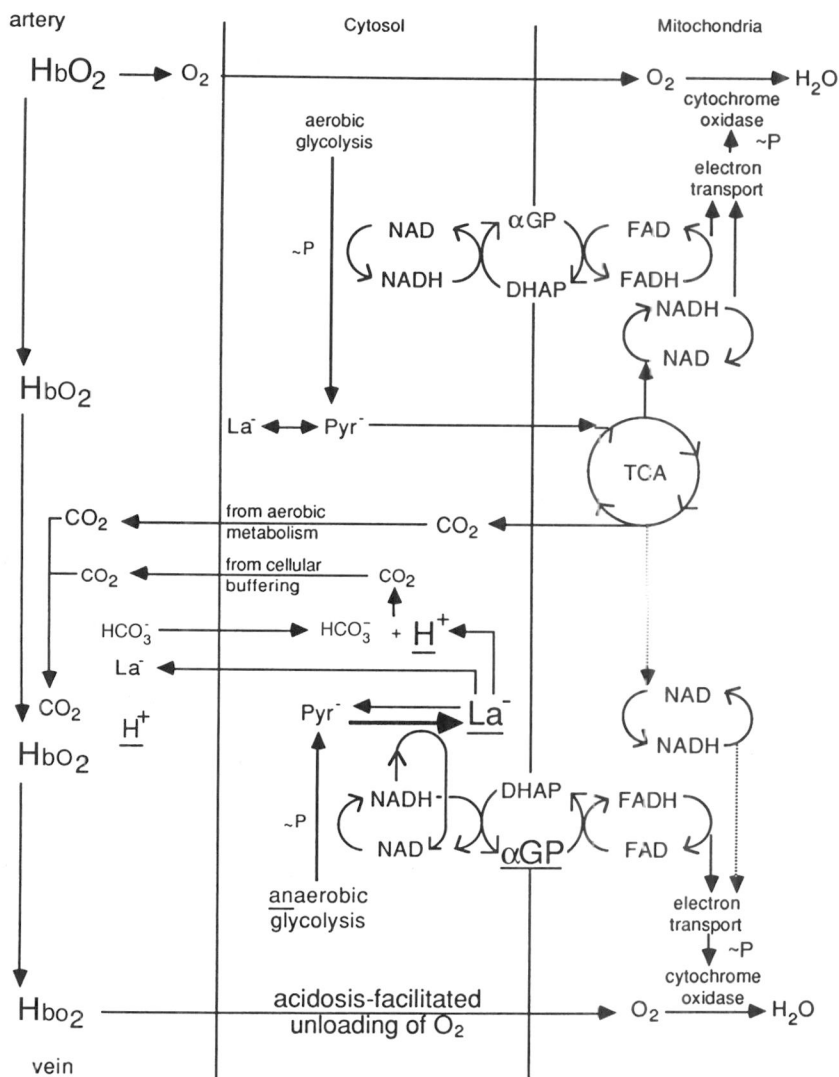

FIGURE 2.28.   Scheme of changing capillary oxyhemoglobin (HbO_2) saturation during blood transit from artery to vein during heavy intensity exercise. At arterial end of capillary, HbO_2 dissociates primarily due to decrease in Po_2. Glycolysis proceeds aerobically, without an increase in lactate (La^-), because mitochondrial membrane redox shuttles (e.g. dihydroxyacetone acetone phosphate, DHAP) regulate cystolic redox state ($NADH+H^+/NAD^+$, abbreviated NADH/NAD). Primary substrate for the triboxylic acid (TCA) cycle is pyruvate (pyr). As pyr is metabolized in the mitochondria, protons and electrons flow through the electron transport chain to O_2, generating $\sim$P with H_2O and CO_2 as by-products. As blood reaches the venous end of capillary where Po_2 becomes critically low, mitochondrial membrane redox shuttle fails to reoxidize NADH to NAD at an adequate rate. Thus the NADH/NAD ratio increases. Accordingly, pyr is converted to La^- and DHAP is converted to glycerol 3-phosphate (G3P) in proportion to the change in cell redox state (90). The effect is an increase in cell La^- with a stoichiometric increase in H^+. The latter is immediately buffered by HCO_3^- in the cell. Decreasing cellular HCO_3^- and increasing cellular La^- results in intracellular-extracellular La^- and HCO_3^- exchange (Fig. 2.2). Simultaneously, CO_2, formed during intracellular buffering, leaves the cell. The sum of aerobically and anaerobically produced CO_2 (from buffering), along with decreasing blood HCO_3^- (see Fig. 2.20) further acidify the capillary blood toward the venous end of the capillary, enhancing dissociation of HbO_2 (Bohr effect). This acidosis-facilitated dissociation of HbO_2 allows aerobic metabolism to proceed at a rate proportional to the rate of acidification of blood, without a further reduction in capillary Po_2. (Modified from Wasserman K. Coupling of external to cellular respiration during exercise: the wisdom of the body revisited. Am J Physiol 1994;266:E519–E539.)

$C(a - \bar{v})o_2$ is relatively small at the exercise work rate that the patient with McArdle's syndrome is forced to stop exercise due to muscle fatigue (85). In healthy subjects, above the AT, end capillary oxyhemoglobin saturation continues to decrease in accordance with the pH decrease, while Po_2 remains constant at its low value (Po_2 may actually increase in chronic heart failure patients, as described in Chapter 4). Thus for normal extraction of O_2 by the muscles, two factors, decreasing Po_2 and increasing H^+ are required. The former appears to play a more important role in oxyhemoglobin dissociation below the AT while the latter has a major role above it (Fig. 2.19).

The biochemical interactions between capillary blood and muscle cell for optimizing the O_2 supply to mitochondria during heavy exercise are summarized in Figure 2.28. At the arterial end of the capillary, as the muscle consumes O_2, capillary P_{O_2} decreases and oxyhemoglobin dissociates. As capillary P_{O_2} falls to its "critical" value for diffusion, lactic acid starts to increase in the cell. Capillary blood H^+ quickly increases because the lactic acid-producing cells generate additional CO_2 from HCO_3^- as it dissociates when buffering lactic acid. Simultaneously, capillary blood HCO_3^- is consumed by the cell as cellular lactate exchanges with interstitial HCO_3^- (Fig. 2.28). While the intracellular buffering of lactic acid by HCO_3^- minimizes the change in cell pH, it acidifies blood more quickly than if a non-HCO_3^- buffer neutralized the cellular lactic acidosis. This is a most remarkable physiological mechanism, since the Bohr effect would not be as great with any other buffer than as with HCO_3^-. Thus, the lactic acidosis-facilitated oxyhemoglobin dissociation assures a higher blood O_2 extraction and thereby a higher maximal $\dot{V}O_2$ than would otherwise be possible.

Plasma Electrolyte Concentrations

During an incremental exercise test, arterial plasma sodium and chloride concentrations and total cation and anion concentrations increase (Fig 2.29) above the LT (86). This suggests that extracellular water volume has decreased. Since the total exercise duration was only about 15 minutes with only a few minutes of heavy exercise, it is unlikely that the extracellular fluid loss is due to sweating. Rather, the most likely cause is the increase in intracellular osmolality due to increase in intracellular lactate and other by-products of metabolism which accompany lactate increase. This increase in intracellular osmotic force must occur and thereby obligate water flux into the cell to balance the osmotic forces on both sides of the cell membrane.

Plasma K^+ differs from Na^+ and Cl^- ions in that its concentration starts to increase below the AT, although its rate of increase is faster above the AT. Wasserman et al. (66) suggested that K^+ release from cells is linked to the hydrolysis of phosphocreatine. When the latter is hydrolyzed, it creates an alkaline reaction in the cell. Thus strong cations are in relative excess compared to the extracellular fluid. Since K^+ is the primary intracellular cation, it would be this cation which would leave the cell to balance the charge across the cell membrane. It has been shown that the anion balancing the K^+ released during early exercise is accounted for by HCO_3^- (66).

Hemoconcentration

That hemoconcentration occurs when humans perform exercise has been described in a number of studies (87–89). While in certain animals, this is due to splenic contraction, this does not appear to be the mechanism in humans. Jung et al. (81) found that the hemoconcentration occurs primarily during

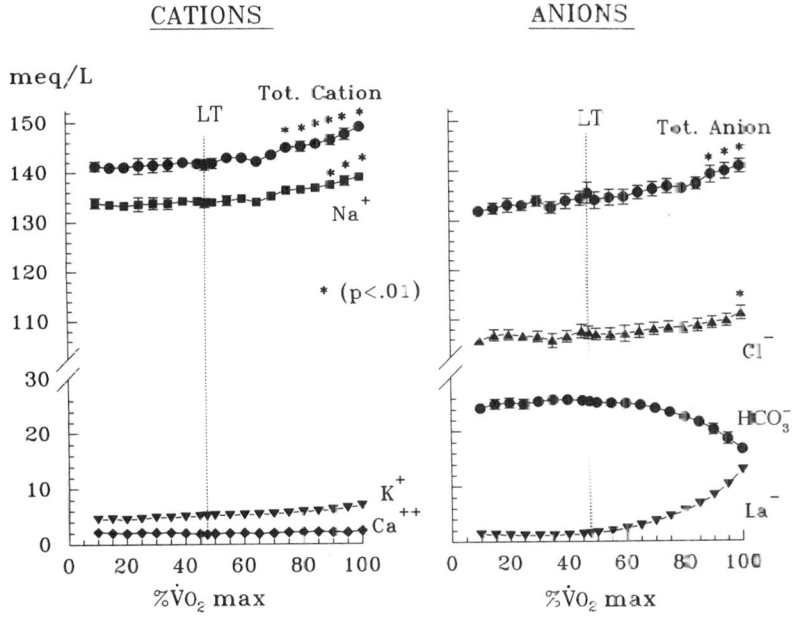

FIGURE 2.29. Change in arterial plasma Na^+, K^+, Ca^{++} and total measured cations (left panel) and Cl^-, HCO_3^-, and La^- and total measured anions (right panel) during a progressively increasing exercise test to maximum level tolerated. Data are the average for 10 normal adult subjects. The vertical bars on points are the SEM. The vertical line passing through all the curves is the average lactate threshold. (Modified from Wasserman K, Nguyen P, Korotzer B, et al. Arterial plasma electrolyte changes above the lactate threshold. FASEB J 1997;11:A214.)

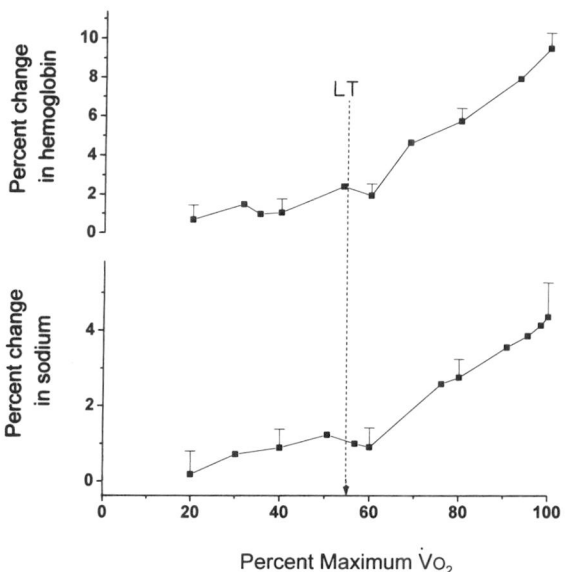

FIGURE 2.30.   Change in arterial hemoglobin, and plasma sodium concentration during progressively increasing work rate exercise. Data are the average for 10 normal adult subjects. The vertical bars on points are the SEM. The vertical line passing through the curves is the average lactate threshold for the group. The standard deviation of the lactate threshold is ±4.8% (Modified from Jung T, Korotzer B, Stringer WW, et al. Lactate concentration increase and transcellular fluid flux during exercise. Am J Respir Crit Care Med 1996;153:A647.)

exercise above the *LT*, as illustrated in Figure 2.30. The clue for the mechanism of hemoconcentration resides in the observation that the concentration of the total extracellular cations and anions increase above the *LT* (Fig. 2.29). Since the cell osmolality must increase above the *LT*, extracellular fluid would move into cells rich in lactate. The shrinkage of the extracellular fluid would increase the red cell and therefore the arterial O_2 concentration, providing more O_2 per ml of blood flow at exercise levels which cause lactate to increase. This could benefit the subject during exercise in which the O_2 supply limits exercise performance.

Metabolic Intermediaries

Katz and Sahlin (90) found, in muscle biopsy studies performed immediately at the cessation of exercise in humans, that cellular alpha-glycerol phosphate increased in proportion to the increase in lactate. Muscle cell pyruvate and alanine also increased above the *LT*. These changes are most likely secondary to the change in cytosol redox state and the accelerated rate of muscle glycolysis which takes place above the *LT*.

$\dot{V}O_2$ and $\dot{V}CO_2$ Kinetics

Figure 1.4 shows the typical onset responses of $\dot{V}O_2$ and $\dot{V}CO_2$ for moderate intensity exercise, i.e., exercise that does not engender lactic acidosis, and heavy intensity exercise, i.e., exercise that results in lactic acidosis. The patterns of gas exchange differ between the exercise performed at work rates associated with and without lactic acidosis (53, 91). In the absence of lactic acidosis, $\dot{V}O_2$ reaches a steady state by 3 minutes, while $\dot{V}CO_2$ increases more slowly, reaching a steady state by 4 minutes. In the steady state of moderate intensity exercise, the $\dot{V}CO_2$ is slightly lower than $\dot{V}O_2$ (Fig. 2.31A) because the metabolic substrate respiratory quotient is less than 1.0.

Panels D, E, and F of Figure 2.31 illustrate that $\dot{V}CO_2$ kinetics are relatively slow during the period of $\dot{V}O_2$ increase within the first minute of exercise. This slow CO_2 output relative to O_2 uptake during this early exercise period can be accounted for, in the main, by the metabolic alkalosis, and increase in blood HCO_3^- which accompanies K^+ increase (66). This early metabolic alkalosis, and relative CO_2 retention without increase in $PaCO_2$, have been attributed to the alkalization of muscle and blood perfusing it, as a result of the rapid phosphocreatine hydrolysis taking place primarily during the first minute of exercise.

For exercise performed above the *AT*, $\dot{V}O_2$ dynamics are slow compared with exercise performed below the *AT*, and a steady state in $\dot{V}O_2$ is often not reached before the subject fatigues (see Fig. 2.6). In contrast to $\dot{V}O_2$ dynamics, $\dot{V}CO_2$ dynamics do not change appreciably during above *AT* exercise (Fig. 2.32), and, usually after 1 minute of such exercise, $\dot{V}CO_2$ exceeds $\dot{V}O_2$ (Figs. 2.31, 2.32), the magnitude depending on the rate of lactate increase (91, 92). The extra CO_2 during heavy intensity exercise can be accounted for by the CO_2 produced as HCO_3^- buffers the H^+ from lactic acid, and to a lesser degree, CO_2 unloading from body stores due to hyperventilation, if $PaCO_2$ is decreased (see Figs. 2.2, 2.25).

Ventilatory Drive

Ventilation tracks the acidity added to the blood as a result of metabolism. Thus the addition of CO_2 from the HCO_3^- buffering of lactic acid, as well as the reduction in plasma HCO_3^- concentration, adds acid equivalents to the blood. The ventilatory control mechanisms are stimulated to provide levels of

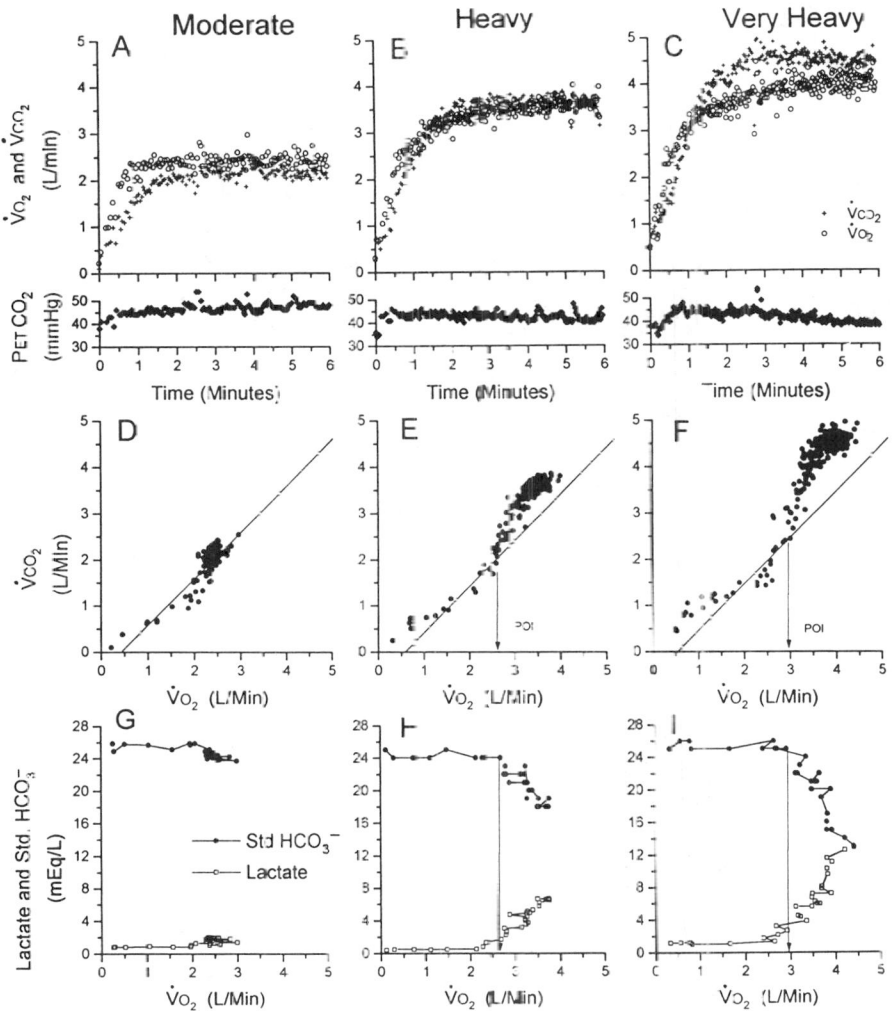

FIGURE 2.31. O_2 uptake ($\dot{V}O_2$), CO_2 output ($\dot{V}CO_2$), $P_{ET}CO_2$ plotted as a function of time (panels A, B and C) and $\dot{V}CO_2$, arterial lactate and standard (Std) HCO_3^- plotted as a function of $\dot{V}O_2$ (panels D-I) for constant work rate tests of moderate, heavy and very heavy work intensity. Steepening of $\dot{V}CO_2$ relative to $\dot{V}O_2$ (arrow in panels E and F) occurs simultaneously with the increase in lactate and decrease in HCO_3^- (arrow in panels H and I) reflecting the buffering of the lactic acid by HCO_3^- (Modified from Stringer WW, Wasserman K, Casaburi R. The $\dot{V}CO_2/\dot{V}O_2$ relationship during heavy, constant work rate exercise reflects the rate of lactate accumulation. Eur J Appl Physiol 1995;72:25–31.)

ventilation that continue to increase during exercise as long as the arterial pH remains reduced. The proposed control mechanisms will be discussed in greater detail below. The magnitude of the added ventilatory drive is illustrated in Figure 2.33 and Table 2.4.

While net lactic acid production, through its H^+, stimulates breathing, causing hyperventilation, it might induce dyspnea in the ventilatory limited subject. However, the lactic acidosis might provide more benefit than hindrance to the normal subject during the performance of high intensity exercise by: 1) facilitating oxyhemoglobin dissociation through the Bohr effect, thereby allowing increased

TABLE 2.4. Increase in Blood Lactate (Δ Lactate), $\dot{V}E$ and Heart Rate at 6 min of Work Rate of 200W

Subject	Δ Lactate (Mmol/L)	$\dot{V}E$ (L/min)	H.R. (Beats/min)
1	1.9	60	156
2	2.7	81	163
3	5.0	79	151
4	5.1	85	153
5	9.7	151	186

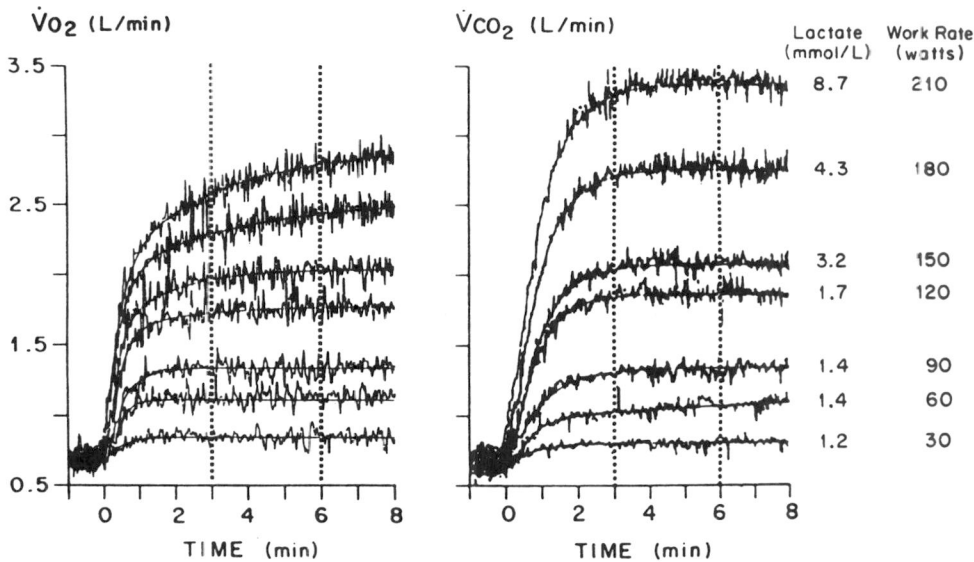

FIGURE 2.32. O_2 uptake ($\dot{V}O_2$) and CO_2 output ($\dot{V}CO_2$) as related to time at seven different levels of work for a healthy subject. The three lowest work rates are below the subject's lactic acidosis threshold (*LAT*) while the four highest work rates are above it. The $\dot{V}O_2$ continues to rise for the 4 work rates above the *LAT*, the rate of rise being more marked the higher the work rate. In contrast, the $\dot{V}CO_2$ kinetics are relatively unchanging, reaching a constant level by 3 to 4 minutes in all 7 tests. (Modified from Casaburi R, Barstow TJ, Robinson T, et al. Influence of work rate on ventilatory and gas exchange kinetics. J Appl Physiol 1989;67:547–555.)

O_2 extraction from blood, 2) the increased arterial O_2 content resulting from the hemoconcentration which takes place above the *AT*, 3) the local vasodilatation caused by the tissue acidosis, and 4) the hyperventilation-induced increase in PaO_2 which can increase PaO_2, particularly important to the subject performing exercise at high altitude.

Catecholamines

The plasma catecholamines increase at work rates above the *LT* (93). We find that the increases in epinephrine and norepinephrine concentrations occur above the *LT* and therefore can not account

for the *LT* itself. The increases might represent a cardiovascular compensatory mechanism for the anaerobic stress. Similar changes are reported to take place, but at lower work rates, in patients with chronic heart failure.

Rate-Pressure Product

The product of heart rate and systolic pressure increases during exercise, becoming more steep above the *AT* (94). The increase in slope suggests that myocardial work is increasing. The increasing catecholamine levels possibly contribute to the steepening in the rate-pressure product. The increasing

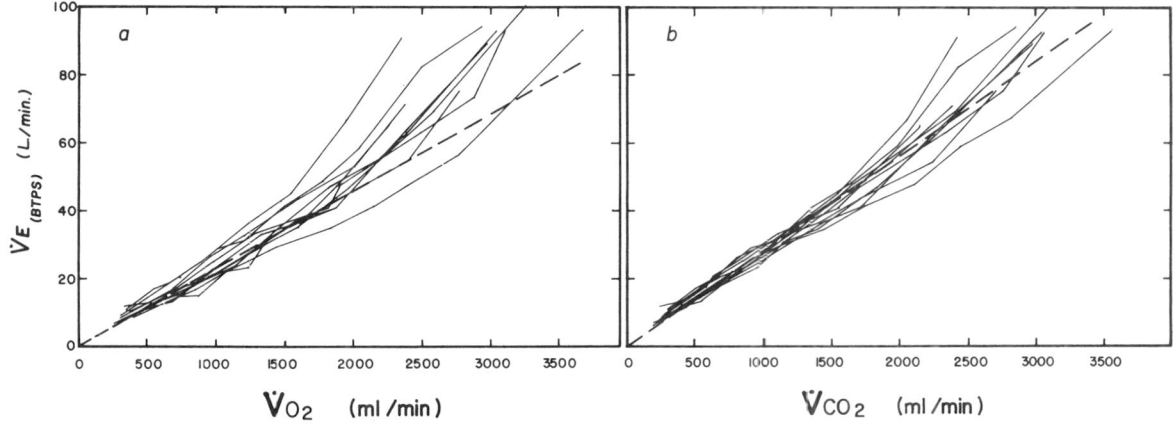

FIGURE 2.33.   Relationship between steady state minute ventilation ($\dot{V}E$) and oxygen consumption ($\dot{V}O_2$), and CO_2 production ($\dot{V}CO_2$) in ten normal subjects. The curvilinear increase in ventilation at high metabolic rates reflects respiratory compensation for the metabolic acidosis. The reduced dispersion noted in the correlation between $\dot{V}E$ and $\dot{V}CO_2$, as compared to $\dot{V}E$ and $\dot{V}O_2$, reflects the functional dependence of ventilation on CO_2 flow to the lungs and the effect of differences in RQ among the subjects. (Reprinted with permission from ref. 33.)

rate-pressure product above the *AT* might be a mechanism which serves to enhance O_2 delivery to muscle when there is an imbalance between O_2 demand and O_2 supply.

Anaerobic, Lactate and Lactic Acidosis Thresholds

The $\dot{V}O_2$ at which arterial lactate and the L/P ratio increase is reproducible for a given subject. The actual value depends primarily on fitness and the form of exercise. The $\dot{V}O_2$ at which the anaerobic supplementation (lactate increase) of the aerobic energy exchange begins, has been termed the anaerobic threshold (*AT*) (95). The mechanistic basis for the anaerobic threshold, and the changes in gas exchange which accompanies it, follows:

1. The increased O_2 required by the metabolically active muscles can create an O_2 supply/demand imbalance so that capillary PO_2 falls to its lowest value compatible with diffusion ("critical" capillary PO_2); this is reflected in a minimum end-capillary PO_2 and an increase in net lactic acid production as work rate or exercise time increases further (Fig. 2.16).
2. The imbalance between the O_2 supply and O_2 requirement causes the proton scavenging mitochondrial membrane proton shuttle (Fig. 2.1) to lose pace with the rate of $NADH + H^+$ production in the cytosol, resulting in a more reduced cytosolic redox state.
3. The lowering of the cytosolic redox state causes pyruvate to react with the increased $NADH + H^+$, and become reduced to lactate while regenerating NAD^+ and allowing glycolysis to continue.
4. The accumulating lactic acid is immediately buffered, intracellularly, predominantly by HCO_3^-, generating additional CO_2 (see Fig. 2.2).
5. HCO_3^- exchanges for lactate across the muscle cell membrane (Fig. 2.2), causing arterial blood HCO_3^- to decrease as lactate increases (Figs. 2.21, 2.22, 2.31, 2.34).
6. The buffering and acid-base disturbances produce predictable changes in gas exchange (Figs. 2.25, 2.27, 2.34).

Because the *AT*, *LT*, and *LAT* are all part of the same phenomenon from a practical point of view, making the distinction only distinguishes the method of measurement and does not dispute their

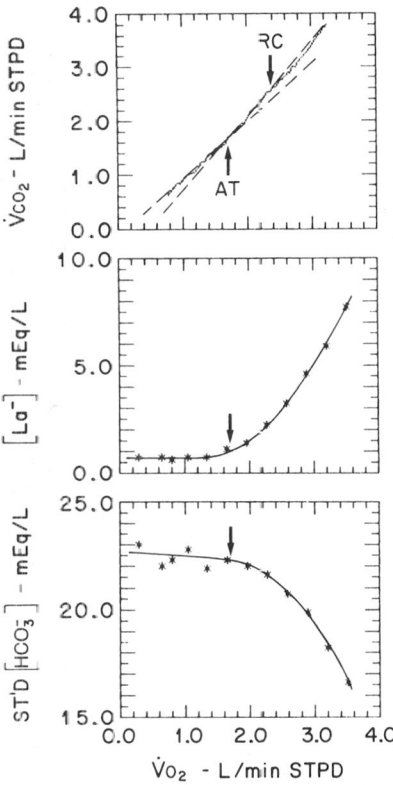

FIGURE 2.34.   Plots of arterial lactate and standard HCO_3^- concentrations and $\dot{V}CO_2$ as a function of $\dot{V}O_2$ for a single subject. Arrows indicate estimates of the anaerobic threshold (*AT*) from the $\dot{V}CO_2$ vs. $\dot{V}O_2$ plot, which are seen to also represent reasonable estimates of lactate increase and HCO_3^- decrease versus $\dot{V}O_2$. RC is the respiratory compensation point.

common underlying mechanism, anaerobic metabolism (96). While these terms are commonly used interchangeably, we regard the technically correct definitions to be as follows.

Anaerobic Threshold (*AT*)

The *AT* is the exercise $\dot{V}O_2$ above which anaerobically-produced high-energy PO_4 supplements the aerobically produced high energy PO_4, with consequent lowering of the cytosolic redox state, increasing L/P ratio and increasing lactate production at the site of cellular anaerobiosis.

Lactate Threshold (*LT*)

The *LT* is the exercise $\dot{V}O_2$ above which a net increase in lactate production is observed to result in a sustained increase in lactate concentration in the circulating blood.

Lactic Acidosis Threshold (*LAT*)

The *LAT* is the exercise $\dot{V}O_2$ above which arterial Std HCO_3^- (the principal buffer of lactic acid) is observed to decrease because of a net increase in lactic acid production. During an increasing work rate exercise test, this can be detected by an increase in CO_2 output above that which would be predicted from aerobic metabolism (because of dissociation of HCO_3^- as it buffers lactic acid).

METABOLIC-CARDIOVASCULAR-VENTILATORY COUPLING

Cellular Respiration and High Energy Phosphate Regeneration

Chemical energy, in the form of high energy phosphate ($\sim$P), is utilized at an increased rate when muscles contract. This is regenerated during exercise when mitochondrial respiration (O_2 consumption and CO_2 production) increases. The rate of regeneration of $\sim$P is proportional to cellular O_2 consumption (O_2). Creatine $\sim$P concentration rapidly decreases in proportion to the work rate performed (97) and its concentration remains reduced as the work is sustained, returning to the pre-exercise resting level within the first few minutes of recovery (98). A scheme describing the gas transport mechanisms for coupling cellular (internal) to pulmonary (external) respiration is shown in Figure 1.1. When exercise is initiated, high-energy phosphate bonds of preexisting ATP are split to support the immediate energy requirements of contracting muscle. The resulting ADP is rapidly rephosphorylated to ATP from creatine phosphate and the conversion of substrate energy to chemical energy ($\sim$P), primarily in muscle mitochondria. Experimental evidence suggests that the increases in concentration of creatine, inorganic phosphate and ADP in the muscle stimulate oxidative phosphorylation, thereby replenishing ATP (47). This keeps the ATP relatively constant during exercise as the metabolic requirement approaches the subject's maximal exercise capacity. Only as maximal work rates are approached does muscle ATP concentration start to decrease and the less phosphorylated adenosine compounds increase (44).

The cardiovascular and the ventilatory systems respond to the increased cellular O_2 requirement as well as the increased CO_2 and H^+ production, major by-products of muscle bioenergetics. For homeostasis, transfer of CO_2 and O_2 between the mitochondria and the external environment requires finely coordinated control of cardiovascular and ventilatory mechanisms which couple cellular to pulmonary respiration.

Cardiovascular Coupling to Metabolism: Muscle O_2 Supply

Cardiac output increases at the start of exercise in the upright position by increasing stroke volume and heart rate. Heart rate increases as vagal tone decreases. Stroke volume increases due to increased cardiac inotropy and increased venous return resulting from pressure gradients caused by compression of veins by contracting muscles and decreased intrathoracic pressure accompanying increased depth of breathing (99). As exercise continues, further increases in cardiac output are achieved predominantly by increasing heart rate, with stroke volume remaining relatively constant, especially at work rates above approximately 30% of $\dot{V}O_2$peak.

The pulmonary vascular bed dilates at the start of exercise in concert with the increase in right ventricular output and pulmonary artery pressure. This dilatation results in the perfusion of previously unperfused and underperfused lung units in the normal pulmonary vascular bed, accounting for the fact that there is only a small increase in pulmonary artery pressure as pulmonary blood flow increases in the normal lung. A low pulmonary vascular resistance is essential for the normal exercise response of the left ventricle. Without it, the weakly-muscled right ventricle could not readily pump the venous blood through the pulmonary circulation to the left side of the heart at a rate fast enough to effect the cardiac output increase needed to support cellular respiration.

Because the cardiac output increase is less than the increase in $\dot{V}O_2$, the extraction of O_2 from and addition of CO_2 to the muscle capillary blood must increase. Muscle blood flow increases according to its metabolic activity (100). Because of the falling capillary PO_2 and the Bohr effect, it is possible to extract 75 to 85% of the O_2 going through the capillary bed of maximally working muscle.

The oxygen supply to the muscle cells is dependent on five factors:

1. Cardiac output
2. Distribution of perfusion to the tissues in need of O_2
3. Partial pressure profile of O_2 in the capillary blood

4. Hemoglobin concentration
5. Hemoglobin's affinity for O_2

The transport of O_2 from blood to mitochondria is dependent on maintaining an adequate diffusion gradient for O_2 as the blood travels through the contracting muscle. The Po_2 gradient between blood and cell is high at the arterial end of the capillary but it decreases as the blood approaches the venous end of the capillary, depending on the O_2 flow/metabolic rate ratio (Fig. 2.14).

Cardiac Output

The cardiac output obviously must play a key role in the O_2 supply to the cells. At the start of exercise in the upright posture, stroke volume increases virtually immediately (101) the magnitude being dependent upon the relative degree of the individual's fitness, age and size (99). In the exceptionally fit young person, the stroke volume can increase by as much as 100%; the increase is much smaller in less fit and elderly people. After the initial increase in stroke volume that takes place at low levels of exercise, cardiac output increase comes about predominantly by increasing heart rate, i.e., heart rate usually increases linearly with $\dot{V}o_2$ (see the case studies of normal subjects in Chapter 9). A method for estimating the stroke volume during exercise from the $\dot{V}o_2$/heart rate relationship will be presented in Chapter 3.

Distribution of Peripheral Blood Flow

If the increase in cardiac output is not distributed appropriately to the sites of $\dot{V}o_2$ requirement, their O_2 supply will be compromised. During exercise, the fraction of the cardiac output diverted to the skeletal muscles increases, while the fraction perfusing organs such as the kidney, liver, and gastrointestinal tract, decreases (99). The increase in blood flow through the working muscles, and a small fraction through the skin to eliminate some of the heat generated during exercise, account for almost all of the increase in cardiac output that takes place during exercise. The mechanism by which blood flow is distributed during exercise depends on the response of the autonomic nervous system and local humoral control. The blood flow–metabolic rate relationship affects the level of local humoral factors, such as increased $[H^+]$, Pco_2, $[K^+]$, osmolarity, adenosine, temperature, and Po_2. These can act locally to regulate blood flow (79).

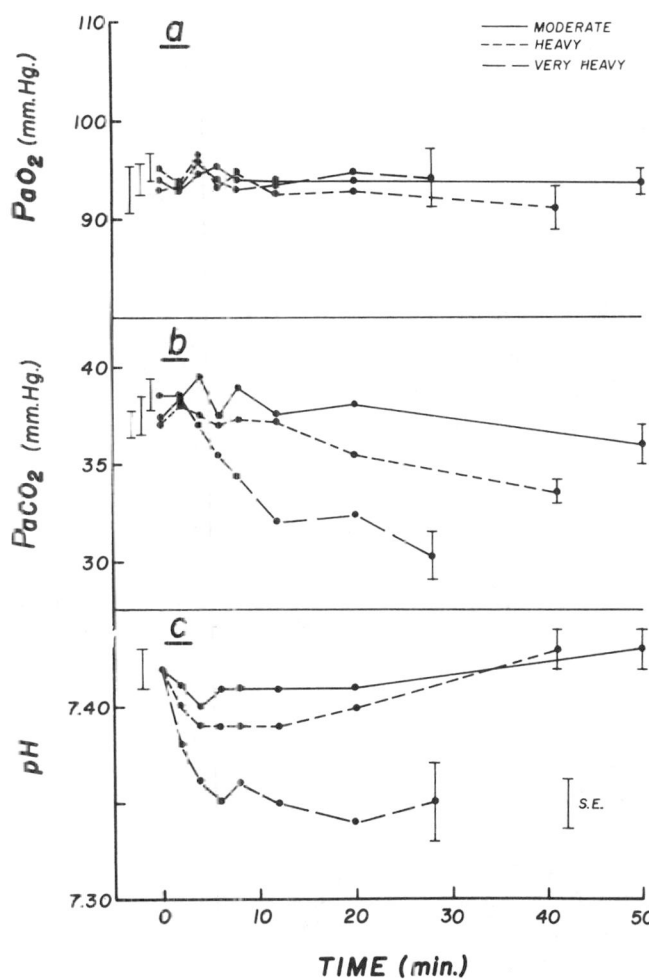

FIGURE 2.35. Effect of prolonged constant work rate exercise of moderate, heavy, and very heavy work intensity on arterial blood gases and pH. Each point is the average of ten subjects. (Reprinted with permission from Wasserman K, VanKessel AL, Burton GB. Interaction of physiological mechanisms during exercise. J Appl Physiol 1967;22:71–85.)

Arterial Po_2

In the normal subject, arterial Po_2 (Pao_2) is a function of mean alveolar Po_2 (Pao_2). For an idealized lung (all lung units having the same ventilation/perfusion ratio and no diffusion impairment) where the gas exchange ratio is 0.8 and $Paco_2$ is equal to 40 mmHg, Pao_2 would equal approximately 102 mmHg at sea level. Reductions in Pao_2 relative to the ideal Pao_2 are due to one or more of the following mechanisms: 1) a right-to-left shunt; 2) O_2 diffusion disequilibrium at the alveolar capillary interface; or 3) maldistribution of alveolar ventilation ($\dot{V}a$) with respect to lung perfusion ($\dot{Q}$). Normal young adults have a Pao_2 of about 92 mmHg (Fig. 2.35) with a $P(a - a)o_2$ of approximately 12 mmHg during exercise (33). This difference between the alveolar and arterial P_{O_2} can be attributed to a small right-to-left shunt (possibly the Thebesian blood vessels in the heart and the bronchial circulation) and the lack of total uniformity of $\dot{V}_A/\dot{Q}$ within the lungs. In highly fit subjects, diffusion impairments have also been described at very high work rates with $P(A - a)_{O_2}$ exceeding 30 mmHg (102).

Oxyhemoglobin Dissociation in Tissue

Oxyhemoglobin dissociation and the essential role played by the Bohr effect on oxygen extraction was discussed above (Figs. 2.19, 2.28). Altered hemoglobin affinity for O_2, as seen with abnormal hemoglobins, either congenital or acquired, may impair muscle O_2 supply. This might be due to either the effect on the arterial O_2 content or on the P_{50} of the hemoglobin (the partial pressure of O_2 in the blood when active hemoglobin is 50% saturated with O_2). Genetic defects causing a shift in the oxyhemoglobin dissociation curve to the left (low P_{50}) can impair O_2 extraction by the exercising muscle, since a "floor" P_{O_2} for diffusion is reached at a reduced $\dot{V}_{O_2}$. This may induce polycythemia (103). Hemoglobinopathies which shift oxyhemoglobin dissociation to the right (high P_{50}) allows O_2 to unload from hemoglobin more readily and are generally associated with anemia (103). Shifts in P_{50} are common even in normal subjects. A rightward shift resulting from acidosis, increased temperature, or high levels of 2,3diphosphoglycerate (2,3DPG) favors diffusion of O_2 from the capillaries into the mitochondria. This contrasts with the leftward shift resulting from alkalosis, carbon monoxide poisoning, or low 2,3DPG concentration, where the O_2 diffusion gradient is reduced.

Hemoglobin and Arterial O_2 Content

The arterial O_2 content depends on the arterial P_{O_2} and hemoglobin concentration that is free to take up O_2. Thus anemia, resulting in a decreased blood O_2 content, can compromise the supply of O_2 to the tissues during exercise. Also hemoglobin that is inactive (methemoglobin) or has carbon monoxide on the O_2-binding sites (as in cigarette smokers) will also result in a reduced O_2 content. All of these conditions will result in a more rapid decrease in capillary P_{O_2} than normal and the minimal capillary P_{O_2} needed for diffusion will take place at a lower metabolic rate than if all of the hemoglobin is available for O_2 transport. In the presence of anemia or increased concentration of inactive hemoglobin, the blood flow/metabolic rate ratio of the muscle ($\dot{Q}m/\dot{V}_{O_2}$ m) must increase.

Ventilatory Coupling to Metabolism

The blood passing through the lungs must be arterialized by: a) eliminating the added CO_2; b) replenishing the O_2 consumed; and c) achieving pH homeostasis. Minute ventilation ($\dot{V}_E$) normally increases at a rate required to remove the CO_2 added to the capillary blood by metabolism, and minimize the increase in H^+ concentration when lactic acidosis develops. Below the AT, the $\dot{V}_E$ increase is generally so precise that arterial P_{CO_2} and pH are regulated at approximately resting values (34). Above the AT, the metabolic acidosis stimulates ventilation, thereby reducing $P_{A CO_2}$ while constraining the fall in pH. The ventilatory increase is usually achieved at low and moderate work rates primarily by an increase in tidal volume and, to a lesser degree, breathing frequency (Fig. 2.36). The latter increases to a greater extent at work rates above the AT.

Carbon Dioxide Elimination

CO_2 production increases during exercise because of the increase in metabolic activity of the exercising muscles. The amount of CO_2 generated by this process is related to O_2 consumption by the RQ of the muscle substrate. As described above and illustrated in Figures 2.31 and 2.32, a substantial amount of additional CO_2 is derived from CO_2 stores when bicarbonate buffers lactic acid at work rates above the AT. CO_2 from stores is also added to the expired gas when the ventilatory control mechanism compensates by hyperventilation for the lactic acidosis. In contrast to tissue oxygen supply, the actual cardiac output needed for CO_2 elimination is not critical. CO_2 elimination is determined by the alveolar ventilation and the arterial P_{CO_2} (Fig. 2.37). However, the cardiac output does determine the venous-arterial CO_2 content difference $C(a - \bar{v})_{O_2}$ for a given metabolic (exercise) activity.

The venous CO_2 content for a given venous P_{CO_2} is dependent on changes in buffer base, and to the O_2 content (Christiansen-Douglas-Haldane effect) (104). The latter changes most over the lower work rate range (below the AT). The former changes most over the heavy intensity range (above the AT) due to HCO_3^- buffering of lactic acid. Since these factors affect the position of the CO_2 dissociation curve, estimates of CO_2 content from mixed venous P_{CO_2} alone must be suspect for work rates above the AT.

FIGURE 2.36. Minute ventilation ($\dot{V}E$) plotted as percentage of its asymptotic value, tidal volume (V_T) breathing rate (f), and end tidal P_{CO_2} (P_{ETCO_2}) for exercise below and above the anaerobic threshold in the same subject. The absolute values of minute ventilation are shown to the left of the vertical dashed line at the transition from unloaded cycling (0 W) to the indicated work rate. For the work rate below the anaerobic threshold, $\dot{V}E$, f, V_T and P_{ETCO_2} reach a constant value after several minutes. For the work rate above the anaerobic threshold, $\dot{V}E$ and f continue to drift upwards and P_{ETCO_2} downwards (without a significant change or slight decrease in V_T), signifying the lack of ventilatory steady-state.

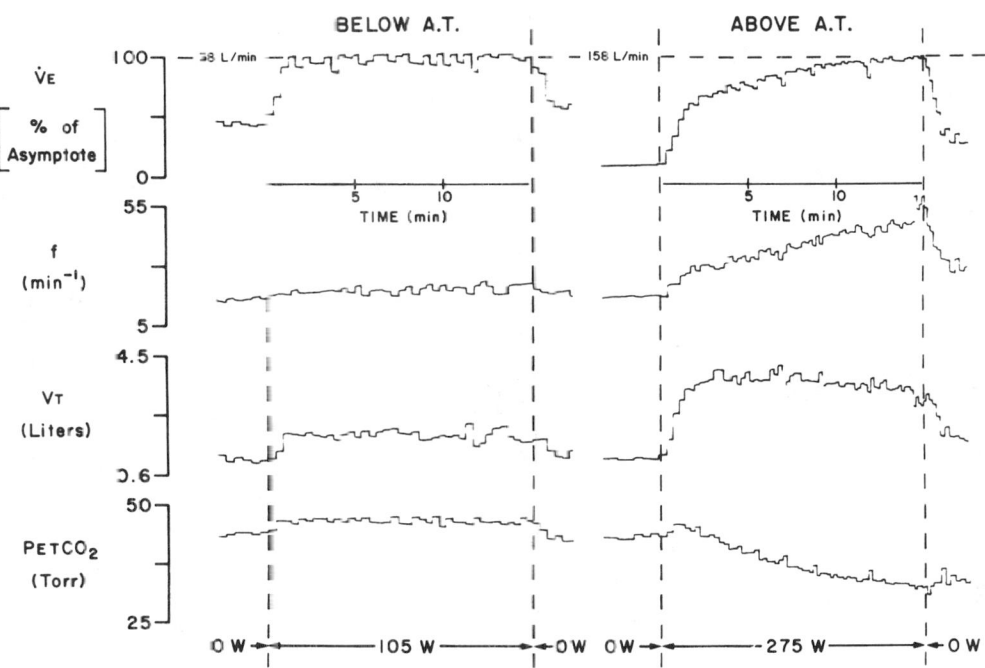

Alveolar Ventilation

The quantity of ventilation required to clear a given amount of CO_2 from the blood ($\dot{V}_{CO_2}$) depends on the CO_2 concentration in the alveolar gas ($F_{ACO_2} = P_{ACO_2}/PB$), where F_{ACO_2} is the concentration of CO_2 in the alveolar volume if the lung was functioning ideally, that is the ventilation-perfusion ratios of all lung units were the same, and PB is barometric pressure. Mass balance considerations dictate that, in an idealized lung, gas concentrations are the same in all alveolar spaces because of uniform $\dot{V}_A/\dot{Q}$

$$\dot{V}_{CO_2} = \dot{V}_A \times P_{ACO_2}/PB$$

This is the alveolar ventilation equation in which $\dot{V}_A$ represents the theoretical alveolar ventilation required for maximally efficient lungs to regulate P_{ACO_2} at a given $\dot{V}_{CO_2}$. This important relationship is plotted in Figure 2.37.

Dead Space Ventilation

Not all respired air effectively ventilates the lungs since some must ventilate the conducting airways, uninvolved in gas exchange, and some ventilates nonperfused or underperfused alveoli. The difference between the ideal alveolar ventilation and the total ventilation is the physiological dead space ventilation. Uneven ventilation relative to perfusion will result in a calculated increase in V_D/V_T and an increase in $\dot{V}E$ to clear a given volume of CO_2 from the lungs. The reason for this can be seen by referring to Figure 2.37. Given a P_{ACO_2} of 40 mmHg, composed of equal blood flow from compartments with P_{CO_2} of 50 and 30 mmHg, the increase in true alveolar ventilation would be dominated by the lung unit with the low alveolar P_{CO_2}, i.e., high $\dot{V}_A/\dot{Q}$ lung unit. Thus, the mixed expired CO_2 would be relatively low with mismatching of $\dot{V}_A/\dot{Q}$ as compared with that

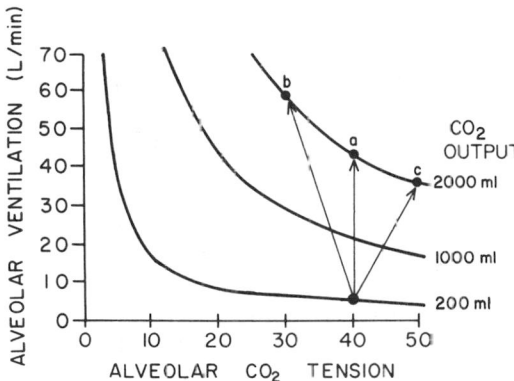

FIGURE 2.37.   Effect of changing ideal alveolar (which is equal to arterial) P_{CO_2} during exercise on alveolar ventilation. The point on the CO_2 output isopleth of 200 ml/min represents the normal resting value. Points a, b and c illustrate the alveolar ventilation for isocapnia, hypocapnia (-10 mm Hg), and hypercapnia ($+10$ mm Hg) for an exercise CO_2 output of 2000 ml/min. (Reprinted with permission from Wasserman K. Breathing during exercise. N Engl J Med 1978;298:780–785.)

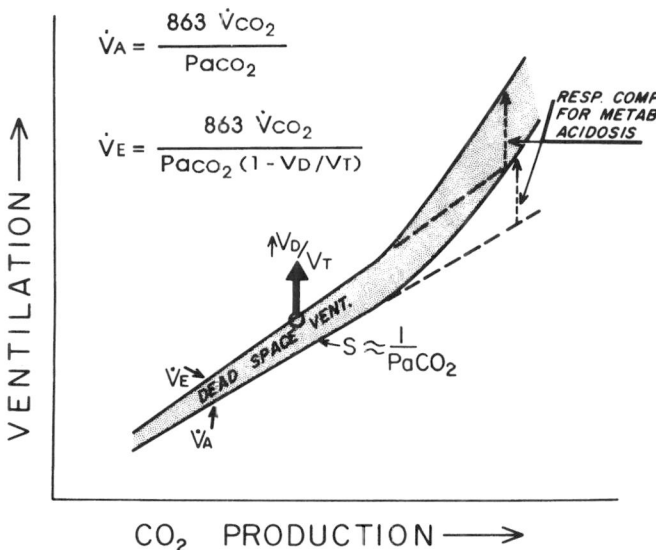

$$\dot{V}_A = \frac{863 \; \dot{V}_{CO_2}}{Pa_{CO_2}}$$

$$\dot{V}_E = \frac{863 \; \dot{V}_{CO_2}}{Pa_{CO_2} \, (1 - V_D/V_T)}$$

FIGURE 2.38.   Factors that determine alveolar and minute ventilation ($\dot{V}_A$ and $\dot{V}_E$, respectively) during exercise are shown in the equations on top of the figure, and the relationships are shown as a graph. V_D/V_T is the physiological dead space/tidal volume ratio and "S" is the slope of the relationship, shown to be proportional to the reciprocal of the Pa_{CO_2}. Respiratory compensation for the metabolic acidosis reduces the Pa_{CO_2} value. As Pa_{CO_2} decreases the ventilatory curves become more steep. (Modified from Wasserman K. Breathing during exercise. N Engl J Med 1978;298:780–785.)

for an ideal lung in which $\dot{V}_A/\dot{Q}$ was perfectly matched. See Figures 2.38 and 2.39 for illustration of the effect of increase in V_D/V_T on $\dot{V}_E$ and section on "Physical Factors" under "Control of Breathing"

for a quantification of the effect of increased dead space on the ventilatory response to exercise.

Acid-base Balance

Because the end products of the bioenergetic pathways for generating $\sim$P are acids, the volatile carbonic and the non-volatile lactic acid, ventilation must keep pace with the acid load if pH homeostasis of body fluids is to be preserved. Figures 2.22 and 2.40 show the acid-base changes in response to constant work rates of moderate, heavy and very heavy intensity exercise. The ventilatory response does not overshoot the ventilation needed to regulate arterial pH. Characteristically, below the *AT* the arterial pH is regulated at resting levels or slightly below because of a small increase in Pa_{CO_2} (75). For above *AT* exercise, the acidosis becomes more marked because of the decrease in HCO_3^- caused by net increase in lactic acid production.

Since the change in pH is minimal during moderate intensity exercise, recovery of pH following exercise is rapid, involving only correcting Pa_{CO_2} to the resting setpoint value (Fig. 2.41). At this exercise intensity only the ventilatory excretion of the exercise-induced increase in CO_2 stores is required. If the exercise is of heavy or very heavy intensity, recovery of pH is slow because it is linked to the rate of regeneration of HCO_3^- which, in turn, is dependent on the rate of lactate catabolism (Fig. 2.41) (34).

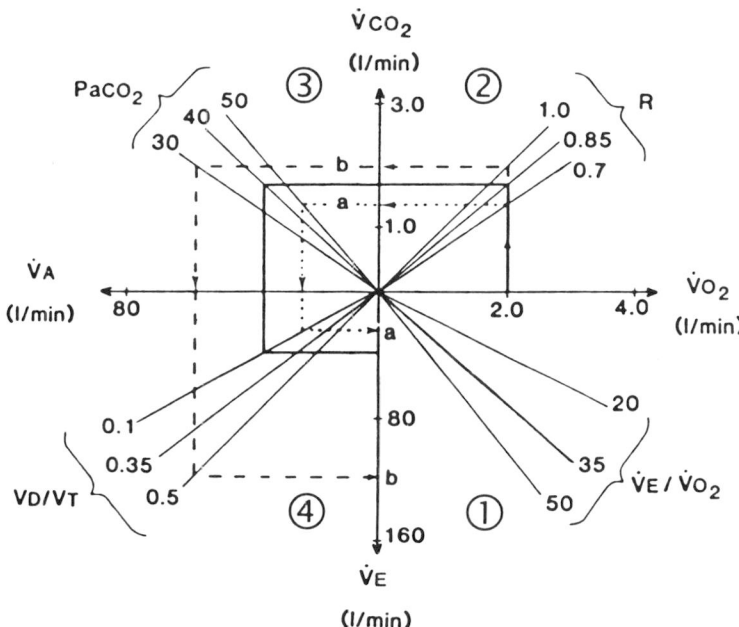

FIGURE 2.39.   Graphic display of influence of respiratory exchange ratio (R), arterial partial pressure of CO_2 (Pa_{CO_2}), and dead-space fraction of the breath (V_D/V_T) on ventilatory requirement ($\dot{V}_E$) for exercise with an O_2 consumption (O_2) = 2 L/min (STPD). The ventilatory requirement can be significantly altered from normal response (solid line), with a particular combination of determining variables leading to reduced (arrow a) or markedly increased (arrow b) $\dot{V}_E$. $\dot{V}_A$: alveolar ventilation. See text for equations showing how the parameter affects the variables in each quadrant. (Modified from Whipp BJ, Pardy RL. Breathing during exercise. American Physiological Society Handbook of Physiology, Bethesda, MD, Sect 3, Vol III, Chapter 34, p. 605.)

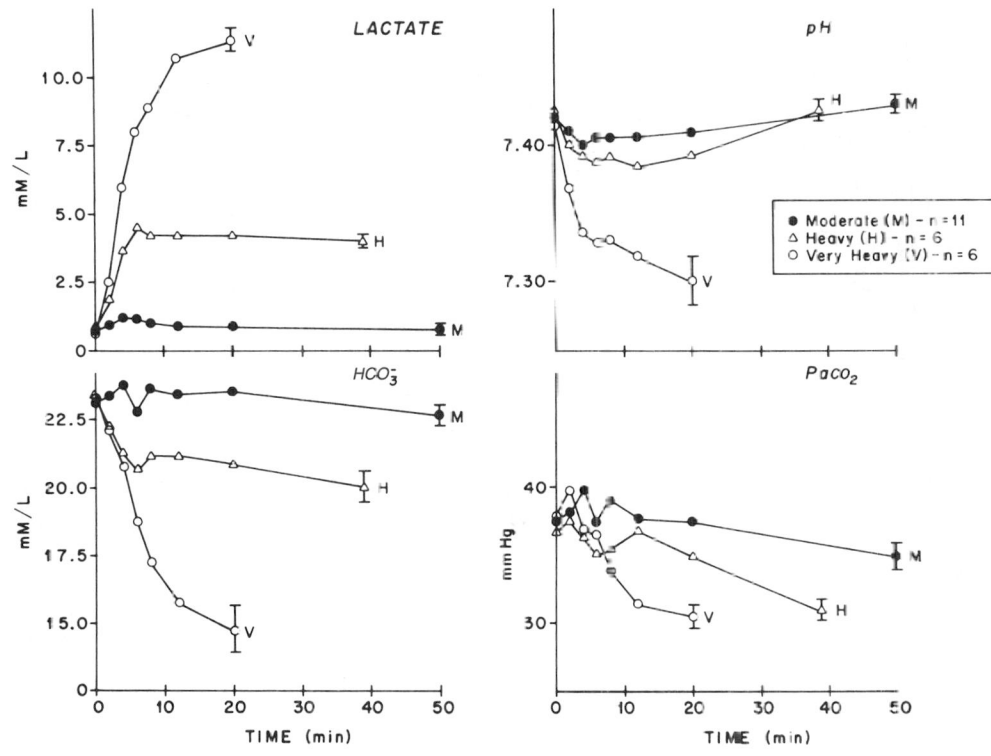

FIGURE 2.40. Time course of change in arterial lactate, bicarbonate, pH and $Paco_2$ for moderate, heavy and very heavy exercise following the onset of constant load cycle ergometer exercise. Moderate exercise intensity (N = 11) refers to an increase in arterial lactate level of less than 0.8 mmol/L above rest. Heavy exercise intensity (N = 6) refers to an arterial lactate increase at the end of exercise of 2.5–4.9 mmol/L above rest. Very heavy intensity exercise (N = 6) refers to a lactate increase of 7 mmol/L or greater above rest at the end of exercise. (Data computed from subjects previously reported in ref. 33.)

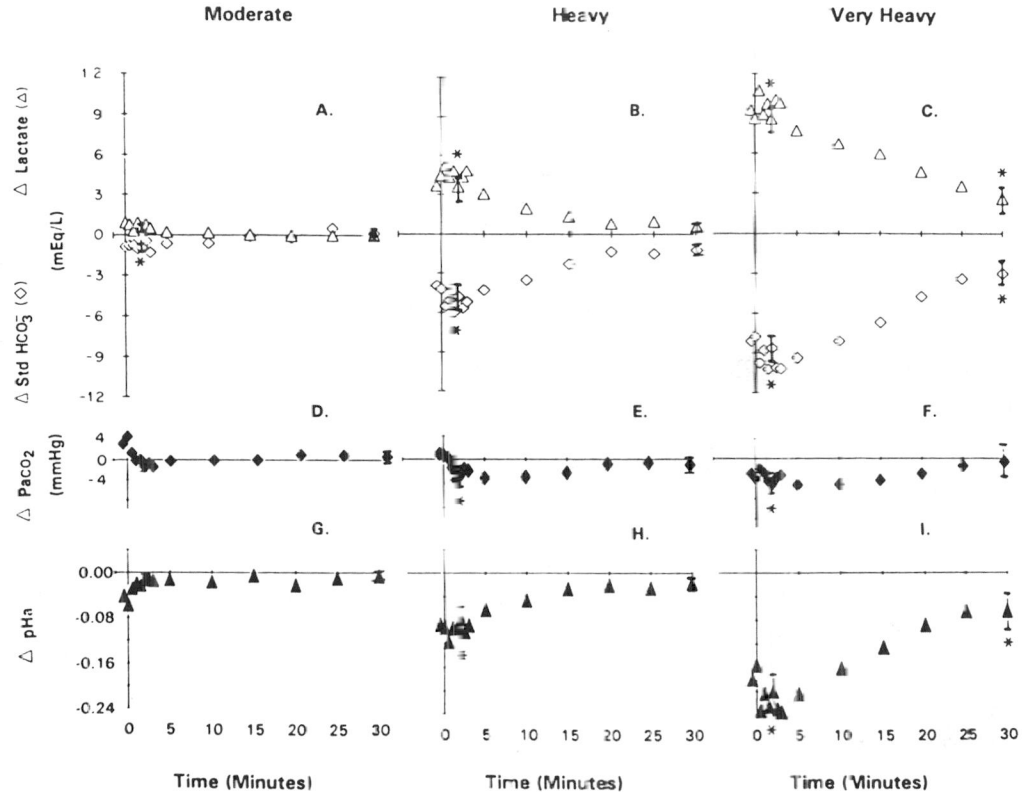

FIGURE 2.41. $\triangle$ lactate, $\triangle$ Std HCO_3^-, $\triangle$ pH_a, and $\triangle$ $Paco_2$ relative to resting values during 30 min of recovery from 6 min of moderate, heavy, and very heavy constant work-rate exercise. Points are the average of 8 subjects. At selected times during recovery (2 and 30 min), SEs and significant differences (*P < 0.05 from resting value) are provided. (Reprinted with permission from Stringer W, Casaburi R, Wasserman K. Acid-base regulation during exercise and recovery in man. J Appl Physiol 1992;72:954–961.)

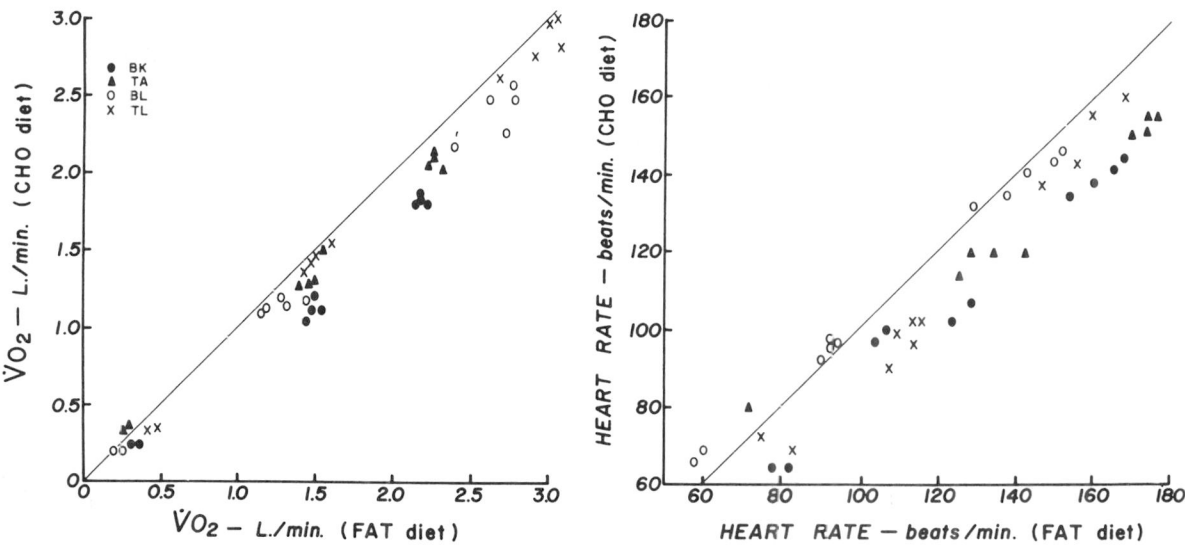

FIGURE 2.42.   Effect of dietary substrate on oxygen consumption and heart rate during exercise. Studies were done on four subjects at rest and two levels of exercise after three days on high carbohydrate diet (RQ at rest = .97) and three days on high fat diet (RQ at rest = .75). The oxygen consumption is higher on the high fat diet than on the high carbohydrate diet during the performance of a given work rate. This is consistent with the biochemical evidence that the high energy phosphate yield from carbohydrate is greater than that from fat for a given O_2 cost. Heart rate during exercise is higher on the high fat diet as compared with the high carbohydrate diet reflecting the link between oxygen consumption and cardiac output.

Effect of Dietary Substrate

O₂ Consumption

Slightly more high energy phosphate compounds are generated per molecule of O_2 utilized when carbohydrate is the substrate compared to fat ($\sim P : O_2 = 6.0$ vs. 5.65, respectively). Consequently, steady-state $\dot{V}_{O_2}$ should be slightly increased for a given work rate when fatty acids are the predominant substrate. The $\dot{V}_{O_2}$ required to perform cycle ergometer work after consuming a high carbohydrate diet for three days as compared to a high fat diet for a similar duration is shown in Figure 2.42. The $\dot{V}_{O_2}$ is slightly increased, as predicted, when the work task is performed with fatty acids as the dominant substrate as compared to carbohydrate.

Table 2.5 shows the theoretical high energy phosphate-gas exchange equivalents for pure carbohydrate and pure fatty acid substrate.

Heart Rate

Because cardiac output increases linearly with $\dot{V}_{O_2}$, the higher $\dot{V}_{O_2}$ required for a given level of exercise when fatty acids are the substrate compared to carbohydrate should predictably demand a higher cardiac output with the former as compared to the latter. This is reflected in a slightly higher heart rate when fatty acids are the dominant exercise substrate, as compared with carbohydrate (see Fig. 2.42).

TABLE 2.5.   Theoretical Gas Exchange and High Energy Phosphate Yield from Carbohydrate and Free Fatty Acid Oxidation for a Standardized Exercise Bout Requiring an O₂ Uptake of 1 L/min

	RQ	$\dot{V}_{O_2}$ (L/min)	$\dot{V}_{CO_2}$ (L/min)	$\sim P : O_2$	$\sim P : CO_2$	$O_2 : \sim P$	$CO_2 : \sim P$
Carbohydrate (glucose)	1.0	1.0	1.0	6.00	6.00	0.17	0.17
Free fatty acid (palmitate)	0.7	1.0	0.7	5.65	8.13	0.18	0.12

Modified from ref. 155.

CO₂ Production

While $\dot{V}O_2$ and heart rate are less at a given work rate when carbohydrate is the major substrate, $\dot{V}CO_2$ decreases when fat is the major source of energy (105, 106). This is predicted on the basis of the lower RQ for fat than for carbohydrate (Table 2.5). However, the effect is more striking at rest than during exercise. Sue et al. (105) found that a low carbohydrate diet affected resting much more than exercise $\dot{V}CO_2$, RQ and $\dot{V}E$. Apparently, the muscles are able to extract carbohydrate from a low carbohydrate diet, making the muscle substrate RQ higher than most other organs in the body except for the brain. Thus, the muscles maintain the most oxygen-efficient fuel possible for aerobic work (see Fig. 2.3).

Ventilation

Ventilation is less for a given work rate with a predominant fat substrate, consistent with the hypothesis that the ventilatory control mechanisms appear to cause $\dot{V}E$ to change in proportion to $\dot{V}CO_2$ (106). However, as with $\dot{V}CO_2$, the effect is more marked at rest than during exercise (105). When $\dot{V}E$ is plotted against $\dot{V}CO_2$, the relationship is the same whether the RQ is high or low. Thus, a consistent relationship is observed among normal subjects when $\dot{V}E$ is plotted against $\dot{V}CO_2$ (see Fig. 2.33). However, when $\dot{V}E$ is plotted against $\dot{V}O_2$, there is less consistency in the responses among subjects. The greater inter-subject variability, with $\dot{V}O_2$ as the independent variable, is due to RQ differences among subjects, with the high RQ subjects having the steeper $\dot{V}E$-$\dot{V}O_2$ slope (Fig. 2.39). The mechanism for the curvilinear steepening of $\dot{V}E$ at the higher metabolic rates is accounted for by the metabolic acidosis of heavy exercise and its ventilatory compensation as described in Figure 2.38.

CONTROL OF BREATHING
Overview

Despite a manifold increase in CO_2 production and O_2 utilization during exercise, the ventilatory control mechanisms normally keep arterial PCO_2 and $[H^+]$ remarkably constant over a wide range of metabolic rates (34, 107). Since the end-products of the bioenergetic pathways for generating the $\sim P$ for muscle contraction are acids, the volatile carbonic and the non-volatile lactic acid, ventilation must respond to this acid load if pH homeostasis of body fluids is

to be preserved. Therefore, before getting into specifics on reflex mechanisms controlling ventilation, it is appropriate to review how the ventilatory control mechanisms regulate acid-base balance during exercise and the physiological demands which this regulation imposes on the ventilatory control mechanism(s).

Acid-Base Regulation

Ventilation appears to be coupled by physiological control mechanisms to CO_2 exchange during exercise. If $\dot{V}E$ did not increase adequately for the increased rate of CO_2 production, a respiratory acidosis with associated disturbances in cellular function would result. Likewise, if ventilation increased proportionally more than the rate of CO_2 production, respiratory alkalosis would result and this would impair cellular function and O_2 unloading from hemoglobin in the muscles. However, exercise usually is an almost isocapnic, isohydric, hypermetabolic state at moderate exercise intensities (Figs. 2.22, 2.40). A metabolic acidosis is normally present only for heavy or higher exercise intensities, due to increased blood lactate accumulation. Respiratory acidosis is usually only present transiently in normal subjects because ventilation increase lags the increase in CO_2 output (108). Patients with abnormal respiratory mechanics or impaired chemoreceptor function, or normal subjects breathing through an apparatus that imparts a high resistive load, can develop a significant respiratory acidosis. However, respiratory alkalosis does not typically develop during exercise in normal subjects and is rarely seen in pathophysiological states. Therefore, the physiological mechanism(s) controlling breathing appear to operate with a small transient pH error to the acid side. The ventilatory control mechanism corrects this by increasing ventilation and regulating $PaCO_2$. The $PaCO_2$ is rarely reduced in response to exercise except when the pH decreases due to metabolic acidosis.

Figures 2.22 and 2.40 show the acid-base changes in response to constant work rates of moderate, heavy and very heavy intensity exercise. The ventilatory response does not overshoot that needed to regulate pH. Characteristically, below the *AT*, the arterial pH is regulated at resting levels or slightly less because of a small increase in $PaCO_2$ (75). For above *AT* exercise, the acidosis becomes more marked due to a net increase in lactic acid production. This has a great effect on ventilatory response to exercise because it increases the CO_2 produced

(22.3 ml of CO_2 for each mmol of HCO_3^- buffering a mmol of lactic acid), while simultaneously reducing the arterial HCO_3^- level. To constrain the fall in arterial pH caused by the elevation in lactate, a large ventilatory increase takes place (Fig. 2.25 and Table 2.4). In recovery, as during exercise, pH homeostasis, rather than the level of Pa_{CO_2}, seems to be the important determinant of ventilatory control (Fig. 2.41).

Physical Factors

The physical factors that determine the alveolar ventilation was discussed under Ventilatory Coupling to Metabolism. In this section we are concerned with the physical factors that determine the actual ventilation ($\dot{V}_E$), the alveolar ventilation plus the respired air that does not participate in normal gas exchange with the pulmonary circulation. $\dot{V}_E$ includes ventilation going to the anatomical dead space (conducting, non-alveoli containing airways) and nonperfused or underperfused alveoli. This is the physiological dead space and is calculated as follows:

$$V_D = V_T \frac{(Pa_{CO_2} - P_{ECO_2})}{Pa_{CO_2}}$$

where P_{ECO_2} is the CO_2 concentration in the mixed expired gas, V_T is the tidal volume and $\dot{V}_D$ is the physiological dead space volume. Thus the difference between the actual volume of air respired during breathing ($\dot{V}_E$) and the theoretical alveolar ventilation ($\dot{V}_A$) is dictated by V_D/V_T as follows:

$$\dot{V}_A = \dot{V}_E (1 - V_D/V_T)$$

To determine the $\dot{V}_E$ needed to eliminate a given quantity of CO_2, substitute $\dot{V}_E (1 - V_D/V_T)$ for $\dot{V}_A$ in the alveolar ventilation equation given earlier and solve for $\dot{V}_E$. The resulting equation is:

$$\dot{V}_E \text{ (BTPS)} = \frac{863 \dot{V}_{CO_2} \text{ (STPD)}}{Pa_{CO_2} (1 V_D/V_T)}$$

where 863 is the product of the barometric pressure, temperature, and water vapor correction factors needed to express $\dot{V}_E$ at BTPS, $\dot{V}_{CO_2}$ in STPD, and CO_2 as a partial pressure. From this equation, the quantity of breathing required for exercise is defined by three factors: 1) the $\dot{V}_{CO_2}$; 2) the level or set-

point at which Pa_{CO_2} is regulated by the ventilatory control mechanisms; and 3) the physiological dead space/tidal volume ratio. The influences of these three factors on $\dot{V}_E$ are graphically illustrated in Figure 2.38. (By substituting values in the equations shown in the figure, the axes in the figure can be scaled.) At work rates above the AT, $\dot{V}_E$ and $\dot{V}_A$ increase nonlinearly and steeply as $\dot{V}_{CO_2}$ increases because of the metabolic acidosis-induced hyperventilation.

Quadrant 1 of Figure 2.39 shows that the exercise $\dot{V}_E$ for a given O_2 cost of exercise (right going horizontal axis) can be quite variable. The cause for this variability can be described by the physiological factors that contribute to $\dot{V}_E$. The first factor is the CO_2 produced as a result of the O_2 cost of work. This is defined by the equation $\dot{V}_{CO_2} = R \times \dot{V}_{O_2}$ and plotted in quadrant 2. The R isopleths describe the ratio of CO_2 output resulting from aerobic metabolism and HCO_3^- buffering of lactic acid, relative to $\dot{V}_{O_2}$. Quadrant 3 is derived from the alveolar ventilation equation, $\dot{V}_{CO_2} = \dot{V}_A \times Pa_{CO_2}$, and takes into account variability in Pa_{CO_2}. Finally $\dot{V}_E$ is determined by adding the dead space ventilation to the alveolar ventilation as described in the equation for $\dot{V}_E$ given above (quadrant 4).

Reflexes Regulating Breathing During Exercise

Despite intensive research, there is no general agreement on the reflexes controlling ventilation during exercise. The observation that arterial pH, P_{CO_2}, and P_{O_2} are essentially unchanged during exercise of moderate intensity exercise has been difficult to explain mechanistically, within the framework of the currently recognized reflexes and their stimuli and manner by which they are thought to operate. Repeated efforts to discover chemoreceptors in locations where potential stimuli are available (e.g., pulmonary circulation or exercising limbs), in order to explain the exercise hyperpnea, have been largely unsuccessful. The only chemoreceptors that have been clearly demonstrated to play an important role in the hyperpnea of exercise are the carotid bodies, and then primarily above the AT and during exercise transients (109, 110). The following is a brief review of the reflex mechanisms proposed to have a role in exercise hyperpnea (see the reviews by Whipp (107) and Wasserman, Whipp, and Casaburi (34) for a more detailed discussion of this subject).

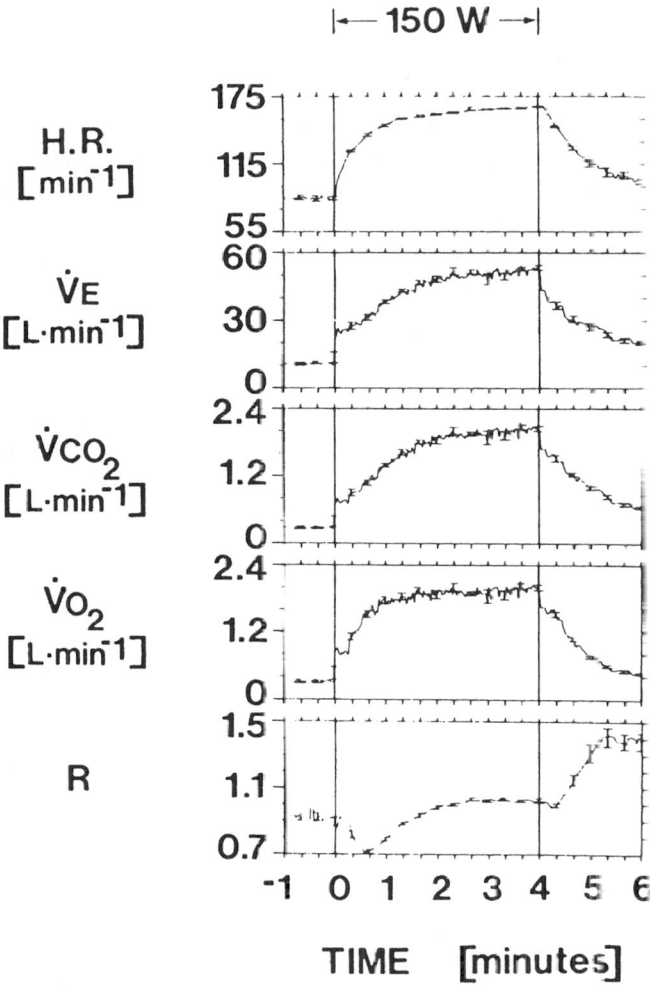

|← 150 W →|

H.R. [min⁻¹]

V̇E [L·min⁻¹]

V̇CO₂ [L·min⁻¹]

V̇O₂ [L·min⁻¹]

R

TIME [minutes]

FIGURE 2.43. Changes in ventilation and gas exchange during cycle ergometer constant work rate exercise starting from rest ("0" time) and ending at four minutes in a normal subject. This study is the average of six similar repetitions in which gas exchange was measured breath-by-breath. The vertical bars are the standard errors of the data. The abrupt increase in V̇E, V̇CO₂, and V̇O₂ at the start of exercise ("0" time) is termed Phase I and thought to be related, mechanistically, to the abrupt increase in cardiac output at the start of exercise. R is usually unchanged from rest for about 15 sec. The start of Phase II is signaled by a decrease in R and is the period of exponential-like increase in V̇E, V̇CO₂, and V̇O₂ to their asymptotes (Phase III). This is the period when increasing cellular respiration is reflected in lung gas exchange. R decreases transiently during Phase II because V̇O₂ increases faster than V̇CO₂ due to gas solubility differences in tissues. It usually then increases to a value higher than rest because the RQ of the muscle substrate, being primarily glycogen, is higher than the average for the body, which depends on the RQ of the diet.

Corticogenic or Conditioned Reflexes

The magnitude of the abrupt increase in V̇E at the start of exercise (Fig. 2.43) varies appreciably from individual to individual. However, high work rates generally result in only a slightly further increase at

the start of exercise over that observed for the lightest loads. Consequently, for a mild work rate, the initial increase in V̇E is a larger fraction of the total ventilatory response than that for a heavy work rate (Fig. 2.44). The magnitude of the initial increase in V̇E is also not appreciably affected by different degrees of arterial oxygenation or if functioning carotid bodies are absent (75). The ventilatory pattern that follows the initial increase is greatly influenced by the work rate in relation to the AT (see Fig. 2.36) and by carotid body chemosensitivity.

Anxiety might account for part of the rapid ventilatory increase at the start of exercise (Phase I) in some subjects. Krogh and Lindhard (111), suggested that the rapid V̇E increase at the start of exercise might originate from the cerebral cortex as a conditioned reflex. Fink and associates (112) suggest that the cerebral cortex may play a role in the exercise hyperpnea beyond the initial ventilatory response. Martin and Mitchell (113) proposed that there may be a strong learning component to the ventilatory response. Eldridge et al. (114) and DiMarco et al. (115) obtained evidence from studies in cats suggesting that the initial ventilatory stimulus for the exercise hyperpnea might involve hypothalamic mediation. Despite these important observations describing a neurogenic link to the initial and sustained ventilatory response to exercise, the patterns of ventilatory and gas exchange responses in humans suggest that the sustained ventilatory response is predominantly metabolically coupled and that the initial ventilatory (Phase I) response might also be linked to the circulatory response to exercise (34, 116–118).

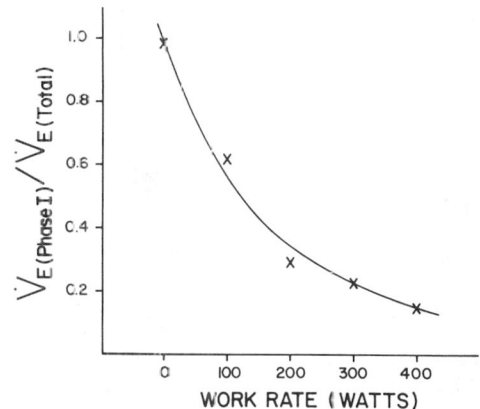

FIGURE 2.44. The magnitude of the Phase I ventilatory response to exercise (from rest) as related to steady state ventilation for various work rates. The higher the work rate, the smaller the fraction of the total ventilatory response attributable to Phase I.

Respiratory Center and Central Chemoreceptors

The respiratory center includes collections of neurons in the brain stem which discharge rhythmically to stimulate motor neurons to the respiratory muscles. Medullary lesions associated with tumors, primary hypoventilation syndromes, or central respiratory depression associated with hypoxia-inducing pulmonary diseases, can cause the respiratory pacemaker mechanisms to depend upon peripheral chemoreceptor input for providing a controlled rhythmic output. The apnea produced by O_2 administration in some patients with arterial hypoxemia is evidence that these pacemaker mechanisms may lose the required rhythmic discharge properties.

The role of the medullary chemoreceptors in ventilatory control during exercise hyperpnea is unclear. Although these chemoreceptors respond to changes in pH, cerebrospinal fluid acidosis does not occur during exercise. In fact a respiratory alkalosis is evident in the cerebrospinal fluid as a consequence of arterial hypocapnia (119). The central chemoreceptors do not appear to respond to the acute exercise-induced metabolic acidosis (75). In adult patients with primary alveolar hypoventilation syndrome (patients with normal pulmonary function but with hypercapnia and markedly diminished or absent ventilatory response to CO_2 breathing), the ventilatory response to exercise is diminished not only because they have rest and exercise hypercapnia (high CO_2 setpoint), but also because their arterial PCO_2 increases further with exercise (120). However, it is difficult to know if this occurs secondary to central insensitivity to CO_2 or if it is due to a failure of the respiratory center to effectively integrate the afferent stimuli to give an appropriate ventilatory output. Furthermore, children with this syndrome have been reported to have normal ventilatory response to exercise despite absence of response to inhaled CO_2 (121).

Carotid Bodies

Much has been learned about the role of carotid bodies during muscular exercise from studies on selected asthmatic patients who had both carotid bodies resected, but whose baroreceptors were left intact (110, 122). The ventilatory response to exercise was studied in these subjects when they: 1) were asymptomatic; 2) had normal, or near normal, respiratory function; and 3) had normal exercise tolerance. Their ventilatory responses to exercise were different from those of normal subjects in three ways:

1. The subjects without carotid bodies did not increase their ventilatory drive in response to hypoxia (109) nor did they decrease their ventilatory drive in response to hyperoxia (122).
2. They failed to develop ventilatory compensation for the exercise-induced metabolic acidosis (75) and consequently evidenced a greater arterial acidemia during high intensity exercise.
3. The rate of increase in ventilation in response to exercise was slow compared to that of normal subjects, causing a transient arterial hypercapnia when $\dot{V}E$ was increasing from rest to the steady-state (75).

The ventilatory response to the transition from low work rate to high work rate exercise is slowed and the amplitude reduced during O_2 breathing in normal subjects (123). Attenuating carotid body drive by breathing high O_2, in normal subjects with altered acid-base status, also slowed the ventilatory response to a constant work rate challenge (124). The more baseline acidosis, the greater was the attenuation of the ventilatory response. Studies on the acute effect of hyperoxia on $\dot{V}E$, support the concept that the carotid bodies have an important role in the normal ventilatory response to exercise (125). While the exact mechanisms mediating this response remain to be elucidated, several potential stimuli of the carotid bodies increase during exercise. These include PCO_2, K^+, adenosine, osmolarity, catecholamines, and H^+. Whatever the precise role of these potential stimuli in the control of breathing during exercise, studies in which exercise ventilation is continuously measured during a switch of the inspired gas from air to 100% O_2, reduces ventilation transiently by only approximately 15 to 20% in normal subjects. However, in patients who develop arterial hypoxemia during exercise, the carotid bodies may account for a much greater proportion of the exercise hyperpnea (see example in Chapter 3).

Aortic Bodies

The aortic bodies seem to be unimportant as ventilatory chemoreceptors in humans, in contrast to some other animal species (e.g., cats and dogs). Removal of the carotid bodies alone has been shown to eliminate the ventilatory response to hypoxia and the acute metabolic acidosis of exercise (75, 109).

Vagal Reflexes

The lungs are richly innervated by branches of the vagus nerve. While investigators have postulated that the vagus nerve might contribute importantly to the exercise hyperpnea, studies on the ventilatory response to exercise in awake dogs by Philipson et al. (126) showed that vagal blockade, induced by bilateral cooling of the cervical vagus nerves, did not change the overall ventilatory response to exercise, although the breathing pattern was altered. The authors concluded that the vagus nerves were not important in the overall ventilatory response to exercise in dogs at the exercise levels studied (up to 4 times resting $\dot{V}O_2$).

Mechanoreceptors in the Extremities

To explain the exercise hyperpnea, it had been widely postulated that stimulation of position receptors or muscle spindles in the exercising muscle play a major role in the genesis of exercise hyperpnea (127). The principal argument in favor of an appreciable role for the neural afferents from exercising muscles stems from the observation of a rapid increase in $\dot{V}E$ at the start of exercise (Phase I) (Fig. 2.43), in advance of the predicted arrival of the products of exercise metabolism in the central circulation.

Some neurophysiological studies have helped clarify the possible role of afferents from the exercising limb in mediating the exercise hyperpnea (128). Studies in which the transmission of stimuli in large, myelinated fibers (e.g., transmitting proprioception) were interrupted (129) demonstrate that these receptors play only a small role, if any. Hornbein et al. (130), Hodgson and Mathews (131), and Waldrop et al. (132) using different approaches to stimulate the muscle spindles, demonstrated no significant role for these organs in the exercise hyperpnea. Stimulation of the type III and IV muscle afferents (i.e., unmyelinated or small-myelinated neurons) have been demonstrated to induce hyperpnea (133). However, recent studies have demonstrated that blocking their afferent transmission does not appreciably impair the exercise hyperpnea (134). This is consistent with work that demonstrates that the coupling of $\dot{V}E$ to metabolic rate ($\dot{V}CO_2$) is not abnormal in human subjects with complete spinal-cord transection caused to "exercise" by means of electrical stimulation of the leg muscles (135, 136). But even if ventilatory stimuli originating in the exercising muscles are active during exercise, the respiratory center is not stimulated with enough intensity by these signals to override the mechanisms that regulate arterial pH.

Cardiodynamic Hyperpnea

Cardiovascular reflexes linked to the ventilatory control mechanism have been put forth as an alternative explanation to that of mechanoreceptors in the extremities for the rapid onset of the exercise hyperpnea (34, 117, 118, 137). The abrupt increase in cardiac output and peripheral blood flow at the start of exercise could deliver increased quantities of blood to receptor sites downstream from the pulmonary capillaries, resulting in an increased PCO_2 and $[H^+]$ and decreased PO_2 at the sites of arterial chemoreceptors, if $\dot{V}A$ did not keep pace with the increase in pulmonary blood flow. These changes could provide feedback stimuli to the respiratory control mechanism in less than the circulation time between the muscles and arterial chemoreceptors. However, Casaburi et al. (138) showed that pulmonary artery O_2 saturation decreased within the first few seconds of the start of upright cycle ergometer exercise, much earlier than had previously been expected from the muscle capillary-pulmonary artery circulation time. This rapid appearance of highly desaturated venous blood at the pulmonary artery at the start of exercise was due to the abrupt increase in venous return containing desaturated, high PCO_2 blood from the dependent legs which already resided in the leg and iliac veins before the start of exercise. Thus, at the start of lower extremity exercise in the upright position, this blood is quickly injected into the pulmonary circulation by compression of the veins of the contracting muscles and increased abdominal pressure and decreased intrathoracic pressure resulting from the relatively large descent of the diaphragm. Both the rapid return of desaturated, high PCO_2 venous blood and the rapid immediate (Phase I) increase in ventilation are attenuated if the same cycling exercise is performed in the supine position so that legs and heart are at about the same level (116, 139).

Linking the Phase I increase in $\dot{V}E$ to the abrupt increase in cardiac output (cardiovascular reflex) rather than involving non-metabolic, neurogenic mechanisms is notionally attractive in that two unlinked neurogenic mechanisms, one for blood flow and one for ventilation, would be unlikely to produce the near-isocapnic hyperpnea so consistently observed from the start through the steady state of moderate intensity exercise. These control mecha-

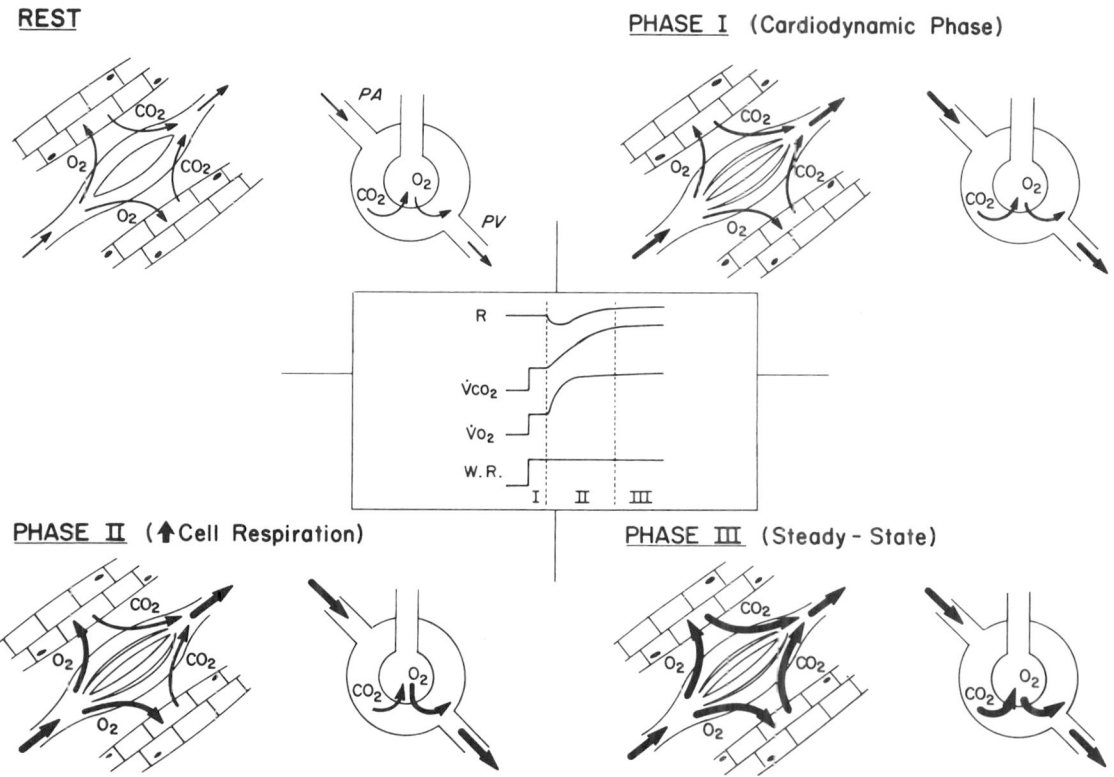

FIGURE 2.45.   Gas exchange at the lungs in response to constant work rate exercise (center diagram). Gas exchange at the cell (left side of each quadrant) couples to cardiorespiratory gas exchange (right side of each quadrant) through cardiovascular adjustments in the lungs and tissues. Phase I gas exchange is postulated to be caused by the immediate increase in cardiac output (pulmonary blood flow) at the start of exercise (cardiodynamic gas exchange). Phase II gas exchange reflects the decreased O_2 content and increased CO_2 content of the venous blood secondary to increased cell respiration as well as a further increase in cardiac output. (See legend to Figure 2.43 for explanation of decrease in R during Phase II). Eventually a steady state is reached between internal and external respiration (Phase III). PA = pulmonary artery, PV = pulmonary vein, W.R. = work rate. (Reprinted with permission from Wasserman K. Coupling of external to internal respiration. Am Rev Resp Dis 1984;129(Suppl.):S21–S24.)

nisms, in some way, regulate pH in a predictable fashion. But how this is achieved is by no means clear.

GAS EXCHANGE KINETICS

The $\dot{V}_E$, $\dot{V}_{O_2}$, or $\dot{V}_{CO_2}$ responses following the onset of constant work rate exercise from rest can be characterized by three time-related phases, as evident by the experimental data in Figure 2.43. The mechanisms of the gas exchange dynamics in response to exercise, as seen in Figure 2.43, are schematized in Figure 2.45.

Phase I is the immediate increase in gas exchange at the start of exercise. It lasts for about 15 seconds and is accounted for by the abrupt increase in pulmonary blood flow consequent to the increase in heart rate and stroke volume at the start of exercise. This is the period before blood from the exercising muscles, modified by cellular metabolism, has appeared in the lungs. Because the composition of this blood was determined under conditions of rest, R characteristically is the same as that at rest (Fig. 2.43).

Phase II for $\dot{V}_{O_2}$ lasts from about 15 seconds after exercise onset to the 3rd minute of exercise. It reflects the period of major increase in cellular respiration. If the exercise is below the AT, a steady state in $\dot{V}_{O_2}$ is achieved by 3 minutes (Fig. 1.4). If the exercise is above the AT, the steady state in $\dot{V}_{O_2}$ is delayed or not achieved before the subject fatigues (Figs. 1.4, 2.6). Phase III starts 3 minutes after exercise onset, and reflects the start of the $\dot{V}_{O_2}$ steady state period if the work rate is below the AT. If the work rate is above the subject's AT, the rate of increase in $\dot{V}_{O_2}$ correlates with the magnitude of the lactate increase (Fig. 2.46) (24, 28, 30).

Oxygen Uptake Kinetics

During the steady state, oxygen uptake from the lungs ($\dot{V}_{O_2}$) reflects the oxygen consumed by the

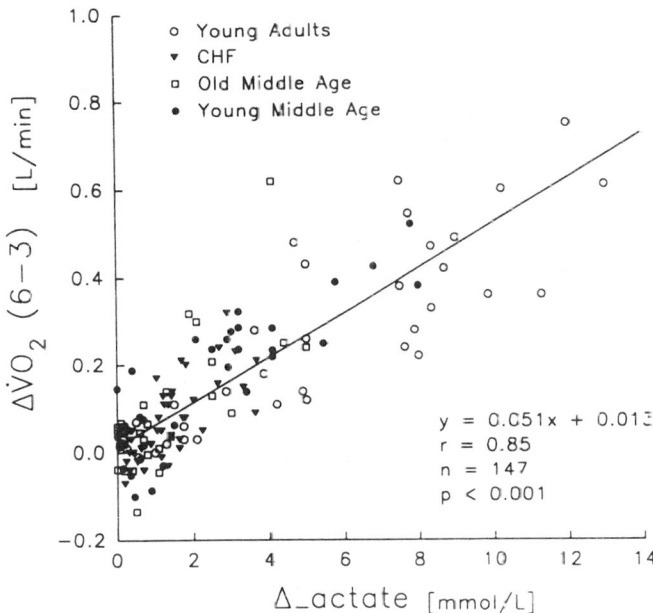

FIGURE 2.46. Increase in blood lactate (above resting value) as related to the difference in oxygen consumption between 3 and 6 minutes of constant work rate exercise in normal, young middle-aged and late middle-aged adults and patients with heart failure. Normally, $\dot{V}O_2$ does not increase after 3 minutes when the work is performed below the anaerobic threshold ($\dot{V}O_2(6-3) = 0$). (Data from ref. 28, 30, with the data of late middle-aged adults added.)

cells (Fig. 2.6). During phase II of exercise, $\dot{V}O_2$ is equal to the O_2 consumed by the cells minus the rate of decrease in blood O_2 stores (oxyhemoglobin of the venous blood, physically dissolved O_2, and oxymyoglobin in muscles) (Fig. 2.43). Change in gas stores in the lungs have little effect on $\dot{V}O_2$ kinetics for two reasons: 1) the concentration of alveolar gas changes very little, increasing only slowly during phase II, and 2) in normal subjects, the functional residual capacity (FRC) may decrease about 1/2 liter. Since 1/2 liter of alveolar gas contains about 75 ml of O_2, a change in FRC during phase I or II can have a small impact on gas exchange kinetics. These are relatively small changes, but an approach has been described to correct for change in both alveolar concentration and change in lung volume (140). The increase in $\dot{V}O_2$ is only transiently determined by the hemodynamic response to exercise (cardiac output and $C(a - \bar{v})O_2$). At the onset of moderate exercise, oxygen uptake from the lungs approximately doubles the resting $\dot{V}O_2$ and then remains relatively unchanged during Phase I. If $C(a - \bar{v})O_2$ did not increase during Phase I, cardiac output could be inferred to have increased two fold. During upright exercise starting from the motionless sitting position, Casaburi et al. (138) has shown that about

1/3 of the Phase I $\dot{V}O_2$ may be accounted for by the increase in $C(a - \bar{v})O_2$. This is apparently due to blood stasis during rest in the upright resting condition. If stasis is prevented with elastic wraps on the legs, the abrupt increase in $C(a - \bar{v})O_2$ at the start of exercise disappears (139). The Phase I increase is greatly reduced when exercise is performed in the supine position (116) or from prior mild exercise (141).

During Phase II, $\dot{V}O_2$ increases as a single exponential with a time constant of approximately 30 seconds for a work rate below the AT (91). If the exercise intensity is heavy or very heavy for a normal subject, or if the subject is so impaired that the cardiovascular response is inadequate to supply the total oxygen need, the increase in $\dot{V}O_2$ can be significantly slowed and a steady state is not achieved by 3 minutes (Figs. 1.4, 2.32). In this metabolic condition, lactate continues to increase until the $\dot{V}O_2$ reaches an asymptote (142). A steady state in $\dot{V}O_2$ is achieved and can be sustained only when all of the cellular energy requirements are derived from reactions using oxygen transferred from the atmosphere.

O_2 Deficit

The O_2 deficit is traditionally computed as the difference between the total oxygen uptake during an exercise bout and the product of the steady-state $\dot{V}O_2$ and the exercise duration (Fig. 2.47). However, if the true steady-state value for $\dot{V}O_2$ is not reached at the time of cessation of exercise, the calculated O_2 deficit will be less than the true O_2 deficit. A correct estimate of O_2 deficit can be obtained for exercise below the AT since a steady state is readily achieved by 3 minutes (143).

O_2 Debt

The oxygen debt is the difference between the total oxygen uptake in excess of the resting oxygen uptake during the recovery period (Fig. 2.47) (82). Once $\dot{V}O_2$ reaches a steady state during exercise, the oxygen debt no longer increases, regardless of the exercise duration (144). In this instance the O_2 debt will be repaid within about 5 minutes of recovery. If the work is above the AT, the O_2 debt can be quite high and may not be repaid for an hour or more. The size of the O_2 debt is linked to the increase in blood lactate concentration (145). As long as the oxygen uptake does not reach a steady state and lactate continues to rise during constant work rate

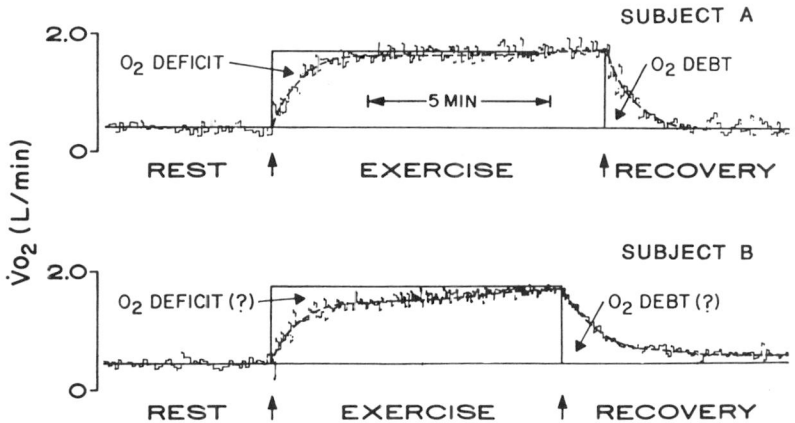

FIGURE 2.47. O_2 uptake kinetics in response to constant work rate exercise of 100 watts in two subjects at different levels of fitness. This figure illustrates the effect of fitness on O_2 deficit and O_2 debt. See text for precise definitions of O_2 deficit and O_2 debt.

exercise, the O_2 deficit and debt will continue to increase. For work levels at which a true steady state in $\dot{V}O_2$ can be achieved, i.e., below the *AT*, the size of the O_2 debt approximates that of the O_2 deficit (143).

Mean Response Time

The average of replicate, second by second, measurements of $\dot{V}O_2$, $\dot{V}CO_2$ and R for four different levels of constant work rate exercise are shown in

Figure 2.48 for a normal subject. For the 25 watt exercise level, it is evident that about 80% of the $\dot{V}O_2$ required to perform the work (steady-state $\dot{V}O_2$) was achieved during phase I (within 15 s of the start of exercise), the cardiodynamic phase of gas exchange. The fraction of the phase I contribution to the steady-state $\dot{V}O_2$ decreases at higher work rates so that Phase II kinetics become more important in achieving the O_2 requirement.

The subject in this example seems to be at his

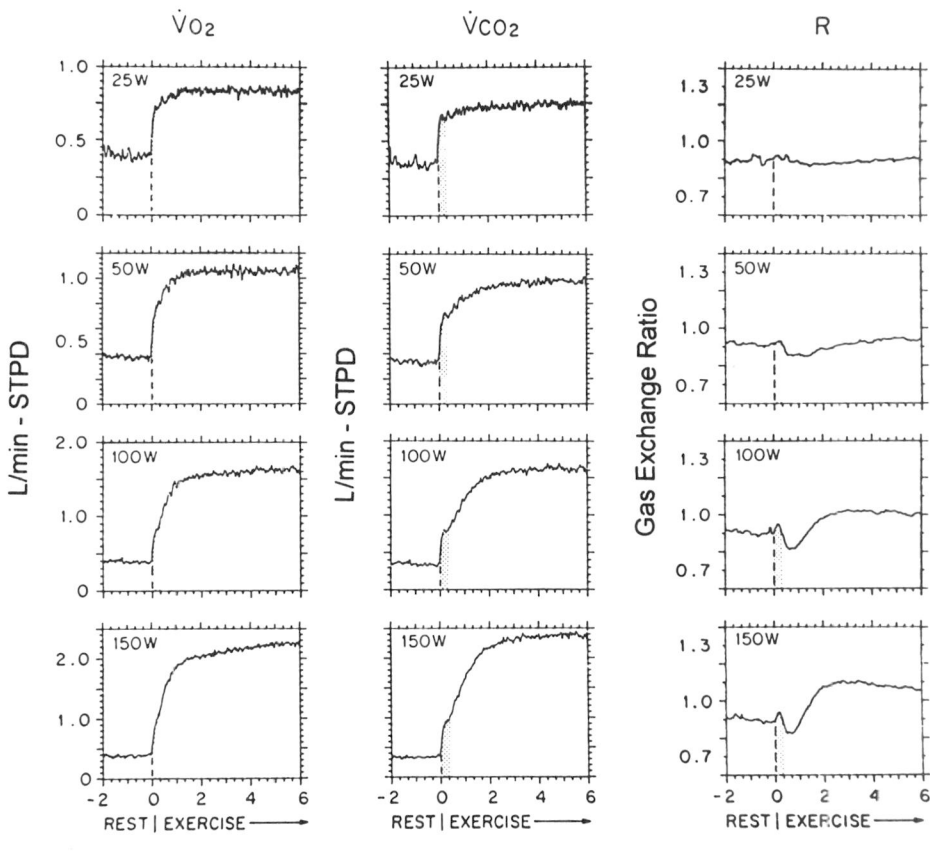

FIGURE 2.48. $\dot{V}O_2$, $\dot{V}CO_2$, and the respiratory gas exchange ratio (R) at four cycle ergometer work rates starting from rest and cycling for 6 minutes at the work rates indicated. The vertical dashed line indicates the time of start of exercise. The shaded area (15 sec) identifies the period of phase I. Each work rate was repeated four times on different days, and the breath-by-breath data were interpolated, second-by-second. These values were then time-aligned to zero and then time-averaged each second to reduce random noise and enhance the reproducible responses. (Data taken from study reported in Sietsema K, Daly JA, Wasserman K. Early dynamics of O_2 uptake and heart rate as affected by exercise work rate. J Appl Physiol 1989;67:2535–2541.)

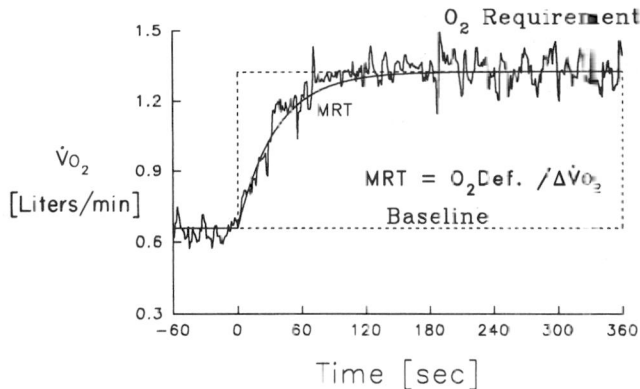

FIGURE 2.49.   Illustration of method for calculating $\dot{V}O_2$ mean response time (MRT) to constant work rate exercise from breath-by-breath data. A single exponential best fit curve is put through the data and the time constant (63% of the asymptotic response) for the increase in $\dot{V}O_2$ above baseline is calculated. If there were no O_2 deficit, the $\dot{V}O_2$ would reach a steady state during the first breath, and the MRT would be "0." As shown in the equation, the O_2 deficit can be calculated from the MRT and the increase in $\dot{V}O_2$ above baseline at steady-state.

AT at about 100 watts, with $\dot{V}O_2$ being in steady-state by 3 minutes. However, the subject is clearly above his *AT* at 150 watts since $\dot{V}O_2$ continues to increase and $\dot{V}CO_2$ increases above $\dot{V}O_2$. Because the $\dot{V}O_2$ kinetics are informative with respect to determining fitness and the presence of disease in the gas transfer function, there has been considerable interest to quantify them. Since the actual data do not conform to a single exponential relationship, the "mean response time" (MRT) is used for quantification of the kinetics of response. The MRT characterizes the combination of the phase I and II complex of $\dot{V}O_2$ dynamics, and is obtained by performing a single exponential fit through the data. The time constant of the exponential (63% of the asymptotic response) is defined as the MRT, as shown in Figure 2.49.

Figure 2.50 gives the $\dot{V}O_2$ MRT of 10 different subjects at five different work rates as related to their fitness ($\dot{V}O_2$max). This figure shows that MRT is similar among subjects of differing fitness at very low work rates (e.g., unloaded cycling) since even unfit individuals can virtually achieve their steady-state response during Phase I. However as work rate is increased, the discrimination becomes more obvious, the subjects with the highest $\dot{V}O_2$max having the lowest MRT.

In summary, if Phase I is a large fraction of the steady-state response for a given work rate, the O_2 deficit (Fig. 2.38) and debt will be small. In contrast, if Phase I is small, the O_2 deficit and debt will be relatively large. The O_2 deficit and debt will also be large if the Phase II $\dot{V}O_2$ kinetics for a given work rate are slow (e.g., the 150 watt work rate in Figure 2.48). Since $\dot{V}O_2$ kinetics are faster for the more fit subject (Fig. 2.50), he/she will have a smaller O_2 deficit and debt for a given work rate.

CO₂ Output Kinetics

For below *AT* exercise, $\dot{V}CO_2$ has slower kinetics than $\dot{V}O_2$ (steady state may not occur until approximately 4 minutes). The time of peak reduction in R (Figs. 2.43, 2.48) identifies a time period in which CO_2 produced aerobically is not being entirely eliminated by the lungs, accounting for the slower CO_2

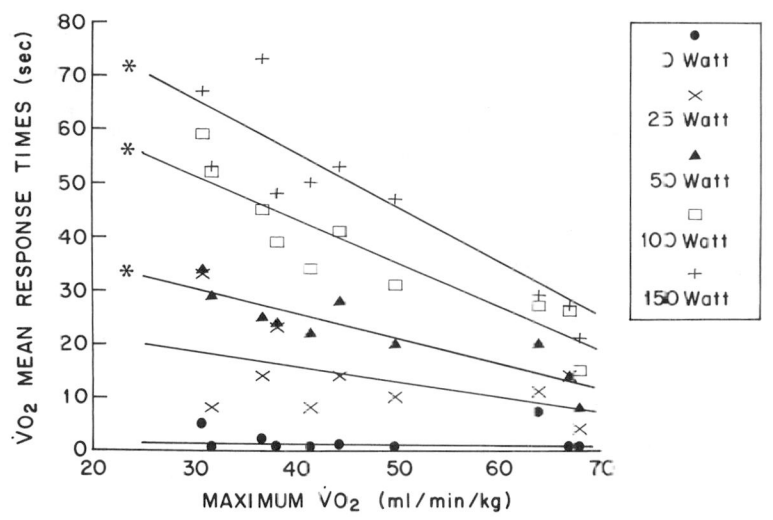

FIGURE 2.50.   Mean response times (MRT) in 10 normal subjects, at the work rates indicated, as related to the subject's maximum $\dot{V}O_2$ (peak $\dot{V}O_2$). At work rates of 50 watts and higher, the MRT is greater, the less fit the subject. (Reprinted with permission from Sietsema K, Daly JA, Wasserman K. Early dynamics of O_2 uptake and heart rate as affected by exercise work rate. J Appl Physiol 1989;67:2535–2541.)

kinetics. This time is between 30 and 45 sec. The relatively slow kinetics for $\dot{V}_{CO_2}$ might be explained by the following reactions: 1) the hydrolysis of phosphocreatine fixes CO_2 as HCO_3^-, 2) as venous oxyhemoglobin saturation decreases, the reduced hemoglobin is capable of holding more CO_2 at the same P_{CO_2} (Haldane effect) and 3) the increase in muscle P_{CO_2}.

Because hydrolysis of phosphocreatine contributes to the $\sim P_{O_4}$ at the beginning of exercise, and this reaction produces an alkalinizing reaction (146), CO_2 produced in the muscle from aerobic metabolism is fixed as HCO_3^-. Thus, $\dot{V}_{CO_2}$ increases more slowly than $\dot{V}_{O_2}$. From approximately 15 to 45 seconds after the onset of constant work rate exercise, R decreases before it increases (Figs. 2.43, 2.48). The increase in R to a constant value, after the decrease, reflects the effect of the substrate RQ in the muscle. If a lactic acidosis occurs during the exercise, $\dot{V}_{CO_2}$ increases faster than $\dot{V}_{O_2}$ due to the additional CO_2 formed as HCO_3^- dissociates during the buffering reaction (Fig. 2.37). This generally starts after about 40 seconds of constant work rate exercise (Fig. 2.31). Thus R will overshoot the steady-state R, as seen at 150 watts for the subject illustrated in Figure 2.48, until lactate stops increasing.

If the work rate being studied is below the AT, true homeostasis occurs in phase III and $\dot{V}_{O_2}$ and $\dot{V}_{CO_2}$ achieve true steady state values (Fig. 1.4, upper panel, three lowest work rates in Figs. 2.32, 2.48). For exercise above the AT, $\dot{V}_{O_2}$ will not achieve a steady state by 3 minutes but will continue to increase (Fig. 1.4, lower panel and four highest work rates of Fig. 2.32 and 150 watts of Fig. 2.48). In contrast, the slow increase observed for $\dot{V}_{O_2}$ is not observed for $\dot{V}_{CO_2}$. The additional CO_2 produced when HCO_3^- buffers the lactate, increases $\dot{V}_{CO_2}$ to a higher value than $\dot{V}_{O_2}$ at a rate proportional to the loss of aerobic CO_2 production (Figs. 2.31, 2.32).

SUMMARY

The physiological responses to exercise are summarized in Figure 1.1. Approximately 28% of the calories generated during work are transformed into useful external work, while the remaining 72% are lost primarily as heat. The oxidative energy obtained from oxygen creditors (hemoglobin, myoglobin, creatine-P_{O_4}, and pyruvate conversion to lactate) during the O_2 deficit period, which must be repaid during the recovery period of exercise as the O_2 debt, varies with the work rate. If the subject is very

fit for the work rate, the O_2 deficit and debt are very small. At moderate work rates, the pyruvate-to-lactate mechanism provides a very small fraction of the credit energy obtained during the O_2 deficit period, while for very heavy work rates the pyruvate-lactate mechanism may account for upwards of 80% of the total credit (33). Gas exchange during exercise should be considered from the standpoint of cellular respiration and how cardiovascular and ventilatory mechanisms are coupled to it. Not only does the magnitude of cellular respiration affect external respiration but, importantly, the degree to which the work rate is above the subject's AT has a major influence on the ventilatory response to exercise. Exercise above the AT causes increased CO_2 and H^+ production, both having powerful effects as ventilatory stimuli of the ventilatory control mechanism. The gas exchange kinetics are also altered and exercise endurance is reduced above the AT.

The peripheral blood flow distribution appears to depend on the work rate and local humoral factors that optimize the O_2 (blood) flow–metabolic rate relationship. Normally, cardiac output is linearly correlated with oxygen consumption. Because of local control mechanisms, uniformity in the ratio of blood flow to O_2 consumption keeps the slope relatively low (approximately 6 L flow/L O_2 consumption). The uniformity enables the muscle end-capillary P_{O_2} to be sufficiently large to allow as much as 85% of the O_2 to be extracted from the capillary blood during maximal exercise.

During exercise, minute ventilation responds to the changing rate of CO_2 delivered to the lungs, including that generated by aerobic oxidation of energy substrate and that generated by the buffering of lactic acid by HCO_3^-. In addition, the carotid bodies are stimulated by H^+, providing further ventilatory drive. Exercise ventilation is also determined by the size of the physiological dead space ventilation, and the level at which arterial P_{CO_2} is regulated. Arterial P_{O_2} remains relatively constant during exercise, despite increasing $\dot{V}_{O_2}$.

Incremental exercise tests, which measure $\dot{V}_{O_2}$ and $\dot{V}_{CO_2}$ dynamically, allow detection of the AT by gas exchange. Also, during constant work rate exercise, breath-by-breath measurements of $\dot{V}_{O_2}$ and $\dot{V}_{CO_2}$ can be used to determine if the exercise is being performed with or without a lactic acidosis. These measurements can be used to estimate the magnitude of the lactate increase, and the exercise duration that might be tolerated at the work rate performed.

$\dot{V}O_2$, $\dot{V}CO_2$, and $\dot{V}E$ abruptly increase at the start of exercise (Phase I). After the first 15 seconds of constant load exercise $\dot{V}O_2$, $\dot{V}CO_2$, and $\dot{V}E$ rise exponentially (Phase II) to a steady-state or an asymptote (Phase III). Their kinetics are influenced by cellular metabolism and the O_2 and CO_2 storage capacities in tissues. During Phase II and III, $\dot{V}E$ closely follows the changing rate of CO_2 delivery to the lungs rather than the actual CO_2 produced or the O_2 consumed, if the exercise is performed without a lactic acidosis. $\dot{V}E$ increases disproportionately to $\dot{V}CO_2$ when the exercise induces a lactic acidosis. Breath-by-breath gas exchange measurements provide insight into mechanisms of respiratory control. The latter appears to be set to regulate arterial $[H^+]$ under a variety of conditions of exercise and recovery by regulating CO_2 excretion.

References

1. Saltin B, Gollnick PD. Skeletal muscle adaptability Significance for metabolism and performance. In: Peachey LD, ed. Handbook of Physiology, Section 10. Skeletal Muscle. Bethesda: Am Physiol Soc, 1983;555.

2. Gibbs CL, Gibson WR. Energy production of rat soleus muscle. Am J Physiol 1972;223:874–881.

3. Henrickson I, Reitman IS. Quantitative measures of enzyme activities in type I and type II muscle fibres of man after training. Acta Physiol Scand 1976;97:392–397.

4. Buller A, Eccles I, Eccles R. Differentiation of fast and slow muscles in the cat hind limb. J Physiol 1960;97:399–416.

5. Karlsson J. Introduction: Basics in human skeletal muscles metabolism. Int J Sports Med 1982;2:15.

6. Essen B. Intramuscular substrate utilization. Ann NY Acad Sci 1977;301:30–44.

7. Lehninger AL. Biochemistry. New York: Worth Publishers, 1971;407.

8. Cooper DM, Wasserman DH, Vranic M, Wasserman K. Glucose turnover in response to exercise during high- and low-FIO_2 breathing in man. Am J Physiol 1986; 251:E209–E214.

9. Idstrom JP, Harihara Subramanian V, Chance B, Schersten T, Bylund-Fellenius AC. Oxygen dependence of energy metabolism in contracting and recovering rat skeletal muscle. Am J Physiol 1985;248:H40–H48.

10. Cooper CB, Beaver W, Cooper DM, Wasserman K. Factors affecting the component of the alveolar CO_2 output-O_2 uptake relationship during incremental exercise in man. Exp Physiol 1992;77:51–64.

11. Beaver WL, Wasserman K. Muscle RQ and lactate accumulation from analysis of the $\dot{V}CO_2$ -$\dot{V}O_2$ relationship during exercise. Clin J Sport Med 1991;1:27–34.

12. Clode M, Campbell EJM. The relationship between gas exchange and changes in blood lactate concentrations during exercise. Clin Sci 1969;37:263–272.

13. Bergstrom J, Hermansen L, Hultman E, Saltin B. Diet, muscle glycogen and physical performance. Acta Physiol Scand 1967;71:140–150.

14. Rosell S, Saltin B. Energy need, delivery, and utilization in muscular exercise. In: Bourne GH, ed. The Structure and Function of Muscle. New York: Academic Press, 1973;vol 3.

15. Simonsen E. Depletion of energy yielding substances. In: Simonsen E, ed. Physiology of Work Capacity and Fatigue. Springfield: Charles C. Thomas, 1971.

16. Ahlborg B, Bergstrom J, Ekelund LG, Hultman E. Muscle glycogen and muscle electrolytes during prolonged physical exercise. Acta Physiol Scand 1967;70:129–142.

17. Jones NL. Exercise testing in pulmonary evaluation: rationale, methods, and the normal respiratory response to exercise. N Engl J Med 1975;293:541–544.

18. Wasserman DH, Lickley LA, Vranic M. Interactions between glucagon and other counterregulatory hormones during normoglycemic and hypoglycemic exercise in dogs. J Clin Invest 1984;74:1404–1413.

19. Wasserman DH, Cherrington AD. Hepatic fuel metabolism during muscular work: role and regulation. Am J Physiol 1991;260:E811–E824.

20. Pozefsky T, Felig P, Tobin ID. Amino acid balance across tissues of the forearm in postabsorptive man. Effects of insulin at two dose levels. J Clin Invest 1969;48:2273–2282.

21. Wahren J. Substrate utilization by exercising muscle in man. In: Yin PN, Goodwin IF, eds. Progress in Cardiology. Philadelphia: Lea & Febiger, 1973;255–280.

22. Wahren J, Felig P, Havel RJ, Jorfeldt L, Pernow B, Saltin B. Amino acid metabolism in McArdle's syndrome. N Engl J Med 1973;288:774–777.

23. Whipp BJ, Mahler M. Dynamics of pulmonary gas exchange during exercise. In: West JB, ed. Pulmonary Gas Exchange. New York: Academic Press, 1980;2:33–96.

24. Whipp BJ, Wasserman K. Oxygen uptake kinetics for various intensities of constant load work. J Appl Physiol 1972;33:351–356.

25. Wasserman K, Whipp BJ. Exercise physiology in health and disease. Am Rev Respir Dis 1975;112:219–249.

26. Astrand PO, Rodahl K. Textbook of Work Physiology, 2nd Ed. New York: McGraw-Hill, 1977;393–411.

27. Whipp BJ, Wasserman K. Efficiency of muscular work. J Appl Physiol 1969;26:644–648.

28. Roston WL, Whipp BJ, Davis JA, Effros RM, Wasserman K. Oxygen uptake kinetics and lactate concentration during exercise in humans. Am Rev Respir Dis 1987; 135: 1080–1084.

29. Koike A, Wasserman K, McKenzie DK, Zanconato S, Weiler-Ravell D. Weiler-Ravell: Evidence that diffusion limitation determines oxygen uptake kinetics during exercise in humans. J Clin Invest 1990;86:1698–1706.

30. Zhang YY, Wasserman K, Sietsema KE, Barstow T, Mizumoto G, Sullivan CS. O_2 uptake kinetics in response to exercise: A measure of tissue anaerobiosis in heart failure. Chest 1993;103:735–741.

31. Wells JG, Balke B, Van Fossan BD. Lactic acid accumulation during work. A suggested standardization of work classification. J Appl Physiol 1957;10:51–55.

32. Wasserman K. The anaerobic threshold measurement

to evaluate exercise performance. Am Rev Respir Dis (Suppl.) 1984;129:535–540.

33. Wasserman K, VanKessel AL, Burton GB. Interaction of physiological mechanisms during exercise. J Appl Physiol 1967;22:71–85.

34. Wasserman K, Whipp BJ, Casaburi R. Respiratory control during exercise. In: Cherniack NS, Widdicombe G, eds. Handbook of Physiology, Vol. 2. Bethesda: American Physiological Society 1986;595–619.

35. Hughson RH, Weisiger KW, Swanson GD. Blood lactate concentration increases as a continuous function in progressive exercise. J Appl Physiol 1987;62:1975–1981.

36. Beaver WL, Wasserman K, Whipp BJ. Improved detection of the lactate threshold during exercise using a log-log transformation. J Appl Physiol 1985;59:1936–1940.

37. Wasserman K, Beaver WL, Whipp BJ. Gas exchange theory and the lactic acidosis 10 (anaerobic) threshold. Circulation 1990;81(Suppl II):II14–II30.

38. Knuttgen HG, Saltin B. Muscle metabolites and oxygen uptake in short-term submaximal exercise in man. J Appl Physiol 1972;32:690–694.

39. Jorfeldt L, Juhlin-Dannfelt A, Karlsson J. Lactate release and relation to tissue lactate and human skeletal muscle during exercise. J Appl Physiol 1978;44:350–352.

40. Lindholm A, Saltin B. The physiological and biochemical response of standardlined horses to exercise of varying speed and duration. Acta Vet Scand 1974;15:310–324.

41. Katz A, Sahlin K. Regulation of lactic acid production during exercise. J Appl Physiol 988;65:509–518.

42. Chwalbinska-Moneta J, Rogbergs RA, Costill DL, Fink WJ. Threshold for muscle lactate accumulation during progressive exercise. J Appl Physiol 1983;55:1178–1186.

43. Wasserman K, Beaver WL, Davis JA, Pu JZ, Heber D, Whipp BJ. Lactate, pyruvate, and lactate-to-pyruvate ratio during exercise and recovery. J Appl Physiol 1985;59:935–940.

44. Bylund-Fellenius AC, Walker PM, Elander A, Holm S, Holm J, Schersten T. Energy metabolism in relation to oxygen partial pressure in human skeletal muscle during exercise. Biochem J 1981;200:247–255.

45. Sahlin K, Harris RD, Nylind B, Hultman E. Lactate content and pH in muscle samples obtained after dynamic exercise. Pflugers Arch 1976;367:143–149.

46. Ivy JL, Withers RT, Van Handel PJ, Elger DH, Costill DL. Muscle respiratory capacity and fiber type as determinants of the lactate threshold. J Appl Physiol 1980;48:523–527.

47. Chance B, Mauriello G, Aubert XM. ADP arrival at muscle mitochondria following a twitch. In: Rodahl K, Horvath SF, eds. Muscle as a Tissue. New York: McGraw-Hill, 1962.

48. Wittenberg BA, Wittenberg JB. Transport of oxygen in muscle. Ann Rev Physiol 1989;51:857–878.

49. Gayeski TEJ, Honig CR. Intracellular Po2 in long axis of individual fibers in working dog gracilis muscle. Am J Physiol 1988, 254 (Heart Circ Physiol 21): H1179–H1186.

50. Roughton FJW. Transport of oxygen and carbon dioxide. In: Handbook of Physiology. 1964;767–825.

51. Stringer WW, Wasserman K, Casaburi R, Porszasz J, Maehara, French W. Lactic acidosis as a facilitator of oxyhemoglobin dissociation during exercise. J Appl Physiol 1994;76:1462–1467.

52. Koike A, Wasserman K, Taniguchi K, Ohtomo N, Hiroe M, Maurumo F. The critical capillary Po2 and the anarobic threshold during exercise in patients with cardiovascular diseases. J Am Coll Cardiol 1994;23:1644–1650.

53. Wasserman K. Coupling of external to cellular respiration during exercise: the wisdom of the body revisited. Am J Physiol 1994;266:E519–E539.

54. Andersen P, Saltin B. Maximal perfusion of skeletal muscle in man. J Physiol 1985;366:233–249.

55. Donald KW, Gloster J, Harris AE, Reeves J, Harris P. The production of lactic acid during exercise in normal subjects and in patients with rheumatic heart disease. Am Heart J 1961;62:273–293.

56. Sullivan MJ, Knight D, Higginbotham MB, Cobb FR. Relation between central and peripheral hemodynamics during exercise in patients with chronic heart failure. Circulation 1989;80:769–781.

57. Beaver WL, Wasserman K, Whipp BJ. Bicarbonate buffering of lactic acid generated during exercise. J Appl Physiol 1986;60:472–478.

58. Stringer W, Casaburi R, Wasserman K. Acid-base regulation during exercise and recovery in man. J Appl Physiol 1992;72:954–961.

59. Owles WH. Alterations in the lactic acid content of the blood as a result of light exercise, and associated changes in the CO_2-combining power of the blood and in the alveolar CO_2 pressure. J Physiol 1930;69:214–237.

60. Bouyhus A, Pool J, Binkhorst RA, vanLeeuwen P. Metabolic acidosis of exercise in healthy males. J Appl Physiol 1966;21:1040–1046.

61. Yoshida T, Udo M, Chida M, Makiguchi K, Ichioka M, Muraoka I. Arterial blood gases, acid-base balance, and lactate and gas exchange variables during hypoxic exercise. Int J Sport Med 1989;10:279–285.

62. Trosper TL, Philipson KD. Lactate transport by cardiac sarcolemmal vesicles. Am J Physiol 1987;252:483–489.

63. Mainwood GW, Worsley-Brown P, Paterson RA. The metabolic changes in frog satorius muscles during recovery from fatigue at different external bicarbonate concentrations. Can J Physiol Pharmacol 1971;50:143–155.

64. Hirsche H, Hombach V, Langhor VD, Wacker U, Busse J. Lactic acid permeation rate in working gastrocnemii of dogs during metabolic alkalosis and acidosis. Pflugers Arch 1975;56:209–222.

65. Korotzer B, Jung T, Stringer WW, Nguyen P, Jones A, Wasserman K. Effect of Acetazolamide on lactate, lactate threshold and acid-base balance during exercise. Am J Respir Crit Care Med 1997;155:171A.

66. Wasserman K, Stringer WW, Casaburi R. Mechanism of the exercise hyperkalemia: an alternate hypothesis. J Appl Physiol 1997;83:631–643.

67. Karlsson J. Pyruvate and lactate ratios in muscle tissue and blood during exercise in man. Acta Physiol Scand 1971;81:455–458.

68. Sahlin K, Katz A, Henriksson J. Redox state and lactate

accumulation in human skeletal muscle during dynamic exercise. Biochem J 1987;245:551–556.

69. Koike A, Weiler-Ravell D, McKenzie DK, Zanconato S, Wasserman K. Evidence that the metabolic acidosis threshold is the anaerobic threshold. J Appl Physiol 1990;68:2521–2526.

70. Koike A, Wasserman K, Armon Y, Weiler-Ravell D. The work-rate-dependent effect of carbon monoxide on ventilatory control during exercise. Respir Physiol 1991; 85:169–183.

71. Vogel JA, Gleser MA. Effect of carbon monoxide on oxygen transport during exercise. J Appl Physiol 1972; 32:234–239.

72. Yoshida T, Udo M, Chida M, Ichioka M, Makiguchi K. Effect of hypoxia on arterial and venous blood levels of oxygen, carbon dioxide, hydrogen ions and lactate during incremental forearm exercise. Eur J Appl Physiol 1989;58:772–777.

73. Lundin G, Strom G. The concentration of blood lactate acid in man during muscular work in relation to the partial pressure of oxygen of the inspired air. Acta Physiol Scand 1947;13:253–256.

74. Beaver WL, Wasserman K, Whipp BJ. A new method for detecting the anaerobic threshold by gas exchange. J Appl Physiol 1986;60:2020–2027.

75. Wasserman K, Whipp BJ, Koyal SN, Cleary MG. Effect of carotid body resection on ventilatory and acidbase control during exercise. J Appl Physiol 1975;39:354–353.

76. Ward SA, Whipp BJ. Influence of body CO_2 stores on ventilatory metabolic coupling during exercise. In: Honda Y, Miyamoto Y, Konno K, and JG Widdicombe, eds. Control of Breathing and Its Modeling Perspective. Widdicombe, New York: Plenum Press, 1992;425–431.

77. Tanaka K, Matsumura Y, Matsuzaka A, Hirakoba K, Kumagai S, Sun O, Asano K. A longitudinal assessment of anaerobic threshold and distance-running performance. Med Sci Sports Exerc 1984;16:278–282.

78. Zoladz JA, Sargeant AJ, Stoklosa J, Zychowski A. Changes in acid-base status of marathon runners during incremental field test. Eur J Appl Physiol 1993;67:71–76.

79. Duling BR. Control of striated muscle blood flow. In: Crystal RG, West JB, eds. The Lung: Scientific Foundations. New York: Raven Press, Ltd, 1991;1497.

80. Kilmartin JV, Rossi-Bernardi L. Interaction of hemoglobin with hydrogen ions, carbon dioxide, and organic phosphates. Physiol Rev 1973;53:836–890.

81. Jung T, Korotzer B, Stringer WW, Jones A, Wasserman K. Lactate concentration increase and transcellular fluid flux during exercise. Am J Respir Crit Care Med 1996; 153:A647.

82. Hill AV, Long CNH, Lupton H. Muscular exercise, lactic acid, and the supply and utilization of oxygen. VI. The oxygen debt at the end of exercise. Proc R Soc Lond 1924;97:127–137.

83. McGilvery RW. Quantitative significance of lactate production. In Biochemistry: A functional approach. Philadelphia: W.B. Saunders Co., 1970;268–270.

84. McArdle B. Myopathy due to a defect in muscle glycogen breakdown. Clin Sci 1951;10:13–35.

85. Lewis SF, Haller RG. The pathophysiology of McArdle's disease: Clues to regulation in exercise and fatigue. J Appl Physiol 1986;61:391–401.

86. Wasserman K, Nguyen P, Korotzer B, Jung T, Fu P, Stringer WW. Arterial plasma electrolyte changes above the lactate threshold. FASEB J 1997;11:A214.

87. Kaltreider N, Menely G. The effect of exercise on the volume of the blood. J Clin Invest 1940;19:637–644.

88. Beaumont W. Red cell volume with changes in plasma osmolarity during maximal exercise. J Appl Physiol 1973;35:47–50.

89. Senay LC, Rogers G, Jooste P. Changes in blood plasma during progressive treadmill and cycle exercise. J Appl Physiol 1980;49:59–65.

90. Katz A, Sahlin K. Effect of decreased oxygen availability on NADH and lactate contents in human skeletal muscle during exercise. Acta Physiol Scand 1987;131:119–127.

91. Casaburi R, Barstow TJ, Robinson T, Wasserman K. Influence of work rate on ventilatory and gas exchange kinetics. J Appl Physiol 1989;67:547–555.

92. Zhang YY, Sietsema KE, Sullivan CS, Wasserman K. A method for measuring bicarbonate buffering of lactic acid during constant work rate exercise. Eur J Appl Physiol 1994;69:309–315.

93. Weltman A, Wood CM, Womack CJ, Davis SE, Blumer JL, Alvarez J, Sauer K, Gaesser GA. Catecholamie and blood lactate responses to incremental rowing and running exercise. J Appl Physiol 1994;76:1144–1149.

94. Riley M, Maehara K, Porszasz J, Engelen M, Barstow T, Tanaka H, Wasserman K. Association between the anaerobic threshold and the breakpoint in the double-product-work rate relationship. Eur J Appl Physiol 1997;75:14–21.

95. Wasserman K, Whipp BJ, Koyal SN, Beaver WL. Anaerobic threshold and respiratory gas exchange during exercise. J Appl Physiol 1973;35:236–243.

96. Patessio A, Casaburi R, Carone M, Appendi L, Donner CF, Wasserman K. Comparison of gas exchange, lactate and lactic acidosis thresholds in COPD patients. Am Rev Resp Dis 1993;148:622–626.

97. Mahler M. First order kinetics of muscle oxygen consumption and an equivalent proportionality between $\dot{Q}O_2$ and phosphorylcreatine level. J Gen Physiol 1985; 86:135–165.

98. Yoshida T, Watari H. ^{31}P-Nuclear magnetic resonance spectroscopy study of the time course of energy metabolism during exercise and recovery. Eur J Appl Physiol 1993;66:494–499.

99. Rowell LB. Human Circulation Regulation During Physical Stress. New York: Oxford University Press, 1986;215.

100. Guyton AC, Jones CE, Coleman TG. Cardiac output in muscular exercise. In: Circulatory Physiology: Cardiac Output and its Regulation. Philadelphia: W.B. Saunders Co., 1973.

101. Loeppky JA, Greene ER, Hoekenga, Caprihan A, Luft UC. Beat-by-beat stroke volume assessment by pulsed Doppler in upright and supine exercise. J Appl Physiol 1981;50:1173–1182.

102. Dempsey JA, Hanson P, Henderson K. Exercise-induced arterial hypoxemia in healthy humans at sea level. J Physiol (London)1984;355:161–175.

103. Bunn HF, Forget BG. Hemoglobin: Molecular, Genetic and Clinical Aspects. Philadelphia: W.B. Saunders Company, 1986;595–616.

104. Christiansen J, Douglas CG, Haldane JS. The absorption and dissociation of carbon dioxide by human blood. J Physiol 1914;48:244–271.

105. Sue DY, Chung MD, Grosvenor M, Wasserman K. Effect of altering the proportion of dietary fat and carbohydrate on exercise gas exchange in normal subjects. Am Rev Respir Dis 1989;139:1430–1434.

106. Brown SE, Wiener S, Brown RA, Maratelli PA, Light RW. Exercise performance following a carbohydrate load in chronic airflow obstruction. J Appl Physiol 1985; 58:1340–1346.

107. Whipp BJ. The control of exercise hyperpnea. In: Hornbein T, ed. Regulation of Breathing. New York: Marcel Dekker, 1981;1069–1139.

108. Casaburi R, Whipp BJ, Wasserman K, Beaver WL, Koyal SN. Ventilatory and gas exchange dynamics in response to sinusoidal work. J Appl Physiol 1977;42:300–311.

109. Lugliani R, Whipp BJ, Seard C, Wasserman K. Effects of bilateral carotid body resection on ventilatory control at rest and during exercise in man. N Engl J Med 1971;285:1105–1111.

110. Wasserman K, Whipp BJ. The carotid bodies and respiratory control in man. In: Paintal AS, ed. Morphology and Mechanisms of Chemoreceptors. Delhi: Vallabhbhai Patel Chest Institute, 1976;156–175.

111. Krogh A, Lindhard J. The regulation of respiration and circulation during the initial stages of muscular work. J Physiol (London) 1913;47:112–136.

112. Fink GR, Adams L, Watson JDG, Innes JA, Wuyam B, Kobayashi I, Corfield DR, Murphy K, Jones T, Frackowiak RSJ, Guz A. Hyperpnea during and immediately after exercise in man. Evidence of motor cortical involvement. J Physiol (London) 1995;489:663–675.

113. Martin PA, Mitchell GS. Long-term modulation of the exercise ventilatory response in goats. J Physiol (London) 1993;470:601–617.

114. Eldridge FL, Millhorn DE, Waldrop TG. Exercise hyperpnea and locomotion: parallel activation from the hypothalamus. Science 1981;211:844–846.

115. DiMarco AF, Romaniuk JR, von Euler C, Yamamoto Y. Immediate changes in ventilation and respiratory pattern associated with onset and cessation of locomotion in the cat. J Physiol (London) 1983;343:116.

116. Weiler-Ravell D, Cooper DM, Whipp BJ, Wasserman K. Control of breathing at the start of exercise as influenced by posture. J Appl Physiol 1983;55:1460–1466.

117. Wasserman K, Whipp BK. Castagna J. Cardiodynamic hyperpnea: hyperpnea secondary to cardiac output increase. J Appl Physiol 1974;36:457–464.

118. Jones PW, Huszczuk A, Wasserman K. Cardiac output as a controller of ventilation through changes in right ventricular load. J Appl Physiol 1982;53:218–224.

119. Bisgard GE, Forester HV, Byrnes B, Stanek K, Klein J, Manohar M. Cerebrospinal fluid acid-base balance during muscular exercise. J Appl Physiol 1978;45:94–101.

120. Lugliani R, Whipp BJ, Brinkman J, Wasserman K. Doxapram hydrochloride: A respiratory stimulant for patients with primary alveolar hypoventilation. Chest 1979;76: 414–419.

121. Shea SA, Andrews LP, Shannon DC, Banzett RB. Ventilatory responses to exercise in humans lacking ventilatory chemosensitivity. J Physiol (London) 1993;469: 623–640.

122. Whipp BJ, Wasserman K. Carotid bodies and ventilatory control dynamics in man. Fed Proc 1980;39:1628–1673.

123. Casaburi R, Stremel RW, Whipp BJ, Beaver WL, Wasserman K. Alteration by hyperoxia of ventilatory dynamics during sinusoidal work. J Appl Physiol 1980;48:1083–1091.

124. Oren A, Whipp BJ, Wasserman K. Effect of acidbase status on the kinetics of the ventilatory response to moderate exercise. J Appl Physiol 1982;52:1013–1017.

125. Griffiths TL, Henson LC, Whipp BJ. Influence of inspired oxygen concentration on the dynamics of the exercise hyperpnea in man. J Physiol 1986;380:387–403.

126. Phillipson EA, Hickey RF, Bainton CR, Nadel JA. Effect of vagal blockade on regulation of breathing in conscious dogs. J Appl Physiol 1970;29:475–479.

127. Dejours P. Control of respiration in muscular exercise. In: Fenn WO, Rahn H, eds. Handbook of Physiology. Washington, DC: American Physiological Society, 1964; 631–638.

128. McCloskey DI, Mitchell JH. Reflex cardiovascular and respiratory responses originating in exercising muscle. J Physiol (London) 1972;224:173–186.

129. Kao FF. An experimental study of the pathways involved in exercise hyperpnea employing crosscirculation techniques. In: Cunningham DJC, Lloyd BB, eds. The Regulation of Human Respiration. Blackwell Scientific Publications, 1961;461–502.

130. Hornbein TF, Sorenson SC, Parks CR. Role of muscle spindles in lower extremities in breathing during bicycle exercise. J Appl Physiol 1969;27:476–479.

131. Hodgson HJF, Mathews PBC. The ineffectiveness of excitation of the primary endings of the muscle spindle by vibration as a respiratory stimulant in the decerebrate cat. J Physiol (London) 1968;194:555–563.

132. Waldrop TG, Rybicki K, Kaufman MP. Chemical activation of group I and group II muscle afferents has no cardiorespiratory effects. J Appl Physiol 1984;56:1223–1228.

133. Kaufman MP, Waldrop TG, Rybicki KJ, Ordway GA, Mitchell JH. Effects of static and rhythmic contractions on the discharge of group III and IV muscle afferents. Cardiovasc Res 1984;18:663–668.

134. Fernandes A, Galbo H, Kjer M, Mitchell JH, Secker NH, Thomas S. Cardiovascular and ventilatory responses to dynamic exercise during epidural anaesthesia in man. J Physiol (London) 1990;420:281–293.

135. Brice AG, Forster HV, Pan LG, Funahashi A, Hoffman MD, Murphy CL, Lowry TF. Is the hyperpnea of muscu-

lar contractions critically dependent on spinal afferents? J Appl Physiol 1988;64:226–233.

136. Adams L, Frankel H, Garlick J, Guz A, Murphy K, Semple SJG. The role of spinal cord transmission in the ventilatory response to exercise in man. J Physiol (London) 1984;355:85–97.

137. Innes JA, Solarte I, Huszczuk A, Yeh E, Whipp BJ, Wasserman K. Respiration during recovery from exercise; effects of trapping and release of femoral blood flow. J Appl Physiol 1989;67:2608–2613.

138. Casaburi R, Daly J, Hansen JE, Effros RM. Abrupt changes in mixed venous blood gas composition following onset of exercise. J Appl Physiol 1989;67:1106–1112.

139. Casaburi R, Cooper C, Effros RM, Wasserman K. Time course of mixed venous oxygen saturation following various modes of exercise transition. FASEB J 1989;3:A849.

140. Beaver WL, Lammara N, Wasserman K. Breath-by-breath measurement of true alveolar gas exchange. J Appl Physiol 1981;51:1662–1675.

141. Whipp BJ, Ward SA, Lamarra M, Davis JA, Wasserman K. Parameters of ventilatory and gas exchange dynamics during exercise. J Appl Physiol 1982;52:1506–1513.

142. Wasserman K, Casaburi R, Beaver WL, Roston W, Whipp BJ. Assessing the adequacy of tissue oxygenation during exercise. In: Bryan-Brown CW, Ayres SM, eds New Horizons: Oxygen Transport and Utilization 1987;109–144.

143. Whipp BJ, Seard C, Wasserman K. Oxygen deficit-oxygen debt relationships and efficiency of anaerobic work. J Appl Physiol 1970;28:452–456.

144. Schneider EG, Robinson S, Newton JL. Oxygen debt in aerobic work. J Appl Physiol 1968;25:58–62.

145. Margaria R, Edwards HT, Dill DB. The possible mechanisms of contracting and paying the oxygen debt and the role of lactic acid in muscular contraction. Am J Physiol 1933;106:689–715.

146. Piiper J. Production of lactic acid in heavy exercise and acid-base balance. In: Moret PR, Weber J, Haissly J, et al. Lactate: Physiologic, Methodologic and Pathologic Approach. New York: Springer-Verlag, 1980;35–45.

147. Lusk G. Science of Nutrition. Johnson Reprint Corp., New York, 1976;65.

148. Severinghaus JW. Simple accurate equations for human blood $\dot{Q}o_2$ dissociation computations. J Appl Physiol 1979;46:599–602.

149. Stringer WW, Wasserman K, Casaburi R. The $\dot{V}co_2/\dot{V}o_2$ relationship during heavy, constant work rate exercise reflects the rate of lactate accumulation. Eur J Appl Physiol 1995;72:25–31.

150. Wasserman K. Breathing during exercise. N Engl J Med 1978;298:780–785.

151. Whipp BJ, Pardy RL. Breathing during exercise. American Physiological Society Handbook of Physiology Sect 3, Vol III, Chapter 34, p. 605.

152. Wasserman K. Coupling of external to internal respiration. Am Rev Resp Dis 1984;129(Suppl.):S21–S24.

153. Sietsema K, Daly JA, Wasserman K. Early dynamics of O2 uptake and heart rate as affected by exercise work rate. J Appl Physiol 1989;67:2535–2541.

154. Whipp, BJ, Ward SA. Coupling of ventilation to pulmonary gas exchange during exercise. In: Exercise: Pulmonary Physiology and Pathophysiology. New York: Marcel Dekker, Inc., 1991;275.

CHAPTER 3

Measurements During Integrative Cardiopulmonary Exercise Testing

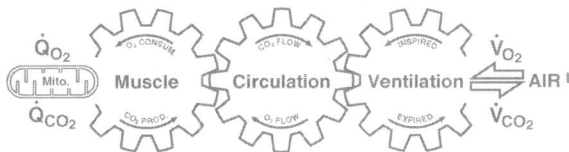

CARDIOPULMONARY EXERCISE testing (CPET) permits simultaneous evaluation of the ability of the cardiovascular and respiratory systems to perform their major functions, i.e., gas exchange. Because exercise requires an integrative cardiopulmonary response to support the increase in muscle respiration required to perform exercise, gas exchange measurements are fundamental to the understanding of the mechanism(s) of exercise limitation. It is evident from the scheme shown in Figure 1.1 that a reduction in $\dot{V}O_2$max (peak $\dot{V}O_2$) can be caused by any disease process affecting skeletal muscle function or the organ systems required to transport O_2 and CO_2 between the air and the muscle cell. Use of CPET only to determine $\dot{V}O_2$max or peak $\dot{V}O_2$, as is commonly done, fails to employ this laboratory test for its unique capability, to define the pathophysiology of exercise limitation. This chapter describes measurements obtained from CPET which are useful when assessing the responses of each of the organ systems coupling external respiration (O_2 uptake and CO_2 output at the airway) to cellular respiration (O_2 consumption and CO_2 production of the cells) during exercise.

WHAT IS AN INTEGRATIVE CARDIOPULMONARY EXERCISE TEST?

The primary function of the cardiovascular and pulmonary systems is to support cellular respiration. The success of the cardiovascular and pulmonary systems in meeting this function is reflected in the O_2 uptake and CO_2 output in response to a specific work rate. An integrative cardiopulmonary exercise test can address many more questions than an exercise test that only assesses the electrocardiogram to address the presence or absence of cardiac ischemia. While also employing electrocardiographic measurements, CPET also addresses a large number of questions about other disorders. These questions are listed in Table 3.1, along with the measurements that can be used to address each question. Because the questions that can be addressed by integrative

TABLE 3.1.   Questions Addressed by Cardiopulmonary Exercise Testing*

Question	Disorder	Markers of Abnormality
1. Is exercise capacity reduced?	Any disorder	Maximal $\dot{V}O_2$—panel 3
2. Is the metabolic requirement for exercise increased?	Obesity	$\dot{V}O_2$–WR relationship—panel 3
3. Is exercise limited by impaired O_2 flow?	Ischemic, myopathic, valvular, congenital heart disease;	ECG; AT; $\Delta\dot{V}O_2/\Delta WR$; $\dot{V}O_2$/HR—panels 2,3,5
	Pulmonary vascular disease;	$\Delta\dot{V}O_2/\Delta WR$; AT; $\dot{V}O_2$/HR; $\dot{V}E/\dot{V}CO_2$—panels 2,3,5,6
	Peripheral arterial disease;	BP; $\Delta\dot{V}O_2/\Delta WR$;—panels 3,5
	Anemia, hypoxemia, elevated COHb	AT; $\dot{V}O_2$/HR—panels 2,3,5
4. Is exercise limited by reduced ventilatory capacity?	Lung; chest wall	BR; ventilatory response—panels 1,7,9
5. Is there an abnormal degree of $\dot{V}/\dot{Q}$ mismatching?	Lung disease; pulmonary vascular disease; heart failure	$P(A - a)O_2$; $P(a - ET)CO_2$; VD/VT; $\dot{V}E/\dot{V}CO_2$—panels 4,6,9
6. Is there a defect in muscle utilization of O_2 or substrate?	Muscle glycolytic or mitochondrial enzyme defect	AT, R, $\dot{V}CO_2$; HR vs $\dot{V}O_2$; lactate; lactate/pyruvate ratio—panels 3,8
7. Is exercise limited by a behavioral problem?	Neurosis	Breathing pattern—panels 7,8
8. Is work output reduced because of poor effort?	Poor effort with secondary gain.	Increased HRR; Increased BR; peak R < 1.1; normal AT, $P(A - a)O_2$ and $P(a - ET)CO_2$—panels 2,5,7,8

* Peak $\dot{V}O_2$ = highest O_2 uptake measured; WR = work rate; AT = anaerobic threshold; $\Delta\dot{V}O_2/\Delta WR$ = increase in $\dot{V}O_2$ relative to increase in work rate; $\dot{V}O_2$/HR = O_2 pulse; $\dot{V}E/\dot{V}CO_2$ = ventilatory equivalent for CO_2; BR (breathing reserve) = maximum voluntary ventilation–ventilation at maximum exercise; $P(A - a)O_2$ = alveolar-arterial PO_2 difference; $P(a - ET)CO_2$ = arterial-end tidal PCO_2 difference; VD/VT = physiologic dead space/tidal volume ratio; R = $\dot{V}CO_2/\dot{V}O_2$ = respiratory exchange ratio; HRR (heart rate reserve) = predicted maximum heart rate–maximum exercise heart rate; Peak R = peak gas exchange ratio; COHb = carboxyhemoglobin. Panel numbers in right column refer to Figure 3.30.

cardiopulmonary exercise testing are so comprehensive, testing at the beginning of a work-up of exercise limitation from any cause reduces the cost and time required to evaluate the patient.

WHEN SHOULD CARDIOPULMONARY EXERCISE TESTING BE USED?

1. **Differential diagnosis.** When the cause of dyspnea or exercise limitation is uncertain (i.e., for differential diagnosis), integrative CPET can serve to define the specific organ system limiting gas transport. This enables a more specific further work-up.
2. **Disability evaluation.** By providing an objective assessment of exercise capacity and degree of impairment, CPET is of considerable, if not essential, value in disability evaluation.
3. **Rehabilitation.** CPET provides information of the level of exercise that the patient can perform without undue stress. Thus the test results guide the physician for exercise prescription in physical rehabilitation. It also furnishes quantitative evidence of the benefit of a rehabilitation program as well as the mechanism(s) of benefit. Improvement in exercise tolerance can not be objectively assessed without CPET.
4. **Assessing pre-operative risk**. CPET is of value for preoperative evaluation of risk for patients about to undergo major surgery (1, 2); such testing enables the examiner to evaluate the stress that the cardiopulmonary system can undergo before anaerobic ATP production, with resulting lactic acidosis, is recruited to complement aerobic ATP production. Predictably, CPET provides much more information about cardiovascular and pulmonary reserve during metabolic stress than measurements of cardiovascular and ventilatory function measured at rest.
5. **Prioritizing patients for heart transplantation.** Peak $\dot{V}_{O_2}$ has been found to be the best predictor of survival time in patients with chronic heart failure (3, 4). A given heart lesion may have a different functional significance in two different patients because of a difference in how the peripheral circulation adapts to the cardiac abnormality. Because CPET addresses the body's global physiological adaptation to exercise, including compensatory mechanisms for the abnormal cardiac function, it has been valuable in the prediction of survival time without heart transplantation. Therefore it is an essential component in the evaluation of chronic heart failure patients for heart transplantation (5).
6. **Effectiveness of therapy.** Measurement of gas exchange has also been useful in evaluating functional improvement resulting from pacemakers in patients with heart block (6) and to objectively assess various forms of medical therapy in patients with a variety of disorders (7, 8).

The measurements and functions that integrative CPET assesses are summarized in Table 3.2. Fortunately, most are noninvasive and can be performed in modern cardiopulmonary function laboratories. The gas exchange variables that provide the most valuable information are described in this chapter, whereas methods of measurement, calculation, calibration, and accuracy are described in the Appendix.

CPET is useful because it enables the examiner to: 1) quantify the level of the subject's exercise limitation; 2) assess the adequacy of the performance of various components in the coupling of pulmonary to cellular gas exchange; 3) determine the organ system limiting exercise; and 4) determine the $\dot{V}_{O_2}$ at which exercise limitation occurs. These evaluations can be addressed during short (approximately 10-minute), progressive, non–steady-state exercise tests, rather than during a more prolonged exercise test with relatively long duration steps. Prolonged testing is more likely to delay recovery of the patient, thereby making it more difficult for the investigator to repeat testing, if required.

MEASUREMENTS
Electrocardiogram (ECG)

Because exercise causes the heart rate to increase and diastolic time to shorten, the time for coronary perfusion is decreased. Thus, coronary artery disease is more likely to be detected while exercising than during rest (9). Myocardial ischemia results from an inadequate O_2 supply to meet the O_2 requirement in support of cardiac work. When the heart muscle contracts without adequate O_2, lactic acid production increases and the muscle cells alter their ionic permeability. Thus the rate of reestablishing the electrical membrane potential during repolarization is slowed in the ischemic areas of the myocardium. This causes the T wave and ST segments to change acutely when the O_2 requirement for the increased cardiac work of exercise exceeds the availability of O_2 (Table 3.3). An increased fre-

TABLE 3.2. Assessing Function with Physiologic Measurements

Measurements	Function
Electrocardiogram	Myocardial O_2 availability–requirement balance
$\dot{V}O_2$	Cardiac output $\times$ C(a − $\bar{v}$)O_2
Peak $\dot{V}O_2$	Highest $\dot{V}O_2$ achieved during presumed maximal effort for an incremental exercise test (specific for type of work), may or may not equal $\dot{V}O_2$max
$\dot{V}O_2$max	Highest $\dot{V}O_2$ achievable as evidenced by failure for $\dot{V}O_2$ to increase despite increasing work rate (specific for type of work); highest cardiac output $\times$ C(a − $\bar{v}$)O_2
$\Delta\dot{V}O_2/\Delta WR$	Aerobic contribution to exercise (low value suggests high anaerobic contribution)
Cardiac output	Useful when related to vascular pressure
Anaerobic threshold (AT)	Highest $\dot{V}O_2$ that can be sustained without developing a lactic acidosis; important determinant of potential for endurance work (specific for form of work)
O_2 pulse	Product of SV and C(a − $\bar{v}$)O_2; under conditions when SV is constant, change in O_2 pulse is proportional to change in C(a − $\bar{v}$)O_2
Heart rate reserve (HRR)	Difference between predicted and measured heart rate at $\dot{V}O_2$ max
Arterial pressure	Detecting systemic hypertension, ventricular outflow obstruction, or myocardial failure (pulsus alternans or decreasing pressure with increasing WR)
$\dot{V}E = \dot{V}A + \dot{V}D$	$\dot{V}D$ is increased due to mismatching of $\dot{V}A$ to Q. $\dot{V}$ is increased inversely with decrease in $PaCO_2$ whether caused by a low CO_2 setpoint, metabolic acidosis, or hypoxemia.
BR = MVV-$\dot{V}E$ at max. exercise or (MVV-$\dot{V}E$ at max. exercise) ÷ MVV	Breathing reserve; theoretical additional $\dot{V}E$ available at cessation of exercise
Exercise VD/VT	Measure of mismatching of ventilation and perfusion
P(a − ET)CO_2	Detects high $\dot{V}A/\dot{Q}$ components of lung with mismatching of $\dot{V}A/\dot{Q}$
P(A − a)O_2	Increased in presence of mismatching of $\dot{V}A/\dot{Q}$, diffusion defect, or right to left shunt
Expired flow pattern	Useful for indicating presence of significant airflow obstruction
VT/IC	Fraction of the inspiratory capacity used in breathing
Immediate $\dot{V}O_2$ increase (Phase I) in response to constant WR	Ability to increase pulmonary blood flow at start of exercise (Phase I)
$\Delta\dot{V}O_2$ (6-3)	Proportional to lactate increase; positive if work rate is above LT
Abrupt decrease in $\dot{V}E$ during hyperoxic switch	Contribution of the carotid body to ventilatory drive during hyperoxic (100% O_2) switch

WR = work rate; $\dot{V}E$ = minute ventilation; HR = heart rate; $\dot{V}D$ = physiological dead space; SV = stroke volume; BR = breathing reserve; C(a − $\bar{v}$)O_2 = arterial-mixed venous O_2 content difference; MVV = maximal voluntary ventilation; VT = tidal volume; $\dot{V}D$ = physiological dead space ventilation per minute; IC = inspiratory capacity; $\dot{V}A$ = alveolar ventilation per minute; $\Delta\dot{V}O_2$ (6-3) = difference between $\dot{V}O_2$ at 6 and 3 minutes during constant work rate exercise.

quency of ectopic beats as the work rate increases is also suggestive of myocardial ischemia. Other patients, however, manifest occasional premature ventricular or atrial contractions at rest that disappear or become less frequent during exercise. We regard these ectopic beats as benign and unrelated to a disturbance in the balance between myocardial O_2 availability and requirement, because they are overridden by the sinus tachycardia of exercise.

In many instances, false-positive and borderline changes occur in the ECG when one relies solely on changes in the T wave and ST segments to detect myocardial ischemia. When these ECG changes are accompanied by myocardial dyskinesis, however, $\dot{V}O_2$ may fail to rise appropriately for the increasing work rate. Thus, a reduction in $\Delta\dot{V}O_2/\Delta WR$, accompanied by ECG changes consistent with myocardial ischemia, with or without angina, strengthens the diagnosis of coronary artery disease involving a significant mass of myocardium. In addition, the diagnosis of ischemic heart disease becomes more likely when ECG changes occur in the presence of a fall in systemic blood pressure.

Maximal Oxygen Uptake ($\dot{V}O_2$max) and Maximum Oxygen Uptake (Peak $\dot{V}O_2$)

The body clearly has an upper limit for O_2 utilization at a particular state of fitness or training. This is determined by the maximal cardiac output (10), the arterial O_2 content, the fractional distribution of the

TABLE 3.3. Electrocardiographic Evidence of Myocardial Ischemia During Exercise (12 Lead)

ST segment depression
T wave changes
PVCs that appear during exercise

cardiac output to the exercising muscle (11) and the ability of the muscle to extract O_2 (12). The ventilatory capacity is of importance in determining the upper limit of $\dot{V}O_2$ only when ventilation is insufficient to eliminate the CO_2 produced by aerobic metabolism and the bicarbonate buffering of lactic acid (13).

Maximal aerobic power (i.e., maximal $\dot{V}O_2$ or $\dot{V}O_2$max) was originally defined as the $\dot{V}O_2$ at which performance of increasing levels of constant work rate exercise failed to increase $\dot{V}O_2$ by 150 ml/min, despite increasing work rate (10). This is illustrated in Figure 3.1A and shown experimentally in Figure 2.6. However, this definition has shortcomings because it is dependent on the exercise protocol and because 150 ml is a large fraction of the highest $\dot{V}O_2$ obtained in many patients.

This upper limit in $\dot{V}O_2$ may also be determined in a progressively increasing exercise test, in which a decreasing rate of increase in $\dot{V}O_2$ is observed just before the subject fatigues, despite further increases in the work rate. However, sometimes the subject can not sustain the work rate to the point of oxygen limitation, and a flattening of the $\dot{V}O_2$-work rate

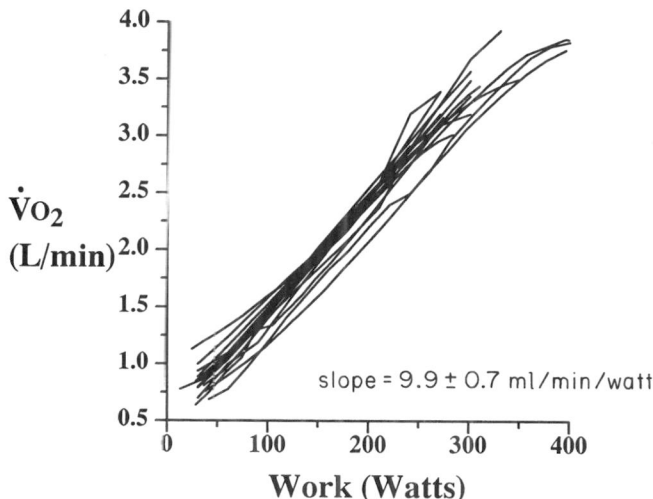

FIGURE 3.2.   The effect of work rate on oxygen uptake ($\dot{V}O_2$) during progressively increasing work rate cycle ergometer exercise for 17 normal subjects. The average regression slope and standard deviation for the subject population is given in the equation in the figure. The slope is consistent among subjects but is displaced upward, depending on body weight as shown in Figure 2.7. (Reprinted with permission from Wasserman K, Sue DY. Coupling of external to cellular respiration. In: Wasserman K, ed. Exercise Gas Exchange in Heart Disease. Arrmonk, NY: Futura Publishing Co., 1996;1–15.)

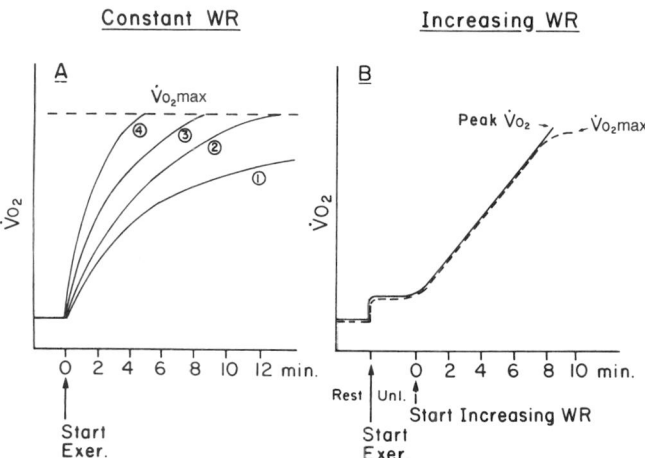

FIGURE 3.1.   Determining the maximal $\dot{V}O_2$ ($\dot{V}O_2$max) from supra-maximal work rate tests (A). The time course of $\dot{V}O_2$ following the onset of exercise is shown for progressively higher work rates. For work rate 1, the $\dot{V}O_2$ asymptote is below $\dot{V}O_2$max. Work rate 2 reaches a $\dot{V}O_2$ which is the same as the highest $\dot{V}O_2$ reached by work rates 3 and 4. Because the maximum $\dot{V}O_2$ for work rates 2, 3 and 4 is the same despite increasing work rate, this identifies $\dot{V}O_2$max for the form of work being studied. Distinguishing between $\dot{V}O_2$max and "peak" or "maximum" $\dot{V}O_2$ from a maximal effort incremental exercise test is shown in B. When the subject's maximum tolerable work rate results in a flattening of the $\dot{V}O_2$-work rate slope, this is the subject's maximal $\dot{V}O_2$ or $\dot{V}O_2$max. When the $\dot{V}O_2$ does not slow its rate of rise with increasing work rate, but the subject has reached his or her maximum tolerable work rate, this is the peak (or maximum) $\dot{V}O_2$ during the test.

relationship is not seen. This is called the peak or maximum $\dot{V}O_2$. Thus, the maximal $\dot{V}O_2$ represents the *highest* $\dot{V}O_2$ attainable for a given form of exercise, as evidenced by a failure for $\dot{V}O_2$ to increase further despite an increase in work rate. Maximal $\dot{V}O_2$ is contrasted with the maximum $\dot{V}O_2$ (peak $\dot{V}O_2$) obtained during a progressively increasing work rate test. It is simply the highest $\dot{V}O_2$ achieved for a presumed maximal exercise effort. While this value does not satisfy the foregoing definition of the *maximal* value determined from repeated constant work rate tests, it is usually equal to the predicted $\dot{V}O_2$max in normal subjects. The distinction between $\dot{V}O_2$max and peak $\dot{V}O_2$ is diagrammed in Figure 3.1. A plateau in $\dot{V}O_2$ during a series of supramaximal constant work rate tests or progressively increasing work rate test shows that a maximal $\dot{V}O_2$ has, in fact, been attained. In actual studies in normal subjects performing progressively increasing exercise to the point of fatigue or dyspnea, only about 1/2 of normal subjects making maximal effort reach a plateau in $\dot{V}O_2$ (Fig. 3.2). After reaching their peak $\dot{V}O_2$, many subjects can not endure the discomfort long enough to achieve a work rate-related plateau in $\dot{V}O_2$. Thus, progressively increasing work rate to the point of fatigue produces a peak $\dot{V}O_2$ that closely approximates the predicted

$\dot{V}O_2$max (14), even when a plateau in $\dot{V}O_2$ is not evident. A plateau in $\dot{V}O_2$ may also fail to occur during a progressively increasing work rate test when the subject stops exercising because of leg or chest pain, shortness of breath, mechanical limitation to breathing, or lack of motivation. In these instances, the peak $\dot{V}O_2$ will be less than the predicted $\dot{V}O_2$max.

Note that, at high exercise intensities, the $\dot{V}O_2$ does not reflect all the high-energy phosphate expended by the subject. It does not account for the energy generated when high energy phosphate is split from phosphocreatine (PCr) and, more importantly, the ATP generated with anaerobic glycolysis, which results in a net increase in lactate. The latter becomes increasingly important as an energy source as work rate increases above the anaerobic threshold (15).

A progressively increasing work rate exercise test, as illustrated in Figure 3.1B, has several advantages: (1) the test starts out at a relatively low work rate, so that it does not require the application of great muscle force or a sudden, large cardiorespiratory stress; (2) the $\dot{V}O_2$max or peak $\dot{V}O_2$ can be determined from an exercise test in which the period of increasing work rate lasts only 8 to 12 minutes; (3) the subject is stressed for only a few minutes at relatively high work rates; and (4) the $\dot{V}O_2$-work rate relationship can be determined if the cycle is the form of ergometry. To obtain the best data for interpreting the measured responses to a progressively increasing work rate exercise test, the work rate increments should be uniform in magnitude and duration. This means that the ergometer must be linear and accurately calibrated.

The peak $\dot{V}O_2$ is the first measurement to be examined because it establishes whether the patient's physiologic responses allow normal maximal aerobic function. Other measurements are then used to differentiate the cause of any exercise limitation whether or not the subject reaches his or her predicted peak $\dot{V}O_2$.

Oxygen Uptake and Work Rate

Although $\dot{V}O_2$ measurements are made from respired gas measured at the mouth, the increase in $\dot{V}O_2$ reflects O_2 utilization by the muscle cells performing the work of exercise. The $\dot{V}O_2$-work rate relationship describes how much O_2 is utilized by the exercising subject in relation to the quantity of external work performed. Because it gives important information concerning the coupling of external to cellular respiration, we find it valuable to graph $\dot{V}O_2$ as a function of work rate.

Pattern of Work Rate Increase and the $\dot{V}O_2$ Response

$\dot{V}O_2$ increases smoothly when cycle ergometer work rate is increased in a continuous ramp pattern or in equal steps of 1-minute duration (Fig. 3.3). This

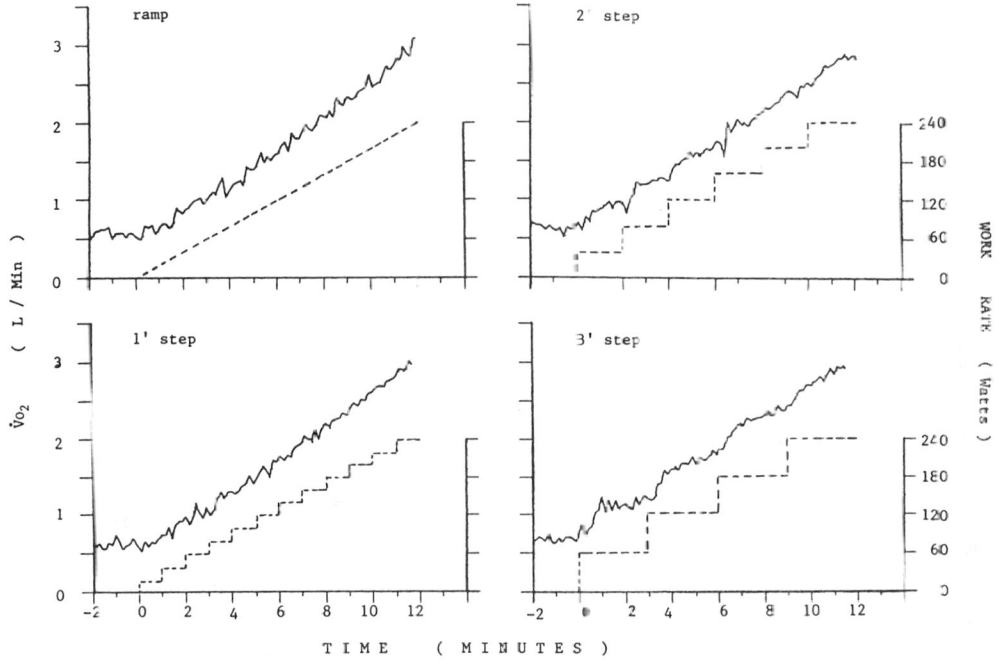

FIGURE 3.3. $\dot{V}O_2$ response in a single subject to four different protocols ramp and 1-, 2- and 3-minute steps. The dashed lines show the work rate and pattern of work rate increase with time. The $\dot{V}O_2$ data are the average of 9-second periods. (Reprinted with permission from Zhang YY, Johnson MC, Chow N, et al. Effect of exercise testing protocol on parameters of aerobic function. Med Sci Sports Exerc 1991;23:625–630.)

type of protocol has advantages in the ease with which the patient perceives the addition of work rate during testing. Increasing work rate in 2- or 3-minute steps results in large abrupt changes in work rate, and the increase in $\dot{V}_{O_2}$ at each interval takes on a step appearance (Fig. 3.3) (16). Because the time constant for $\dot{V}_{O_2}$ at work intensities below the anaerobic threshold is 35 to 45 seconds in healthy subjects, steps at 1-minute increments give smooth increases in $\dot{V}_{O_2}$. Thus the slope of increase in $\dot{V}_{O_2}$ as a function of work rate can be calculated with either the ramp or 1-minute step increase (16). For 3-minute step increases in work rate, the step appearance in $\dot{V}_{O_2}$ is damped at the higher work intensity because of the slowing of $\dot{V}_{O_2}$ kinetics as the subject approaches $\dot{V}_{O_2}$max (17). The loss of the step change in $\dot{V}_{O_2}$ depends on fitness (Fig. 3.4).

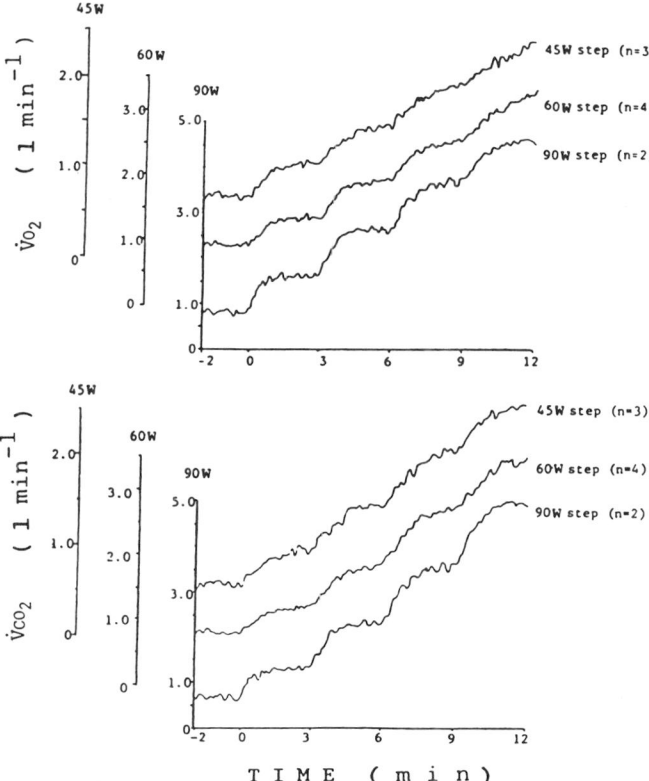

FIGURE 3.4. The average time course of $\dot{V}_{O_2}$ and $\dot{V}_{CO_2}$ for each quarter of a subject's work capacity, assessed in 3-minute work rate steps, is shown for normal subjects at three fitness levels. The greater the size of the step increases in work rate (90-, 60-, or 45-W steps), the greater the subject's fitness ($\dot{V}_{O_2}$peak). At higher work rates, the gas exchange kinetics slow and thereby appear to be more damped. Because the subjects with the larger step increases are more fit, their kinetics are faster and there is less damping of gas exchange. (Reprinted with permission from reference 17.)

Upward Displacement of $\dot{V}_{O_2}$ as a Function of Work Rate

The position of the $\dot{V}_{O_2}$-work rate relationship depends on body weight (see Fig. 3.5A). Obese subjects require increased $\dot{V}_{O_2}$ to do a given amount of external work (see Chapter 2, "Oxygen Cost of Work"). Compared with a non-obese individual, the increase in $\dot{V}_{O_2}$ during exercise is considerably greater than the increase in $\dot{V}_{O_2}$ at rest in obese subjects. This is because of the added O_2 cost to move the limbs during cycling ergometry and the cost of moving the entire body during treadmill exercise. Based on two separate studies of cycle ergometer exercise on adults, the $\dot{V}_{O_2}$ during unloaded cycling at 60 rpm was displaced upward by approximately 5.8 ml/min per kilogram of body weight (18, 19). Although upwardly displaced, the $\dot{V}_{O_2}$-work rate relationship in obesity parallels that of the normal weight subject during cycle ergometry. For treadmill exercise, a predictable adjustment for body weight is not possible because of complex mechanical factors such as varying center of gravity as the angle of the treadmill is changed and the variable length of the stride as the speed and grade are altered. These variables make it difficult to estimate the subject's actual power output during treadmill ergometry.

Slope of $\dot{V}_{O_2}$ as a Function of Work Rate

The slope of $\dot{V}_{O_2}$ as a function of work rate is important because it measures the aerobic work efficiency. The slope for the ramp or 1-minute incremental cycle ergometer progressively increasing work rate test is 10.2 ± 1.0 ml O_2/min/watt(W) for normal subjects by Hansen et al. (18) and 9.9 ± 0.7 ml/min/W obtained by Wasserman and Sue (20) (Fig. 3.2). These values are similar to the 10.1 ml O_2/min/W value previously obtained from steady-state measurements in sedentary subjects (19). Riley et al. (21) obtained an average slope of 11.5 ml O_2/min/W with a standard deviation of 0.78 for 12 trained cyclists.

If the muscles are unable to extract the O_2 required to perform the exercise, then the slope will be shallower than normal (see Fig. 3.5B) and the predicted $\dot{V}_{O_2}$max will not be reached. Although there may be several reasons for this slope to be reduced, a reduction is most commonly due to conditions that impair O_2 flow to the exercising extremities, such as heart disease, pulmonary vascular disease or peripheral arterial occlusive disease. In peripheral arterial occlusive disease, the fixed steno-

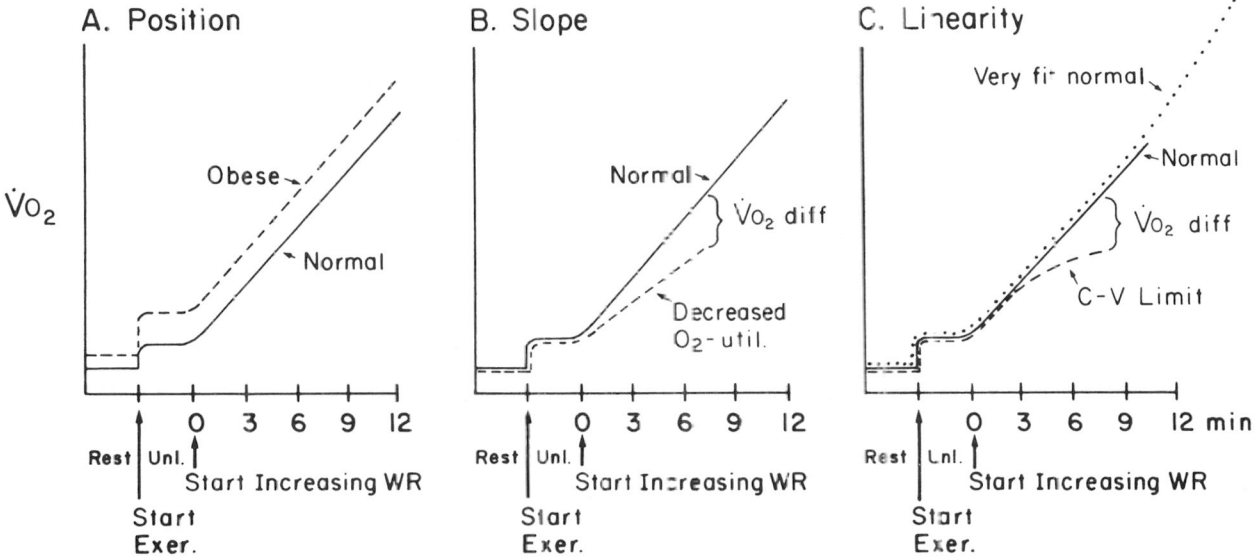

FIGURE 3.5.   Position displacement (A), slope (B), and linearity (C) of the $\dot{V}O_2$-work rate relationship. Obesity displaces the $\dot{V}O_2$-work rate relationship upward, but the slope is unchanged (A). A decreased slope of the $\dot{V}O_2$-work rate relationship (B) reflects inadequate O_2 availability to the exercising muscles, such as when peripheral blood flow is impaired. The linearity of the $\dot{V}O_2$-work rate relationship (C) can be altered in patients with cardiovascular diseases (slope becomes more shallow) because of impaired O_2 flow to the exercising muscles or in very fit people (slope becomes steeper; see text). The difference between the expected $\dot{V}O_2$ for the work rate performed and the actual $\dot{V}O_2$ at the maximum work rate of the subject is referred to as the $\dot{V}O_2$ difference.

sis restricts the blood flow and $\dot{V}O_2$, resulting in a linear but a relatively shallow increase in $\dot{V}O_2$ such as shown in Figure 3.5B. In contrast to other cardiovascular disorders, $\dot{V}CO_2$ slope relative to work rate increase is also relatively shallow in such patients (22).

Linearity of $\dot{V}O_2$ as a Function of Work Rate

Because O_2 uptake kinetics are a more complex function of work rate than a single exponential at work rates above the anaerobic threshold (AT) (23, 26), the slope of the $\dot{V}O_2$-work rate relationship is not necessarily constant as work rate is increased above the AT (Fig. 3.5C). If the rapidity of the work rate increase is large relative to the subject's degree of fitness, then a relatively large proportion of energy generated is from anaerobic sources and the slope would be expected to become more shallow (Fig. 3.6, 60 W/min). In contrast, when the rate of increase in work rate is small, at least four factors can cause an augmented O_2 uptake and thereby cause the $\dot{V}O_2$-work rate slope to be steeper above the AT: (1) subjects often use additional muscle groups when performing heavy exercise, e.g., pulling on cycle handlebars during leg cycling to brace one's trunk on the ergometer as the pedals get harder to turn; this leads to additional and unmeas-

ured arm work; (2) breathing work is increased nonlinearly as high levels of ventilation are reached, causing increased O_2 consumption by the breathing muscles; (3) significant lactate conversion to glycogen (Cori cycle) by tissues actively involved in gluconeogenesis (liver) requires additional oxygen; and (4) anaerobic work is less efficient than aerobic work.

In view of the foregoing considerations, the finding of a deviation in the $\dot{V}O_2$-work rate slope above the AT, such as illustrated in Figure 3.6, is understandable. If the rate of the work rate increase were relatively small for a fit subject, then the anaerobic contribution to energy generation (as assessed by the rate of lactate increase) at a given $\dot{V}O_2$ would be relatively small. Consequently, the four factors noted previously would contribute to a more rapid increase in $\dot{V}O_2$ relative to work rate (26, 27) than that observed below the AT. In contrast, rapid work rate increases result in a sizable fraction of anaerobic work above the AT (as assessed by a high rate of lactate increase), and $\dot{V}O_2$ would rise more slowly relative to the work rate increase (28). Thus, in the same subject, the $\dot{V}O_2$-work rate relationship above the AT can be more steep (slow work rate increase) or less steep (rapid work rate increase), as compared to that observed below the AT (Fig. 3.6). Regardless of the rate of work rate increase, however, the maximum $\dot{V}O_2$ is not affected to an appreciable degree.

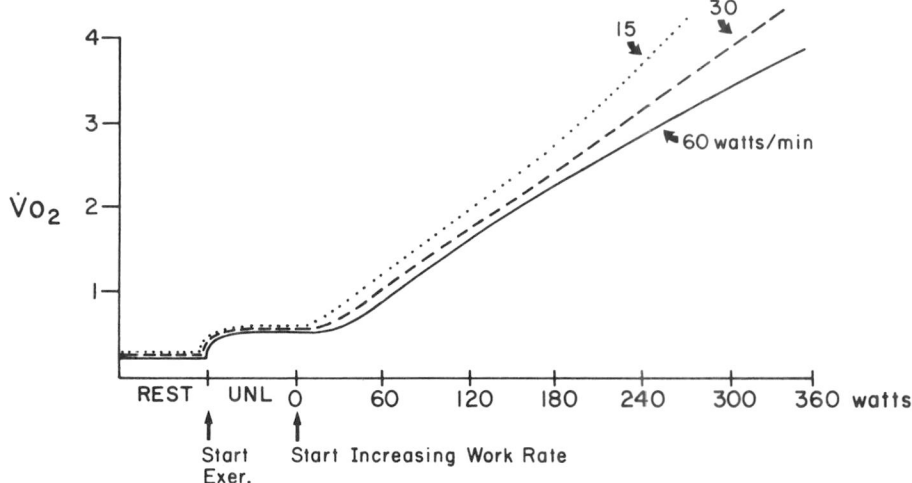

FIGURE 3.6.   Effect of work rate increment on the slope of the plot of $\dot{V}_{O_2}$ versus work rate in a normal subject. A work rate increment for which the time from the start of the incrementing period to the maximum $\dot{V}_{O_2}$ is between 8 and 12 minutes (30 watts/min) generally results in a linear $\dot{V}_{O_2}$-work rate relationship to the subject's maximum. For work rate increments that are relatively large (60 watts/min), causing the subject to fatigue in less than 8 minutes, $\dot{V}_{O_2}$ may slow its rate of rise relative to work rate before the peak $\dot{V}_{O_2}$ is reached. In contrast, for relatively small work rate increments in which it takes 15 minutes or more before the subject fatigues (15 watts/min), $\dot{V}_{O_2}$ generally increases more steeply at high work rates. The effect of the rate of increase in work rate affects the slope only above the *AT*. (Reprinted with permission from Hansen JE, Casaburi R, Cooper DM, et al. Oxygen uptake as related to work rate increment during cycle ergometer exercise. Eur J Appl Physiol 1988;57:140–145.)

In general, work rate increments of 15 to 25 W per minute in normal men and 10 to 20 W in normal women give a similar rate of rise in $\dot{V}_{O_2}$ both above and below the *AT*. A method for selecting the work rate increment for progressively increasing work rate exercise testing of normal subjects and patients is described in Chapter 5.

In disorders of the cardiovascular system, the linearity of the $\dot{V}_{O_2}$-work rate relationship is commonly abnormal regardless of the rate at which work rate is increased (see Fig. 3-5C). The $\dot{V}_{O_2}$ may increase normally as the work rate is increased at low levels, but $\dot{V}_{O_2}$ may slow its rate of increase as the maximum $\dot{V}_{O_2}$ is approached. The non-linearity or decreasing slope of the $\dot{V}_{O_2}$-work rate relationship (Fig. 3.5C) is usually accompanied by a persistently steep $\dot{V}_{CO_2}$-work rate slope, reflecting the CO_2 released from the HCO_3^- buffering of simultaneously generated lactic acid (29, 30). In these situations, the subject's $\dot{V}_{O_2}$ max is clearly reduced.

Can $\dot{V}_{O_2}$ or Mets Be Predicted from the Work Rate?

Some laboratories estimate $\dot{V}_{O_2}$ from work rate during exercise rather than directly measuring $\dot{V}_{O_2}$. This practice is potentially inaccurate and should be discouraged. A unit called a "met" was derived from the average resting $\dot{V}_{O_2}$ for a 70 kg, 40-year-old man. It is equal to 3.5 ml/min per kilogram of body weight. By assuming that a known fixed relationship exists during exercise between the ergometer work rate and the subject's $\dot{V}_{O_2}$, some laboratories report an *estimate* of $\dot{V}_{O_2}$ in ml/min. After obtaining this derived $\dot{V}_{O_2}$ and expressing it per kilogram of body weight, the $\dot{V}_{O_2}$ per kg is divided by 3.5 to obtain the number of mets performed by the subject.

Under certain conditions, however, $\dot{V}_{O_2}$ cannot be accurately predicted from the estimated work rate for the reasons summarized in Table 3.4. For instance, if the ergometer is not accurately calibrated, the $\dot{V}_{O_2}$ estimated could be in serious error. In addition, if $\dot{V}_{O_2}$ is not in a steady state, the $\dot{V}_{O_2}$ is commonly less than that extrapolated from the work rate. Moreover, the $\dot{V}_{O_2}$ often does not increase linearly with increasing work rate in patients with

TABLE 3.4.   **Conditions in Which Work Rate Fails to Predict $\dot{V}_{O_2}$**

Faulty ergometer calibration
Steady state not reached
Obesity
Valvular heart disease
Coronary artery disease
Cardiomyopathy
Peripheral arterial disease
Pulmonary vascular disease

cardiovascular diseases (31) (see Fig. 3-5C and the cardiovascular cases in Chap. 9). Thus, using work rate to calculate $\dot{V}O_2$ or mets will usually lead to overestimates in these patients.

In addition, work rate fails to predict $\dot{V}O_2$ if body weight is not taken into account. This factor is often ignored, or incorrect estimates of the effect of body weight are used. The $\dot{V}O_2$ to perform a given amount of external work will be higher in an obese as compared to lean subject. This is because of the need to expend additional energy to move a large body when effecting external work. For cycle ergometer work, we have found that the O_2 cost of cycling an unloaded ergometer at 60 rpm is an additional 5.8 ml/min for each kg body weight (18, 19).

Analysis of the $\dot{V}O_2$-work rate relationship is of value only if the ergometer and the measurement system are accurately calibrated. Unfortunately, many cycle ergometers are not accurate, particularly over the low work rate range. We calibrate our cycle ergometer at regular intervals and have added a motor to the flywheel to obviate the initial work of overcoming the flywheel inertia (see Appendix). The accuracy and consistency of gas exchange measurements are also checked on a regular basis (see Appendix).

$\dot{V}O_2$ Difference

This term refers to the difference between the expected and measured $\dot{V}O_2$ at the subject's maximum work rate (see Fig. 3.5). The $\dot{V}O_2$ difference calculation assumes that $\dot{V}O_2$ increases linearly with an expected slope with the work rate and that, at the subject's maximum work rate, there should be no difference between the expected $\dot{V}O_2$ for that work rate and the measured $\dot{V}O_2$, i.e., a $\dot{V}O_2$ difference of zero. The expected $\dot{V}O_2$ in milliliters per minute for cycle ergometry in which the work rate is increased in ramp pattern, or in 1-minute steps, is estimated from the equation:

$$\text{expected } \dot{V}O_2 = \dot{V}O_{2\,\text{unloaded}} + 10 \times (T - 0.75) \times S$$

where $\dot{V}O_{2\,\text{unloaded}}$ is $\dot{V}O_2$ measured after 3 minutes of unloaded pedaling, T is the total time in minutes of incremental work until maximum $\dot{V}O_2$ is reached, 0.75 min is the assumed time displacement between the start of the linear increase in work rate and the linear increase in $\dot{V}O_2$ (determined from studies on normal subjects), i.e., the functional time constant for $\dot{V}O_2$, and S is the slope of the work rate increment in watts per minute.

Cardiac Output and Stroke Volume

Cardiac output measurement may be useful when trying to assess whether the patient's reduced O_2 uptake is due to reduced O_2 transport or failure of the muscles to extract O_2, for whatever cause. However, cardiac output measurement, by itself, even if accurate, may not reveal whether it is adequate for the work rate performed. The major concern of exercise testing should be to determine whether the heart is capable of providing the exercise-stressed muscles with enough oxygen. To answer this important question, measurement of the AT and $\Delta\dot{V}O_2/\Delta WR$ during a progressively increasing work rate test and the measurement of $\dot{V}O_2$ and $\dot{V}CO_2$ kinetics during a constant work rate may be more useful. Furthermore, all of these measurements are made noninvasively and, therefore, can be repeated easily.

Thermodilution

If a catheter of the Swan-Ganz type is introduced into the pulmonary artery, the cardiac output and stroke volume can be determined by the direct Fick method. If a thermistor-tip catheter is used, a thermodilution curve can be obtained from the thermistor in the pulmonary artery, following the injection of iced saline into the lumen of the catheter opening into the right atrium. From this curve, and the volume of iced saline injected, blood flow through the right atrium can be calculated (36). Right heart catheterization is an invasive procedure, however.

Indirect Fick Using $\dot{V}CO_2$ and Estimated $C\bar{v}CO_2$

Estimates of cardiac output (C.O.) during exercise are sometimes made with the indirect Fick method (C.O. = $\dot{V}CO_2/C(a - \bar{v})CO_2$) from a measurement of $\dot{V}CO_2$ and an estimate of arterial PCO_2 ($PaCO_2$) from end-tidal PCO_2 ($PETCO_2$) and mixed venous PCO_2 by the CO_2 rebreathing method (32) (see Appendix A for definitions of symbols and Appendix D for description of rebreathing method). This approach has many potential errors. First, estimation of $PaCO_2$ from $PETCO_2$ measurements, as commonly done, is unreliable especially in patients (33, 34). $PETCO_2$ is less than $PaCO_2$ in patients with lung disease, heart failure and pulmonary vascular disease and greater than $PaCO_2$ in normal subjects (See Chapter 4). Second, the assumption is made that mixed venous CO_2 content can be determined accu-

TABLE 3.5. Arteriovenous O_2 Difference $C(a - \bar{v})CO_2)$ and Extraction Ratio (ER) ± Standard Deviation at Rest, *AT* and Peak $\dot{V}O_2$

	$\dot{V}O_2$ (L/min)	$C(a - \bar{v})CO_2$ (ml/dl)	ER[‡]
		Normal Men[*]	
Rest		6.14 ± 1.7	0.30 ± 0.09
AT	1.84 ± 0.36	11.3 ± 0.87	0.53 ± 0.04
Peak $\dot{V}O_2$	3.77 ± 0.61	16.2 ± 1.2	0.74 ± 0.07
		Chronic Heart Failure[†]	
Rest	0.28 ± 0.07	7.8 ± 2.6	0.43 ± 0.11
AT	0.83 ± 0.25	13.0 ± 2.4	0.68 ± 0.09
Peak $\dot{V}O_2$	1.26 ± 0.39	15.0 ± 2.7	0.77 ± 0.07

[*] Data from Stringer W, Hansen J, Wasserman K. Cardiac output estimated non-invasively from oxygen uptake ($\dot{V}O_2$) during exercise. J Appl Physiol 1997;82: 908–912.
[†] Data from Agostoni PG, Wasserman K, Perego G, et al. Stroke volume (SV) measured, non-invasively at anaerobic threshold (*AT*) in heart failure (HF). Am J Resp Crit Care Med 1997;155: A171.
[‡] ER = extraction ratio = fractional difference between CaO_2 and $C\bar{v}O_2$.

rately from mixed venous PCO_2, using a standard CO_2 dissociation curve in which blood CO_2 content is plotted as a function of blood PCO_2. If the work is above the *AT*, however, the CO_2 content will be decreased for the same mixed venous PCO_2 as below the *AT* (35) because of a shift downward in the subject's CO_2 dissociation curve. This shift downward results from the decrease in CO_2 content for a given PCO_2 of blood when HCO_3^- buffers lactic acid. Third, the assumption is made that the CO_2 dissociation curve is linear, although in actuality it gets less steep the higher the PCO_2.

Measuring $\dot{V}O_2$ and Estimating $C(a - \bar{v})O_2$

Stringer et al. (37) pointed out that cardiac output can be calculated during exercise by the direct Fick principle (C.O. = $\dot{V}O_2/C(a - \bar{v})O_2$), with reliability as good as generally reported by other methods, from the $\dot{V}O_2$ measurement alone if the measurement is made at a work rate at which $C(a - \bar{v})O_2$ can be estimated with relative accuracy. They showed that in normal humans, as has been reported in heart failure (38), $C(a - \bar{v})O_2$ increases relatively linearly to peak $\dot{V}O_2$, achieving a value of approximately 15 ml/dl. Agostoni et al. (39) found that patients with chronic heart failure, on average, had slightly higher values for $C(a - \bar{v})O_2$ at the *AT*, the worse the exercise tolerance. However, they had similar values to normal at peak $\dot{V}O_2$ (Table 3.5). From the shape of the $\dot{V}O_2$ curves shown in Figure 3.7, variability in the $C(a - \bar{v})O_2$ has less influence on the cardiac output determination, in absolute terms, as $C(a - \bar{v})O_2$ increases.

Normal subjects had a standard deviation for $C(a - \bar{v})O_2$ of 7.6% and 7.4% and for extraction ratio of 7.5% and 9.4% at the *AT* and peak $\dot{V}O_2$, respectively (Table 3.5) (37). Patients with heart failure had a standard deviation for $C(a - \bar{v})O_2$ of 18% and 18% and an extraction ratio of 13% and 9% at *AT* and peak $\dot{V}O_2$, respectively (Table 3.5) (39). The higher standard deviation for $C(a - \bar{v})O_2$ at the *AT* for the patients, as compared with normal subjects, is because of the tendency for these values to increase, the worse the heart failure (Fig. 3.7).

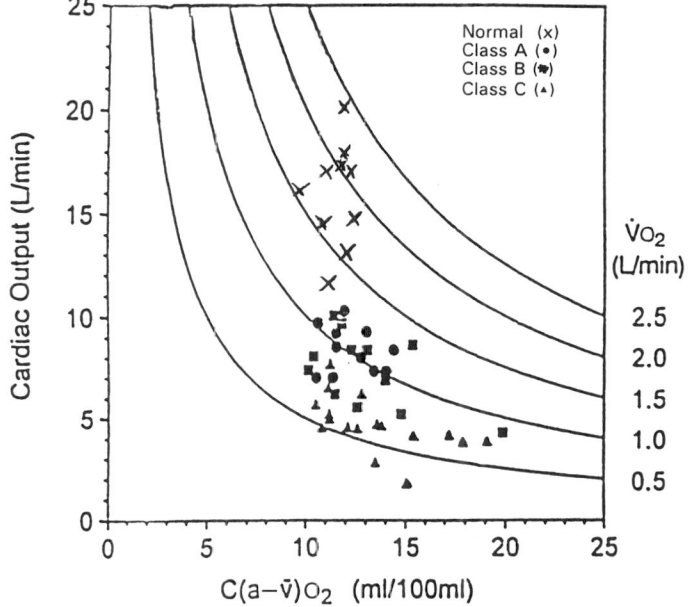

FIGURE 3.7. Cardiac output, calculated by the Direct Fick method) is plotted as a function of arterial venous O_2 difference ($C(a - \bar{v})O_2$) at the *AT* for normal and heart failure subjects in physiological class A (peak $\dot{V}O_2 > 20$ ml/min/kg), B (peak $\dot{V}O_2 = 15$–20 ml/min/kg), and C (peak $\dot{V}O_2 = 10$–15 ml/min/kg). Superimposed are $\dot{V}O_2$ isopleths. See text for further discussion of the application of these plots in estimating cardiac output. (Data taken from references 37 and 39.)

Fick cardiac outputs are plotted as a function of $C(a - \bar{v})O_2$ at the *AT* in normal subjects and patients with stable chronic heart failure, taken from the work of Stringer et al. (37) and Agostoni et al. (39), respectively. For the heart failure subjects, the higher $C(a - \bar{v})O_2$ values in the distribution are dominated by the more exercise limited patients. From Figure 3.7, it is evident that the variability in $C(a - \bar{v})O_2$ has a relatively small effect, in absolute values, on estimating exercise cardiac output at the *AT*, particularly in patients with low *AT* values. Whether using a value for $C(a - \bar{v})O_2$ at *AT* or peak $\dot{V}O_2$ for a given population, the stroke volumes derived from the respective cardiac outputs and heart rates should be similar. Thus, provided the subject is not anemic, C.O. and stroke volume can be estimated, noninvasively from the measurement of $\dot{V}O_2$ at the *AT* and peak $\dot{V}O_2$ in those subjects who are exercise limited by their cardiovascular system (see Oxygen Pulse and Stroke Volume later in this chapter).

Anaerobic (Lactate, Lactic Acidosis) Threshold (*AT, LT, LAT*)

The *AT* is defined as the level of exercise $\dot{V}O_2$ above which aerobic energy production is supplemented by anaerobic mechanisms and is reflected by an increase in lactate and lactate/pyruvate ratio in muscle and arterial blood (see Figs. 2.11, 2.12). The biochemical and physiologic basis of the *AT* hypothesis and its relationship to lactate increase and the development of lactic acidosis are described in Chapter 2. The underlying mechanism for its measurement depends on the onset of anaerobic glycolysis leading to a net increase in lactic acid production (see pathway B of Fig. 2.1). At work rates below the *AT*, the muscle (40, 41) and blood (42) lactate/pyruvate ratio is the same as at rest and no metabolic acidosis develops. Above the *AT*, a lactic acidosis develops. Thus, the threshold can be defined physiologically as the $\dot{V}O_2$ above which the critical capillary PO_2 has been reached and production of ATP through anaerobic glycolysis supplements the aerobic ATP production. It can also be defined in terms of changing redox state within the cell as the $\dot{V}O_2$ at which lactate and lactate/pyruvate ratio increase (*LT*); or in terms of acid base balance change as the $\dot{V}O_2$ at which lactic acidosis develops (*LAT*). Like the $\dot{V}O_2$max, the threshold measurement is influenced by the size of the muscle groups involved in the activity.

Major Physiological Effects

In Chapter 2, the significance of the *AT* and the major changes that take place during the performance of exercise above as compared to below the *AT* were discussed. These include the development of metabolic acidosis with a sustained increase in blood lactate and lactate/pyruvate ratio. Plasma bicarbonate decreases reciprocally to the lactate increase at a $\dot{V}O_2$ which depends on the level of fitness and wellness for aerobic work as shown in Figure 3.8.

The *AT* also demarcates the exercise $\dot{V}O_2$ above which $\dot{V}O_2$ kinetics slow and above which exercise can no longer be performed in a true steady state. Ventilatory drive is stimulated by the metabolic acidosis resulting from lactate accumulation. Thus $\dot{V}E$ increases, primarily by increasing breathing frequency, as work rates above the *AT* are sustained (see Fig. 2.36). The rate of increase depends on the magnitude of the lactic acidosis and the work rate. Also of great importance is that endurance time in

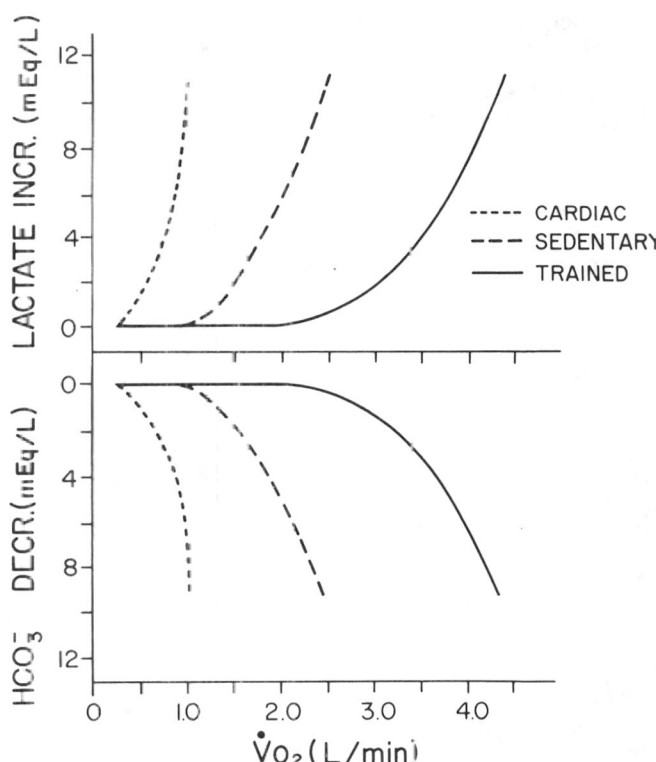

FIGURE 3.8.   Lactate increase and bicarbonate decrease during incremental exercise in trained and sedentary normal subjects and in patients with primary cardiac disease of class II to III severity as defined by the New York Heart Association Classification. (Modified from Wasserman K, Whipp BJ. Exercise physiology in health and disease (State of the art). Am Rev Respir Dis 1975;112:219–249.)

the performance of a specific work task is reduced above the *AT* in proportion to the increase in lactate evoked by the exercise (Fig. 2.10). The higher the lactate concentration, the shorter the endurance time and the steeper the rate of increase of $\dot{V}O_2$ during Phase III (43).

Methods of Measurement

H^+ is produced, stoichiometrically, when lactate is produced in the cell. At the pH of cell water, virtually all of the increase in H^+ production must be buffered. The H^+ produced with the first 0.5 mmol/L increase in lactate appears to be buffered by non-HCO_3^- buffering mechanisms (30, 45, 46). Above that, HCO_3^- buffers the newly produced H^+ stoichiometrically (30, 45, 47). Thus, an obligatory increase occurs in CO_2 production above that produced by aerobic metabolism at work rates above the threshold. It is relatively easy to detect the development of cellular lactic acidosis by measuring the rate of increase in $\dot{V}CO_2$ relative to that of $\dot{V}O_2$ during a progressively increasing exercise test. Beaver et al. (29) used a statistical regression method. Sue et al. (48) simplified the method, observing that the $\dot{V}CO_2$ versus $\dot{V}O_2$ relationship below the threshold had a slope consistently at or slightly less than 1.0, and

that the slope changed to a value greater than 1.0 above the threshold.

A relatively short, progressive work rate test can rapidly determine the $\dot{V}O_2$ at which lactic acidosis develops when gas exchange is measured breath-by-breath, or as the average of several breaths. The reason that gas exchange is so effective in detecting the development of cellular metabolic acidosis is that the time delay is only a few seconds between the HCO_3^- buffering of lactic acid in the cell and the increase in CO_2 derived from the buffering reaction in the respired air. A flow diagram describing the sequence of gas exchange and ventilation changes in response to lactic acidosis for a progressively increasing work rate exercise test is shown in Figure 3.9. The changes in gas exchange which take place above the *AT* are illustrated in Figure 3.10.

V-Slope Method (Fig. 3.9, Mechanism I). When the net increase in lactate accumulation produces an acidosis, $\dot{V}CO_2$ accelerates relative to $\dot{V}O_2$. When these variables are plotted against each other, the relationship is composed of two apparently linear components, the lower of which (S_1) has a slope of slightly less than 1.0, whereas the upper component (S_2) has a slope steeper than 1.0 (see Fig. 2.27). The intercept of these two slopes is the *AT* as measured by gas exchange (Fig. 3.10). The buffering of lactic

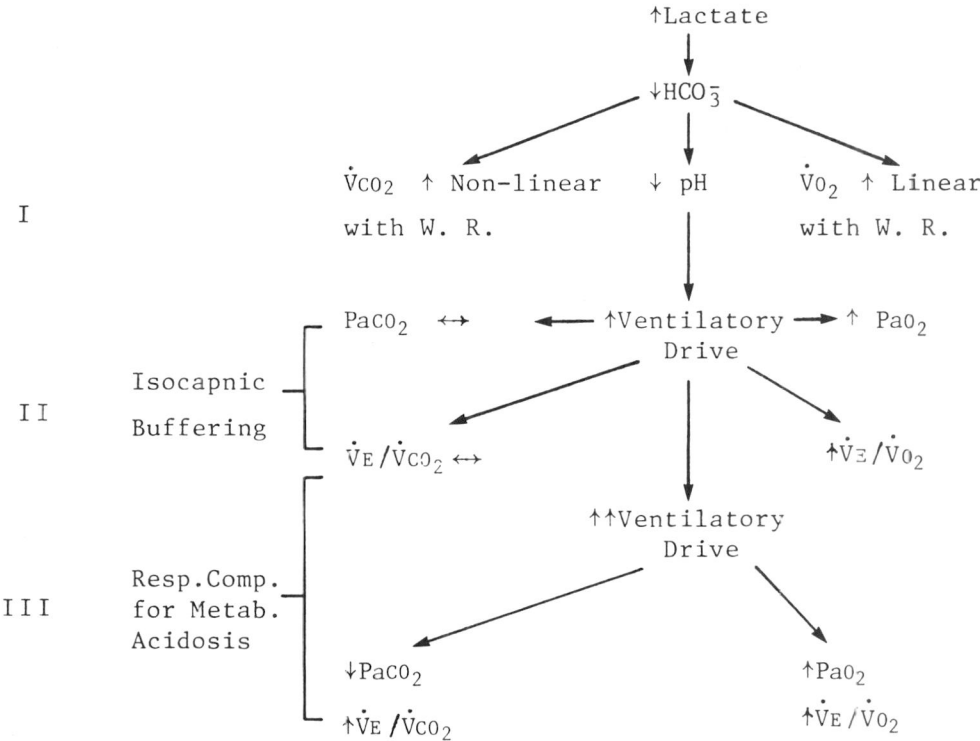

FIGURE 3.9. Diagram of effects on gas exchange of increased lactate accumulation during a progressive incremental exercise test. Small arrows directed upward indicate increases, small arrows directed downward indicate decreases, and horizontal arrows indicate no change. Mechanism I describes gas exchange that results solely from buffering of newly formed lactic acid (lower left panel of Figure 3.10). Mechanism II describes changes in alveolar and end-tidal PCO_2 and PO_2 and ventilatory equivalents for O_2 and CO_2 that result from increased ventilatory drive consequent to CO_2 generated by buffering reaction (right upper and lower panels of Figure 3.10). Mechanism III describes changes caused by further increase in ventilatory drive consequent to respiratory compensation for metabolic acidosis (changes to the right of *AT* lines in right upper and lower panels of Figure 3.10).

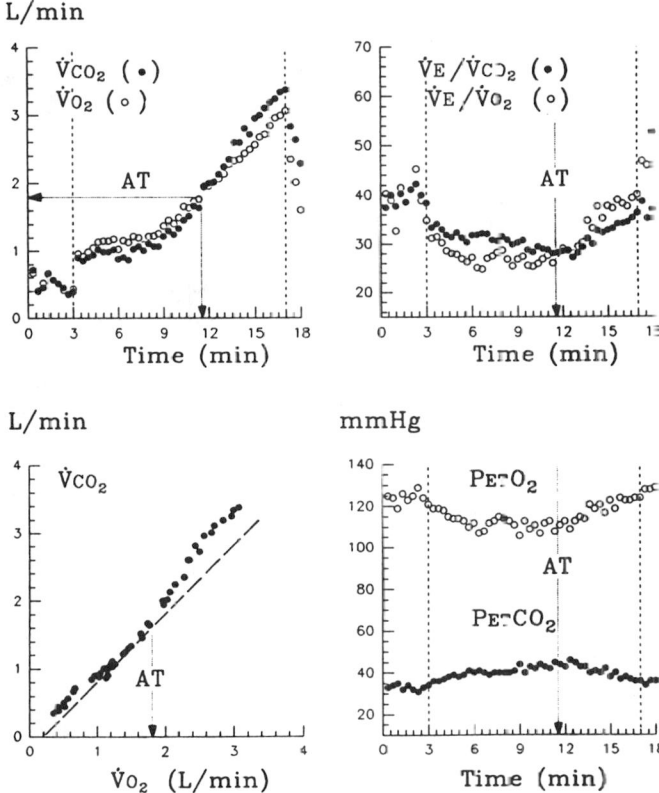

FIGURE 3.10.   Gas exchange for a normal subject during a progressively increasing work rate exercise test to illustrate the gas exchange changes that take place at the *AT*. In each panel, the far-left vertical dashed line indicates the start of work rate increase after a 3-minute period of unloaded cycling. The work rate was increased 25 watts/min. The right vertical dashed line indicates the end of exercise. The V-slope plot of the data shown in the upper left panel is shown in the lower left panel. The diagonal line is at 45° or a slope of 1. The *AT* is where the $\dot{V}_{CO_2}$ starts to increase faster than $\dot{V}_{O_2}$ so the slope of the plot becomes steeper than 1. This is shown as the vertical dashed line marked *AT*. The *AT* can also be located where the $\dot{V}_E/\dot{V}_{O_2}$ curve (right upper panel) inflects upward (vertical dashed line labeled *AT*). The nadir of the $\dot{V}_E/\dot{V}_{CO_2}$ curve occurs at a higher work rate and reflects the start of ventilatory compensation for the metabolic acidosis. Because of the hyperventilation with respect to O_2, $P_{ET}O_2$ increases at the *AT* (right lower panel) whereas $P_{ET}CO_2$ does not start to decrease systematically until approximately 2 minutes later, coinciding with the increased ventilatory drive which serves to partially compensate for the decrease in arterial pH which takes place above the *AT*.

acid causes an obligatory increase in $\dot{V}_{CO_2}$ relative to $\dot{V}_{O_2}$ from the CO_2 produced when HCO_3^- buffers lactic acid. This technique is referred to as the V-slope method because it relates the increase in volume of CO_2 output to volume of O_2 uptake. As shown in Figure 2.27, S_1 and S_2 can be determined from statistically derived regression slopes of $\dot{V}_{CO_2}$ versus $\dot{V}_{O_2}$ in the respective regions of interest. The break-point or intercept of the two slopes can be selected by a computer program that defines the

$\dot{V}_{O_2}$ above which $\dot{V}_{CO_2}$ increases faster than $\dot{V}_{O_2}$, without hyperventilation. The values obtained by this method agree closely with the lactate and, more precisely the $[HCO_3^-]$ threshold (29, 48). If a patient develops a lactic acidosis with only slight activity, only S_2 may be evident; in this case, the *LAT*, and therefore the *AT*, will be less than the lowest exercise $\dot{V}_{O_2}$.

Sue et al. (48) pointed out that, because S_1 must have a slope value of 1.0 or less and S_2 a slope value of greater than 1.0, the break-point representing the *AT* can be determined by placing a 45° right triangle on the $\dot{V}_{CO_2}$ versus $\dot{V}_{O_2}$ plot (plotted on equal scales). The $\dot{V}_{O_2}$ at which the data points start to increase at an angle greater than 45° is the *AT*. Whereas this method uses simultaneous measurements of $\dot{V}_{CO_2}$ and $\dot{V}_{O_2}$, it is independent of the subject's ventilatory response and insensitive to irregularities in breathing. It is erroneously called the "ventilatory threshold" by many investigators. This is clearly wrong. Because $\dot{V}_E$ is an equal factor on both the x and y axes, the breakpoint can not be due to ventilation. The V-slope plot is actually a plot of moles of CO_2 output to O_2 uptake. It is also the same as a plot of C.O. × C(a − v̄)CO_2 versus C.O. × C(a − v̄)O_2. Therefore the threshold is due to an increase in C(a − v̄)CO_2 relative to C(a − v̄)O_2 as a result of the addition of CO_2 to the venous blood as shown in Figures 2.20 and 2.28.

Ventilatory Equivalent Method (Fig. 3.9, Mechanism II). As the work rate is increased in a progressive exercise test (ramp or 1-minute steps), the linear pattern of increase in $\dot{V}_{CO_2}$ and $\dot{V}_E$ seen at low work rates (see Fig. 2.25) changes to a curvilinear pattern at high work rates while $\dot{V}_{O_2}$ continues to increase relatively linearly. $\dot{V}_E$ and $\dot{V}_{CO_2}$ initially accelerate in a proportional manner above the *AT*. Therefore, $\dot{V}_E/\dot{V}_{O_2}$ and $P_{ET}O_2$ increase, whereas $\dot{V}_E/\dot{V}_{CO_2}$ and $P_{ET}CO_2$ remain constant for a brief period (isocapnic buffering; see Figs. 2.25, 3.10). Thus, hyperventilation occurs with respect to O_2 but not CO_2 as the *AT* is exceeded. This isocapnic buffering period normally lasts about 2 minutes. It is referred to as the isocapnic buffering period because of the lack of hyperventilation with respect to CO_2 despite the development of metabolic acidosis (49). The increase in $\dot{V}_E/\dot{V}_{O_2}$ without an increase in $\dot{V}_E/\dot{V}_{CO_2}$ is typical of HCO_3^- buffering metabolic acid rather than other factors causing ventilation to increase out of proportion to $\dot{V}_{O_2}$, e.g., hypoxemia, pain, or psychogenic hyperventilation. When $\dot{V}_E/\dot{V}_{O_2}$ is observed to increase without a simultaneous increase in $\dot{V}_E/\dot{V}_{CO_2}$ during a progressively increasing work rate test, it is a specific gas exchange demonstration that the *AT* has been surpassed.

One reason for increasing work rate relatively rapidly during the progressively increasing work rate test is to take advantage of the finding that the CO_2 contribution from buffering is observed only during the buffering process (the period of decreasing bicarbonate) and not after the lactate has been buffered. Thus CO_2 generated from buffering is evident in the expired gas only when lactate and HCO_3^- are changing. Increasing the work rate at a relatively fast rate will result in a higher rate of lactate accumulation and steeper S_2 above the *AT*, than when the rate of increase in work rate is relatively slow (54).

As the work rate is increased further above the *AT*, the carotid bodies respond to the decreasing pH, and ventilatory stimulation is intensified (see Fig. 3.9, mechanism III and Figs. 2.25, 3.10). This causes Pa_{CO_2} to decrease, preventing pH from falling as much as would be predicted by the addition of lactic acid to a closed system. This ventilatory compensation for the lactic acidosis is reflected in an increase in $\dot{V}_E/\dot{V}_{CO_2}$ and a decrease in $P_{ET_{CO_2}}$, as well as by further increases in $\dot{V}_E/\dot{V}_{O_2}$ and $P_{ET_{O_2}}$ (see Figs. 2.25, 3.8). When ventilatory compensation for metabolic acidosis starts, the $\dot{V}_{O_2}$ is well above the *AT* or *LAT*. This $\dot{V}_{O_2}$ is referred to as the respiratory compensation (RC) point.

The *AT* is measured as a metabolic stress, i.e., in units of O_2 uptake, not work rate. In contrast to the RC point, it is unaffected by the rate at which the work rate is incremented (50, 51) or by metabolic substrate (52–54).

Improving Estimation of the Anaerobic Threshold

Occasionally, the *AT* cannot be reliably detected by the ventilatory equivalent method (see Fig. 3.9, mechanism II) because of atypical records caused by irregular breathing, an inappropriate rate of increase in work rate, suboptimal plotting scales, or a poor ventilatory response by the patient to the metabolic acidosis. To obviate these problems, one can measure blood lactate or standard bicarbonate directly. Beaver et al. (55) found that the *LT* during exercise can be most reliably selected by plotting log blood lactate against log $\dot{V}_{O_2}$. Similarly, the start of the [HCO_3^-] fall, indicating the start of developing lactic acidosis (*LAT*), can be most reliably detected from a plot of log standard [HCO_3^-] against log $\dot{V}_{O_2}$ (45). A slight difference exists in the $\dot{V}_{O_2}$ for these

thresholds. *LT* precedes *LAT*, because of non-HCO_3^- buffering of the initial lactate increase (30, 45). Although we distinguish between *LT* and *LAT* for scientific correctness, the difference is not of clinical significance.

When the break-point between S_1 and S_2 is not clear using the V-slope method, it is likely that the CO_2 released from HCO_3^- buffering of lactic acid was small because work rate was increased too slowly during the progressively increasing work rate test (56), the patient did not produce a substantial amount of lactic acid (e.g., some patients with COPD) or the patient did not produce lactic acid (e.g., because of muscle phosphorylase deficiency, McArdle's syndrome) (57). In the former instance, the test should be repeated with a faster rate of increase in work rate. If the break-point ($\dot{V}_{CO_2}$ increasing faster than $\dot{V}_{O_2}$) is still not observed, it can be concluded that the patient is unable to raise blood lactate levels substantially.

Heart Rate-Oxygen Uptake Relationship and Heart Rate Reserve

Both cardiac output and heart rate normally increase linearly with $\dot{V}_{O_2}$ during increasing work rate exercise (58) (Fig. 3.11). In many types of heart disease, the heart rate increase is relatively steep for the increase in $\dot{V}_{O_2}$ because the stroke volume is low. In addition, $\dot{V}_{O_2}$ commonly slows its rate of increase with work rate when the myocardium becomes ischemic in patients with coronary artery disease. Because heart rate typically continues to increase in these patients, the rate of increase in heart rate relative to $\dot{V}_{O_2}$ becomes steeper, deviating from the linearity established at lower work rates (Fig. 3.11). This implies that cardiac output increase is not keeping pace with the work rate increase because stroke volume is decreasing. Although this curvilinear increase in the heart rate-$\dot{V}_{O_2}$ relationship is not uniformly seen in patients with heart disease, it is a useful diagnostic observation and suggests a significant worsening in left ventricular function with increasing work rate (59).

Pulmonary vascular disease is also associated with a steep heart rate response because venous return to the left side of the heart and therefore left ventricular output are low in this disorder. Patients with airflow obstruction (Fig. 3.11) commonly have a moderately elevated heart rate response at a given $\dot{V}_{O_2}$ resulting from a reduced stroke volume. Heart rate increases linearly with work rate in this disorder, however. The maximum heart rate in the pa-

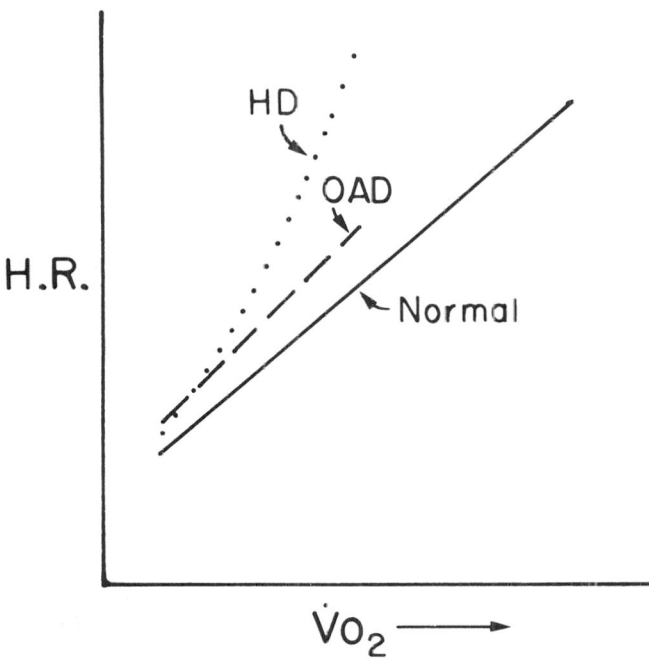

FIGURE 3.11.   Characteristic changes in heart rate (H.R.) relative to $\dot{V}O_2$ for normal subjects, for patients with chronic obstructive airway disease (OAD), and for those with heart disease (HD). The steeper heart rate-$\dot{V}O_2$ relationship for the patient with obstructive airway disease may reflect relative unfitness or reduced stroke volume secondary to disturbed lung mechanics or pulmonary circulation. In contrast, the relatively low maximum heart rate reflects respiratory limitation to the maximum level of exercise. The steepening heart rate-$\dot{V}O_2$ relationship seen in some patients with heart disease reflects the failure of $\dot{V}O_2$ to increase in response to the increasing work rate, as illustrated in Figure 3.5C.

tient with ventilatory limitation is usually below the predicted value for the normal subject because the patient reaches the point of ventilatory limitation before the cardiovascular system is maximally stressed (60).

The estimated *heart rate reserve* is an expression of the potential further heart rate increase at the end of a maximal effort exercise test. We define this simply as the difference between the age-determined predicted maximal heart rate and the actual maximum exercise heart rate (see the section on maximal heart rate and heart rate reserve in Chapter 6).

Although the predicted maximal heart rate has considerable variation, as determined from population studies, the heart rate reserve is still a useful concept for differential diagnosis. Table 3.6 lists disorders in which the heart rate reserve may be increased. Normally, the heart rate reserve is relatively small (less than 15 beats/min). It is also usually normal in patients with silent myocardial ischemia and valvular heart disease and in patients with disorders of the pulmonary circulation. In contrast,

patients with peripheral arterial disease and patients with coronary artery disease with angina may discontinue exercise because of pain before the normal maximal heart rate is reached. Patients with disorders of the conducting system of the heart, or sinoatrial node disease such as seen with certain cardiomyopathies, may also have a low maximum heart rate. Patients who take β-adrenergic blocking drugs or patients who are limited in exercise because of primary lung disease usually have a large heart rate reserve. Finally, those patients who make a poor effort have an increased heart rate reserve because they fail to maximally stress their cardiovascular system at the time they stop exercising.

Oxygen Pulse ($\dot{V}O_2/HR$) and Stroke Volume

The O_2 pulse is calculated by dividing the $\dot{V}O_2$ by the simultaneously measured heart rate. It depends on the volume of O_2 extracted by the peripheral tissues and is the volume of O_2 taken up by the pulmonary blood during the period of a heart beat. This measurement is useful because it equals the product of stroke volume and the arterial-mixed venous O_2 difference ($C(a - \bar{v})O_2$). The initial upward deflection of the curve depends primarily on the size of the stroke volume. As the work rate is increased, the O_2 pulse increases (Fig. 3.12), primarily because of an increasing $C(a - \bar{v})O_2$. If the stroke volume is reduced, the $C(a - \bar{v})O_2$ and, therefore, the O_2 pulse reach maximal values at a relatively low work rate. In this situation, the O_2 pulse has a low asymptote (60) (see the heart disease (HD) curve in Fig. 3.12). The maximum O_2 pulse is also low in anemia, high levels of carboxyhemoglobin, or severe arterial hypoxemia, all because of reduced arterial O_2 content and therefore a reduced $C(a - \bar{v})O_2$ at maximal exercise. When arterial O_2 content and therefore $C(a - \bar{v})O_2$ at maximal exercise can be assumed to be normal, (approximately 15 ml/dl) stroke volume can be estimated from the

TABLE 3.6.   Disorders Associated with Increased Heart Rate Reserve

Claudication limiting exercise
Angina limiting exercise
"Sick sinus" syndrome
β-adrenergic blockade
Lung disease
Poor effort
Skeletal muscle weakness or atrophy

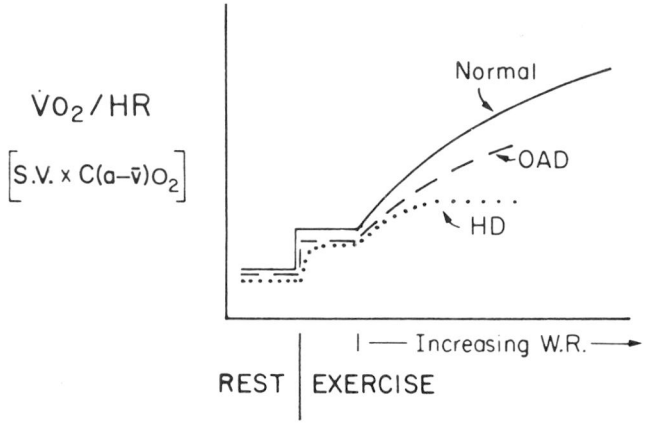

FIGURE 3.12.   Characteristic changes in $\dot{V}O_2$/heart rate (HR) (O_2 pulse) as related to increase in work rate (W.R.). The O_2 pulse is equal to stroke volume X $C(a - \bar{v})O_2$. Thus, patients with low stroke volumes (e.g., heart disease [HD]) will tend to have low O_2 pulse values at maximal exercise. In contrast, patients with obstructive airway disease (OAD) have a pattern similar to that in normal subjects, although the values are lower at each work rate, reflecting the relatively low stroke volume in these patients.

O_2 pulse by the following equation:

$$SV = O_2 \, pulse/15 \times 100$$

where SV is in ml and O_2 pulse is in ml/beat.

The O_2 pulse measured breath-by-breath in the transition from rest to exercise and exercise to recovery is also informative. The immediate increase in O_2 pulse at the start of exercise depends on the size of the stroke volume increase and the increase in

$C(a - \bar{v})O_2$. It will be low in patients who can not increase their stroke volume in response to exercise. While the O_2 pulse promptly decreases in the normal subject when stopping exercise, as expected, it commonly increases temporarily in patients with heart failure. The explanation for this paradoxical response is that the afterload of the left ventricle is abruptly decreased when stopping exercise because of the immediate decrease in systemic arterial blood pressure. This allows improved ventricular ejection and increased stroke volume as exercise stops in the patient with the failing heart (61).

Arterial Blood Pressure

Arterial pressure measurements, particularly when directly measured, are helpful diagnostically as well as for patient safety. The normal responses of systolic, diastolic, and pulse pressures are described in Chapter 6 (section on Brachial Artery Blood Pressure). The systolic pressure increases to a much greater degree than the diastolic pressure and in proportion to the work rate increase. A decrease in systolic and pulse pressures with increasing work rate suggests cardiac dysfunction. The development of a pulsus alternans may also be seen in patients with cardiomyopathies. Finally, the direct arterial pressure tracing, made at a fast recorder speed, which shows either a slow rise time or an abrupt slowing in the arterial pressure rise, may provide evidence for ventricular outflow obstruction, such as seen with aortic stenosis or hypertrophic cardiomyopathy.

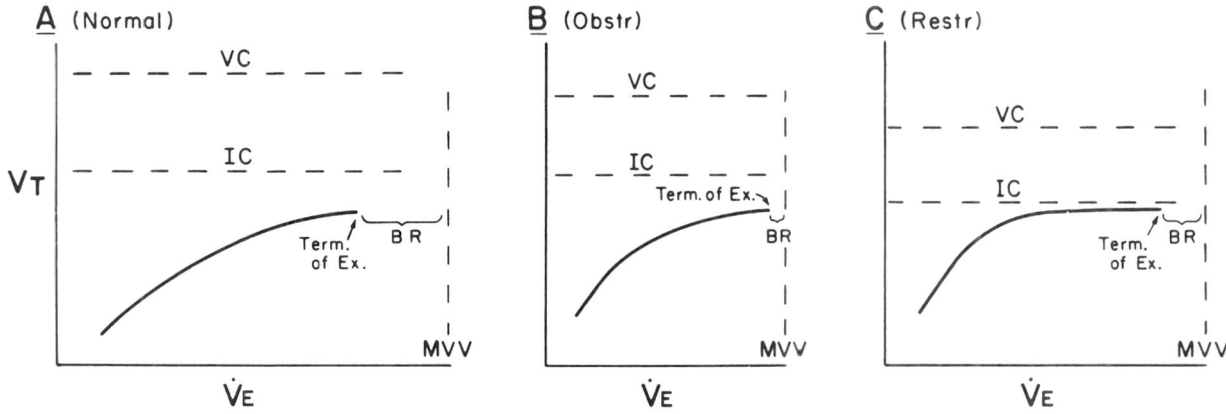

FIGURE 3.13.   Examples of tidal volume change as related to minute ventilation during incremental exercise testing in a normal subject (A), and patients with obstructive (B) and restrictive (C) lung disease. The curve ends at the subject's maximal exercise performance. The vertical dashed line indicates the subject's maximum voluntary ventilation (MVV). The horizontal dashed lines represent the vital capacity (VC) and inspiratory capacity (IC). The distance between the highest $\dot{V}E$ and MVV is the subject's breathing reserve (BR). In the case of patients with obstructive lung disease, the BR is quite small. In restrictive lung diseases, the IC is reduced and V_T closely approximates the IC.

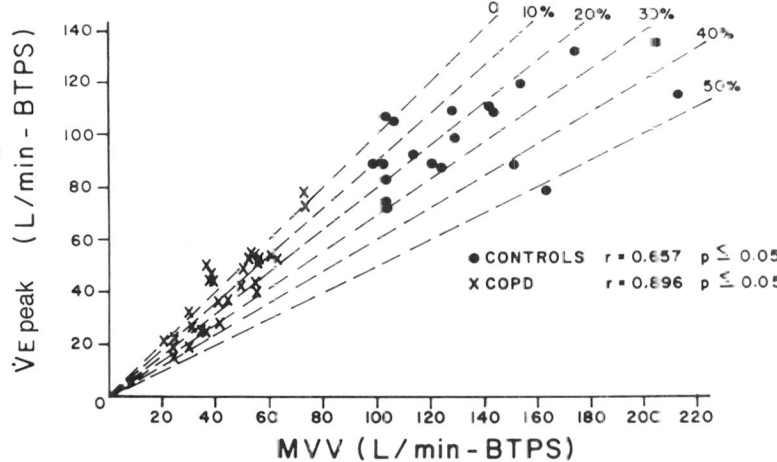

FIGURE 3.14.   Maximum exercise ventilation ($\dot{V}$Epeak) as related to MVV in patients with chronic obstructive pulmonary disease (COPD) and in normal subjects. The dashed-line isopleths indicate the percentage of breathing reserve (MVV-$\dot{V}$Epeak)/MVV X100. The "r" values are the correlation coefficients for the control and the COPD groups.

Breathing Reserve

The breathing reserve is expressed either as the difference between the maximal voluntary ventilation (MVV) and the maximum exercise ventilation in absolute terms or this difference as a fraction of the MVV (see Table 3.2; Fig. 3.13). Except in extremely fit individuals who can attain high levels of $\dot{V}$E, normal males have a breathing reserve of at least 11 L per minute or 10 to 40% of the MVV (Fig. 3.14) (62). A low breathing reserve is characteristic of patients with primary lung disease who have ventilatory limitation. The breathing reserve is also high when cardiovascular or other diseases limit exercise performance.

Expiratory Flow Pattern

The expiratory flow pattern can be useful in detecting airway obstruction during exercise. The peak expiratory flow rate is near the middle of the expiratory phase of respiration in normal subjects and has an appearance of 1/2 sine wave. In contrast, the expiratory flow pattern of the patient with obstructive airway disease has an early peak and appears trapezoidal because exhalation is sustained until the next inspiration is initiated. Thus, expiration is abruptly terminated without an end-expiratory pause (Fig. 3.15). This pattern can acutely normalize in asthmatics after inhaled bronchodilators (Fig. 3.15). Although the expiratory flow pattern gives only qualitative evidence of airflow obstruction during exercise, it is obtained simply by recording expired airflow with a flow meter. More complex approaches, such as flow-volume analysis (63, 64) and increase in functional residual capacity (65), might add further information on disturbances in lung mechanics during exercise.

Tests of Uneven $\dot{V}$A/$\dot{Q}$

Wasted Ventilation and Dead Space/Tidal Volume Ratio

Alveolar ventilation ($\dot{V}$A) is the theoretical ventilation involved in pulmonary gas exchange that would exist for a given $\dot{V}CO_2$ if the ventilation/perfusion ratios and therefore the PCO_2 of all alveolar units were the same and equal to the arterial PCO_2. This is the "ideal" alveolar ventilation. However, the actual minute ventilation includes ventilation to non-gas exchange conducting airways and alveoli which may not be ideally perfused. The difference between the actual minute ventilation and the ideal alveolar ventilation is the physiologic dead space ventilation. A valuable estimate of the degree of mismatching of ventilation to perfusion during exercise is the physiologic dead space/tidal volume ratio (VD/VT). The VD/VT is lowest when alveolar ventilation relative to perfusion is uniform.

At rest, the physiologic dead space volume is normally about one third of the breath. During exercise, it is reduced to about one fifth of the breath (Fig. 3.16) (66), the major decrement occurring at

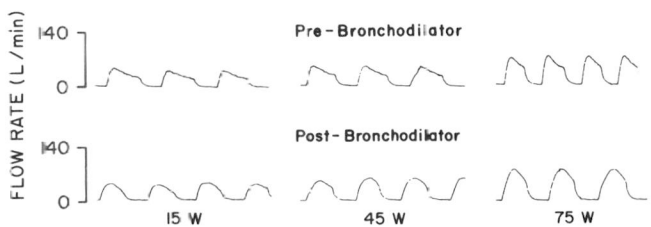

FIGURE 3.15.   Expiratory flow pattern in an asthmatic subject at increasing work rates before and after acute bronchodilator therapy. (Reprinted with permission from Brown HV, Wasserman K, Whipp BJ. Strategies of exercise testing in chronic lung disease. Bull Euro Physiopathol Resp 1977;13:409-423.)

the lowest work rates. In patients with pulmonary disorders in whom ventilation–perfusion relationships are uneven, however, or in patients with pulmonary vascular disease whose alveoli are poorly perfused or unperfused, the V_D/V_T is increased at rest and fails to decrease normally during exercise.

The V_D/V_T is a valuable measurement because it is typically abnormal in patients with primary pulmonary vascular disease or pulmonary vascular disease secondary to obstructive or restrictive lung disease and patients with heart failure. This is discussed in greater detail in the chapter on pathophysiology of disease (Chapter 4). An elevated V_D/V_T is sometimes the only gas exchange abnormality evident during exercise testing (34). Figure 3.16 illustrates the pattern of change in V_D/V_T as the work rate is increased in the normal individual and in patients with alveolar ventilation-perfusion ratio ($\dot{V}_A/\dot{Q}$) non-uniformity resulting from lung or pulmonary vascular diseases. In patients with non-uniform $\dot{V}_A/\dot{Q}$, the V_D/V_T may be only slightly elevated at rest, but it remains relatively unchanged during exercise or even increases if a right to left shunt develops during exercise (opening a foramen ovale). Thus, exercise brings out the abnormality in ventilation–perfusion relationships.

When V_D/V_T is increased, $\dot{V}_E$ is typically inordinately high for the work rate performed. $\dot{V}_E$ may also be high in conditions in which the P_{aCO_2} is relatively low (low CO_2 set-point) such as with a chronic metabolic acidosis. In this setting, V_D/V_T

will be normal if the lungs are normal, despite hyperventilation. Therefore, a high $\dot{V}_E$ at a given work rate (high $\dot{V}_E/\dot{V}_{CO_2}$) is indicative of either high V_D/V_T or hyperventilation. The two pathophysiologic mechanisms can be differentiated by simultaneously measuring gas exchange and arterial P_{CO_2}.

Figure 3.17 shows the $\dot{V}_E$ required for various metabolic rates ($\dot{V}_{CO_2}$) at designated values of P_{aCO_2} and V_D/V_T. This plot is useful for demonstrating the relationships among $\dot{V}_E$, P_{aCO_2}, $\dot{V}_{CO_2}$, and V_D/V_T. It also serves as a nomogram for determining V_D/V_T when the three other variables are known.

Arterial P_{O_2} (P_{aO_2}) and Alveolar-Arterial P_{O_2} Difference ($P(A - a)O_2$)

Normally, P_{aO_2} does not decrease during exercise, and $P(A - a)O_2$ remains under 20 mm Hg (Fig. 3.18A) (18, 66, 67). In patients with airway disease, a reduced P_{aO_2} and an increased $P(A - a)O_2$ during progressively increasing work rate exercise testing (Fig. 3.18B) typically result from underventilation of regions of lung relative to their perfusion, i.e., low alveolar ventilation to perfusion ratio lung units (66, 69). During exercise, when cardiac output increases, causing more desaturated blood to flow through low $\dot{V}_A/\dot{Q}$ areas of the lungs, arterial hypoxemia becomes more marked. Fortunately, the blood vessels in the poorly ventilated low $\dot{V}_A/\dot{Q}$ areas of the lung constrict normally under the influence of decreasing alveolar P_{O_2} (70). This diversion of blood flow to areas of relatively good ventilation is a protective mechanism in that it reduces the degree of hypoxemia and often prevents progressive hypoxemia as the work rate is increased in most patients with COPD (see Fig. 3.18B). Hypoxemia will also worsen in patients with obstructive lung disease when a potentially patent foramen ovale opens as right atrial pressure exceeds left atrial pressure, causing part of the venous return to shunt from right to left at the atrial level. A simple, sensitive test to diagnose a right to left shunt that develops during exercise uses 100% O_2 breathing. For example, when breathing 100% O_2, the P_{aO_2} is reduced approximately 100 mmHg below normal (600 mmHg) for each approximate 3–5% right to left shunt until the P_{aO_2} reaches a low value of 150 mmHg. Then the decrease in P_{aO_2} is smaller for a given shunt size.

Exercise hypoxemia may also develop in patients with pulmonary fibrosis or pulmonary vascular disease who have a reduced pulmonary capillary bed with all recruitable pulmonary blood vessels func-

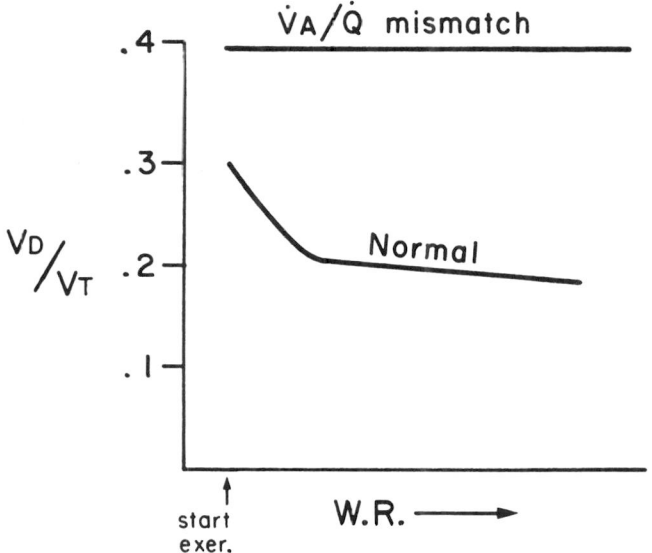

FIGURE 3.16. Example of the change in the physiologic dead space/tidal volume ratio (V_D/V_T) during rest and at increasing work rate (W.R.) for a normal subject and a patient with ventilation-perfusion ($\dot{V}_A/\dot{Q}$) mismatching.

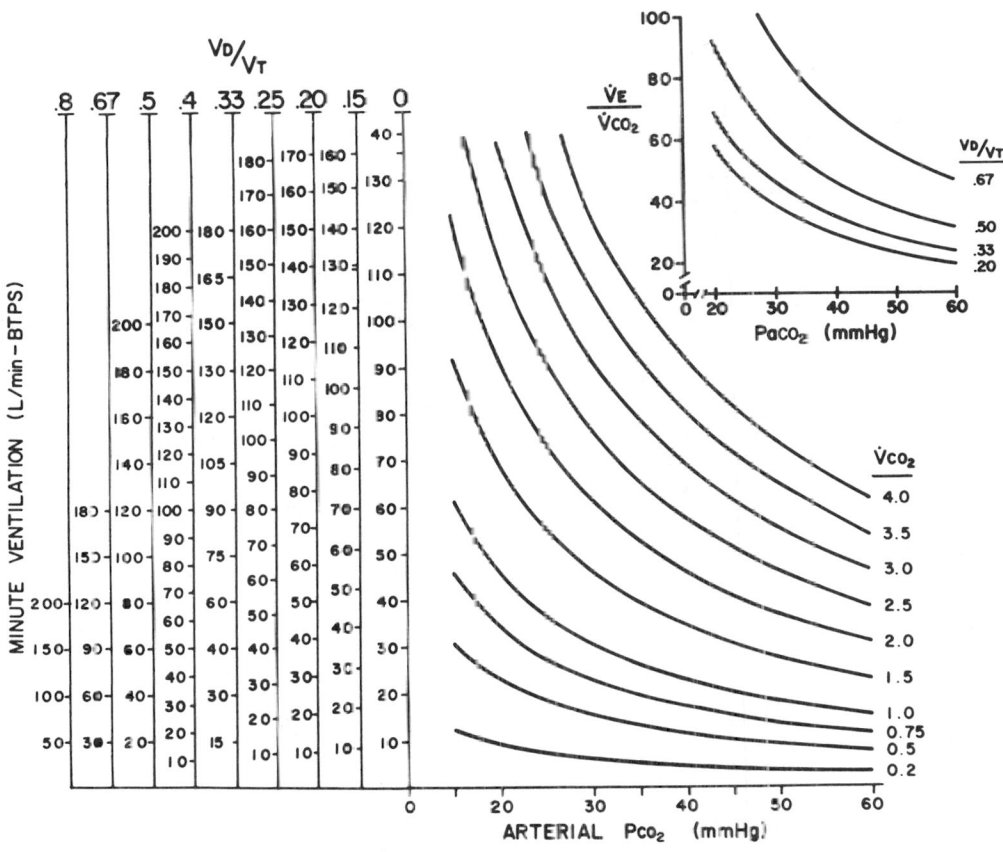

FIGURE 3.17.   Minute ventilation ($\dot{V}E$) required for various values of $\dot{V}CO_2$, as influenced by $PaCO_2$ for various physiologic dead space/tidal volume (VD/VT) fractions. If any three of the foregoing values are known, the fourth can be determined. For instance, if $\dot{V}E$, $\dot{V}CO_2$, and $PaCO_2$ are measured, then VD/VT can be determined from the ordinate that agrees with the measured $\dot{V}E$. The inset shows the effect of changing $PaCO_2$ on the $\dot{V}E/\dot{V}CO_2$ ratio during exercise with a constant VD/VT. (Reprinted with permission from Wasserman K, Whipp BJ. Exercise physiology in health and disease (State of the art). Am Rev Respir Dis 1975;112:219–249.)

tioning at rest. When cardiac output increases, no additional blood vessels are available to accommodate for the increase in pulmonary blood flow needed to supply the muscles with their increased O_2 requirement. Therefore, these disorders are char-

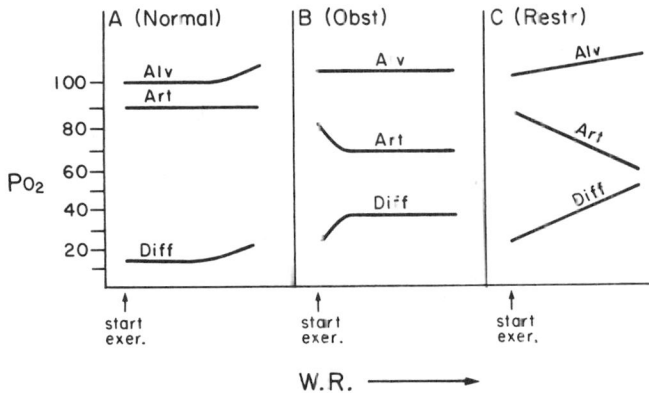

FIGURE 3.18.   Pattern of arterial and alveolar PO_2 and alveolar-arterial PO_2 differences in a normal subject (A) and in patients with obstructive (B) and restrictive (C) lung diseases as related to increasing work rate (W.R.).

acteristically associated with exercise-induced hypoxemia which becomes systematically more pronounced as the work rate is increased (see Fig. 3.18C). This pattern of decreasing PAO_2 and increasing $P(A - a)O_2$ with increasing work rate reflects a decrease in residence time of red cells in the pulmonary capillaries when the pulmonary capillary blood volume is critically reduced. Thus, pulmonary capillary PO_2 does not have enough time to equilibrate with the alveolar PO_2; the disequilibrium becomes more marked as pulmonary blood flow increases.

PaO_2 also usually decreases as the work rate is increased in conditions in which the alveoli are filled with material in which O_2 is relatively insoluble (e.g., as in pulmonary alveolar proteinosis). When the perfusion increases in these lung units, O_2 in the gas space fails to equilibrate with O_2 in the red cell, and hypoxemia becomes more marked as the blood flow increases (a diffusion defect). At rest, however, when pulmonary blood flow is low, PaO_2 may be normal because red cell residence time in the pulmonary capillary is adequate.

When a patient hyperventilates, PaO_2 may appear to be normal even in patients with pulmonary disease. Calculation of $P(A - a)O_2$ may reveal abnormalities in blood oxygenation masked by hyperventilation. An abnormally elevated $P(A - a)O_2$ is indicative of uneven $\dot{V}A/\dot{Q}$, a diffusion defect, and/or a right to left shunt.

Arterial-End-Tidal PCO_2 Difference ($P(a - ET)CO_2$)

Ventilation of underperfused or unperfused alveoli is wasted or dead space ventilation (alveolar dead space). Since only perfused alveoli can get CO_2, underperfused alveoli relative to ventilation have a low CO_2 concentration. Thus the expired PCO_2, and most specifically the $PETCO_2$ is reduced relative to the $PaCO_2$. By measuring the $P(a - ET)CO_2$, we have another measurement that can be used as evidence of increased alveolar dead space or uneven $\dot{V}A/\dot{Q}$ (33, 34, 66) (Fig. 3.19). In the healthy lung, at rest, $PaCO_2$ is approximately 2 mm Hg greater than $PETCO_2$. During exercise, however, $PETCO_2$ increases relative to $PaCO_2$ and normally exceeds it (Fig. 3.19A and data in Chapter 6). The mechanism for this is relatively straightforward. Because of the increased rate of CO_2 delivery to the lung, associated with the high rate of CO_2 production during exercise, alveolar PCO_2 continues to rise during exhalation. $PETCO_2$ is the highest alveolar PCO_2 during the respiratory cycle, approaching the mixed venous value. On the other hand, the $PaCO_2$ reflects the average alveolar PCO_2 during the entire respiratory cycle. Therefore, provided that the functioning alveoli are relatively uniformly perfused, the end of breath PCO_2 ($PETCO_2$) will exceed the average of the changing alveolar PCO_2 during the respiratory cycle ($PaCO_2$). Direct measurements of continuously measured PCO_2 in the expired air and $PaCO_2$ are shown in Figure 3.20. The slope of instantaneously measured exhaled PCO_2 during the alveolar phase of the breath increases as work rate increases. Because the $PETCO_2$ is the highest PCO_2 in the alveolus during the respiratory cycle, and the arterial PCO_2 represents the average alveolar PCO_2, $PETCO_2$ exceeds $PaCO_2$ during exercise. In contrast, $PETCO_2$ is normally less than the $PaCO_2$ at rest because of the low resting rate of CO_2 production and hypoperfusion of the apical areas of the healthy lung in the upright position.(see Figs. 3.19, 3.20). Thus, $P(a - ET)CO_2$ is slightly positive at rest but negative during exercise (on average, by about -4 mm Hg). Subjects with a slow breathing rate will have a $PETCO_2$ closer to the mixed venous value and therefore have a higher $PETCO_2$ relative to $PaCO_2$.

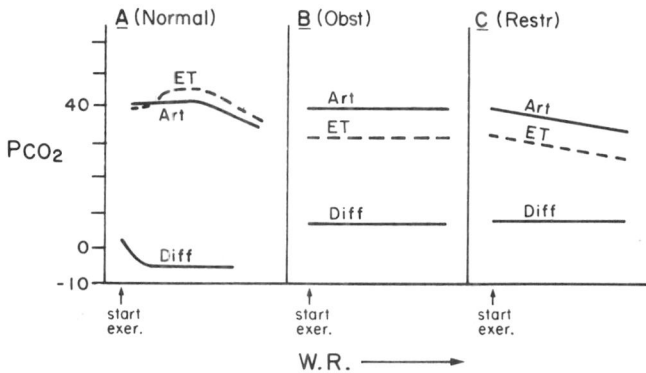

FIGURE 3.19.   Pattern of arterial and end-tidal (ET) PCO_2 values and arterial-end-tidal PCO_2 difference in the normal subject (A) and in patients with obstructive (B) and restrictive (C) lung disease as related to increasing work rate. All have normal resting $PaCO_2$ values.

If the $P(a - ET)CO_2$ remains positive during exercise, this is evidence for decreased perfusion to ventilated alveoli (uneven $\dot{V}A/\dot{Q}$ with high $\dot{V}A/\dot{Q}$ units) (see Fig. 3.19B, C). An extreme situation may be seen when CO_2-rich venous blood is diverted to the left side of the circulation without passing through the lungs during exercise (right to left shunt). In this case, $PaCO_2$ is much higher than $PETCO_2$ because the blood perfusing the lung is hyperventilated to compensate for the CO_2 load entering the arterial circulation through the shunt (71). In this situation, $P(a - ET)CO_2$ is markedly positive because of a decreased $PETCO_2$ during exercise. The magnitude of the increased $P(a - ET)CO_2$ depends on the size of the right to left shunt.

Sue et al. (34) compared the resting D_{LCO} with arterial blood gases during maximal exercise in 276 male shipyard workers. Fourteen of 16 subjects with $D_{LCO} < 70\%$ had abnormal gas exchange, measured as an increase in $P(A - a)O_2$, VD/VT, and $P(a - ET)CO_2$, during exercise. However eighty-eight subjects had abnormal gas exchange with a normal D_{LCO}. Increases in VD/VT and $P(a - ET)CO_2$ occurred when there was a major component of uneven, high $\dot{V}A/\dot{Q}$ lung units. Both were abnormal in the same subjects. In contrast, an increase in $P(A - a)O_2$ was abnormal when there was a major component of uneven, low $\dot{V}A/\dot{Q}$ lung units. An increased $P(a - ET)CO_2$ and VD/VT occurred more frequently than an increased $P(A - a)O_2$. When $P(A - a)O_2$ was increased, $P(a - ET)CO_2$ and VD/VT were also increased. In many instances, however, only $P(a - ET)CO_2$ and VD/VT were abnormal.

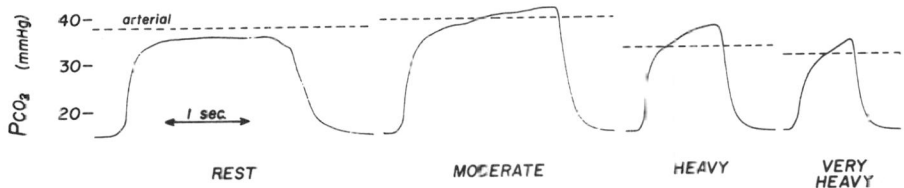

FIGURE 3.20.   Mean arterial (dashed lines) compared with instantaneous alveolar (solid lines) P_{CO_2} for the resting state and at increasing intensities of exercise. The end-tidal P_{CO_2} is normally less than Pa_{CO_2} at rest but greater than Pa_{CO_2} during exercise. (Reprinted with permission from Wasserman K, Van Kessel A, Burton GB. Interaction of physiological mechanisms during exercise. J Appl Physiol 1967;22:71–85.)

Ventilatory Equivalents as Indices of Uneven $\dot{V}_A/\dot{Q}$

Because the measurements of V_D/V_T, $P(a - a)_{O_2}$, and $P(a - _{ET})_{CO_2}$ require arterial blood sampling, it is helpful to get a clue to a possible abnormality in $\dot{V}_A/\dot{Q}$ from noninvasive techniques. The nadir of the ventilatory equivalent for CO_2 ($\dot{V}_E/\dot{V}_{CO_2}$) can be used as a noninvasive guide to $\dot{V}_A/\dot{Q}$ unevenness during a progressively increasing work rate test. Normally, $\dot{V}_E/\dot{V}_{CO_2}$ and $\dot{V}_E/\dot{V}_{O_2}$ change as illustrated in Figure 3.21A. The $\dot{V}_E/\dot{V}_{O_2}$ normally decreases to its nadir at the AT, and the $\dot{V}_E/\dot{V}_{CO_2}$ decreases to its nadir at the respiratory compensation point, i.e., when ventilatory compensation begins in response to metabolic (lactic) acidosis. The normal $\dot{V}_E/\dot{V}_{O_2}$ at the nadir is between 22 and 27 and $\dot{V}_E/\dot{V}_{CO_2}$ is between 26 and 30. Normal values for these ventilatory equivalents with a $P_{ET CO_2}$ of approximately 40 mmHg suggest a normal V_D/V_T and uniform matching of $\dot{V}_A$ to $\dot{Q}$ (see inset in Fig. 3.17). Elevated ventilatory equivalent values at the AT (Fig. 3.21 B, C) reflect either hyperventilation or an increase in V_D/V_T (uneven $\dot{V}_A/\dot{Q}$). Acute hyperventilation is supported by an R > 1. To distinguish between chronic hyperventilation and increased V_D/V_T as a cause of high ventilatory equivalents, it is necessary to measure Pa_{CO_2} with respiratory gas exchange during exercise (see Fig. 3.17).

Patients with chronic obstructive lung disease usually have uneven $\dot{V}_A/\dot{Q}$. Therefore, their $\dot{V}_E/\dot{V}_{CO_2}$ is high (Fig. 3.21B). Because of their mechanical limitation to breathing, however, they usually do not hyperventilate in response to metabolic acidosis. Thus, despite a metabolic acidosis, the $\dot{V}_E/\dot{V}_{CO_2}$ at the terminal work rate does not usually increase (Fig. 3.21B).

In a progressive exercise test, the $\dot{V}_E/\dot{V}_{O_2}$ normally increases at work rates above the AT, the amount depending on the magnitude of the lactic acidosis and the sensitivity of the chemoreceptor response to the acidosis (Fig. 3.21A). The ventilatory equivalent for O_2 will fail to increase above the AT if the chemoreceptors for detecting increased H^+ are insensitive or inoperable. These subjects may not reach the nadir for $\dot{V}_E/\dot{V}_{O_2}$ until their terminal work rate.

Arterial Bicarbonate and Acid-Base Response

Subjects making a maximal effort during a progressively increasing work rate exercise test normally develop a significant metabolic acidosis by the time the terminal work rate is reached. This is observed even for an increasing work rate exercise testing protocol of relatively short duration (8 to 12 minutes) (see Figs. 2.21, 2.25, 3.22). The greatest increase in arterial lactate and reductions in arterial $[HCO_3^-]$ and pH are noted about 2 minutes after

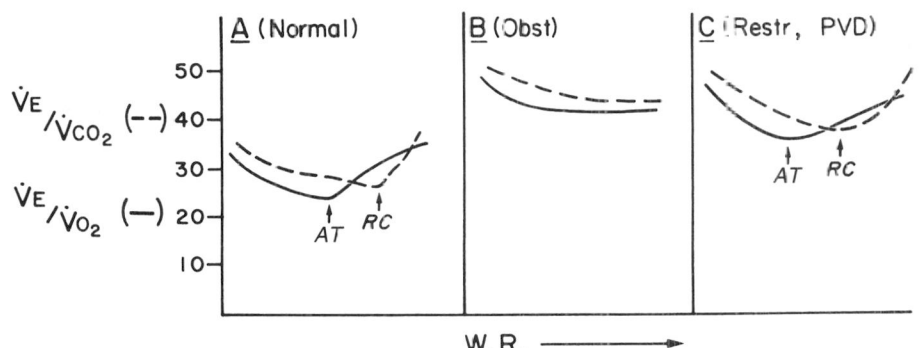

FIGURE 3.21.   Ventilatory equivalent for CO_2 ($\dot{V}_E/\dot{V}_{CO_2}$) and O_2 ($\dot{V}_E/\dot{V}_{O_2}$) for a normal subject (A) and for patients with obstructive (B) and restrictive lung or pulmonary vascular disease (C), as related to increasing work rate (WR). The nadir in $\dot{V}_E/\dot{V}_{O_2}$ reflects the anaerobic threshold (AT), and the nadir of the $\dot{V}_E/\dot{V}_{CO_2}$ curve reflects the respiratory compensation point (RC).

the cessation of the increasing work rate exercise test (see Chapters 6, 9). We find that the 2-minute recovery [HCO_3^-] decreases by at least 6 mmol/L below the resting value if the effort is good and the patient is not limited by a ventilatory or mechanical disorder.

Tidal Volume/Inspiratory Capacity Ratio (VT/IC)

Normally, VT increases during exercise, but it rarely exceeds 80% of the inspiratory capacity (IC), measured during standard resting pulmonary function tests. This ratio is usually abnormal in patients with restrictive lung diseases such as pulmonary fibrosis. Patients with restrictive lung diseases have a reduced IC and therefore have a limited ability to increase their VT in response to exercise (see Fig. 3.13). Thus, in patients with pulmonary fibrosis, as the work rate is increased the VT/IC ratio reaches a value close to 1.0 at a relatively low work rate. The reduced VT requires a high breathing rate to achieve the V̇E needed for CO_2 elimination. While we routinely relate VT to both the VC and the IC (see Chapter 9), we find the VT/IC ratio to be more helpful than the VT/VC ratio.

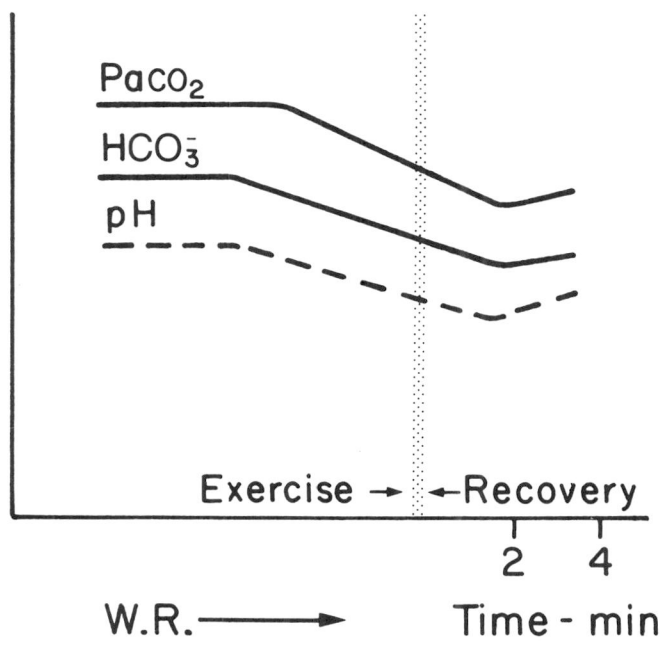

FIGURE 3.22.   Arterial P_{CO_2}, bicarbonate and pH as related to increasing work rate and recovery. The stippled vertical bar indicates the point at which exercise stops. Note that the decrease in $P_{a CO_2}$ is delayed relative to the decrease in [HCO_3^-] and pH (the period of isocapnic buffering). The arterial P_{CO_2}, [HCO_3^-] and pH continue to decrease in the recovery period, before starting to increase back toward normal.

Measurements Unique to Constant Work Rate Exercise Testing

Whereas the absolute V̇O2 required to perform a given work rate should be predictable from the principles established in Chapter 2, the ability to supply the O_2 needed to perform exercise depends on the cardiovascular response. In addition, the increase in V̇CO2 depends on the rate of aerobic metabolism measured as V̇O2 times the muscle substrate RQ, as well as the rate of buffering of lactic acid by HCO_3^- (see Figs. 1.4, 2.31).

Constant work rate tests permit the study of physiologic responses by specific organ systems to transport O_2 and CO_2. They also facilitate investigation of control mechanisms. If the constant work rate performed is above the *AT*, then V̇O2 kinetics are slowed and the relationship between V̇O2 and V̇CO2 kinetics change relative to the kinetics for below *AT* exercise (see Figs. 1.4, 2.31). These changes in kinetics reflect the patient's cardiovascular status during exercise at the specific work rate studied. The following are useful measurements that can be obtained from the time course of the response to the onset of a constant work rate.

Increase in V̇O2 During Phase I

Normally, oxygen uptake abruptly increases at the start of exercise (Phase I) because of the immediate increase in flow of venous blood through the lungs resulting from the increased venous return. The latter is enhanced at the start of exercise by increased cardiac inotropy, compression of veins by contracting muscles and increased heart rate (see Figs. 2.43, 2.45, 2.48). Increased pulmonary blood flow is the predominant mechanism accounting for the increase in V̇O2 during the first 15 seconds of exercise. Under conditions in which pulmonary blood flow fails to increase abruptly at the start of exercise, the Phase I increase in oxygen uptake is attenuated (72–75). A reduced Phase I increase in oxygen uptake is found in disorders that limit the increase in pulmonary blood flow at the start of exercise (73–75). A reduced ventilatory response in Phase I does not discernibly mask the normal rapid increase in V̇O2 (76).

Oxygen Uptake Kinetics: Is the Work Rate Above or Below the *AT*?

After the immediate increase (first 15 seconds of exercise) in V̇O2 and V̇CO2 in a constant work rate test, V̇O2 and V̇CO2 increase as exponential functions

(Phase II). Because of this, their rates of rise have been described by time constants, i.e., the time for 63% of the final response to be reached. Although this single exponential approach has been used by some investigators (15, 23–25, 27), it is not a totally accurate measurement because $\dot{V}O_2$ has first order exponential kinetics only for work rates below the AT. Above the AT, the $\dot{V}O_2$ kinetics must be defined by at least two exponential functions, the second becoming more prominent the higher the work above the threshold (24, 25).

Mean Response Time. Sietsema et al. (77) performed multiple 6-minute constant work rate tests in normal subjects at work rates ranging from unloaded cycling to 150 W. These investigators assumed single exponential kinetics and calculated a *mean response time* (MRT) for the data. The MRT measurement at the higher work rates allowed discrimination of the subject's fitness to perform a progressively increasing work rate test. Thus, the subjects with the highest $\dot{V}O_2$ max/kg body weight had the lowest MRTs for the 75-, 100-, and 150-W work rates (Fig. 2.50).

Figure 3.23 shows the application of the measurements of oxygen uptake kinetics. For the same relatively low work rate (40-W cycling work), $\dot{V}O_2$ for a patient with chronic obstructive pulmonary disease (COPD) had a longer time constant than for a normal subject, matched for age and gender. When compared with the time constants for normal subjects at 50 W in Figure 2.50, the consumption of oxygen by the exercising muscles is slow to increase in the patient with COPD. This indicates that the O_2 deficit is increased and implies the development of a lactic acidosis by the subject in response to this work rate.

Simultaneous Assessment of $\dot{V}O_2$ and $\dot{V}CO_2$ Kinetics. $\dot{V}CO_2$ initially rises more slowly than $\dot{V}O_2$ during Phase II. $\dot{V}O_2$ measured at the airway does not reflect all of the increase in aerobic metabolism at the start of exercise because O_2 is also consumed from the blood O_2 stores. This is seen as a decrease in mixed venous O_2 content and an increase in the arteriovenous O_2 difference. There is also a small amount of O_2 physically dissolved in tissue fluid and O_2 combined with myoglobin that can be consumed as tissue PO_2 decreases. Venoarterial CO_2 difference increases in a like amount to the increase in arteriovenous O_2 difference. Therefore, the increase in CO_2 stores in the blood compartment would not cause the $\dot{V}CO_2$ kinetics to be disparate with the $\dot{V}O_2$ kinetics evidenced by the early decrease in R (see Fig 2.48). However, there are several

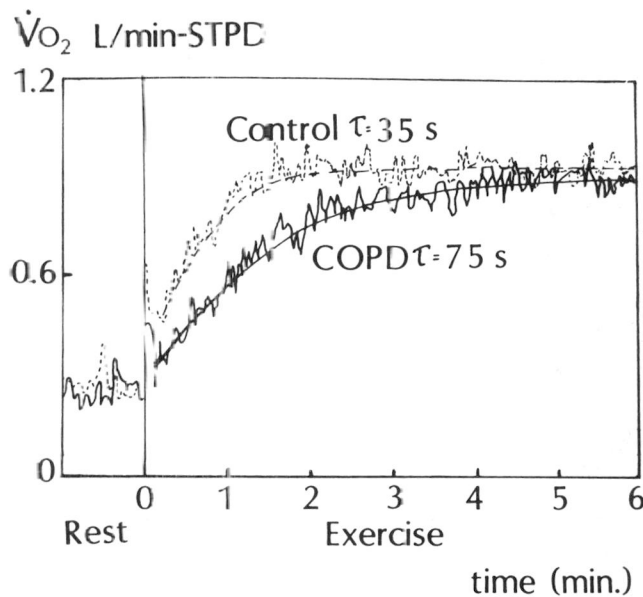

$\dot{V}O_2$ L/min-STPD

FIGURE 3.23.   Pattern of oxygen uptake ($\dot{V}O_2$) in a patient with chronic obstructive pulmonary disease (COPD) and a matched normal subject during the performance of a constant 40-W cycle ergometer exercise. Note that $\dot{V}O_2$ during Phase I (the first 15 seconds of exercise) is less in this patient with COPD, and the rate of rise of $\dot{V}O_2$ to its asymptote during Phase II is slower, as shown by the longer time constant (τ), as compared with a normal "control" subject. (Data from Nery LE, Wasserman K, Andrews JD, et al. Ventilatory and gas exchange kinetics during exercise in chronic airways obstruction. J Appl Physiol 1982;53:1594–1602.)

other reactions that take place at the start of exercise that result in CO_2 retention in the tissues. These are: 1) the hydrolysis of phosphocreatine, which creates an alkaline reaction in muscle thereby converting CO_2 into HCO_3^- (78); 2) the Haldane "effect," which results from the acute desaturation of venous oxyhemoglobin; and 3) increase in physically dissolved CO_2 as tissue PCO_2 increases. Quantitatively, the first appears to be the most important of these three factors.

For above AT constant work rate exercise, $\dot{V}CO_2$ increases more rapidly than $\dot{V}O_2$ after about 1–2 minutes (see Fig. 1.4). This is primarily due to the buffering of newly-formed lactic acid by HCO_3^-. Thus, from the simultaneous analysis of $\dot{V}CO_2$ and $\dot{V}O_2$, it is possible to determine whether the work rate is accompanied by a lactic acidosis.

$\Delta\dot{V}O_2$ (6-3). $\dot{V}O_2$ after 3 minutes (Phase III) is constant when the exercise work rate is below the subject's AT, i.e., the subject is in metabolic homeostasis. However, $\dot{V}O_2$ increases after 3 minutes in proportion to the increase in lactate for work rates above the AT (24, 43, 79, 80). The increase in oxygen uptake between 3 and 6 minutes of exercise ($\Delta\dot{V}O_2$ (6-3)) can be determined by linear regression

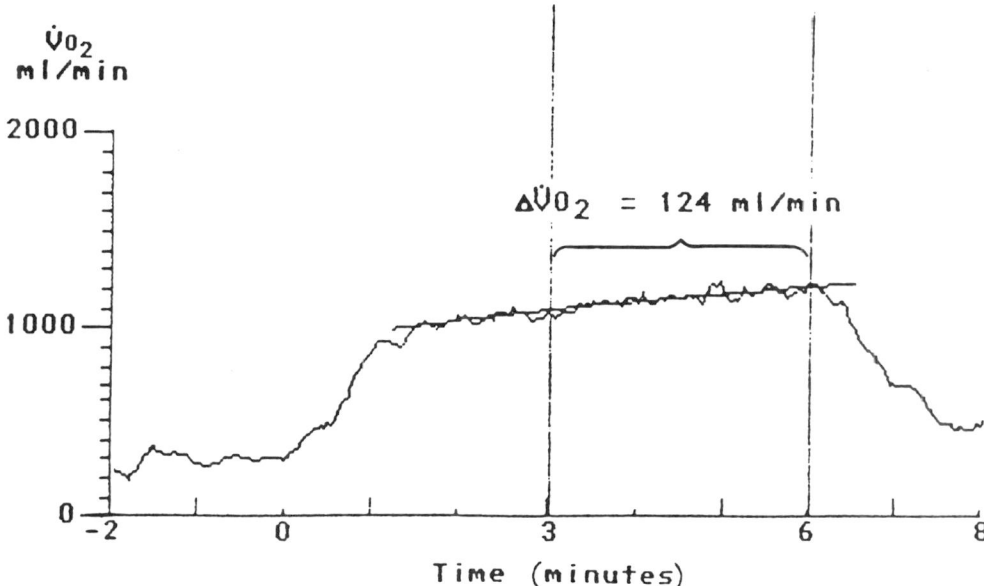

FIGURE 3.24. Method illustrating the measurement of the difference in oxygen uptake ($\dot{V}O_2$) between 3 and 6 minutes [$\Delta\dot{V}O_2$ (6-3)] of constant work rate exercise (70 W) in a patient with cardiac disease. The straight line drawn on the plot between 3 and 6 minutes was determined by the best least square fit for the breath-by-breath data. The difference in $\dot{V}O_2$ at the 6- and 3-minute points is calculated from the 3- and 6-minute intercepts of the linear regression of the data between 3 and 6 minutes.

of the oxygen uptake between 3 and 6 minutes of exercise (Fig. 3.24). When $\Delta\dot{V}O_2$ (6-3) is correlated with the increase in lactate above rest, a good correlation is found for both patients and normal subjects (Fig. 3.25). The regression of the relationship goes through the origin, suggesting that confounding factors do not override the importance of lactate increase in the development of this slow component when performing constant work rate exercise above the *AT*.

Combining $\dot{V}O_2$ and $\dot{V}CO_2$ Kinetics for Detecting Anaerobic Metabolism and Lactic Acid Buffering. By measuring CO_2 output and O_2 uptake breath-by-breath for work above unloaded cycling exercise, Zhang et al. (81) demonstrated that the cumulative output of CO_2 progressively increases relative to the cumulative increase in O_2 uptake for constant work rate exercise associated with a lactic acidosis, in contrast to work for which a lactic acidosis was not found (Fig. 3.26). By multiplying $\dot{V}O_2$ by the muscle substrate respiratory quotient (on average approximately 0.95), the aerobic CO_2 production was calculated. The difference between the total CO_2 output and the aerobic CO_2 output should represent the CO_2 output from buffering lactic acid plus CO_2 from hyperventilation, if any (Fig. 3.26). The latter accounted for only about 6% of the excess CO_2 over that derived from aerobic metabolism in the 50% of subjects who hyperventilated in response to the exercise-induced lactic acidosis at 6 minutes of exercise. When the number of millimoles of CO_2 output derived from the buffering of lactic

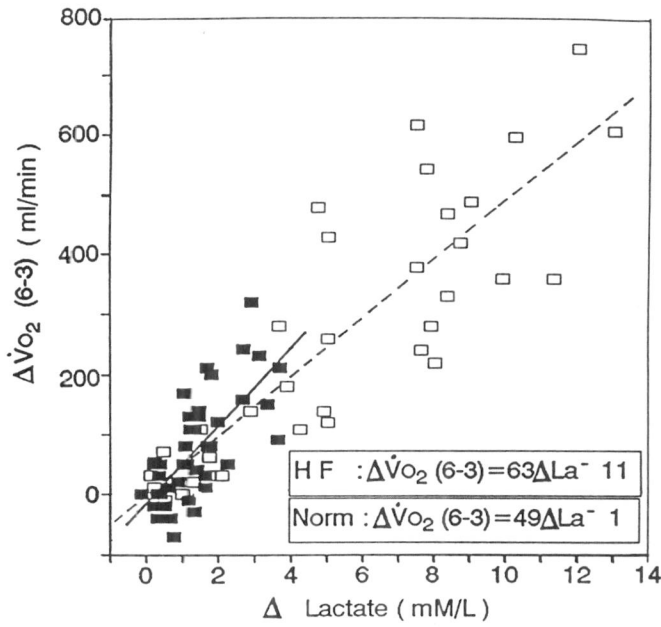

FIGURE 3.25. Degree of unsteady-state in oxygen uptake ($\dot{V}O_2$), expressed as the increase in $\dot{V}O_2$ between 3 and 6 minutes [$\dot{V}O_2$ (6-3)], as a function of the increase in blood lactate above rest in normal subjects (open squares) and in patients with heart failure (solid squares). The blood was sampled from the antecubital vein at 2 minutes of recovery (exercise) as well as at rest. Neither the slopes nor the intercepts of the regression equations differed significantly between the two groups. (Reprinted with permission from Roston, et al. Oxygen uptake kinetics and lactate concentration during exercise in man. Am Rev Respir Dis 1987;135:1080–1084 and Zhang, et al. O_2 uptake kinetics in response to exercise: A measure of tissue aerobiosis in heart failure. Chest 1993;103:735–741.)

acid at 6 minutes of constant work rate exercise was calculated, this quantity correlated closely with the lactate concentration increase determined from antecubital vein blood sampled 2 minutes into recovery (Fig. 3.27). This method, therefore, describes a noninvasive estimate of the *magnitude* of HCO_3^- decrease or lactate increase at the end of 6 minutes of constant work rate exercise. The slope of the regression line defines the volume of distribution of lactate (25 liters or about 1/3 body weight for the population of adults subjects studied).

In a steady state below the *AT*, no anaerobic mechanisms support bioenergetics, and the O_2 debt has reached a maximum (82). However, constant work rate exercise performed at a level above the *AT* results in a delay or an inability to reach a constant $\dot{V}O_2$ (see Fig. 2.32). Thus $\dot{V}O_2$ continues to increase for exercise above *AT* after 3 minutes, the rate of increase depending on the fractional distance between *AT* and $\dot{V}O_2$max (Fig 3.28). To determine if a specific work rate is above the *AT*, measurement of $\dot{V}O_2$ at 3 and 6 minutes

during a 6-minute constant work rate test is helpful. If the 6-minute $\dot{V}O_2$ is greater than the 3-minute $\dot{V}O_2$, the work rate is above the *AT*. The $\Delta\dot{V}O_2$ (6-3) correlates well with the lactate increase (Fig. 3.25). Measurement of $\dot{V}CO_2$ simultaneously with $\dot{V}O_2$ provides added confirmation that the work rate is above the *AT*.

Carotid Body Contribution to Ventilation. Several techniques (83, 84) have been proposed to study the contribution of the carotid bodies to the ventilatory response to breathing stimuli. We find a modified Dejours test (85), performed during moderate constant work rate exercise (86, 87), to be informative and applicable to patients with lung diseases. In the steady state of an air breathing exercise test, the surreptitious switch to 100% oxygen results in an almost immediate decrease in ventilation (within one or two breaths) if the carotid bodies actively contribute to ventilatory drive. By continuously monitoring ventilation breath-by-breath, the magnitude of the decrement in ventilation can be measured (Fig. 3.29). Ventilation decreases to a nadir by 15 seconds. This decrease reflects the carotid body contribution to the ventilatory drive and can be expressed as a percentage of the pre-O_2 breathing ventilation. Once the nadir is reached, ventilation starts increasing back toward its control value despite continued breathing of 100% O_2, but usually does not reach it. The most likely explanation for this rebound in $\dot{V}E$ is the $PaCO_2$ stimulus to ventilation caused by the abrupt drop in $\dot{V}E$ following the start of O_2 breathing. That is, whereas hyperoxia continues to inhibit carotid body drive to ventilation, the increase in $PaCO_2$ resulting from the transient ventilatory decrease stimulates the central chemoreceptors. Thus, part of the carotid body contribution to ventilatory drive is masked if ventilation is not measured dynamically breath-by-breath.

The very nice feature of this test is that it is done rapidly, lasting only about 1 to 2 minutes of exercise, and is safe. It can be performed at work rates below or above *AT* to determine the separate contribution of the exercise-induced lactic acidosis to carotid body ventilatory control.

DATA DISPLAY AND INTERPRETATION

CPET studies have taught us that different defects in the coupling of external (airway) to cellular (mitochondrial) respiration will affect gas exchange in different ways. Thus the pattern of gas exchange at the airway can be used to diagnose pathophysiology

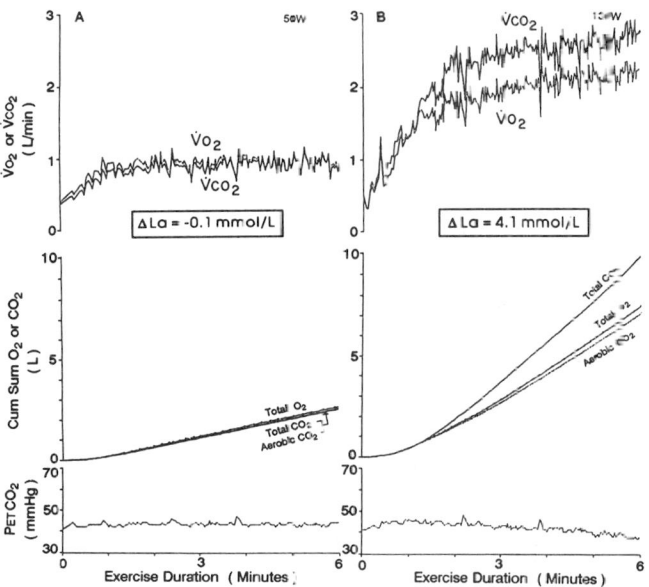

FIGURE 3.26. Breath-by-breath changes in $\dot{V}O_2$, $\dot{V}CO_2$, total or accumulated O_2 uptake (Cum Sum O_2), total or accumulated CO_2 output (Cum Sum CO_2), aerobic CO_2 output ($\dot{V}O_2 \times 0.95$), and $PETCO_2$ in response to 50-W (panel A) and 130-W (panel B) work rate tests for one subject. The difference between the accumulated total CO_2 output and aerobic CO_2 output is the accumulated buffer CO_2 output. In panel A, the total and aerobic Cum Sum CO_2 curves overlap and cannot be distinguished. The increase in antecubital vein lactate at the end of 6 minutes of exercise for each study is shown. (Reprinted with permission from Zhang YY, Sietsema KE, Sullivan CS, et al. A method for estimating bicarbonate buffering of lactic acid during constant work rate exercise. Eur J Appl Physiol 1994;69:309–315.)

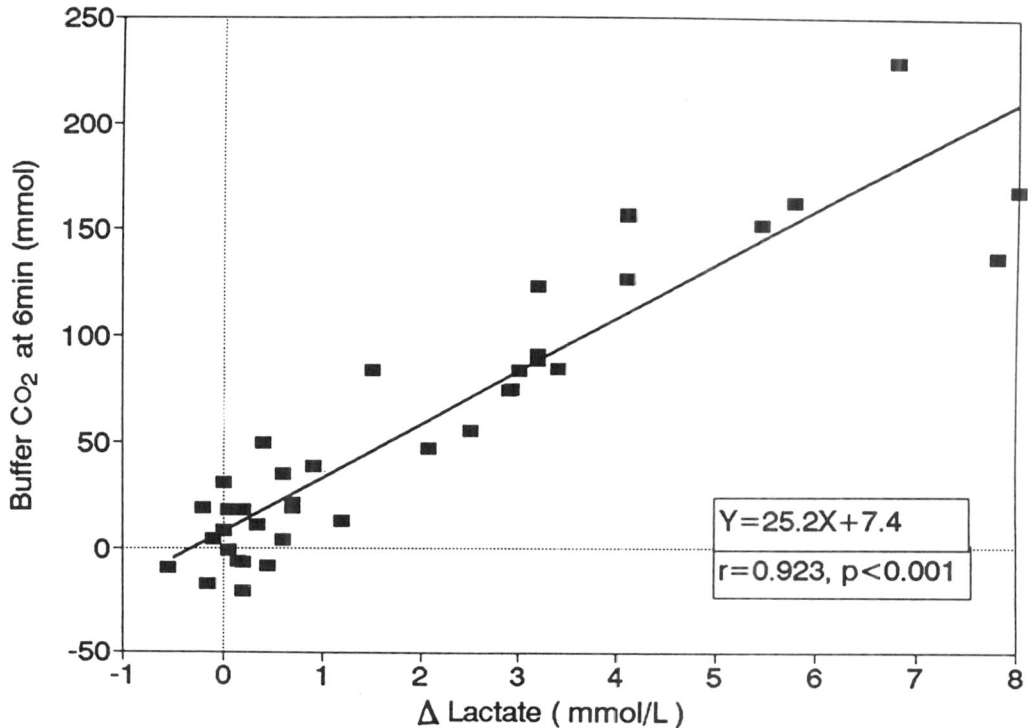

FIGURE 3.27.   Buffer CO_2 (mmol) as a function of the increase in blood lactate concentration (La^-) at the end of 6 minutes of exercise. The correlation coefficient, significance of the correlation and the equation for the regression are shown. (Reprinted with permission from Zhang YY, Sietsema KE, Sullivan CS, et al. A method for estimating bicarbonate buffering of lactic acid during constant work rate exercise. Eur J Appl Physiol 1994;69:309–315.)

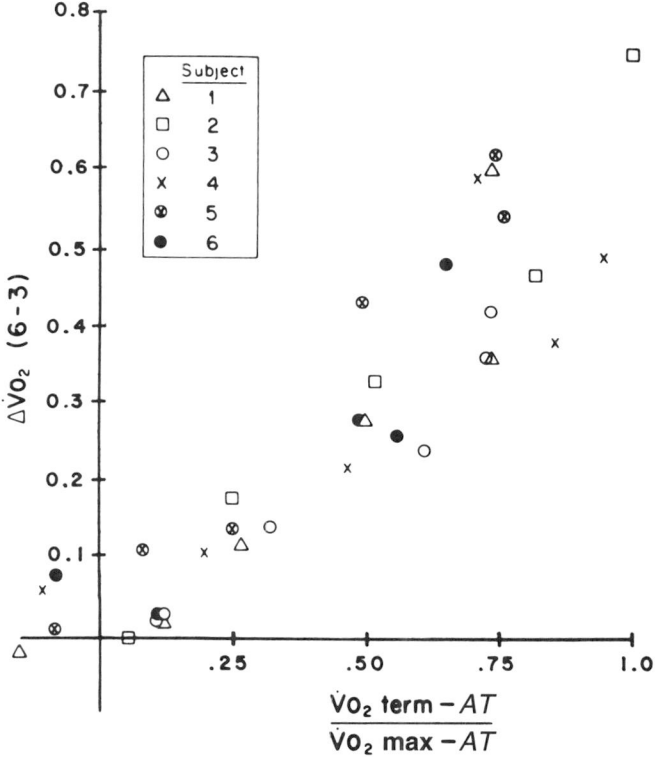

FIGURE 3.28.   Difference between 6- and 3-minute $\dot{V}O_2$ for constant work rate exercise ($\Delta\dot{V}O_2$ (6-3)) as related to the ratio of the difference between the $\dot{V}O_2$ asymptote at the termination of exercise ($\dot{V}O_2$ term) and the AT and the differences between the $\dot{V}O_2$max and the AT. (Modified from Roston WL, Whipp BJ, Davis JA, et al. Oxygen uptake kinetics and lactate concentration during exercise in man. Am Rev Respir Dis 1987;135:1080–1084.)

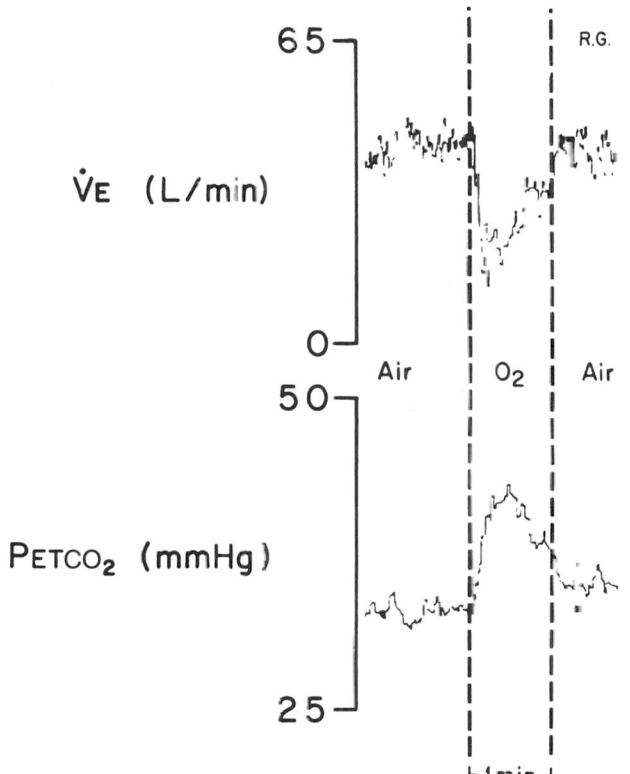

FIGURE 3.29.   Illustration of a safe test for assessing carotid body contribution to ventilation during exercise. The study is that of a patient with pulmonary alveolar proteinosis with a PaO_2 of 54 during exercise. A work rate is selected at which the patient can perform without difficulty and for which a steady state in ventilation is reached by 4 to 5 minutes. When $\dot{V}E$ is constant, the inspired gas is switched from air to 100% oxygen for 1 minute. $\dot{V}E$ decreases to a nadir within several breaths, and, as a consequence, $PETCO_2$ rises. After 15 seconds, $\dot{V}E$ spontaneously starts to rebound toward the air-breathing value, presumably because of CO_2 stimulation of central chemoreceptors. By 45 seconds, $\dot{V}E$ becomes relatively constant at a reduced value, and $PETCO_2$ levels off at an elevated value as compared to the control period. Thus, three phases in ventilation are observed when switching to 100% oxygen breathing: the first 15 seconds when the carotid bodies are attenuated maximally; the period between 15 and 45 seconds which shows a rebound in $\dot{V}E$ presumably caused by the increase in arterial PCO_2, and the period after 45 seconds when $\dot{V}E$ and $PETCO_2$ reach constant values. The abrupt changes in $\dot{V}E$ in response to the O_2 switch and return to air breathing reflect the rapid control exerted by the carotid bodies in the regulation of ventilation. (Reprinted from Wasserman K, Whipp BJ, Davis JA. Respiratory physiology of exercise: metabolism, gas exchange, and ventilatory control. In: Widdicombe JG, ed. International Review of Physiology III. Baltimore: University Park Press, 1981;149–211.)

and to support or refute the correctness of a clinical diagnosis. With an appropriate display of the data, it is possible to determine, noninvasively, the functional status of the cardiovascular system, the ventilatory system and the uniformity of matching of ventilation to perfusion. Because graphical display is much easier to read than a tabular data display,

we transform the CPET data into a graphic display. Furthermore, to avoid interrelating multiple pages of graphs and overburdening the medical record with pages of tedious data, almost all of the data are displayed on a single page of 9 graphs containing 15 plots. These plots are systematically arranged to assess cardiovascular, ventilatory, ventilation-perfusion matching and the metabolic responses to exercise (Fig. 3.30). Normal target values such as $\dot{V}O_2$max and maximum heart rate (HR) are displayed on specific plots. Normal values for all the measurements in the 9-panel graphical array are summarized in Chapter 6.

Evaluation of Systemic Function from the 9-Panel Graphical Array

The questions that could be asked of exercise tests are shown in Table 3.1. Using Figure 3.30 to illustrate the use of the 9-panel graphical array, the answer to the first question relating to exercise capacity is addressed in panel 3 from the measurement of maximum (peak) $\dot{V}O_2$. If peak $\dot{V}O_2$ is reduced, we ask if the reduction is due to a cardiovascular limitation (panels 2, 3, 5), ventilatory limitation (panels 1, 3, 4, 7), ventilation-perfusion mismatching (panels 3, 6, 9) or abnormality in use of metabolic substrate (panels 3, 8). The 9 panels describe the following physiology:

Panel 1. $\dot{V}E$ vs work rate. This plot normally becomes curvilinear as work rate is increased above the anaerobic threshold, except when ventilatory work is excessive such as observed in some patients limited by obesity or obstructive lung disease.

Panel 2. Heart rate (HR) and $\dot{V}O_2$/HR (O_2-pulse) vs work rate. HR is high and $\dot{V}O_2$/HR is low for a given work rate in patients with certain cardiovascular defects except with chronotropic incompetence or heart block or in the presence of β-adrenergic blockade.

Panel 3. $\dot{V}O_2$ and $\dot{V}CO_2$ vs work rate and slope showing predicted rate of increase in $\dot{V}O_2$ for the work rate increase (diagonal line). This is the first panel to address when interpreting if a patient is limited in exercise performance, because this plot gives a global assessment of the presence of exercise limitation. The $\Delta\dot{V}O_2/\Delta$WR is commonly abnormal in patients with cardiovascular disease, the pattern varying with the defect, e.g., heart disease, peripheral arterial disease, pulmonary vascular disease. The $\dot{V}CO_2$ increases

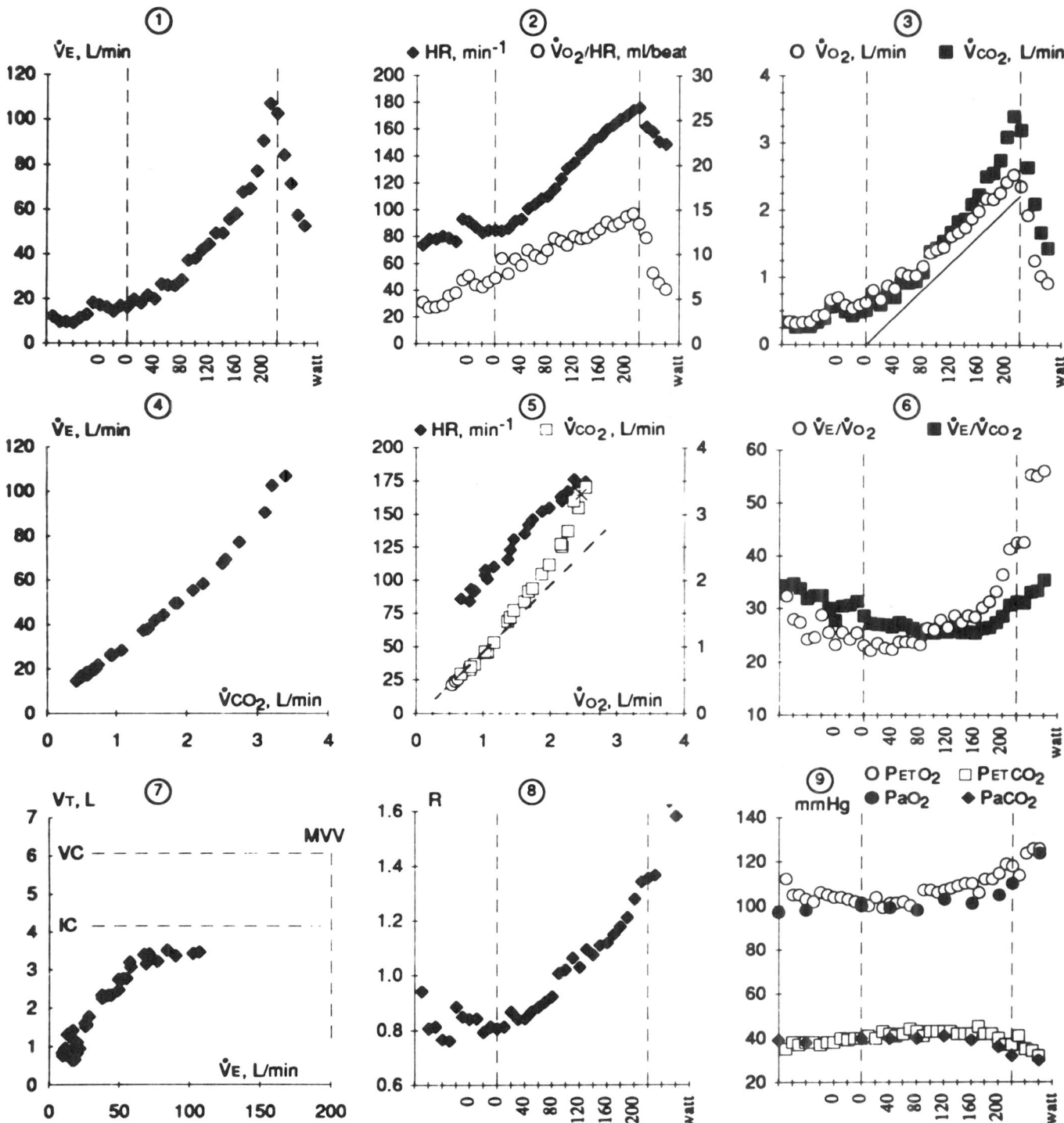

FIGURE 3.30.   Nine panel graphical array used to describe the cardiovascular , ventilatory, ventilation/perfusion matching and metabolic responses to exercise. Study is from a 55-year-old male patient. The responses are normal. The diagonal line drawn on panel 3 is the slope of the normal increase in $\dot{V}O_2$ for the work rate increase (10 ml/min/watt). The "x" in panel 5 is the predicted peak $\dot{V}O_2$ and predicted peak HR. $\dot{V}E$ = minute ventilation; watt = unit of power output (work rate); HR = heart rate; $\dot{V}O_2$/H.R. = O_2 pulse; MVV = maximal voluntary ventilation; IC = inspiratory capacity; VC = vital capacity; R = respiratory exchange ratio ($\dot{V}CO_2/\dot{V}O_2$); $PETO_2$ = end tidal PO_2; $PETCO_2$ = end tidal PCO_2; PaO_2 = arterial PO_2; $PaCO_2$ = arterial PCO_2. (Modified from case 1 in Chapter 9.)

above $\dot{V}_{O_2}$ after a lactic acidosis develops and continues to increase steeply despite a constant or actual slowing of the rate of $\dot{V}_{O_2}$ increase.

Panel 4. $\dot{V}_E$ vs $\dot{V}_{CO_2}$ plotted in a ratio of 30:1. This plot yields a linear relationship until ventilatory compensation for metabolic acidosis steepens the plot or CO_2 retention makes it more shallow. The slope of the linear part is steep with hyperventilation or an increase in the exercise physiological dead space/tidal volume ratio.

Panel 5. HR vs $\dot{V}_{O_2}$ and $\dot{V}_{CO_2}$ vs. $\dot{V}_{O_2}$. HR increases linearly with $\dot{V}_{O_2}$ to their predicted maximums in normal subjects. In patients with heart failure or pulmonary vascular disease, the increase is steep. The relationship may lose its linearity, with HR increasing progressively more rapidly than $\dot{V}_{O_2}$ in patients with myocardial ischemia. Up to the *AT*, $\dot{V}_{CO_2}$ increases linearly with $\dot{V}_{O_2}$ with a slope of one, or slightly less than one. Then $\dot{V}_{CO_2}$ increases more rapidly, the steepening of the slope depending on the rate of buffering of lactic acid. The breakpoint describes the *AT*. This is the V-slope method for determining *AT* (29). It will be low in patients with poor cardiovascular function.

Panel 6. Ventilatory equivalent for O_2 and CO_2 ($\dot{V}_E/\dot{V}_{O_2}$ and $\dot{V}_E/\dot{V}_{CO_2}$) vs work rate. $\dot{V}_E/\dot{V}_{O_2}$ decreases to a nadir at the *AT*. $\dot{V}_E/\dot{V}_{CO_2}$ decreases to a nadir at the ventilatory compensation point. Both values are high in diseases in which pulmonary blood flow is abnormally reduced to ventilated lung gas exchange units.

Panel 7. Tidal volume (V_T) vs $\dot{V}_E$. The patient's vital capacity (VC) and inspiratory capacity (IC) are shown on the vertical axis and actually measured maximum voluntary ventilation (MVV) or FEV_1 times 40 is shown on the horizontal axis. Ventilatory frequency can be plotted as isopleths through the origin. With airflow limitation, maximal exercise $\dot{V}_E$ approximates the MVV. Thus the breathing reserve (MVV-$\dot{V}_E$ at maximal exercise) is approximately zero. The breathing reserve can not be predicted from resting pulmonary function measurements alone. With restrictive lung disease, V_T may approximate the IC at low work rates and respiratory rate may ultimately increase above 50 or 60.

Panel 8. Respiratory exchange ratio ($\dot{V}_{CO_2}/\dot{V}_{O_2}$, R) vs work rate. This plot usually starts at approximately 0.8 and increases to above 1.0 above the *AT*, although these values may be lower after long fasting resulting in glycogen depletion. Inability or failure to produce an exercise lactic

acidosis would mitigate an increase in R to values above 1.0, except when accompanied by acute hyperventilation (decreased Pa_{CO_2}). Acute hyperventilation at rest or low work rates, as reflected by a decreasing $P_{ET_{CO_2}}$, yields an R greater than 1.0.

Panel 9. $P_{ET_{CO_2}}$ and $P_{ET_{O_2}}$ vs work rate. Low $P_{ET_{CO_2}}$ signals either hyperventilation or high $\dot{V}_A/\dot{Q}$ mismatching. "R" (panel 8) reveals if hyperventilation is acute. Arterial blood gases or knowledge of plasma HCO_3^- differentiates chronic hyperventilation from $\dot{V}_A/\dot{Q}$ abnormality in patients with a low $P_{ET_{CO_2}}$. Arterial blood gases are plotted on this graph to detect the presence of high and low $\dot{V}_A/\dot{Q}$ mismatching.

Factors Confounding Interpretation of CPET

Three physiological derangements, not usually considered as diseases of the cardiorespiratory system, may contribute significantly to exercise intolerance. These physiological derangements are: 1) obesity; 2) anemia; and 3) carboxyhemoglobinemia secondary to cigarette smoking.

Obesity adds to the O_2 and cardiac output cost of exercise. It may also restrict the ventilatory system and increase the work of breathing. The restriction or ventilatory capacity and the work of breathing become more marked as the $\dot{V}_E$ requirement increases.

Anemia reduces the arterial O_2 content and the maximal arteriovenous O_2 content difference. Therefore, to achieve a given $\dot{V}_{O_2}$, a greater cardiac output is required than if anemia were not present. Also because the O_2 content of the arterial blood is reduced, the capillary P_{O_2} decreases to its critical value, inducing anaerobic metabolism and lactic acidosis to take place at a reduced work rate and $\dot{V}_{O_2}$.

The carboxyhemoglobin of the heavy cigarette smoker is often about 10–12%. This not only reduces the arterial O_2 content to a level that would be found in patients with an arterial P_{O_2} of about 50–55 mmHg, but also shifts the oxyhemoglobin dissociation curve to the left making it more difficult for O_2 to dissociate from hemoglobin at a given P_{O_2}. Thus the capillary P_{O_2} falls more rapidly to its critical value, resulting in a lactic acidosis at a reduced level of work (88).

The net effect of each of these complicating factors is a reduction in the amount of external work that the patient can accomplish. However, in obesity, the maximal $\dot{V}_{O_2}$ and *AT* are normal or high when referenced to their ideal body weight. In contrast, the maximal $\dot{V}_{O_2}$, AT and peak work rate are reduced in patients with anemia and increased carboxyhemoglobinemia.

SUMMARY

Changes in O_2 uptake and CO_2 output by the lungs reflect changes in cell respiration induced by exercise. While the source of the increased gas exchange with exercise is the increase in cell respiration, cardiac output and ventilation modulate the gas exchange at the airway. Thus diseases of the cardiovascular and ventilatory systems will affect the gas exchange pattern at the airway, depending on the disease pathophysiology. Measurements that assess these functions following controlled work rate perturbations define the physiologic state of the organ systems that participate in gas transport. Defects in the coupling of external to internal respiration result in gas exchange abnormalities characteristic of the limiting organ system. For example, whereas diseases of the heart, the lungs, and the peripheral and pulmonary circulations all result in demonstrable abnormalities in gas exchange, each type of disorder manifests specific and relatively unique abnormalities that are amplified by exercise testing. The effects of various disease states on these measurements are described in Chapter 4.

References

1. Older P, Smith R, Courtney P, Hone R. Preoperative evaluation of cardiac failure and ischemia in elderly patients by cardiopulmonary exercise testing. Chest 1993;104:701–704.
2. Smith TP, Kinasewitz GT, Tucker WY, Spillers WP, George WP. Exercise capacity as a predictor of post-thoracotomy morbidity. Am Rev Respir Dis 1984;129:730–734.
3. Mancini D, Eisen H, Kussmaul W, Mull R, Edmunds L, Wilson J. Value of peak exercise oxygen consumption for optimal timing of cardiac transplantation of ambulatory patients with heart failure. Circulation 1991;83:778–786.
4. Stevenson LW. Role of exercise testing in the evaluation of candidates for cardiac transplantation. In: Wasserman K, ed. Exercise gas exchange in heart disease. Arrmonk, NY: Futura Publishing Co., 1996;271–286.
5. Mudge GH, Goldstein S, Addonizio LJ, Caplan A, Mancini D, Levine TB, Ritsch ME, Stevenson LW. Task Force 3: Recipient Guidelines/Prioritization. J Am Coll Cardiol 1993;22:21–26.
6. Treese N, MacCarter D, Akbulut O, Coutinho M, Baez M, Liebrich A, Meyer J. Ventilation and heart rate response during exercise in normals: relevance for rate variable pacing. Pacing Clin Electrophysiol 1993;16:1693–1700.

7. Koike A, Itoh H, Doi M, Taniguchi K, Marumo F, Umehara I, Hiroe M. Effects of isosorbide dinitrate on exercise capacity in cardiac patients. Relationship between oxygen uptake responses and hemodynamic effects. Japanese Circ J 1990;54:1535–1545.
8. Weber KT. What can we learn from exercise testing beyond the detection of myocardial ischemia? Clin Cardiol 1997;20:684–696.
9. Gibbons RJ, Balady GJ, Beasley JW, Bricker T, Duvernoy WFC, Froelicher VF, Mark DB, Marwick TH, McCallister BD, Thompson PD, Winters WL, Yanowitz FG. ACC/AHA Guidelines for Exercise Testing: A report of the American College of Cardiology/American Heart Association Task Force on Practice Guidelines (Committee on Exercise Testing). J Am Coll Cardiol 1997;30:260–315.
10. Taylor HL, Buskirk E, Henschel A. Maximal oxygen intake as an objective measure of cardiorespiratory performance. J Appl Physiol 1955;8:73–80.
11. Andersen P, Saltin B. Maximal perfusion of skeletal muscle in man. J Appl Physiol 1985;366:233–249.
12. Vogel JA, Gleser MA. Effect of carbon monoxide on oxygen transport during exercise. J Appl Physiol 1972;32:234–239.
13. Whipp BJ, Ward SA. Coupling of Ventilation to Pulmonary Gas Exchange During Exercise. In: Whipp BJ, Wasserman K, eds. Exercise: Pulmonary Physiology and Pathophysiology. New York, Marcel Dekker, Inc., 1991;275.
14. Cooper DM, Weiler-Ravell D, Whipp BJ, Wasserman K. Aerobic parameters of exercise as a function of body size during growth in children. J Appl Physiol 1984;56:628–634.
15. DiPrampero PE. Energetics of muscular exercise. Rev Physiol Biochem Pharmacol 1981;89:143–222.
16. Zhang YY, Johnson MC, Chow N, Wasserman K. Effect of exercise testing protocol on parameters of aerobic function. Med Sci Sports Exerc 1991;23:625–630.
17. Zhang YY, Johnson MC, Chow N, Wasserman K. The role of fitness on $\dot{V}_{O_2}$ and $\dot{V}_{CO_2}$ kinetics in response to proportional step increases in work rate. Eur J Appl Physiol 1991;63:94–100.
18. Hansen JE, Sue DY, Wasserman K. Predicted values for clinical exercise testing. Am Rev Respir Dis 1984;129(Suppl):S49–S55.
19. Wasserman K, Whipp BJ. Exercise physiology in health and disease (State of the art). Am Rev Respir Dis 1975;112:219–249.
20. Wasserman K, Sue DY. Coupling of external to cellular respiration. In: Wasserman K, ed. Exercise Gas Exchange in Heart Disease. Arrmonk, NY: Futura Publishing Co., 1996;1–15.
21. Riley M, Wasserman K, Fu PC, Cooper CB. Muscle substrate utilization from alveolar gas exchange in trained cyclist. Eur J Appl Physiol 1996;72:341–348.
22. Wasserman K. Diagnosing cardiovascular and lung pathophysiology from exercise gas exchange. Chest 1997;112:1091–1101.
23. Linnarsson D. Dynamics of pulmonary gas exchange and heart rate changes at start and end of exercise. Acta Physiol Scand 1974;415(Suppl. 1):5–68.

24. Whipp BJ, Wasserman K. Oxygen uptake kinetics for various intensities of constant load work. J Appl Physiol 1972;33:351–356.

25. Barstow TJ, Casaburi R, Wasserman K. Oxygen uptake kinetics and the O_2 deficit as related to exercise intensity and blood lactate. J Appl Physiol 1993;75:755–762.

26. Whipp BJ, Mahler M. Dynamics of Pulmonary Gas Exchange During Exercise. In: West JB, ed. Pulmonary Gas Exchange, Vol. II. New York: Academic Press, Inc., 1980;33–96.

27. Hesser CM, Linnarsson D, Bjurstedt H. Cardiorespiratory and metabolic responses to positive, negative and minimum-load dynamic leg exercise. Respir Physiol 1977;30: 51–67.

28. Haouzi P, Fukuba Y, Casaburi R, Stringer W, Wasserman K. O_2 uptake kinetics above and below the lactic acidosis threshold during sinusoidal exercise. J Appl Physiol 1993;75:1644–1650.

29. Beaver WL, Wasserman K, Whipp BJ. A new method for detecting the anaerobic threshold by gas exchange. J Appl Physiol 1986;60:2020–2027.

30. Stringer W, Casaburi R, Wasserman K. Acid-base regulation during exercise and recovery in man. J Appl Physiol 1992;72:954–961.

31. Koike A, Hiroe M, Adachi H, Yajima T, Nogami A, Ito H, Takamoto T, Taniguchi K, Marumo F. Anaerobic metabolism as an indicator of aerobic function during exercise in cardiac patients. J Am Coll Cardiol 1992;20: 120–126.

32. Jones NL, Campbell EM. Clinical Exercise Testing. Philadelphia: W.B. Saunders Company, 1982;130–138.

33. Jones NL, McHardy CJR, Naimark A. Physiological dead space an alveolar-arterial gas pressure differences during exercise. Clin Sci 1966;31:19–29.

34. Sue DY, Oren A, Hansen JE, Wasserman K. Diffusing capacity for carbon monoxide as a predictor of gas exchange during exercise. N Engl J Med 1987;316:1301–1306.

35. Rubin SA, Brown HV. Ventilation and gas exchange during exercise in severe chronic heart failure. Am Rev Respir Dis 1984;129(Suppl.):S63–S64.

36. Weisel RD, Berger RL, Hechtman HB. Measurement of cardiac output by thermodilution. N Engl J Med 1975;292: 682–684.

37. Stringer W, Hansen J, Wasserman K. Cardiac output estimated non-invasively from oxygen uptake ($\dot{V}O_2$) during exercise. J Appl Physiol 1997;82:908–912.

38. Weber KT, Janicki JS. Cardiopulmonary exercise (CPX) testing in heart and lung disease. In: Cardiopulmonary Exercise Testing: Physiologic Principles and Clinical Applications. Philadelphia: W.B. Saunders, 1986;200.

39. Agostoni PG, Wasserman K, Perego G, Marenzi GC, Cattadori G, Guazzi M, Assanelli E, Lauri G, Guazzi MD. Stroke volume (SV) measured, non-invasively at anaerobic threshold (AT) in heart failure (HF). Am J Resp Crit Care Med 1997;155:A171.

40. Bylund-Fellenius AC, Walker PM, Elander A, Holm S, Holm J, Schersten T. Energy metabolism in relation to oxygen, partial pressure in human skeletal muscle during exercise. Biochem J 1981;200:247–255.

41. Sahlin K, Katz A, Henriksson J. Redox state and lactate accumulation in human skeletal muscle during dynamic exercise. Biochem J 1987;245:551–556.

42. Wasserman K, Beaver WL, Davis JA, Pu J-Z, Heber D, Whipp BJ. Lactate, pyruvate, and lactate-to-pyruvate ratio during exercise and recovery. J Appl Physiol 1985;59: 935–940.

43. Roston WL, Whipp BJ, Davis JA, Effros RM, Wasserman K. Oxygen uptake kinetics and lactate concentration during exercise in man. Am Rev Respir Dis 1987;135:1080–1084.

44. DiPrampero PE. Energetics of muscular exercise. Rev Physiol Biochem Pharmacol 1981;88:143–222.

45. Beaver WL, Wasserman K, Whipp BJ. Bicarbonate buffering of lactic acid generated during exercise. J Appl Physiol 1986;60:472–478.

46. Wasserman K, Stringer W, Casaburi R. Mechanism of the exercise hyperkalemia: An alternate hypothesis. J Appl Physiol 1997;83:631–643.

47. Osnes J-B, Hermansen L. Acid-base balance after maximal exercise of short duration. J Appl Physiol 1972;32: 59–63.

48. Sue DY, Wasserman K, Moricca RB, Casaburi R. Metabolic acidosis during exercise in patients with chronic obstructive pulmonary disease. Chest 1988;94:931–938.

49. Wasserman K. Breathing during exercise. (Physiology in Medicine series). N Engl J Med 1978;298:780–785.

50. Davis JA, Whipp BJ, Lamarra N, Huntsman DJ, Frank MH, Wasserman K. Effect of ramp slope on determination of aerobic parameters from the ramp exercise test. Med Sci Sports Exerc 1982;14:339–343.

51. Buchfuhrer MJ, Hansen JE, Robinson TE, Sue DY, Wasserman K, Whipp BJ. Optimizing the exercise protocol for cardiopulmonary assessment. J Appl Physiol 1983; 55:1558–1564.

52. Yoshida T. Effect of dietary modifications on lactate threshold and onset of blood lactate accumulation during incremental exercise. Eur J Appl Physiol 1984;53:200–205.

53. McClellan TM, Gass GC. The relationship between the ventilation and lactate thresholds following normal, low and high carbohydrate diets. Eur J Appl Physiol 1989;58: 568–576.

54. Cooper CB, Beaver WL, Cooper DM, Wasserman K. Factors affecting the components of the alveolar CO_2 output-O_2 uptake relationship during incremental exercise in man. Exp Physiol 1992;77:51–64.

55. Beaver WL, Wasserman K, Whipp BJ. Improved detection of the lactate threshold during exercise using a log-log transformation. J Appl Physiol 1985;59:1936–1940.

56. Wasserman K. Determinants and detection of anaerobic threshold and consequences of exercise above it. Circulation 1987;81(Suppl VI):VI-29–VI-39.

57. Riley M, Nicholls P, Patterson VH. Anaerobic threshold: the problem of McArdle's disease. J Appl Physiol 1993;75: 745–754.

58. Donald KW, Bishop JM, Cumming C, Wade OL. The effect of exercise on the cardiac output and central dynamics of normal subjects. Clin Sci 1955;14:37–73.

59. Koike A, Itoh H, Taniguchi K, Hiroe M. Detecting abnormalities in left ventricular function during exercise by

respiratory measurement. Circulation 1989;80:1737–1746.

60. Nery LE, Wasserman K, French W, Oren A, Davis JA. Contrasting cardiovascular and respiratory responses to exercise in mitral valve and chronic obstructive pulmonary diseases. Chest 1983;83:446–453.

61. Koike A, Itoh H, Doi M, Taniguchi K, Marumo F, Umehara I, Hiroe M. Beat-to-beat evaluation of cardiac function during recovery from upright bicycle exercise in patients with coronary artery disease. Am Heart J 1990; 120: 316–323.

62. Sue DY, Hansen JE. Normal values in adults during exercise testing. Exercise: Physiology and Clinical Applications. Clin Chest Med 1984;5:89–97.

63. Gallagher CG. Exercise limitation and clinical exercise testing in chronic obstructive pulmonary disease. Clinical Exercise Testing. Clin Chest Med 1994;15:305–326.

64. Babb TG, Rodarte JR. Estimation of ventilatory capacity during submaximal exercise. J Appl Physiol 1993;74:2016–2022.

65. Babb TG, Rodarte JR. Exercise capacity and breathing mechanics in patients with airflow limitation. Med Sci Sports Exerc 1992;24:967–974.

66. Wasserman K, Van Kessel A, Burton GB. Interaction of physiological mechanisms during exercise. J Appl Physiol 1967;22:71–85.

67. Whipp BJ, Wasserman K. Alveolar-arterial gas tension differences during graded exercise. J Appl Physiol 1969; 27:361–365.

68. West JB. Ventilation/Perfusion and Gas Exchange. Oxford, Blackwell Scientific Publications. 1965;8.

69. Farhi LE. Ventilation perfusion relationship and its role in alveolar gas exchange. In: Caro C, ed. Advances in Respiratory Physiology. London: Edward Arnold, 1966;177.

70. Fishman AP: Hypoxia on the pulmonary circulation. How and where it acts. Circulation Res 1976;38:221–231.

71. Sietsema KE, Cooper DM, Perloff SK, Child JS, Rosove MH, Wasserman K, Whipp BJ. Control of ventilation during exercise in patients with central venous-to-systemic arterial shunts. J Appl Physiol 1988;64:234–242.

72. Weiler-Ravell D, Whipp BJ, Cooper DM, Wasserman K. The control of breathing at the start of exercise as influenced by posture. J Appl Physiol 1983;55:1460–1466.

73. Nery LE, Wasserman K, Andrews JD, Huntsman DJ, Hansen JE, Whipp BJ. Ventilatory and gas exchange kinetics during exercise in chronic airways obstruction. J Appl Physiol 1982;53:1594–1602.

74. Sietsema KE, Cooper DM, Rosove MA, Perloff JK, Child JS, Canobbio MM, Whipp BJ, Wasserman K. Dynamics of oxygen uptake during exercise in adults with cyanotic congenital heart disease. Circulation 1986;73:1137–1144.

75. Sietsema K. Oxygen uptake kinetics during exercise in patients with pulmonary vascular disease. Am Rev Respir Dis 1992;145:1052–1057.

76. Weissman ML, Jones PW, Oren A, Lamarra N, Whipp BJ, Wasserman K. Cardiac output increase and gas ex-

change at the start of exercise. J Appl Physiol 1982; 52:236–244.

77. Sietsema KE, Daly JA, Wasserman K. Early dynamics of O_2 uptake and heart rate as affected by exercise work rate. J Appl Physiol 1989;67:2535–2541.

78. Wasserman K, Stringer W, Casaburi R, Zhang YY. Mechanism of the exercise hyperkalemia. J Appl Physiol 1997; 83:631–643.

79. Zhang YY, Wasserman K, Sietsema KE, Barstow TJ, Mizumoto G, Sullivan CS, Ben-Dov I. O_2 uptake kinetics in response to exercise: A measure of tissue anaerobiosis in heart failure. Chest 1993;103:735–741.

80. Wasserman K, Casaburi R, Beaver WL, Roston WL, Whipp BJ. Assessing the adequacy of tissue oxygenation during exercise. New Horizons: Oxygen Transport and Utilization. Fullerton, CA: Soc Crit Care Med 1987; 109–144.

81. Zhang YY, Sietsema KE, Sullivan CS, Wasserman K. A method for estimating bicarbonate buffering of lactic acid during constant work rate exercise. Eur J Appl Physiol 1994;69:309–315.

82. Schneider EG, Robinson S, Newton JL. Oxygen debt in aerobic work. J Appl Physiol 1968;25:58–62.

83. Rebuck AS, Slutsky AS. Measurement of ventilatory responses to hypercapnia and hypoxia. Regulation of Breathing. New York: Marcel Dekker, 1991;745–772.

84. Severinghaus JW. Proposed standard determination of ventilatory responses to hypoxia and hypercapnia in man. Chest 1976:70(Suppl.):129–131.

85. Dejours P. Control of respiration by arterial chemoreceptors. Ann NY Acad Sci 1963;109:682–695.

86. Whipp BJ, Wasserman K. Carotid bodies and ventilatory control dynamics in man. Fed Proc 1980;39:1623–1673.

87. Springer C, Cooper DM, Wasserman K. Evidence that maturation of the peripheral chemoreceptors is not complete in childhood. Respir Physiol 1988;74:55–64.

88. Koike A, Wasserman K, Taniguchi K, Hiroe M, Marumo F. Critical capillary oxygen partial pressure and lactate threshold in patients with cardiovascular disease. J Am Coll Cardiol 1994;23:1644–1650.

89. Hansen JE, Casaburi R, Cooper DM, Wasserman K. Oxygen uptake as related to work rate increment during cycle ergometer exercise. Eur J Appl Physiol 1988;57:140–145.

90. Pardee HB, DeGraff AG, Della Chapelle CE, Eggleston C, Kossman CE, Maynard E, Schwedel JB, Stewart HJ, Wright IS. Functional capacity classification of patients. Nomenclature and criteria for diagnosis of diseases of the heart and blood vessels. New York: New York Heart Association, 1953;81.

91. Brown HV, Wasserman K, Whipp BJ. Strategies of exercise testing in chronic lung disease. Bull Euro Physiopathol Resp 1977;13:409–423.

92. Wasserman K, Whipp BJ, Davis JA. Respiratory physiology of exercise: Metabolism, gas exchange, and ventilatory control. In: Widdicombe JG, ed. International Review of Physiology III. Baltimore: University Park Press, 1981; 149–211.

CHAPTER 4

Pathophysiology of Disorders Limiting Exercise

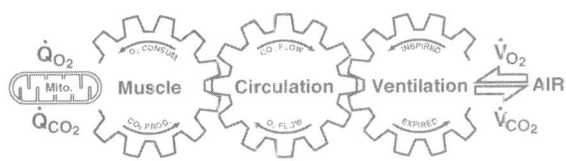

THE COUPLING of external to cellular respiration to perform exercise involves many organ systems. From Figure 4.1, it is evident that diseases of the blood, peripheral circulation, the heart, the pulmonary circulation, the lungs, the chest wall, respiratory control, and metabolic pathways in bioenergetics influence the normal coupling of external to cellular respiration. Thus, defects of any might limit exercise performance. The objective of this chapter is to describe the changes in external respiration that characterize the pathophysiology brought about by diseases of the organ systems that participate in supporting the bioenergetic mechanisms to perform exercise (Table 4.1). Individually or in combination, these disorders limit exercise by causing symptoms of dyspnea, fatigue, and/or pain.

OBESITY (TABLE 4.2)

Whereas the obese subject has some increase in resting metabolic rate ($\dot{V}_{O_2}$) relative to lean body mass, the increase is more marked during dynamic exercise (see Figs. 2.7, 3.5). Additional energy is needed to move heavy legs in leg cycling exercise or the large body mass while ambulating. This adds to the O_2 needed to perform external work (Fig. 4.2) (1, 2). Because the metabolic rate is increased to perform a given amount of external work, obese people require an increased cardiorespiratory response to exercise. However, the heart, blood vessels, lungs and muscles do not usually increase in size commensurate with the subject's added weight.

Consequently, for the obese individual to do any amount of physical work, there must be greater than normal cardiovascular and ventilatory response. Therefore the maximal level of effective *external* work that a subject, who is overweight because of obesity, will be able to perform must be reduced because a greater part of the subject's cardiovascular and ventilatory reserve will be consumed to support the energy required to move the enlarged body mass.

Constraints are imposed on the maximal exercise performance because of altered cardiovascular and ventilatory mechanics in obesity, especially in the extremely obese subject. Because of the large mass, resting cardiac output per kilogram of lean body weight is already high. Thus the cardiac output reserve available to support the increased muscle O_2 requirement for exercise is reduced (3). Furthermore, the added mass on the chest wall and the increased pressure in the abdomen cause increased ventilatory work. In obese subjects, the increased abdominal pressure may constrain diaphragmatic descent during inspiration, reducing the vital capacity. Both the increased abdominal pressure and the added weight to the chest wall effectively "chest strap" (4–7) the patient, causing the resting end-expiratory lung volume (FRC) to be reduced (in extreme cases, close to the residual volume) (8). This can lead to atelectasis of peripheral lung units and hypoxemia at rest. In addition, pulmonary vascular resistance may be increased, primarily as a result of pulmonary insufficiency. Thus, cor pulmo-

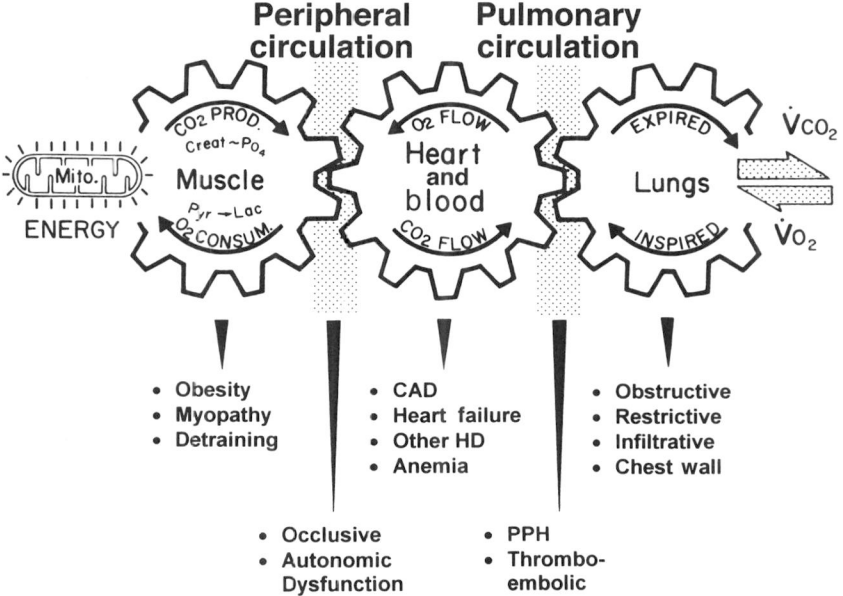

FIGURE 4.1. Sites of interference in the metabolic-cardiovascular-ventilatory coupling for various disease states.

TABLE 4.1. Disorders and Mechanisms Impairing Work Tolerance

Disorder	Pathophysiology	Primary Limitation
Obesity	Increased metabolic requirement; respiratory restriction	Decreased cardiorespiratory reserve
Peripheral arterial disease	Prevents normal vasodilatation; exercise hypertension	Impaired muscle O_2 supply; increased cardiac work.
Heart diseases	Reduced ability to increase cardiac output (stroke volume); ventilation-perfusion mismatching and lung restriction in heart failure	Reduced tissue O_2 delivery (fatigue); increased ventilatory requirement (dyspnea)
Pulmonary vascular diseases	Limited cardiac output increase; decreased gas exchange efficiency	Impaired tissue O_2 delivery (fatigue); increased ventilatory requirement (dyspnea)
Ventilatory disorders Airflow obstruction	Increased airway resistance; abnormal $\dot{V}_A/\dot{Q}$	Reduced ventilatory capacity; increased ventilatory requirement
Restrictive lung disease	Inability to increase pulmonary blood flow; reduced lung distensability; decreased efficiency of gas exchange; exercise-induced hypoxemia	Reduced tissue O_2 delivery (fatigue); increased drive to breathe (dyspnea)
Chest wall defect	Abnormal rib cage mechanics; respiratory muscle weakness	Reduced ability to breathe (dyspnea)
Defects in hemoglobin content and quality	Reduced blood O_2 capacity; increased O_2 affinity for hemoglobin (left shifted HbO_2 dissociation curve)	Impaired tissue O_2 delivery
Smoking	Increased carboxyhemoglobin; hypertension; increased airway resistance	Reduced tissue O_2; increased cardiac output demand; reduced ventilatory capacity
Metabolic acidosis	Reduced buffering capacity; low Pa_{CO_2} setpoint	Increased ventilatory drive (dyspnea)
Neuromuscular disease	Musculoskeletal coupling inefficiency	Reduced mechanical efficiency; pain
Glycolytic enzyme defect	Deficiency in carbohydrate substrate; inability to support metabolism with anaerobiosis	Muscle pain; reduced aerobic and anaerobic ATP regeneration (fatigue)
Electron transport defect	Inability to regenerate ATP aerobically	Low work rate metabolic acidosis
Anxiety	Non-physiological breathing patterns	Shortness of breath
Poor effort or manipulated performance	Secondary gain; chaotic breathing; no or little metabolic acidosis at peak exercise	Self

TABLE 4.2. Discriminating Measurements during Exercise in Obesity*

High O_2 cost to perform external work

Upward displacement of $\dot{V}_{O_2}$-work rate relationship

Peak $\dot{V}_{O_2}$/body weight and *AT*/body weight are low

Peak $\dot{V}_{O_2}$/height and *AT*/height are normal or high (with active life style)

Normal to high O_2 pulse when "normal" is determined from predicted weight

Low Pa_{O_2} at rest that normalizes during exercise

Normal V_D/V_T

Failure to develop normal ventilatory compensation for metabolic acidosis

$\dot{V}_E$ maintains a linear increase with work rate and $\dot{V}_{CO_2}$

* See Table 3.2 for a definition of symbols.

male may develop with secondary erythrocytosis, hepatomegaly, peripheral edema, and right ventricular hypertrophy.

The increased O_2 cost of performing mechanical work is predictable and well worked out for cycle ergometer work (1, 2). The $\dot{V}_{O_2}$-work rate relationship is displaced upward, depending on the degree of obesity, by 5.8 ml/min/kg. However obesity causes no discernable change in the slope of the $\dot{V}_{O_2}$-work rate relationship (1, 2). The effect of adipose tissue distribution in the body, i.e., legs or trunk, on $\dot{V}_{O_2}$ has not been investigated.

The maximum $\dot{V}_{O_2}$ and *AT* are low when related to actual body weight, but usually normal when related to height (2) or to predicted weight or lean body mass (9). Because of the high metabolic cost to do even modest levels of exercise, an active,

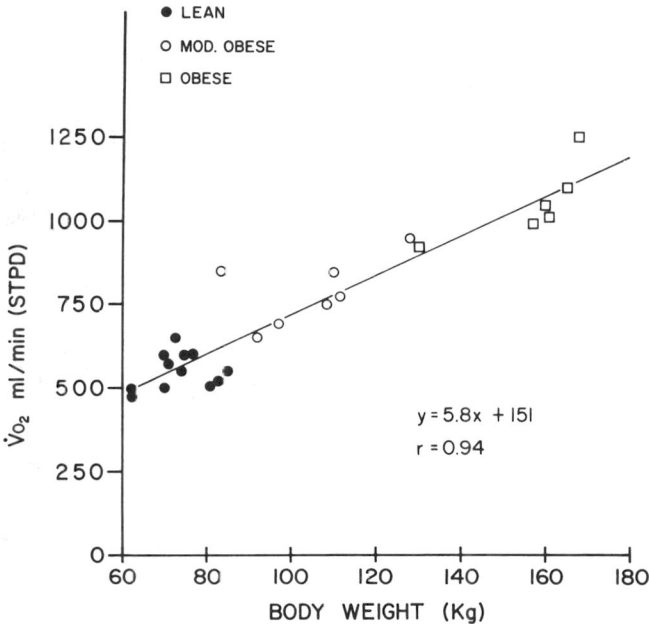

FIGURE 4.2. O_2 cost of performing unloaded cycling as related to body weight. (Reprinted with permission from Wasserman K, Whipp BJ. Exercise physiology in health and disease (State of the art). Am Rev Resp Dis 1975;112:219–249.)

otherwise healthy, obese subject may have good cardiovascular fitness but reduced work capacity. Thus, the actual $\dot{V}_{O_2}$ max, based on height or lean body weight, may be greater than that predicted for a normal, sedentary subject. The hypoxemia commonly present at rest in the obese subject results from atelectasis of peripheral lung units. This usually improves during exercise, presumably because the deep breathing re-expands atelectatic lung units. It is the only pulmonary condition in which arterial oxygenation improves during exercise. Because ventilation-perfusion relationships usually normalize during exercise in the patient with uncomplicated obesity, exercise V_D/V_T, $P(A - a)_{O_2}$, and $P(a - ET)_{CO_2}$ values are normal.

TABLE 4.3. Discriminating Measurements during Exercise in Peripheral Arterial Disease*

Low $\Delta\dot{V}_{O_2}/\Delta WR$
Low maximum $\dot{V}_{O_2}$
Low *AT*
Leg pain
Exercise-induced hypertension

* See Table 3.2 for a definition of symbols.

PERIPHERAL ARTERIAL DISEASES (TABLE 4.3)

Because of the pathologic changes that reduce the internal diameter of the conducting arteries to the limbs, peripheral arterial diseases impair the ability to increase blood flow appropriately to meet the increased metabolic demand of exercise. Thus, O_2 flow fails to increase sufficiently to satisfy the O_2 requirement for performing exercise totally aerobically (Fig. 2.14). The inability to supply sufficient O_2 to the exercising muscles to meet the O_2 requirement may result in a reduced $\Delta\dot{V}_{O_2}/\Delta WR$ ratio at even low work levels. Although a compensatory increase in mitochondrial number in the ischemic muscle may occur with time, the improved O_2 extraction, which this mechanism portends, is inadequate to make up for the deficiency in O_2 flow (10). Consequently, the ischemic muscles produce lactic acid at relatively low work rates with subsequent leg pain and fatigue. When the lactic acidosis is evident in the central circulation, breathing is further stimulated. If the patient also has lung disease, dyspnea may be an important symptom.

With peripheral arterial disease, the maximum $\dot{V}_{O_2}$ and the lactic acidosis threshold are reduced, although the latter may not be detectable because lactate may enter the central circulation very slowly as a result of reduced muscle perfusion. Thus the lactic acidosis of the ischemic muscles may not always be obvious.

Many patients with peripheral arterial disease have excessively elevated blood pressure responses at the low work rates performed. The heart rate at maximum exercise is usually relatively low because the patient stops exercise from claudication at a work rate too low to provide a maximal cardiac stimulus.

HEART DISEASES

Because gas transport is the major and most immediate role of the cardiovascular system, cardiac dysfunction of all four primary types of heart disease (i.e., coronary artery, cardiomyopathic, valvular, and congenital) will cause changes in the pattern of $\dot{V}_{O_2}$, $\dot{V}_{CO_2}$, and heart rate responses to exercise. Before discussing each major class of heart disease, it is noteworthy to consider features in common with all forms of heart disease.

In nearly all heart defects, the increase in HR as a function of $\dot{V}_{O_2}$ is steeper than normal. This reflects the increased dependence on heart rate to increase

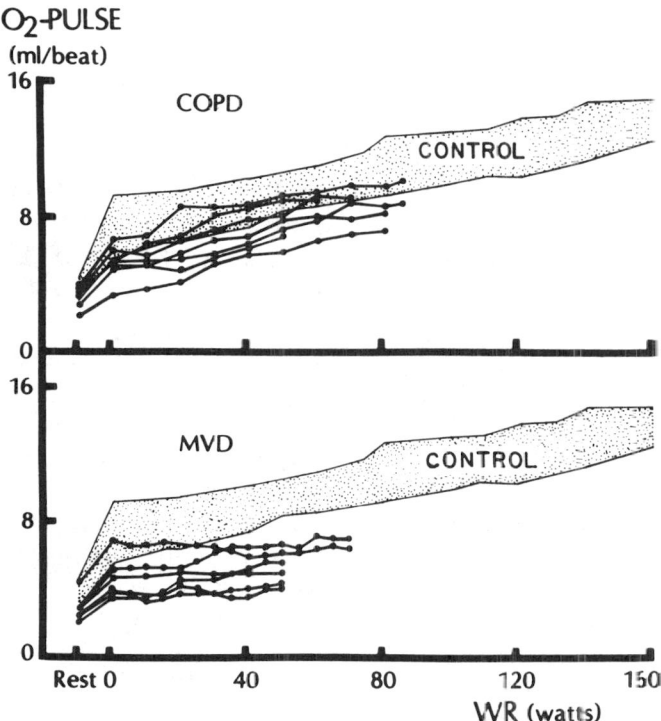

O₂-PULSE
(ml/beat)

FIGURE 4.3.   O₂-pulse response to incremental exercise in patients with chronic obstructive pulmonary disease (COPD) (upper panel) and mitral valve disease (MVD) (lower panel) compared with the range of values of a control group (stippled area). (Modified from Nery LE, Wasserman K, French W, et al. Contrasting cardiovascular and respiratory responses to exercise in mitral valve and chronic obstructive pulmonary diseases. Chest 1983;83:446–453.)

cardiac output, because stroke volume is reduced consequent to the disease. Although the heart rate–$\dot{V}O_2$ relationship is usually relatively steep in heart disease, exceptions occur when the heart rate response to exercise is inappropriately low. These include patients taking β-adrenergic blocking drugs, some patients with cardiomyopathies whose sinoatrial node fails to respond appropriately with tachycardia to the low cardiac output state, and patients with heart block.

Because of the relatively low cardiac output response, mixed venous oxygen reaches its lowest value, and the arterial-mixed venous oxygen difference ($C(a - \bar{v})O_2$) its highest value, at a low work rate (11). Consequently, the O₂ pulse ($C(a - \bar{v})O_2 \times SV$) reaches a constant value that is abnormally low and occurs at an unusually low work rate compared to normal (Fig. 4.3). The increase in $\dot{V}O_2$ as WR increases commonly becomes smaller near the maximum work rate (see Fig. 3.5C), reflecting an increased contribution of energy from anaerobic metabolism presumably because of impaired O₂ transport (12) or utilization (13).

Patients with heart diseases develop metabolic acidosis at low work rates (1, 14–16); this may become chronic and evident at rest and is accompanied by a low $PaCO_2$ (17). This disorder necessitates a high minute ventilation that becomes more marked the higher the work rate (see Chapter 2, "Determinants of the Ventilatory Requirement"). A number of studies have shown that patients with chronic heart failure develop mismatching of ventilation relative to pulmonary perfusion, particularly of the high $\dot{V}A/\dot{Q}$ type. This results in an increased VD/VT and a further increase in the breathing requirement to maintain blood pH homeostasis (18–22). This increase in VD/VT is a major factor, along with the increase in $\dot{V}CO_2$ in response to developing lactic acidosis, in stimulating the increased ventilatory response to exercise (19), and likely contributes to the symptom of dyspnea in patients with chronic heart failure.

Constant work rate tests may be helpful for evaluating the cardiovascular response to specific levels of exercise in heart disease. If the work rate is above the lactic acidosis threshold, $\dot{V}O_2$ will not reach a steady-state by 3 minutes. The magnitude of the increase in $\dot{V}O_2$ between 3 and 6 minutes ($\Delta\dot{V}O_2$ (6–3)) is correlated to the exercise lactic acidosis (see Fig. 3.24).

Coronary Artery Disease (Table 4.4)

Although mild coronary artery disease may only be manifest in the laboratory by electrocardiographic (ECG) changes at high work rates, more significant coronary artery disease will cause the peak $\dot{V}O_2$ and the AT to be reduced. Patients with coronary artery disease may or may not experience chest pain. ECG changes consistent with ischemia occur when the exercise-induced increase in myocardial oxygen requirement is not met by the myocardial oxygen

---

TABLE 4.4.   Discriminating Gas Exchange Measurements during Exercise in Coronary Artery Disease*

$\Delta\dot{V}O_2/\Delta WR$ normal at low work rates, but may change to more shallow slope above AT

Reduced maxima O₂ pulse

Heart rate–$\dot{V}O_2$ relationship may become abnormally steep as peak $\dot{V}O_2$ is approached

High breathing reserve

Metabolic acidosis at end exercise

Immediate post-exercise O₂ pulse increase

* See Table 3.2 for a definition of symbols.

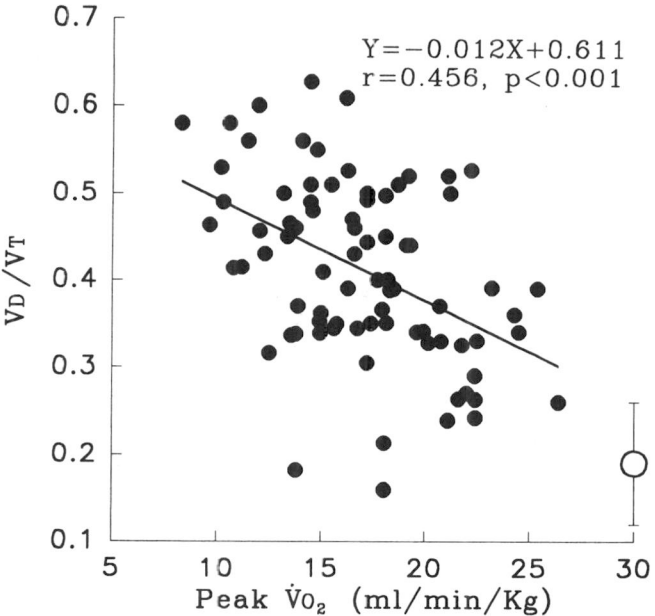

$$Y = -0.012X + 0.611$$
$$r = 0.456, \; p < 0.001$$

FIGURE 4.4.   Physiological dead space/tidal volume ratio (V_D/V_T) as a function of peak $\dot{V}_{O_2}$ on a cycle ergometer in 78 patients with chronic stable heart failure. The open circle on the right is the mean $V_D/V_T \pm$ SD for normal subjects. (Reprinted with permission from Wasserman K, Zhang YY, Gitt A, et al. Lung function and exercise gas exchange in chronic heart failure. Am J Respir Crit Care Med 1997;96:2221–2227.)

supply. Myocardial ischemia may result in ventricular ectopic beats during exercise with increasing frequency as the work rate is increased.

Characteristically, the $\Delta\dot{V}_{O_2}/\Delta WR$ ratio is normal at low work rates of an incremental exercise test but may abruptly decrease when myocardial ischemia prevents the myocardium from contracting with the synchrony required to maintain stroke volume. The ECG usually becomes abnormal, whether or not angina develops, when $\Delta\dot{V}_{O_2}/\Delta WR$ decreases. When the slope of rise in $\dot{V}_{O_2}$ versus work rate becomes abnormally shallow, however, $\dot{V}_{CO_2}$ continues to increase steeply, creating a large disparity between $\dot{V}_{CO_2}$ and $\dot{V}_{O_2}$ increase. With myocardial ischemia, heart rate as a function of $\dot{V}_{O_2}$ usually becomes steeper, developing a curvilinear relationship rather than the linear relation normally found.

The O_2 pulse fails to increase to its normal predicted value when myocardial ischemia develops, or it may remain constant, similar to that shown in Figure 4.4. This is likely due to a decrease in stroke volume secondary to asynchronous contraction of the left ventricular wall in the region of ischemia. The reduced stroke volume may be compensated for by an increase in $C(a - \bar{v})_{O_2}$, thereby maintaining the O_2 pulse.

In normal persons, the O_2 pulse decreases immediately after exercise. However, a paradoxical increase in O_2 pulse commonly occurs in patients who develop myocardial ischemia or heart failure in response to exercise. This paradoxical increase in O_2 pulse may be due to an immediate increase in stroke volume in these patients because of the abrupt decrease in left ventricular afterload and improved ventricular contractility when exercise stops (23).

Metabolic acidosis usually develops because of impaired O_2 transport resulting from the failure to increase cardiac output commensurate with the increasing work rate when a significant portion of the left ventricle stops contracting normally. How much metabolic acidosis develops depends on the number of minutes the subject exercises with the ischemic myocardium and the area of ischemia.

The breathing reserve is normal or high because the subject is forced to stop exercise from symptoms at a relatively low metabolic rate. The ventilatory equivalents are normal, manifesting relatively uniform ventilation-perfusion relationships in contrast to that observed in patients with chronic stable heart failure.

Myopathic Heart Disease (Table 4.5)

Because patients with cardiomyopathies have difficulty in transporting oxygen to the skeletal muscle, the increase in skeletal muscle $\dot{V}_{O_2}$ relative to the increase in work rate is usually slower than normal. This slowing, however, is not abrupt, in contrast to the slowing of $\dot{V}_{O_2}$ increase relative to work rate seen in patients who develop acute myocardial ischemia

TABLE 4.5. Discriminating Gas Exchange Measurements during Exercise in Chronic Heart Failure*

$\dot{V}_{O_2}$ increase with WR may *gradually* slow near peak $\dot{V}_{O_2}$
Reduced peak $\dot{V}_{O_2}$
Reduced *AT*
Reduced maximal O_2 pulse
Steep HR–$\dot{V}_{O_2}$ relationship with low maximal HR
Possible development of oscillatory breathing and gas exchange pattern of 45- to 90-second periods at low WR; oscillatory pattern is less evident as peak WR is reached
O_2 pulse increases paradoxically immediately post-exercise
Slow $\dot{V}_{O_2}$ kinetics and high $\Delta\dot{V}_{O_2}$ (6-3) above *AT* during constant work rate test
Increased V_D/V_T and slope of $\dot{V}_E$ vs $\dot{V}_{CO_2}$ are related to degree of severity

* See Table 3.2 for a definition of symbols.

during exercise. The failure to transport O_2 at the rate needed to regenerate the ATP used for muscular contraction makes it impossible to sustain muscular contraction; consequently the muscle fatigues and the subject must stop.

The peak $\dot{V}O_2$ is reduced consequent to the low cardiac output response to exercise. The AT is also commonly reduced. The peak O_2 pulse is low because of the reduced stroke volume. The heart rate increase is steep relative to the increase in $\dot{V}O_2$. The maximal heart rate may be reduced in these patients, however, because cardiomyopathy is commonly accompanied by chronotropic incompetence.

Because of the relatively low cardiac output response to exercise, mixed venous oxygen reaches its lowest value, and $(C(a − \bar{v})O_2)$ reaches its highest value, at a low work rate (11). Consequently, the O_2 pulse $(C(a − \bar{v})O_2 \times SV)$ reaches a constant value that is both low and occurs at an unusually low work rate compared to normal (Fig. 4.3). As described earlier, $\Delta\dot{V}O_2/\Delta WR$ is often reduced as the maximum work rate is approached. This can be viewed as a reflection of an increased contribution of energy from anaerobic metabolism, presumably because of impaired O_2 transport (12) or utilization (24).

Patients with heart failure have a high ventilatory requirement relative to the metabolic rate of the subject. Three factors might contribute to this high ventilatory requirement (see Chapter 2, "Determinants of the Ventilatory Requirement"). A metabolic acidosis occurs at lower work rates in heart failure patients compared to normal (1, 14, 15); this may become chronic and be evident at rest and be accompanied by a low $PaCO_2$ (17). A low $PaCO_2$ setpoint will necessitate a high minute ventilation that becomes more marked with exercise (25). Also, as described earlier, patients with chronic heart failure develop mismatching of ventilation relative to pulmonary perfusion, particularly of the high $\dot{V}A/\dot{Q}$ type, resulting in an increased VD/VT. The latter correlates with the degree of functional impairment in exercise performance (Fig. 4.4). This reduced gas exchange efficiency is a major factor accounting for the increased ventilatory drive in heart failure. Finally the increase in CO_2 produced at low work rates because of the buffering of lactic acid by HCO_3^- increases the acid load to the ventilatory system. All three factors dictate a larger breathing requirement to maintain arterial H^+ homeostasis in response to exercise (19) and likely contribute to the symptom of dyspnea in patients with chronic heart failure.

TABLE 4.6. Discriminating Gas Exchange Measurements in Valvular Heart Disease*

$\Delta\dot{V}O_2/\Delta WR$ commonly low
Low peak $\dot{V}O_2$
Low AT
Low and unchanging O_2 pulse
Steep linear increase in HR–$\dot{V}O_2$ relationship
Slow $\dot{V}O_2$ kinetics and high $\Delta\dot{V}O_2$ (6-3) during constant work rate test

* See Table 3.2 for a definition of symbols

A regular oscillatory pattern of breathing in which the magnitude of $\dot{V}O_2$, $\dot{V}CO_2$, and $\dot{V}E$ varies up and down with a period of approximately 45 to 90 seconds, depending on the individual, is often observed in some patients with chronic heart failure. This oscillatory pattern in gas exchange is more marked at lower work rates and tends to diminish as the subject nears the maximum work rate. Because the $\dot{V}O_2$ changes prior to the periodic changes in $\dot{V}CO_2$ and particularly $\dot{V}E$ (26), it is likely that flow through the pulmonary circulation is oscillating. This could account for oscillatory changes in arterial blood gases and pH which, in turn, oscillate ventilation. These changes in pulmonary blood flow likely reflect the behavior of the failing heart to the regular rhythmic changes in systemic arterial resistance originating from the vasomotor center. This behavior contrasts with that of the normal heart in which the forward output adjusts to changes in the venous return (pre-load), rather than to changes in systemic arterial resistance (after-load).

Valvular Heart Disease (Table 4.6)

Because the stroke volume is reduced in patients with valvular heart disease, the increase in $\dot{V}O_2$ relative to increase in work rate is usually reduced, i.e., low $\Delta\dot{V}O_2/\Delta WR$. Both the AT and the peak $\dot{V}O_2$ are reduced. The O_2 pulse is reduced and reaches a plateau value at a relatively low work rate (Fig. 4.3). Heart rate increases steeply relative to $\dot{V}O_2$, with the maximal heart rate achieved at a relatively low work rate. As with other cardiac conditions that lead to heart failure, $\dot{V}O_2$ kinetics are slow.

Congenital Heart Disease (Table 4.7)

Constant work rate tests are of particular value in patients with congenital heart disease. Because the

TABLE 4.7. Discriminating Gas Exchange Measurements during Exercise in Congenital Heart Disease*

Low peak $\dot{V}O_2$

Low *AT*

Phase I $\dot{V}O_2$ reduced when accompanied by increased pulmonary vascular or valvular resistance

Slow $\dot{V}O_2$ kinetics and high $\Delta\dot{V}O_2$ (6-3) during constant work rate test

Immediate hyperpnea and decrease in P_{ETCO_2} in cyanotic type; magnitude of increase in $\dot{V}E$ and decrease in P_{ETCO_2} related to size of right to left shunt

Immediate worsening of hypoxemia at start of exercise in cyanotic type

* See Table 3.2 for a definition of symbols.

increase in $\dot{V}O_2$ and $\dot{V}CO_2$ are determined by the increase in flow of O_2-desaturated, CO_2-rich blood through the pulmonary circulation, the pattern of increase in blood flow through the lungs can be measured from the O_2 uptake and CO_2 output kinetics. Thus, patients with pulmonary outflow obstruction (27) or patients with an increase in right to left shunt may fail to demonstrate a normal increase in blood flow at the start of exercise, resulting in a reduced or absent Phase I increase in $\dot{V}O_2$ and $\dot{V}CO_2$ (28). Phase II kinetics are also inappropriately slow, and the magnitude of Phase II becomes a relatively large portion of the total O_2 requirement at low work rates (29). A slowly rising $\dot{V}O_2$ is also evident at relatively low work rates during Phase III. Thus $\Delta\dot{V}O_2$ between 3 and 6 minutes of exercise is increased, indicating that lactate is increasing in response to the exercise. As in other cardiovascular disorders, the peak $\dot{V}O_2$ and *AT* are reduced.

A markedly elevated ventilatory response is noted at the start of exercise in patients with cyanotic congenital heart disease (30). In this disorder, the blood flowing through the lungs is hyperventilated to compensate for the blood that bypasses the lungs and enters the left side of the circulation through the right to left shunt. Hyperventilation of the blood passing through the lungs results in an immediate decrease in P_{ETCO_2} at the start of exercise, and this decrease is sustained until the start of recovery. $PaCO_2$ and pH remain relatively unchanged in patients with a right to left shunt, whereas the PO_2 decreases (30). The relatively unchanged acid-base status suggests that the respiratory control mechanism is sensitive to the regulation of arterial $[H^+]$, and is not greatly influenced by the high pulmonary artery pressures in this population of patients.

PULMONARY VASCULAR DISEASES (TABLE 4.8)

Causes of Increased Ventilation

Diseases of the pulmonary circulation, such as pulmonary emboli, idiopathic pulmonary fibrosis and idiopathic pulmonary vascular occlusion (Primary Pulmonary Hypertension), characteristically cause reduced perfusion to ventilated alveoli. Consequently, alveoli with unoccluded capillaries must accept a greater than normal perfusion and must be ventilated to a proportionately greater degree than normal to remove the metabolic CO_2 and to maintain $PaCO_2$ and pH at appropriate levels. The over-ventilation of the poorly perfused alveoli is wasted (alveolar dead space). Because minute ventilation is the sum of the "ideal" or effective alveolar ventilation and the physiologic dead space ventilation, minute ventilation is increased in patients with pulmonary vascular diseases at rest and to a greater degree during exercise. The increased dead space ventilation results in a high V_D/V_T and a persistently positive $P(a - _{ET})CO_2$.

An additional cause of increased ventilatory drive during exercise in patients with pulmonary vascular occlusive disease is arterial hypoxemia which gets worse during exercise. The decrease in PaO_2 stimulates the carotid bodies, the chemoreceptors that stimulate ventilation in the presence of arterial hypoxemia (31).

Causes of Exercise Arterial Hypoxemia

PaO_2 may be near normal at rest but manifest striking arterial oxyhemoglobin desaturation during exercise. Several mechanisms may play a role. First, the time available for diffusion equilibrium of O_2,

TABLE 4.8. Gas Exchange Abnormalities during Exercise in Diseases of the Pulmonary Circulation*

High $\dot{V}E$ at submaximal work rates

High V_D/V_T

Positive $P(a - _{ET})CO_2$ during exercise

PaO_2 decreases as WR is increased

$P(A - a)O_2$ increases with increasing WR

Low peak $\dot{V}O_2$

Low *AT*

$\Delta\dot{V}O_2/\Delta$WR more shallow toward maximum WR

Low O_2 pulse

* See Table 3.2 for a definition of symbols.

already shortened at rest by the reduced size of the functional capillary bed, is further shortened by the exercise-induced increase in pulmonary blood flow. In the normal capillary bed, the red cell residence time is about 0.8 seconds at rest (32). Despite increasing cardiac output as much as 5-fold at maximal exercise in the fit normal subject, the red cell residence time is still above 0.3 seconds (the time required for O_2 equilibration between capillary and alveolar space in a normal lung unit) because of recruitment of pulmonary capillaries (approximately doubling the resting capillary blood volume). However, in the presence of pulmonary vascular occlusive disease, functional capillary bed is destroyed and capillary bed reserved for recruitment to perform exercise is already recruited at rest. These phenomena necessarily result in critically short transit times in the pulmonary capillary during exercise. Consequently, the desaturated red cell arriving from the systemic venous circulation can not remain in the reduced pulmonary capillary bed long enough for diffusion equilibrium of O_2 between the alveolar gas and red cell, especially if pulmonary capillary blood velocity increases in response to exercise. This pathophysiological state is probably the most common cause of worsening arterial hypoxemia as $\dot{V}O_2$ increases during exercise.

Another cause of hypoxemia during exercise in patients with increased pulmonary vascular resistance is the development of a right to left shunt resulting from the opening of a potentially patent foramen ovale. Approximately 20% of the population is thought to have an "unsealed" foramen ovale. In the healthy subject, this is of no importance because left atrial pressure is normally higher than right atrial pressure and blood does not shunt in either direction. However, if pulmonary vascular resistance is increased so that the right ventricle cannot pump the venous return into the pulmonary circulation as fast as it is delivered (right ventricular failure), right ventricular end-diastolic pressure and, therefore, right atrial pressure will rise. If the right atrial pressure exceeds that of the left atrium, some of the right atrial flow will pass through the unsealed foramen ovale, creating a right to left shunt. This can cause marked exercise hypoxemia and be only evident during exercise. The development of a right to left shunt can easily be identified by repeating the exercise test while the subject breathes 100% oxygen. If this shunt develops, the arterial PO_2 should decrease well below that predicted during O_2 breathing (> 550 mmHg). The PaO_2 will decrease approximately 100 mmHg for every 3 to 5% of

cardiac output passing through the right to left shunt.

Finally, hypoxemia from low $\dot{V}A/\dot{Q}$ lung units is common in acute pulmonary embolism. However, low $\dot{V}A/\dot{Q}$ lung units are a less important cause of arterial hypoxemia in patients with chronic pulmonary vascular occlusive disease. High $\dot{V}A/\dot{Q}$ lung units predominate in chronic pulmonary vascular occlusive disease in patients without airflow obstruction.

Effect on Systemic Hemodynamics

Pulmonary vascular occlusion disease causes a hemodynamic stenosis in the central circulation, making it difficult for the right ventricle to deliver blood to the left atrium at a rate sufficient to meet the increased cardiac output needed for exercise. Because the cardiac output increase in response to exercise is reduced, the AT and peak $\dot{V}O_2$ and O_2 pulse are reduced in patients with pulmonary vascular disease, similar to that seen in patients with heart failure. However, additional physiological measurements during exercise which distinguish primary pulmonary vascular occlusive diseases (including those secondary to pulmonary fibrosis) from primary heart disease are a very high physiological dead space, high ventilatory equivalents for CO_2 and O_2, and abnormalities in blood gases including a high $P(A - a)O_2$ and a positive $P(a - ET)CO_2$. Thus, physiologic measurements during exercise are particularly helpful in diagnosing chronic pulmonary vascular occlusive disease. The abnormalities are those associated with a low cardiac output state and disturbances in gas exchange, especially during exercise (33). Abnormal ventilatory mechanics are a less common cause of exercise intolerance in patients with pulmonary fibrosis (33).

TABLE 4.9. Discriminating Measurements during Exercise in Patients with Obstructive Lung Disease*

Low peak $\dot{V}O_2$
High VD/VT
Positive $P(a - ETCO_2)$ during exercise
Usually high $P(A - a)O_2$
Increased O_2 cost of work
Failure to develop respiratory compensation for metabolic acidosis
Low breathing reserve
High heart rate reserve
Abnormal (trapezoidal) expiratory flow pattern

* See Table 3.2 for a definition of symbols.

TABLE 4.10. Effect of Airway Obstruction Due to Emphysema on Average Blood Lactate Concentration, Minute Ventilation, and Work Rate at an O_2 Consumption of Approximately 1.0 L/min

$FEV_1(L)$	$\dot{V}O_2(L/min\ STPD)$	WR (watts)	$\dot{V}E$ (L/min BTPS)	$\dot{V}E/\dot{V}O_2$	La^- (mmol/L)	$La^-/\dot{V}O_2$
1.02	0.90	35	35	39	3.03	3.37*
1.80	1.05	34	36	34	2.95	2.80**
Normal	~1.0	50	25	25	<1.0	1.0†

* Mean data from reference 34.
** Mean data from reference 35.
† Mean data from chapter 2.
FEV_1 = forced expiratory volume in 1 second; WR = work rate; $\dot{V}E$ = minute ventilation; La^- = blood lactate concentration; STPD = standard temperature and pressure, dry; BTPS = body temperature, ambient pressure, saturated.

VENTILATORY DISORDERS

Obstructive Lung Diseases (Table 4.9)

Patients with chronic obstructive pulmonary diseases (COPD), including emphysema, chronic bronchitis, bronchial asthma, and mixtures of these disease entities are usually limited during exercise by dyspnea or fatigue. Dyspnea generally results from difficulty in achieving the ventilation needed to eliminate the additional CO_2 generated during exercise at the level of Pa_{CO_2} regulated by the patient (patient's P_{CO_2} setpoint) and because many of these patients are highly sedentary and develop a lactic acidosis at a relatively low work rate (Table 4.10).

Ventilatory Capacity–Ventilatory Requirement Imbalance

Figure 4.5 conceptualizes the pathophysiologic features leading to dyspnea in patients with COPD. The two major contributing factors are the decreased ventilatory capacity and the increased ventilatory requirement. In emphysema, the decreased ventilatory capacity is due to increased airflow obstruction combined with reduced lung elastic recoil, whereas in chronic bronchitis and asthma, the decreased ventilatory capacity is due to increased airway resistance.

The increased ventilatory requirement in patients with COPD is primarily due to inefficient ventilation of the lungs consequent to the mismatching of ventilation to perfusion; i.e., certain regions of the lungs are hypoventilated, whereas others are hyperventilated. This has the effect of increasing the fraction of the breath that is wasted (increased $\dot{V}D/\dot{V}T$), thereby requiring an increased ventilation to eliminate the

CO_2 produced by the patient to maintain the arterial P_{CO_2} at its set-point (see Fig. 2.38).

As shown in Figure 4.6, ambulatory patients with stable obstructive lung disease regulate Pa_{CO_2} at a reasonably constant level despite increasing work rates. However, ventilatory compensation for the exercise-induced lactic acidosis rarely occurs in these patients (see Fig. 3.20B and cases of patients with COPD in Chap. 9). With severe airway obstruction, Pa_{CO_2} often increases, worsening the exercise acidosis (17). Hypoxemia results from the underventilation of perfused lung units. Despite increasing ventilatory drive through the carotid body chemoreceptors (31), the hypoxic stimulus rarely is sufficient to induce a respiratory alkalosis in these patients. Although regulation of Pa_{O_2} is less precise

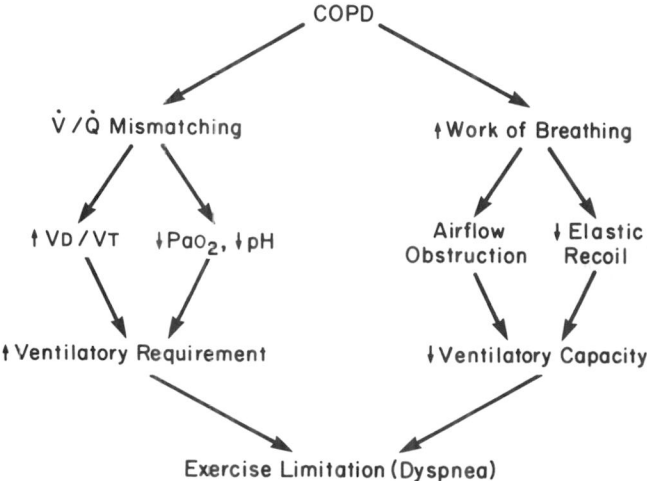

FIGURE 4.5. Factors that play a role in exercise limitation and dyspnea in patients with chronic obstructive pulmonary disease (COPD). These patients have both an increase in ventilatory requirement to perform exercise and a reduction in ventilatory capacity. See text for a detailed discussion of each of the factors shown. $\dot{V}/\dot{Q}$ = ventilation-perfusion ratio; $\dot{V}D/\dot{V}T$ = dead space-tidal volume ratio.

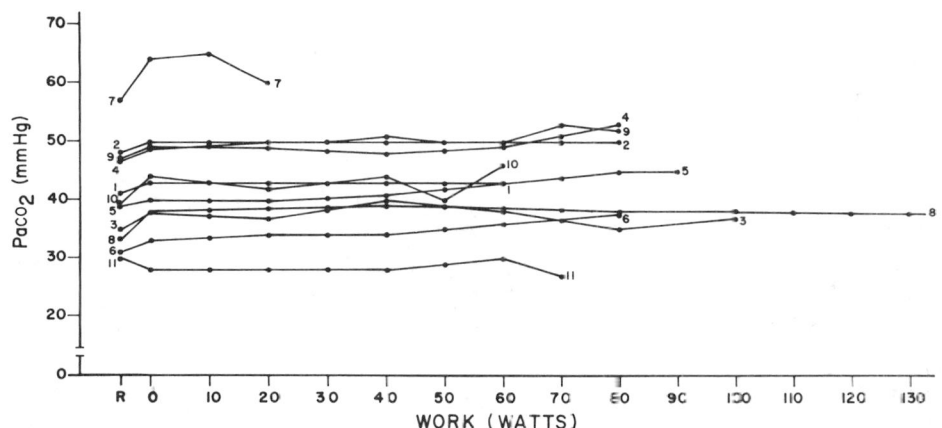

FIGURE 4.6   PaCO₂ as related to work rate in 11 patients with stable chronic airflow obstruction (each point is a different work rate). The numbers on each curve identify the patient.

than PaCO₂ in these patients (Fig. 4.7), PaO₂ usually does not fall to extremely low levels, even at the patient's maximum work rate. The shape of the oxyhemoglobin dissociation curve generally allows arterial O₂ content to be maintained at satisfactory levels despite a moderate decrease in PaO₂.

The $P(A - a)O_2$ is usually increased as a consequence of the perfusion of relatively poorly ventilated airspaces. The increase in $P(A - a)O_2$ is usually not systematic with increasing work rate, in contrast to patients with primary pulmonary vascular diseases or pulmonary fibrosis. $P(a - ET)CO_2$ is also increased, reflecting over-ventilation relative to perfusion. But, $P(a - ET)CO_2$ remains relatively constant and elevated as work rate is increased, rather than decreasing and becoming negative as in normal subjects (see Chapter 6).

Although one may predict that the O₂ cost of breathing will be increased in patients with COPD, this has been difficult to demonstrate. That these patients do have an increased metabolic cost becomes evident, however, when one examines the work that could be performed for a given $\dot{V}O_2$ (Table 4.10). We found that the work output was reduced at a $\dot{V}O_2$ of 1 L/min in two studies on patients with COPD. Moreover, patients with COPD may develop a lactic acidosis at a relatively low work rate (34, 35) (Table 4.10). This is most likely due to the sedentary life style of these patients. When training these patients, their lactate level for a given work rate and the ventilatory requirement for exercise decreased (35).

Dyspnea depends on a balance between how much air *must* be breathed to keep pace with metabolism and how much *can* be breathed. Patients with COPD, because of their increase in VD/VT, low work rate lactic acidosis and hypoxemia, must breathe more to maintain blood gases and pH, but they cannot breathe as much as a normal subject. Although many approaches have been taken to determine if patients with COPD are ventilatory limited, the breathing reserve has served this role very well. The maximal voluntary ventilation (MVV) measured at rest is a reasonable measure of the patient's ventilatory capacity. Work tasks requiring ventilation rates in excess of this value cannot be sustained. Thus, the breathing reserve, defined as the difference between the MVV and $\dot{V}E$ at the maximum level of exercise that the subject could perform, is decreased to values close to zero in patients with COPD (Fig. 4.8). This contrasts with the large ventilatory reserve at the end of exercise found in most normal subjects (36–38) and in patients with heart disease.

Examining the expiratory flow pattern can be use-

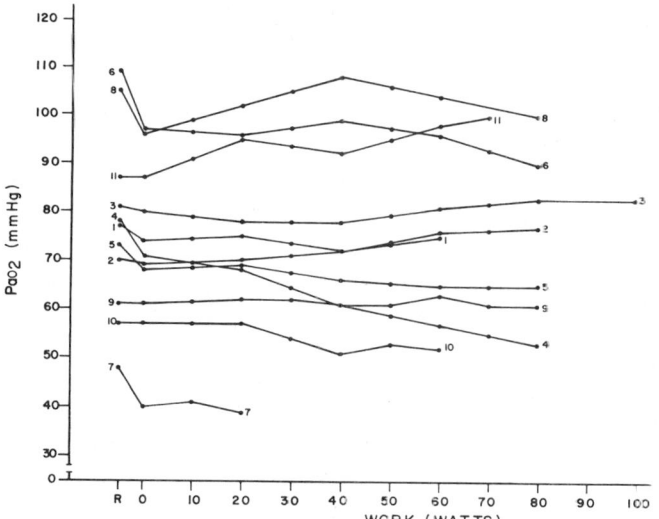

FIGURE 4.7.   PaO₂ as related to increase in work rate for the same 11 patients shown in Figure 4.6 (each point is a different work rate). The numbers on each curve identify the patient and allow cross-correlation with each patient's PaCO₂ shown in Figure 4.6.

ful in documenting airflow limitation. Typically, as shown in Figure 3.15, the pattern has an early expiratory peak and then a sustained expiratory flow until the point of inhalation, giving a trapezoidal appearance to the recorded pattern. No apneic pause occurs at the end of exhalation, in contrast to the finding in normal subjects when work rate is not excessively hard. After effective bronchodilatation, the expiratory flow pattern normalizes with the peak flow moving to the middle of the expiratory phase of respiration (see Fig. 3.15).

When patients develop air-trapping with exercise, the FRC increases as evidenced by a reduction in the inspiratory capacity. The inspiratory capacity can be measured during exercise by instructing the patient to take a maximum breath after a normal exhalation. This can be done without difficulty after a little practice in patients with obstructive lung disease and normal subjects. In contrast to the decrease in inspiratory capacity in patients with airflow obstruction, normal subjects have an increase in inspiratory capacity suggesting that their FRC had decreased during exercise.

Whereas the peak $\dot{V}O_2$ is reduced in patients with uncomplicated obstructive lung disease, the $\dot{V}O_2$ usually does not decrease its rate of rise as work rate is increased in response to a progressively increasing work rate test, in contrast to the frequent finding in patients with circulatory limitation. This is because ambulatory patients with stable obstructive lung

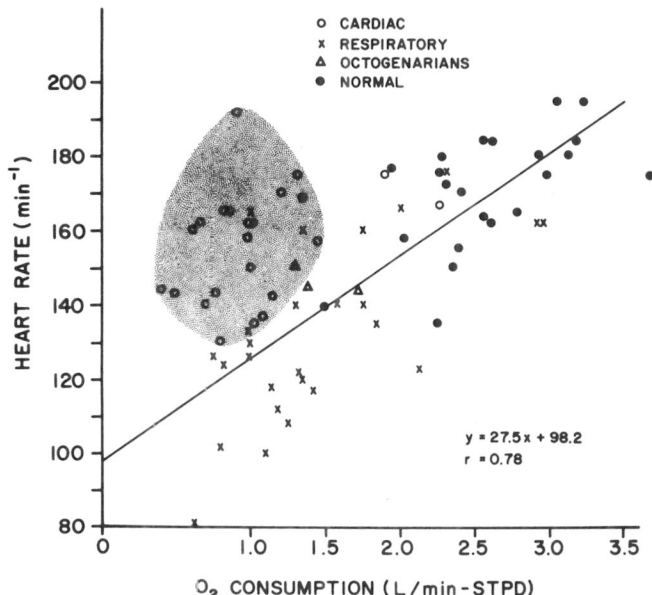

FIGURE 4.9. Heart rate at maximal exercise for normal subjects, octogenarians, and patients with chronic respiratory disease or cardiac disease. The normal subjects reach a higher maximum heart rate and $\dot{V}O_2$. Note that the octogenarians fall on the same slope as the younger normal subjects, although their maximum heart rate and maximum oxygen uptake are less. Similarly, the patients with respiratory defects have a still lower maximum oxygen uptake and heart rate. The cardiac patients (stippled area) have a higher maximum heart rate relative to the maximum O_2 uptake than that of the other subjects. (Reprinted with permission from Wasserman K, Whipp BJ. Exercise physiology in health and disease (State of the art). Am Rev Resp Dis 1975;112:219–249.)

disease are usually more limited in their ability to eliminate CO_2 (ventilatory limitation) than in their ability to make O_2 available to the mitochondria.

Often, patients with COPD develop a lactic acidosis at relatively low work rates because of their relatively untrained state (Table 4.10). Other patients with more severe airflow obstruction may not be able to exercise sufficiently to reach their AT, however, and they may not develop a lactic acidosis during exercise. Whether they reach their AT, and at what $\dot{V}O_2$, may be important clues as to the relative value of exercise training in rehabilitation of the patient. Those patients with a significant lactic acidosis at a relatively low work rate should benefit from skeletal muscle training, reduction in the magnitude of lactic acid increase and, therefore, reduced ventilatory drive.

The heart rate at maximum work rate is generally low (high heart rate reserve) (Fig. 4.9), but maximum heart rate can be increased if the patient's maximum work rate can be improved through O_2 breathing or bronchodilatation. In contrast to cardiac disor-

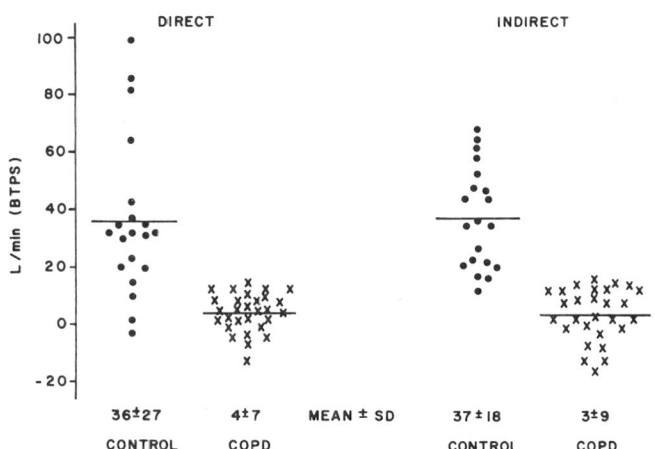

FIGURE 4.8. Breathing reserve (MVV—maximum $\dot{V}E$) for a group of normal subjects and a group of patients with stable chronic obstructive pulmonary disease (COPD). The values under each column show the mean ± standard deviation. Measurements are made using the directly measured MVV and the indirectly measured MVV calculated by multiplying FEV_1 by 40. Note that the breathing reserve in patients with COPD is small and the standard deviation is narrow, reflecting the importance of airflow limitation in determining exercise intolerance.

ders, O_2-pulse continues to increase normally with increasing work rate, although the final absolute values are usually reduced (see Fig. 4.3).

O_2 Transport–O_2 Requirement Imbalance

To sustain exercise, ATP must be regenerated, aerobically. Failure of the left ventricular output to meet the muscle O_2 demand for ATP regeneration at the rate required for the increasing work rate, will force the patient to stop exercise due to muscular fatigue. An imbalance in the circulatory transport of O_2 to muscles and its requirement, will be reflected in a decreased peak $\dot{V}O_2$ and AT and a reduced rate of increase in $\dot{V}O_2$ as work rate increases. The following mechanisms underlie the failure of left ventricular output to keep pace with the increased O_2 requirement of a progressively increasing work rate test:

1. Positive intrathoracic pressure. Large positive pressures develop in the chest during exhalation in patients with poor lung elastic recoil and hyperinflation (patients with emphysema). Thus left ventricular output may be impaired during exercise because of the development of high intrathoracic pressures during exhalation as expiratory muscles contract to accelerate exhaling respired gases (partial Valsalva maneuver) to achieve the increased breathing rate required to maintain arterial blood gas homeostasis. These high intrathoracic pressures impede venous return to the heart and probably account for the relatively low exercise cardiac output observed in emphysema patients.

2. Increased pulmonary vascular resistance. Increased pulmonary vascular resistance might also cause left ventricular output to be inadequate to meet the increased O_2 needed for aerobic regeneration of ATP during exercise. Many patients with emphysema have significantly elevated pulmonary vascular resistance that, while not limiting at rest, prevents the right ventricle from increasing blood flow through the pulmonary circulation at the rate needed to meet the muscle O_2 requirement during exercise.

3. Primary heart disease and reduced arterial O_2 content. Patients with lung diseases might also have primary heart disease that limits the ability of the circulation to increase O_2 transport at the rate needed to perform exercise. Other mechanisms that contribute to the impairment of O_2 flow to the muscles, such as reduced arterial O_2 content due to reduced PaO_2, anemia and carboxyhemoglobinemia, when combined with the pathophysiology of COPD, might cause severe symptoms in patients with only moderate or even mild disease.

Physiological Markers of Inadequate O_2 Transport

A failure for the left ventricular output to meet the muscle O_2 demand is likely to force the patient to stop exercise, prematurely, because the rate of ATP is not able to be regenerated at the rate required for the increasing work rate. In the presence of reduced O_2 transport, the AT and $\Delta\dot{V}O_2/\Delta WR$ as well as the peak $\dot{V}O_2$ are likely to be reduced. Thus $\Delta\dot{V}O_2/\Delta WR$ will be below the expected rate of 10 ml/min/W, and $\dot{V}CO_2$ will be inappropriately high relative to $\dot{V}O_2$.

While respiratory mechanics are significantly impaired in COPD patients, it is imperative to evaluate exercise gas exchange in these patients in order to determine if reduced O_2 transport is caused by impaired ventilatory mechanics or metabolic changes with increased ventilatory drive characteristic of heart failure. The increased ventilatory drive in these patients results from the increased H^+ accompanying the increased lactate as well as the CO_2 released by the increased rate of buffering lactic acid.

Restrictive Lung Diseases (Table 4.11)

Patients with pulmonary fibrosis generally are exercise limited because of dyspnea and/or fatigue. Study of the pathophysiology of these patients reveals that they have disturbed lung mechanics and a reduction in the functional pulmonary capillary bed (Fig. 4.10). Hansen and Wasserman (33), in a study of a population of patients with restrictive lung disease of mixed etiology, found that most of the patients were limited by their inability to increase pulmonary blood flow adequately in response to exercise (right pathway leading to exercise limitation in Fig. 4.10). Not only did their patients have a reduced peak $\dot{V}O_2$, but the AT was also commonly reduced. In contrast to COPD patients,

TABLE 4.11. Discriminating Measurements during Exercise in Patients with Restrictive Lung Diseases*

Low peak $\dot{V}O_2$
High V_T/IC
Breathing frequency > 50 at max WR
Low breathing reserve
High V_D/V_T
High $P(a - ET)CO_2$
PaO_2 decreases and $P(A - a)O_2$ increases as WR is increased
$\Delta\dot{V}O_2/\Delta WR$ is reduced

*See Table 3.2 for a definition of symbols.

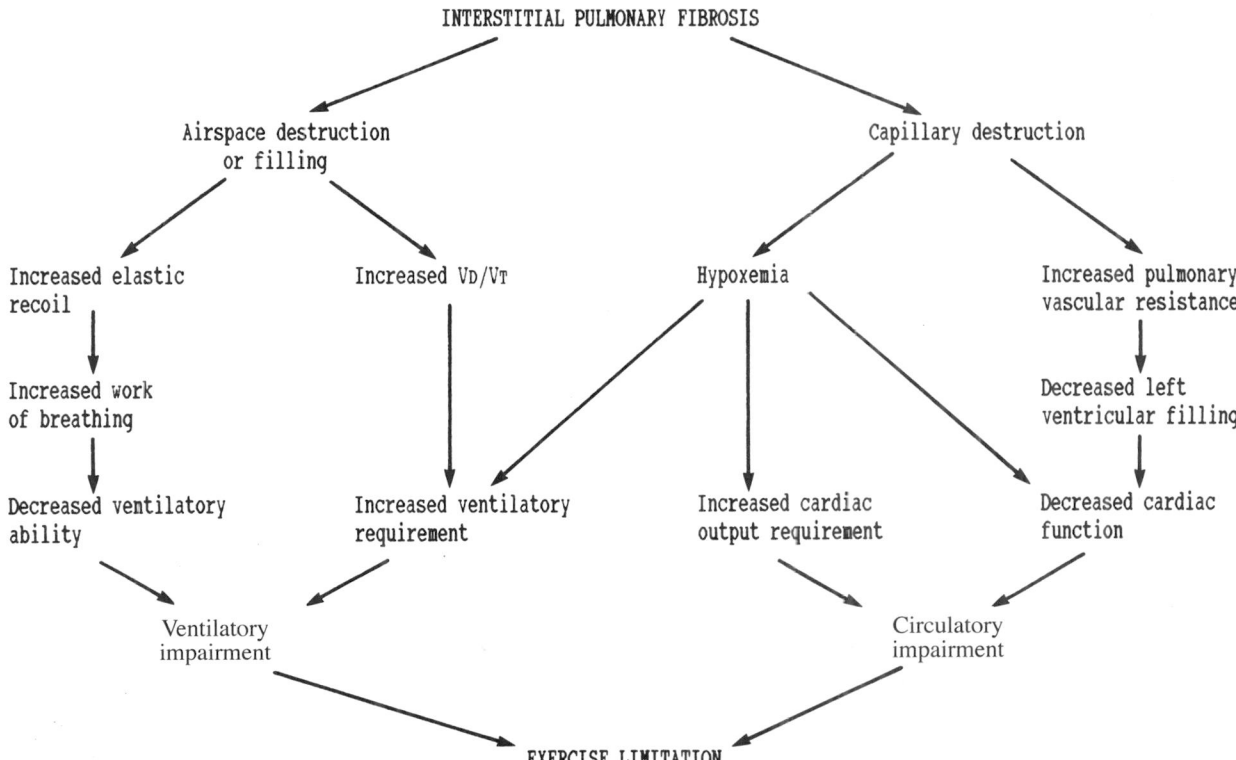

FIGURE 4.10.   Pathophysiology of exercise limitation in patients with interstitial lung disease and idiopathic pulmonary fibrosis. (Reprinted with permission from Hansen JE, Wasserman K. Pathophysiology of activity limitation in patients with interstitial lung disease. Chest 1996;109:1566–1576.)

$\Delta\dot{V}O_2/\Delta WR$ was reduced with the slope of the relationship becoming more shallow as peak $\dot{V}O_2$ was approached.

Pulmonary fibrosis of the idiopathic type (IPF) develops from chronic lung inflammation (39). The pathologic features are usually nonuniform so some acini, including their blood supply, are completely replaced by scar tissue. In contrast neighboring units less or uninvolved may undergo compensatory hyperinflation. From the point of view of lung mechanics, the net effect of the pathophysiology of IPF is a reduction in the total number of functioning acini and, consequently, a relatively poorly compliant, small lung (40). Whereas both the total lung capacity and its subcompartments are reduced, the predominant reduction is that of the inspiratory capacity. Thus, the extent to which the tidal volume can increase with exercise is limited, and the patient must increase breathing frequency to a value higher than normal to meet the ventilatory requirement for exercise. Consequently, the V_T/IC ratio is high and approaches 1, and the breathing frequency at maximum exercise often exceeds 50 breaths/min. Ventilation at the maximum work rate may approach the MVV, if the patient is not limited by

inability to increase cardiac output because of the restricted pulmonary capillary bed. However, often, the pathophysiological picture is mixed, reflecting both a failure to increase $\dot{V}O_2$ appropriate for the work rate performed, and an increased ventilatory response due to exercise lactic acidosis, hypoxemia, and increased V_D/V_T.

Early in the pathophysiologic development of interstitial lung diseases, it appears as though the pulmonary capillary bed is functionally reduced and normal recruitment of more capillary bed in response to exercise fails to occur. This restricted capillary bed results in a shortened red cell transit time in the pulmonary capillaries as the exercise work rate is increased. The progressive reduction of the red cell residence time in the pulmonary capillary, as work rate and cardiac output increase, results in a systematic decrease in PaO_2 as $\dot{V}O_2$ increases similar to that seen in pulmonary vascular occlusive disease. This systematic change in PaO_2 is usually not seen in obstructive lung disease (see Fig. 4.6). Low $\dot{V}A/\dot{Q}$ ratios might also contribute to the hypoxemia in patients with pulmonary fibrosis (39). The ventilatory response of patients with pulmonary fibrosis is steep, partly because of a reduced $PaCO_2$

set-point in some subjects, but mainly because of an increased V_D/V_T in all subjects. Worsening hypoxemia as work rate is increased, elevated dead space ventilation caused by nonuniform ventilation-perfusion ratios, increased lactic acidosis from impaired systemic O_2 transport and a reduced ability to expand the lungs leading to rapid, shallow breathing, contribute to dyspnea in these patients (Fig. 4.10). In addition, exercise fatigue might be brought about by the inability to provide O_2 to the muscles at a rate sufficient for the exercise work rate performed.

Pulmonary alveolar proteinosis is a good example of exercise hypoxemia that is primarily due to a diffusion defect (41). This disease results in alveolar filling by a semi-solid proteinaceous material. Pulmonary fibrosis is minimal or nonexistent. Frequently, the vital capacity and total lung capacity are only slightly reduced, and FEV_1 is normal. Because the mean path length from lung gas to capillaries is increased considerably in this disorder by a medium unfavorable for permeation by O_2, this diffusion barrier limits the mass flow of O_2 into the pulmonary capillaries. During exercise, when red cell transit time in the capillary bed is reduced and its residence time shortened, less time is available for diffusion equilibrium. Thus the major findings in this disorder are a systematic decrease in PaO_2 and increase in $P(A - a)O_2$ with increasing work rate (42).

Chest Wall (Respiratory Pump) Disorders (Table 4.12)

Disorders of the respiratory pump include muscle weakness, chest deformities, rigidity of the thoracic cage (as in ankylosing spondylitis), muscle and motor nerve disorders, and extreme obesity. Patients with these disorders, like those with restrictive pulmonary disorders, have a limited ability to increase V_T. Although their lungs are essentially normal, the maximal intrapleural pressure available to expand the lungs is insufficient to allow V_T to increase normally as work rate is increased. Therefore, to obtain the increase in $\dot{V}_E$ required for exercise, these patients must predominantly increase breathing frequency.

The reduced maximum $\dot{V}O_2$ defines the degree of exercise limitation. The $\dot{V}O_2$ increases normally with increasing work rate. Because the lung parenchyma is essentially normal, PaO_2 is usually normal and does not decrease as the work rate is increased. The breathing reserve is low at the termination of exercise, a characteristic of conditions in which the breathing mechanics limit maximal exercise performance. Because of the impaired ventilatory mechanics, these patients usually do not develop normal ventilatory compensation for the lactic acidosis of exercise. Heart rate reserve is high at the maximal exercise tolerated because the cardiovascular system is not fully stressed due to the breathing limitation.

DEFECTS IN HEMOGLOBIN CONTENT AND QUALITY (TABLE 4.13)

As shown in Figure 1.1, a considerable increase in O_2 flow from the atmosphere to the mitochondria is essential for the normal exercise response. This function is critically dependent on the ability of the circulation to carry a large quantity of O_2, as well as to pick up O_2 in the lungs and unload O_2 in the exercising muscles. Therefore, it is appropriate to consider how changes in the properties of blood might impair O_2 delivery to the mitochondria and thereby reduce exercise capacity.

The patient with a reduced blood O_2 carrying capacity commonly has a relatively high cardiac output, with a higher than expected heart rate for a given work rate, i.e., a relative tachycardia. The stroke volume is normal or even increased, in contrast to patients with cardiac diseases and disorders of the pulmonary circulation. Because the arterial

---

TABLE 4.12. Discriminating Measurements during Exercise in Patients with Chest Wall Disorders*

Low peak $\dot{V}O_2$
High V_T/IC
High breathing frequency
Low breathing reserve
High heart rate reserve

* See Table 3.2 for a definition of symbols.

TABLE 4.13. Discriminating Measurements during Exercise in Patients with Anemia, Increased COHb, or Conditions Associated with a Low P_{50}*

Low peak $\dot{V}O_2$
Low AT
Low O_2 pulse
Normal V_D/V_T, $P(a - ET)CO_2$ and $P(A - a)O_2$

* See Table 3.2 for a definition of symbols.

O_2 content is low, the potential for the arterial-venous O_2 difference to increase in response to exercise is reduced. Consequently, the maximum O_2 pulse (product of stroke volume and $C(a - \bar{v})O_2$) is reduced in patients with reduced arterial O_2 content. As in other disorders of O_2 flow, the maximum $\dot{V}O_2$ and AT are also likely to be reduced. Measurements that reflect ventilation-perfusion mismatching are normal. In addition to the above changes in gas exchange evident in patients with reduced arterial blood O_2 content, specific mechanisms of reduced arterial O_2 content are described below.

Anemia

Because anemia results in a reduced blood O_2 carrying capacity, it compromises O_2 delivery to the mitochondria (see Fig. 4.1). With anemia, the systemic capillary PO_2 falls more rapidly than normal during the transit of blood from artery to vein (see Fig. 2.14). Thus, the diffusion gradient of O_2 from the blood to the mitochondria decreases more rapidly than in non-anemic conditions. Consequently, a critically low capillary PO_2 may be reached at a reduced $\dot{V}O_2$. This necessitates invoking anaerobic mechanisms for ATP generation with increasing lactate concentrations and metabolic acidosis taking place at a lower $\dot{V}O_2$ than normal (see Fig. 2.1).

Subjects with anemia alone commonly experience breathlessness with increased ventilatory drive during exercise. Whereas the arterial O_2 content is low, the arterial PO_2 is not reduced. Because the carotid bodies respond to arterial PO_2 and not O_2 content the reduced O_2 content is not itself the cause of the increased ventilatory drive and therefore cannot account for the symptom of breathlessness. More likely, the breathlessness and increased ventilatory drive with exercise in the more anemic patient are the consequence of the metabolic acidosis that accompanies the patient's low anaerobic threshold. The acidemia results in an increased ventilatory drive (mediated by the carotid bodies) and a relatively high minute ventilation at a low maximum work rate.

Left-Shifted Oxyhemoglobin Dissociation Curve

Conditions that cause a leftward shift in the oxyhemoglobin dissociation curve (reduced P_{50}), such as some hemoglobinopathies, a decrease in 2,3-DPG due to a defect in red cell metabolism, an increase in carboxyhemoglobin, or increased glycosylated hemoglobin found in poorly controlled diabetic pa-

tients, should cause the capillary blood PO_2 to decrease more rapidly than normal for a given O_2 extraction across the circulation (43). Thus, at a reduced work rate, the PO_2 difference between capillary and mitochondrion may reach a critical value below which it cannot fall despite an increased bioenergetic demand for O_2. Consequently, O_2 flow through the exercising muscle does not provide all the O_2 needed by the mitochondria to support ATP regeneration aerobically, and anaerobic regeneration of ATP will be required to support the energy requirement. Exercise studies on patients with a left-shifted hemoglobinopathy support the concept that these disorders lead to anaerobic glycolysis and increased net lactate production at reduced work rates (44).

Carboxyhemoglobinemia and Cigarette Smoking

Carboxyhemoglobinemia from exposure to carbon monoxide results in a reduced O_2 carrying capacity without the reduced blood viscosity found in anemia. When the carboxyhemoglobin level is increased, arterial oxygen content is reduced. In addition, carbon monoxide causes a leftward shift in the oxyhemoglobin dissociation curve. This reduces the peak $\dot{V}O_2$ and AT (45–47). Cigarette smoking adversely affects exercise tolerance by its effects on the blood, the cardiovascular system, and the lungs. Heart rate, blood pressure, and the double product (heart rate times systolic blood pressure) are increased when one performs exercise immediately after smoking (47). Ventilation-perfusion relationships become abnormal, as evident from the increased $P(a - ET)CO_2$ during exercise. The effect of short-term smoking on airway resistance was not detected in normal young male subjects who did, however, experience acute cardiovascular changes and changes consistent with worsened $\dot{V}A/\dot{Q}$ matching immediately after cigarette smoking (47).

CHRONIC METABOLIC ACIDOSIS (TABLE 4.14)

Chronic metabolic acidosis can result from poorly controlled diabetes, chronic renal failure, renal tubular acidosis, or from certain drugs, such as a carbonic anhydrase inhibitor (acetazolamide) in the treatment of glaucoma. These conditions reduce blood $[HCO_3^-]$. To restore normal arterial blood and central chemoreceptor pH, ventilation is stimulated by H^+ until arterial PCO_2 is reduced to a new lower PCO_2 set-point (25, 48). The magnitude of the in-

TABLE 4.14. Discriminating Measurements during Exercise in Patients with a Chronic Metabolic Acidosis*

Low [HCO_3^-]
Steep $\dot{V}E/\dot{V}CO_2$ relationship
Normal $P(A - a)O_2$ and $P(a - ET)CO_2$
Normal VD/VT
Low breathing reserve

---

* See Table 3.2 for a definition of symbols.

crease in ventilation is approximately proportional to the reduction in [HCO_3^-] and $PaCO_2$. However, during exercise, the $\dot{V}CO_2$ increases. Thus to maintain the lower $PaCO_2$, ventilation must increase proportionately. The higher the work rate, the higher the additional ventilation. The higher ventilatory requirement to maintain the arterial pH when [HCO_3^-] is reduced leads to an apparent increase in "sensitivity" of the respiratory control mechanisms.

The presence of a chronic metabolic acidosis before exercise begins is evident from the resting arterial blood gases. The [HCO_3^-] and $PaCO_2$ are reduced and pH is only slightly reduced or normal. During exercise, $\dot{V}E$ increases proportionally with the increase in CO_2 production. Because the slope of the $\dot{V}E-\dot{V}CO_2$ relationship is steeper the lower the $PaCO_2$, the effect of the metabolic acidosis on ventilation is amplified progressively as work rate is increased (see Fig. 2.37). Without measuring arterial blood gases, a relatively steep slope relationship between $\dot{V}E$ and $\dot{V}CO_2$ during exercise, with R in the normal range, signifies either chronic hyperventilation or increased VD/VT. Arterial blood gas and pH measurements differentiate these two potential causes of the high ventilatory response.

By itself, chronic metabolic acidosis is not a prominent cause of dyspnea, but in conjunction with other diseases such as obstructive airways disease, it may lower the CO_2 set-point to such a marked degree that the ventilatory requirement to perform a given work rate may exceed the subject's MVV. In this case, the dyspnea sensation would be high. Correction of the metabolic acidosis might reduce the ventilatory requirement below the subject's MVV and relieve the dyspnea sensation.

MUSCLE DISORDERS AND ENDOCRINE ABNORMALITIES

Little information is available concerning the metabolic cost of exercise in patients with primary muscle disorders. Because of reduced motor efficiency, patients with neuromuscular disorders with accompanying spasticities and motor incoordination presumably have an increased O_2 requirement for performing physical work. We have not had the opportunity to evaluate these patients in the exercise laboratory.

Certain muscle enzyme deficiencies limit exercise performance. For example, patients with inability to use muscle glycogen because of myophosphorylase deficiency (McArdle's syndrome) (49) or other disease of the glycolytic pathway (50) are unable to exercise to work levels that require anaerobic mechanisms to supplement the energy generated by aerobic mechanisms. These patients experience severe muscle pain and the release of myoglobin and creatine kinase from muscle when attempting to exercise at levels that normally induce a lactic acidosis. The $\dot{V}O_2$-work rate relationship (work efficiency) appears to be normal for work rates below the level that induces pain in these patients (51). The maximum work capacity of these patients is limited to work rates near the anaerobic threshold of normal sedentary subjects. Thus, their peak $\dot{V}O_2$ is of the order of 1 L/min. Their ventilatory response to exercise is generally normal (52), although it has also been reported to be high (53). The heart rate and cardiac output responses of these patients are inordinately high for the metabolic rate, and the arterial-venous O_2 difference at maximal work rate is low (54). Studies suggest that the failure to extract O_2 normally results from the failure of muscles to produce lactic acid. The reduced production of H^+ ions does not allow the full rightward shift in the oxyhemoglobin dissociation curve in the capillary bed that allows the normal O_2 unloading from hemoglobin (Bohr effect). The Bohr effect is needed for the normal maximal O_2 extraction from blood during exercise (55).

Patients with mitochondrial electron transport chain defects develop lactic acidosis at exceptionally low work rates (56, 57). In contrast with myophosphorylase deficient patients, however, the gas exchange abnormalities accompanying these metabolic defects have not been well studied. Nevertheless, it is recognized that the gas exchange abnormalities likely differ from those seen with defects in the glycolytic pathway and resemble those found in patients with heart failure, demonstrating increased CO_2 output relative to O_2 uptake (56).

Diabetes mellitus affects large arteries (atherosclerosis), small blood vessels, and capillaries. When the disease is poorly controlled, diabetic patients also have a leftward shift in the oxyhemoglobin dissociation curve (glycosylated hemoglobin). Any one of these abnormalities could cause a reduction in AT and $\dot{V}O_2$max. Studies in diabetic children suggest that the AT and peak $\dot{V}O_2$ are reduced even when the patient's diabetes is under good control (58–60).

Poorly regulated diabetics increase their use of fatty acids for energy. During exercise, use of fatty acids by muscle, in contrast to the normally preferred carbohydrate, should make the poorly-controlled patient less efficient, metabolically. Figure 2.3 illustrates the effect of the proportion of carbohydrate to fatty acid substrate on metabolic efficiency with respect to O_2 consumption.

The ventilatory response to exercise has been demonstrated to be increased and the $PaCO_2$ reduced in women during the progestational phase of the menstrual cycle. The effect of this increased ventilatory drive on maximal exercise performance in women is unknown.

PSYCHOGENIC CAUSES OF EXERCISE LIMITATION AND DYSPNEA

Anxiety

Anxiety reactions occasionally cause dyspnea during exercise. One manifestation of anxiety is intense hyperventilation with development of acute respiratory alkalosis. The hyperventilation pattern is unique in that the breathing frequency is quite regular. In addition, the tachypnea starts abruptly, as though "switched on," rather than gradually, as is normally seen during progressive exercise. Hyperventilation might actually start at rest, in anticipation of the exercise. Psychogenic dyspnea might also be evident as rapid and unusually shallow breathing

Another manifestation of an anxiety reaction described as shortness of breath may, in fact, be irregular breathing or breath-holding. Observing the behavior pattern and the patient's facial expression may be helpful in detecting this problem.

Poor Effort and Manipulated Exercise Performance

It is important to distinguish manipulated exercise performance for secondary gain from other disorders. An exercise test in which both heart rate reserve (see panel 2, Fig. 3.30) and breathing reserve (see panel 7, Fig. 3.30) are high and the AT is not reached (see panel 5, Fig. 3.30) strongly suggests poor effort. However, inadequate effort may be evident from a normal AT with a high heart rate reserve and breathing reserve without a progressive increase in R above 1.1 during a progressively increasing work rate test (panel 8, Fig. 3.30). A chaotic breathing pattern evident in panel 7 of the 9-panel graphical array supports manipulation of the exercise test since ventilation, tidal volume, and breathing frequency increase in a distinct pattern. A chaotic breathing pattern and psychogenic dyspnea would be most evident during breath-by-breath monitoring.

It is often necessary to sample arterial blood sequentially for measurement of lactate increase, as well as to confirm a normal $P(A - a)O_2$, $P(a - ET)CO_2$ and VD/VT during exercise before stating that a claimant for disability is not impaired on a pulmonary basis. Also arterial blood gas and pH measurements are needed to document whether they change in response to exercise as would be observed in a normal person, a person with disease or a person who is manipulating ventilation so that the changes are non-physiological. Variable and inconsistent changes in breath-by-breath measurements of $PETCO_2$ and $PETO_2$ are also a clue to this diagnosis (see panel 9, Fig. 3.30).

Combinations of Defects

A patient's symptoms may be more marked than predicted from the non-exercise assessment of the severity of the patient's disease. This might be noted particularly when the primary disease is combined with a complicating problem, e.g., cigarette smoking or use of a drug that affects ventilatory drive directly or indirectly through a metabolite, e.g., H^+. Thus, patients with coronary artery disease who have hypertension or who smoke might be less symptomatic and have improved exercise tolerance if their blood pressure were under adequate control or if they did not smoke. Patients with chronic airflow obstruction may be more symptomatic if they also have chronic metabolic acidosis or obesity. Because coronary artery disease and chronic airflow obstruction are so common, both defects may be present in the same patient and may therefore make the patient's symptoms more pronounced than if the two diseases did not coexist. When more than one disease is present that can cause the same symptom(s) during exercise, a cardiopulmonary exercise test is probably the best way to identify which disease is the primary contributor to the patient's symptoms, as well as to provide a noninvasive, relatively inexpensive method to assess therapy.

SUMMARY

The major function of the cardiovascular and ventilatory systems is gas exchange between the cells and the atmosphere. Therefore, impairments in cardiovascular and respiratory function are most apparent during exercise because cell respiration is stimulated and defects are amplified. Because each component of the gas transport system that couples external to internal respiration has a different role, the pattern of the gas exchange abnormality differs according to the pathophysiology. Recognition of these differences allows the examiner to distinguish which organ system in the patient most likely accounts for his/her exercise limitation. Thus, whereas primary heart disease and primary lung disease both cause a reduction in work capacity, the patterns of the gas exchange response differ. By making measurements that address the gas transport function at each site in the coupling of external to cellular respiration, it is possible to deduce the physiologic status of each component

References

1. Wasserman K, Whipp BJ. Exercise physiology in health and disease (State of the art). Am Rev Resp Dis 1975; 112:219–249.
2. Hansen JE, Sue DY, Wasserman K. Predicted values for clinical exercise testing. Am Rev Resp Dis 1984;129 (Suppl):S49–S55.
3. Alexander JK, Amad KH, Colebatch HJH. Observations on some clinical features of extreme obesity, with particular reference to circulatory effect. Am J Med 1962; 32:512–524.
4. Bates DV, Macklem PT, Christie RJ. Respiratory Function in Disease, 2nd Ed. Philadelphia: W.B. Saunders, 1971; 100–101.
5. Gilbert R, Sipple JH, Auchincloss JH. Respiratory control and work or breathing in obese subjects. J Appl Physiol 1961;16:21–26.
6. Sharp JG, Henry JP, Sweany SK, Meadows WR, Pietras RJ. The total work of breathing in normal and obese men. J Clin Invest 1964;43:728–739.
7. Cherniack RM. Respiratory effects of obesity. Can Med Assoc J 1959;80:613–616.
8. Ray CS, Sue DY, Bray G, Hansen JE, Wasserman K. Effects of obesity on respiratory function. Am Rev Resp Dis 1983;128:501–506.
9. Buskirk E, Taylor HL. Maximal oxygen intake and its relation to body composition, with special reference to chronic physical activity and obesity. J Appl Physiol 1957;11:72–78.
10. Bylund-Fellenius AC, Walker PM, Elander A, Holm S, Holm J, Schersten T. Energy metabolism in relation to oxygen, partial pressure in human skeletal muscle during exercise. Biochem J 1981;200:247–255.
11. Weber KT, Janicki JS. Cardiopulmonary Exercise Testing Physiological Principles and Clinical Applications. Philadelphia: W.B. Saunders, 1986;183.
12. Wasserman K, Stringer W. Critical capillary PO_2, net lactate production, and oxyhemoglobin dissociation: Effects on exercise gas exchange. In: Wasserman K, ed. Exercise Gas Exchange in Heart Disease. Armonk, NY: Futura Publishing Company, Inc., 1998,157–181.
13. Sullivan MJ, Duscha B, Slentz AC. Peripheral determinants of exercise intolerance in patients with chronic heart failure. In: Wasserman K, ed. Exercise Gas Exchange in Heart Disease. Armonk, NY: Futura Publishing Company, Inc., 1996;209–227.
14. Wilson JR, Martin JL, Schwartz D, Ferraro N. Exercise intolerance in patients with chronic heart failure: role of impaired nutritive flow to skeletal muscle. Circulation 1984;69:1079–1087.
15. Sullivan MJ, Knight D, Higginbotham MB, Cobb FR. Relation between central and peripheral hemodynamics during exercise in patients with chronic heart failure. Muscle blood flow is reduced with maintenance of arterial perfusion pressure. Circulation 1989;80:769–781.
16. Kitzman DW, Higginbotham MB, Cobb FR, Sheikh KH, Sullivan MJ. Exercise intolerance in patients with heart failure and preserved left ventricular systolic function: failure of the Frank-Starling mechanism. J Am Coll Cardiol 1991;17:1065–1072.
17. Nery LE, Wasserman K, French W, Oren A, Davis JA. Contrasting cardiovascular and respiratory responses to exercise in mitral valve and chronic obstructive pulmonary diseases. Chest 1983;83:446–453.
18. Rubin SA, Brown HV. Ventilation and gas exchange during exercise in severe chronic heart failure. Am Rev Resp Dis 1984;129(Suppl.):S63–S64.
19. Wasserman K, Zhang YY, Gitt A, Belardinelli R, Koike A, Lubarsky L, Agostoni PG. Lung function and exercise gas exchange in chronic heart failure. Circulation 1997; 96:2221–2227.
20. Metra M, Raccagni D, Carini G, Orzan F, Papa A, Nodari S, Cody RJ, Dejours P. Ventilatory and arterial blood gas changes during exercise in heart failure. In: Wasserman K, ed. Exercise Gas Exchange in Heart Disease. Armonk, NY: Futura Publishing Co., 1996;125–143.
21. Sullivan MJ, Higginbotham MB, Cobb FR. Increased exercise ventilation in patients with chronic heart failure: intact ventilatory control despite hemodynamic and pulmonary abnormalities. Circulation 1988;77:552–559.
22. Kobayashi T, Itch H, Kato K. The role of increased dead space in the augmented ventilation of cardiac patients. In: Wasserman K, ed. Exercise Gas Exchange in Heart Disease. Armonk, NY: Futura Publishing Co., 1996; 145–156.
23. Koike A, Itoh H, Doi M, Taniguchi K, Marumo F, Umehara I, Hiroe M. Beat-to-beat evaluation of cardiac function during recovery from upright bicycle exercise in patients with coronary artery disease. Am Heart J 1990; 120: 316–323.
24. Sullivan MJ, Green HJ, Cobb FR. Altered skeletal muscle metabolic response to exercise in chronic heart failure: relation to skeletal muscle aerobic enzyme activity. Circulation 1991;84:1597–1607.

25. Oren A, Wasserman K, Davis JA, Whipp BJ. Effect of CO_2 set point on ventilatory response to exercise. J Appl Physiol 1981;51:185–189.

26. Ben-Dov I, Sietsema K, Casaburi R, Wasserman K. Evidence that circulatory oscillations accompany ventilatory oscillations during exercise in patients with heart failure. Am Rev Resp Dis 1992;145:776–781.

27. Sietsema K. Oxygen uptake kinetics during exercise in patients with pulmonary vascular disease. Am Rev Resp Dis 1992;145:1052–1057.

28. Sietsema KE, Cooper DM, Rosove MA, Perloff JK, Child JS, Canobbio MM, Whipp BJ, Wasserman K. Dynamics of oxygen uptake during exercise in adults with cyanotic congenital heart disease. Circulation 1986;73:1137–1144.

29. Wasserman K. New concepts in assessing cardiovascular function. The Dickinson W. Richards Lecture. Circulation 1988;78:1060–1071.

30. Sietsema KE, Cooper DM, Perloff SK, Child JS, Rosove MH, Wasserman K, Whipp BJ. Control of ventilation during exercise in patients with central venous-to-systemic arterial shunts. J Appl Physiol 1988;64:234–242.

31. Comroe JH. Section 3: Respiration. Handbook of Physiology. Washington D.C., American Physiological Society, 1964;557–583.

32. Comroe JH Jr., Forster II RE, Dubois AB, Briscoe WA, Carlsen E. Diffusion. The Lung: Clinical Physiology and Pulmonary Function Test. 2, 125–133. 1962. Chicago: Year Book Medical Publishers, Inc. 1962;125–133.

33. Hansen JE, Wasserman K. Pathophysiology of activity limitation in patients with interstitial lung disease. Chest 1996;109:1566–1576.

34. Cooper CB, Daly JA, Burns MR, et al. Lactic acidosis contributes to the production of dyspnea in chronic obstructive pulmonary disease. Am Rev Resp Dis 1991;143:A80.

35. Casaburi R, Patessio A, Ioli F, Zanaboni S, Donner C, Wasserman K. Reductions in exercise lactic acidosis and ventilation as a result of exercise training in patients with obstructive lung disease. Am Rev Resp Dis 1991;143:9–18.

36. Wasserman K, Brown HV. Exercise performance in chronic obstructive pulmonary diseases. Med Clin North Am 1981;65:525–547.

37. Bye PTP, Farkas GA, Roussos CH. Respiratory factors limiting exercise. Am Rev Physiol 1983;45:439–451.

38. Pierce AK, Luterman D, Loundermilk J, Blomquist G, Johnson RL, Jr. Exercise ventilatory patterns in normal subjects and patients with airway obstruction. J Appl Physiol 1968;25:249–254.

39. Fulmer JD. An introduction to the interstitial lung diseases. Clin Chest Med 1982;3:457–473.

40. Keogh BA, Lakatos E, Price D, Crystal RG. Importance of the lower respiratory tract in oxygen transfer. Am Rev Resp Dis 1984;129(Suppl.):S76–S80.

41. Wagner PD, Dantzker DR, Dueck R, de Polo JR. Distribution of ventilation-perfusion ratios in patients with interstitial lung disease. Chest 1976;69:256–257.

42. Wasserman K, Mason GR. Pulmonary alveolar proteinosis. In: Murray JF, Nadel JA, eds. Textbook of Respiratory Medicine. Philadelphia: W.B. Saunders, 1988; 1535–1548.

43. Bunn HF, Forget BG. Molecular, genetic and clinical aspects. In: Philadelphia: W.B. Saunders Co., 1986;595–616.

44. Butler WM, Spratling LS, Kark JA, Shoomaker EB. Hemoglobin Osler: report of a new family with exercise studies before and after phlebotomy. Am J Hematol 1982;13: 293–301.

45. Pirnay S, Dujardin J, Deroanne R, Petit JM. Muscular exercise during intoxication by carbon monoxide. J Appl Physiol 1971;31:573–575.

46. Vogel JA, Gleser MA. Effect of carbon monoxide on oxygen transport during exercise. J Appl Physiol 1972; 32:234–239.

47. Hirsch GL, Sue DY, Wasserman K, Robinson TE, Hansen JE. Immediate effects of cigarette smoking on cardiorespiratory responses to exercise. J Appl Physiol 1985; 58:1975–1981.

48. Jones NL, Sutton JR, Taylor R, Toews CJ. Effect of pH on cardiorespiratory and metabolic responses to exercise. J Appl Physiol 1977;43:959–964.

49. McArdle B. Myopathy due to a defect in muscle glycogen breakdown. Clin Sci 1951;10:13–35.

50. Lewis SF, Vora S, Haller RG. Abnormal oxidative metabolism and O_2 transport in muscle phosphofructokinase deficiency. J Appl Physiol 1991;70:391–398.

51. Davis JA, Wasserman K, Anderson T. O_2 consumption as related to work-rate in McArdle's syndrome. Unpublished observations.

52. Riley M, Nugent A, Steele IC, Bell N, Trimble ER, Nicholls DP, Patterson VH. Gas exchange during exercise in McArdle's disease. J Appl Physiol 1993;75:745–754.

53. Haller RG, Lewis SF. Abnormal ventilation during exercise in McArdle's syndrome: Modulation by substrate availability. Radiology 1986;36:716–719.

54. Lewis SF, Haller RG. The pathophysiology of McArdle's disease: Clues to regulation in exercise and fatigue. J Appl Physiol 1986;61:391–401.

55. Wasserman K, Hansen JE, Sue DY. Facilitation of oxygen consumption by lactic acidosis during exercise. News Physiol Sci 1991;6:29–34.

56. Bogaard JM, Scholte HR, Busch FM, Stam H, Versprille A. Anaerobic threshold as detected from ventilatory and metabolic exercise responses in patients with mitochondrial respiratory chain defect. In: Tavassi L, DiPrampero PE, eds. Advances in Cardiology. The Anaerobic Threshold: Physiological and Clinical Significance. Basel: Karger, 1986;135–145.

57. Haller RG, Lewis SF, Estabrook RW, DiMauro S, Servidei S, Foster DW. Exercise intolerance, lactic acidosis, and abnormal cardiopulmonary regulation in exercise associated with adult skeletal muscle cytochrome c oxidase deficiency. J Clin Invest 1989;84:155–161.

58. Berger M, Berchtold P, Cuppers HJ, Drost H, Kley HK, Muller WA, Wiegelmann W, Zimmerman H. Metabolic and hormonal effects of muscular exercise in juvenile type diabetics. Diabetologia 1977;13:355–365.

59. Rubler S, Arvan S. Exercise testing in young symptomatic diabetic patients. Angiology 1976;27:539–548.

60. Storstein L, Jervell J. Response to bicycle exercise testing in long-standing juvenile diabetes. Acta Med Scand 1979;205:277–280.

CHAPTER 5

Clinical Exercise Testing

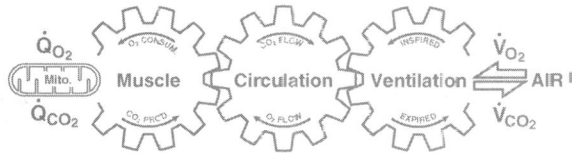

EXERCISE LABORATORY AND EQUIPMENT

General (Laboratory) Environment

The proper interpretation of exercise test data depends on accurate data collection and correct calculations. Admittedly, useful exercise testing can be performed with little or no equipment. A measured course, stairway, or hallway can provide a reproducible and functional exercise stress. After review of symptoms and physical examination, information collected might include heart and ventilatory rate and blood pressure at the conclusion of exercise. However, a properly equipped laboratory provides a site for more complete data collection, where the patient can be relatively stationary on an ergometer with a controlled and reproducible stress, blood pressure and heart rate may be measured repeatedly, gas exchange can be measured, the electrocardiogram may be continuously monitored, and blood may be sampled. Figure 5.1 diagrams the devices and measurements that are generally available in a modern exercise laboratory.

The laboratory should be air-conditioned and regulated at a comfortable temperature and humidity. The patient's view should be pleasant and not cluttered with tubing, wires, or a bulletin board with distracting papers. If blood is to be sampled, the syringes should be prepared and placed in a convenient location to avoid confusion or extra motion during the time of the study. The number of people in the laboratory should be limited to those needed for making the measurements and for patient safety. Finally, extra sounds should be kept to a minimum. Soft background music helps to dampen noise but does not interfere with communication between the examiner and the technician. In summary, a pleasant, professional environment is needed to obtain the maximum confidence and therefore performance by the patient.

Measuring Gas Exchange

Although exercise testing can be performed with little or no equipment, the more sophisticated and potentially useful analysis of cardiopulmonary function during exercise necessitates gas exchange measurement. A variety of systems, measuring devices, recorders, and other equipment have been put together for these purposes, and there are several commercial systems that make considerable use of computerization to determine gas exchange using a gas mixing chamber or from breath-by-breath analysis of expired gas.

Mixing Chambers

In systems using a mixing chamber, expired ventilation is determined using a flow or volume measurement device, while expired gas is passed into a fixed- or variable-sized mixing chamber from which gas is sampled and analyzed for O_2 and CO_2 concentra-

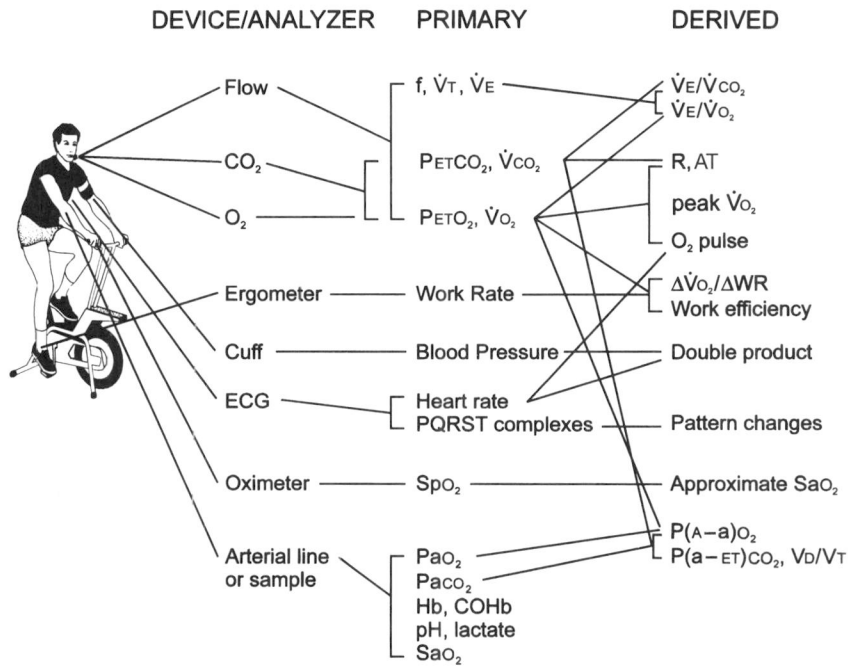

FIGURE 5.1.   Devices and analyzers used to measure variables during exercise on a cycle ergometer. Devices and analyzers individually or collectively may measure a single or several primary variables. The variables in the right-hand column are usually calculated from two or more primary variables.

tions. With proper mixing of expired gas from each breath, differences in O_2 and CO_2 concentration from the beginning to the end of each breath are minimized, and the resultant O_2 and CO_2 concentrations are equal to the volume-weighted average concentrations or "mixed expired" O_2 and CO_2 concentrations. These are equivalent to the O_2 and CO_2 concentrations that would have been obtained by collecting the expired gas in a bag.

In an ideal mixing chamber, with instantaneous and complete mixing, the introduction of a constant flow of a given gas eventually results in the gas in the mixing chamber having a composition identical to that of this gas. The time course by which the concentration of the gas approaches that of the input gas is approximately exponential, and for an ideal chamber, the mixing characteristics can be described by a time constant = V_{mc}/V, where V_{mc} is the volume of the mixing chamber and V is the constant flow of gas into and out of the chamber. A large gas flow (or minute ventilation) or a mixing chamber of small size has a short time constant. Under these conditions, this chamber would respond rapidly to a change in gas concentration; however, the small volume means that a subject with a large tidal volume will produce marked fluctuations in gas concentrations in the chamber. On the other hand, too large a mixing chamber volume compared to tidal volume results in an impractically long time to reach any new equilibrium, making the mixing chamber poorly responsive to changes in gas concentration. A fixed volume mixing chamber may be satisfactory during exercise in which $\dot{V}_E$, F_{ECO_2} and F_{EO_2} change slowly, but may not be satisfactory when rapid changes are expected. If ventilation is continuously measured, a time or volume adjustment must be made to match the correct mixed expired gas concentrations with the correct ventilation.

Breath-by-Breath

A breath-by-breath system measures airflow or volume continuously and simultaneously determines instantaneous expired CO_2 and O_2 concentrations. The CO_2 output and O_2 uptake during each breath are calculated, and the cumulated totals of all breaths over a measured time period are reported as $\dot{V}CO_2$ and $\dot{V}O_2$. To make accurate measurements, ventilation and gas concentrations must be determined as near to continuously as possible. The number of different measurements and the large number and frequent sampling of data make a breath-by-breath system impractical without the aid of computer-controlled sampling and calculation.

We have used breath-by-breath systems for both research applications and for evaluation of patients (1–3). These systems make it possible to determine gas exchange rapidly and accurately under many conditions. By interpolating breath-by-breath expired volume, O_2 uptake, and CO_2 output second-by-second, it is possible to reduce the variability in breath-by-breath measurements. The second-by-second values can then be time-averaged using replicate studies (1–3), thereby reducing the noise in measurement and enhancing the physiologic responses to rapid changes in work rate.

Measurement of Volume, Flow Rate, or Ventilation

Several methods of measuring respired gas volume and flow rates during exercise are used. Each has advantages and disadvantages that make them suitable for different types of systems. Whereas expired ventilation or flow is usually measured, physiologic variables can be calculated from inspired volume or flow with the appropriate adjustments. Devices for measuring volume or flows may be used directly as part of the breathing circuit, or they may be used to measure volumes from a collecting container. If the device is used directly, then flow resistance, linearity, and frequency response may be important considerations (4). If flow is measured rather than volume, e.g., with a pneumotachograph or Pitot tube flowmeter, then flow is integrated over time to determine volume per unit time. Volume can be measured directly using a gas meter, spirometer, or volume transducer. Although, theoretically, flow can be determined from the volume signal by differentiation, this is usually not done because such a method is inherently noisy compared to integration.

Pneumotachograph

The most commonly used pneumotachograph consists of a number of parallel tubes (Fleisch type) that offer a small resistance to gas flow. Gas flow is directly proportional to pressure drop across the resistance when flow is laminar, and the relationship is given by Poiseuille's law. With laminar flow, the only energy loss from the moving gas occurs because of friction from the walls of the tube and a small amount of frictional loss caused by differences in velocity for adjacent gas molecules. The inverse of the proportionality coefficient between flow and pressure is resistance, which is constant for constant dimensions of the resistive element for a given gas viscosity. When flow becomes nonlaminar or turbulent, the relationship between flow and pressure becomes nonlinear. In a Fleisch pneumotachograph, laminar flow is encouraged by small flow channels and low gas velocities. Small flexible plastic tubes are connected at each end of the resistance element, and these two tubes are connected to a differential pressure transducer. The pressure transducer must be highly sensitive because the pressure difference at the usually recommended maximal flow rate is only 1.2 to 1.3 cm H_2O. The pneumotachograph, by definition, introduces additional resistance into the breathing circuit, but this is not usually detectable by the subject (about 0.2 to 0.6 cm $H_2O/L/sec$).

The pneumotachograph is linear within a range of flows but becomes non-linear when flow exceeds a particular value based on the size of the device. For exercise testing in adults, flows encountered generally indicate that a No. 3 Fleisch pneumotachograph is appropriate. This device has a linear response for flows up to 5 to 10 L per second. Finucane et al. (4) found that the pressure-flow relationship was linear over the widest gas flow range when the immediate upstream geometry was a tube of the same diameter as the pneumotachograph. Compensation for documented nonlinearities in the pressure-flow relationship can be made by altering the output of the differential pressure transducer either electrically or, in computer-based systems, mathematically. The linear flow range has been increased by as much as 50 to 100% with, generally, less than 2% inaccuracy at recommended maximal flow. In commercial systems, empiric calibration curves may be used to optimize pneumotachograph performance. Finucane et al. (4) found that, for Fleisch pneumotachographs, flow values lagged behind pressure changes for sinusoidal flow at frequencies up to 10 Hz; however, the lag was small and insignificant compared to the frequency response of other parts of the breathing circuit.

Because expired gas is usually warmer and contains more water vapor than ambient air, contact of expired gas with an ambient temperature pneumotachograph could result in condensation and obstruction of the pneumotachograph resistance elements. Pneumotachographs, therefore, are often used with an electric heater to warm the pneumotachograph to a temperature slightly above expired gas. However, a heated pneumotachograph not only warms the expired gas, but warms it by a variable amount depending on the flow. Warming the gas increases its volume and thereby alters the pressure-flow relationship. Whereas theoretic methods can be used to estimate the degree of warming, two practical methods may eliminate the problem. In the first method the expired gas is kept warm, and the temperature of the pneumotachograph is only slightly warmer (0.5°C) than the temperature of the gas passing through it. Another way is for the pneumotachograph to be kept at ambient temperature and the expired gas allowed to cool.

Oxygen is significantly more viscous than nitrogen. Because viscosity is a direct factor in Poiseuille's law relating pressure difference and flow rate, room air and 100% O_2 have different pressure-flow relationships. For 100% O_2 breathing, flows are measured approximately 11% higher for a pneumotachograph calibrated with air. In systems that use a pneumotachograph, appropriate adjustment at the time of calibration or during calculation of ventilation and gas exchange is necessary. Although only gas viscosity is a direct factor in Poiseuille's law, gas density is a determinant of whether laminar or turbulent flow will exist at a given gas velocity in a given straight tube.

Other Flowmeters

One relatively new device for measurement of flow uses the principle of the Pitot tube (5), a device for measuring flow velocity in fluids. The Pitot tube measures the difference in pressure at an opening placed directly facing the fluid stream compared to the pressure at an opening perpendicular to the fluid stream (static pressure). From Bernoulli's law, the velocity of fluid movement is proportional to the square root of the pressure difference, and, from the cross-sectional area of the device, the flow can be calculated. The Pitot tube has the advantage of being non-resistive. It is also dependent on turbulent flow rather than on laminar flow conditions. A flowmeter suitable for exercise gas exchange measurements based on the Pitot tube principle uses a differential pressure transducer to determine the pressure difference between the static and midstream ports. A suitable algorithm calculates the flow from the pressure signal and could also correct for any nonlinearities over the flow measurement range. Advantages of such a device compared to a conventional pneumotachograph include low resistance and lack of a requirement for laminar flow. Problems with heating or cooling of expired gas are minimized with such a device.

The mass of gas rather than the volume or flow is measured using a hot-wire anemometer (6, 7). This device determines the change in amount of electrical current, compared to baseline, needed to maintain a constant temperature of a wire placed in the air stream. The wire material is selected so the wire resistance is strongly influenced by the wire temperature. The rate of mass movement of gas and its thermal capacity relate to the current change and, by using an appropriate model, the flow of gas can be calculated. This method is inherently nonlinear, but this can be adjusted using suitable digital computer algorithms.

Calibration

Validation of any flowmeter is essential for confidence in the ability of the device to measure accurately and reproducibly under testing conditions. A water-sealed spirometer is recommended as a primary standard for volume measurements, and spirometer volume changes over a timed period can be used as a flow standard. Secondary standards include calibrated large-volume syringes of 1 to 4 L and various gas flowmeters. These secondary standards should be calibrated against a spirometer before use. If flow or volume signals are further processed by analog or digital means, the results will be subject to the response characteristics and calculation methods of these instruments (8). The accuracy of flow and volume can also be determined using a calibrated pump calibrator.

Pneumotachographs have special calibration considerations related to the problems of temperature, water vapor, viscosity, and geometry. The ideal method is to calibrate the pneumotachograph under conditions identical to those of the testing process. A known flow of gas of essentially identical temperature, relative humidity, and gas composition to the anticipated measured gas should be delivered to the pneumotachograph through identical upstream geometry. In practice, simpler methods using a calibrated syringes are used for day to day calibration and verification.

Breathing Valves, Mouthpieces, and Masks

Most gas exchange measurement systems require the use of a breathing valve to separate inspired from expired gas flows so expired gas can be collected and analyzed. The ideal valve prevents contamination of either gas flow by the other. The ideal valve also has no resistance to breathing, low rebreathed volume (low valve dead space), and operates silently. Other advantages include low size and weight, lack of generation of turbulence in the air stream, ease of cleaning and sterilization, and low cost.

No single valve design is ideal. For testing healthy, fit adults, however, a low resistance valve is preferred because of the high levels of ventilation that must be accommodated. These valves usually consist of two or three sets of one-way "J valves" each for inspiration and expiration. The small "J valves" allow rapid opening and closing. All of these have dead space volumes of 100 to 320 ml that must be considered if calculation of V_D/V_T is intended. A high-capacity Rudolph valve may also be suitable for high flow applications. At lower flow rates, Koegel and Hans-Rudolph valves with smaller dead space volumes and slightly higher flow resistances may be used.

Dead space can be determined for the valve plus attached mouthpiece by measuring the amount of water it can contain. Valve resistance can be determined during constant airflow using a pressure transducer and flowmeter. This value may be different between inspiration and expiration, or underestimated during exercise testing because the valve flaps can require additional pressure to open when wet or when gas flow is pulsatile. Finally, valves may develop back-leaks, especially when subjected to high flows and pressures during heavy exercise. These leaks should be suspected for any valve, but especially after prolonged use, infrequent cleaning, excessive secretions, or damage to component parts. Errors in ventilation or gas exchange measurements may be important clues to a leaking breathing valve. If a leak is suspected, simultaneous recording of inspiratory and expiratory flow during exercise may reveal the presence and location of the leak.

Traditionally, patients have had nose clips applied so that all inspired and expired gases are routed through rubber or soft plastic mouthpieces. Now there are available face masks of differing sizes and shapes so that they can be sealed comfortably over the patient's nose and mouth. Dead space is usually slightly more with masks than with a mouthpiece and nose clip.

Gas Analyzers

O_2 and CO_2 Analyzers

For gas exchange measurements, the concentration of O_2 and CO_2 in the expired gas must be determined. Although few laboratories perform them, Scholander and Haldane methods for gas analysis are accurate, but time consuming, tedious, and impractical. Details of Scholander and Haldane analysis of expired gases can be found in standard references (9). They may be useful for initial calibration of gas analyzers and primary analysis of stored gases used for calibration purposes.

Carbon dioxide analyzers measure absorption by CO_2 of appropriate wavelengths of infrared light. Infrared light is passed through a cell containing the gas to be measured, and the amount of light transmitted is compared to a reference value. Absorption is proportional to the fractional CO_2 concentration. The measurement cell must be kept clean and free of water condensation.

Oxygen analyzers use several different principles. The paramagnetic analyzer measures the change in a magnetic field introduced by differences in oxygen concentration. Because other respiratory gases have little paramagnetic susceptibility, these will not affect the magnetic field. More commonly used, the electrochemical O_2 analyzer depends on chemical reactions between O_2 and a substrate that generates a small electrical current. This current is proportional to the rate of O_2 molecules reacting with the substrate and thus to the concentration of O_2.

These CO_2 and O_2 analyzers measure partial pressure of the gas and are affected by water vapor, pressure in the sampling systems, and changes in barometric pressure and altitude. Thus, for a given fractional concentration of gas, changes in any of these conditions at the sensor location will erroneously result in different measured gas fractions. Because the sample flow rate delivering gas to the analyzer is held constant, a change in sampling site pressure may result from changes in resistance of the delivery tubing. This effect can be minimized by using a high-pressure suction pump and a large resistance in the connection between the analyzer and the pump. Care must be taken to ensure that sample tube resistance is identical during calibration and measurement, and water condensation, saliva, or foreign bodies are not trapped in the delivery tubing.

Both CO_2 and O_2 analyzers report the fraction of CO_2 or O_2 of the total gas, including any water vapor present. This is especially important to consider during calibration because ambient air usually contains some water vapor. Expired gas is saturated with water vapor at the lowest temperature that it reaches before being analyzed. Because temperature determines the partial pressure of water in a saturated gas, this temperature must be accurately known or estimated if expired CO_2 and O_2 are to be accurately determined. An alternative is to pass the gas over anhydrous calcium sulfate or cool the gas to remove water vapor. These methods can introduce a substantial delay between the time the gas is exhaled and the time the sample reaches the analyzer. Recently, tubing has been developed that selectively transports water vapor through its walls out of the sample into the ambient air. In effect, the water vapor partial pressure of the gas delivered to the analyzer is equal to that of ambient air and is not influenced by temperature of the gas at the point of sampling. Additional consideration of the significance of water vapor in calculating $\dot{V}O_2$ can be found in Appendix C.

Mass Spectrometer

In a mass spectrometer of the fixed collector type, sampled gases are converted to positively charged ions by an electron beam. Then, in a near vacuum, the ions are accelerated by an electric field and are then subjected to a magnetic field. The direction the ions take in the magnetic field is dependent on their mass/charge ratios. The different ions representing different gases are detected by appropriately located detectors that each produce a voltage output proportional to the number of ions that strike the collector per unit time. The individual detector voltages can be electronically divided by the total voltage. This quotient is the fractional concentration of each gas. Note that, because the total voltage is dependent on the sum of the individual detector voltages, any gas for which there is no detector does not contribute to the total. For respiratory mass spectrometry, detectors for O_2, CO_2, and N_2 are typically used; ordinarily there are no detectors for water vapor, argon, or other inert gases present in trace amounts in air. Thus, the O_2, CO_2, and N_2 concentrations given by a mass spectrometer are concentrations relative to a dry gas whether or not water vapor was a component of the originally sampled gas.

Calibration and Quality Control

Gas analyzers, including mass spectrometers, should be checked for linearity within the range of needed values. This can be done by analyzing gases of known concentration of O_2 and CO_2. If an analyzer is nonlinear, a calibration curve can be constructed by observing the analyzer output at several gas concentrations (10). Calibration of gas analyzers should be performed using gases of known concentration. The analyzers should be warmed up for sufficient time to ensure against electrical drift, an identical sampling arrangement to that used during testing should be used, and the sample cells should be clean. A two-point calibration can be used if the analyzer is sufficiently linear. It is convenient to use dry room air as one calibration point, assuming an O_2 of 20.93% and CO_2 of 0.04% (essentially zero). A calibration gas of approximately 15% O_2, 5% CO_2, and balance N_2 (but whose actual values are accurately known) is appropriate for the second point because these concentrations are in the middle of the anticipated range of expired gas concentrations. The concentrations of the calibration gas mixture may be analyzed independently by Haldane or Scholander techniques or by a carefully calibrated mass spectrometer. Alternatively, gas having O_2 and CO_2 concentrations of acceptable precision can be obtained from a reliable gas supplier, but these high precision gases are expensive. A useful procedure is to keep for long-term use a tank of gas for which O_2 and CO_2 are accurately known (high precision), then to use this gas periodically to compare with less expensive gases used for day-to-day calibration. After long storage, it is best to roll the tank to avoid gas stratification.

The gas transport delay time and the response time of each analyzer to the introduction of a new gas are important aspects of breath-by-breath exercise systems. This is further addressed in Appendix C.

Ergometers: Treadmills and Cycles

Treadmill

Treadmills allow subjects to perform familiar walking and running exercise at measured speeds and grades of incline. A variety of protocols for increasing work performed have been designed, and both low and high work rates may be obtained. Treadmills have some advantages over cycle ergometers. A subject performing on a treadmill generally has a peak $\dot{V}O_2$ approximately 5 to 10% higher than on a cycle ergometer, and some subjects and patients are simply not able to cycle because of problems of coordination or inexperience.

On the other hand, treadmills require more space than a cycle ergometer, demand somewhat more caution during use, and may introduce movement artifacts in measurement of ventilation and pulmonary gas exchange. If the subject holds on to any part of the treadmill, such as a hand railing, or to the arm of a technician or physician, the $\dot{V}O_2$ may be decreased because work requirement is lessened. Work efficiency during treadmill walking cannot be precisely determined because of the difficulty in estimating work rate. We prefer a treadmill protocol using constant speed with a fixed increase in grade per time interval (e.g., 1–3% per minute) to produce close to a linear increase in work rate with time. However, this treadmill protocol may not be optimal for all subjects. Treadmill speed and grade should be routinely checked for accuracy and reproducibility. Grade may be determined by using a plumb line and tape measure. Speed can be accurately determined by using a stopwatch to time the movement of a mark made on the treadmill belt.

Cycle Ergometer

Cycle ergometers enable a precise estimation of the work rate. Leg cycling may be performed sitting or supine. Advantages of the cycle ergometer over the treadmill include the ability to vary the work rate in step, incremental, or ramp fashion; the ability to determine work efficiency; smaller size; potentially greater safety because the subject is supported at all times; and less effect of movement artifact on measurements. Some subjects and patients, however, may not be able to pedal the cycle because of lack of coordination and experience, and the seat may become uncomfortable during a long study.

When the patient is in the upright position, seat height is important and should be carefully adjusted. When the patient is seated, the foot at the lowest point of the pedaling cycle should be such that the knee is almost but not completely straight. It is useful to record the seat height in the subject's records so future studies may be done identically. Subjects should be asked to wear tennis shoes suitable for the types of pedals on the cycle. Toe clips may or may not be used, as desired. Because subjects must cycle at a relatively constant rate, a metronome or tachometer can be used to assist subjects' performance.

Two types of cycle ergometers are in general use. Mechanically braked devices use an adjustable brake to increase or decrease contact of a friction belt with a moving flywheel attached to the pedals. The work rate achieved is proportional to the cycling frequency or speed of the flywheel, but a particular work rate is only achieved if the subject cycles within a narrow range of pedaling rate. An electrically braked cycle ergometer uses a variable electromagnetic field to produce a resistance to pedaling that varies with flywheel speed, changing the resistance to cycling to maintain work rate at the set level regardless of pedaling speed. A work rate set on this type of cycle ergometer is thereby present over a wide range of cycling speeds. The work rate on the electrically braked devices may be set by a remote controller, or it may be adjusted automatically by a digital computer controller.

Calibration of the cycle is highly desirable both during initial setup of the laboratory and periodically thereafter. Manufacturers' specifications and calibration procedures should be followed. Commercially available or specially built devices that generate known amounts of power can act as standards for calibration and verification (11). Other methods have been devised to provide for cycle calibration and validation (12–14). In addition, because $\dot{V}O_2$ in an individual maintains a constant relationship to work rate, a group of readily available subjects (e.g., laboratory staff) may be used for periodic checks of the cycle work rate.

When a subject pedals on the cycle with "no resistance added" or "unloaded," some work is obviously being performed. In addition to the work rate necessary to move the legs, the work rate needed to keep the cycle flywheel in motion is usually about 10–15 W for electromagnetically braked ergometers, but it may be as much as 20 to 30 W for mechanically braked cycle ergometers (and may vary considerably with pedaling rate). This work rate may exceed the maximal capacity of some severely limited patients. Manufacturer specifications may provide information on the work rate of "unloaded cycling," but users should make this determination for themselves. We have used a special protocol (see Selecting the Work Rate Increment) that takes advantage of an accessory motor attached to our cycle flywheel. This motor keeps the flywheel spinning at a rate sufficient to minimize the "unloaded" work rate.

Cycle versus Treadmill

Whether the treadmill or the cycle ergometer is the preferable mode of exercise for exercise testing has been a subject of considerable debate (Table 5.1). The treadmill has been in common use for decades. It allows one to exercise most ambulatory patients except those who are severely dyspneic, uncoordinated, or confused, or those who have significant lower extremity musculoskeletal disease. The treadmill uses an activity familiar to everyone and allows

TABLE 5.1. Comparison of Treadmill and Cycle Ergometers for Exercise Testing

Feature	Treadmill	Cycle
Higher maximum $\dot{V}O_2$ and maximum O_2 pulse	+	
Similar maximum HR and maximum $\dot{V}E$	+	+
Familiarity of exercise	++	+
Quantitation of external work	−−	++
Freedom from artifacts in ECG, air flow, and pressure tracing	−−	++
Ease of obtaining arterial blood specimens	−−	++
Safety (fewer musculoskeletal injuries)		+
Usefulness in supine position		+
Use of less vertical and horizontal laboratory space		+
Less noise		+
Lower cost		+
Portability	−	+
Greater experience in the United States	+	
Greater experience in Europe		+

More important advantage (++) or disadvantage (−−); less important advantage (+) or disadvantage (−).

the investigator the opportunity to vary both speed and grade to change the work rate. It has several disadvantages, however. The treadmill is frightening to some patients and may be noisy, bulky, and expensive. Moreover, the laboratory ceiling may be too low for use at the higher treadmill grades. Repeated experience on the treadmill may lead to some increase in the efficiency of walking. Probably the greatest disadvantage of the treadmill is the difficulty in quantifying work rate. Any connection between the patient and the treadmill, except that between the patient's shoes and the treadmill belt, can decrease the expected energy requirement for body movement at that grade and speed. Railings, arm boards, mouthpieces, blood pressure measuring devices, and steadying hands all have the potential to reduce the patient's actual work rate. Length of stride as speed or grade is changed, shift of center of gravity, and change from walking to jogging all can affect the patient's metabolic requirement.

Even the most athletic patients require several minutes of practice in starting and ending the treadmill exercise before beginning measurement. Although injuries are rarely reported, careful surveillance is necessary. Because patients can lose their balance on the moving belts, it is wise to have additional help immediately available on the sideboard of the treadmill, particularly for elderly patients.

The cycle ergometer allows a more accurate quantifying of external work rate and can be used when patients are in the supine or upright position. A minor disadvantage is that most individuals have a lower peak $\dot{V}O_2$ and AT on the cycle than on the treadmill, even though their maximum HR, maximum $\dot{V}E$, and maximum blood lactate are similar on both ergometers. In 8 studies of male subjects, the mean peak $\dot{V}O_2$ on the cycle varied from 89 to 95% of treadmill values (15). The cycle is less expensive, less bulky, and less noisy than the treadmill. None of our patients have been injured using the cycle or treadmill, but we believe that the cycle is safer for those patients who are less well coordinated. We place the patient's feet in toe clips and sometimes, if necessary, bind their shoes to the pedals with tape, so they do not slip out.

Because of less arm and torso movement on the cycle than on the treadmill, one finds fewer artifacts in ventilatory and circulatory measurements and has greater ease in obtaining blood samples. Because the tubular post supporting our cycle seat once buckled while being used by a very obese patient, we now use a stainless steel rod to support a conventional bicycle seat (covered with sheepskin or gel) or a platform-type seat. "Seat pain" can be a problem with prolonged repeated testing, but it is uncommon with the clinical protocols described previously. In agreement with Astrand (16), we prefer the cycle to the treadmill for clinical testing because we can accurately quantify external work rate and thereby establish the patient's work rate-$\dot{V}O_2$ relationship, a critical measurement in assessing cardiovascular function.

Work and Work Rate (Power)

In basic physical units, force (kg-m/sec^2 or newton) = mass (kg) × acceleration (m/sec^2). When this force is applied over a distance, work is performed. Thus, work (kg-m^2/sec^2 or newton-m or joule) = force (kg-m/sec^2 or newton) × distance (m). However, we are most often interested in the rate of work or power = work (kg-m^2/sec^2 or newton-m or joule) per sec. The unit of power is the watt, and one watt (W) is defined as 1 joule/sec = 1 newton-m/sec = 1 kg-m^2/sec^3.

During exercise against the resistance of a cycle ergometer, the work rate is the distance traveled by a point on the circumference of the wheel × the rotational frequency of the flywheel × the restraining force. This restraining force can be expressed as newtons or, commonly, as kiloponds, where 1 kilopond (kp) = 1 kg × 9.81 m/sec^2. In practice, cycle ergometer work rate (power) is expressed as watts or kilopond-m/min. To convert from kp-m/min to W, divide by 6.12. For example, a work rate of 612 kp-m/min equals 100 W.

Electrocardiogram and Systemic Blood Pressure

Exercise ECG

Silver/silver chloride ECG electrodes with circumferential adhesive provide good electrical contact and minimize movement artifacts. These are similar to those used in the ICU for ECG monitoring. The skin is shaved if necessary and is wiped with rubbing alcohol before the patches are applied on areas of the body that will not be subject to great motion during exercise. A net vest may reduce artifacts due to movement.

For those patients for whom we use ECG for rate and rhythm monitoring, three electrodes are used as shown in Figure 5.2. However, we do not hesitate to move the electrodes to obtain an optimal tracing.

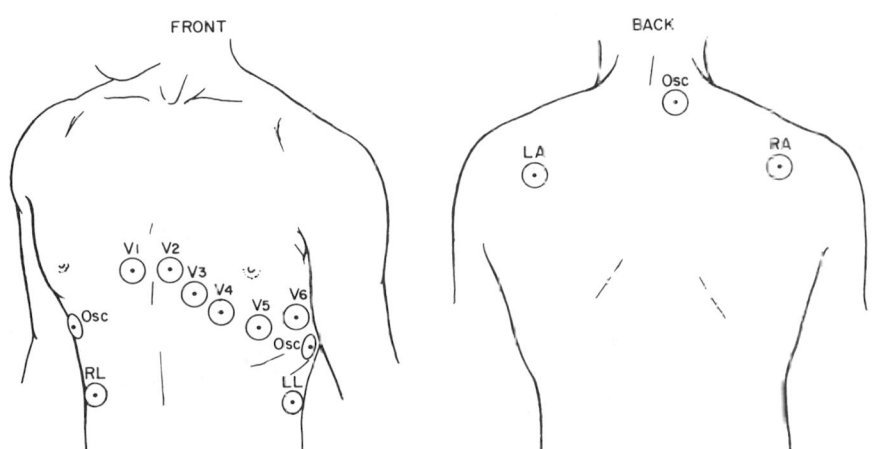

FIGURE 5.2. ECG lead placement for upright ergometry. The V1 and V2 electrodes are placed more caudad than usually done for supine tracings, whereas V3, V4, V5, and V6 are in their usual locations. The "arm" electrodes (LA and RA) are placed posterior to the shoulders, whereas the "leg" electrodes (LL and RL) are placed anterolaterally near the lower rib margins. The three oscilloscope (Osc) electrodes are placed separately to minimize electrical interference.

We use the 12-lead ECG in addition for patients in whom we suspect myocardial ischemia, but we find these to be useful in many patients undergoing clinical exercise testing. The positions of the electrodes are shown in Figure 5.2. The arm electrodes are placed close to the monitoring patches on the back above the scapulae; the leg electrodes are placed on the low back above the iliac crests. These locations minimize movement artifact. The chest electrodes (V-leads) are positioned in standard locations on the anterolateral chest. Commercial systems allow computer processing of summarized signals to reduce motion artifacts.

Systemic Blood Pressure

Blood pressure should be measured frequently during exercise to be aware of extreme hypertension or to detect impending hypotension. Indwelling arterial catheters allow nearly continuous direct measurement of systemic arterial blood pressure and wave contours, and afford optimal patient safety. The pressure transducer should be located at the level of the left atrium (approximately the fourth intercostal space in the upright position) and the transducer carefully calibrated. More commonly, blood pressure is measured with a manometer, inflatable arm cuff, and auscultation. Blood pressure can also be measured and recorded using several recently developed commercial devices: a) mechanically controlled or automated inflatable cuffs and auscultation; b) pulse oximeters; or c) pressure transducers placed over the radial artery. Such devices should be validated against sphygmomanometer measurements made in the opposite arm.

Oximetry, Blood Sampling and Arterial Catheters

Valid measurements of Pa_{O_2}, Pa_{CO_2}, or pH for calculation or measurement of Sa_{O_2}, $P(A - a)_{O_2}$, $P(a - ET)_{CO_2}$, or V_D/V_T, are often essential for the interpretation of clinical exercise tests. However, on many occasions correct diagnoses and interpretations can be made using less invasive measurements.

Pulse Oximetry

Pulse oximetry estimates arterial blood oxygen saturation using pulsatile changes in light absorption. In the past, *in vivo* oximetry using transmission spectrophotometry through the antihelix of the ear required multiple wavelengths of light, a heater to increase blood flow, and a heavy, complex device attached to the subject's ear. Since the late 1970s, the principle of pulse oximetry has been widely used (17). Using this technique, an estimate of arterial oxygen saturation is derived from a combination of spectrophotometry and pulse plethysmography. These devices use two wavelengths of light produced by light-emitting diodes, one in the red and one in the infrared spectrum, and a detector that measures light intensity passing through the ear lobe or fingertip. Differential absorption of light at these two wavelengths provides enough information to determine the ratio of oxyhemoglobin to total hemoglobin, assuming that all the pulsatile change is due to the effects of arterial blood. Pulse oximetry is theoretically independent of skin pigmentation and the thickness of the ear lobe or finger; however, some studies have shown that dark skin pigmentation may affect results (18, 19). Pulse oximeters cannot distinguish carboxyhemoglobin and methemoglobin from oxyhemoglobin; it may be convenient to think of the percentage of oxygen saturation reported from a pulse oximeter as being equal to (100 − % deoxyhemoglobin). In general, pulse oximetry becomes more inaccurate when oxygen saturation is less than 75% (17).

During exercise, movement artifact and stray incidental light may interfere with pulse oximeter accuracy; these may be particularly bothersome during vigorous exercise. Although some studies have found acceptable accuracy of pulse oximeters during exercise (18–21), Hansen and Casaburi (22) have shown that overestimation and underestimation of arterial blood oxygen saturation may occur near the patient's maximum work rate. Reasons for this may include dependence of the pulse oximeter on sufficient blood flow to the vascular bed measured, a change in the shape of the arterial pulse waveform, a change in empirically determined calibration factors, movement artifact, or other problems. Another study using two different pulse oximeters, however, concluded that pulse oximetry was accurate in normal subjects breathing hypoxic gas during exercise (21). Escourrou and co-workers (23) found significantly different pulse oximetry estimates of oxygen saturation compared to measured values with three models of pulse oximeters. The authors concluded, however, that changes in pulse oximeter O_2 saturation from rest to exercise were sufficiently useful for clinical decision making.

The major disadvantage of pulse oximetry is that

saturation rather than arterial P_{O_2} is measured. Thus, although the correlation between measured arterial O_2 saturation and pulse oximetry O_2 saturation is very good, significant decreases in arterial P_{O_2} in the range of P_{O_2} above 60 mmHg result in only small decreases in O_2 saturation. For patients whose Pa_{O_2} decreases to below 60 mmHg during exercise, pulse oximetry proves useful. For other patients whose resting and exercise Pa_{O_2} is greater than 60 mmHg but who are suspected of significant decreases in Pa_{O_2} during exercise, one approach is to use pulse oximetry during a preliminary test. If arterial oxygen saturation decreases by more than 3 to 5%, then an arterial catheter is placed for direct measurement of Pa_{O_2} and $P(A - a)_{O_2}$ during a repeat exercise study. It is emphasized that clinically important decreases in Pa_{O_2} may occur that could be undetectable by pulse oximetry alone.

Single Samples of Arterial Blood

Arterial blood samples allow direct measurement of Sa_{O_2}, Pa_{O_2}, Pa_{CO_2}, pH, lactate, and other important values. Often, a single sample of arterial blood is obtained during an exercise test to assess blood gases. If this is done, the sample must be obtained before the end of the exercise rather than during recovery because rapid changes in Pa_{O_2} occur immediately after the patient stops exercising (24–26). Each sample should be drawn over a specific 10- to 20-second period, so that it can be well-matched with concurrent gas exchange measurements involving several breaths. The radial artery is the more common site for a single sample; local anesthesia to that site administered before exercise reduces patient discomfort.

Some investigators use free-flowing ear capillary blood or heated hand vein blood as a substitute for arterial blood. Blood values from these sites are likely to approximate arterial P_{CO_2} values for measurement of V_D/V_T but are less likely to approximate arterial P_{O_2} values.

Systemic Arterial Catheter

An indwelling arterial catheter makes repeated sampling of arterial blood for blood gases simple and fast, and it provides continuous monitoring of blood pressure during exercise as well. The most common insertion sites are the brachial and radial arteries, and the same kinds of small-bore catheters used in the ICU for arterial catheterization can be used. The radial artery site has the theoretic advan-

tage that the ulnar artery can supply blood to the hand if the radial artery is blocked, whereas the brachial artery is the sole blood supply of the lower arm. With meticulous care, however, we have never had a serious complication of brachial artery catheterization in several thousand insertions over a 30-year period. A disadvantage of the radial artery site is that it may interfere with gripping of the cycle ergometer handlebars; in addition, referring direct blood pressure measurements to the left atrial level may be more difficult. Figure 5.3 demonstrates the brachial artery catheter in place while Appendix D describes its insertion.

Arterial punctures and catheterization are rarely complicated by bleeding, arterial spasm, distal arterial thromboembolism, thrombosis, or infection, or by significant pain or discomfort. Most frequently,

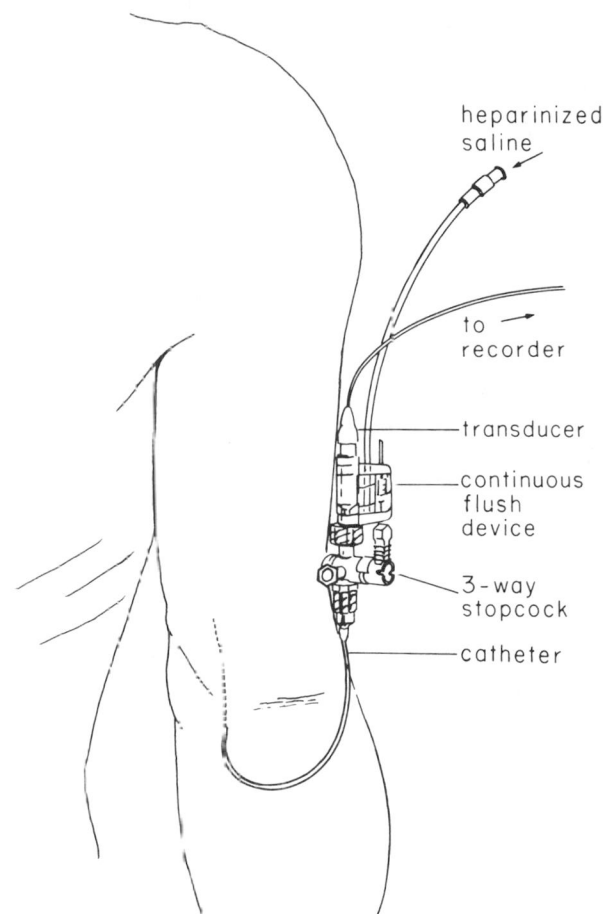

FIGURE 5.3. Brachial artery catheter placement. A 25-cm polyvinyl catheter has been placed percutaneously in the left brachial artery. The dressings have been removed to show catheter placement. The hub of the catheter connects to a continuous flush device, a three-way stopcock, and a transducer, the last located parallel to the fourth intercostal space in the mid-clavicular line (at the mid-atrial level in the sitting position).

subjects complain of mild discomfort and discoloration from bleeding following puncture. Arterial catheters should be used with special care or avoided in a patient with known peripheral arterial disease.

Pulmonary Artery Catheter

For some patients, a pulmonary artery catheter can add valuable information during exercise testing. For example, it may be useful in selected patients with suspected or known primary or secondary pulmonary hypertension or cardiac disease, or for research purposes. Pulmonary artery pressure, pulmonary artery wedge pressure, mixed venous blood gases, and cardiac output by thermal indicator dilution can be measured. The Swan-Ganz pulmonary artery catheter is balloon-tipped and flow-directed, and a physician can pass it through a large vein in the arm through the right atrium, right ventricle, and into the pulmonary artery with or without fluoroscopic guidance. Because arrhythmia and heart block potentially occur during placement, insertion should be done only with ECG monitoring and appropriate resuscitation equipment and medications standing by. For pressure measurements, a calibrated transducer and recorder are used. During exercise, especially with patients with lung disease, large swings in intrathoracic pressure with respiration may be transmitted to the pulmonary artery and wedge pressures, and pressure measurements will be subject to large respiratory variation. Intravascular pressures at end-exhalation are selected by convention and are usually most relevant. Blood samples can be drawn from the pulmonary artery distal port to be analyzed for mixed venous P_{O_2} and O_2 content needed for the calculation of cardiac output using the Fick equation or calculation of venous admixture.

Cardiac output can also be determined by thermodilution, i.e., by rapidly injecting a bolus of physiologic fluid (usually 5% dextrose in water) of known volume, temperature (usually 0°C), specific heat, and specific gravity into the right atrial port of the pulmonary artery catheter and measuring the temperature change with a thermistor or temperature sensor at the catheter tip in the pulmonary artery. The temperature change downstream reflects the volume of dilution of the bolus and cardiac output can be calculated using an automated system. The integral of temperature over time is inversely proportional to cardiac output. Stetz et al. (27) reviewed several studies and concluded that thermodilution cardiac outputs in catheterization laboratories and intensive care units were of comparable accuracy to Fick or dye-dilution methods. These authors suggested, however, that a 20 to 26% difference in cardiac output should be found before concluding that two single determinations were different. Advantages of thermodilution include safety, speed, and repeatability.

Disadvantages of using a pulmonary artery catheter include increased risks, costs, and preparation time. Uncommon complications can include arrhythmia, heart block, bleeding, perforation of the right ventricle or pulmonary artery, and infections. Under specific circumstances, however, the benefits gained from information obtained from these catheters may outweigh the risks.

Data Sampling and Computation

Automated exercise gas exchange systems make intensive use of computers to control data collection, perform calculations, store results, and display information. The speed and capability of computerized calculations can correct data from non-linear analyzers and make adjustments for different environmental or subject characteristics. The computer can also be used to control the ergometer using preprogrammed protocols. Many commercial systems come with a variety of different data displays and printed tables and graphs that should serve most needs. Some systems allow the user to design customized formats for reports. In addition, the system may allow data to be transferred to database and spreadsheet applications for use on personal computers.

Typically, data sampled from a flow meter and transducer, gas analyzers, pulse oximeter, heart rate monitor, or other device undergo analog-to-digital conversion under computer control. Accurate calculations require a sufficiently high sampling rate; for most gas exchange data, a sampling rate in the range of 50 to 100 Hz appears to be adequate. This is easily in the range of available analog-to-digital converters and computer systems.

Validation and Maintenance

In the past, systems of analyzers and computers for determination of gas exchange during exercise were developed and assembled in individual laboratories. Validation often comprised the majority of the time required for development of these systems. Now, most often, commercial exercise systems are used by clinicians and investigators. Though it is tempting to consider these automated systems accurate, precise, and reproducible, they should undergo validation and should have periodic monitoring for accuracy and reproducibility of results.

Validation can be performed by simultaneous collection of mixed expired gas while the exercise system is collecting data (1, 2, 28). For mixing chamber and breath-by-breath systems, extremes of tidal volume and flow are particularly challenging. It is easiest to collect expired gas during the steady-state of constant work exercise; but such validation may not provide evidence of accurate measurement during rapidly changing exercise protocols or when the major focus is on the short-term time course of gas exchange.

A particularly useful device is an automated calibrator that simulates gas exchange at a known and reproducible rate. One type of simulator uses a sinusoidal pump of known volume and measurable frequency to provide an accurate "expired minute ventilation" (29). Gas exchange (O_2 uptake and CO_2 output) is simulated by the introduction of a gas mixture containing 21% CO_2 in N_2 into a reservoir bag which mixes with room air pumped into the gas exchange measurement system. $\dot{V}O_2$ and $\dot{V}CO_2$ measured by the system should be equal to 0.21 × the flow rate of the 21% CO_2 in N_2 flowing into the reservoir bag of the pump calibrator. The respiratory gas exchange ratio should equal 1; however, adjustment of the exercise system algorithms may be necessary to accommodate the nearly dry, room temperature gas delivered by the calibrator to the gas exchange measuring device which is set up to measure body temperature, saturated expirate. The pump calibrator has been demonstrated to provide an accurate simulation of gas exchange that can be used for validation. In addition, the device is useful for routine periodic checks of reproducibility. If an error (or change) in measured minute ventilation, $\dot{V}O_2$, or $\dot{V}CO_2$ is found, analysis of the differences in the measurements may also suggest the nature of the problem.

An inexpensive and relatively simple way to test the entire system together is for an individual to cycle at a constant mild to moderate work intensity, such as 50 W, for 6 minutes. On repeated testing, the $\dot{V}O_2$ after 3 minutes should be in a steady state and within 5 to 10% of previously measured values (approximately 1.0 L/min for an individual of average size exercising at 50 W). Values significantly deviant from prior tests suggest errors in flow, gas analyzer or delay measurements, or ergometer

calibration. If the tested individual can control his breathing frequency appropriately, there should be less than 5% difference in $\dot{V}O_2$ whether breathing at a frequency of 15, 30, or 60 per minute. Greater variation in $\dot{V}O_2$ values at different breathing frequencies suggests errors in delay or response times in the gas analyzers.

Validation and reproducibility data should be kept for future reference. Many commercial systems have an option to print a listing of the current status of gas analyzers, environmental conditions, calibration gas concentrations, temperature, and other important system variables. This information can be helpful in identifying a problem and in resolving problems with the help of the manufacturer.

PREPARING FOR THE EXERCISE TEST

The objective of a clinical exercise test should be to learn the maximum about the patient's pathophysiologic causes of exercise limitation 1) with the greatest accuracy; 2) with the least stress to the patient; and 3) in the shortest period of time. The optimal examination allows the simultaneous evaluation of the adequacy of the muscles, heart, lungs, and the peripheral and pulmonary circulations to meet the gas exchange requirements of exercise. The test should enable the investigator to distinguish disorders in these systems from inadequate effort, obesity, anxiety, or unfitness. For the differential diagnosis of exercise limitation caused by cardiovascular or respiratory disease, relatively complete gas exchange measurements should be made. Exercise with large muscle groups is needed to stimulate internal respiration sufficiently to stress the cardiovascular and pulmonary systems adequately; therefore, either a cycle ergometer or a treadmill should be used for testing. Isometric exercise is of limited value because it is largely anaerobic, providing little information about the ability of the cardiovascular and respiratory systems to support the energy requirements of exercise. The protocol selected for exercise testing depends on the purpose of the test.

Requesting the Test and Notifying the Patient

We use a pre-printed request form for exercise tests. On this form the referring physician gives us the following information:

1. Patient's name, address, and telephone number
2. Patient's weight, height, sex, and age

3. Tentative diagnosis and the reason for the study
4. Type of test requested and special requirements

Most often, the exercise test should be discussed with the referring physician so the type of test and the reason for doing it are clear beforehand. In addition, the discussion helps one to decide whether the cycle or treadmill is the preferable form of ergometry, whether an arterial catheter is desired, and whether supplemental O_2 should be given during the exercise test. This is also a time at which the patient's medications, previous studies, special needs or limitations, and other details can be discussed. Other important information include the specific complaints of the patient during exercise, results of pertinent studies (chest radiographs, resting respiratory function, resting electrocardiograms, echocardiograms), and potential risks and contraindications to exercise.

At the time the exercise test is scheduled, the patient is advised to wear comfortable clothes and low heeled or athletic shoes, adhere to his or her usual medical regimen, eat a light meal two or more hours before arrival, and avoid cigarettes and coffee for at least two hours. The patient is given a brief description of the exercise test, and told how long it will take and what to expect.

The Patient in the Exercise Laboratory

Preliminary Tests

Recently obtained spirometric data can be used unless the patient has variable obstructive lung disease or performed erratically when spirometry was obtained. In these conditions, and in most cases, the vital capacity (VC), inspiratory capacity (IC), forced expiratory volume in 1 second (FEV_1), and maximal voluntary ventilation (MVV) should be obtained when the patient arrives at the exercise laboratory. The American Thoracic Society has published detailed instructions for performing spirometry (30). The direct MVV is calculated from a 12-second maneuver of rapid and deep breathing; the indirect MVV is calculated by multiplying the FEV_1 by 40 (31). The MVV values are needed for determination of the exercise breathing reserve. In patients with severe interstitial lung disease, the indirect MVV is often more appropriate than the direct MVV if the patient breathed at extremely high frequency during the MVV because these frequencies will be unattainable during cycle or treadmill exercise. On the other hand, in patients with inspiratory obstruction, neu-romuscular disorders, and severe obesity, the direct MVV should be used even if considerably less than the indirect MVV. In other patients with poor spirometric efforts, the indirect MVV is usually a more reliable measure of ventilatory capacity. The hemoglobin and carboxyhemoglobin levels should be known or measured and the D_LCO measured in those patients with lung disease or dyspnea.

Physician Evaluation

The physician should obtain relevant clinical information from the patient with particular emphasis on medications, tobacco use, accustomed activity level, and the presence of angina pectoris or other exercise-induced symptoms. It is worthwhile ascertaining the patient's understanding of the tests and the amount of effort that will be required. The physician should perform a focused examination with particular attention to the heart, lungs, peripheral pulses, and musculoskeletal system, measure blood pressure in each arm, and obtain an accurate shoeless height and weight. The physician determines the type of exercise test and protocol on the basis of the exercise request, the clinical evaluation, review of the current ECG and other preliminary tests, and any other special considerations.

Informed consent for the exercise test must be obtained. The patient is told that he or she will be asked to make a maximal effort (for most studies) but is advised that exercise can be stopped at any time. The patient is warned of potential discomfort and risks associated with the procedure and the kinds of information that will be obtained and how this may benefit the patient. Finally, the patient is encouraged to ask questions about the testing before giving consent.

Equipment Familiarization

We find it particularly useful to familiarize the patient with the exercise testing equipment before starting the actual test. If the treadmill is used, time is provided for practice trials so the patient can get on and off the moving treadmill belt with confidence. If the cycle is used, the seat height is adjusted so the legs are nearly completely extended when the pedals are at their lowest point. Because a mouthpiece or mask interferes with the ability of the patient to communicate verbally, the patient is taught to use the signal "thumb up" if everything is satisfactory and "thumb down" if he or she is experiencing any difficulty. The patient is advised to point to the site of discomfort if chest pain or pressure or leg pain is experienced. The code of finger signals for intensity that we use is: one finger if mild, two fingers if moderate, and three fingers if severe. We advise the patient that they are in charge and can stop exercise if they feel distressed. Alternatively, we stop the exercise if we note important abnormalities.

The mask or mouthpiece and nose clip are tried before the actual test. The patient is advised that it is acceptable to swallow with the mouthpiece in place or moisten the inside of the mouth with the tongue. We explain the importance of having a good seal of the lips around the mouthpiece or the mask about the face.

Arterial Catheter

If the study requires repeated arterial blood sampling, a catheter is inserted into a radial or brachial artery (see Appendix D for detailed description of how to place the catheter) (32). It is important to check radial and ulnar artery pulsations before and after catheter insertion. The catheter is attached to a stopcock and a blood pressure transducer via a continuous flush device that provides a slow infusion of a heparin-containing solution (10 units/ml). When one uses a brachial artery catheter, the catheter should be long enough (20 to 25 cm) so that its hub can be brought around to the lateral aspect of the lower part of the upper arm (Fig. 5.3). The transducer is positioned on the upper arm at a height corresponding to the fourth interspace of the mid-clavicular line (mid-atrial level when the patient is upright). To avoid spurious dilution of the blood specimen with heparin-containing solution, about 0.5 ml of fluid is discarded before collecting each arterial blood sample (usually by letting the blood flow into gauze under arterial pressure before the syringe is connected to the stopcock). Each sample is collected over approximately 20 seconds so the gas tensions are representative of the mean arterial value and minimally influenced by respiratory variations in alveolar gas tensions. Immediately after sampling, the catheter lumen is flushed with heparin-containing solution.

Post-Exercise Care

At the conclusion of the test and soon after removal of the mouthpiece, the physician should question the patient in a non-leading fashion about what symptoms caused him or her to stop exercise. This is especially important in a maximum or symptom-limited exercise study. A series of questions may be required to assess just what the patient means by his or her description of limiting symptoms. For example, it is important to differentiate calf from thigh pain and to determine the exact character of any chest discomfort. In particular, it is always worthwhile to find out if the symptoms reproduce the complaints of exertional dyspnea or exertional chest pain or other discomfort experienced by the patient outside the laboratory.

If, on review of the data, it appears that a symptom-limited test was terminated prematurely because of inadequate patient effort, a repeat test after a recovery period of 30 to 45 minutes may be indicated. For instance, if the patient made an insufficient effort, as suggested by the combination of high breathing and heart rate reserves, a low R, and only a slight fall in bicarbonate, the test bears repeating with greater encouragement from the examiner.

After use, the arterial catheter is removed while keeping direct pressure over the puncture site for at least 5 to 10 minutes. When the pressure is removed, the site is inspected carefully for evidence of bleeding. With adequate pressure and observation after removal of the catheter, hematomas can be avoided. With any evidence of extra-vascular bleeding, pressure is continued for at least another 3 minutes. A light dressing covered with a tight elastic bandage is then applied over the puncture site, and the peripheral pulses are checked. The patient is advised not to use that arm for heavy exercise for the next 24 hours. The dressing and elastic bandage can be removed by the patient at home after several hours have elapsed.

After an exercise test with blood sampling, it is advisable to review the blood gas results before discarding any remaining blood in the sampling syringes. This makes it possible to reanalyze samples in which the results are questionable.

PERFORMING THE EXERCISE TEST

The following sections describe several different protocols that are used for addressing various clinical questions. Most often we use a maximum (symptom-limited) incremental exercise test on a cycle ergometer, and this protocol is described in detail. However, if the patient is being evaluated for other reasons such as exercise-induced bronchospasm, oxygen supplementation, myocardial ischemia, fitness, or other reasons, then other protocols or special considerations may be appropriate.

Incremental Exercise Test to Symptom-Limit Maximum

In this protocol, the patient exercises on a cycle ergometer (or a treadmill) while measurements of gas exchange are made at rest, during 3 minutes of very low level exercise, and then while the work rate is increased each minute or continuously (ramp). In general, the patient is encouraged by the technician and physician in attendance to continue as long as safely possible.

Selecting the Increment Size

We select the increment size after considering the patient's history (especially the amount and intensity of his or her daily activity), physical examination (notably obesity and evidence of cardiac or respiratory disease), and pulmonary function evaluation (particularly the FEV_1 and MVV). If we expect the patient to have a near-normal power output, we estimate the $\dot{V}O_2$ at unloaded pedaling from the patient's body weight and the peak $\dot{V}O_2$ from the patient's age and height. We then calculate the work rate increment necessary to reach the patient's estimated peak $\dot{V}O_2$ in 10 minutes. The steps that we use to approximate the correct increment for the cycle are as follows.

1. $\dot{V}O_2$ unloaded in ml per minute = 150 + (6 × weight, kg)
2. Peak $\dot{V}O_2$ in ml per minute = (height, cm—age, years) × 20 for sedentary men and × 14 for sedentary women
3. Work rate (W) increment per minute = (peak $\dot{V}O_2$, ml/min—$\dot{V}O_2$ unloaded, ml/min)/100

For example, given an apparently healthy sedentary man 180 cm in height, 100 kg in weight, and 50 years of age, his anticipated $\dot{V}O_2$ unloaded, ml/min = 150 + 6 × 100 kg = 750 ml/min; his anticipated peak $\dot{V}O_2$ = (180 − 50) × 20 = 2600 ml/min. To achieve an incremental test duration of 10 minutes, we would use a work rate increment of (2600 − 750)/100 = 18.5 W per minute. Practically, we would select an increment of 20 W per minute and expect the test duration to be slightly less than 10 minutes.

If we know that the patient has an MVV, FEV_1, or D_LCO less than 80% of that predicted, we would consider reducing the expected peak $\dot{V}O_2$ proportionally. For example, an MVV or D_LCO that is 50% of predicted will reduce the expected peak $\dot{V}O_2$ to roughly one half to two thirds of normal. If the patient has resting tachycardia, symptoms suggestive of angina, or evidence of chronic heart failure, we also reduce the expected peak $\dot{V}O_2$, the amount being judged by our pre-exercise assessment of impairment. In each case we reduce the size of the work rate increment in an attempt to keep the total incremental exercise time at about 10 minutes. Given a choice, we would rather overestimate than underestimate the work rate increment. With too large an increment, the test will be too brief, but the patient will recover quickly, an advantage if retesting is necessary. With too small an increment, however, the patient may stop for ambiguous reasons and may feel too fatigued for re-testing.

When we expect patients to have extremely severe exercise limitation, we use a special protocol in which, after the rest period, the external work load is incremented less rapidly than usual in the initial portion of the test. With this protocol, for the first 3 minutes of unloaded pedaling, the patient cycles at 20 rpm; for the fourth minute at 40 rpm; and for the fifth minute at 60 rpm. Throughout this portion of the test, an accessory motor attached to the cycle rotates the cycle flywheel at a speed of slightly over 60 rpm so that the exercise performed is truly unloaded exercise. At the sixth minute, the accessory motor is turned off while the patient continues pedaling at 60 rpm, giving a slight load to the cycle. Starting with the seventh minute, the work rate is increased by 5 to 10 W per minute. This protocol allows the accumulation of more data at a very low metabolic rate, and frequently allows delineation of very low AT values which are otherwise unmeasureable. This problem may be found in patients with very obese legs, in whom unloaded pedaling at 60 rpm may cause the $\dot{V}O_2$ to exceed 1.0 L per minute. Using this protocol, we do not insist that the patient cycle smoothly at 20 and 40 rpm; intermittent movement of the pedals is satisfactory.

Resting Measures (Fig 5.1)

A 12-lead ECG is obtained with the patient in the supine position. If an arterial catheter is placed, we obtain a blood specimen in the sitting position before the patient goes on the mouthpiece to avoid effects on the breathing pattern and blood gases induced by the mouthpiece. After the patient is moved to the cycle or treadmill and made comfortable, a nose clip is put on and checked for leaks, and the mouthpiece is inserted. We measure (and

$\dot{V}O_2/HR$) are printed out breath-by-breath, every 10 seconds, or every quarter to half minute by averaging an integral number of whole breaths. HR, $\dot{V}E$, $\dot{V}O_2$, and $\dot{V}CO_2$ are viewed on a screen as the data are collected. The measured and calculated variables are plotted out after the test, as shown in Chapter 9. With an arterial catheter, arterial blood pressure is recorded continuously and arterial blood is sampled for blood gases, pH, lactate, cooximetry, and hemoglobin values at rest. If an arterial catheter is not used, blood pressure is obtained with a pressure cuff and pulse oximeter values are recorded.

Unloaded Exercise and Cycling Rate

To overcome the inertia of the cycle flywheel with an electromagnetically braked cycle, an accessory motor (33) can be used to rotate the flywheel at a rate of slightly over 60 rpm while the patient's feet are motionless on the pedals. As soon as the patient starts pedaling, the accessory motor is turned off. This is particularly helpful for testing patients with limited strength in their legs. At a verbal signal, the patient begins 3 minutes of unloaded pedaling. The patient is advised to look at the rpm meter and to maintain a cycling speed of 60 rpm. A metronome may be used to assist the patient in maintaining cadence, i.e., one leg stroke for each beat of the metronome. A 12-lead ECG, blood pressure measurement, and, if the patient has an arterial catheter, a blood sample are obtained near the end of the 3 minutes of unloaded pedaling.

Incremental Exercise

Measurements are continued while the work rate is increased continuously (ramp) (34) or by a uniform amount each minute until the patient is limited by symptoms or is unable to continue safely (Fig. 5.4). An increment rate is selected depending on the expected performance of the patient. A 12-lead ECG and arterial samples for blood gas and pH measurement are ordinarily obtained every 2 minutes. The technician and physician work cooperatively in observing the patient's facial expression, checking the blood pressure and ECG recordings for untoward changes and arrhythmia, looking for leaks at the nose or mouthpiece, observing for signals from the patient, and verbally encouraging the patient to maximize his or her performance. The resistance of the cycle is removed if the patient evidences distress, if there is a fall in systolic or mean blood pressure greater than 10 mmHg, if a significant arrhythmia

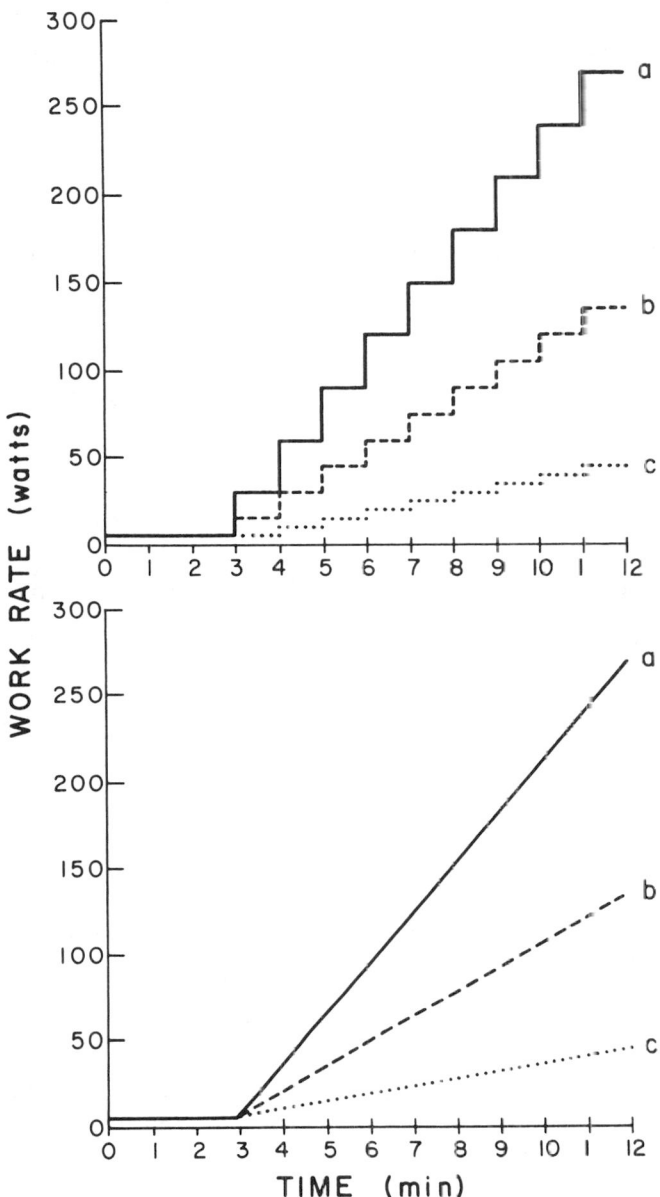

FIGURE 5.4. One-minute incremental (upper) and ramp incremental (lower) protocols for cycle ergometry. In both cases, the subject initially cycles for 3 minutes of unloaded pedaling. In the example shown, the work rate is incremented 30 (a), 15 (b), or 5 (c) W per minute depending on the height, age, gender, and health of the subject. The increment is added at the start of each minute for the 1-minute test, whereas the increment is completed at the end of each minute for the ramp test. Larger or intermediate increments can also be used. The cycle is returned to the unloaded setting when the cycling frequency cannot be maintained over 40 rpm or when the physician or subject decides to terminate the incremental exercise.

frequently record) expiratory and inspiratory airflow, O_2 and CO_2 tension at the mouthpiece, oximetry, and a single-lead ECG on a multi-channel recorder. Heart rate (HR), breathing frequency (f), $\dot{V}E$, $\dot{V}O_2$, $\dot{V}CO_2$, R, $PETO_2$, $PETCO_2$, and O_2 pulse develops, or if the patient has ST segment depression of 3 mm or greater. The exercise is also terminated if the patient is unable to maintain cycling frequency above 40 rpm. If practical and indicated, an arterial blood sample is obtained during the last half minute of exercise.

Recovery

We ask the patient to continue to breathe through the mouthpiece during 2 minutes of recovery. In the immediate post-exercise period, the patient is advised to continue to pedal at a slow frequency without a load on the ergometer. This prevents the precipitous fall in blood pressure that is occasionally experienced when vigorous exercise is abruptly terminated. A final arterial blood sample is obtained at 2 minutes of recovery.

Critique

Duration of Test and Incremental Size. Balke and colleagues introduced the use of 1-minute incremental treadmill tests for the study of fitness in a large military population (35, 36). Although Balke initially used a 1% increment in grade per minute with a constant treadmill speed of 3.3 mph, he also used a 2% increment in grade every minute. Several investigators, including Consolazio (37), Jones (38), and Spiro (39), and their colleagues, used the cycle ergometer with the work rate increment increased by an equal amount every minute or half minute. Increments of 8, 15, 17, or 25 W per minute, 10 W per half minute, or 4 W every 15 seconds have been reported (40). We introduced the use of a continuously incrementing (ramp pattern) exercise protocol (34, 41), (Fig. 5.3) and we have used it extensively in adults and children (42). In comparing the ramp test with 1-, 2-, and 3-minute step increments at the same overall average work rate increase, Zhang et al. (43) have shown that no significant differences were found in the $\dot{V}O_2$max, AT, $\dot{V}E$peak, HRpeak, $\Delta\dot{V}O_2/\Delta WR$, or exercise duration among the four protocols in healthy subjects. Step patterns in some measures could be seen in the 2- and 3-minute step protocols, however (see Fig. 3.3). Thus, although any of these protocols might be used, either the ramp or the 1-minute incremental test seems practical and preferable for patients.

Several investigators (44, 45) have stressed the desirability of adjusting the work rate increment according to the patient's cardiorespiratory status. Tests that are too brief, that is, with the work rate increased too rapidly, may not allow a sufficient quantity of data to be accumulated. Tests that are too long, that is, with too small a work rate increase, are likely to be terminated prematurely because of boredom or "seat discomfort." We found that tests in which the incremental part of the protocol is completed in 6 and 12 minutes give the highest peak $\dot{V}O_2$ in normal subjects (46). Longer or shorter duration tests are likely to give slightly lower values. We know of no similar study in patients with heart or lung disease; consequently, we can only assume that the findings with patients would be similar. Therefore, we attempt to select a work rate increment that will result in termination of the incremental part of the exercise test in 8 to 10 minutes.

Validity of Measurement. Some investigators have expressed concern whether the peak $\dot{V}O_2$ is as high in continuous incremental protocols as in discontinuous protocols and whether the highest $\dot{V}O_2$ reached (peak $\dot{V}O_2$) should be identified as the $\dot{V}O_2$max. Taylor et al. (47) defined the $\dot{V}O_2$max from a series of progressively higher constant work rate tests. They defined the $\dot{V}O_2$max as the $\dot{V}O_2$ when an increase in work rate resulted in an increase of $\dot{V}O_2$ of less than 150 ml per minute above the $\dot{V}O_2$ from the previous lower work rate. This criterion is appropriate for tests in fit subjects using large work rate increments, such as 2.5% grade change at a treadmill speed of 7 mph. In tests featuring a 15-W per minute increase in work rate, however, the rate of increase in $\dot{V}O_2$ is normally only 150 ml per minute. Therefore, at increments of 15 W per minute or less, it is invalid to use the criterion of Taylor et al. to determine whether the peak $\dot{V}O_2$ is indeed the $\dot{V}O_2$max. A single study (48) reported an approximately 10% lower peak $\dot{V}O_2$ using a continuous rather than a discontinuous graded work rate test; however, the long duration (20 to 30 minutes) of these continuous tests could have accounted for the reduction (45). In contrast, Maksud (49), Wyndham (50), and McArdle (51) and their associates found no difference in peak $\dot{V}O_2$ measured in continuous incremental tests compared with discontinuous constant work rate treadmill tests. Pollock and colleagues (52) found a plateau in $\dot{V}O_2$ in 59 to 69% of the continuous incremental treadmill tests they administered. We found a similar peak $\dot{V}O_2$ in normal men using a ramp-pattern increase in cycle ergometer tests, whether the increase was 20, 30, or 50 W per minute (41). Thus, we believe that the $\dot{V}O_2$max can be approximated with continuous incremental protocols of the proper duration.

Using the ramp pattern test, we also found that the *AT*, time constant for $\dot{V}O_2$, work efficiency, maximum $\dot{V}E$, and maximum HR were comparable to values found with constant work rate tests (34, 41). Because we were concerned that non–steady-state incremental exercise tests might give different values for $\dot{V}E$, $\dot{V}O_2$, $\dot{V}CO_2$, $P(A - a)O_2$, $P(a - ET)CO_2$, and HR as compared to steady state, we studied 23 men (11 normal, 9 with obstructive lung disease, and 3 with restrictive lung disease) during steady state constant work rate and 1-minute incremental exercise tests (Table 5.2) (53). The steady-state exercise $P(A - a)O_2$ values ranged from 1 to 43 mmHg, and the V_D/V_T values ranged from 0.12 to 0.44. We found that $\dot{V}CO_2$, $\dot{V}E$, PaO_2, and R were slightly lower during incremental exercise than constant work rate exercise at the same $\dot{V}O_2$. These differences were anticipated and can be fully explained by the differences in kinetics of $\dot{V}O_2$, $\dot{V}CO_2$, and $\dot{V}E$ in incremental versus constant work exercise. The $P(A - a)O_2$, $P(a - ET)CO_2$, $PaCO_2$, $\dot{V}E/\dot{V}CO_2$, and V_D/V_T values were in close agreement in both protocols for both the normal subjects and the patients, however. Thus, it is possible to make measurements of gas exchange and ventilation-perfusion matching equally well during incremental or steady-state exercise.

With rapid incremental tests, frequent and accurate measurements are needed. Blood pressure and HR are not difficult to measure. Accurate measurement of $\dot{V}E$, $\dot{V}CO_2$, and $\dot{V}O_2$ requires special thought and understanding of the properties of the measuring devices. The reader is referred to Beaver et al.

(1, 54), and Sue et al. (2) for an analysis of potential errors.

Constant Work Rate Exercise Tests

Exercise tests performed with the patient or subject exercising at a constant work rate may be useful in particular situations compared with an incremental work rate test. The selection of the appropriate work rate depends on the question being addressed and the number of different work rates that are chosen. Constant work rate exercise tests may be helpful in determining $\dot{V}O_2$peak or the lactic acidosis threshold, measuring gas exchange kinetics, diagnosing exercise-induced bronchospasm, and assessing the contribution of the carotid bodies to exercise hyperpnea.

Determining $\dot{V}O_2$max

Historically, discontinuous constant work rate tests, each with a large increase in work rate with intervening rest periods, were used to measure $\dot{V}O_2$max (55) as described. Advantages of determining $\dot{V}O_2$max from progressively greater constant work rate tests are: 1) the higher intensity work rates selected can be based on the patient's cardiovascular and ventilatory responses to the lower work rate tests; 2) timed manual bag collection of mixed expired gas for measurement of $\dot{V}CO_2$ and $\dot{V}O_2$ near the end of each exercise does not require rapidly responding gas analyzers; and 3) failure of the $\dot{V}O_2$ to increase despite and increase in work rate provides unequivocal identification of $\dot{V}O_2$max. Disadvantages are the following 1) the repeated tests take

TABLE 5.2.   Effect of Protocol on Measurements of PaO_2, $P(A - a)O_2$ and V_D/V_T During Cycling at the Same Mean $\dot{V}O_2$ (0.92 ± 0.03 L/min)

	N	PaO_2, mmHg		$P(A - a)O_2$, mmHg		V_D/V_T	
		Incr.*	Constant†	Incr.	Constant	Incr.	Constant
Normal	11	89	94	14	13	0.26	0.25
Restrictive lung disease	3	87	89	18	21	0.21	0.19
Obstructive lung disease	9	79	83	25	22	0.32	0.32
All subjects	23	85‡	89	19	17	0.27	0.28

* 1-minute incremental exercise protocol.
† Constant work rate protocol; measurements made at 6 minutes.
‡ Indicates significant difference between 1 minute incremental (Incr.) and constant work rate test at p < 0.05 by paired t test; other measurements are not significantly different.
(Data from reference 53).

considerable time for patient, physician, and technician; 2) these tests are tiring and exhausting and may be more likely to result in injury to the patient; and 3) although such tests are often considered "steady-state" tests, this cannot be true at work rates at or above that necessary to ensure a $\dot{V}O_2$max.

Measuring Gas Exchange Kinetics

Constant work rate tests are ideal for measuring cardiovascular, ventilatory, and gas exchange kinetics. Measurement of these variables, especially $\dot{V}O_2$, during the transition from rest to low level exercise or between two levels of exercise using breath-by-breath analysis allows measurements of time constants or half-times of response (56). Averaging the data obtained from several breath-by-breath tests may be necessary for adequate precision (57, 58). Sietsema et al. (3) used such a protocol to demonstrate striking reductions in the $\dot{V}O_2$ increase during the first 20 seconds after exercise onset in patients with cyanotic congenital heart disease. In normal subjects, the magnitude and mean response time (MRT) of $\dot{V}O_2$ correlated well with the fitness (peak $\dot{V}O_2$/kg) of the individual; the lower peak $\dot{V}O_2$/kg, the longer the MRT for constant work rates of 100 W or higher (59). Similarly, Ben-Dov et al. (60) demonstrated significantly lower increases in $\dot{V}O_2$ in the first 20 seconds of constant work rate exercise in hyperthyroidism, despite the overall higher metabolic requirement of the disease. At higher constant work rates, Koike et al. (61) demonstrated the lengthening of the $\dot{V}O_2$ time constant as carboxyhemoglobin levels were increased.

Determining Anaerobic Threshold

The measurement of $\dot{V}O_2$ kinetics over a 6-minute period of constant work rate can also be useful. If the AT is uncertain after incremental testing, a constant work rate test can be performed at a work level expected to approximate the individual's AT. If the work rate turns out to be above the individual's AT, the $\dot{V}O_2$ will not plateau by the end of the third minute, but will continue to rise (62). The degree of rise will be greater the further the work level is above the AT and correlates highly with the extent of the developed lactic acidosis (see Figs. 2.46, 3.25) (63, 64). A repetition of the test at one or two other constant work rate levels should allow an accurate determination of the AT.

Several studies have shown the utility of precisely assessing the AT and the sensitivity of the $\Delta\dot{V}O_2$(6-3) to disorders in O_2 transport. Casaburi et al. (65) showed the advantage of training patients with chronic obstructive pulmonary disease with constant work rates above rather than below their AT. Koike et al. (61) demonstrated increases in the $\Delta\dot{V}O_2$(6-3) with reductions in hemoglobin availability, whereas Zhang et al. (66) showed the positive correlation between the $\Delta\dot{V}O_2$(6-3) and the severity of heart failure in patients with chronic stable heart failure.

Detecting Exercise-induced Bronchospasm

Although exercise-induced bronchospasm can often be demonstrated after the usual incremental testing in the afflicted individual, it may be more evident after 6 minutes of near maximal constant load exercise (67). It is necessary to obtain good baseline measurements of FEV_1, or some other index of airway obstruction, immediately before exercise. Most investigators prefer the treadmill to the cycle ergometer for inducing post-exercise bronchospasm, although we have used both successfully. To induce post-exercise bronchospasm, it is our practice to increase the work rate to approximately 80% of the predicted maximal work rate after a 1-minute warm-up at a lower work rate. The patient inspires dry air from a bag filled with compressed air rather than room air because, according to current concepts, dry air aids in the induction of bronchospasm and reduces day-to-day variability if repeated tests are necessary (68). After 6 minutes of heavy exercise, the mouthpiece is immediately removed. Spirometric tracings are obtained as soon as possible and at 3, 6, 10, 15, and 20 minutes after exercise.

Measuring Carotid Body Contribution to Exercise Ventilation

The effect of carotid body input to the medullary respiratory centers can be assessed by altering the PO_2 of the blood reaching the carotid bodies (69). Normally, if the carotid bodies are contributing significantly to ventilatory drive, a rise in carotid artery PO_2 will immediately reduce the carotid body neural outflow and depress ventilation transiently. This can be detected by an immediate fall in $\dot{V}E$, VT, and f and a rise in $PETCO_2$ approximately 6 to 10 seconds after an unobtrusive switch of inspiratory gas from room air to 100% O_2 (see Fig. 3.29). After 1 minute of 100% O_2 breathing, a switch back to room air results in a return to baseline $\dot{V}E$ and $PETCO_2$ values. Because ventilation is less variable during exercise than at rest, we prefer to perform these measurements during constant work rate exercise of moderate intensity. Steady-state levels of $\dot{V}E$ at moderate exercise are usually attained in less than 5 minutes. Thus, the effect of the change in F_{IO_2} can be more clearly detected and quantified. Maximal effect is usually seen with an increase in Pa_{O_2} to 250 mmHg or more. If the patient has a normal arterial O_2 saturation and response, VE will decrease transiently by about 15%. If a pneumotachograph is used to determine ventilation, an adjustment must be made in calculating the ventilatory decrease to account for the 11% higher gas viscosity of 100% O_2 than air. The flow meters of some commercial systems automatically correct for this difference in gas viscosity. On-line recording of breath-by-breath ventilation, V_T, f, and gas concentrations is desirable.

Treadmill Test for Detecting Myocardial Ischemia

Protocols

Bruce (70), Ellestad (71), Naughton (72), and their colleagues and other cardiologists have developed and popularized several incremental treadmill protocols for detecting ECG changes of myocardial ischemia.

The Bruce protocol (Fig. 5.5C) begins with 3-minute stages of walking at 1.7 mph at 0, 5, or 10% grade (70). The 0 and 5% grades are omitted in more fit individuals. Thereafter, the grade is incremented 2% every 3 minutes, and the speed is incremented 0.8 mph every 3 minutes until the treadmill reaches 18% grade and 5 mph. After this, the speed is increased by 0.5 mph every 3 minutes.

Ellestad's protocol (Fig. 5.5E) uses 7 periods, each of 2 or 3 minutes' duration, at progressively increasing speeds of 1.7, 3, 4, 5, 6, 7, and 8 mph. The grade is 10% for the first 4 periods, with durations of 3, 2, 2, and 3 minutes, respectively, and 15% for the last 3 periods, each of 2 minutes' duration (71).

Naughton's protocol (Fig. 5.5A) uses 10 exercise periods of 3 minutes' duration, each separated by rest periods of 3 minutes (72). The grade and speed of each period are as follows: 0% and 1 mph; 0% and 1.5 mph; 0% and 2 mph; 3.5% and 2 mph; 7% and 2 mph; 5% and 3 mph; 7.5% and 3 mph; 10% and 12.5% and 3 mph; and 15% and 3 mph.

In each of the foregoing treadmill protocols, blood pressure is measured and a multiple-lead ECG is recorded at each work rate and during recovery. The patient is carefully observed, and the test is terminated at the physician's discretion (e.g., for decline in blood pressure, significant ventricular arrhythmia, progressive ST segment changes, attainment of a given HR) or by the patient's symptoms.

Critique

These treadmill tests have the advantage of extensive clinical use. A survey in 1977 concluded that the complication rate for such "exercise stress testing" was 3.6 myocardial infarctions, 4.8 serious arrhythmias, and 0.5 deaths per 10,000 tests (73). In this survey, the treadmill was the ergometer used most often (71%), whereas the favorite protocol (65%) was that of Bruce. The peak $\dot{V}O_2$ is generally 5 to 11% higher with treadmill as compared with cycle ergometer testing (1), whereas maximum HR is similar. As usually performed, $\dot{V}E$, breathing pattern, $\dot{V}O_2$, and gas exchange are not measured during these tests so other important information on cardiovascular and pulmonary system function is not available. Bruce et al. have shown a high correlation of maximum $\dot{V}O_2$ and duration of treadmill exercise in their normal population (74). Nevertheless, it is invalid to consider the duration of exercise a measure of peak $\dot{V}O_2$ in patients suspected of having cardiovascular disease. The unequal duration of increment and variability in increment size are disadvantages of these tests, although interpretation is usually not based on measurements of $\dot{V}O_2$. In addition, HR itself is a poor measure of exercise intensity in many patients with heart disease. Administration of β-adrenergic blocking drugs also modifies the HR-work rate relationship and must be taken into account when interpreting the results of exercise tests.

Rather than using the foregoing protocol for treadmill testing, Jones (38) and we (46) prefer to use a constant treadmill speed and increment the grade by a constant amount each minute for the entire study. After 3 minutes of warm-up at zero grade and a comfortable walking speed (which may range from 1 to 4.5 mph, depending on our fitness assessment), we use a constant grade increment of 1, 2, or 3% each minute to the patient's maximum tolerance. We scale speed and grade so the test will end approximately 10 minutes after we begin to increment the treadmill grade (Fig. 5.4F). We also make measurements of $\dot{V}E$, $\dot{V}CO_2$, and $\dot{V}O_2$. Following an initial delay of about one minute after the increment begins, this protocol gives a relatively

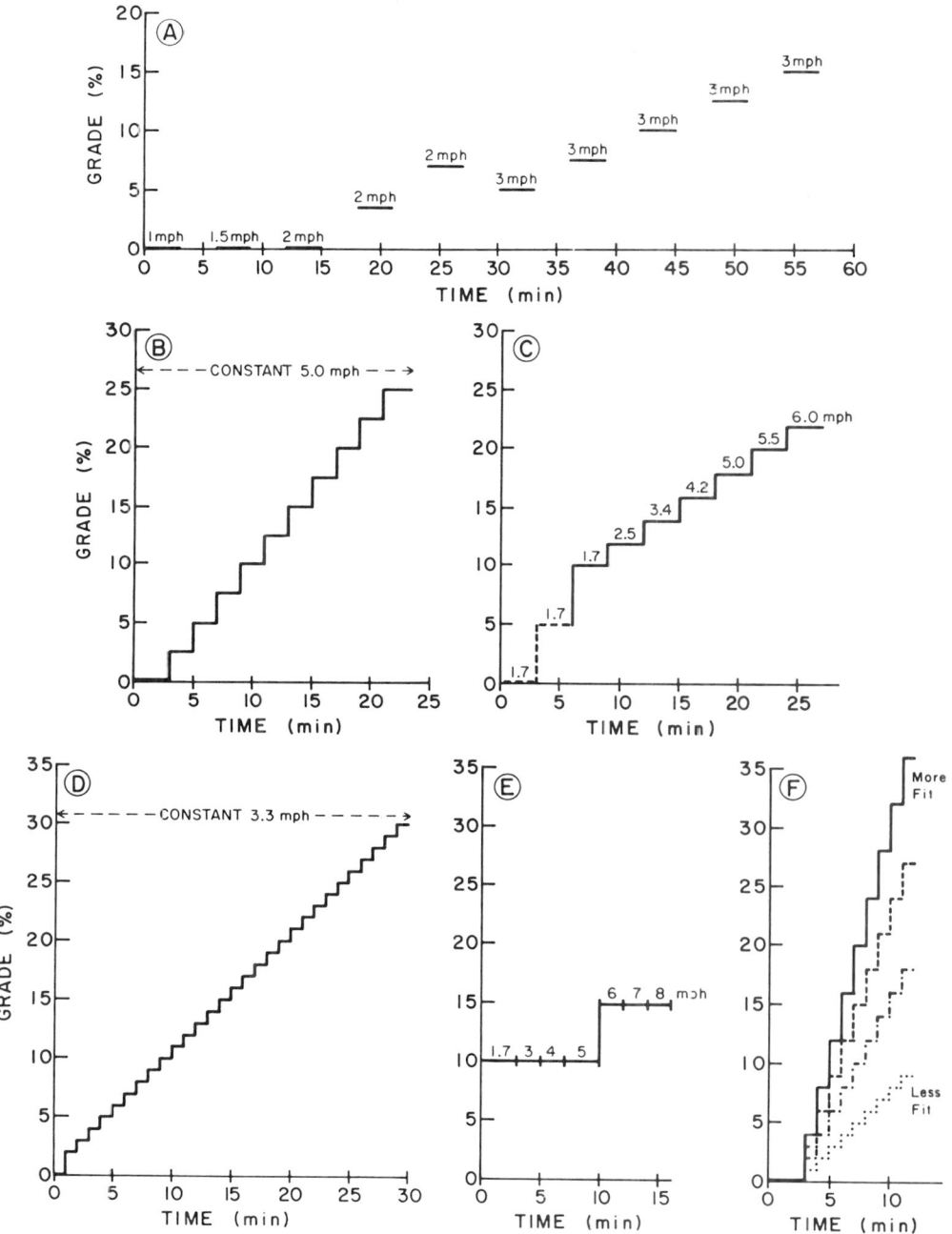

FIGURE 5.5.   Several treadmill protocols. A, Naughton protocol. Three-minute exercise periods of increasing work rate alternate with 3-minute rest periods. The exercise periods vary in grade and speed. B, Astrand protocol. The speed is constant at 5 mph. After 3 minutes at 0% grade, the grade is increased 2½% every 2 minutes. C, Bruce protocol. Grade and speed are changed every 3 minutes. The 0% and 5% grades are omitted in healthier subjects. D, Balke protocol. After 1 minute at 0% grade and 1 minute at 2% grade, the grade is increased 1% per minute, all at a speed of 3.3 mph. E, Ellestad protocol. The initial grade is 10% and the later grade is 15%, while the speed is increased every 2 or 3 minutes. F, Harbor protocol. After 3 minutes of walking at a comfortable speed, the grade is increased at a constant preselected amount each minute: 1%, 2%, or 3%, so the subject reaches his or her peak V̇O₂ in approximately 10 minutes.

linear increase in $\dot{V}O_2$ in normal subjects. The additional measures allow us to calculate values such as peak $\dot{V}O_2$, AT, R, maximum $\dot{V}E/MVV$, $\dot{V}E/\dot{V}O_2$, $\dot{V}E/\dot{V}CO_2$, and O_2 pulse, thus adding considerable insight into gas exchange, ventilatory, and cardiovascular function.

Arm Ergometry

Method

Arm exercise protocols similar to those for lower extremity exercise are usually done because of dysfunction of the lower extremities. The usual technique is to use a converted cycle ergometer with the axle placed at or below the level of the shoulders while the subject sits or stands and moves the pedals so the arms are alternately fully extended. The most common frequency is 50 rpm. Occasionally, upper extremity exercise is performed using wheelchair wheels coupled to a cycle ergometer or by rowing, paddling, or swimming. These modes may be particularly useful for paraplegics, oarsmen, or athletes. To obtain maximal cardiovascular and respiratory stress, arm cycling must be done concurrently with lower extremity exercise.

If the person performing the test is healthy and has not undergone specific upper extremity training, the peak $\dot{V}O_2$ for arm cycling will approximate 50 to 70% of that for leg cycling (75–78). Further, the AT for most healthy subjects is also lower. Maximum $\dot{V}E$ is similarly reduced, whereas maximum HR is only 2 to 12% less than with leg cycle exercise. Thus, the maximum O_2 pulse is less with arm than with leg cycling.

Critique

Although arm cycling exercise has occasional uses, it does not stress the cardiovascular and respiratory systems as much as leg cycling or treadmill exercise. As such, it is a poor substitute when one assesses the cardiovascular and respiratory systems, except when lower extremity exercise is impossible.

Other Tests Suitable for Fitness or Serial Evaluations

A variety of tests have been used to evaluate individuals or groups without attempting to ascertain whether a particular system (e.g., cardiovascular, respiratory, or musculoskeletal) or motivation of the performer is limiting exercise. Such tests are likely to be used for children, young adults, military personnel, or laborers exposed to environmental stress or pollutants (Fig. 5.5B, D). These tests are often considered measures of cardiovascular fitness and may allow division of the population studied into several levels of fitness, but they can also be used to serially evaluate patients with known disorders. Formerly, these tests could be repeated frequently only with simple equipment. Now, gas exchange measurements with telemetry are possible.

Harvard Step Test and Modifications

The original Harvard Step Test consisted of having the subject step up and down at a uniform rate of 30 step-ups per minute onto a stool, bench, or platform 20 inches high for a period of 5 minutes, if possible, with measurements of pulse rate for 30 seconds after 1 minute of recovery (9). Modifications include: 1) the addition of backpacks which add approximately one third to the subject's weight; 2) reduction in the duration of the test to 3 minutes; 3) change in the step height to 17 inches for women; 4) measurement of HR during exercise; 5) change in the time of measurement of recovery pulse; 6) change in test scoring; and 7) use of a gradational step in which the height of the platform could be raised 2 cm every minute or 4.5 cm every 2 minutes (9, 79, 80).

600-Yard Run-Walk

The 600-yard run-walk requires that the subject cover a 600-yard level distance in the shortest possible time (81). He or she may intersperse running with walking but must try to finish as quickly as possible. A properly marked track or football field is suitable. For 37 male university staff and faculty members, time for completion showed a moderately good correlation (r = 0.644) with their peak $\dot{V}O_2$ measured by an incremental cycle ergometer test (which ranged from 25 to 50 ml/min/kg).

12-Minute Field Test

In the 12-minute field performance test, the subjects, dressed in running attire, cover as much distance as possible by running or walking (82). The distance covered was shown to correlate well (r = 0.897) with $\dot{V}O_2$max measured during an intermittent incremental treadmill test in 115 military personnel ($\dot{V}O_2$max range of 30 to 60 ml/min/kg) (82).

12-Minute Walking Test

The distance covered in 12 minutes of walking (equivalent to the original 12-minute field test described by Cooper) has been used for assessing disability in patients with chronic bronchitis (83). Each patient is instructed to cover as much distance as possible on foot in 12 minutes, for example, walking over a marked course in a hospital corridor. The patient is told to try to keep going, but not to be concerned if he or she has to slow down or stop to rest. The aim is for the patient to feel that at the end of the test he or she could not have covered more ground in the time given. A physician or therapist accompanies the patient, acting as timekeeper and giving encouragement as necessary.

Daily repetitions of the 12-minute test in 12 hospital in-patients on 3 different days showed a significant improvement in distance on day 2 over day 1, but not on day 3 over day 2 (60). In 35 patients with lung disease, the distance correlated significantly with peak $\dot{V}O_2$ (r = 0.52), maximum exercise $\dot{V}E$ (r = 0.53), FVC (r = 0.406), but not with FEV_1 (r = 0.283) (83).

PREPARING THE REPORT

In our laboratory, after entry of blood gas and blood pressure values, the computer system produces graphic and tabular displays of the results of the exercise study similar to those shown in Chapter 10. Consistency of format facilitates interpretation. The layout of the 9-panel graphic array allows one to quickly review the cardiovascular and ventilatory systems, ventilation-perfusion relationships, and exercise metabolism. The addition of ECG and blood pressure data usually leads to a pathophysiological diagnosis. The textual report we prepare includes brief summaries of relevant clinical information and medications, specific exercise related complaints, pulmonary function test results, a brief description of the methods and procedure, a table of key gas exchange variables, and a narrative analysis and interpretation. We also include a glossary of terms found on the report that may be unfamiliar to some referring physicians. Our recommendations and examples of what to include in the final report are listed in Table 5.3.

SUMMARY

Numerous exercise devices, protocols, and physiologic measuring systems are available for the safe and economical evaluation of normal individuals, athletes, or patients suspected of having, or known to have, respiratory, cardiovascular, or neuromuscular disease. The specific exercise performed can be tailored to the diagnostic or therapeutic questions

TABLE 5.3. What Should Be Included in a Report on an Exercise Test Patient and Pre-Test Information

A. Patient and Pre-Test Information

Recommendation for the Report	Example
Patient's exercise related complaint or the limitation being addressed by the exercise test	"Patient experiences shortness of breath while walking up hills."
The specific question being addressed by the requested exercise test (often raised by a referring physician)	"What is the degree of exercise limitation?" "Can my patient tolerate a pneumonectomy?" "Should oxygen be prescribed for my patient during exercise?" "Has the new medication improved exercise capacity?"
Pertinent clinical information that may be helpful in relating to the interpretation	Type of exercise limitation noted by the patient (fatigue, chest pain, dyspnea). Level of physical activity in a normal day's routine. Medications. Occupational history.
Findings from a focused physical examination	Blood pressure, chest and heart examination. Patient's actual height and weight.
Results of other studies relevant to exercise capacity, especially if they contribute to developing the interpretation and conclusions	Resting electrocardiograms, chest roentgenograms, pulmonary function tests, echocardiograms.
Recent information	Recent food or medications? VC, IC, FEV_1, MVV on day of testing.
Pre-test diagnosis	COPD, coronary artery disease, asthma, claudication

(continued)

TABLE 5.3. What Should Be Included in a Report on an Exercise Test Patient and Pre-Test Information

B. Information about the Exercise Laboratory to be Included in the Report

Recommendation for the Report	Example
Exercise laboratory equipment	Type of ergometer used. Measurements made.
Exercise protocol	Progressive or constant-work. Defined protocol (e.g., Bruce) or specify progression and time of exercise protocol. Was oxygen supplementation used?
Environmental conditions	Room temperature, barometric pressure
Documentation of other procedures performed in the laboratory, if any	Arterial catheter, pulmonary artery catheter, pulse oximetry, electrocardiograms, post-exercise spirometry, non-invasive blood pressure measurements

C. Observations during and after the Exercise Test

Recommendation for the Report	Example
Patient's performance during exercise test	Symptoms limiting exercise
Reason(s) for stopping exercise	Why did the patient stop? Was the test stopped by the patient or the physician? Ask whether the symptoms duplicated the symptoms that ordinarily limit exercise.
Data displays	Graphs and tables of data obtained during exercise test. Summary tables of most important information.

D. Exercise Test Interpretation and Recommendations

Recommendation for the Report	Example
Maximum exercise capacity.	Absolute $\dot{V}O_2$, ml/min, $\dot{V}O_2$ relative to size ($\dot{V}O_2$, ml/min/kg) and relative to normal subject (%-predicted).
Observations leading to mechanistic or diagnostic conclusions	Which variables when compared to normal led you to reach a conclusion about the cause of exercise limitation.
Comment regarding the patient's symptoms at end of exercise Answer(s) to specific question(s) asked by referring physician	"The shortness of breath experienced was similar to symptoms limiting normal activity." "This exercise test is consistent with the presence of impaired cardiac response to exercise."
Assessment of patient's effort during test	Subjective assessment of effort. Heart rate or breathing reserve. Recovery R. Change in blood HCO_3^- or lactate levels.
Normal or reference values used	Normal values for patient's size, gender, or age. References to the literature for normal values used.
Complications during exercise test	Arrhythmia, chest pain, hyper- or hypotension, extremity pain or discomfort
Recommendations, if any, to referring physician	Change management or order additional tests such as exercise with arterial blood gases

being asked and the facilities and technical and professional expertise available. Ordinarily, a maximum amount of information can be obtained by making ventilatory, gas exchange, ECG, blood pressure, and blood gas measurements during a cycle or treadmill test that includes: 1) sitting or standing at rest; 2) unloaded cycling or treadmill walking for 3 minutes; 3) 1-minute incremental exercise with an increment size enabling the subject to reach his or her maximally tolerated work rate in about 10 minutes; and 4) early recovery. Less frequently, constant work rate tests, arm ergometry, or timed walking tests may be useful.

References

1. Beaver WL, Wasserman K, Whipp BJ. On-line computer analysis and breath-by-breath graphical display of exercise function tests. J Appl Physiol 1973;34:128–132.

2. Sue DY, Hansen JE, Blais M, Wasserman K. Measurement and analysis of gas exchange during exercise using a programmable calculator. J Appl Physiol 1980;49:456–461.

3. Sietsema KE, Cooper DM, Rosove MH, Perloff JK, Child JS, Canobbio MM, Whipp BJ, Wasserman K. Dynamics of oxygen uptake during exercise in adults with cyanotic congenital heart disease. Circulation 1986;73:1137–1144.

4. Finucane KE, Egan BA, Dawson SV. Linearity and frequency response of pneumotachographs. J Appl Physiol 1972;32:121–126.

5. Porszasz J, Barstow T, Wasserman K. Evaluation of a symmetrically disposed Pitot tube flowmeter for measuring gas flow during exercise. J Appl Physiol 1994;77:2659–2665.

6. Yoshiya I, Nakajima T, Nagai I, Jitsukawa S. A bidirectional respiratory flowmeter using the hot-wire principle. J Appl Physiol 1975;38:360–365.

7. Yoshiya I, Shimada Y, Tanaka K. Evaluation of a hot-wire respiratory flowmeter for clinical applicability. J Appl Physiol 1979;47:1131–1135.

8. Jackson AC, Vinegar A. A technique for measuring frequency response of pressure, volume, and flow transducers. J Appl Physiol 1979;47:462–467.

9. Consolazio CF, Johnson RE, Pecora LI. Physiological Measurements of Metabolic Function in Man. New York: McGraw-Hill, 1963;368–401.

10. Gabel RA. Calibration of nonlinear gas analyzers using expotential washout and polymonial curve fitting. J Appl Physiol 1973;34:400–401.

11. Clark JH, Greenleaf JE. Electronic bicycle ergometer: a simple calibration procedure. J Appl Physiol 1971;30:440–442.

12. Van Praagh E, Bedu M, Roddier P, Coudert J. A simple calibration method for mechanically braked cycle ergometers. Int J Sports Med 1992;13:27–30.

13. Russell JC, Dale JD. Dynamic torquemeter calibration of bicycle ergometers. J Appl Physiol 1986;61:1217–1220.

14. Giezendanner D, Di Prampero PE, Cerretelli P. A programmable electrically braked ergometer. J Appl Physiol 1983;55:578–582.

15. Hansen JE. Exercise instruments, schemes, and protocols for evaluating the dyspneic patient. Am Rev Respir Dis 1984;129(Suppl.):S25–S27.

16. Astrand I. Aerobic work capacity in men and women with special reference to age. Acta Physiol Scand 1960;49(Suppl. 169):1–9.

17. Clark JS, Votteri B, Arriagno RL, Cheung P, Eichhorn JH, Fallat RJ, Lee SE, Newth CJL, Sue DY. Noninvasive assessment of blood gases. Am Rev Respir Dis 1992;145:220–232.

18. Zeballos RJ, Weisman IM. Reliability of ear oximetry during exercise and hypoxia in black subjects. Chest 1989;96:162S.

19. Smyth RJ, D'Urzo AD, Slutsky AS, Galdo BM, Rebuck AS. Ear oximetry during combined hypoxia and exercise. J Appl Physiol 1986;60:716–719.

20. Ries AL, Farrow JT, Clausen JL. Accuracy of two ear oximeters at rest and during exercise in pulmonary patients. Am Rev Respir Dis 1985;132:685–689.

21. Powers SK, Dodd S, Freeman J, Ayers GD, Samson H, McKnight T. Accuracy of pulse oximetry to estimate HbO_2 fraction of total Hb during exercise. J Appl Physiol 1989;67:300–304.

22. Hansen JE, Casaburi R. Validity of ear oximetry in clinical exercise testing. Chest 1987;91:333–337.

23. Escourrou PJL, Delaperche MR, Visseaux A. Reliability of pulse oximetry during exercise in pulmonary patients. Chest 1990;97:635–638.

24. Ries AL, Fedullc PF, Clausen JL. Rapid changes in arterial blood gas levels after exercise in pulmonary patients. Chest 1983;83:454–456.

25. Frye M, DiBenedetto R, Lain D, Morgan K. Single arterial puncture vs. arterial cannula for arterial gas analysis after exercise. Chest 1988;93:294–299.

26. O'Neill AV, Johnson DC. Transition from exercise to rest. Ventilatory and arterial blood gas responses. Chest 1991;99:1145–1150.

27. Stetz CW, Miller RG, Kelly GE, Raffin RA. Reliability of the thermodilution method in the determination of cardiac output in clinical practice. Am Rev Respir Dis 1982;126:1001–1004.

28. Versteeg PG, Kippersluis GJ. Automated systems for measurement of oxygen uptake during exercise testing. Int J Sports Med 1989;10:107–112.

29. Huszczuk A, Whipp BJ, Wasserman K. A respiratory gas exchange simulator for routine calibration in metabolic studies. Eur Respir J 1990;3:465–468.

30. American Thoracic Society. Standardization of spirometry: 1987 update. Am Rev Respir Dis 1987;136:1285–1307.

31. Campbell SC. A comparison of the maximum volume ventilation with forced expiratory volume in one second: an assessment of subject cooperation. J Occup Med 1982;24:531–533.

32. Seldinger SI. Catheter replacement of the needle in percutaneous arteriography: a new technique. Acta Radiol 1953;39:368–376.

33. Huszczuk A. Personal Communication, 1985.
34. Whipp BJ, Davis JA, Torres F, Wasserman K. A test to determine parameters of aerobic function during exercise. J Appl Physiol 1981;50:217–221.
35. Balke B. Correlation of static and physical endurance. 1. A test of physical performance based on the cardiovascular and respiratory response to gradually increased work. Project No. 21-32-004, Report No. 1. 1952. San Antonio, TX, United States Air Force School of Aviation Medicine.
36. Balke B, Ware RW. An experimental study of "physical fitness" of Air Force personnel. US Armed Forces Med J 1959;10:675–688.
37. Consolazio CF, Nelson RA, Matoush LO, Hansen JE. Energy metabolism at high altitude (3,475). J Appl Physiol 1966;21:1732–1740.
38. Jones NL. Clinical Exercise Testing, 3rd Ed. Philadelphia: W.B. Saunders, 1988.
39. Spiro SG. Exercise testing in clinical medicine. Br J Dis Chest 1977;71:145–172.
40. Fairshter RD, Walters J, Salvess K, Fox M, Minh VD, Wilson AF. Comparison of incremental exercise test during cycle and treadmill ergometry. Am Rev Respir Dis 1982;125(Suppl.):254 (Abstract).
41. Davis JA, Whipp BJ, Lamarra N, Huntsman DJ, Frank MH, Wasserman K. Effect of ramp slope on determination of aerobic parameters from the ramp exercise test. Med Sci Sports Exerc 1982;14:339–343.
42. Cooper DM, Weiler-Ravell D. Gas exchange response to exercise in children. Am Rev Respir Dis 1984; 129(Suppl.):S47–S48.
43. Zhang YY, Johnson MC, Chow N, Wasserman K. Effect of exercise testing protocol on parameters of aerobic function. Med Sci Sports Exerc 1991;23:625–630.
44. Arstilla M. Pulse-conducted triangular exercise-ECG test. Acta Med Scand 1972;529(Suppl.):103–109.
45. Redwood DR, Rosing DR, Goldstein AR, Beiser G, Epstein SE. Importance of the design of an exercise protocol in the evaluation of patients with angina pectoris. Circulation 1971;43:618–628.
46. Buchfuhrer MJ, Hansen JE, Robinson TE, Sue DY, Wasserman K, Whipp BJ. Optimizing the exercise protocol for cardiopulmonary assessment. J Appl Physiol 1983; 55:1558–1564.
47. Taylor HL, Buskirk E, Henschel A. Maximal oxygen intake as an objective measure of cardiorespiratory performance. J Appl Physiol 1955;8:73–80.
48. Froelicher VF, Brammel H, Davis GD, Noguera I, Stewart A, Lancaster MD. A comparison of three maximal treadmill exercise protocols. J Appl Physiol 1974;36:720–725.
49. Maksud MG, Coutts KD. Comparison of a continuous and discontinuous graded treadmill test for maximal oxygen uptake. Med Sci Sports Exerc 1971;3:63–65.
50. Wyndham CH, Strydom NB, Leary WP, Williams CG. Studies of the maximum capacity for men for physical effort. Arbeitsphysiologie 1966;22:285–295.
51. McArdle WD, Katch FI, Pechar GS. Comparison of continuous and discontinuous treadmill and bicycle tests for max $\dot{V}O_2$. Med Sci Sports Exerc. 1972;5:156–160.
52. Pollack ML, Bohannon RL, Cooper KM, Ayres J, Ward A, White SR, Linnerud ND. A comparative analysis of four protocols for maximal treadmill stress testing. Am Heart J 1976;92:39–46.
53. Furuike AN, Sue DY, Hansen JE, Wasserman K. Comparison of physiologic dead space/tidal volume ratio and alveolar-arterial PO_2 difference during incremental and constant work exercise. Am Rev Respir Dis 1982;126:579–583.
54. Beaver WL. Water vapor corrections in oxygen consumption calculation. J Appl Physiol 1973;35:928–931.
55. Astrand PO, Rodahl K. Textbook of Work Physiology, 2nd Ed. New York: McGraw-Hill, 1977;333–365.
56. Nery LE, Wasserman K, Andrews JD, Huntsman DJ, Hansen JE, Whipp BJ. Ventilatory and gas exchange kinetics during exercise in chronic airways obstruction. J Appl Physiol 1982;53:1594–1602.
57. Lamarra N, Whipp BJ, Blumenberg M, Wasserman K. Model-order estimation of cardiorespiratory dynamics during moderate exercise. Modelling and control of breathing. New York: Elsevier Science, 1983;338–345.
58. Whipp BJ, Ward SA, Lamarra N, Davis JA, Wasserman K. Parameters of ventilatory and gas exchange dynamics during exercise. J Appl Physiol 1982;52:1506–1513.
59. Sietsema KE, Daly JA, Wasserman K. Early dynamics of O_2 uptake and heart rate as affected by exercise work rate. J Appl Physiol 1989;67:2535–2541.
60. Ben-Dov I, Sietsema KE, Wasserman K. O_2 uptake in hyperthyroidism during constant work rate and incremental exercise. Eur J Appl Physiol 1991;62:261–267.
61. Koike A, Wasserman K, McKenzie DK, Zanconato S, Weiler-Ravell D. Evidence that diffusion limitation determines oxygen uptake kinetics during exercise in humans. J Clin Invest 1990;86:1698–1706.
62. Whipp BJ, Wasserman K. Oxygen uptake kinetics for various intensities of constant load work. J Appl Physiol 1972;33:351–356.
63. Roston WL, Whipp BJ, Davis JA, Effros RM, Wasserman K. Oxygen uptake kinetics and lactate concentration during exercise in man. Am Rev Respir Dis 1987;135:1080–1034.
64. Casaburi R, Barstow T, Robinson T, Wasserman K. Influence of work rate on ventilatory and gas exchange kinetics. J Appl Physiol 1989;67:547–555.
65. Casaburi R, Wasserman K, Patessio A, Ioli F, Zanaboni S, Donner CF. A new perspective in pulmonary rehabilitation; anaerobic threshold as a discriminant in training. Eur J Respir Dis 1989;2:618–623.
66. Zhang YY, Wasserman K, Sietsema KE, Barstow TJ, Mizumoto G, Sullivan CS, Ben-Dov I. $\dot{Q}O_2$ uptake kinetics in response to exercise: A measure of tissue anaerobiosis in heart failure. Chest 1993;103:735–741.
67. Cropp GIA. The exercise bronchoprovocation test: standardized of procedures and evaluation of response. J Allergy Clin Immunol 1979;64:627–633.
68. Deal EC Jr, McFadden ER Jr, Ingram RH, Strauss RH, Jaeger JJ. Role of respiratory heat exchange in production of exercise-induced asthma. J Appl Physiol 1979;46:467–475.
69. Wasserman K. Testing regulation of ventilation with exercise. Chest 1976;70(Suppl):173–178.

70. Bruce RA. Exercise testing of patients with coronary artery disease. Ann Clin Res 1971;3:323–332.

71. Ellestad MH. Stress Testing, 2nd Ed. Philadelpha: F.A. Davis, 1980.

72. Patterson JA, Naughton J, Pietras RJ, Gumar RN. Treadmill exercise in assessment of patients with cardiac disease. Am J Cardiol 1972;30:757–762.

73. Stuart RJ, Ellestad MH. National survey of exercise stress testing facilities. Chest 1980;77:94–97.

74. Bruce RA, Kusimi F, Hosmer D. Maximal oxygen intake and nomographic assessment of functional aerobic impairment in cardiovascular disease. Am Heart J 1973;85:546–562.

75. Bar-Or O, Zwiren LD. Maximal oxygen consumption test during arm exercise-reliability and validity. J Appl Physiol 1975;38:424–426.

76. Vokac Z, Bell H, Bautz-Holter E, Rodahl K. Oxygen uptake/heart rate relationship in leg and arm exercise, sitting and standing. J Appl Physiol 1975;39:54–59.

77. Davis JA, Vodak P, Wilmore JH, Vodal J, Kurtz P. Anaerobic threshold and maximal aerobic power for three modes of exercise. J Appl Physiol 1976;41:544–550.

78. Casaburi R, Barstow T, Robinson T, Wasserman K. Dynamic and steady-state ventilatory and gas exchange responses to arm exercise. Med Sci Sports Exerc 1992;24:1365–1374.

79. Nagle FJ, Balke B, Naughton JP. Gradational step tests for assessing work capacity. J Appl Physiol 1965;21:745–748.

80. Nagle FJ, Balke B, Baptista G, Alleyia J, Hawley E. Compatability of progressive treadmill, bicycle and step tests based on oxygen uptake responses. Med Sci Sports Exerc 1971;3:149–154.

81. Fleishman EA. The Structure and Measurement of Physical Fitness. Englewood Cliffs, NJ: Prentice-Hall, 1964; 171–172.

82. Cooper KM. A means of assessing maximal oxygen intake. JAMA 1968;203:201–204.

83. McGavin CR, Gupta SP, McHardy GJR. Twelve minute walking test for assessing disability in chronic bronchitis. Br Med J 1976;1:822–823.

CHAPTER 6

Normal Values

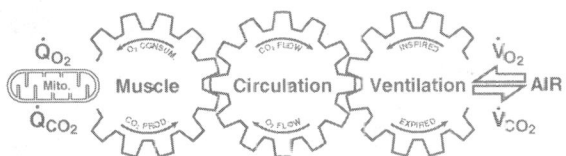

INTERPRETATION OF the results of exercise tests requires knowledge of the normal responses. In this chapter, we present values for important physiologic variables that we think represent the best data available for sedentary normal subjects during exercise. In some instances, several sets of normal values for the same measurement are included. When doing so, we have made a recommendation.

PEAK OXYGEN UPTAKE

The selection of peak $\dot{V}_{O_2}$ predicted values (both mean and at the 95% confidence level) is a challenging problem, especially because the geographic area, body sizes and activity levels of a specific clinical population may differ from those of reference populations. It is relevant to note that the measurement of $\dot{V}_{O_2}$ during heavy exercise may be technically difficult. Peak $\dot{V}_{O_2}$ in normal subjects during exercise varies with age, gender, body size, level of ordinary activity, and type of exercise. When comparing the peak $\dot{V}_{O_2}$ of an individual to the predicted peak $\dot{V}_{O_2}$, a predicted value generated for the same form of exercise must be used. It is preferable if the population from which the predicting equations were obtained included a large number of individuals with similar characteristics to the patient being tested.

Astrand and Rodahl (1) have pointed out that peak $\dot{V}_{O_2}$ expressed as (ml/min) $\times$ kg^{-1} is higher in smaller than larger top athletes, even when obesity is not a factor. However, when expressed as (ml/min) $\times$ kg$^{-2/3}$, peak $\dot{V}_{O_2}$ does not differ between smaller and larger athletes. They argued against the practice of using weight as a primary variable in predicting peak $\dot{V}_{O_2}$. Despite their rational explanation and the obvious bias introduced by obesity on peak values when expressed as (ml/min) $\times$ kg^{-1}, many exercise physiologists and clinicians continue to estimate cardiovascular function by comparing actual to predicted values based on age, gender, and weight, even in obese individuals. However, this practice will predict too high a peak $\dot{V}_{O_2}$ in obese individuals. We believe that sufficient evidence now exists to assert that, even though peak $\dot{V}_{O_2}$ values may still be expressed as (ml/min) $\times$ kg^{-1} in many publications, this practice is not optimal for the clinical evaluation of the cardiorespiratory function of patients (2–4).

AGE AND GENDER

Many investigators have reported that peak $\dot{V}_{O_2}$ declines with age and is smaller for women than men (5–7). Although cross-sectional studies of change in peak $\dot{V}_{O_2}$ with age are easier to perform than longitudinal studies, they may be misleading on account of selection bias. This is because older subjects included in a study are more likely to be active, relative to their peers, than their younger counterparts; hence the peak $\dot{V}_{O_2}$ values in older subjects tend to decrease more slowly than peak $\dot{V}_{O_2}$ values in longitudinal studies (8). In a longitudinal study, Astrand et al. (9) measured $\dot{V}_{O_2}$ max during cycling exercise in 66 well-trained, physically active men and women aged 20 to 33 years and studied them again 21 years later. The mean decrease in $\dot{V}_{O_2}$ max was 22% for the 35 women and 20% for the 31 men.

Bruce et al. (10) used stepwise multiple regression analysis to identify whether gender, age, physical activity, weight, height, or smoking aided in the prediction of $\dot{V}_{O_2}$ max during treadmill exercise in adults. They found that gender and age were the two most important factors. The $\dot{V}_{O_2}$ max of women was approximately 77% of $\dot{V}_{O_2}$ max of men when adjusted for body weight and activity. Astrand (11) reported 17% lower $\dot{V}_{O_2}$ max for 18 women students compared with 17 male students of comparable size.

Activity Level

Investigators generally agree that values obtained from athletes, physical education teachers, servicemen, or participants in organized exercise groups should be modified before being considered for use as reference values for a clinical population. Balke and Ware (12) found the peak $\dot{V}_{O_2}$ of Air Force personnel to be strongly related to their activity pattern. Drinkwater et al. (6) found that the peak $\dot{V}_{O_2}$ of extremely active women did not decline over two decades despite a gradual increase in body weight. The decline in peak $\dot{V}_{O_2}$ with age is more rapid in habitually inactive men, even allowing for greater weight gain in the inactive group (8). Importantly, even brief periods of physical training can increase peak $\dot{V}_{O_2}$ by 15 to 25% or more (5, 13).

Adults of Normal (Predicted) Body Weight

It is logical to assume that physical size would be a factor in peak $\dot{V}_{O_2}$ because the mass of the exercising muscles as well as the dimensions of the cardiovascular and pulmonary systems should determine the maximum quantity of O_2 that can be delivered and used. As previously noted, Astrand and Rodahl found that peak $\dot{V}_{O_2}$ expressed as (ml/min) $\times$ kg^{-1}

was higher in smaller than in larger athletes. When expressed as (ml/min) $\times$ kg$^{-2/3}$, however, peak $\dot{V}O_2$ did not. These data would argue against the traditional practice of using weight as a primary variable in predicting peak $\dot{V}O_2$ or defining fitness.

Despite the variability related to activity levels, relatively good agreement among series exists for mean predicted peak $\dot{V}O_2$ values of non-obese, sedentary populations, if one uses age, gender, and height rather than age, gender, and weight. Pulmonologists are accustomed to predicting most respiratory function values using height rather than weight. Jones et al. (4) found, in a population of over 1000 patients referred to their laboratory, that maximum work capacity was best related to gender, height, and age rather than gender, weight, and age. In 204 volunteers between 20 and 70 years of age, Davis (14) also found that the prediction of peak $\dot{V}O_2$ was not improved by adding weight as a variable to gender, age, and height. However, variance in the series could be reduced by considering factors such as body mass index, lean body weight, or activity level.

We have reviewed the similarities and differences in peak $\dot{V}O_2$ in several series of men and women

of relatively normal body weight (2, 10, 14–17). Figures 6.1 and 6.2 show values of three North American, one Japanese (16), and one Brazilian series (17) for sedentary men and women of normal body proportions.

For men, all five series show reasonably similar parallel declines with age at all heights. The variability is least at 170 cm (less than 0.5 L/min) and greatest at the extremes of height. Jones' values are lowest at 160 cm and highest at 190 cm. On average, Itoh et al. (16) series of Japanese men tends to be higher than others while Neder et al. series (17) of Brazilian men tends to be lower than others.

The values in the women's series also show reasonably similar parallel declines with age at all heights (Fig. 6.2A–D). The values for Japanese women (16) are generally higher and the Brazilian women (17) generally lower. The North American series agree remarkably well at a height of 160 cm (Fig. 6.2B). Davis and Bruce/Hansen formulae also agree well at other heights, with Jones et al. (15) series having lesser values at shorter heights and greater values at taller heights.

For both genders, the close agreement in peak $\dot{V}O_2$ in North American series at average heights

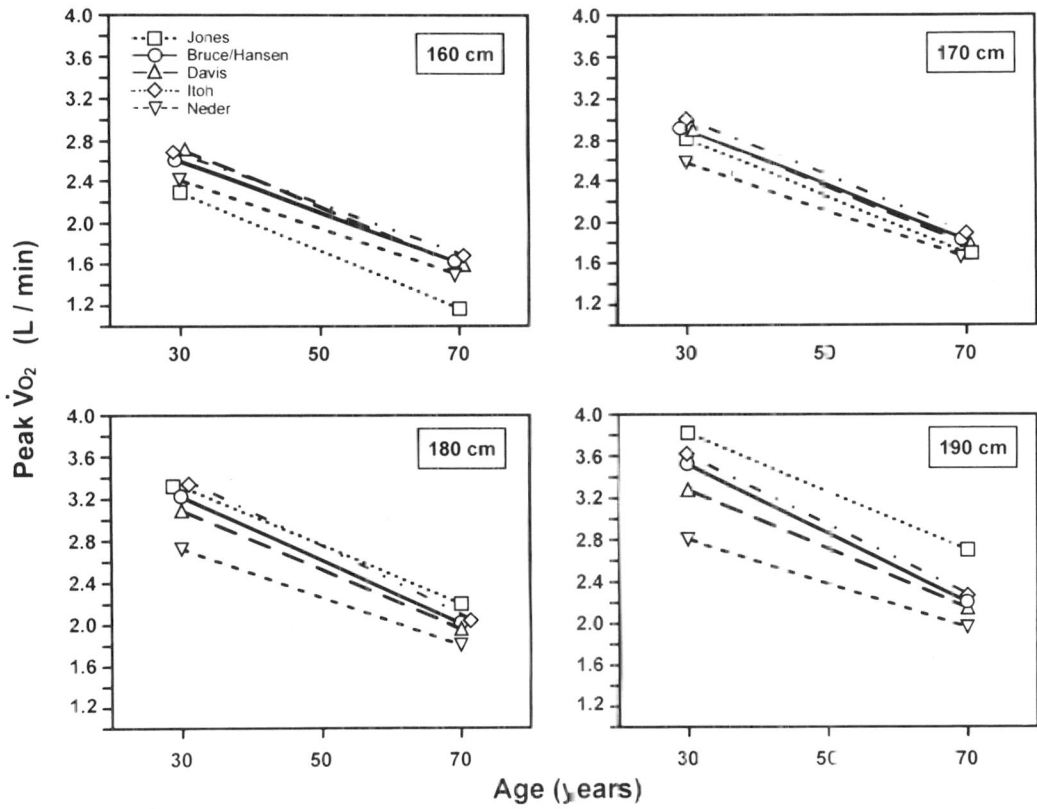

FIGURE 6.1.   Comparison of predicted peak $\dot{V}O_2$ for cycle ergometry of sedentary men of normal (predicted) weight calculated from five reference series for ages 30 to 70 for four different heights and weights: 160 cm and 66 kg, 170 cm and 74 kg, 180 cm and 82 kg, and 190 cm and 89 kg. Data are from Jones et al. (15), Bruce et al. (10) as modified by Hansen et al (2), Itoh et al. (16), Davis (14) and Neder et al. (17).

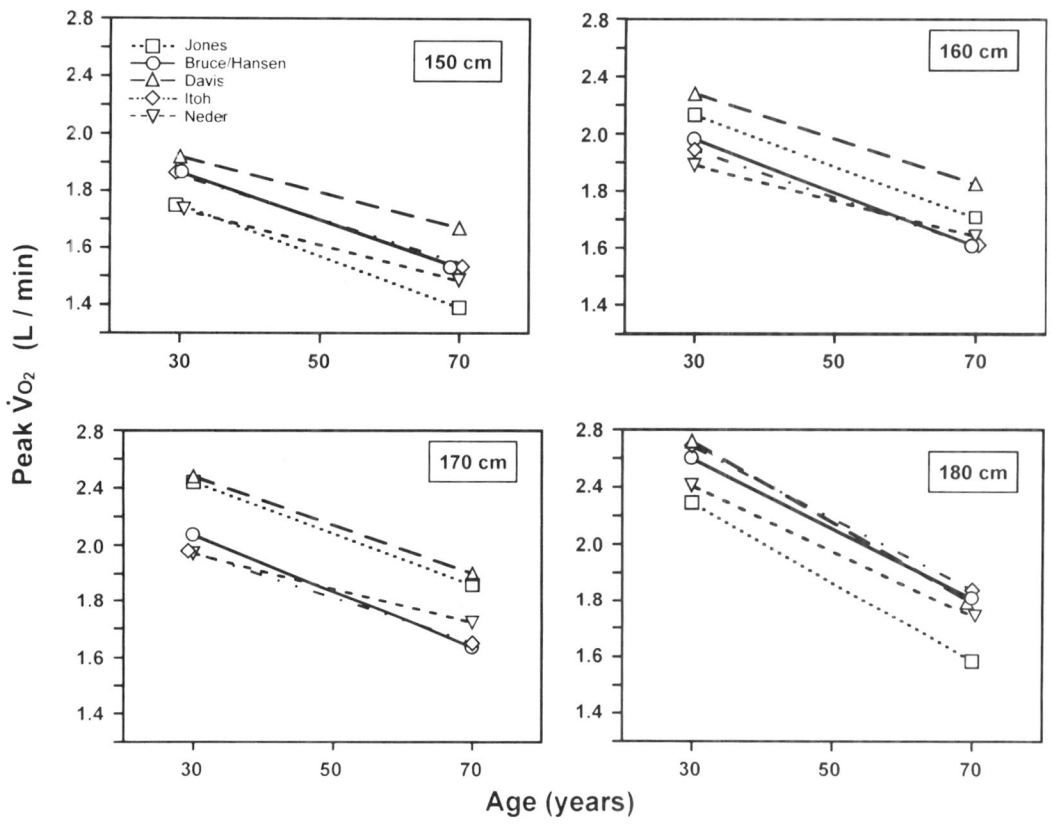

FIGURE 6.2.   Comparison of predicted peak $\dot{V}O_2$ for cycle ergometry of sedentary women of normal (predicted) weight calculated from five reference series for ages 30 to 70 for four different heights and weights: 150 cm and 55 kg, 160 cm and 62 kg, 170 cm and 68 kg, and 180 cm and 74 kg. Data are from Jones et al.(15), Bruce et al. (10), as modified by Hansen et al. (2), Itoh et al. (16), Davis (14) and Neder et al. (17).

suggests confidence in these values at these heights, with lesser confidence at the extremes of height. We have no clear methodologic or other reasons to justify discarding any of these series. The diversity of values for both genders at different locales suggests differences in physical activity levels or selection criteria. Therefore it is a good policy for each laboratory to measure peak $\dot{V}O_2$ in a group of "average" sedentary persons in their vicinity to see how well they match the "normal" values from other series.

Overweight Patients

The selection of an appropriate predicted peak $\dot{V}O_2$ in the overweight patient is difficult. This is largely because the overweight individual is likely to have predominantly an increase in adipose tissue rather than an increase in potential exercising muscle mass. Thus, it is difficult to envision that peak $\dot{V}O_2$ increases in direct proportion to increased body weight for that reason. Furthermore, it is unlikely that cardiovascular and pulmonary function scale with total body weight.

In a cycle ergometer study of 77 middle-aged men (mean age 54 years, range 34 to 74) whom we judged to have normal cardiovascular and respiratory systems and good motivation, we compared peak $\dot{V}O_2$ with the predicted values of Bruce et al. (10) data for $\dot{V}O_2$ max modified for cycle ergometry. There was good agreement for normal weight subjects, but when a subject was overweight (2, 3), there was better agreement using normal weight (weight predicted from height) rather than actual weight. Buskirk and Taylor (18) found that $\dot{V}O_2$max correlated better with a measure of fat-free body weight (r = 0.85) than total body weight (r = 0.63) in 43 healthy students and in 13 soldiers performing treadmill exercise.

Although Jones et al. (4) did not report peak $\dot{V}O_2$ for their 1000 normal individuals, they found that adding weight as a variable to height, age, and gender did not improve the prediction of cycle ergometry exercise capacity. Thus, weight alone did not appreciably influence external work capacity on the cycle. Yet we know that, in healthy individuals, peak $\dot{V}O_2$ correlates highly with maximum external

TABLE 6.1.   Comparison of Physical Characteristics of Healthy Reference Populations and a Clinical Population*

Men				
Series	*Number*	*Age*	*Height*	*Weight*
Bruce et al.[10]	138	43.6 ± 11.1	177.5 ± 6.6	78.6 ± 8.6
Jones et al.[4]	732	48.0 ± 12.0	174.0 ± 6.5	81.8 ± 12.6
Davis[14]	103	43.4 ± 14.6	178.7 ± 7.1	82.8 ± 12.1
Harbor-UCLA†	750	54.2 ± 11.7	172.8 ± 7.4	83.4 ± 17.1

Women				
Series	*Number*	*Age*	*Height*	*Weight*
Bruce et al.[10]	157	41.4 ± 11.2	166.0 ± 6.3	62.1 ± 9.8
Jones et al.[4]	339	47.0 ± 13.5	162.0 ± 6.2	67.3 ± 12.8
Davis[14]	101	44.6 ± 14.6	164.4 ± 6.6	63.6 ± 10.4
Harbor-UCLA†	240	49.1 ± 13.5	160.5 ± 8.4	71.2 ± 21.6

* Values are mean ± SD.
† All groups but the Harbor-UCLA series are healthy reference populations.

work performed. At all external work levels on the cycle, those with larger legs have higher measured $\dot{V}O_2$ than those with smaller legs. On average, we estimate that unloaded $\dot{V}O_2$ while cycling will increase approximately 6 ml/min/kg of extra body weight (19). In addition, overweight individuals can be expected to have slightly higher peak $\dot{V}O_2$ and anaerobic threshold (*AT*) values than others of the same age, gender, and height because in walking the same distances they expend more energy and their muscles become more trained. Thus, body weight can change predicted peak $\dot{V}O_2$ without affecting maximum external work capacity on the cycle ergometer.

We recently reviewed our experience of approximately 1000 clinical cardiopulmonary exercise tests performed in our laboratories. Our clinical population is, on average, shorter, more obese, and more variable in weight than any of the reference populations in standard series of healthy, relatively sedentary North American older adults (Table 6.1, Fig. 6.3). This is especially true of the women tested. For men, 70% exceeded normal (predicted) weight (see Table 6.2 equations), 45% exceeded 110% of normal weight, 26% exceeded 120% of normal weight, 6% exceeded 140% of normal weight, and 2% exceeded 160% of normal weight. For women, 70% exceeded normal weight, 56% exceeded 110% of normal weight, 42% exceeded 120% of normal weight, 25% exceeded 140% of normal weight, and 12% exceeded 160% of normal weight. These findings emphasize the importance of not using pre-

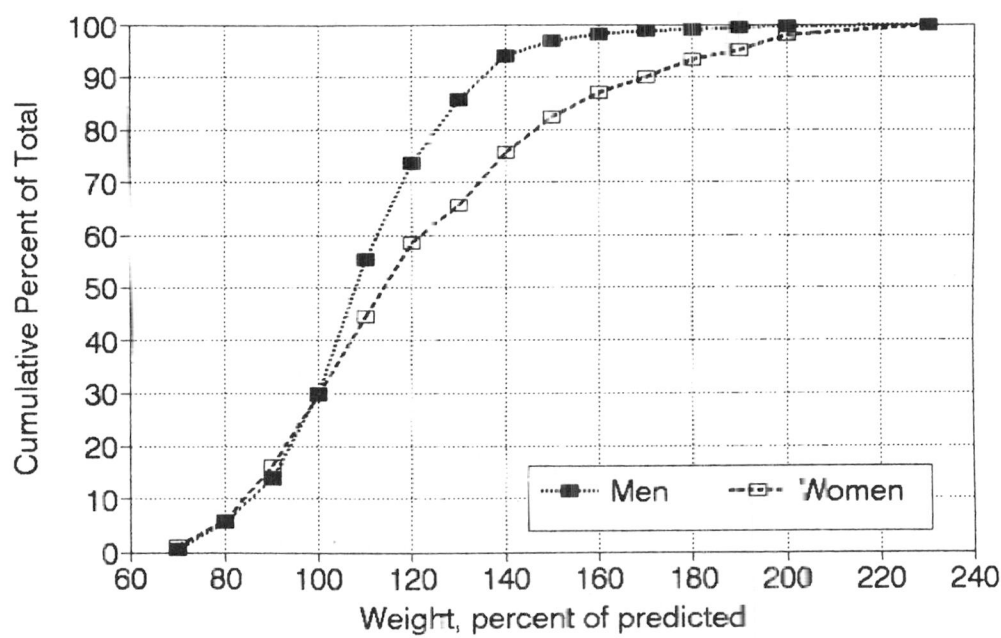

FIGURE 6.3.   Relationship of actual with normal (predicted) weight in approximately 1000 consecutive patients who were presented to our laboratory for diagnostic exercise testing. Normal (predicted) weight for men in kilograms = 0.79 × height in cm −60.7, for women in kilograms = 0.65 × height in cm −42.8. Our patient population can be seen to include a high proportion of overweight individuals. (Formula from Bruce RA, Kusumi F, Hosmer D. Maximal oxygen intake and nomographic assessment of functional aerobic impairment in cardiovascular disease. Am Heart J 1973;85:546–562.)

TABLE 6.2. Calculation of Predicted Peak $\dot{V}_{O_2}$ ml/min

A. Sedentary Men
Cycle factor = 50.72 − 0.372 × A
Step 1. Measure man's weight (W, kg) and height (H, cm) in light clothes without shoes and record age (A, yr)
Step 2. Calculate man's normal (predicted) W in kg as follows:
Normal (predicted) W = 0.79 × H − 60.7
Step 3A. If man's actual W equals normal W:
Predicted peak $\dot{V}_{O_2}$ (ml/min) = actual W × cycle factor
Step 3B. If patient's actual W is less than normal W:
Predicted peak $\dot{V}_{O_2}$ (ml/min) = [(normal W + actual W)/2] × cycle factor
Step 3C. If patient's actual W exceeds normal W:
Predicted peak $\dot{V}_{O_2}$ (ml/min) = (normal W × cycle factor) + 6 × (actual W − normal W)
Step 4. If treadmill is used rather than cycle:
Multiply predicted $\dot{V}_{O_2}$ by 1.11

B. Sedentary Women
Cycle factor = 22.78 − 0.17 × A
Step 1. Measure woman's weight (W, kg) and height (H, cm) in light clothes without shoes and record age (A, yr)
Step 2. Calculate woman's normal (predicted) W in kg as follows:
Normal (predicted) W = 0.65 × H − 42.8
Step 3A. If woman's actual W equals normal W:
Predicted peak $\dot{V}_{O_2}$ (ml/min) = (actual W + 43) × cycle factor
Step 3B. If patient's actual W is less than normal W:
Predicted peak $\dot{V}_{O_2}$ (ml/min) = [(normal W + actual W + 86)/2] × cycle factor
Step 3C. If patient's actual W exceeds normal W:
Predicted peak $\dot{V}_{O_2}$ (ml/min) = [(normal W + 43) × cycle factor] + 6 × (actual W − normal W)
Step 4. If treadmill is used rather than cycle: Multiply predicted peak $\dot{V}_{O_2}$ by 1.11

Modified from references 2 and 10.

dicted peak $\dot{V}_{O_2}$ values expressed as (ml/min) × kg^{-1} in populations of this make-up.

Although it is difficult to be certain of correct predicted values in patients that are overweight, we recommend increasing the predicted peak $\dot{V}_{O_2}$ by 6 ml/min for each kg of weight above normal (predicted) weight, whether the cycle or treadmill is used for exercise testing.

In our analysis, it is clear that the predicted peak $\dot{V}_{O_2}$ in obese patients using weight normalized to height will be less than that expected using actual weight. Therefore, although an overweight patient may have a "normal" peak $\dot{V}_{O_2}$ value, this does not mean that person is necessarily capable of performing the same amount of external work as a non-overweight person of the same height, age, and gender. A greater proportion of the $\dot{V}_{O_2}$ is needed to move the heavier legs and body of the overweight person; a smaller amount of $\dot{V}_{O_2}$ is thereby available to be allocated toward performing external work. For example, on the cycle ergometer, an overweight and a non-overweight patient may have the same peak $\dot{V}_{O_2}$, but the work rate at which the non-overweight patient reaches this $\dot{V}_{O_2}$ value is substantially higher than that of the overweight patient.

Underweight Patients

In the first edition of this book, we suggested decreasing the predicted peak $\dot{V}_{O_2}$ in direct proportion to the decrease in body weight for those patients whose weight was less than normal (as if muscle mass were primarily reduced). As there is likely to be reduction in muscle as well as fat in most underweight persons, we now prefer to use the average of the actual weight and normal weight to predict peak $\dot{V}_{O_2}$ and in related calculations in such patients, as noted in Figure 6.4.

Children

Cooper and colleagues (20, 21) reported peak $\dot{V}_{O_2}$ for 109 children, aged 6 to 17 years, who performed cycle ergometry using a continuously increasing work rate protocol (Fig. 6.5). Because these subjects were not obese, peak $\dot{V}_{O_2}$ correlated similarly with either weight or height. These investigators found, in addition, that their data were similar to those of Astrand (7) for the boys, but the girls studied by Astrand had a significantly higher $\dot{V}_{O_2}$ max versus height relationship. Cooper et al. (20) suggested that cultural or societal differences might account for this difference.

Exercise Mode

The type of exercise is an important determinant of peak $\dot{V}_{O_2}$. Peak $\dot{V}_{O_2}$ during arm cranking ergometer exercise (which is inappropriate to use in evaluating most patients) is about 70% of that of leg cycling exercise (22) because of the smaller mass of muscle and lower maximum work rate achievable. Many studies (7, 23–28) have shown that the peak $\dot{V}_{O_2}$ of leg cycling is approximately 89 to 95% of the maximal values achieved with treadmill exercise. Thus, the form of ergometry and muscle groups involved must be considered when predicting peak $\dot{V}_{O_2}$.

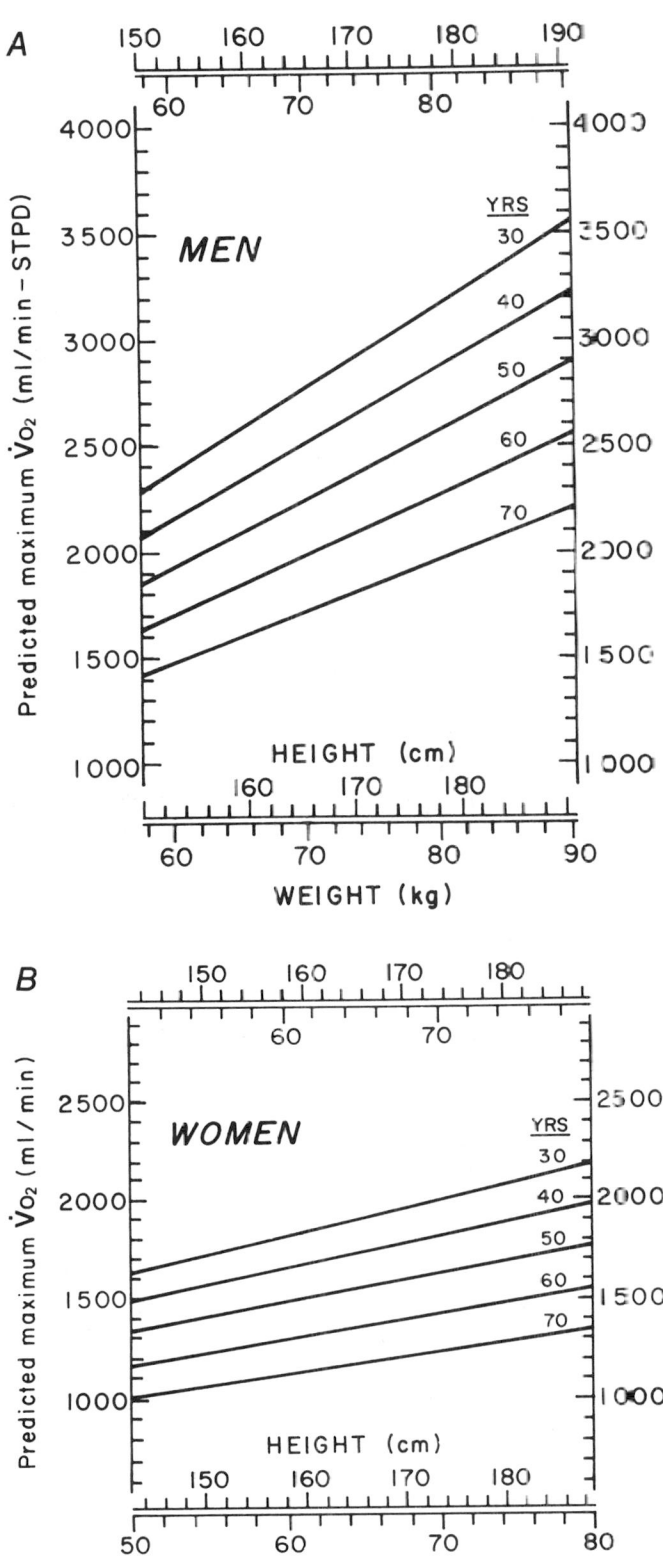

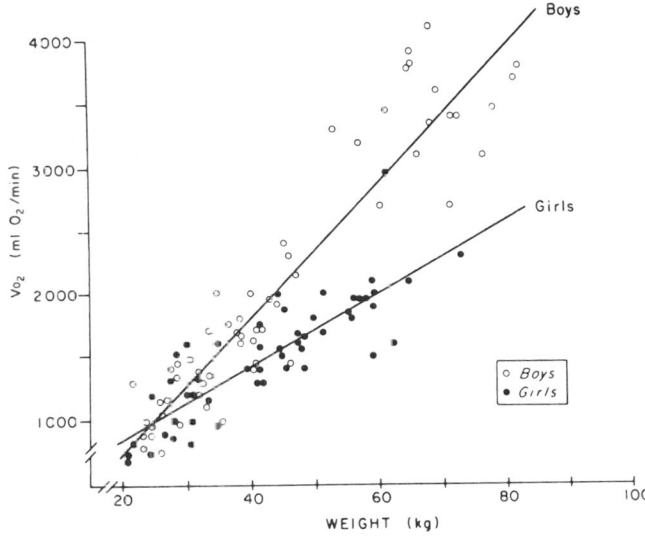

FIGURE 6.5. Peak O_2 uptake of 109 normal North American boys and girls for leg cycling. Regression equations for peak $\dot{V}O_2$ (ml/min) as function of body weight (kg) were: for boys, $\dot{V}O_2 = 52.8 \times$ weight $- 303$ (r = 0.94); for girls, $\dot{V}O_2 = 28.5 \times$ weight $+ 238$ (r = 0.84). (Reprinted with permission from Cooper DM, Weiler-Ravell D, Whipp BJ, et al. Aerobic parameters of exercise as a function of body size during growth in children. J Appl Physiol 1984;56:628–634.)

Recommendation

1. Recommended mean values for peak $\dot{V}O_2$ are given for sedentary men and women in Table 6.2 and children of average activity levels in Table 6.3 performing cycle and, in the case of adults, treadmill exercise. Figure 6.4 gives mean predicted peak $\dot{V}O_2$ values for sedentary men and women of normal (predicted) weight. Figure 6.5 gives mean predicted peak $\dot{V}O_2$ values for leg cycling for children.

2. In overweight patients, increase the predicted peak $\dot{V}O_2$ by 6 ml/min for each kg of weight

FIGURE 6.4. Mean peak $\dot{V}O_2$ values for sedentary men (A) and women (B) of normal (predicted) weight using the cycle ergometer. To use, locate the patient's height and weight on the horizontal axis. *If the patient is underweight* (i.e., the patient's actual weight is to the left of that directly above the patient's height), draw a line half-way between the marks vertically to the line that indicates

the patient's age. From this intersection draw a line horizontally to the vertical axis and read off the predicted peak $\dot{V}O_2$ in liters per minute STPD. *If the patient is overweight* (i.e., the patient's actual weight is to the right of that directly above the patient's height), draw a line vertically from the height marker to the line that indicates the patient's age. From this intersection draw a line horizontally to the vertical axis and read off the preliminary predicted peak $\dot{V}O_2$ in liters/min STPD. To obtain the actual predicted peak $\dot{V}O_2$ for the obese patient, add 6 ml/min for each kilogram the patient is overweight. Finally, if the treadmill is used, predicted cycle values should be increased 11%. (Formula from Bruce RA, Kusumi F, Hosmer D. Maximal oxygen intake and nomographic assessment of functional aerobic impairment in cardiovascular disease. Am Heart J 1973;85:546–562 and data are from Hansen JE, Sue DY, Wasserman K. Predicted values for clinical exercise testing. Am Rev Respir Dis 1984;129(Suppl):S49–S55.)

TABLE 6.3. Predicted Peak $\dot{V}_{O_2}$ and *AT* in Normal Children for Cycle Ergometry

	Boys ≤ 13	Boys > 13	Girls ≤ 11	Girls > 11
Number studied	37	21	24	27
Peak $\dot{V}_{O_2}$, ml/min/kg (mean ± SD)	42 ± 6	50 ± 8	38 ± 7	34 ± 4
lower 95% confidence limit	32	37	26	27
AT, ml/min/kg (mean ± SD)	26 ± 5	27 ± 6	23 ± 4	19 ± 3
lower 95% confidence limit	18	17	16	14

From Copper DM, Weiler-Favell D. Gas exchange response to exercise in children. Am Rev Respir Dis 1984;129(Suppl.):S47–S48.

above normal (predicted) weight, if the cycle is used for exercise testing.

Sample Calculation

Find the predicted peak $\dot{V}_{O_2}$ for treadmill exercise for an overweight 60-year-old sedentary man who is 180 cm tall and weighs 110 kg. Using Table 6.2A, step 2, or the horizontal axis of Figure 6.3A, we ascertain that he is overweight, his predicted weight being 81.5 kg (normal W = 0.79 × 180 − 60.7 = 142.2 − 60.7 = 81.5). Using Table 6.2A, step 3C, we find his predicted peak $\dot{V}_{O_2}$ for cycle ergometry is 81.5 × (50.72 − 0.372 × 60) + 6 × (110 − 81.5) = 81.5 × 28.4 + 6 × 28.5 = 2315 + 171 = 2486 ml/min. Using step 4, the predicted peak $\dot{V}_{O_2}$ for treadmill ergometry is 2486 × 1.11 = 2760 ml/min. Using Figure 6.4A, by extending a line vertically from 180 cm to the 60-year line, we find that the predicted peak $\dot{V}_{O_2}$ for cycle ergometry is 2320 ml/min for a non-obese man. This amount, plus 6 ml/kg × 28.5 kg (for overweight), yields a predicted peak $\dot{V}_{O_2}$ of 2490 ml/min for cycle ergometry for this patient. This value times 1.11 yields a predicted value of 2750 ml/min for treadmill ergometry.

3. In underweight patients, reduce the predicted peak $\dot{V}_{O_2}$ values for normally sized persons by using the average of the actual and normal weight for the peak $\dot{V}_{O_2}$ in such patients.

Sample Calculation

Find the predicted peak $\dot{V}_{O_2}$ for a 50-year-old sedentary woman who is 160 cm tall and weighs 45 kg. Using Table 6.2B, step 2, or Figure 6.4B, we find that she is underweight and that her normal weight is 61 kg (normal W = 0.65 × 160 − 43 = 104 − 43 = 61). Using Table 6.2B, step 3B, her predicted peak $\dot{V}_{O_2}$ is [(45 + 61 + 86)/2] × (22.78 − 0.17 × 50) = 94 × 14.28 = 1342 ml/min. Using Figure

6.4B, by extending a line vertically from 53 kg (which is the average of her actual and normal weight) to the 50-year line, we find that the predicted peak $\dot{V}_{O_2}$ is 1350 ml/min.

4. Use 83% of mean predicted value as a reasonable approximation for the lower 95% confidence limit in the patient of average height. Patients at extremes in height, weight, or age, especially in women, are likely to have an even lower 95% confidence limit. As pointed out by Jones et al. (4), peak exercise values tend to be skewed even in relatively sedentary populations because training increases values above the mean considerably more than inactivity decreases values below the mean.

MAXIMUM HEART RATE (HR) AND HEART RATE RESERVE (HRR)

The maximum heart rate achieved declines with age in all studies. No consistent differences have been found between men and women or among the types of exercise used, i.e., leg cycling, stepping, or inclined treadmill, walking or running.

The two most common formulae for predicting maximum HR in adults are: 220 − age (years) and 210 − 0.65 × age (years) (29). Data from this laboratory fit the former equation slightly better. The standard deviation for each formula is 10 beats/min. As reported by Sheffield et al. (30) and Astrand and Rodahl (1), the maximum heart rates derived from fit individuals approximate either formula reasonably well. The study of K.H. Cooper et al. (31) shows a lower maximum HR in the less fit than the more fit individual. Our finding that the maximum HR was reduced in obese men is consistent with the suggestion that a sedentary existence may reduce maximum HR even in well-motivated subjects (2).

Scandinavian children were found to have an average maximum HR of 205 beats/min (1), whereas North American children aged 8 to 18 had an average maximum heart rate of 187 beats/min with a lower 95% confidence limit of 160 (32).

The concept of HRR can be useful for estimating the relative stress of the cardiovascular system during exercise, but it should be used with caution. A normal HRR is zero. The mean predicted maximum HR may not be reached because of normal population variability, poor motivation, medications such as beta-adrenergic blockers, or because of heart, peripheral vascular, lung, endocrine, or musculoskeletal diseases.

Recommendation

The following equations can be used to estimate the maximum heart rate (HR) and the heart rate reserve (HRR) for adults and children:

1. Maximum heart rate (beats/min) = 220 − age (years)
2. Heart rate reserve (HRR) = Predicted maximum HR − observed maximum HR

RELATIONSHIP OF $\dot{V}O_2$ AND HEART RATE: THE MAXIMUM OXYGEN PULSE

In a given individual, a consistent relationship exists between $\dot{V}O_2$ and HR during exercise (see Fig. 3.11). The quotient of the $\dot{V}O_2$ and HR is the O_2 pulse (see Fig. 3.12); its values are dependent on the stroke volume and the difference between the arterial and mixed venous blood O_2 content. This arterial-venous O_2 difference is, in turn, dependent on the availability of hemoglobin, blood oxygenation in the lung, and extraction of oxygen in the periphery. Examples of the normal and abnormal $\dot{V}O_2$ versus HR response and O_2 pulse response are shown in Figure 6.7. The normal relationship of $\dot{V}O_2$ with HR (patients 1 and 2) is linear over a wide range with a positive intercept on the HR axis. Although sedentary patients 1 and 2 differ considerably in their predicted maximum values (because they differ in age and gender or size), both have normal responses. An exercise response with a higher $\dot{V}O_2$/HR than predicted indicates better than average cardiorespiratory function, whereas a response with a lower $\dot{V}O_2$/HR indicates poorer than average cardiorespiratory function (patient 3). In our clinical population, this latter response is most com-

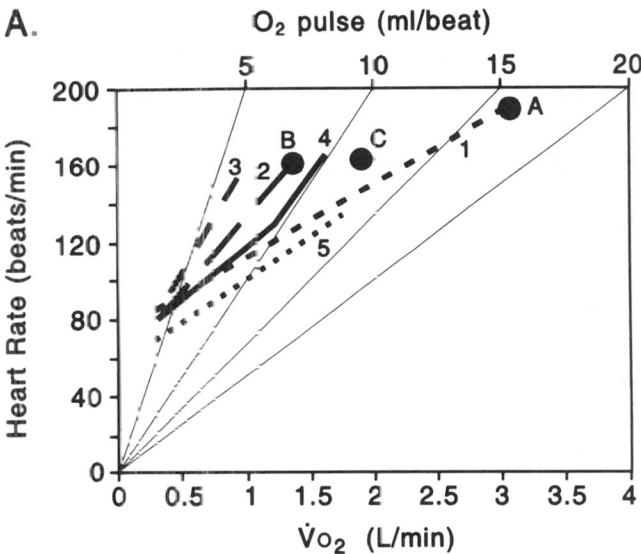

A.

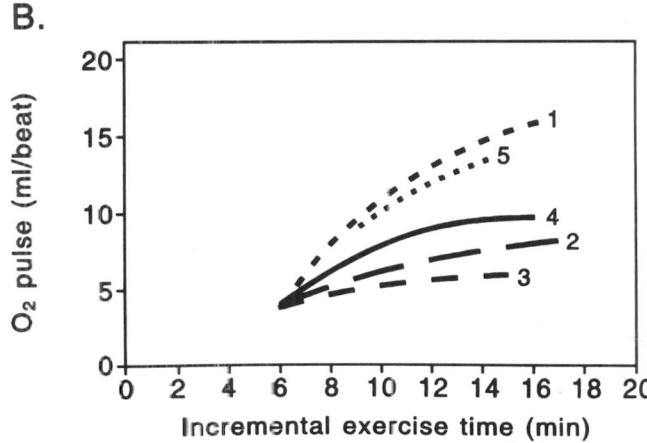

B.

FIGURE 6.6.   Values of $\dot{V}O_2$, heart rate, and O_2 pulse for five individuals during incremental cycle ergometer tests. For clarity, resting, unloaded pedaling, and recovery data are not shown. The upper figure has isopleths for O_2 pulse at 5, 10, 15, and 20 ml/beat. The three large solid circles are maximal exercise target values (each of which depended on each patient's age, gender, size, activity level, and exercise mode) and are labeled A for patients 1 and 5, B for patients 2 and 3, and C for patient 4. The responses for patients 1 and 2 are normal. Patient 3 had decreased cardiovascular function throughout the test and would not have reached target values even if able to exercise longer. Patient 4 manifested decreased cardiovascular function about 2 minutes before the cessation of exercise. Patient 5 stopped exercise prematurely for other than cardiovascular causes. B plots the same O_2 pulse data against time for the five patients. Patients 1 and 2 reach their target values, whereas patients 3, 4, and 5 do not. The plateau in O_2 pulse seen for patient 4 is abnormal.

monly due to low stroke volume, but it could be due to anemia or carboxyhemoglobinemia, poor blood oxygenation in the lung, right to left shunt, or (rarely) low peripheral oxygen extraction. In patient 4, the increasing slope of the HR versus $\dot{V}O_2$ relationship for the last several minutes of exercise is abnormal, indicating that the rise in $\dot{V}O_2$ is dispro-

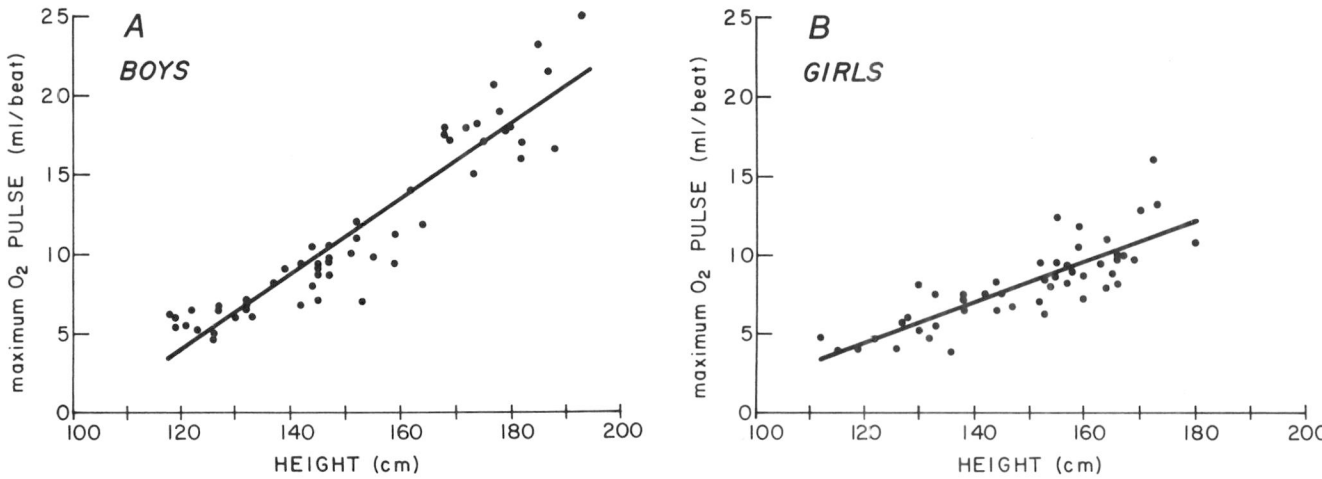

FIGURE 6.7.   Maximum O_2 pulse for normal North American boys (A) and girls (B). For boys, the best fit regression line is O_2 pulse (ml/beat) = 0.23 × height (cm) − 24.4. The lower 95% confidence limit is 3.8 ml/beat below the regression line. For girls, the equation is O_2 pulse (ml/beat) = 0.128 × height (cm) − 10.9 with a lower 95% confidence limit of 3.0 ml/beat below the regression line. (Modified from Cooper DM, Weiler-Ravell D, Whipp BJ, et al. Growth-related changes in oxygen uptake and heart rate during progressive exercise in children. Pediatr Res 1984;18:845–851.)

portionately slower than that of heart rate as work rate increases. In patient 5, the rate of rise of the HR versus $\dot{V}O_2$ is normal, but exercise ends at a relatively low work rate. If the cessation of incremental exercise is due to pain, musculoskeletal disease, ventilatory insufficiency, or other such factors, these factors (rather than circulatory disease) may be the cause of an abnormally low maximum O_2 pulse.

These differing responses can be seen in Figure 6.6A, which has $\dot{V}O_2$ and HR axes and O_2 pulse isopleths. Figure 6.6B plots the O_2 pulse versus time for the same responses. Normally, the rate of increase in O_2 pulse declines gradually as the O_2 pulse approaches maximum values. (This is a necessary consequence of a linear $\dot{V}O_2$ versus HR response with a positive intercept on the HR axis.) This curvilinear response of the O_2 pulse during incremental exercise is clearly demonstrated in Figure 6.6B. Thus, both the absolute values of $\dot{V}O_2$, HR, and O_2 pulse and their patterns of change are important; one or several may be abnormal in various disease states.

The predicted O_2 pulse at any given work rate is strongly dependent on the individual's body size, gender, age, degree of fitness, and hemoglobin concentration. Normal values for the predicted maximum O_2 pulse on the cycle ergometer range from approximately 5 ml/beat in a 7-year-old child to 8 ml/beat in a 150 cm, 70-year-old woman to 17 ml/beat in a 190 cm, 30-year-old man. The actual O_2 pulse may be considerably higher than predicted in the cardiovascularly fit person or in the patient receiving beta-adrenergic blocking drugs.

Recommendation

1. The predicted maximum O_2 pulse should be calculated from the equations selected to predict peak $\dot{V}O_2$ and maximum HR.
2. Predicted maximum O_2 pulse (ml/beat) = Predicted peak $\dot{V}O_2$ (ml/min)/Predicted maximum HR (beats/min).
3. Both the pattern of change as well as the absolute values of O_2 pulse should be considered.
4. Mean values, confidence limits, and graphic data for children are given in Figure 6.7.

BRACHIAL ARTERY BLOOD PRESSURE

Blood pressure can be measured by auscultation during exercise by skilled technicians or physicians, but assessing the fourth Korotkoff phase diastolic pressure (muffling of sound) and the fifth Korotkoff phase diastolic pressure (disappearance of sound) may be difficult because of the background noise of the ergometer. A recent American Heart Association Statement (33) addresses the problems related to the measurement of blood pressure by sphygmomanometry. However, intra-arterial pressures can be accurately and continuously measured by means of a pressure transducer attached to an indwelling catheter whenever arterial blood specimens are not being drawn.

Jones et al. (15) report an average increase of 19 mmHg in systolic pressure as cycle work increased from 50 to 100 Watts. Blood pressure measurements recorded in Table 6.4 are from a predominantly cigarette-smoking and sedentary normal population (2, 34). Values may be lower in non-smoking, more active individuals. Noteworthy are the striking rise in systolic (by both cuff and direct intra-arterial recording) and mean pressures, the considerable rise in intra-arterial diastolic pressures, the modest rise in fourth phase cuff diastolic pressures, and the gradual decline in fifth phase cuff diastolic pressures during incremental exercise. Although resting pressures are higher in older men, the mean maximum exercise systolic and diastolic pressures are similar in both groups. Note that the true mean arterial pressure closely approximates the diastolic pressure plus half the pulse pressure, rather than one third the pulse pressure during exercise when using a cuff (34).

Accurate intra-arterial blood pressure values are more difficult to obtain during treadmill ergometry because of movement artifacts. When the subject is using the cycle, the arm and transducer are stabilized by the hand on the handlebar, but tight gripping should be avoided to minimize the hypertensive effect of isometric exercise.

Recommendation

The brachial artery blood pressure values of non-hypertensive men, measured directly (intra-arterially) or by cuff and sphygmomanometer during 1-minute incremental exercise, are given in Table 6.4.

ANAEROBIC (LACTATE, LACTIC ACIDOSIS) THRESHOLD

The AT is expressed in units of O_2 uptake, but it can also be related to the predicted peak $\dot{V}O_2$. The $\dot{V}O_2$ at which the blood lactate level begins to rise has been used to define the AT in normal subjects (35, 36) and noninvasively is best measured by the V-slope method (37–39). A useful way to define abnormality is to multiply the lower 95% confidence limit of the predicted AT/predicted peak $\dot{V}O_2$ (Table 6.5) by the predicted peak $\dot{V}O_2$ of the subject. Thus, although the mean AT for men ranged between 49 and 63% of peak $\dot{V}O_2$ in several series (13, 40–42), the lowest value in our study of 77 middle-aged (34 to 74 years) normal sedentary men was 40% of peak $\dot{V}O_2$ (2). This lower limit of normal agrees reasonably well with the lowest value for AT in normal men suggested by Wasserman et al. (40) of 1 L/min of $\dot{V}O_2$, approximately the cost of maintaining a moderate walking pace.

Jones et al. (15) and Davis et al. (43) have studied the effect of age on AT. Jones' ratios of AT/peak $\dot{V}O_2$ are slightly higher than Davis' ratios. Though different AT detection methods were used (Jones et al. used ventilatory equivalents and Davis et al. used V-slope), both groups found that the absolute AT declines with age in both sexes, but less than the decrease in predicted peak $\dot{V}O_2$; thus the ratio of AT/peak $\dot{V}O_2$ tends to increase with age. In addition to the gradual increase in the ratio with age, the ratios tend to be higher in women than men.

TABLE 6.4.   Blood Pressure during 1-Minute Incremental Cycle Exercise Measured Directly from Catheter in Brachial Artery and in Opposite Arm by Cuff*

	Prior Exam, at Rest	Rest on Cycle	Exercise Near AT	Exercise Near Maximum
Sedentary, Non-Hypertensive Men, Ages 34 to 74				
Systolic intra-arterial		142 ± 18	182 ± 23	207 ± 27
Systolic cuff	124 ± 11	131	171	200
Diastolic intra-arterial		86 ± 10	92 ± 11	99 ± 12
Diastolic fourth phase	79 ± 7	84	86	88
Diastolic fifth phase		81	80	77
Mean intra-arterial		107	128	142
Sedentary, Non-Hypertensive Men, Ages 19 to 24				
Systolic intra-arterial		129		203
Diastolic intra-arterial		78		106
Mean intra-arterial		96		141

* Values are mean or mean ± SD in mmHg.
(Data are from references 2 and 34.)

Cooper et al. (20) tested 51 girls and 58 boys between the ages of 6 and 17 years. They were healthy and non-obese, but did not participate in vigorous sports. Mean AT was 58% of peak $\dot{V}O_2$, but again, the lower limit of normal for this sample of normal children was approximately 44% of peak $\dot{V}O_2$ (Fig. 6.8).

The mode of exercise may affect the value of AT in normal subjects. Davis et al. (44) studied 39 healthy college-age men. Mean $\dot{V}O_2$ at the AT was $46 \pm 9\%$ of peak $\dot{V}O_2$ for arm cycling, $64 \pm 9\%$ of peak $\dot{V}O_2$ for leg cycling, and $59 \pm 6\%$ of peak $\dot{V}O_2$ for treadmill exercise. A substantial difference was noted between the AT during arm cycling and either form of leg exercise, but no significant difference existed between the AT obtained from cycle exercise and that obtained from treadmill exercise. Buchfuhrer et al. (45) found similar ratios of AT/peak $\dot{V}O_2$ for treadmill and for cycle exercise, $50 \pm 9\%$ and $47 \pm 11\%$, respectively. Withers et al. (46), however, comparing highly trained cyclists and runners, found a higher AT for the total group on the treadmill (mean 76% of peak $\dot{V}O_2$) than on the cycle (mean 64% of peak $\dot{V}O_2$), with the cyclists reaching higher AT and AT/peak $\dot{V}O_2$ on the cycle and runners reaching higher AT and AT/peak $\dot{V}O_2$ on the treadmill.

Recommendation

1. The mean values and confidence limits for the AT in normal children are given in Table 6.3, with the ratios of AT/peak $\dot{V}O_2$ in Figure 6.8. It can be seen in the latter that the lower 95% confidence limit for the AT/peak$\dot{V}O_2$ is about 44%.

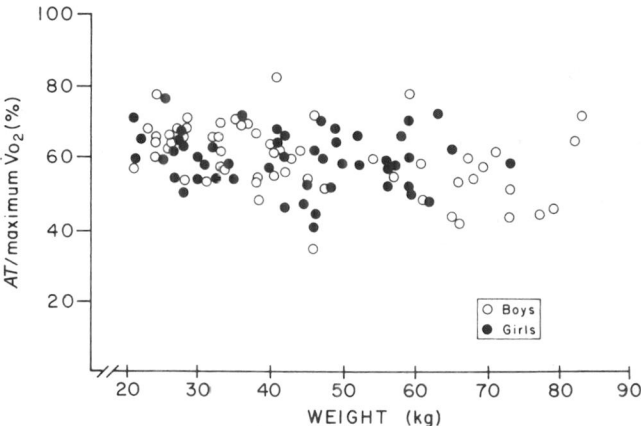

FIGURE 6.8. The ratio of anaerobic threshold to peak $\dot{V}O_2$ (AT/maximum $\dot{V}O_2$), as a percentage, for 109 normal North American boys and girls. (Reprinted with permission from Cooper DM, Weiler-Ravell D, Whipp BJ, et al. Aerobic parameters of exercise as a function of body size during growth in children. J Appl Physiol 1984;56:628–634.)

2. Table 6.5 gives the mean and lower 95% confidence limit for the AT/peak $\dot{V}O_2$ in normal adult men and women.

OXYGEN UPTAKE-WORK RATE RELATIONSHIP ($\Delta\dot{V}O_2$/ΔWR)

When a progressively increasing work rate test is initiated, a delay occurs before oxygen uptake begins to increase in a linear fashion. This delay must be considered in the calculation of the overall value of the $\Delta\dot{V}O_2$/ΔWR. This kinetic delay is equal to the time constant of $\dot{V}O_2$ following a stepwise increase and is between half and three quarters of a minute. Thus, the formula used in calculation is:

$$\Delta\dot{V}O_2/(\Delta WR = (\text{peak } \dot{V}O_2 - \text{unloaded } \dot{V}O_2)/[(T - 0.75) \times S]$$

where $\dot{V}O_2$ is measured in ml per minute, T is the time of incremental exercise, and S is the slope of work rate increment in watts per minute (47). The overall $\Delta\dot{V}O_2$/ΔWR during incremental cycle ergometer exercise varies modestly with the slope of work rate increase, the cardiovascular fitness of the individual, and the duration of the test (47, 48). In 10 normal young men, tests of approximately 15 minutes' duration (15-W/min increment) gave higher $\Delta\dot{V}O_2$/ΔWR values (11.2 ± 0.15 ml/min/W) than tests of approximately 5 minutes' duration (60-

TABLE 6.5. Mean and Lower 95% Confidence Limits for Predicted AT/Predicted Peak $\dot{V}O_2$ in Adults, as a Percentage*

Age (yr)	Men		Women	
	Mean	Lower 95% Limit	Mean	Lower 95% Limit
20	53	42	52	41
30	54	43	55	44
40	55	44	58	47
50	56	45	60	49
60	57	46	63	52
70	58	47	65	54

(Data from references 15 and 43.)

W/min increment) (8.8 ± 0.15 ml/min/W). In tests of long duration, a lower fraction of the total energy cost of the work is supported from body stores of oxygen and anaerobic sources (e.g., lactate production), and a larger fraction is supported by oxygen extracted from the inspired air. The reverse allocation of energy support occurs in maximal tests of short duration. In tests of intermediate duration; however, the mean ± SE of $\Delta\dot{V}O_2/\Delta WR$ found in 10 normal young men was 10.2 ± 0.16 ml/min/W (48), and in 54 older sedentary normal men the mean ±SD was 10.3 ± 1.0 ml/min/W (47). Jones et al. (15) also found a $\Delta\dot{V}O_2/\Delta WR$ of 10.3 ml/min/Watt in 100 healthy adult men and women. This range is small enough so the $\Delta\dot{V}O_2/\Delta WR$ is clinically useful in identifying patients with circulatory disorders.

In patients with circulatory disease (pulmonary, cardiac, or peripheral), the $\Delta\dot{V}O_2/\Delta WR$ may be reduced because of either abnormally slow O_2 extraction kinetics at the muscle or the inability to raise muscle blood flow appropriately to provide oxygen rapidly enough to satisfy muscle requirements (47, 49, 50). Many persons with coronary artery disease manifest a low $\Delta\dot{V}O_2/\Delta WR$ relationship, primarily evident during the latter portion of their maximal exercise tests because of an inability to increase cardiac output. Many, but not all, men with circulatory disorders have a significantly reduced $\Delta\dot{V}O_2/\Delta WR$ (47). We have not analyzed data to describe the mean and range of $\Delta\dot{V}O_2/\Delta WR$ for normal children, but we have seen that many athletes have a higher than average $\Delta\dot{V}O_2/\Delta WR$ (in the range of 11 to 12 ml/min/W).

Recommendation

For incremental cycle ergometry exercise of 6 to 12 minutes duration, the overall $\Delta\dot{V}O_2/\Delta WR$ for sedentary adults is 10.3 ml/min/W, with an SD of 1.0 ml/min/W and a lower limit of normal at the 95% confidence level of 8.6 ml/min/W.

BREATHING RESERVE, TIDAL VOLUME, AND BREATHING FREQUENCY AT MAXIMUM EXERCISE

Exercise Ventilation and Breathing Reserve

Maximum exercise ventilation (maximum exercise $\dot{V}E$) is similar for leg cycling or treadmill walk-

running (7, 45), but is less for arm cycling (44), because the maximal metabolic rate is lower when smaller muscle groups are used. The breathing reserve relates the ventilatory response during such maximum exercise to the maximum ability to breathe. Because normal, untrained subjects do not ordinarily have ventilatory limitations on their ability to perform work (19), some ability to increase ventilation further is usually present during maximal exercise. This potential increase in ventilation is generally estimated from the direct MVV, a test performed at rest. The MVV is highly dependent on the subject's motivation and effort. Normal values for MVV lasting 12 and 15 seconds are available (51, 52). The difference between the measured MVV and the maximum $\dot{V}E$ during exercise is used as a measure of the ventilatory or breathing reserve. A low breathing reserve suggests that a subject's exercise capacity may be limited by his or her ventilatory capacity. The breathing reserve is usually reduced in patients with moderate to severe restrictive or obstructive lung disease (see Fig. 4.8).

Many investigators have examined the normal relationship between MVV and the maximum exercise $\dot{V}E$. Maximum exercise $\dot{V}E$ averages 50 to 80% of the 12- or 15-second MVV, indicating a breathing reserve of 20 to 50% of the MVV. Because the direct MVV is dependent on the subject's cooperation, effort, and technique of performance, the MVV is sometimes indirectly estimated from the FEV_1 or $FEV_{0.75}$. Gandevia and Hugh-Jones (53) suggested that the indirect MVV could be estimated as $FEV_1 \times 35$, whereas Cotes (54) suggested $FEV_{0.75} \times 40$ or $36.8 \times FEV_1 - 2.3$. Miller and colleagues (55) found that $FEV_1 \times 41$ or $FEV_{0.75} \times 46$ estimated MVV. Our data (2) and those of Campbell (56) indicate that $FEV_1 \times 40$ provides an optimal estimate of the direct MVV both in normal subjects and in patients with obstructive lung disease. If the direct MVV is less than the indirect MVV ($FEV_1 \times 40$), poor cooperation or understanding in the performance of the maneuver, extreme obesity, neurologic disorders, or inspiratory obstruction may be possible causes. If one is uncertain regarding a discrepancy between the direct MVV and the indirect MVV, or if the patient has variable obstruction, it may be necessary to have the patient repeat the direct MVV before performing the exercise test. We believe it preferable to use the indirect MVV ($FEV_1 \times 40$) rather than the direct MVV for calculation of the breathing reserve in patients with interstitial disease who have used inordinately high frequencies (e.g., over 100 breaths/min) in the MVV maneuver, frequencies that are unrealistic for the patient to maintain during exercise.

In 77 normal middle-aged subjects during an incremental cycle ergometer exercise test (2, 3), the mean direct MVV was 131 ± 23.6 L/min (range 81 to 203 L/min). The mean maximum exercise $\dot{V}E/MVV$ was $71.5 \pm 14.6\%$; only 13 subjects had a value greater than 80%. When we used $FEV_1 \times 40$ as an indirect estimate of the MVV, the mean maximum exercise $\dot{V}E$/indirect MVV was $71.5 \pm 15.3\%$, i.e., the same percentage as for the directly measured MVV. Expressing breathing reserve as MVV − maximum exercise $\dot{V}E$, we obtain an average of 38.1 ± 22.0 L/min using the directly measured MVV and 38.0 ± 21.5 L/min for the indirect MVV. We consider it likely that the patient is ventilatory limited when the breathing reserve is less than 11 L/min.

Tidal Volume and Breathing Frequency

We consider that patients have ventilatory limitation if the exercise tidal volume (V_T) reaches the resting inspiratory capacity, particularly at submaximal work rates, or if the breathing frequency exceeds approximately 55 breaths/min. The expected maximum exercise V_T, like VC and other resting pulmonary function measurements, depends on the subject's height, age, and gender. In addition, the dead space or re-breathed volume of the breathing apparatus influences ventilation (57–59).

Hey et al. (60) recommended that V_T be related to $\dot{V}E$ to analyze the breathing pattern, such as is shown in Figure 3.13. At low exercise intensity, the increase in $\dot{V}E$ is accomplished primarily by an increase in V_T. After the V_T reaches approximately 50 to 60% of the VC, further increases in $\dot{V}E$ are accomplished primarily by increasing breathing frequency (f) (54, 61). Thus, f is a curvilinear function of $\dot{V}E$. Spiro et al. (61) found that the maximum V_T reached in normal subjects was approximately 55% of VC in normal men and 45% in normal women, whereas Cotes (62) suggested that maximum V_T is about 50% of VC for VC values between 2.0 and 5.0 L in normal men and women of European descent. Astrand (1) found that, at maximal exercise, the V_T averaged between 1.9 and 2.0 L, or 52 to 58% of the VC, whereas f at maximal exercise ranged between 34 and 46 breaths/min. Little difference in V_T/VC was noted among age groups, but f was lower in the older subjects studied.

Wasserman and Whipp (19) compared exercise

V_T to IC. They found that V_T does not usually exceed approximately 70% of the IC during exercise, but it increases to a value approaching 100% in patients with restrictive lung disease, suggesting that the IC may limit the increase in V_T (see Fig. 3.13). In a series of 77 healthy middle-aged men, the mean resting V_T of 0.71 ± 0.26 L increased to 1.44 ± 0.43 L at the AT and 2.28 ± 0.43 L at maximum exercise (2, 3). Maximum f was 41.6 ± 9.6 min^{-1}. Maximum V_T averaged $70.0 \pm 10.7\%$ of the IC and $55.0 \pm 8.7\%$ of the VC. No one had a maximum exercise V_T greater than their resting IC, and only 3 had a $f > 60$ min^{-1}.

Partitioning the duration of the ventilatory cycle (T_{TOT}) into inspiratory (T_I) and expiratory (T_E) components may also prove useful, but to date this measurement is not commonplace in clinical exercise testing, in part because most commercial exercise systems measure expiratory airflow only.

Recommendation

Resting spirometry values must be reliable. At maximum work rates, the following values (mean $\pm$ SD) have been found for normal adult men, ages 34 to 74, for cycle ergometry using a breathing valve with a dead space of 64 ml (2, 3).

1. Maximum exercise $\dot{V}E$/maximum voluntary ventilation (MVV), $\% = 72 \pm 15$
2. Breathing reserve = (MVV − maximum exercise $\dot{V}E$) = 38 ± 22 L/min; lower limit of normal 11 L/min
3. Maximum tidal volume (maximum V_T) < inspiratory capacity (IC) in all subjects
4. Maximum breathing frequency (f) < 55/min in over 95% of all subjects

VENTILATORY MEASURES AT THE ANAEROBIC THRESHOLD: $\dot{V}E/\dot{V}CO_2$, $\dot{V}E/\dot{V}O_2$, AND THE BREATHING RESERVE INDEX

The $\dot{V}E$ of a given patient is linked to the metabolic demand, the efficiency of ventilation, the degree of respiratory compensation for metabolic acidosis, the appropriateness of the ventilatory control mechanisms, and the mechanical capabilities of the lungs, chest wall, and respiratory muscles. In normal men below the AT, ventilation is linked to metabolic requirements within a narrow range. During sea level exercise below the *AT*, mean $\dot{V}_E$ (L/min, BTPS) = 24.6 × $\dot{V}_{CO_2}$ (L/min, STPD) + 3.2, with an SEE of 2.4 L/min, in normal adult men (63). Fairbarn et al. (64) found this relationship to change with age as follows: $\dot{V}_E$ (L/min, BTPS) = 22.6 × $\dot{V}_{CO_2}$ (L/min, STPD) − 4.4 with an SEE of 5.3 L/min at age 30, $\dot{V}_E$ = 25.8 × $\dot{V}_{CO_2}$ + 4.3 at mean age 55 with an SEE of 5.0, and $\dot{V}_E$ = 29.5 × $\dot{V}_{CO_2}$ + 4.3 with an SEE of 7.5 at mean age 75. Consistent with this Cotes also found the $\dot{V}_E/\dot{V}_{CO_2}$ to increase approximately 1.0 for each decade of age (54).

The normal values for $\dot{V}_E/\dot{V}_{CO_2}$ and $\dot{V}_E/\dot{V}_{O_2}$ (mean ± SD) during sea level exercise near the *AT* for middle-aged, normal, sedentary men are: 29.1 ± 4.3 and 26.5 ± 4.4, respectively, where the $\dot{V}_E$ is expressed at BTPS with apparatus dead space ventilation subtracted, and $\dot{V}_{CO_2}$ and $\dot{V}_{O_2}$ are expressed as STPD (2). Wasserman et al. (65) found that $\dot{V}_E/\dot{V}_{CO_2}$ declined to approximately 28 during cycle ergometer exercise in 10 healthy young men before it increased with the onset of ventilatory compensation for the exercise lactic acidosis. In steady-state exercise unaccompanied by a lactic acidosis, the $\dot{V}_E/\dot{V}_{O_2}$ is lower than the $\dot{V}_E/\dot{V}_{CO_2}$ because the respiratory quotient is less than one (19). Both $\dot{V}_E/\dot{V}_{O_2}$ and $\dot{V}_E/\dot{V}_{CO_2}$ are necessarily increased at high altitudes at which there is hyperventilation in response to hypoxia.

The ratio $\dot{V}_E/\dot{V}_{CO_2}$ gives an index of the dead space ventilation, but this inference must be made with care. The following equation is a modification of the alveolar mass balance equation:

$$\dot{V}_E/\dot{V}_{CO_2} = k/[P_{aCO_2} \times (1 - V_D/V_T)]$$

Thus, $\dot{V}_E/\dot{V}_{CO_2}$ is expected to be higher than normal when the physiologic dead space/tidal volume ratio (V_D/V_T) is high, but it also can be high when the patient hyperventilates (i.e., P_{aCO_2} is lower than normal) (see inset in Fig. 3.17). In an invasive exercise test, V_D/V_T can be calculated if P_{aCO_2} is measured. Importantly, P_{ETCO_2} cannot be assumed to be equal to P_{aCO_2} in a noninvasive test. In fact, as explained later, a low P_{ETCO_2} does not necessarily indicate hyperventilation because it also can be seen with a normal P_{aCO_2} combined with a high V_D/V_T. Situations where P_{aCO_2} is substantially lower than P_{ETCO_2} are uncommon, however. Thus, when $\dot{V}_E/\dot{V}_{CO_2}$ is high and P_{ETCO_2} is not low (i.e., 40 mm Hg or above), it is likely that V_D/V_T is high.

The breathing reserve index (BRI) at the lactate threshold (*LT*), defined as the ($\dot{V}_E$ at the *LT*)/MVV, was hypothesized and successfully utilized as a method of contrasting pulmonary mechanical limitation to exercise from the limitations of patients with cardiovascular disease and normal control subjects by Medoff et al. (66). They found in these persons that the $\dot{V}_E$ at the *LT* correlated highly (r = 0.85) with the $\dot{V}_E$ at maximum exercise. Further they found a BRI of 0.73 ± 0.03 (SEM) in 32 COPD patients considered to be ventilatory limited at maximum exercise, as contrasted with a BRI of 0.27 ± 0.02 in 29 patients with a cardiovascular limit and BRI of 0.24 ± 0.03 in 12 normal controls. Finally, a BRI ≥0.42 predicted a pulmonary limitation at maximum exercise with sensitivity, specificity, and positive and negative predictive values all exceeding 93%. *LT* measured from blood lactate values should correlate highly with *AT* measured from gas exchange by the V-slope method, as noted in Chapter 3, but the investigators did not report their *AT* data. This analysis has not been reported for patients with restrictive lung disease.

Recommendations

1. Normal values (mean ± SD) for $\dot{V}_E/\dot{V}_{CO_2}$ and $\dot{V}_E/\dot{V}_{O_2}$ at the *AT* (expressed as L/min BTPS/L/min STPD) for sedentary middle-aged men are 29.1 ± 4.3 and 26.5 ± 4.4, respectively. Mean values for women and men over 60 should be slightly higher (1–2); for men under 30, slightly lower (1–2).
2. The BRI at the *AT* for normal controls and cardiovascularly limited patients near the *AT* approximates 0.25 ± 0.03 (SEM). A value exceeding 0.42 appears to be highly predictive of ventilatory limitation in patients with obstructive lung disease (66).

PHYSIOLOGIC DEAD SPACE/TIDAL VOLUME RATIO (V_D/V_T)

The physiologic dead space (V_D) is dependent on anatomic and physiologic factors, whereas the V_D/V_T is also dependent, even in normal subjects, on the pattern of breathing. At rest, the V_D/V_T may be elevated because of the rapid, shallow breathing of anxiety. Physiologic control mechanisms usually stabilize ventilation at a slower and more efficient breathing pattern soon after the onset of exercise unless anxiety is extreme. Calculation of the V_D and V_D/V_T must be carefully performed, making an adjustment for the apparatus dead space (see

Appendix C). In addition, gas exchange measurements must be synchronous with arterial blood sampling for measuring P_{aCO_2}.

All studies have shown a fall in V_D/V_T during exercise in normal subjects. Thus, whereas mean V_D/V_T at rest ranged from 0.28 to 0.35 in several studies of normal subjects, mean V_D/V_T decreased to between 0.20 and 0.25 near the *AT* and to less than 0.21 at maximum exercise (2, 58, 65, 67).

Figure 6.9 shows the effect of exercise on V_D/V_T at various levels of cycle exercise in young men. Cotes (54) suggested that V_D (ml) $= 140 + 0.07\ V_T$ (ml) with an SD $= 90$ ml in young men during exercise. Jones et al. (58) found the following relationship during exercise in 17 normal young men: V_D (ml) $= 138 + 0.077\ V_T$ (ml), with r $= 0.69$. Lifshay et al. (59) showed that men aged 50 to 81 had a significantly higher V_D than men and women aged 18 to 37. The prediction equations of Bradley et al. (68) for V_D use sex, age, height, $\dot{V}_{CO_2}$, $\dot{V}_E$, f, and temperature as factors.

The practice of some manufacturers of offering a calculation of "noninvasive V_D/V_T" is invalid in patients. This calculation substitutes P_{ETCO_2} for P_{aCO_2} in the foregoing alveolar mass balance equation rearranged to allow V_D/V_T calculations. Because the difference between P_{ETCO_2} and P_{aCO_2} is influenced by V_D/V_T, this calculation involves a heavy dose of circular reasoning.

Recommendation

Normal values for V_D/V_T at rest and during upright exercise after allowance for valve dead space are:

1. For men under age 40: V_D/V_T (mean $\pm$ SD) $= 0.29 \pm 0.06$ at rest, 0.17 ± 0.05 at *AT* and 0.16 ± 0.04 at maximum exercise.
2. For men over age 40: V_D/V_T (mean $\pm$ SD) $= 0.30 \pm 0.08$ at rest, 0.20 ± 0.07 at *AT* and 0.19 ± 0.07 at maximum exercise (2).
3. Upper 95% confidence limits for men over 40: $V_D/V_T = 0.45$ at rest, 0.33 at *AT*, and 0.30 at maximum exercise (2).
4. The V_D/V_T of patients should not be reported using P_{aCO_2} calculated from expired gas measures. Blood P_{CO_2} from a systemic artery or well-heated hand vein should be used.

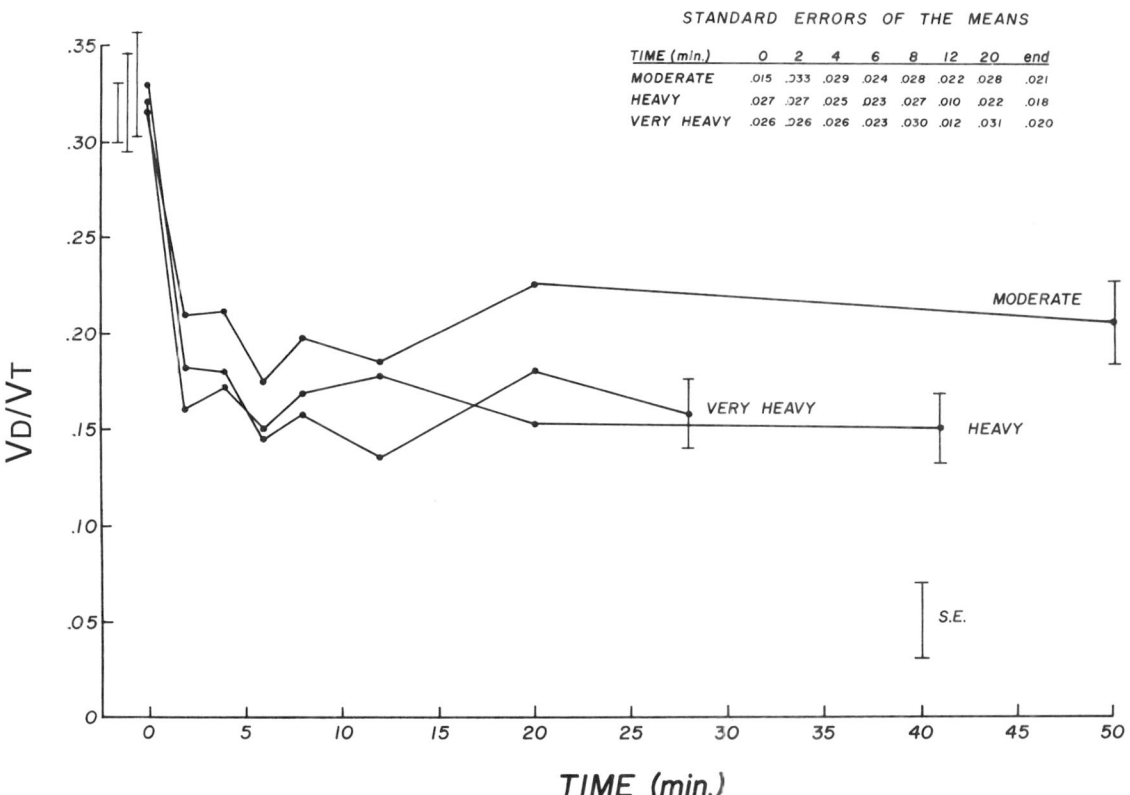

FIGURE 6.9.   The physiologic dead space/tidal volume ratio (V_D/V_T) in 10 normal young men at rest and during 3 intensities of cycle ergometer exercise as related to exercise duration. The SEM are given in the table inset. (Reprinted with permission from Wasserman K, VanKessel A, Burton GB. Interaction of physiological mechanisms during exercise. J Appl Physiol 1967;22:71–85.)

ARTERIAL AND END-TIDAL CARBON DIOXIDE TENSIONS [Paco₂, Petco₂, and P(a − et)co₂]

Resting Petco₂ and Paco₂ values are dependent on the degree of apprehension, anxiety, and training of the subject. Many anxious individuals have a strong tendency to hyperventilate, especially while breathing through a mouthpiece and awaiting the signal to begin exercise (Fig. 6.10). Once exercise starts, however, the blood gases and pH are not discernibly different, whether performing the work while breathing through a low resistance breathing valve or breathing normally without a mouthpiece (69). In more apprehensive individuals, the Paco₂ values rise from rest to moderate exercise as physiologic control mechanisms suppress psychogenic hyperventilation. In the relaxed individual, Paco₂ values remain relatively stable at rest and during mild and moderate exercise. Although Paco₂ values cannot be predicted accurately from Petco₂ values in an individual person, particularly in a patient with lung disease, measurement of Petco₂ is often valuable for following trends in Paco₂.

Wasserman et al. (65) found that P(a − et)co₂ changed from approximately +2.5 mmHg at rest to −4 mmHg during heavy work in 10 normal men (Fig. 6.11). Jones et al. (58) found that, in 17 normal subjects at the highest work rates reached, Petco₂ was always more than 2 mmHg higher than Paco₂. In 5 normal men, Whipp and Wasserman (67) found P(a − et)co₂ was 2.8 ± 1.6 mmHg at rest and −2.8 ± 0.6 mmHg at a work rate of 220 W. All P(a − et)co₂ values were negative for work rates above 115 W. In five normal young men near the AT, Jones et al. (70) found that Paco₂ = 5.5 + 0.9 Petco₂ − 0.0021 Vt (SE = 1.4). These relationships are unlikely to be valid in patients with lung disease or with disorders affecting the ventilation/perfusion relationships. In 77 asbestos-exposed healthy men (2, 3), P(a − et)co₂ at rest was −0.3 ± 2.9 mmHg (mean ± SD) and decreased to −4.1 ± 3.2 mmHg at maximum exercise. At the peak of exercise, a positive P(a − et)co₂ was rare.

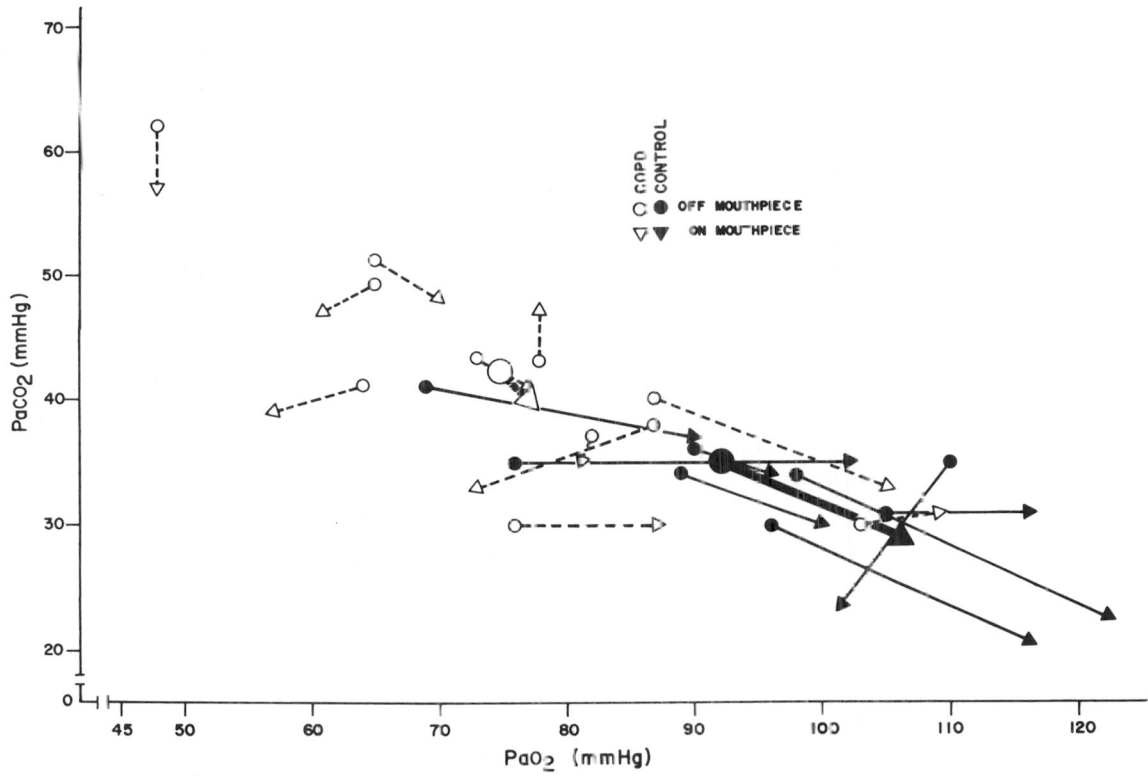

FIGURE 6.10.   Resting arterial partial pressures of CO_2 (Paco₂) and O_2 (Pao₂) in normal control subjects and in patients with chronic obstructive pulmonary disease (COPD) off and acutely on the mouthpiece while awaiting cycle ergometer exercise. Small arrows show individual values and large arrows show mean values. Note the small mean decline in Paco₂ and the increase in Pao₂ in the patients with COPD while breathing on the mouthpiece, whereas the controls show a larger decline in Paco₂ and a much larger rise in Pao₂ with the same mouthpiece at rest. (Courtesy of Dr. J.D. Andrews.)

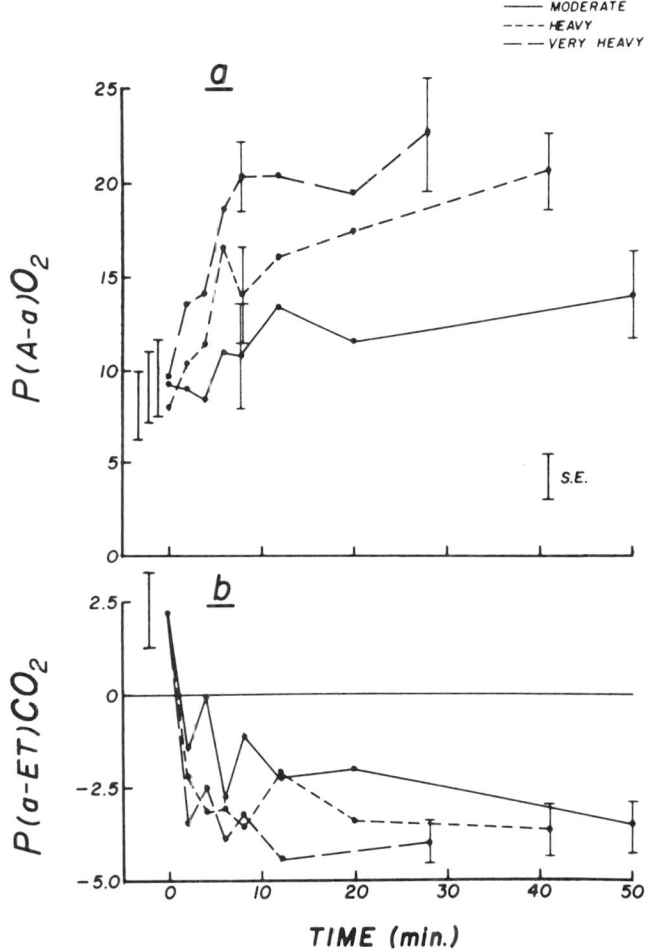

FIGURE 6.11.   The $P(A - a)O_2$ and $P(a - ET)CO_2$ in 10 normal young men at rest and during 3 intensities of cycle ergometer exercise as related to exercise duration. The mean and SEM are depicted. (Reprinted with permission from Wasserman K, VanKessel A, Burton GB. Interaction of physiological mechanisms during exercise. J Appl Physiol 1967;22:71–85.)

Recommendation

Normal values at sea level during upright exercise in adult men are:

1. $PaCO_2$: resting value = 36 to 42 mmHg; stable during mild and moderate exercise, declining with heavy exercise.
2. $PETCO_2$: resting value = 36 to 42 mmHg; increases normally by 3 to 8 mmHg during mild and moderate exercise (depending on breathing pattern), and decreases with heavy exercise.
3. $P(a - ET)CO_2$ (mean ± SD) at the AT = −3 ± 3 mmHg. At maximum exercise the $P(a - ET)CO_2$ = −4 ± 3 mmHg and is negative in more than 95% of normal men.

ARTERIAL, ALVEOLAR, AND END-TIDAL OXYGEN TENSIONS (PaO_2, PAO_2, $PETO_2$), AND ARTERIAL OXYHEMOGLOBIN SATURATION (SaO_2)

The normal resting PaO_2 is dependent on age, body position, and nutritional status. Values are lower with increasing age, obesity, fasting, and in the supine position. Nevertheless, sea level values less than 80 mmHg are not seen in normal persons less than 70 years of age in the sitting position except in those who are obese. The $PETO_2$ and PaO_2 (the latter calculated from the alveolar air equation; see Appendix C) are normally similar, but they may differ by 10 or more mmHg in patients with severe maldistribution of ventilation. The PaO_2 and PAO_2 decrease transiently soon after the start of exercise (because the rise in $\dot{V}E$ is slower than the rise in $\dot{V}O_2$, i.e., R decreases) and then increase back to approximately resting values (see Chapter 2 on O_2 uptake kinetics, O_2 deficit, and O_2 debt).

The SaO_2 normally changes less than 2% from rest to maximal exercise. In highly motivated athletes, the SaO_2 has been reported to fall below resting values (71), but this is uncommon.

The $PETO_2$ normally increases 10 to 30 mmHg for exercise above the AT because of metabolic acidosis-induced hyperventilation and rising R at maximal exercise.

Many reports show that the $P(A - a)O_2$ increases during heavy exercise in normal subjects. Lilienthal et al. (72) and Asmussen and Nielsen (73) found a mean $P(A - a)O_2$ of 30 mmHg at high work rates. Jones et al. (58) found, in 17 normal active men not in physical training, a mean $P(A - a)O_2$ of 12 mmHg at rest, with an increase to approximately 20 mmHg at work rates with a $\dot{V}O_2$ over 1.5 L/min. Whipp and Wasserman (67), in 5 healthy young men, found a $P(A - a)O_2$ of 7.4 ± 4.2 mmHg (mean ± SD) at rest and 10.8 ± 3.6 mmHg at heavy exercise. Cruz et al. (74) studied 4 subjects at rest and at work rates approximating 50%, 75%, and 100% of peak $\dot{V}O_2$ at sea level and found $P(A - a)O_2$ values of 11.5 ± 5.4, 11.0 ± 4.2, 16.3 ± 2.6, and 20 ± 8.8 mmHg, respectively. Hansen et al. (75) studied 16 healthy young men, aged 18 to 24, during sea level exercise on a cycle ergometer and found that the mean $P(A - a)O_2$ was 8 mmHg while sitting at rest, 7 mmHg during mild exercise, 11 mmHg during moderate exercise, and 15 mmHg during maximum exercise. Similar results were obtained by Wasserman et al. (65) in 10 healthy young men, and values are shown at rest and at 3 work intensities as related to time in Figure 6.11. We found, in 77 normal older men (ages 34 to 74 years), $P(A - a)O_2$ values (mean $\pm$ SD) of 12.8 $\pm$ 7.4 mmHg at rest and 19.0 $\pm$ 8.8 mmHg at maximum exercise (2, 3). At maximum exercise, $P(A - a)O_2$ was greater than 35 mmHg in only 3 of these 77 men.

Recommendation

The normal arterial blood and $PETO_2$ values at sea level during upright exercise in adult men are:

1. PaO_2 at rest = 80 mmHg or greater; usually increasing slightly with heavy exercise
2. SaO_2 at rest = 95% or greater; no decrease with exercise
3. $PETO_2$ at rest = 90 mmHg or greater; increases with heavy exercise
4. $P(A - a)O_2$ (mean $\pm$ SD) for age 20 to 39 at rest = 8 mmHg, at AT = 11 mmHg, and at maximum exercise = 15 mmHg. For age 40 to 69 $P(A - a)O_2$ at rest = 13 $\pm$ 7 mmHg, at AT = 17 $\pm$ 7 mmHg, and at maximum exercise = 19 $\pm$ 9 mmHg. The upper limit of normal (95% confidence level) at AT = 28 mmHg and at maximum exercise = 35 mmHg

FEMORAL AND MIXED VENOUS VALUES AND ESTIMATION OF CARDIAC OUTPUT

Muscle blood flow and oxygen extraction both increase strikingly with exercise. Near maximum leg exercise femoral vein values in normal subjects reach the following mean $\pm$ SE values: PO_2 = 20 $\pm$ 2 mmHg, SO_2 = 17 $\pm$ 3%, pH = 7.00 $\pm$ .04 units, PCO_2 = 80 $\pm$ 5 mmHg, and lactate = 10 $\pm$ 1 mmol/L (76). In patients with heart disease, minimum mean femoral vein values are similar: PO_2 = 18 mmHg and SO_2 = 18–21% (77, 78). Concurrent mixed venous values in the same patients are 2 mmHg and 4% higher, respectively.

The usual values found for $S\bar{v}O_2$ at peak treadmill or cycle exercise approximate 25%. In normal subjects, as well as in patients with heart failure, the $S\bar{v}O_2$, $C\bar{v}O_2$, $C(a - \bar{v})O_2$ and O_2 extraction ratio $[C(a - \bar{v})O_2/CaO_2]$ change in relatively linear fashion as $\dot{V}O_2$ changes from rest to peak values. In five normal men, the $C(a - \bar{v})O_2$ values, in ml/100 ml

blood, were 5.72 + 0.1 $\times$ % peak $\dot{V}O_2$, with a SD of 1.08 ml/100 ml, r = 0.94. Combining the data from three studies (79–81) involving normals and patients with congestive heart failure, the $C(a - \bar{v})O_2$ values, in ml/100 ml blood, were 5.55 + 0.085 $\times$ % peak $\dot{V}O_2$, with a SD of 1.09, r = 0.97. Absolute CaO_2 values are dependent on the hemoglobin concentration, which usually rises 5–8% at peak exercise in healthy individuals, and, of course, the SaO_2. The consistency in mixed venous oxyhemoglobin saturation at peak exercise, allows a non-invasive estimate of cardiac output and stroke volume in patients who are able exercise to their peak $\dot{V}O_2$ unlimited by ventilatory, musculoskeletal, or other non-cardiovascular dysfunction.

Historically, it has been suggested that cardiac output could be measured noninvasively during exercise with the Fick principle by estimating mixed venous CO_2 content using rebreathing techniques (29). This estimate of cardiac output depends on the premise that mixed venous PCO_2 values estimated by rebreathing techniques are highly correlated with mixed venous CO_2 content, even without knowing mixed venous pH or oxyhemoglobin saturation. Data obtained in our exercise laboratories indicate that the correlative relationships between serial measures of mixed venous PCO_2 and CO_2 content during incremental exercise tests are poor, predominantly because of the acidemia that occurs above the AT. These data are strong evidence that cardiac output cannot be accurately measured by CO_2 rebreathing techniques except during rest or light exercise.

Recommendation

1. In the normal person and the person with heart disease femoral vein mean $\pm$ SE values are PO_2 = 19 $\pm$ 3 mmHg and SO_2 = 19 $\pm$ 3 % at maximum leg exercise, when such exercise is not limited by other than cardiovascular factors.
2. Mixed venous values are PO_2 = 21 $\pm$ 3 mmHg and SO_2 = 23 $\pm$ 3%. In such individuals, the $S\bar{v}O_2$, $C\bar{v}O_2$, $C(a - \bar{v})O_2$ and O_2 extraction ratio change in near linear fashion from rest to maximum exercise.
3. In the absence of anemia, hypoxemia, or significant carboxhemoglobinemia, $C(a - \bar{v})O_2$ in ml/100 ml of blood is 5.55 + 0.085 $\times$ peak $\dot{V}O_2$ with a SD = 1.1 ml/100 ml blood. These values can be used to estimate cardiac output and stroke volume, especially at maximum exercise (79).

ACID-BASE BALANCE

In the normal individual, an intense metabolic acidosis is induced by heavy exercise. Measurements of the acid-base status and R at the termination of an incremental exercise test are valuable in deciding whether the subject has made a good effort and perform maximally. Resting venous and arterial lactate values are normally less than 1 mmol/L and typically rise substantially before the termination of maximal exercise. During exercise, venous lactate values can be dependent on the site of lactate production and the sampling site (82), whereas arterial lactate gives a better indication of the total body lactate burden. As previously described, the rise in blood lactate during exercise is accompanied by a nearly equimolar decline in bicarbonate and a decrease in pH. This metabolic acidosis results in hyperventilation, a decline in Pa_{CO_2}, and a further increase in $\dot{V}_{CO_2}$ so that R increases. The arterial lactate and R reach their peak and the pH and bicarbonate reach their nadir at about 2 minutes of recovery after an incremental exercise test. The magnitude of these changes indicates the severity of exercise-induced metabolic acidosis. Normal values for younger (83) and older (2) men for incremental cycle exercise tests are given in Table 6.6. Small changes signify a mild degree of exercise stress secondary to low motivation or disorders that preclude the performance of exercise at a significant level above the *AT*.

Recommendation

1. R values (mean ± SD) in normal older men at end-exercise are 1.21 ± 0.12 while at 2 minutes of recovery are 1.59 ± 0.19.
2. Decline in HCO_3^- and increase in lactate (both in mmol/L) at end-exercise are approximately 6 ± 2 in younger men and 4 ± 2.5 in older men; at 2 minutes of recovery are approximately 8.4 ± 2.5 in all men.

SUMMARY

Normal exercise values for peak $\dot{V}_{O_2}$, *AT*, HR, HRR, O_2 pulse, arterial blood pressure, ventilatory pattern, breathing reserve, ventilatory equivalents, arterial blood gases, $P(A - a)_{O_2}$, $P(a - ET)_{CO_2}$, V_D/V_T, femoral and mixed venous blood gases, and acid-base balance for use in assessment of patients are presented and critiqued.

References

1. Astrand PO, Rodahl K. Textbook of Work Physiology, 3rd Ed. New York: McGraw-Hill, 1986.
2. Hansen JE, Sue DY, Wasserman K. Predicted values for clinical exercise testing. Am Rev Respir Dis 1984; 129(Suppl):S49–S55.
3. Sue DY, Hansen JE. Normal values in adults during exercise testing. Clin Chest Med 1984;5:89–97.
4. Jones NL, Summers E, Killian KJ. Influence of age and structure on exercise during incremental cycle ergometry in men and women. Am Rev Respir Dis. 1989;140:1373–1380.
5. Astrand I. Aerobic work capacity in men and women with special reference to age. Acta Physiol Scand 1960;49(Suppl. 169):1–9.
6. Drinkwater BL, Horvath SM, Wells CL. Aerobic power of females, ages 10 to 68. Gerontology 1975;30:385–394.
7. Hermansen L, Saltin B. Oxygen uptake during maximal treadmill and bicycle exercise. J Appl Physiol 1969; 26:31–37.
8. Dehn MM, Bruce RA. Longitudinal variations in maximal oxygen intake with age and activity. J Appl Physiol 1972;33:805–807.
9. Astrand I, Astrand PO, Hallback I, Kilborn A. Reduction in maximal oxygen uptake with age. J Appl Physiol 1973;35:649–654.
10. Bruce RA, Kusumi F, Hosmer D. Maximal oxygen intake

TABLE 6.6. **Metabolic Acidosis at the End of and during Recovery from Maximum Incremental Cycle Ergometer Exercise in Normal Sedentary Men**

| Time | At End of Exercise | | 2 Minutes into Recovery | |
Age (Years)	18–24	34–74	18–24	34–74
Number studied	10	77	10	77
Average exercise duration (min)	18	9	18	9
Arterial lactate increase (mmol/L*)	6.6 ± 1.4		7.6 ± 1.8	
Arterial HCO_3^- decline from rest (mmol/L*)	6.2 ± 2.3	4.0 ± 2.5	8.7 ± 2.6	8.5 ± 2.9
Arterial pH*	7.31 ± 0.04	7.37 ± 0.04	7.29 ± 0.04	7.33 ± 0.03
Gas exchange ratio (R)*		1.21 ± 0.12		1.59 ± 0.19

* Values are mean ± SD.
(Data are from references 2 and 83.)

and nomographic assessment of functional aerobic impairment in cardiovascular disease. Am Heart J 1973;85:546–562.

11. Astrand PO. Human physical fitness with special reference to sex and age. Physiol Rev 1956;36:307–335.

12. Balke B, Ware RW. An experimental study of "physical fitness" of Air Force personnel. US Armed Forces Med J 1959;10:675–688.

13. Davis JA, Frank MH, Whipp BJ, Wasserman K. Anaerobic threshold alterations caused by endurance training in middle-aged men. J Appl Physiol 1979;46:1039–1046.

14. Davis JA. Personal Communication.

15. Jones NL, Makrides L, Hitchcock C, McCartney N. Normal standards for an incremental progressive cycle ergometer test. Am Rev Respir Dis 1985;131:700–708.

16. Itoh H, Koike A, Taniguchi K, Marumo F. Severity and pathophysiology of heart failure on the basis of anaerobic threshold (AT) and related parameters. Jpn Circ J 1989;53:146–154.

17. Neder JA, Nery LE, Castello A, Sachs A, Silva AC, Whipp BJ. Normal values for clinical exercise testing: a prospective and randomized study. Am J Respir Crit Care Med 1998;157:A89.

18. Buskirk E, Taylor HL. Maximal oxygen intake and its relation to body composition, with special reference to chronic physical activity and obesity. J Appl Physiol 1957;11:72–78.

19. Wasserman K, Whipp BJ. Exercise physiology in health and disease (State of the art). Am Rev Respir Dis 1975;112:219–249.

20. Cooper DM, Weiler-Ravell D, Whipp BJ, Wasserman K. Aerobic parameters of exercise as a function of body size during growth in children. J Appl Physiol 1984;56:628–634.

21. Cooper DM, Weiler-Ravell D. Gas exchange response to exercise in children. Am Rev Respir Dis 1984;129(Suppl.):S47–S48.

22. Astrand PO, Saltin B. Maximal oxygen uptake and heart rate in various types of muscular activity. J Appl Physiol 1961;16:977–981.

23. Wyndham CH, Strydom NB, Leary WP, Williams CG. Studies of the maximum capacity for men for physical effort. Arbeitsphysiologie 1966;22:285–295.

24. Dempsey JA, Reddan W, Rankin J, Balke B. Alveolararterial gas exchange during muscular work in obesity. J Appl Physiol 1966;21:1807–1814.

25. Shephard RJ, Allen C, Benade AJS, Davies CTM, DiPrampero PE, Hedman R, Merriman JE, Myhre K, Simmons R. The maximum oxygen intake. Bull WHO 1968;38:757–764.

26. Faulkner JA, Roberts DE, Elk RL, Conway J. Cardiovascular responses to submaximum and maximum effort cycling and running. J Appl Physiol 1971;30:457–461.

27. McArdle WD, Katch FI, Pechar GS. Comparison of continuous and discontinuous treadmill and bicycle tests for max Vo₂. Med Sci Sports Exerc 1972;5:156–160.

28. Davis JA, Kasch FW. Aerobic and anaerobic differences between maximal running and cycling in middle-aged males. Aust J Sports Med 1975;7:81–84.

29. Jones NL. Clinical Exercise Testing, 3rd Ed. Philadelphia: W.B. Saunders, 1988.

30. Sheffield LT, Maloof JA, Sawyer JA, Roitman D. Maximal heart rate and treadmill performance of healthy women in relation to age. Circulation 1978;57:79–84.

31. Cooper KH, Purdy J, White S, Pollack M, Linnerud AC. Age-fitness adjusted maximal heart rates. Med Sci Sports 1977;10:78–86.

32. Cooper DM, Weiler-Ravell D, Whipp BJ, Wasserman K. Growth-related changes in oxygen uptake and heart rate during progressive exercise in children. Pediatr Res 1984;18:845–851.

33. American Heart Association. Human blood pressure determination by sphygmomanometry. Circulation 1993;88:2460–2470.

34. Robinson TR, Sue DY, Huszczuk A, Weiler-Ravell D, Hansen JE. Intra-arterial and cuff blood pressure responses during incremental cycle ergometry. Med Sci Sports Exerc 1988;20:142–149.

35. Wasserman K, McIlroy MB. Detecting the threshold of anaerobic metabolism in cardiac patients during exercise. Am J Cardiol 1964;14:844–852.

36. Wasserman K. The anaerobic threshold measurement to evaluate exercise performance. Am Rev Respir Dis 1984;129(Suppl.):S35–S40.

37. Beaver WL, Wasserman K, Whipp BJ. A new method for detecting the anaerobic threshold by gas exchange. J Appl Physiol 1986;60:2020–2027.

38. Sue DY, Wasserman K, Morrica RB, Casaburi R. Measurement of anaerobic threshold by V-slope method in patients with chronic obstructive lung disease. Chest 1988;94:931–938.

39. Wasserman K, Beaver WL, Whipp BJ. Gas exchange theory and the lactic acidosis (anaerobic) threshold. Circulation 1990;81(Suppl II) II-14–II-30.

40. Wasserman K, Whipp BJ, Koyal S, Beaver WL. Anaerobic threshold and respiratory gas exchange during exercise. J Appl Physiol 1973;35:236–243.

41. Nery LE, Wasserman K, French W, Oren A, Davis JA. Contrasting cardiovascular and respiratory responses to exercise in mitral valve and chronic obstructive pulmonary diseases. Chest 1983;83:446–453.

42. Orr GW, Green HJ, Hughson RL, Bennett GW. A computer linear regression model to determine ventilatory anaerobic threshold. J Appl Physiol 1982;52:1349–1352.

43. Davis JA, Storer TW, Caiozzo VJ. Prediction of normal values for lactate threshold estimated by gas exchange in men and women. J Appl Cardiol 1997;76:157–164.

44. Davis JA, Vodak P, Wilmore JH, Vodal J, Kurtz P. Anaerobic threshold and maximal aerobic power for three modes of exercise. J Appl Physiol 1976;41:544–550.

45. Buchfuhrer MJ, Hansen JE, Robinson TE, Sue DY, Wasserman K, Whipp BJ. Optimizing the exercise protocol for cardiopulmonary assessment. J Appl Physiol 1983;55:1553–1564.

46. Withers RT, Sherman WM, Miller JM, Costillo DL. Specificity of the anaerobic threshold in endurance trained cyclists and runners. Eur J Appl Physiol 1981;47:93–101.

47. Hansen JE, Sue DY, Oren A, Wasserman K. Relation of oxygen uptake to work rate in normal men and men with circulatory disorders. Am J Cardiol 1987;59:669–674.

48. Hansen JE, Casaburi R, Cooper DM, Wasserman K. Oxy-

gen uptake as related to work rate increment during cycle ergometer exercise. Eur J Appl Physiol 1988;57:140–145.

49. Auchincloss JH, Ashutosh K, Rana S, Peppi D, Johnson LW, Gilbert R. Effect of cardiac, pulmonary, and vascular disease on one-minute oxygen uptake. Chest 1976;70: 486–493.

50. Sietsema KE, Cooper DM, Rosove MH, Perloff JK, Child JS, Canobbio MM, Whipp BJ, Wasserman K. Dynamics of oxygen uptake during exercise in adults with cyanotic congenital heart disease. Circulation 1986;73:1137–1144.

51. Kory RC, Callahan R, Boren NC, Syner JC. The veterans administration-army cooperative study of pulmonary function. 1. Clinical spirometry in normal men. Am J Med 1961;30:243–258.

52. Lindall A, Medine A, Grismor JT. A re-evaluation of normal pulmonary function measurements in the adult female. Am Rev Respir Dis 1967;95:1061–1064.

53. Gandevia B, Hugh-Jones P. Terminology for measurements of ventilatory capacity. Thorax 1957;1:290–293.

54. Cotes JE. Lung Function: Assessment and Application in Medicine. Oxford: Blackwell Scientific Publications, 1975;104.

55. Miller WF, Johnson RL Jr, Wu N. Relationships between maximal breathing capacity and timed expiratory capacities. J Appl Physiol 1959;14:510–516.

56. Campbell SC. A comparison of the maximum volume ventilation with forced expiratory volume in one second: an assessment of subject cooperation. J Occupat Med 1982;24:531–533.

57. Bradley PW, Younes M. Relation between respiratory valve dead space and tidal volume. J Appl Physiol 1980;49:528–532.

58. Jones NL, McHardy GJR, Naimark A, Campbell EJM. Physiological dead space an alveolar-arterial gas pressure differences during exercise. Clin Sci 1966;31:19–29.

59. Lifshay A, Fast CW, Glazier JB. Effects of changes in respiratory pattern on physiological dead space. J Appl Physiol 1971;31:478–483.

60. Hey EN, Lloyd BB, Cunningham DJC, Jukes MGM, Bolton DPG. Effects of various repiratory stimuli on the depth and frequency of breathing in man. Respir Physiol 1966;1:193–205.

61. Spiro SC, Juniper E, Bowman P, Edwards RHT. An increasing work rate test for assessing the physiological strain of submaximal exercise. Clin Sci Molec Med 1974; 46:191–206.

62. Cotes JE. Lung Function: Assessment and Application in Medicine. Oxford: Blackwell Scientific Publications, 1975; 394.

63. Davis JA, Whipp BJ, Wasserman K. The relation of ventilation to metabolic rate during moderate exercise in man. Eur J Appl Physiol 1980;44:97–108.

64. Fairbarn MS. Personal communication.

65. Wasserman K, VanKessel A, Burton GB. Interaction of physiological mechanisms during exercise. J Appl Physiol 1967;22:71–85.

66. Medoff BD, Oelberg DA, Kanarek DJ, Systrom DM. Breathing reserve at the lactate threshold to differentiate a pulmonary mechanical from cardiovascular limit to exercise. Chest 1998;113:913–918.

67. Whipp BJ, Wasserman K. Alveolar-arterial gas tension differences during graded exercise. J Appl Physiol 1969;27:361–365.

68. Bradley CA, Harris EA, Seelye ER, Whitlock RML. Gas exchange during exercise in healthy people. I. The physiological dead-space volume. Clin Sci Molec Med 1976; 51:323–333.

69. Ward SA, Wasserman K, Davis JA, Whipp BJ. Breathing-valve encumbrance and arterial blood gas and acid-base homeostasis during incremental exercise. Fed Proc 1984; 43:634.

70. Jones NL, Robertson DG, Kane JW. Difference between end-tidal and arterial P_{CO_2} in exercise. J Appl Physiol 1979;47:954–960.

71. Dempsey JA, Hanson P, Henderson K. Exercise-induced arterial hypoxemia in healthy humans at sea-level. J Physiol (Lond) 1984;355:161–175.

72. Lilienthal JL, Riley RL, Proemmel DD, Frank RE. An experimental analysis in man of the oxygen pressure gradient from alveolar air to arterial blood during rest and exercise at sea level and at altitude. Am J Physiol 1946;147:199–216.

73. Asmussen E, Nielsen M. Alveolo-arterial gas exchange at rest and during work at different O_2 tensions. Acta Physiol Scand 1960;50:153–166.

74. Cruz JC, Hartley LH, Vogel JA. Effect of altitude relocations upon A_aDO_2 at rest and during exercise. J Appl Physiol 1975;39:469–474.

75. Hansen JE, Vogel JA, Stelter GP, Consolazio CF. Oxygen uptake in man during exhaustive work at sea level and high altitude. J Appl Physiol 1967;23:511–522.

76. Stringer W, Wasserman K, Casaburi R, Porszasz J, Maehara K, French W. Lactic acidosis as a facilitator of oxyhemoglobin dissociation during exercise. J Appl Physiol 1994;76:1462–1467.

77. Agostini PG, Wasserman K, Perego GB, Marenzi GC, Guazzi M, Assanelli E, Lauri G, Guazzi MD. Oxygen transport to muscle during exercise in chronic conjestive heart failure secondary to idiopathic dilated cardiomyopathy. Am J Cardiol 1997;79:1120–1124.

78. Koike A, Wasserman K, Taniguchi K, Hiroe M, Marumo F. The critical capillary P_{O_2} and the lactate threshold in patients with cardiovascular disease. J Am Coll Cardiol 1994;23:1644–1650.

79. Stringer W, Hansen J, Wasserman K. Cardiac output estimated non-invasively from oxygen uptake ($\dot{V}_{O_2}$) during exercise. J Appl Physiol 1997;82:908–912.

80. Weber KT, Janicki JS. Cardiopulmonary exercise testing for evaluation of chronic cardiac failure. Am J Cardiol 1985;55:22A–31A.

81. Sullivan MJ, Knight D, Higginbotham MB, Cobb FR. Relation between central and peripheral hemodynamics during exercise in patients with chronic heart failure. Muscle blood flow is reduced with maintenance of arterial perfusion pressure. Circulation 1989;80:769–781.

82. Yoshida T, Nagata A, Maro M, Takeuchi N, Sada Y. The validity of anaerobic threshold determination by a Douglas bag method compared with arterial blood lactate concentration. Eur J Appl Physiol 1981;46:423–430.

83. Beaver WL, Wasserman K, Whipp BJ. Bicarbonate buffering of lactic acid generated during exercise. J Appl Physiol 1986;60:472–478.

CHAPTER 7

Principles of Interpretation:
A Flow Chart Approach

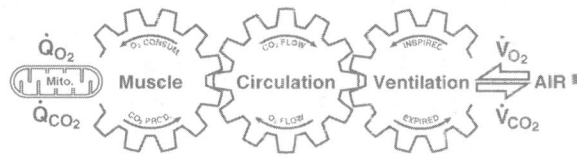

INTRODUCTION TO FLOW CHARTS

When patients complain of exercise intolerance, it is usually because they are unable to accomplish a task that they expect to complete with comparative ease and without unusual effort or undue feelings of fatigue or shortness of breath. Identifying the cause of this exercise intolerance is a major objective of integrative cardiopulmonary exercise testing.

The measurements needed for physiologic assessment are discussed in Chapter 3, and their patterns of change in response to the pathophysiology of specific diseases are described in Chapter 4 and further in the next two chapters. Once one has chosen the optimal exercise protocol (see Chapter 5) and has carefully selected the predicted values for the discriminating physiologic variables (see Chapter 6), the task of identifying the probable cause(s) of the exercise intolerance still remains. In this chapter, we introduce a *flow chart* strategy to show how the measurements made during exercise may be used to deduce pathophysiology, systematically. Although the analytic method presented here is not necessarily ideal in all instances, the flow charts serve to establish a discipline for interpreting cardiopulmonary exercise tests. The flow charts are also of considerable value in providing a foundation for reaching a physiologically based interpretation, as well as providing instruction on the pathophysiology of different diseases that limit exercise tolerance.

In the flow charts, the patient's peak $\dot{V}O_2$ is referred to the predicted $\dot{V}O_2$ max values provided in Chapter 6. Thus, a reduced peak $\dot{V}O_2$ identified at the start of flow charts 3 to 5 means that the value is below the 95% confidence limits of the predicted $\dot{V}O_2$ max.

The first question to address is whether the peak $\dot{V}O_2$ is normal or decreased. The second question is whether the AT is normal or decreased. The answer to these two questions puts the interpreter into the correct subsequent flow chart. By this time the diagnostic possibilities are considerably focused. Other measurements then lead to the single pathophysiological state most consistent with the exercise data. From knowledge of the pathophysiological state, anatomical corollaries may be sought, if deemed necessary, through other studies.

To facilitate description of each decision based on physiologic measurements, each branchpoint is numbered on the flow charts. The symbol -R refers to the right branch of the numbered branchpoint

and -L to the left branch of the numbered branchpoint. Each final branchpoint leads to a box containing a diagnosis that can account for the parameters or measurements reached in the decision-making process. Under the diagnosis is a list of additional measurements that lend further support to that diagnosis.

Each branchpoint decision and the choice of which flow chart to use for data analysis should not be regarded as rigid. If the physiologic variable addressed at a particular branchpoint does not strongly favor one branch, or if the measurements described in the diagnosis box do not support the diagnosis, both branches of a branchpoint should be considered. Similarly, if flow charts 3 or 4 (see Figs. 7.3, 7.4) lead the clinician to a conclusion about pathophysiology that appears unwarranted or difficult to support, flow chart 5 (see Fig. 7.5), using an alternative strategy of reasoning, may be used. The flow charts should be used with some degree of flexibility and always with consideration of sound physiologic principles.

ESTABLISHING THE PATHOPHYSIOLOGIC BASIS OF EXERCISE INTOLERANCE

Maximum Exercise Capacity and Anaerobic Threshold (Flow Chart 1)

Analysis of data obtained during the exercise test begins on flow chart 1 (Fig. 7.1), which separates patients based on their measured peak $\dot{V}O_2$ and anaerobic threshold (AT). Patients are divided into those with normal or reduced exercise capacity (normal or reduced maximum $\dot{V}O_2$). Patients with a reduced maximum exercise capacity are further divided into those with normal, reduced, or indeterminate AT. The analysis then proceeds to a separate flow chart (flow charts 2 to 5; see Figs. 7.2 to 7.5) for each of these groups.

Only a few conditions are associated with exercise intolerance and normal maximum $\dot{V}O_2$; these are considered in flow chart 2 (Fig. 7.2). For those with a low peak $\dot{V}O_2$, a normal AT suggests that O_2 flow at submaximal exercise levels is within normal limits and maximum exercise capacity is limited by one of a variety of other causes considered in flow chart 3 (Fig. 7.3). The combination of both low peak $\dot{V}O_2$ and AT leads to flow chart 4 (Fig. 7.4), in which disorders that limit the capacity to transport oxygen are described. Finally, it is recognized that the AT

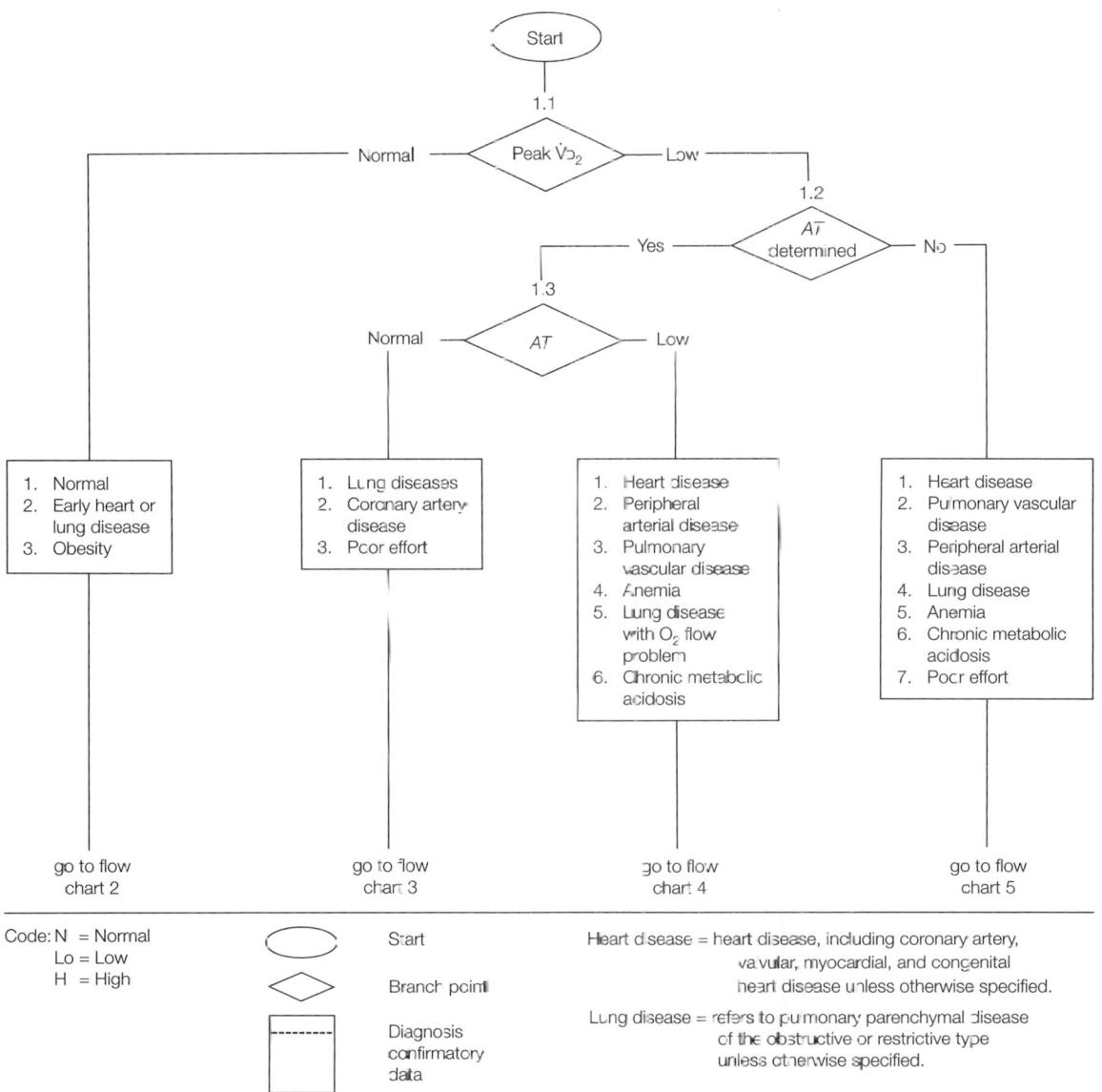

FIGURE 7.1.   Flow chart 1 for the differential diagnosis of the cause of exercise limitation. Analysis starts with the measurement of peak V̇o₂. Ellipsoids indicate starting points, diamonds indicate branchpoints, and boxes indicate diagnoses. Branchpoints are numbered to correspond to text. Measurements listed under diagnoses are used to support the diagnosis. If the supporting measurements do not fit well, try a closely related branchpoint leading to a different diagnosis in which the supporting measurements fit better. The code shown at the bottom of this figure pertains to all five flow charts.

Exercise Intolerance with Normal Peak V̇o₂ (Flow Chart 2)

When peak V̇o₂ is normal, but the patient complains of exercise intolerance, the diagnostic possibilities are 1) that the patient is actually normal but has anxiety about failing health, 2) that the patient is excessively obese, thereby requiring an increased metabolic and cardiopulmonary response to do minimal activity, or 3) that the patient, previously fit, has developed early cardiovascular or lung disease. Thus despite a reduced ability to do the physical work to which he/she is accustomed, the peak V̇o₂ still falls within the normal range of the subject's predicted V̇o₂ max. The diagnostic flow chart leading to each of these diagnoses is shown in Figure 7.2. A normal peak V̇o₂ (equal to the predicted V̇o₂ max) with a low AT is unusual in normal subjects. However, it might be found in unusually sedentary

may not always be determined; a diagnostic scheme for this circumstance is described in flow chart 5 (Fig. 7.5).

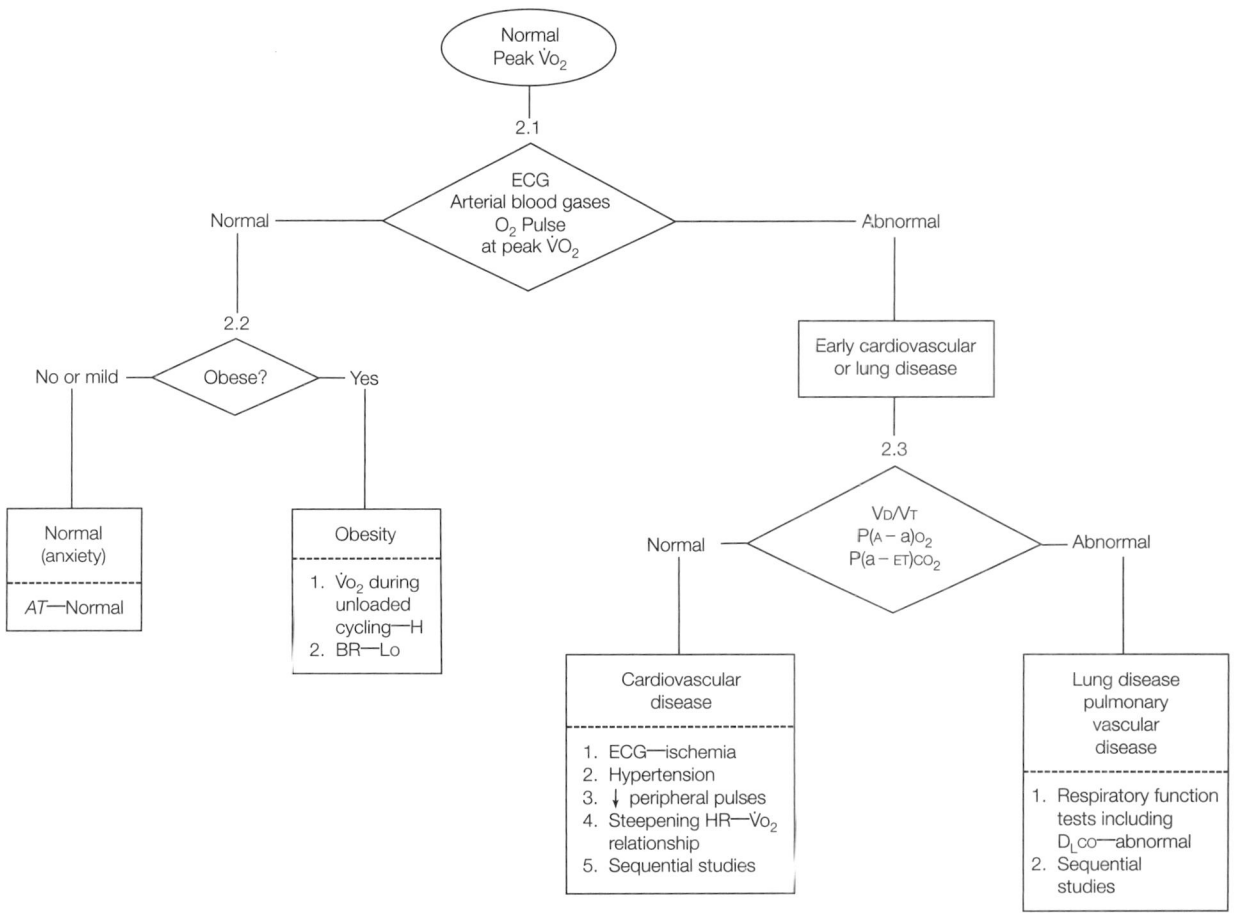

FIGURE 7.2.   Flow chart 2 for conditions in which peak $\dot{V}O_2$ is normal but the patient feels limited during exercise. If the supporting measurements do not fit well, try a closely related branchpoint leading to a different diagnosis in which the confirmatory measurements fit better. Symbols and use of flow chart are as described in Introduction to Flow Charts and Figure 7.1.

subjects or patients with early disease that compromises O_2 transport to muscle cells.

Normal with Anxiety State (Branchpoint 2.1-L, 2.2-L)

People with this condition tend to be physically active and try to maintain their general state of health; otherwise, they would not be concerned. Therefore, their peak $\dot{V}O_2$ is generally on the high side of normal, and they are not obese. If the exercise electrocardiogram, O_2 pulse, and arterial blood gases are normal at all work rates, including the maximum, the patient is probably normal. The breathing reserve is also normal, but it may be on the low side of normal if the subject has a peak $\dot{V}O_2$ that is considerably better than the predicted normal value, i.e., the subject is in good physical condition. A confirmatory measurement is a normal AT that is above the mean predicted value. A patient with

these findings would benefit from reassurance (see Cases 1 and 13 in Chap. 9).

Obesity (Branchpoint 2.1-L, 2.2-R)

Obese subjects require an increased metabolic rate ($\dot{V}O_2$ and $\dot{V}CO_2$) to perform a given physical activity compared to non-obese subjects. The increased metabolic rate results in increased cardiac output (cardiac output $= \dot{V}O_2/C(a - \bar{v})O_2$) and minute ventilation ($\dot{V}E = \dot{V}CO_2/[(1\text{-}V_D/V_T) \times (PaCO_2/P_B)]$) requirements compared with the non-obese subject for a given level of work. When the obese individual is relatively young, the increased oxygen cost for work caused by the large body mass is generally well tolerated (see Case 15, Chapter 9). When the normal deteriorating effects of aging on maximal ventilatory capacity are combined with the extra ventilatory cost of moving the large body to perform work, however, a reduced breathing reserve results.

In addition, because a higher cardiac output is needed to support the increased O_2 to perform work by the obese subject, the cardiac reserve is low. Although the *AT* (when expressed as a percentage of predicted $\dot{V}O_2$peak) is normal, the O_2 cost of walking may be too great to perform this activity without developing a metabolic acidosis. The patient's heart rate reserve is normal at maximum exercise, although the breathing reserve is usually reduced because of ventilatory restriction and increased ventilatory requirement.

Early Cardiovascular or Lung Disease (Branchpoint 2.1-R, 2.3)

In early mild cardiovascular or lung disease, the disorder may not be severe enough to cause the peak $\dot{V}O_2$ to be less than predicted, the latter based on a relatively sedentary population. Specific physiologic variables may become abnormal, however, depending on the site of the defect in the metabolic-cardiovascular-ventilatory coupling. Thus, a patient may have a recently developed mild abnormality of the heart or lungs but still have a peak $\dot{V}O_2$ value that falls within the normal range. It may be difficult to document such a developing abnormality except by sequential studies demonstrating a decline in the peak $\dot{V}O_2$ or *AT*. The most important problems that should be identified or excluded are those related to ischemic heart disease. Also to be excluded are subtle abnormalities in gas exchange that might suggest pulmonary vascular disease that limits the ability to recruit capillary bed in response to exercise. Thus the most important findings during maximal effort exercise are the ECG and arterial blood gases.

A frequent problem of the middle-aged adult is coronary artery disease; therefore, examination of the electrocardiogram (ECG) along with gas exchange measurements that relate the increase in $\dot{V}O_2$ and $\dot{V}CO_2$ to the increase in work rate are helpful and may be diagnostic. The ECG may provide evidence of myocardial ischemia. When it is accompanied by an abrupt decrease in the rate of $\dot{V}O_2$ increase despite a sustained increase in work rate, strong evidence exists that the ECG changes are associated with changes in ventricular function due to myocardial dyskinesis. In addition, a faster rise in heart rate than $\dot{V}O_2$ toward the end of exercise may be an indicator of heart disease; and flattening of the O_2 pulse at submaximal exercise levels also suggests the presence of a reduced stroke volume consistent with heart disease. These changes, associated with evidence of myocardial ischemia on the ECG, make a strong case for the diagnosis of coronary artery disease (2.3-L) (see Case 18, Chapter 9).

Measuring arterial blood gases during incremental exercise testing is also important because the changes in the V_D/V_T, $P(a - ET)CO_2$, and $P(A - a)O_2$, as work rate is increased to the subjects maximum, are the most sensitive markers of lung disease (see Case 46, Chapter 9). Normal values usually rule out mild or developing pulmonary vascular, lung parenchymal, or airway diseases because these measurements are almost always abnormal in these conditions (2.3-R), even when resting pulmonary function tests, such as vital capacity, FEV_1, total lung capacity, and D_LCO are within the normal range.

Low Peak $\dot{V}O_2$ with Normal *AT* (Flow Chart 3)

The breathing reserve provides a good first branchpoint for the differential diagnosis of disorders characterized by a low peak $\dot{V}O_2$ and a normal *AT* (branchpoint 3.1; Fig. 7.3). Patients with a normal or high breathing reserve (3.1-R) include those making a poor effort, those who are limited by muscular and skeletal diseases, or those with myocardial ischemia at relatively low work rates. On the other hand, a low breathing reserve (3.1-L) identifies those patients with lung diseases.

Normal or High Breathing Reserve (3.1-R)

Poor Effort or Muscular-Skeletal Disorder (3.3-L). Perhaps for secondary gain, the subject may make a poor effort and may thereby have a low peak $\dot{V}O_2$ during exercise testing. Both the breathing reserve and heart rate reserve are high, indicating that the patient has not used the full potential of either the cardiovascular or the ventilatory system. The absence of metabolic acidosis at the end of exercise is also evidence of poor effort. Additional confirmatory measures that the lungs and pulmonary circulation are functionally normal include normal exercise V_D/V_T, $P(A - a)O_2$, and $P(a - ET)CO_2$. These demonstrate that the distribution of ventilation relative to perfusion is uniform, virtually ruling out primary lung or pulmonary vascular disease. Simultaneous measurement of lactate and acid-base balance should confirm if an adequate effort was made during the exercise test. Every one who makes a sufficient effort should develop a significant metabolic acidosis during exercise with a $[HCO_3^-]$ decrease of at least 4 mmol/L at peak $\dot{V}O_2$. The rare

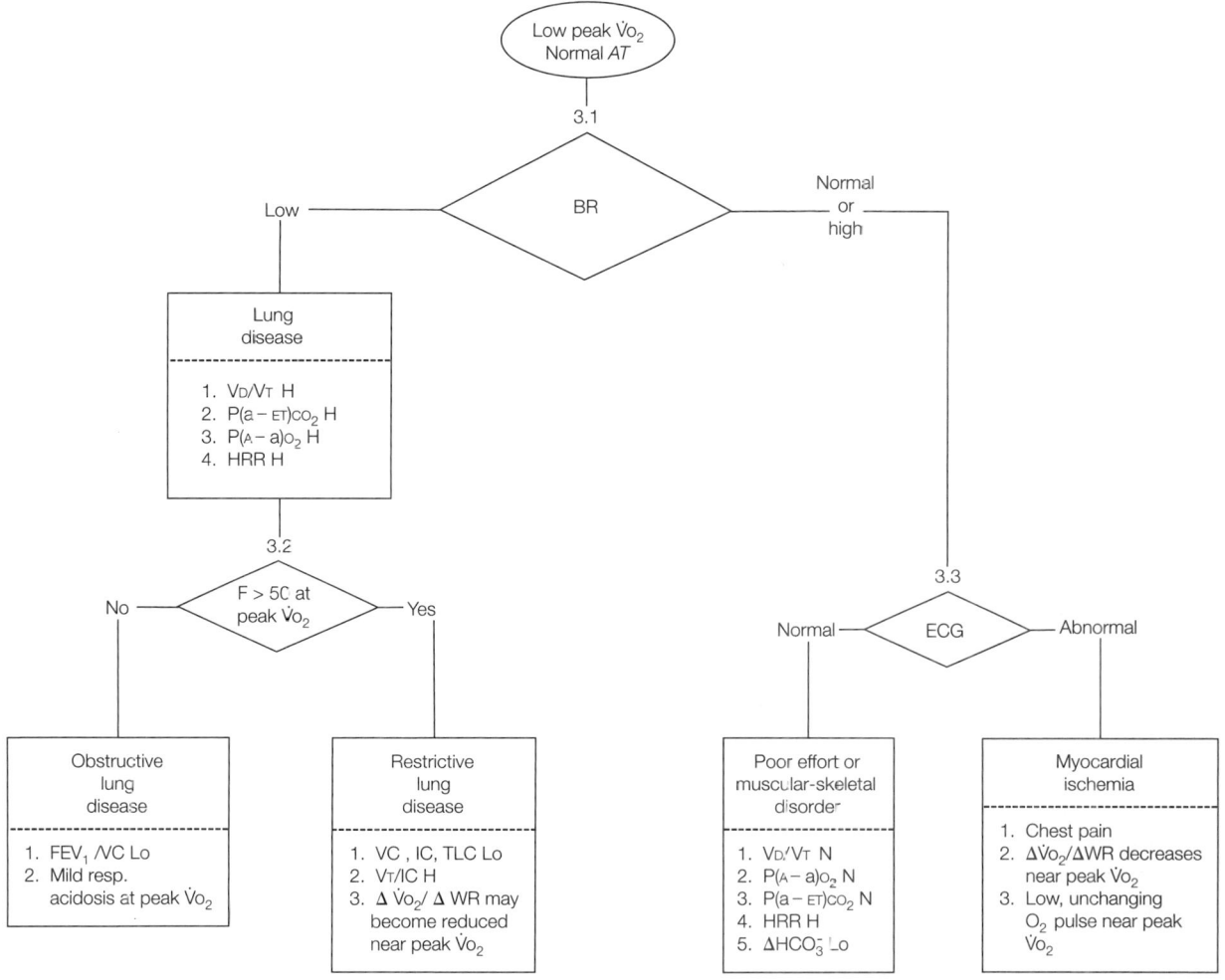

FIGURE 7.3.   Flow chart 3 for conditions in which peak $\dot{V}_{O_2}$ is low but the anaerobic threshold (*AT*) is normal. If the supporting measurements do not fit well, try a closely related branchpoint leading to a different diagnosis in which the supporting measurements fit better. Symbols and use of flow chart are as described in Introduction to Flow Charts and Figure 7.1.

exceptions are patients who have a defect in skeletal muscle myophosphorylase or enzymatic defect in the glycolytic pathway. Also, patients limited during exercise due to severe airflow obstruction may not be able to increase work rate sufficiently to develop a lactic acidosis during exercise.

Optimal cardiovascular and pulmonary evaluation is impossible when arthritis or neuromuscular disease limits exercise. The reason for this is the difficulty in performing enough exercise to stress the cardiovascular or respiratory system. Occasionally, however, a patient with exercise limitation is not suspected of having a muscular-skeletal cause of decreased exercise tolerance (Cases 68–70, Chapter 9).

Myocardial Ischemia (3.3-R). The ECG usually becomes abnormal if the myocardium becomes ischemic as the work rate is increased to the pa-

tient's symptom-limited maximum. The ECG abnormality may be evident only at high work rates, and the patient may or may not experience angina. Whereas coronary artery disease is the most frequent cause of myocardial ischemia, it may also occur in aortic stenosis or marked systemic hypertension without coronary artery disease (Cases 21 and 33, Chapter 9). When myocardial ischemia develops, the $\dot{V}_{O_2}$ may fail to increase normally as the work rate is increased, despite a normal rate of $\dot{V}_{O_2}$ increase at lower work rates before the myocardium becomes ischemic (Cases 18 and 22, Chapter 9).

Low Breathing Reserve (3.1-L)

Low breathing reserve suggests lung disease. The breathing frequency may be a useful next branchpoint to distinguish the dominance of obstructive from restrictive lung disease in mixed disorders. The confirmatory data listed under each diagnosis should be used to further support the diagnosis.

Obstructive Lung Diseases (3.2-L). Although the peak $\dot{V}O_2$ achieved during incremental exercise testing is low in this disorder, the *AT* is often normal. The normal *AT* suggests that the patient does not have a problem with oxygen transport to the tissues at these submaximal work rates (see Case 37, Chapter 9). Characteristically, these patients have abnormalities in PaO_2, VD/VT, $P(a - ET)CO_2$, and $P(A - a)O_2$ during exercise consequent to ventilation-perfusion mismatching. Decreases in PaO_2 commonly occur in a single step at low work rates with little further change as the work rate is increased (see Fig. 4.5). This is probably because the increased perfusion during exercise goes predominantly to normal and high $\dot{V}A/\dot{Q}$ regions of the lungs. Except in mild obstructive lung disease, the breathing reserve is decreased, indicating a ventilatory limitation during exercise. In contrast to O_2 flow limiting disorders, the $\dot{V}O_2$ continues to increase linearly as the work rate is increased to the patient's peak $\dot{V}O_2$, i.e., there is no decrease in $\Delta\dot{V}O_2/\Delta WR$ as the peak $\dot{V}O_2$ is approached. The heart rate reserve is commonly increased because the cardiovascular capacity cannot be fully challenged as a result of the breathing limitation. Finally, expiratory flow frequently has an obstructive pattern (trapezoidal in appearance, with an early peak) as illustrated in Figure 3.15.

In patients with marked airflow obstruction, the *AT* may need to be determined by the V-slope method rather than methods that rely on the increase in ventilatory equivalent for O_2. Although CO_2 output will increase when HCO_3^- buffers lactic acid, the ventilatory response to the increased CO_2 load from buffering is often poor in these patients, and the ventilatory equivalent for O_2 may not increase measurably at the *AT* (see Cases 40 and 42, Chapter 9).

Restrictive Lung Diseases (3.2-R). Pathophysiologic responses seen in restrictive lung diseases have much in common with those of the obstructive lung diseases, but clear differences exist. The VD/VT and $P(a - ET)CO_2$ are increased in both physiological types of lung disorders as reflections of ventilation-perfusion mismatching. In contrast to obstructive lung diseases, however, the $P(A - a)O_2$ usually increases systematically at each work rate during the incremental test. Moreover, the VT increases to its

maximum at a relatively low work rate, and the VT/IC ratio nears a value of one. Because VT cannot increase normally in patients with restrictive lung diseases, the ventilatory response to the increasing work rate is achieved primarily by increasing the breathing frequency, usually exceeding 50 breaths/min at the end of exercise. Patients with restrictive lung diseases often manifest an O_2 flow problem (Cases 49 to 53, Chapter 9). This is shown by the failure of $\dot{V}O_2$ to increase normally as the work rate is progressively increased to the patient's maximum. This may be caused both by the falling arterial O_2 content and by the increased pulmonary vascular resistance (resulting from destruction of pulmonary blood vessels by the fibrosing process) that limits the rate of increase in cardiac output. Thus, these patients commonly have a reduced *AT* with a low peak $\dot{V}O_2$. This diagnosis will be analyzed in greater detail in flow chart 4 (Fig. 7.4).

Low Peak $\dot{V}O_2$ with Low *AT* (Flow Chart 4)

The breathing reserve serves as a good primary branchpoint (4.1) for the differential diagnosis of disorders having a low peak $\dot{V}O_2$ and low *AT*, as shown in flow chart 4 (Fig. 7.4), but further questions about pathophysiology need to be addressed to distinguish among the various conditions that cause a low *AT*. The $\Delta\dot{V}O_2/\Delta WR$ is a good second branchpoint (4.2) for the conditions that have a low breathing reserve; $\dot{V}E/\dot{V}CO_2$ at the *AT* is a useful second branchpoint (4.3) for the conditions with a normal or high breathing reserve.

Normal or High Breathing Reserve (4.1-R)

Normal $\dot{V}E/\dot{V}CO_2$ at *AT* (4.3-L). If the breathing reserve is normal or high and the $\dot{V}E/\dot{V}CO_2$ at *AT* is normal (4.3-L), then we must consider an O_2 flow problem of non-pulmonary vascular disease origin. Myocardial ischemia, cardiomyopathy, valvular heart disease, peripheral arterial disease, and anemia or hemoglobinopathy are diagnoses that should be seriously considered. Hematocrit (4.4) and O_2 pulse ($\dot{V}O_2/HR$) (4.6) are further branchpoints that distinguish these diagnoses.

ANEMIA (4.4-R) Because of the reduced O_2 carrying capacity of the blood, the *AT* and lactic acidosis occur at a relatively low work rate. The low oxygen content of the arterial blood caused by the anemia results in decreased $C(a - \bar{v})O_2$. Thus the maximal

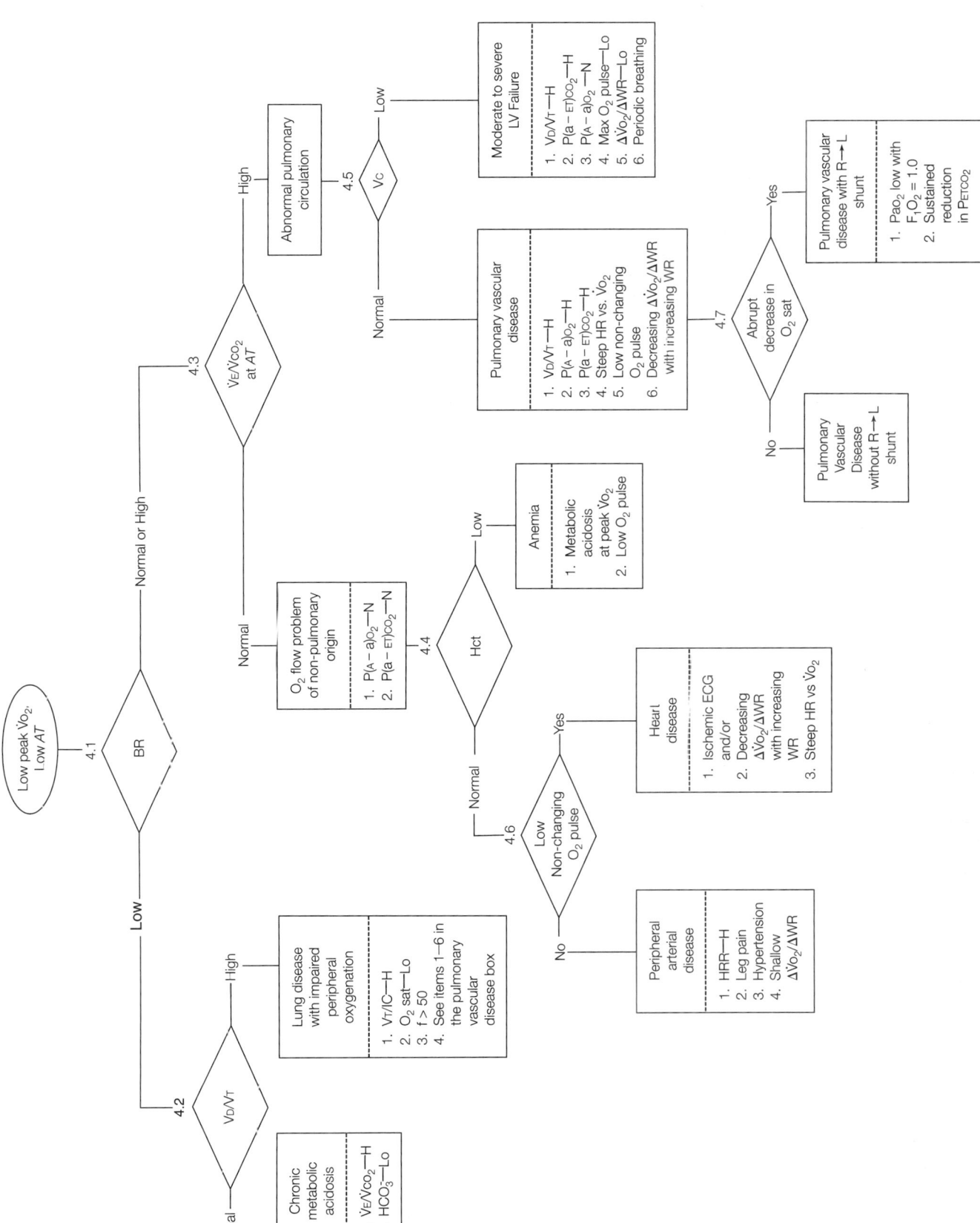

FIGURE 7.4. Flow chart 4 for conditions in which both peak $\dot{V}O_2$ and anaerobic threshold (AT) are low. If the supporting measurements do not fit well, try a closely related branchpoint leading to a different diagnosis in which the supporting measurements fit better. Symbols and use of flow chart are as described in Introduction to Flow Charts and Figure 7.1.

O_2 pulse is reduced, reflecting the decreased $C(a - \bar{v})O_2$. A high cardiac output and heart rate are required to meet the tissue O_2 requirement. The arterial blood gas tensions and the $\dot{V}D/\dot{V}T$ are normal, even at maximal exercise (Case 76, Chapter 9).

HEART DISEASES (4.6-R)   Patients with primary heart diseases (myocardial ischemia secondary to coronary artery disease, cardiomyopathy secondary to any cause, and valvular heart disease) usually have a low peak $\dot{V}O_2$ with a low *AT*. In these disorders, $\dot{V}O_2$ usually slows its rate of rise relative to the work rate as the peak $\dot{V}O_2$ is approached (see Cases 16–28, Chapter 9). However, the pattern of slowing differs according to diagnosis. The contrasting patterns of change will be described in the next chapter. The heart rate often continues to increase as the work rate is increased despite the slower increase of $\dot{V}O_2$. This results in a steepening of the heart rate–$\dot{V}O_2$ relationship as the maximum work rate is approached. Also, the O_2 pulse reaches a constant value at subnormal values (Fig. 3.12). Changes in the ECG consistent with myocardial ischemia during exercise, combined with the concurrent failure for $\dot{V}O_2$ to increase normally, provide support for the diagnosis of exercise-induced myocardial ischemia (see Table 4.4).

In mild to moderate forms of heart failure, regardless of cause, an acute metabolic acidosis occurs at relatively low levels of exercise. In more severe forms of heart failure (NYHA class 3 to 4), $\dot{V}D/\dot{V}T$ becomes elevated because of ventilation-perfusion mismatching. In such patients, the $\dot{V}E/\dot{V}CO_2$ is increased at the *AT* and the flow chart leads to the right at branchpoint 4.3. Consequently, chronic stable advanced heart failure is accompanied by pulmonary vascular changes that must be distinguished from diseases in which the pulmonary circulation is the primary site of disease (see Tables 4.5 and 4.8).

PERIPHERAL ARTERIAL DISEASE (4.6-L) In contrast to primary heart diseases, the heart rate reserve is generally high in this condition since the patient stops exercising because of claudication before the heart can be maximally stressed. Because of obstruction in major conducting arteries, normal arteriolar vasodilatation cannot take place during exercise. Thus systemic arterial hypertension often develops beyond that expected with exercise. The increase in oxygen uptake relative to the increase in work rate may be diminished, resulting in a relatively shallow slope for the $\dot{V}O_2$–work rate relationship (low $\Delta\dot{V}O_2/\Delta WR$). In contrast to other cardiovascular disorders, the $\dot{V}CO_2$–work rate relationship is also

shallow. Finally, in the absence of concomitant lung disease, measurements of $\dot{V}D/\dot{V}T$, $P(a - ET)CO_2$, and $P(A - a)O_2$, which reflect the distribution of ventilation relative to perfusion, are normal (see Cases 30 and 31, Chapter 9).

High $\dot{V}E/\dot{V}CO_2$ at *AT* (4.3-R). If the breathing reserve is normal or high (4.1-R) but the $\dot{V}E/\dot{V}CO_2$ at *AT* is high (4.3-R), then the most likely disorder is disease originating in the pulmonary circulation or moderate to severe left ventricular failure.

PULMONARY VASCULAR DISEASE ORIGINATING IN PULMONARY CIRCULATION (4.5-L). What distinguishes patients with pulmonary vascular disorders that originate in the pulmonary circulation from pulmonary vascular changes that accompany left ventricular failure are the normal vital capacity and FEV_1 (branchpoint 4.5) and abnormal PaO_2 and $P(A - a)O_2$. Patients with disorders that originate in the pulmonary vascular bed and cause pulmonary vascular resistance to be increased include pulmonary thromboembolic disease, primary pulmonary hypertension, and diseases that cause a pulmonary vasculitis. These disorders, when chronic, have little effect on pulmonary mechanics. Thus they have a normal VC and FEV_1 (left branch of 4.5), but they develop abnormalities of lung gas exchange commonly resulting in a reduced PaO_2 and increased $P(A - a)O_2$.

If the pulmonary circulation, interposed between the right and left sides of the heart, does not dilate or recruit pulmonary blood vessels normally during exercise, the increased venous return that accompanies exercise cannot be readily transmitted to the left ventricle. When the right side of the heart cannot "feed" blood to the left side at a rate commensurate with that required for normal exercise, cardiac output cannot respond appropriately to the exercise stimulus. Because the cardiac output can not increase normally, the $\dot{V}O_2$ increase relative to increase in work rate progressively slows below the normal rate of increase of 10 ml/min/Watt. In addition to the abnormal slowing in the rate of rise in $\dot{V}O_2$, the *AT* and peak $\dot{V}O_2$ are reduced. Because the increase in $\dot{V}O_2$ with work rate slows but heart rate continues to increase with work rate, heart rate increases steeply relative to $\dot{V}O_2$ and gets steeper as the peak $\dot{V}O_2$ is approached. Thus, the O_2 pulse fails to increase as the work rate is increased and is reduced at maximum work.

Patients with pulmonary vascular disease have a high $\dot{V}D/\dot{V}T$ and a positive value for $P(a - ET)CO_2$. These provide evidence of poor perfusion of ventilated air spaces. Moreover, the $P(A - a)O_2$ increases abnormally as the work rate is increased, probably because of the shortened red cell transit time due to a reduced capillary bed as described in Chapter 4. Although these changes are similar to those seen in primary lung diseases, other measurements made during exercise distinguish these disorders. For instance, the breathing reserve is usually normal. In addition, metabolic acidosis develops with pulmonary vascular diseases in response to exercise rather than the respiratory acidosis that commonly accompanies severe obstructive lung diseases.

Primary lung diseases can cause major disturbances in function of the pulmonary circulation, which may become the dominant pathophysiologic feature limiting exercise (Cases 41, 44, and 53, Chapter 9). In such instances, the abnormalities noted in the "Pulmonary Vascular Disease" diagnostic box of flow chart 4 (Fig. 7.4) become evident during exercise testing. Limitations in exercise caused by the pulmonary circulation cannot be reliably predicted from resting measurements.

PULMONARY VASCULAR DISEASE WITH A RIGHT TO LEFT SHUNT OR CYANOTIC CONGENITAL HEART DISEASE (4.7-R). Patients with pulmonary vascular disease who open a potentially patent foramen ovale, or have congenital heart disease with a right to left shunt, may demonstrate marked reductions in PaO_2 during air and O_2 breathing in response to exercise (see Case 51, Chapter 9). The VD/VT, $P(a - ET)CO_2$, and $P(A - a)O_2$ values become extremely abnormal in response to exercise, depending on the degree of pulmonary hypoperfusion and the size of the shunt. These values generally become more abnormal as the work rate is increased. Patients with these disorders can be distinguished from those with other pulmonary vascular diseases by an abrupt and sustained decrease in arterial O_2 saturation and $PETCO_2$ as soon as exercise begins. $\Delta \dot{V}O_2 / \Delta WR$ is reduced, and $\dot{V}CO_2$ may exceed $\dot{V}O_2$ at the lowest exercise work rates.

Repeating the exercise test while the patient breathes 100% O_2 is particularly helpful in distinguishing a right to left shunt from other causes of hypoxemia. With no shunt, the arterial PaO_2 will be in the range of 550 to 650 mmHg at rest and all levels of exercise. If a right to left shunt develops during exercise, PaO_2 will fall precipitously. It can be calculated that the arterial PaO_2 will decrease by approximately 100 mmHg for each 3 to 5% of the venous return that shunts from right to left while breathing O_2.

PULMONARY VASCULAR CHANGES SECONDARY TO MODERATELY SEVERE LEFT VENTRICULAR FAILURE (4.5-R). Patients with moderate to severe left ventricular failure have an increase in VD/VT and increase in $P(a - ET)CO_2$, but without hypoxemia or an increase in $P(A - a)O_2$ at peak $\dot{V}O_2$. This indicates that they have an increase in high $\dot{V}A/\dot{Q}$ lung units without low $\dot{V}A/\dot{Q}$ lung units. This is consistent with these patients having developed pulmonary vasoconstriction. In contrast to patients with pulmonary vascular disease originating in the pulmonary circulation, patients with moderately severe left ventricular failure have a reduced VC and a normal FEV_1/VC suggestive of a restrictive pulmonary mechanics. The latter finding, and a normal PaO_2 and $P(A - a)O_2$ at peak $\dot{V}O_2$ distinguishes them from pulmonary vascular disease originating in the pulmonary circulation. Because of the increase in VD/VT, the slope of $\dot{V}E$ versus $\dot{V}CO_2$ is abnormally steep. It should be stressed that these increases in VD/VT and slope of $\dot{V}E$ versus $\dot{V}CO_2$ are not present in more mild forms of left ventricular failure.

Low Breathing Reserve (4.1-L)

In the category of patients with a low peak $\dot{V}O_2$ and low AT accompanied by a low breathing reserve and a high VD/VT (4.2-R), the most likely disorder is a primary lung disease such as pulmonary fibrosis (restrictive lung disease) or COPD in a sedentary patient. In contrast, a low breathing reserve with a normal VD/VT can be caused by diseases associated with a chronic metabolic acidosis and hyperventilation (4.2-L). The following discussion describes further physiologic measurements that help confirm the diagnosis of each of these disorders.

Lung Disease with Impaired Peripheral Oxygenation (4.2-R). In certain pulmonary patients the AT as well as the peak $\dot{V}O_2$ are reduced. Moreover, $\Delta \dot{V}O_2 / \Delta WR$ may be reduced as work rate is increased. These are usually pulmonary patients with severe interstitial lung disease or COPD patients in whom the pulmonary circulation is markedly impaired (Table 4.11). Oxyhemoglobin desaturation may, but not necessarily, contribute to the impairment in O_2 flow to the exercising muscles. Commonly, the reduced $\Delta \dot{V}O_2 / \Delta WR$ is accompanied by a gradual reduction in the rate of increase in $\dot{V}O_2$ as work rate is increased. The physiological explanation for this finding is that patients with restrictive lung diseases have a significant loss of pulmonary capillary bed caused by the disease process. Thus, the pulmonary capillary bed is maximally recruited at rest, and blood flow can only increase during exercise to match the increase in O_2 required if pulmonary artery pressure increased sufficiently to provide a normal pulmonary blood flow response. While there is pulmonary hypertension in many patients with lung diseases, the increase in pulmonary artery pressure is insufficient to provide an adequate increase in pulmonary blood flow (cardiac output) to support the O_2 required by the exercising muscle. Because the dominant pathophysiology in patients with restrictive lung diseases and some patients with COPD often resides in the pulmonary circulation, the abnormalities described in the "Pulmonary Vascular Disease" box also apply to these lung diseases (Cases 51 and 53, Chapter 9).

Chronic Metabolic Acidosis (4.2-L). Patients with chronic renal failure with a renal tubular acidosis, those with poorly controlled diabetes mellitus, and patients taking medications such as acetazolamide, e.g., patients with glaucoma, may have a chronic metabolic acidosis. Because $Paco_2$ is reduced in these conditions (low $Paco_2$ set-point), exercise alveolar and minute ventilation are elevated; i.e., a higher than normal alveolar ventilation is needed to clear the increased metabolic CO_2 generated during exercise. This causes the ventilatory equivalents for O_2 and CO_2 to be increased and reduces the breathing reserve. Because of the high ventilatory requirement, these patients may experience exertional dyspnea before reaching their predicted peak $\dot{V}o_2$ and AT, particularly if they have lung or heart disease, anemia, or obesity. The chronic metabolic acidosis is easily identified from arterial blood gas and pH measurements.

Low Peak $\dot{V}o_2$ with AT Not Determined (Flow Chart 5)

The importance of the AT in deciding the cause of exercise limitation is demonstrated in the previous flow charts. However, in some patients, the AT may not be able to be determined or the interpreter feels that the AT is unreliable. Failure to identify an AT may result from an irregular breathing pattern or because the patient stopped exercise before the AT was reached. Also, the AT might have occurred at such a low work rate that the dynamics of gas exchange at the start of exercise already reflect the presence of a lactic acidosis. In this case, the examiner knows that the AT occurred at a $\dot{V}o_2$ below the

O_2 cost of the lowest work rate imposed during the test, but does not know the exact value.

An alternative strategy to using the AT as the second major branchpoint (flow chart 1) in the decision-making process is described in flow chart 5 (Fig. 7.5). Given a reduced peak $\dot{V}o_2$, tests that detect mismatching of ventilation to perfusion make it possible to distinguish disorders associated with inefficiency of lung gas exchange from disorders with normal lung function and pulmonary circulation. Thus, branchpoint 5.1 uses arterial blood gas and pulmonary gas exchange measurements to identify the presence of mismatching of ventilation-perfusion relationships. Diseases associated with abnormal ventilation-perfusion relationships include restrictive lung diseases, obstructive lung diseases, pulmonary vascular diseases, and moderately severe left heart failure. Patients with coronary artery, valvular and congenital heart disease, and mild to moderate left ventricular failure, anemia, peripheral arterial disease, and poor effort fit into the disorders with normal ventilation-perfusion relationships. The simplest and cheapest way to detect the presence of ventilation-perfusion mismatching is the measurement of V_D/V_T, $P(a - ET)co_2$, and $P(A - a)o_2$ during exercise. As shown in flow chart 5 (Fig. 7.5), if V_D/V_T, $P(a - ET)co_2$, and $P(A - a)o_2$ are normal (5.1-L), we examine the heart rate reserve (HRR) (5.2); if V_D/V_T, $P(a - ET)co_2$, and $P(A - a)o_2$ values are abnormal (5.1-R), we examine the breathing reserve (5.3). The possible diagnoses at each of these branchpoints separate into two major groups, depending on whether the heart rate reserve is normal or high or the breathing reserve is normal or low.

Whereas the first step in flow chart 5 (5.1) depends on knowledge of V_D/V_T and arterial Pco_2 and Po_2, it may not be feasible to collect arterial blood under some circumstances. An alternative is to approximate $Paco_2$ from venous blood drawn from a superficial vein of a warmed hand or from capillary blood from a finger or ear lobe. From these measurements, V_D/V_T and $P(a - ET)co_2$ can be calculated. Normal values would direct the analysis to the left (5.1-L), and abnormal values would direct the analysis to the right (5.1-R).

Normal V_D/V_T, $P(a - ET)co_2$, and $P(A - a)o_2$ (5.1-L)

Heart diseases, anemia, poor effort, and peripheral arterial disease are all associated with a low peak $\dot{V}o_2$, but have normal indices of gas exchange effi-

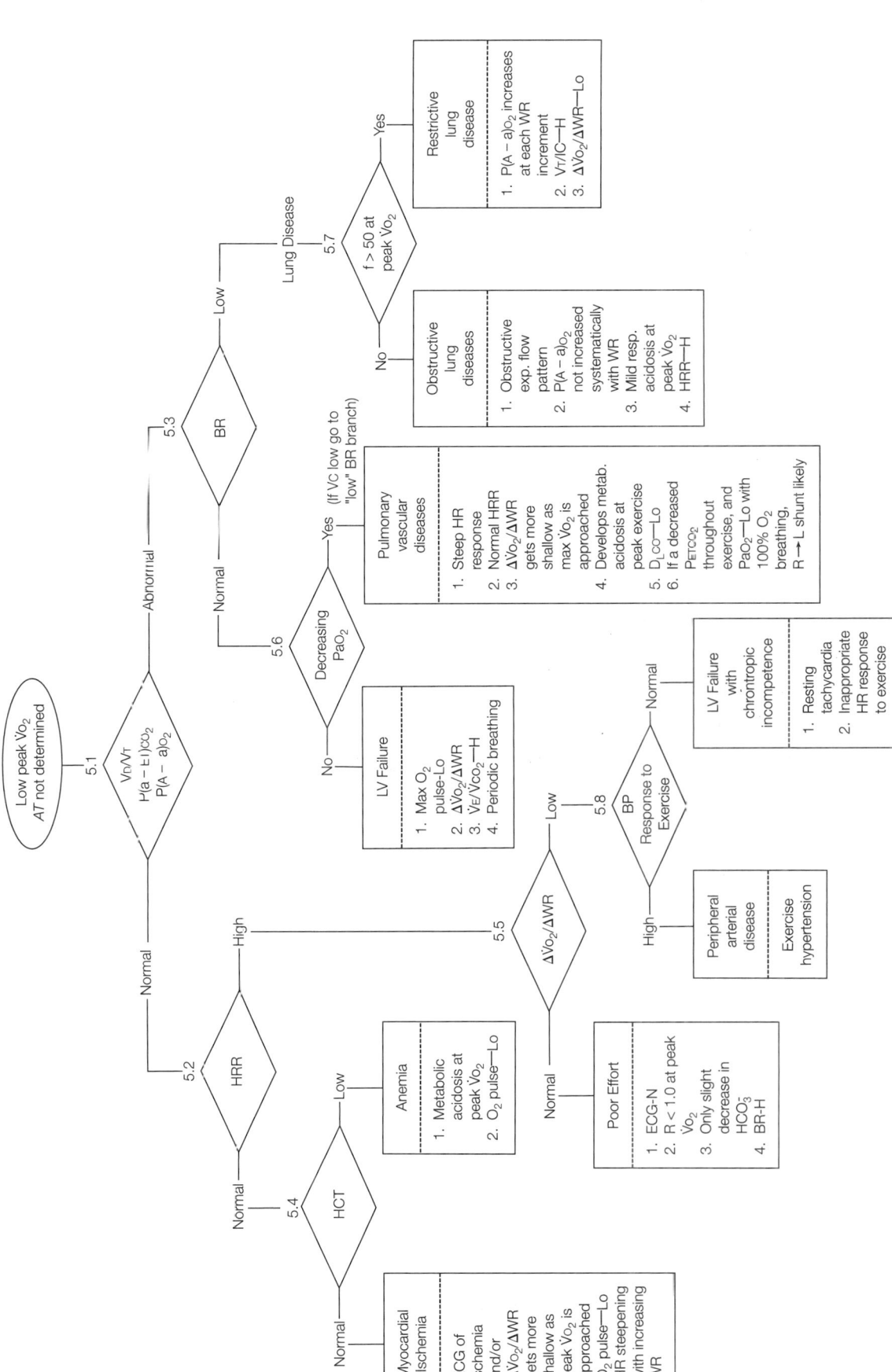

FIGURE 7.5.   Flow chart 5 for conditions in which peak V̇o₂ is low but the anaerobic threshold (AT) has not been measured or cannot be reliably determined. If the supporting measurements do not fit well, try a closely related branchpoint leading to a different diagnosis in which the supporting measurements fit better. Symbols and use of flow chart are as described in Introduction to Flow Charts and Figure 7.1.

ciency (V_D/V_T, $P(a - ET)CO_2$, and $P(A - a)O_2$). The HRR allows this group to be further subdivided into those with a normal HRR (5.2-L) (heart diseases and anemia) and a high HRR (5.2-R) (poor effort, peripheral arterial disease, and heart failure with chronotropic incompetence).

Anemia can be distinguished from the heart disorders with a low peak$\dot{V}O_2$, uniform $\dot{V}A/\dot{Q}$, and normal HRR (5.2-L) by a low hematocrit (5.4). Ischemic, valvular, cardiomyopathic, or non-cyanotic congenital heart diseases are usually characterized by a greater rise in heart rate and lesser rise in $\dot{V}O_2$ than expected for the work rate performed.

Poor effort, peripheral arterial disease, or chronic heart failure with chronotropic incompetence are associated with a low peak $\dot{V}O_2$, uniform $\dot{V}A/\dot{Q}$, and *high* HRR (5.2-R). The $\Delta\dot{V}O_2/\Delta WR$ (5.5) is a useful branchpoint to distinguish poor effort (normal branch) from peripheral arterial disease and chronic heart failure with chronotropic incompetence (low branch). Poor effort can be confirmed by other measurements, including a high breathing reserve, failure to develop a significant metabolic acidosis at end-exercise, an R < 1.0 at the peak $\dot{V}O_2$, a normal ECG, and possibly a very irregular breathing pattern.

Peripheral arterial disease and patients with left ventricular failure with chronotropic incompetence usually have a low $\Delta\dot{V}O_2/\Delta WR$ (5.5-R). Further distinguishing these diagnoses is a pronounced systolic hypertension in response to exercise in the former, but normal or low systolic pressure response in the latter (branchpoint 5.8).

Abnormal V_D/V_T, $P(a - ET)CO_2$, and $P(A - a)O_2$ (5.1-R)

Pulmonary vascular diseases, moderately severe chronic left ventricular heart failure, and obstructive and restrictive lung diseases are associated with a low peak $\dot{V}O_2$ and abnormal indices of gas exchange efficiency (non-uniform $\dot{V}A/\dot{Q}$). The breathing reserve (5.3) allows this group to be further subdivided into those with a normal breathing reserve (heart failure and pulmonary vascular diseases) and those with a low breathing reserve (obstructive and restrictive lung diseases).

The two disorders with a low peak $\dot{V}O_2$ and non-uniform $\dot{V}A/\dot{Q}$, but a normal breathing reserve (5.3-L), can usually be distinguished by the PaO_2 or arterial oxyhemoglobin (O_2Hb) saturation in response to exercise (5.6). The patient with pulmonary vascular disease may have a mildly reduced PaO_2 or arterial O_2Hb saturation at rest that decreases progres-

sively as the work rate increases (5.6-R). If the pulmonary vascular disease is accompanied by a right to left shunt, such as in cyanotic congenital heart disease or the opening of an unsealed foramen ovale, then the decrement in PaO_2 at the start of exercise will be marked. Item 6 in the diagnostic box for pulmonary vascular diseases (Fig. 7.5) describes simple measurements that can support the development of a right to left shunt during exercise. The patient with moderately severe left ventricular failure will have a normal PaO_2 even at maximum exercise, although their V_D/V_T will be elevated (5.6-L).

The two lung disorders with a low peak $\dot{V}O_2$ and a non-uniform $\dot{V}A/\dot{Q}$, but with a low breathing reserve (5.3-R), can generally be distinguished by the breathing frequency and the measurements listed in the respective diagnostic boxes for obstructive and restrictive lung diseases. A breathing frequency > 50 at the patient's peak $\dot{V}O_2$ is commonly associated with restrictive lung disease (5.7-R), whereas a breathing frequency < 50 at the peak $\dot{V}O_2$ is characteristic of the patient with obstructive lung disease (5.7-L). Although this distinction is generally evident from standard pulmonary function measurements, the question addressed by exercise testing is whether or not the resting pulmonary function abnormalities account for the patient's exercise intolerance.

SUMMARY

To determine the likely pathophysiologic causes of exercise limitation, we have found that a logical approach can be developed in a series of five flow charts. Each flow chart starts with a different observation based on whether the maximum or peak $\dot{V}O_2$ and *AT* are normal or abnormal. Physiologic measurements relating heart rate, ventilation, and gas exchange to work rate are used in the further decision-making process. The first flow chart separates four major categories of patients; the second addresses the cause of exercise limitation in patients with a normal peak $\dot{V}O_2$; the third considers the diagnosis in patients with a reduced peak $\dot{V}O_2$ but with a normal *AT*; the fourth considers the diagnosis in patients with a reduced peak $\dot{V}O_2$ and reduced *AT*; and the fifth addresses the diagnosis of the patient with a reduced peak $\dot{V}O_2$ but with the *AT* not determined. These flow charts usually enable the examiner to make a specific organ-related physiologic diagnosis. The flow charts are designed only as guides to an orderly decision-making process. The final judgment must be made by the examiner.

CHAPTER 8

Clinical Applications of Cardiopulmonary Exercise Testing

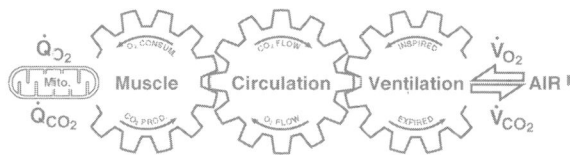

THE INCREASING number of applications for which cardiopulmonary exercise testing is currently employed attests to its growing importance in medicine. In this chapter, applications of cardiopulmonary exercise testing are described. In some instances, these applications are well established. In others, the applications are inadequately recognized and appreciated. These applications are of great value in patient care, and have the potential of reducing health care costs by streamlining diagnosis and facilitating treatment decisions.

DIFFERENTIAL DIAGNOSIS OF DISORDERS CAUSING EXERCISE INTOLERANCE

The physician is sometimes at a loss to determine and understand the pathophysiological mechanism and, therefore, the major disease accounting for symptoms (e.g., fatigue, dyspnea, or pain) causing exercise intolerance. Because different defects in the coupling of external (airway) to cellular respiration affect gas exchange in different ways (see Fig. 4.1), gas exchange responses of cardiopulmonary exercise testing differ according to the defect. Thus the pattern of gas exchange at the airway can be used to identify pathophysiology and also to support or refute the correctness of a specific clinical diagnosis. With an appropriate display of gas exchange data obtained during exercise testing, it is possible to determine the functional status of the cardiovascular and ventilatory systems.

There are also certain diagnoses for which cardiopulmonary exercise testing is the unique diagnostic tool. That is, these diagnoses cannot be made very easily with other diagnostic modalities, but can be inferred from the gas exchange responses to exercise. These include: 1) exercise intolerance due to silent myocardial ischemia; 2) chronic heart failure due to diastolic dysfunction; 3) pulmonary vascular occlusive disease without overt pulmonary hypertension; 4) the development of a right to left shunt during exercise; 5) pulmonary vascular disease limiting exercise in COPD; 6) disorders of muscle that impair muscle bioenergetic function; and 7) psychogenic dyspnea and behavioral causes (anxiety or malingering) of exercise intolerance.

Because a graphic display of data is easier to read than a tabular display, it is advantageous to transform the data into graphs that describe the essential physiological responses to exercise. We find it particularly useful when these data are in the form of 9 strategically positioned panels containing 15 graphs on a single page (see Fig. 3.30). These graphs enable the examiner, knowledgeable in physiology and pathophysiology of exercise, to assess systematically cardiovascular, ventilatory, ventilation-perfusion matching, and metabolic responses to exercise. Armed with this information, the cause of exercise intolerance can usually be made with considerable certainty.

A major reason why the patterns of data for different diseases can be recognized on the 9-panel graphic display is that gas exchange responses are very uniform in healthy subjects. Normal values for all measurements on the 9-panel graphic display are summarized in Chapter 6. For example, the increase in $\dot{V}o_2$ as related to work rate is 10 ml/min/watt with relatively small standard deviation (approximately $\pm$ 0.7). The heart rate response and therefore the heart rate-$\dot{V}o_2$ relationship and O_2 pulse are highly predictable. The normal ventilatory response to exercise is closely coupled to $\dot{V}co_2$ (slope = 24.6 $\pm$ 2.4), because of the uniformity with which $Paco_2$ and Vd/Vt are regulated (Chapter 6).

In Chapter 7, we show how a diagnosis is reached using a deductive reasoning strategy. After it is determined that peak $\dot{V}o_2$ is reduced, a series of questions are asked in a systematic manner about other physiological measurements. In the following section, specific panels from the 9-panel graphical display will be used to contrast the responses seen in several common disorders. By examining the response patterns of a set of variables in several different diseases, it will become clearer how cardiopulmonary exercise testing helps in the differential diagnosis of disorders limiting exercise. However, it must be stressed that a diagnosis is not made by examining one panel or variable: a specific diagnosis is often contingent not only on abnormalities in certain panels but with normal responses in others.

PATHOPHYSIOLOGICAL RESPONSES IN COMMON DISORDERS

O_2 Uptake and CO_2 Output as Related to Work Rate

The basic requirement to sustain muscular exercise is an increase in cellular respiration for regeneration of adenosine triphosphate (ATP). To support the increase in cellular respiration, O_2 and CO_2 transport between the cells and the environment must match the rate of cellular respiration (except for transient lags allowed by the capacitance in the transport system). The increases in O_2 and CO_2 transport are functions of the peripheral circulation, heart, pulmonary circulation, blood, lungs and respiratory muscles. Any defect in this interactive system could result in failure of the muscle to take up and use the O_2 normally for aerobic regeneration of ATP. On the 9-panel graphical display, $\dot{V}O_2$ and $\dot{V}CO_2$ are plotted against work rate (WR) in panel 3 (upper right) and the slope of $\Delta\dot{V}O_2/\Delta WR$ can be seen.

In Figure 8.1, we contrast the characteristic findings for $\dot{V}O_2$ and $\dot{V}CO_2$ plotted against WR for a normal subject with those of 8 patients with different disorders. The predicted $\dot{V}O_2$, age and gender of each subject are shown in the upper left part of the figure. The smaller number under the age is the case number of the subject in Chapter 9. Figure 8.1a (case 1 of chapter 9) shows the responses of a 55-year-old male who was diagnosed as normal. It is the only subject shown in Figure 8.1 with a normal peak $\dot{V}O_2$, $\dot{V}CO_2$ response, and $\Delta\dot{V}O_2/\Delta WR$. The $\Delta\dot{V}O_2/\Delta WR$ can be compared with the normal response by contrasting the slope of $\dot{V}O_2$ increase versus work rate with the diagonal line drawn with a slope of 10 ml/min/watt, the predicted normal slope. Figure 8.1b shows a 47-year-old man who developed depressed ST segments on the ECG starting at the work rate where $\dot{V}O_2$ stopped increasing. The failure of $\dot{V}O_2$ to increase normally with increasing work rate, despite the increase being normal at lower work rates, is not uncommon when myocardial ischemia impairs the heart's ability to increase cardiac output normally. Figure 8.1c displays the data for a 65-year-old male diabetic and cigarette smoker with peripheral arterial disease. Both the $\dot{V}O_2$ and $\dot{V}CO_2$ increase more slowly, but linearly, beginning at the lowest work rate, as might be predicted for someone with a fixed stenosis of the conducting arteries to exercising extremities.

The study shown in Figure 8.1d is of a 35-year-old man with dilated cardiomyopathy. He had a significantly reduced peak $\dot{V}O_2$ and a very low *AT* reflected by a relatively high CO_2 output at a low work rate. The study shown in Figure 8.1e is of a 54-year-old male with vasculitis that affected primarily his pulmonary circulation. The rate of rise in $\dot{V}O_2$ decreases progressively as the peak $\dot{V}O_2$ is approached. Thus the average $\Delta\dot{V}O_2/\Delta WR$ is quite low. The abnormal gas exchange efficiency accompanying this pulmonary vasculitis is addressed in Figures 8.5 and 8.6. The high O_2 cost of exercise during treadmill walking in an obese subject can be seen in Figure 8.1f, which demonstrates the large increase in $\dot{V}O_2$ following the onset of walking at

zero grade at 3 miles per hour. Because the actual work rate performed on a treadmill is very difficult to determine, $\Delta\dot{V}O_2/\Delta WR$ can not be readily calculated.

The data in Figure 8.1g are that of a 50-year-old man with COPD. The $\Delta\dot{V}O_2/\Delta WR$ is normal but the peak $\dot{V}O_2$ is reduced. Confirmatory evidence of abnormal ventilatory mechanics and reduced gas exchange efficiency limiting his exercise capacity is shown in Figures 8.4g and 8.6g, respectively. Exercise data from a 29-year-old man with sarcoidosis resulting in severe pulmonary hypertension are shown in Figure 8.1h. The low peak $\dot{V}O_2$ and reduced $\Delta\dot{V}O_2/\Delta WR$ place him in the severely impaired category. Finally, the study shown in Figure 8.1i is of a 20-year-old male with severe interstitial pulmonary fibrosis, but without pulmonary hypertension. His failure to increase $\dot{V}O_2$ despite increasing work rate reflects nearly complete inability to increase pulmonary blood flow. This finding represents very severe disease and a loss of ability to sustain even mild exercise. The lack of pulmonary hypertension in this patient is due to failure of the right ventricle to hypertrophy and does not connote the absence of severe loss of pulmonary vascular bed. The high $\dot{V}CO_2$ relative to $\dot{V}O_2$ reflects the substantial lactic acidosis which the patient developed during this short exercise test.

Heart Rate and $\dot{V}CO_2$ as a Function of $\dot{V}O_2$

Panel 5 of the 9-panel graphical display illustrated in Figure 3.30 shows heart rate (solid squares) and $\dot{V}CO_2$ (open squares) as functions of $\dot{V}O_2$. These relationships are shown in Figure 8.2 for the same nine patients depicted in Figure 8.1. Heart rate normally increases linearly with $\dot{V}O_2$ to the predicted maximum values for both variables as indicated by the "X" in the figure and illustrated by case 1 of Chapter 9 shown in Figure 8.2a. The heart rate-$\dot{V}O_2$ slope is steeper and often becomes non-linear in the patients with cardiovascular diseases, including those in which the diseases affect the pulmonary circulation, such as pulmonary vasculitis (Fig. 8.2e), sarcoidosis and interstitial pulmonary fibrosis (IPF) (Fig. 8.2h, i).

$\dot{V}CO_2$ increases as a function of $\dot{V}O_2$ with a slope of 1, or slightly less than 1, until the *AT* is reached (Fig. 8.2a). At that point, $\dot{V}CO_2$ increases more steeply than $\dot{V}O_2$ in all of the patients except in the patient with peripheral arterial disease (Fig. 8.2c), presumably due to the relatively small contribution

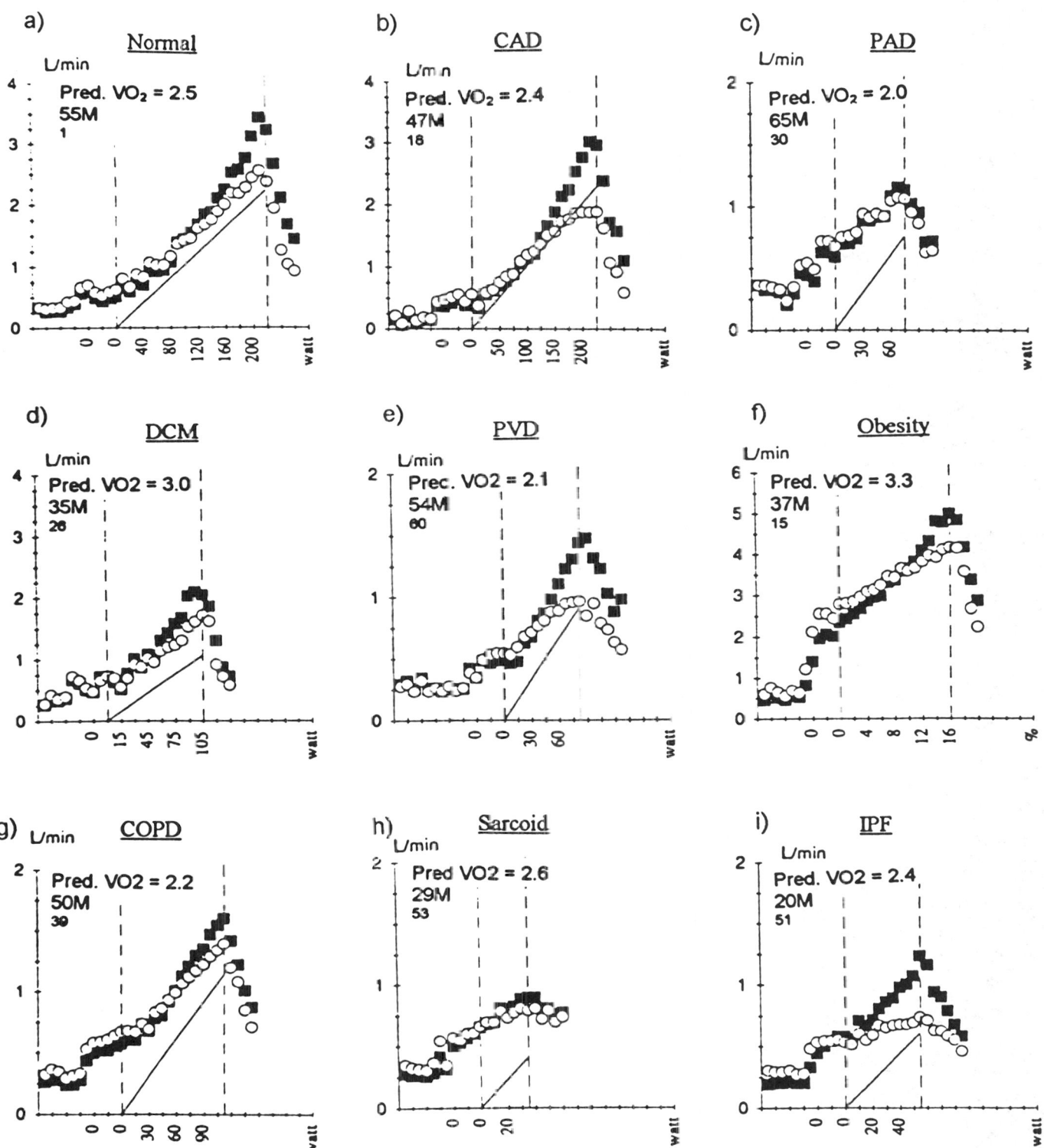

FIGURE 8.1. Plot of $\dot{V}_{O_2}$ and $\dot{V}_{CO_2}$ (STPD) as a function of work rate (watts) for patients with normal exercise performance (a), coronary artery disease (b), peripheral arterial disease (c), dilated cardiomyopathy (d), pulmonary vascular disease (e), obesity (abscissa is % treadmill grade) (f), chronic obstructive pulmonary disease (g), sarcoidosis (h) and interstitial pulmonary fibrosis (i). The data to the left of the first "0" is the rest period. "0" work rate is unloaded cycling. The period of increasing work rate starts at the left vertical dashed line and ends at the right vertical dashed line. The diagonal line between the vertical dashed lines is the normal rate of rise for $\dot{V}_{O_2}$ against work rate with a slope of 10 ml/min/W. The predicted peak $\dot{V}_{O_2}$ is shown in the upper left of each panel. Just below the predicted peak $\dot{V}_{O_2}$ are the age and gender of the patient, and just below that is the case number of the subject in Chapter 9. Further history and data can be found for each patient in Chapter 9.

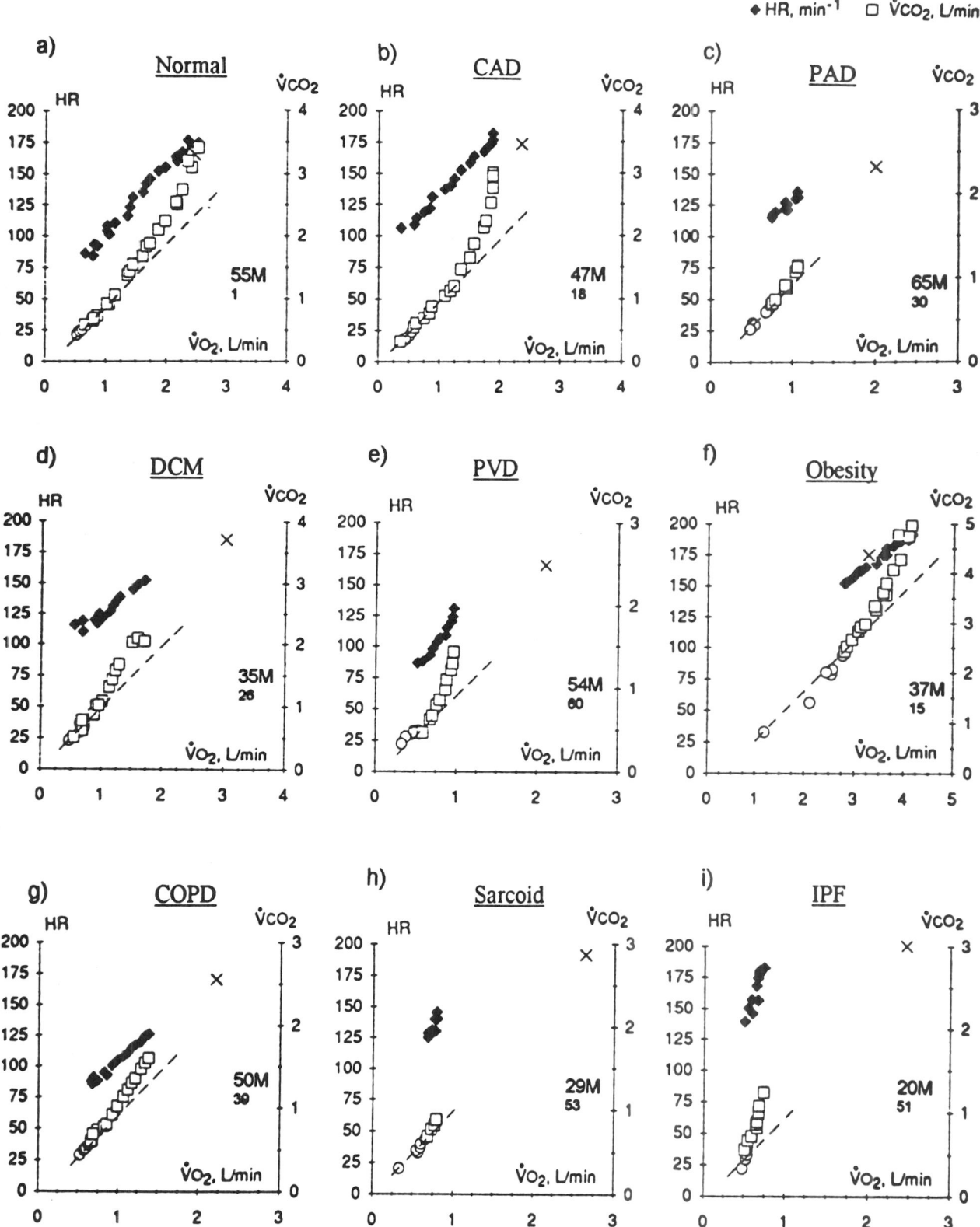

FIGURE 8.2.   Plot of heart rate and $\dot{V}CO_2$ plotted as functions of $\dot{V}O_2$ for the same 9 patients shown in Figure 8.1. Age, gender, and case number (Chapter 9) are shown at lower right. The diagonal dashed line has a slope of 1. The AT is read as the $\dot{V}O_2$ at which $\dot{V}CO_2$ starts increasing at a slope greater than 1.

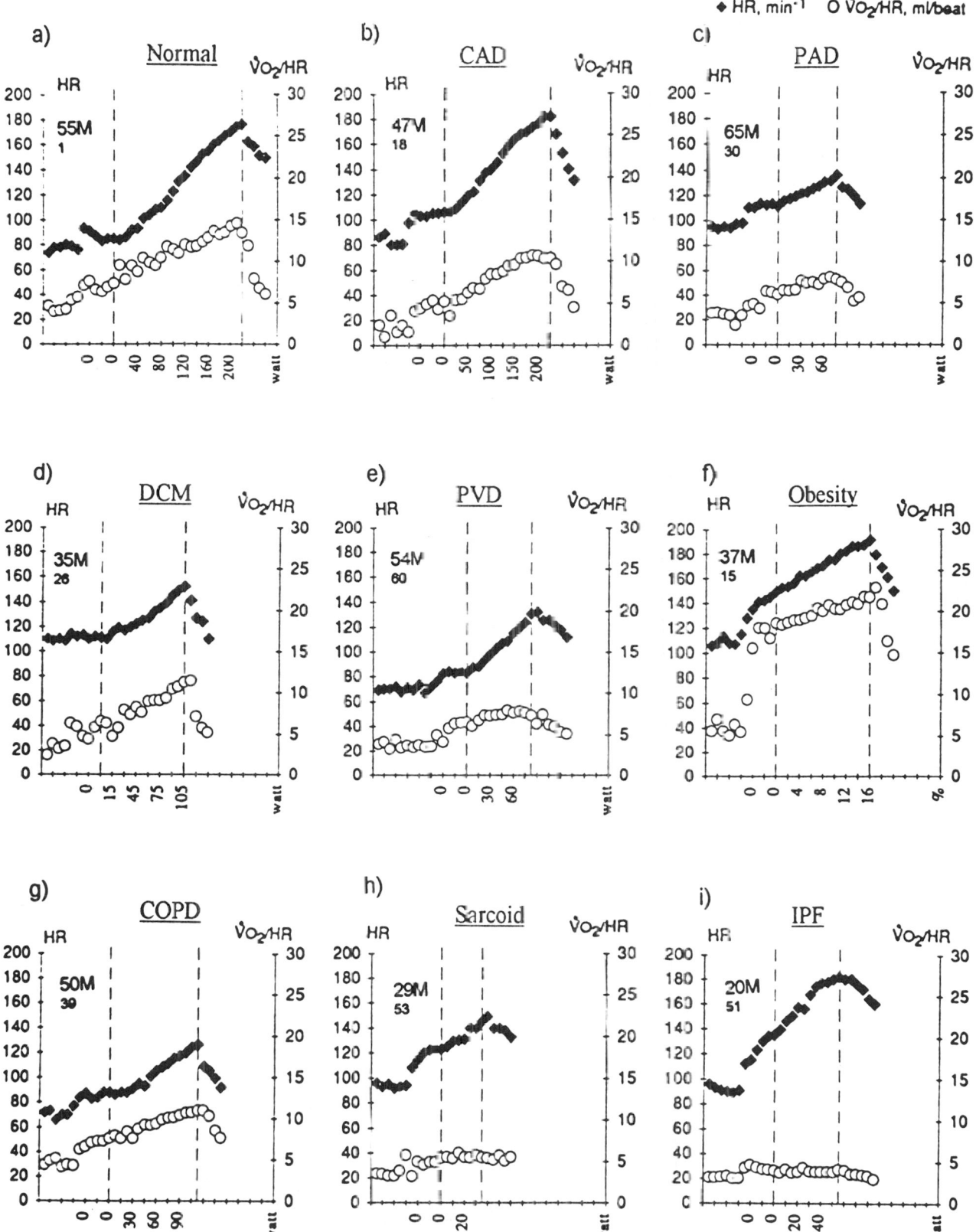

FIGURE 8.3.   Plot of heart rate and O_2 pulse plotted as functions of work rate (watts) for the same 9 patients shown in Figure 8.1. The period of increasing work rate starts at the left vertical dashed line and ends at the right vertical dashed line. Age, gender, and case number (Chapter 9) are shown at upper left.

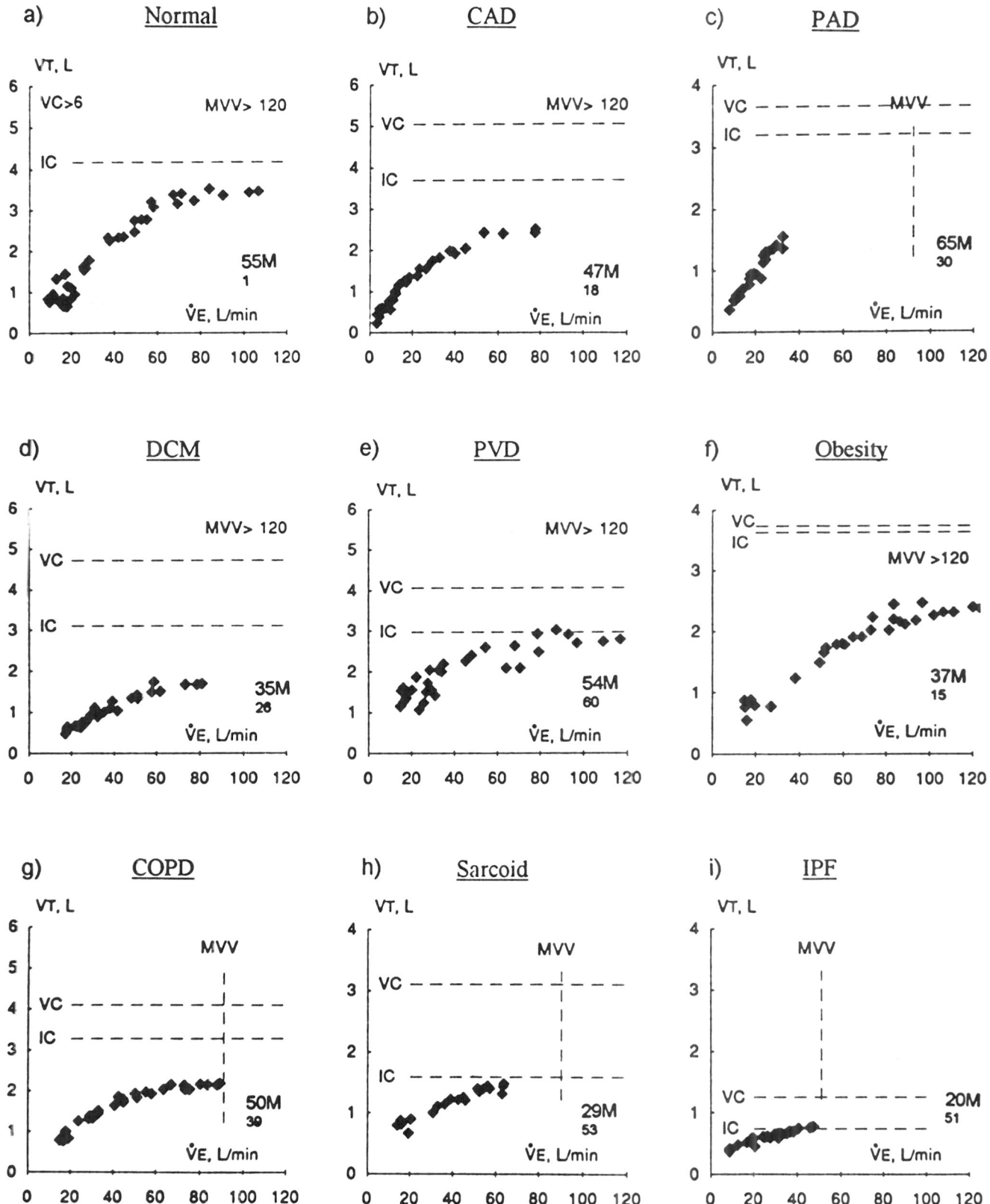

FIGURE 8.4.   Plot of exercise tidal volume plotted as a function of minute ventilation (V̇E) for the same 9 patients shown in Figure 8.1. Age, gender, and case number (chapter 9) are shown at lower right. Also shown are the subject's maximal voluntary ventilation (MVV) on the abscissa (vertical dashed line) and the subject's resting inspiratory capacity (IC) and vital capacity (VC) on the ordinate (horizontal dashed lines) unless above scale.

of blood flow coming from the ischemic lower limbs. In the patient with coronary artery disease (CAD) (Fig. 8.2b), the obese patient (8.2f), and the COPD patient (8.2g), the AT is normal. In the patient with heart failure (8.2d) and the three other patients (vasculitis—Figure 8.2e, sarcoidosis—Figure 8.2h and interstitial lung disease—Figure 8.2i), the AT is significantly reduced to below the 95% confidence limit of normal.

Heart Rate and O_2 Pulse as a Function of Work Rate

Panel 2 of the 9-panel graphic display (Figure 3.30) shows the heart rate (solid squares) and O_2 pulse (open squares) plotted against work rate. Figure 8.3 shows panels for the same nine patients included in Figure 8.1. Heart rate normally increases abruptly at the start of unloaded cycling and then increases approximately linearly with work rate to the predicted maximal heart rate in the normal subject (Fig. 8.3a). Deviation from the normal heart rate response is seen in patients with chronotropic incompetence (Fig. 8.3d) or when the patient is stopped in the performance of exercise because of non-cardiac or non-pulmonary vascular disease problems. The latter is exemplified by the patients with peripheral arterial disease (Fig. 8.3c) and COPD (Fig. 8.3g).

The O_2 pulse, the product of stroke volume and arteriovenous O_2 difference, also shown in panel 2, normally increases with a gradually decreasing rate of rise to the predicted normal value (Fig. 8.3a). However, O_2 pulse fails to increase normally in patients with CAD in which myocardial ischemia reduces exercise capacity (Fig. 8.3b). The O_2 pulse also fails to increase normally in heart failure (Fig. 8.3d), as well as in the three patients in whom the pulmonary circulation is seriously deranged (pulmonary vasculitis, sarcoidosis and interstitial lung disease). As shown in Figures 8.3e, 8.3h and 8.3i, the value of peak O_2 pulse during exercise is abnormally low in these patients.

As noted in Chapter 6, the O_2 pulse can also be discerned from the panels shown in Figure 8.2. The O_2 pulse is low when the extension of the heart rate-$\dot{V}O_2$ relationship is to the left of the target "X" (e.g., Fig. 8.2 b–e, h, and i).

V_T as a Function of $\dot{V}E$

Tidal volume (V_T) is plotted as a function of $\dot{V}E$ in panel 7 of the 9-panel graphic display (Fig. 3.30).

Figure 8.4 shows panel 7 for the same nine patients illustrated in Figure 8.1. Tidal volume normally increases preferentially to breathing frequency during low and moderate intensity exercise to account for the early increase in $\dot{V}E$ in normal subjects (Fig. 8.4a). Above the AT, breathing frequency is the primary factor accounting for the increase in $\dot{V}E$. At peak exercise, there is normally a breathing reserve of greater than 11 L/min, the latter calculated as the difference between the maximal voluntary ventilation and the peak exercise $\dot{V}E$. The tidal volume may increase to the inspiratory capacity (IC), but not above it.

However, patients limited in their exercise tolerance by lung mechanics characteristically have no or a very small breathing reserve. Thus, despite only a mild to moderate reduction in MVV, the patient with COPD has no breathing reserve at his maximal tolerated exercise when ventilatory limited (Fig. 8.4g). This is also true of the patient with IPF (Fig. 8.4i). Further, the patient with IPF has a tidal volume that reaches inspiratory capacity early in exercise, characteristic of restrictive lung disease. The breathing reserves in the other patients are normal.

$\dot{V}E$ as a Function of $\dot{V}CO_2$

$\dot{V}E$ as a function of $\dot{V}CO_2$ is plotted in panel 4 of the 9 panel graphical display (Fig. 3.30). Figure 8.5 shows panel 4 for the 9 patients illustrated in Figure 8.1. $\dot{V}E$ normally increases linearly with $\dot{V}CO_2$ with a slope of 24.6 ± 2.4 in normal subjects up to the point where ventilatory compensation for the developing lactic acidosis develops (Fig. 8.5a). This slope is not increased in the patient with CAD (Fig. 8.5b), peripheral arterial disease (Fig. 8.5c), and obesity (Fig. 8.5f). However, it is usually increased in the patient with chronic heart failure (Fig. 8.5d), pulmonary vasculitis (Fig. 8.5e), COPD (Fig. 8.5g), sarcoidosis (Fig. 8.5h), and IPF (Fig. 8.5i), diseases associated with an increase in V_D/V_T. The slope of the linear component of the plot of $\dot{V}E$ versus $\dot{V}CO_2$ is steeper, the more extensive the disease.

Ventilatory Equivalents for O_2 and CO_2

$\dot{V}E/\dot{V}O_2$ and $\dot{V}E/\dot{V}CO_2$ are plotted against work rate in panel 6 of the 9-panel graphic display (Fig. 3.30). Figure 8.6 shows panel 6 for the nine patients illustrated in Figure 8.1. When $PaCO_2$ is normal, $\dot{V}E/\dot{V}O_2$ decreases and reaches a nadir at the AT with a value less than 28, and $\dot{V}E/\dot{V}CO_2$ reaches a nadir at the

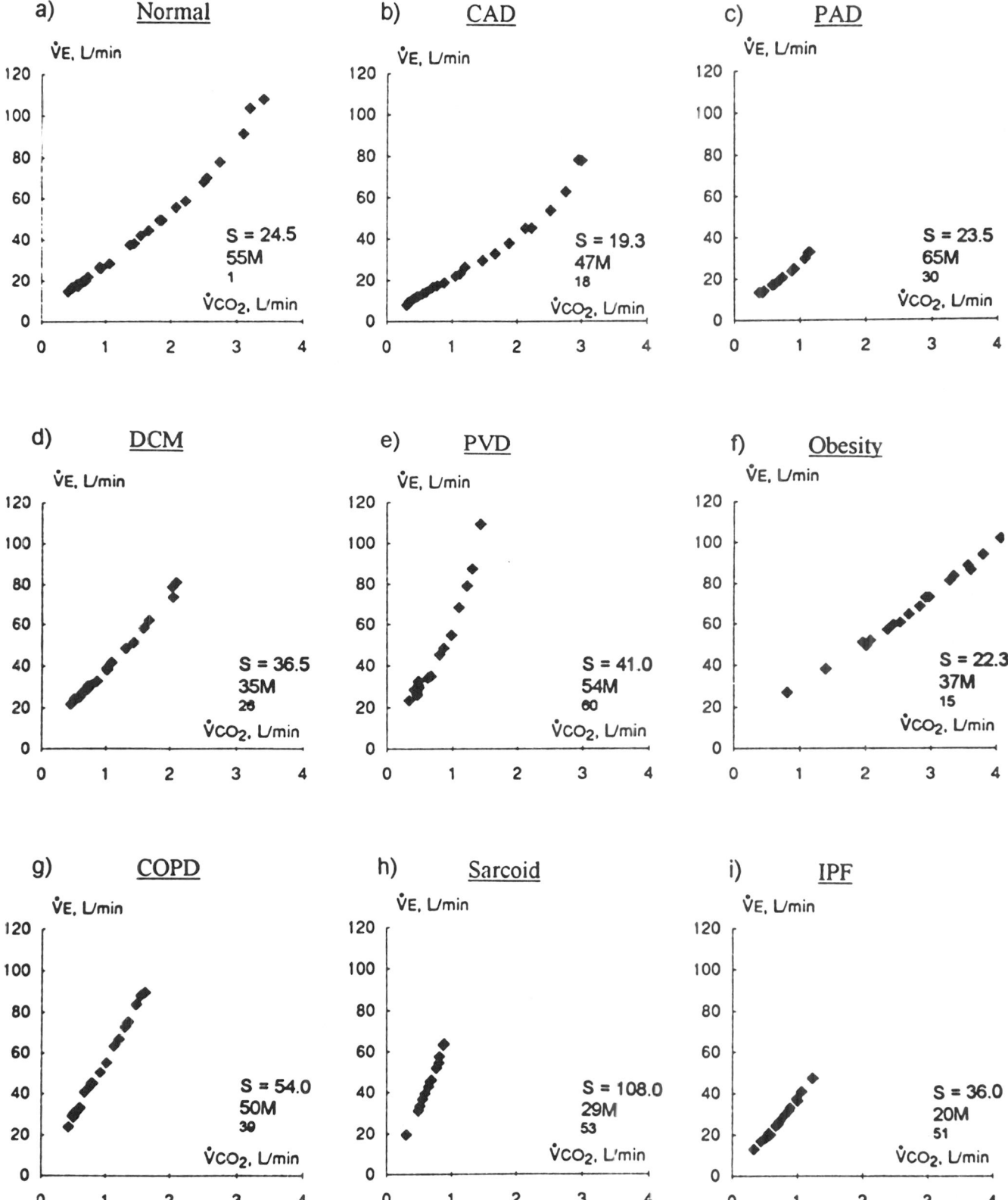

FIGURE 8.5.   Plot of exercise minute ventilation ($\dot{V}E$) plotted as a function of CO_2 output ($\dot{V}CO_2$) for the same 9 patients shown in Figure 8.1. At lower right in each panel is the slope (S) of the linear component of the $\dot{V}E$ versus $\dot{V}CO_2$ relationship. The age, gender, and case number, as presented in Chapter 9, are shown below the slope values.

O V̇E/V̇O₂   ■ V̇E/V̇CO₂

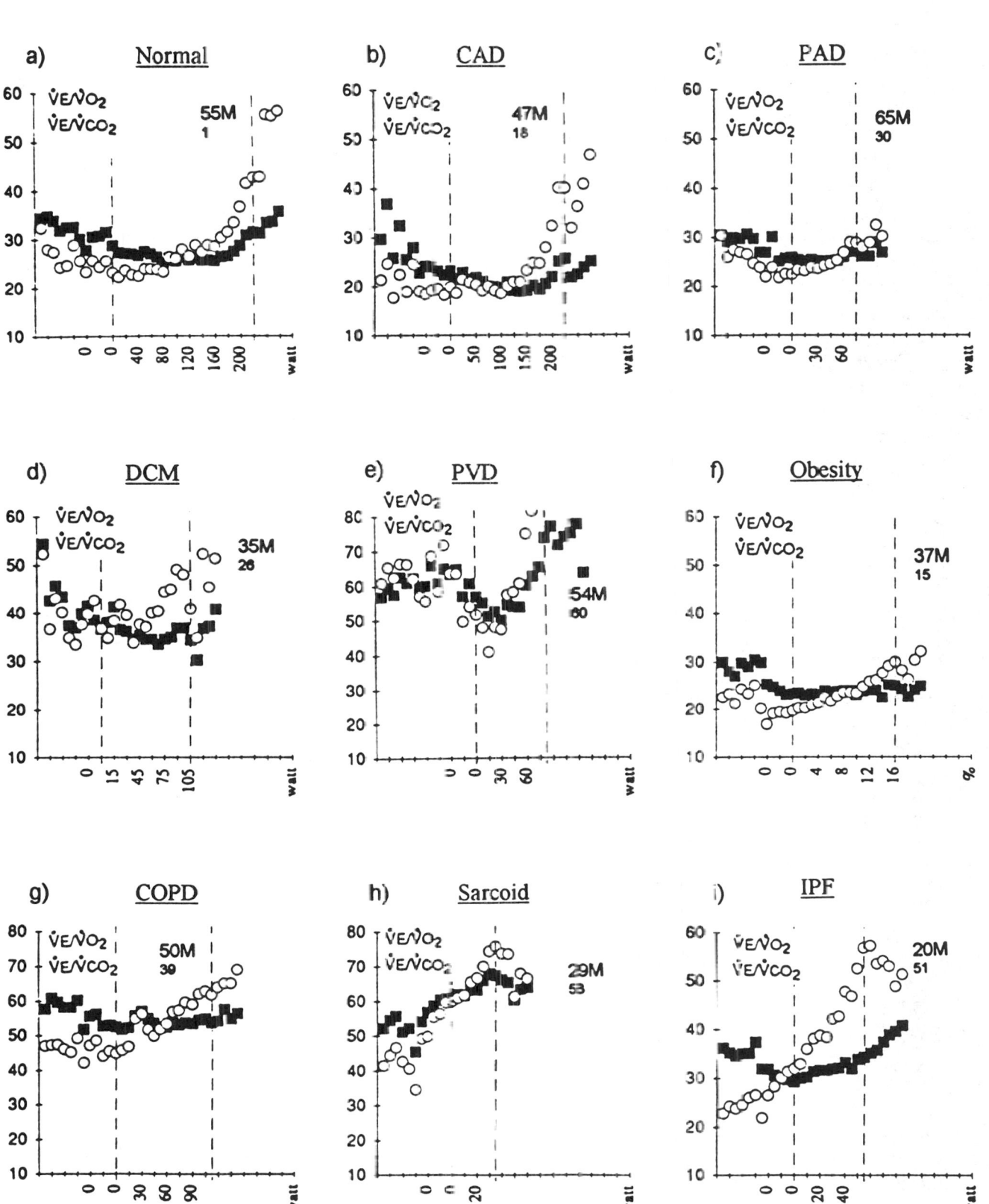

FIGURE 8.6.   Plot of ventilatory equivalent for O_2 ($\dot{V}_E/\dot{V}_{O_2}$) (open circles) and CO_2 ($\dot{V}_E/\dot{V}_{CO_2}$) (closed squares) as functions of work rate (watts) for the same 9 patients shown in Figure 8.1. The age, gender, and case number, as presented in Chapter 9, are shown in the upper right in each panel. The period of increasing work rate starts at the left vertical dashed line and ends at the right vertical dashed line.

ventilatory compensation point with a value less than 32 as shown in Figure 8.5a. The nadir values of $\dot{V}_E/\dot{V}_{O_2}$ and $\dot{V}_E/\dot{V}_{CO_2}$ are normal for the patient with CAD (Fig. 8.6b), peripheral arterial disease (Fig. 8.6c), and obesity (Fig. 8.6f), but increased for patients with chronic heart failure (Fig. 8.6d), pulmonary vasculitis (Fig. 8.6e), COPD (Fig. 8.6g), sarcoidosis (Fig. 8.6h) and IPF (Fig. 8.6i), diseases associated with an increase in V_D/V_T. The more severe the disease or the lower the Pa_{CO_2}, the higher the values of $\dot{V}_E/\dot{V}_{O_2}$ and $\dot{V}_E/\dot{V}_{CO_2}$.

The patterns of change of $\dot{V}_E$, R and $P_{ET_{O_2}}$ and $P_{ET_{CO_2}}$ as a function of work rate (panels 1, 8 and 9, respectively, of Figure 3.30) are not presented for the 9 cases selected here in the interest of space and because these changes can be reviewed in Chapter 9. They provide important correlative data, but probably not as revealing information by themselves as those reviewed above. With arterial blood gases, panel 9 is particularly valuable. All of the panels have greater meaning when reviewed in relation to each other.

DIAGNOSES UNIQUELY MADE BY CARDIOPULMONARY EXERCISE TESTING

Development of Myocardial Ischemia with Myocardial Dyskinesis during Exercise

The normal contraction of the myocardium depends on the ability of all the myofibrils of the heart muscle to contract synchronously in response to the electrical depolarization set off by the sino-atrial pacemaker. With each heart beat, ATP is primarily consumed by the heart during systole and regenerated in diastole when the myocardium is resupplied with oxygenated blood. For normal regeneration of ATP, the O_2 supply must be adequate. Since the diastolic period shortens as heart rate increases, exercise is a useful way to precipitate myocardial ischemia in regions of the heart that have impaired ability to increase blood flow commensurate with the increased myocardial O_2 demand. In addition, the increase in cardiac output during exercise induces an increase in myocardial work as the left ventricle must contract against the higher systemic arterial pressure seen during exercise.

Asynchronous contraction of the myocardium could result in a reduction in stroke volume and the failure of $\dot{V}_{O_2}$ to increase in proportion to the work rate increase, as illustrated in cases 16 to 22 in Chapter 9. The slowing or failure of $\dot{V}_{O_2}$ to increase with increasing work rate indicates that cardiac output is not increasing appropriately. When $\dot{V}_{O_2}$ reaches a plateau despite increasing work rate, cardiac output has reached a maximum. When heart rate continues to increase even though cardiac output has apparently stopped increasing (cases 16–22), stroke volume must be decreasing, reflecting the myocardial dyskinesis of ischemia.

In some patients, ST segment depression on the ECG and chest pain will confirm the development of myocardial ischemia during exercise. However, ECG changes suggestive of myocardial ischemia without chest pain makes the diagnosis of myocardial ischemia questionable. By measuring gas exchange, the physician can confirm the $\dot{V}_{O_2}$ at which myocardial dyskinesis occurs during exercise.

Chronic Heart Failure Due to Diastolic Dysfunction

Systolic dysfunction resulting in heart failure is usually easily diagnosed by the finding of a low ejection fraction and usually cardiomegaly. On the other hand, detecting heart failure due to diastolic dysfunction, a problem not uncommon in the elderly, patients with myocardial ischemia, heart transplant recipient patients and patients with hypertrophic cardiomyopathy (1), is difficult because heart size is usually normal and the ejection fraction is also normal. Thus without cardiopulmonary exercise testing, the cardiologist can only make this diagnosis objectively by making measurements of left ventricular pressure-volume relationships during cardiac catheterization. On the other hand, in patients with chronic heart failure, whether due to systolic or diastolic dysfunction, non-invasive cardiopulmonary exercise testing will identify a reduced peak $\dot{V}_{O_2}$ and AT, reflecting reduced O_2 transport, and when dysfunction is moderate to severe, an increase in $\dot{V}_E/\dot{V}_{CO_2}$ (see Chapter 4). Because the increase in $\dot{V}_E/\dot{V}_{CO_2}$ is due to an increased V_D/V_T in proportion to the reduction in exercise tolerance and is not accompanied by hypoxemia, Wasserman et al. (2) pointed out that these findings must reflect decreased perfusion of ventilated lung (abnormal pulmonary circulation—Fig. 7.4) and not airway dysfunction. Other noninvasive tests such as echocardiography and radionuclide ventriculography at rest are likely to be normal. Thus the diagnostic test best suited for making the diagnosis of chronic heart failure secondary to diastolic dysfunction is cardiopulmonary exercise testing with gas exchange measurements.

Pulmonary Vascular Occlusive Disease without Pulmonary Hypertension

Most patients limited in exercise because of pulmonary vascular disease have exertional dyspnea well before they have resting signs of pulmonary hypertension. Once signs of pulmonary hypertension are present, the patient has recruited all the pulmonary blood vessels normally reserved for recruitment during exercise. By this time, the patient's clinical condition has seriously deteriorated and the patient is no longer able to exercise. Also, the opportunity to intervene at an early stage of the disease process with some potential pulmonary vasodilator or anti-inflammatory treatments may be lost.

There is no diagnostic method in medicine other than exercise gas exchange that is capable of identifying a patient with abnormal pulmonary circulation in an early stage before pulmonary hypertension develops. This is because the patient's symptoms are present only during exercise but not at rest. While the pulmonary blood flow may be adequate at rest, these patients have difficulty in increasing pulmonary blood flow appropriately in response to exercise, resulting in exercise-induced symptoms.

In patients with pulmonary vascular disease, $\dot{V}o_2$ usually does not continue to increase with a normal slope of 10 ml/min/watt during progressively increasing work rate exercise. In fact, the slope progressively decreases up to the point of fatigue, when there may be no further rise in $\dot{V}o_2$ (Fig 8.1e). The peak $\dot{V}o_2$ (panel 3) and *AT* (panel 5) probably best quantify the severity of the illness and will probably prove to be the best guides in the selection of patients with pulmonary vascular disease for lung transplantation. Of course, the steep heart rate rise and low O_2-pulse will be evident in panels 2 and 5. The slope of $\dot{V}e$ plotted as a function of $\dot{V}co_2$ (panel 4), which is about 25 in the normal individual, will be much higher in patients with pulmonary vascular disease (Fig. 8.5e,g–i). This increase depends almost entirely on the increase in V_D/V_T. Panel 6 shows high values for $\dot{V}e/\dot{V}co_2$ at the *AT*, reflecting decreased perfusion to ventilated lung (high $\dot{V}_A/\dot{Q}$), again quantitatively related to the degree of pulmonary vascular occlusion. Arterial blood gases, displayed on panel 9, along with end-tidal

O_2 and CO_2, and calculation of V_D/V_T, further characterize the abnormal physiological state of the pulmonary circulation.

Patent Foramen Ovale with Development of a Right to Left Shunt During Exercise

About 25% of the population have a potentially patent foramen ovale, but this finding is unimportant unless right atrial pressure exceeds left atrial pressure. However, this situation can develop in patients with primary pulmonary vascular disease or pulmonary vascular disease secondary to lung disease. It must be kept in mind that attempts at detecting a patent foramen ovale at rest may be unsuccessful. The patient may only shunt right atrial blood into the left atrium during exercise.

During exercise, if the increase in venous return exceeds the rate that the right ventricle can pump blood into the pulmonary circulation, right ventricular end-diastolic pressure and right atrial pressure will rise. Simultaneously, left atrial filling from the pulmonary circulation is inadequate because of the resistance to blood flow in the lungs and left atrial pressure falls. When right atrial pressure exceeds left atrial pressure, and there is a potentially patent foramen ovale, venous return forced from the right to the left atrium causes a rapid decrease in systemic arterial Po_2. This phenomenon can occur despite normal or near normal arterial oxyhemoglobin saturation at rest (Case 61, Chapter 9). An exercise test with arterial blood sampling during 100% O_2 breathing allows this diagnosis to be confirmed.

The diagnosis of a right-to-left shunt developing during exercise can be suspected by finding characteristic changes of a right-to-left shunt in gas exchange in panels 4 (an abrupt steepening in slope) and 6 (an increasing $\dot{V}e/\dot{V}co_2$ rather than the normal decrease after exercise starts) (Fig. 8.7). Also, panel 9 may reveal an abrupt drop in $Petco_2$ and increase in $Peto_2$ after the start of exercise reflecting hyperventilation of the blood flowing through the lungs, along with an abrupt decrease in arterial oxyhemoglobin saturation. The state of the shunt during exercise can be followed over time, without sampling of arterial blood for measurement of blood gases, by repeat cardiopulmonary exercise testing with particular attention paid to panels 4, 6, and 9.

An example of gas exchange abnormalities revealing the development of a right-to-left shunt during exercise is shown in Figure 8.7; these abnor-

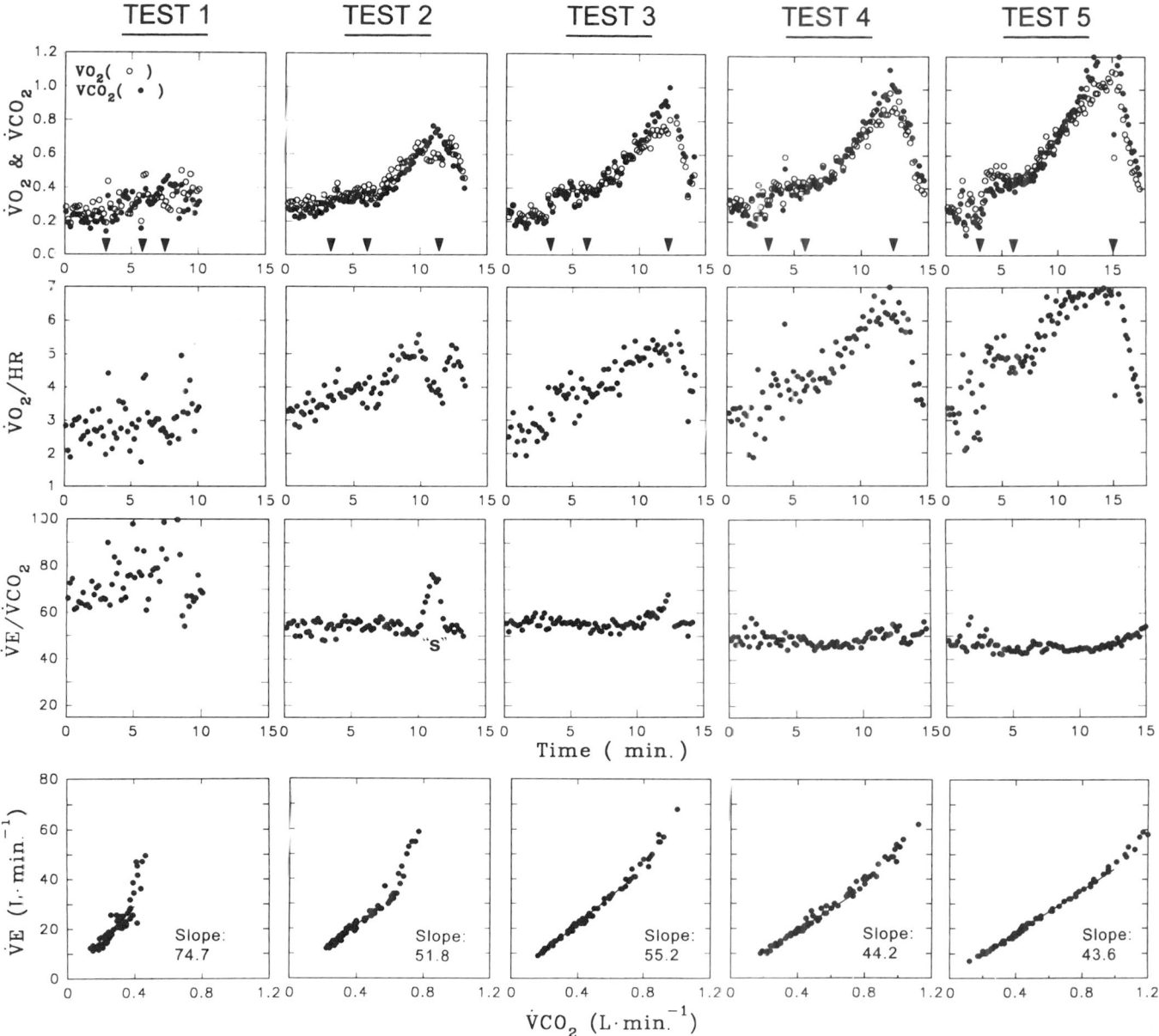

FIGURE 8.7. Five tests in a patient with primary pulmonary hypertension, each done at four month intervals. Test 1 was done as a control before the start of continuous intravenous epoprostenol, a preparation of prostacyclin. Test 2 was done after 4 months of treatment and test 3 was done 4 months later, etc., for a total of 16 months. Although the full 9 panel plots were obtained, for ease of comparing the physiological changes with time, only 4 panels of data are shown for each test. The top panel contain plots of $\dot{V}O_2$ and $\dot{V}CO_2$ (L/min) against time. On the abscissa of this plot are three arrows, the left indicating the transition from rest to unloaded cycling, the middle arrow indicating the start of the increasing exercise period and the arrow on the right indicating the end of exercise. As is evident from this panel in test 1, the patient was very restricted and could perform very little exercise. At that time, her O_2 pulse (ml/beat) (second panel down) could not increase in response to exercise, indicating that the product of her stroke volume and arteriovenous O_2 difference was fixed. The ventilatory equivalents for CO_2 (third panel down) are very high at rest (first 3 minutes) and increase further after exercise starts due to the opening of a right to left shunt, presumably through the foramen ovale. This is reflected in a large change in the slope of $\dot{V}E$ versus $\dot{V}CO_2$ in the fourth panel down. The slope value shown in this panel is that for the lower slope before the diverting of blood through the right to left shunt. The slope value of 74.7 is very high, normal being about 25 (see chapter 6). This steep slope reflects the poor perfusion to ventilated lung (increased VD/VT). The abrupt steepening of this slope reflects an increase in right to left shunt. The repeat study four months after the start of treatment (Test 2) shows a significant increase in peak $\dot{V}O_2$ and O_2 pulse and a reduced ventilatory response as evident from the decrease in $\dot{V}E/\dot{V}CO_2$ and in the lower slope of $\dot{V}E$ versus $\dot{V}CO_2$ (51.8 versus 74.7). The latter two indicate that perfusion to ventilated lung had become more uniform, although still quite abnormal. Just before the end of exercise, a right to left shunt developed, reflected in the abrupt decrease in $\dot{V}O_2$ and O_2 pulse and the increase in $\dot{V}E/\dot{V}CO_2$, designated by "S" in the third panel down, and the abrupt steepening of the slope of $\dot{V}E$ versus $\dot{V}CO_2$ in the fourth panel down. The next three tests show improvement in all measurements, reaching a plateau response by the fifth test. Two more tests at 4 month intervals were done and are not shown because there was no significant change from test 5. Thus the patient is considerably improved and has become stable, but still has significant inability to increase cardiac output as reflected by a reduced peak $\dot{V}O_2$ and O_2 pulse (60 and 70% of predicted, respectively) and elevated $\dot{V}E$ versus $\dot{V}CO_2$ slope and $\dot{V}E/\dot{V}CO_2$ at AT.

malities are from a patient with primary pulmonary hypertension who was tested at 4-month intervals over a 16-month period during treatment with continuous intravenous epoprostenol. When blood begins to shunt from right to left during exercise, $\dot{V}_E$ abruptly increases with an increase in $\dot{V}_E/\dot{V}_{CO_2}$ rather than the usual decrease that takes place when exercise starts. The slope of $\dot{V}_E$ as a function of $\dot{V}_{CO_2}$ sharply increases at the work rate at which the blood starts to shunt right to left (the $\dot{V}_E/\dot{V}_{CO_2}$ versus time and the $\dot{V}_E$ versus $\dot{V}_{CO_2}$ in tests 1 and 2 of Fig. 8.7). The reason that ventilation increases so steeply when the shunt develops is that arterial P_{CO_2} is regulated tightly. Thus, when shunt blood containing high CO_2 from the venous system bypasses the lungs and reaches the chemoreceptors, ventilation is stimulated in proportion to the shunt. Ventilation will increase as the chemoreceptors attempt to regulate P_{CO_2}.

By test 3 (after 8 months of treatment), the pulmonary hypertension was much reduced, peak $\dot{V}_{O_2}$ and O_2 pulse had increased, and the evidence for exercise-induced right-to-left shunt had disappeared. This information was obtained noninvasively and could not have been obtained as successfully even with more complicated invasive tests. Such invasive and more complex tests could not be repeated with the frequency and at the low cost of exercise testing. In this case, exercise testing with gas exchange measurements allowed the cardiologist to recognize that the patient, who was extremely ill when first seen, had improved sufficiently to be taken off the list of patients awaiting lung transplantation.

Pulmonary Vascular Disease Limiting Exercise in COPD

Although patients with COPD usually are exercise limited because of abnormal lung mechanics, as reflected by a low exercise breathing reserve, some are limited primarily by a reduced pulmonary capillary bed, which limits the increase in blood flow. In such a patient, lung reduction surgery might improve the lung mechanics, but not improve exercise tolerance because pulmonary blood flow cannot increase beyond that achieved before surgery. Case 44 in Chapter 9 is an example of this problem. Exercise testing should be done before lung reduction surgery with the objective of confirming that impaired lung mechanics is the primary cause of exercise limitation.

Impaired Muscle Bioenergetic Function

Skeletal muscle myopathy that affects bioenergetic function has effects on exercise gas exchange that depend on the site of the muscle enzyme defect. Thus a patient with a myopathy that affects myophosphorylase or one of the glycolytic enzymes, e.g. phosphofructokinase, could have a reduced maximum exercise tolerance because the patient cannot develop a lactic acidosis and the benefits therefrom, as described in Chapter 2. The effect of the failure to produce an exercise lactic acidosis is reflected in gas exchange and the failure to produce extra CO_2 from the buffering of lactic acid as described by Riley et al (3). In contrast, enzyme defects in the electron transport chain cause a lactic acidosis at a very low work rate, with accompanying gas exchange abnormalities similar to that observed in patients with heart failure (4, 5). Published studies of gas exchange in skeletal muscle enzyme defects affecting other sites in the bioenergetic process are difficult to find. Exercise studies are a good screening technique for detecting muscle enzyme defects affecting bioenergetics and useful to objectively assess therapeutic modalities.

Psychogenic Dyspnea and Behavioral (Anxiety or Malingering) Causes of Exercise Intolerance

How do physicians diagnose psychogenic dyspnea or behavioral causes, volitional or nonvolitional, of exertional intolerance? Usually they are unable to reliably make these diagnoses unless they perform cardiopulmonary exercise testing with quantitative gas exchange measurements.

It appears from our limited experience that such patients often undergo extensive *indirect* diagnostic assessment of exercise tolerance in which large sums of money are spent on tests yielding negative results. Then, rather than performing the *direct* diagnostic assessment, the physician may prescribe an irrelevant drug that only adds to the patient's problem (Chapter 9, cases 13 and 83). Obviously, to diagnose exercise intolerance beyond that due to, and including myocardial ischemia, cardiopulmonary exercise testing is the most specific test. Logically, it should be done before the patient undergoes an expensive imaging and invasive work-up searching for a diagnosis which has little likelihood of being supported.

Volitional behavioral causes of exercise intolerance also require cardiopulmonary exercise testing to make or confirm this diagnosis (Chapter 9, cases 65 and 66). Thus these diagnoses are only available to those physicians who learn how to use cardiopulmonary exercise testing and interpret the results.

GRADING SEVERITY OF HEART DISEASE

The severity of a disease can be assessed either from symptoms of functional capacity or objective measurements of cardiac dysfunction. The New York Heart Association provided a valuable classification system, based on symptoms, which has been almost universally used for about a half of a century (6). It has four functional classifications (Class I–IV) based on the perceived activity level of the patient. Matsumura found it to correlate reasonably well with the anaerobic threshold, showing that symptoms and ability to transport O_2 were correlated (7). Weber and Janicki found that a more objective assessment than the NYHA classification was one based on peak $\dot{V}O_2$ and AT (8). They established a classification of A through D, which describes the peak $\dot{V}O_2$/kg descending in value with advancing letters (Table 8.1). They found that this classification was superior to the New York Heart Association classification to objectively assess cardiac dysfunction. A consensus conference on heart failure for prioritizing patients for heart transplantation based on predicted survival time also agreed with this more objective assessment (9).

Stelken et al. (10) felt that the Weber-Janicki approach, while an advance, would be more satisfactory if it were normalized for age and gender as well as body size. They analyzed the normal predictive values based on size, age and gender, as described

in Chapter 6, and found that percent of predicted peak $\dot{V}O_2$ was a better predictor of survival than peak $\dot{V}O_2$/kg. However, Stevenson compared the classification according to peak $\dot{V}O_2$ without normalizing for age and gender and after adjusting for age and gender (11) to predict survival in patients with heart failure. She found both methods to be good predictors of survival without a clear benefit of one method over the other for the population of patients with heart failure. Importantly, the physiologic assessment has been determined to be the best way to classify patients with heart failure because it provides a better independent predictor of survival than the NYHA symptom classification or measurements of ejection fraction (10, 12, 13).

ESTIMATING PEAK CARDIAC OUTPUT DURING EXERCISE FROM O_2 UPTAKE AT PEAK $\dot{V}O_2$

Cardiac Output Estimated by the Direct Fick Method

Cardiac output, calculated by the direct Fick method, is equal to $\dot{V}O_2/C(a - \bar{v})O_2$. Because $\dot{V}O_2$ can increase over a greater multiple of its resting value than $C(a - \bar{v})O_2$, it has a greater influence on the cardiac output increase measured during exercise than $C(a - \bar{v})O_2$. For instance, $C(a - \bar{v})O_2$ can increase only about threefold in a normal subject whereas $\dot{V}O_2$ can change tenfold or more. Consequently, measurement of $\dot{V}O_2$ increase provides critical information about the cardiac output increase.

But, importantly, $C(a - \bar{v})O_2$ changes almost linearly from a predictable low value of 5 (normal) to 6 (heart failure) ml/dl at rest to about 15 to 16 ml/dl in fit normal subjects (14) and 13 to 14 ml/dl in patients with heart failure (8, 15) at maximal exercise when the hemoglobin concentration is normal. If we knew the change in $C(a - \bar{v})O_2$ over the range of $\dot{V}O_2$ increase from rest to peak, or at specific levels of exercise such as at the anaerobic threshold or peak $\dot{V}O_2$, we could estimate cardiac output from the $\dot{V}O_2$ at these levels of exercise, as shown in Chapter 3. For instance, if the $C(a - \bar{v})O_2$ were reproducibly 12 ml/dl and 15 ml/dl, respectively at the AT and peak $\dot{V}O_2$, we could calculate the cardiac output and the stroke volume from the $\dot{V}O_2$ values at these two levels of exercise. Variation of the $C(a - \bar{v})O_2$ is small among normal subjects (14) and among patients with heart failure (8, 15, 16) when the hemoglobin is normal. But despite the sys-

TABLE 8.1. Weber's Exercise Functional Classification Based on Maximal O_2 Uptake and Anaerobic Threshold*

Class	$\dot{V}O_2$ max (ml/min/kg)	AT (ml/min/kg)	CImax (L/min/m²)
A	>20	>14	>8
B	16–20	11–14	6–8
C	10–15	8–11	4–6
D	<10	<8	<4

$\dot{V}O_2$ max = maximal or peak $\dot{V}O_2$.
AT = anaerobic threshold.
CImax = maximal exercise cardiac index (cardiac output/meter² of body surface area.
* From reference 18.

tematic change in $C(a - \bar{v})O_2$ that takes place during exercise, the absolute value of $C(a - \bar{v})O_2$ must vary with factors that affect oxyhemoglobin content in arterial and mixed venous blood. These factors are considered next.

Behavior of Changing Arterial-Venous O_2 Difference during Exercise

As noted in Chapter 3, cardiac output can be estimated noninvasively at peak exercise using the Fick principle. Calculation depends on the measurement of peak $\dot{V}O_2$ and a concurrent estimate of $C(a - \bar{v})O_2$. Stroke volume is estimated by dividing cardiac output by heart rate. The measurement of $\dot{V}O_2$ and heart rate and estimate of CaO_2 are straightforward. Because $C(a - \bar{v})O_2$ changes in a relatively linear and predictable way from rest to peak $\dot{V}O_2$ (8, 14–16), it is possible to estimate $C(a - \bar{v})O_2$ in normal persons and those with cardiac disorders because they reach similar pulmonary artery O_2 content values ($C\bar{v}O_2$) at peak $\dot{V}O_2$ with an average oxyhemoglobin percent saturation ($S\bar{v}O_2$) equal to 24% at the time of maximal exertion during upright cycle or treadmill exercise. $S\bar{v}O_2$ is slightly lower (perhaps as low as 18%) (14) in the very fit because leg blood flow is a high proportion of the total cardiac output. It tends to be slightly higher (perhaps as high as 30%) (8) in those with severe cardiac failure because the leg blood flow is a smaller portion of total cardiac output in the latter group. Also persons with high peak $\dot{V}O_2$ values seem to have a greater increase in hemoglobin than those with low peak $\dot{V}O_2$ values.

These assumptions appear to be valid unless exercise is terminated by other factors, such as ventilatory limitation, musculoskeletal disorders, poor motivation, or peripheral arterial disease. In the latter instance, blood flow to the legs is unable to increase appropriately and remains a smaller portion of total cardiac output than in the patient without peripheral arterial disease.

Initial and Final Estimate of $C(a - \bar{v})O_2$

Initial Estimate

The initial estimate of $C(a - v)O_2$ (Table 8.2) takes into account the resting hemoglobin concentration and assumes a hemoconcentration at peak exercise of 5%, an arterial oxyhemoglobin (O_2Hb) saturation of 95% (normal), a carboxyhemoglobin (COHb) saturation of 1% (normal) and a mixed venous O_2Hb saturation at maximal exercise of 24% (8, 14, 16) in the calculation. From the values above, recognizing that the O_2 capacity is 1.34 ml/gm Hb, the $C(a - v)O_2$ at peak exercise would be the same as the hemoglobin concentration (Table 8.2).

Final Estimate

To make a final estimate of $C(a - v)O_2$ in subjects who are exceptionally fit or have disease, corrections must be made for how fitness and disease affect 1) hemoconcentration and 2) mixed venous O_2Hb saturation at peak exercise. Also, corrections must be made for the effect of change in arterial O_2Hb

TABLE 8.2.   Estimation of Arteriovenous O_2 Difference ($C(a - \bar{v})O_2$) at Peak Exercise

Hb gm/100 ml*	O_2 cap ml/100 ml	Art. O_2 Sat (%)	Mixed Ven. O_2 Sat (%)	Art. O_2 Cont. (ml/100 ml)	Mixed Ven. O_2 Cont. (ml/100)	$C(a - \bar{v})O_2$+ (ml/100 ml)
16	22.5	96	24	21.4	5.4	16.0
15	21.1	96	24	20.0	5.0	15.0
14	19.7	96	24	18.7	4.7	14.0
13	18.3	96	24	17.4	4.4	13.0
12	16.9	96	24	16.0	4.0	12.0
11	15.5	96	24	14.7	3.7	11.0
10	14.1	96	24	13.4	3.4	10.0

Assumptions: *1. This column identifies the resting hemoglobin concentration. The hemoglobin concentration at peak exercise is considered to be 5% higher than the resting hemoglobin, i.e. a fitness factor of 1.05 (see text for definition). 2. The carboxyhemoglobin concentration is assumed to be 1%.
+Modifications: 1. If the person is very unfit, decrease the $C(a - \bar{v})O_2$ by up to 6%; if the person is very fit, increase the $C(a - \bar{v})O_2$ by up to 6%. 2. Reduce the $C(a - \bar{v})O_2$ by 1% for each 1% increase in carboxyhemoglobin above 1%. 3. Reduce the $C(a - \bar{v})O_2$ by 1% for each 1% decrease in arterial oxyhemoglobin saturation below 96%.

content resulting from 3) arterial O_2 desaturation (e.g., patients with lung diseases) and 4) increased COHb (e.g., cigarette smokers).

Exercise Hemoconcentration. The degree of hemoconcentration (up to 10%) varies with the peak $\dot{V}O_2$ or fitness of the subject. The initial estimate shown in Table 8.2 is for a subject of average fitness and hemoconcentration (5%). For an exceptionally fit subject, the $C(a - v)O_2$ obtained from Table 8.2 should be increased by up to 5%. In contrast, the $C(a - v)O_2$ should be decreased by up to 5% in the very unfit subject or a patient who has a very low peak $\dot{V}O_2$.

Mixed Venous Oxyhemoglobin Saturation. The $C(a - v)O_2$ shown in Table 8.2 is calculated for a subject with average fitness whose mixed venous O_2Hb saturation at peak exercise is 24%. However mixed venous O_2Hb saturation can decrease at peak exercise to as low as 18% and be as high as 30% in disease. To apply the data in Table 8.2 to patients with different levels of fitness, increase $C(a - v)O_2$ up to 6% in the very fit subject and decrease $C(a - v)O_2$ by up to 6% according to their disease limitation.

Oxyhemoglobin Saturation. If the subject has hypoxemia, the $C(a - v)O_2$ determined from Table 8.2 should be decreased by 1% for each 1% decrease in arterial O_2Hb saturation below 96%.

Carboxyhemoglobin Saturation. If the subject has a COHb saturation greater than 1%, decrease the $C(a - v)O_2$ by the percent of COHb saturation minus 1.

Examples of Estimating $C(a - v)O_2$

The following examples illustrate how the initial estimate of $C(a - v)O_2$ from Table 8.2 is modified to take into account unusual fitness, arterial oxyhemoglobin desaturation and increased COHb concentration:

Example A. If the resting Hb were 14 gm/100 ml of blood, the first estimate of $C(a - \bar{v})O_2$ is 14 ml O_2/100 ml blood (Table 8.2). If we considered the person to be very fit, we might find more hemoconcentration (from 5% to 8%) and a slightly lower $S\bar{v}O_2$ (from 24% to 20%). In this case, the final estimate of $C(a - \bar{v})O_2$ would be $14 \times 1.07 = 15.0$ ml O_2/100 ml blood. Further, in this example, where the $C(a - \bar{v})O_2$ is 150 ml O_2 per liter and the $\dot{V}O_2$ is 3500 ml/min and heart rate is 170 beats/minute

at peak exercise, the cardiac output at peak exercise is $3500/150 = 23.3$ L/min and the concurrent stroke volume is $23{,}300/170 = 137$ ml/beat.

Example B. If the resting Hb were 12 gm/100 ml of blood, the initial estimate of $C(a - \bar{v})O_2$ is 12 ml O_2/100 ml blood. For an extreme example, if we considered the person to be quite ill, we might estimate that there was less hemoconcentration (from 5% to 3%) and less decline in $S\bar{v}O_2$ (from 24% to 30%). If, in addition the SaO_2 were only 90% (a 6% decrease in $C(a - \bar{v})O_2$) and if the COHb were 5% (a 4% for a total decrease in $C(a - \bar{v})O_2$). Thus the final estimate of $C(a - \bar{v})O_2$ would be $0.82 \times 12 = 9.8$ ml O_2/100 ml blood. In this example, where $C(a - \bar{v})O_2$ is 98 ml O_2 per liter and the $\dot{V}O_2$ is 900 ml/min and heart rate is 160 at peak exercise, the cardiac output at peak exercise is $900/98 = 9.2$ L/min and the concurrent stroke volume is $9200/160 = 58$ ml/beat.

Short-Cut Estimate of Stroke Volume from O_2 Pulse

The O_2 pulse is equal to the product of $C(a - \bar{v})O_2$ and stroke volume (SV). Therefore stroke volume can be estimated at peak exercise by dividing the O_2 pulse at that time by the concurrent $C(a - \bar{v})O_2$ as shown in Table 8.2. Thus if the arterial oxyhemoglobin saturation were 96% (normal at sea level) and the resting hemoglobin concentration were 15 gm/dl, and the maximum O_2 pulse were 15, the maximum stroke volume would be 100 ml (SV = $15/15 \times 100$). If the O_2 pulse were 25, the stroke volume would be 167 ml (SV = $25/15 \times 100$). Thus the maximum O_2 pulse provides a convenient short-cut to estimating the concurrent stroke volume.

PRIORITIZING PATIENTS FOR HEART TRANSPLANTATION

Exercise testing makes a variety of contributions to the understanding of exercise impairment and exertional dyspnea in chronic congestive heart failure (17). A number of investigators have found that measurements of cardiac function at rest, both invasive and noninvasive, are poorly predictive of patients' symptoms, exercise capacity, prognosis, or need for heart transplantation. Weber and colleagues compared resting cardiac function with exercise capacity in heart failure patients (18) and found that such variables as cardiac index, left ven-

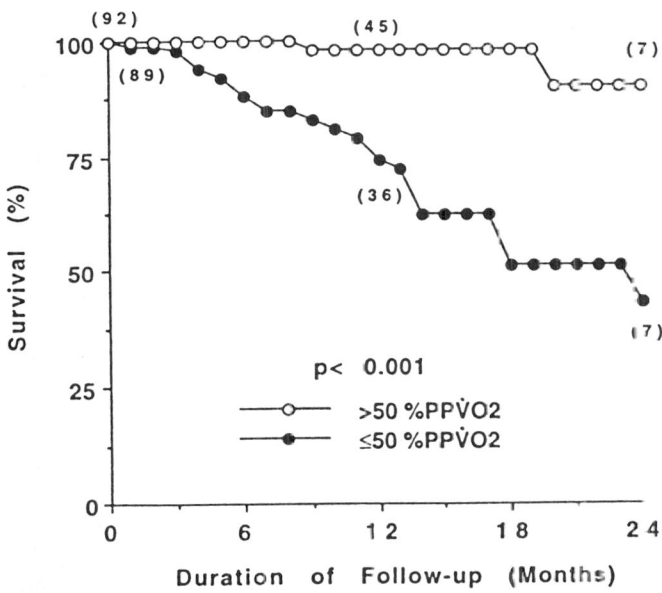

FIGURE 8.8.   Survival time of chronic heart failure patients as related to percent of predicted peak $\dot{V}O_2$ of less than 50% (closed circles) and equal to or greater than 50% (open circles) of predicted peak $\dot{V}O_2$. Reprinted with permission from Stelken AM, Youris LT, Jennison SH, et al. Prognostic value of cardiopulmonary exercise testing using percent achieved of predicted peak oxygen uptake for patients with ischemic and dilated cardiomyopathy. J Am Coll Cardiol 1996;27:345–352.

tricular ejection fraction, wedge pressure, and radiographic heart size correlated poorly with measured peak $\dot{V}O_2$. Neither resting nor exercise pulmonary capillary wedge pressure correlated significantly with peak $\dot{V}O_2$. However, peak $\dot{V}O_2$ did correlate with maximum cardiac output during exercise. Itoh and coworkers (19) showed that peak $\dot{V}O_2$ and anaerobic threshold (AT) correlated with symptom scores, as measured by NYHA class, in 382 heart failure patients. Mean AT was 90 ± 15%, 77 ± 14%, and 60 ± 12% of the predicted values for NYHA class I, class II and class III, respectively. AT correlated only weakly with resting left ventricular ejection fraction measured by echocardiogram or angiography. Weber and colleagues have suggested a classification of heart failure patients based on maximum oxygen uptake and anaerobic threshold as shown in Table 8.1 (18). Koike and colleagues (20) have similarly linked exercise capacity to symptom score. In these patients, peak $\dot{V}O_2$, AT, $\Delta\dot{V}O_2/\Delta WR$, and maximum WR decreased with NYHA symptom scores. NYHA III patients had a maximum $\dot{V}O_2$ averaging 17 ± 3 ml/min/kg, AT of 11 ± 2 ml/min/kg, $\Delta\dot{V}O_2/\Delta WR = 6.2 ± 2$ ml/watt, and maximum work rate of 98 ± 22 watts.

A study by Stelken et al. (10) confirmed the prognostic value of exercise testing in those patients with ischemic and dilated cardiomyopathies. In 181 ambulatory patients with symptoms putting them into NYHA II-III, peak $\dot{V}O_2$, % predicted peak $\dot{V}O_2$, and AT were significantly different when survivors and non-survivors were compared at 12 and 24 months. Differences were often large. For example, for peak $\dot{V}O_2$, the mean value for survivors was 17 ± 6 ml/min/kg; for non-survivors, only 12 ± 4 ml/min/kg. Eighty-nine patients with a peak $\dot{V}O_2$ <50% predicted had 1- and 2-year survivals of 74% and 43%, respectively, compared with 98% and 90% for the 92 patients who achieved >50% predicted peak $\dot{V}O_2$ during exercise testing (Fig 8.8). In fact, peak $\dot{V}O_2$ <50% predicted was the most significant predictor of cardiac death in multivariate analysis. Although most studies normalized their $\dot{V}O_2$ to body weight and ignored the variables of age and gender, Stelken et al. (10) compared the sensitivity of percent of predicted peak $\dot{V}O_2$ based on weight, age, and gender, as described in Chapter 6, to the peak $\dot{V}O_2$ based on body weight alone. Although both were sensitive predictors of survival, they found percent predicted to be a better predictor of survival.

In a study by Rickenbacher et al. (21), 116 consecutive patients with severe but stable congestive heart failure referred for heart transplantation were included in close follow up with medical management. This group demonstrated a very good prognosis, with actuarial survival at 1 year of 98% and at 4 years of 84%. The mean peak $\dot{V}O_2$ was 17.4 ± 4.3 ml/kg/min for the group as a whole. These authors concluded that stable symptoms and a relatively high peak exercise $\dot{V}O_2$ identified patients with a favorable prognosis despite a very low resting ejection fraction. In an earlier study (22), patients with peak $\dot{V}O_2$ < 10 ml/min/kg had a 77% 1-year mortality; if peak $\dot{V}O_2$ was between 10–18 ml/min/kg, mortality at 1 year was only 14%.

The severity of lung gas exchange abnormality has also been used as a prognostic indicator. Some investigators have shown that an abnormally high $\dot{V}E$ versus $\dot{V}CO_2$ slope is associated with worse prognosis (2, 23). For example, Chua et al. (23) found that the slope of the $\dot{V}E$ versus $\dot{V}CO_2$ relationship was helpful in determining prognosis. Of 173 patients with chronic heart failure, a normal slope (defined from 68 healthy age-matched subjects) was associated with 95% survival at 18 months, whereas there was only a 69% survival for those with an abnormally high slope.

On the other hand, Opasich and colleagues (24)

found that NYHA class III and IV patients did not have a prognosis closely linked to peak $\dot{V}_{O_2}$, although class I or II patients did. A peak $\dot{V}_{O_2}$ >18 ml/kg/min was usually associated with good outcome with aggressive medical therapy; those with a value less than or equal to 10 ml/kg/min were at high risk of complications or death.

Some remarkable clinical trials have led to exercise testing providing the critical criteria in predicting survival and therefore in prioritizing patients for cardiac transplantation (25). A prospective study by Mancini et al. (26) randomized patients referred for heart transplant into: 1) those with peak $\dot{V}_{O_2}$ >14 ml/kg/min (considered too well for transplant); 2) those with peak $\dot{V}_{O_2}$ <14 ml/kg/min and accepted for transplant; and 3) those with peak $\dot{V}_{O_2}$ < 14 ml/kg/min but not accepted for surgery because of non-cardiac reasons. If peak $\dot{V}_{O_2}$ > 14 ml/kg/min, then survival was excellent with medical management (1 year survival: 94%; 2 year survival: 84%), whereas those with low peak $\dot{V}_{O_2}$ and who were transplant candidates had a 70% 1-year survival. The prognostic value of these criteria was not appreciably improved when maximum $\dot{V}_{O_2}$ as a percentage of predicted value was used to predict prognosis (27). Deaths and complications were also predicted by a peak $\dot{V}_{O_2}$ <14 ml/kg/min in a study by Roul et al (28).

Osada et al. (29) recently reported 500 patients with severe congestive heart failure referred for transplantation. A total of 154 patients (31%) had a peak $\dot{V}_{O_2}$ equal to or less than 14 ml/min/kg. They found 77 of these patients had a peak systolic blood pressure <120 mmHg, and these had a 55% 3-year survival rate. On the other hand, 74 patients from this group had a peak systolic blood pressure >120 mmHg; survival was significantly greater (83%). In contrast, Kao et al. (30) did not find sufficient discrimination ability to identify the most likely transplant candidates for patients with peak $\dot{V}_{O_2}$ between 12 and 17 ml/kg/min.

Stevenson et al. (31) presented data on 68 heart transplant candidates (peak $\dot{V}_{O_2}$ < 14 ml/min/kg) who had repeat exercise tests at a mean 6 ± 5 months after initial evaluation to examine the possibility of the patient being able to be removed from the transplant list. Thirty were without "major" improvement, but 38 had an increase in peak $\dot{V}_{O_2}$ of more than 2 ml/min/kg, to a value > 12 ml/kg/min. Of these, 7 had no clinical improvement, but 31 were clinically improved. The major improvement group also had improved AT, peak O_2 pulse, and exercise heart rate reserve, and a decrease in resting

heart rate. In the 31 patients taken off the active waiting list, the actuarial survival rate was 100% and the survival rate without relisting for transplant was 85%. All of these patients were vigorously treated with diuretics after afterload reduction and were advised to become involved in informal exercise rehabilitation training. Meyers et al. (32) reported the results of studies on the evaluation of 644 patients with chronic heart failure over a 10 year period. They found that peak $\dot{V}_{O_2}$ outperformed right heart catheterization data, exercise time, and the usual clinical variables used to assess heart failure patients in predicting outcome. They concluded that direct measurement of $\dot{V}_{O_2}$ should be done when clinical or surgical decisions need to be made in patients referred for evaluation of heart failure or for consideration of transplantation.

In summary, peak $\dot{V}_{O_2}$ (and possibly AT) is the most important measurement that a physician can obtain to objectively assess probable survival time of patients with heart failure. Thus, a consensus conference of cardiologists expert in treating patients with heart failure and responsible for selecting and prioritizing patients for heart transplantation acknowledged in their guidelines the importance of peak $\dot{V}_{O_2}$ as the major measurement criterion for including or excluding patients for heart transplantation (9).

PREOPERATIVE EVALUATION OF SURGICAL RISK

Evaluation of perioperative risk has been an area of considerable interest for application of integrative cardiopulmonary exercise testing. In addition to using this technique to quantify cardiac, pulmonary, and circulatory function, similarities have been noticed between the increase in metabolic rate and oxygen delivery seen during exercise and increases in these same variables in the postoperative state. Thus, a patient's capacity to increase oxygen delivery during exercise may correlate with capacity to maintain organ system function after surgery. Exercise testing, especially determination of peak $\dot{V}_{O_2}$ and $\dot{V}_{O_2}$ at the anaerobic threshold, might prove useful in identifying high risk surgical patients, including those judged to have normal cardiopulmonary function by other clinical measurements. Such testing might prove particularly useful in the elderly, those with unsuspected heart or lung disease, and those with marginal organ system function who might otherwise not be offered surgery.

Thoracotomy

Patients being considered for thoracotomy, usually for resection of lung cancer, are at particular risk of postoperative complications. Cardiopulmonary exercise testing has been suggested as a valuable adjunct because spirometry, radionuclide scanning, and arterial blood gases have not been completely successful in identifying all high-risk patients, and, most importantly, may miss patients with significant cardiovascular disease (33–39). In addition, because resectional surgery remains the most effective therapy for lung cancer, exercise testing may identify patients who are likely to tolerate resection even though their poor resting lung function would otherwise preclude surgery. Smith et al. (40) retrospectively reported 22 patients who underwent elective thoracotomy and found 11 who had postoperative respiratory failure, myocardial infarction, arrhythmias, lobar atelectasis, pulmonary embolism, or death. These 11 patients had a significantly lower mean peak $\dot{V}O_2$ than those without complications after surgery, and, if patients who had a peak $\dot{V}O_2$ during cycle exercise < 20 ml/kg/min had not been offered surgery, 91% of patients with complications would have been eliminated. In this study, six of six patients who had a peak $\dot{V}O_2$ < 15 ml/min/kg and four of six patients 15–20 ml/min/kg had complications. Similarly, a peak $\dot{V}O_2$ < 10 ml/kg/min identified the two patients who died and the majority of postoperative complications among 50 patients reported by Bechard and Wetstein (41). Bolliger and coworkers (42) found that peak $\dot{V}O_2$, expressed as percent predicted during cycle ergometry, was predictive of post-resection complications, such as CO_2 retention, prolonged mechanical ventilation, myocardial infarction, pneumonia, pulmonary embolism, and death. In a group of 80 patients, if peak $\dot{V}O_2$ was < 60% predicted, 8 of 9 patients had complications, whereas only 8 of 71 other patients had complications. Thus, this value for peak $\dot{V}O_2$, while identifying only 50% of those with complications, was highly predictive of a postoperative problem. The authors also showed that when patients had a maximum $\dot{V}O_2$ > 75% of predicted, 90% were complication-free. The same group (43) found that a maximum $\dot{V}O_2$ < 10 ml/kg/min was associated with 100% mortality. Patients with complications had a lower mean maximum $\dot{V}O_2$ (10.6 ± 3.6 ml/kg/min vs. 14.8 ± 3.5 ml/kg/min).

A prospective study by Morice and co-workers (44) provided additional evidence for the value of exercise testing in "high-risk" patients undergoing thoracotomy. Thirty-seven patients had been considered inoperable because of a low FEV_1 (<40% predicted), an anticipated post-surgical FEV_1 < 33% predicted using radionuclide scanning, or an arterial PCO_2 >45 mmHg. Thirteen patients who performed exercise testing had a maximum $\dot{V}O_2$ >15 ml/kg/min. Eight of these patients subsequently had resectional surgery. Although mean FEV_1 was poor in this group (mean 40% of predicted), six of eight patients had an uncomplicated course, and all patients were discharged within 22 days of surgery. This study suggests that even some "high-risk" patients can be more fairly assessed with data from exercise testing.

A study by Nakagawa et al. (45) found that resting pulmonary function and predicted postoperative lung function could not clearly separate those with complications or death after thoracotomy from those without these complications. However, if the $\dot{V}O_2$ at an arterial lactate level of 2.2 mmol/L was more than 400 ml/min/m^2, patients were more likely to have a complication-free postoperative course. The criterion of Nakagawa and colleagues is approximately equivalent to an anaerobic threshold value of at least 600–800 ml/min in most adult patients. Pate et al. (46) provided some other potentially useful criteria from a small study of lung resection patients. They concluded that resection was safe if patients had an FEV_1 >1.6 L or >40% of predicted, had a post-resection FEV_1 >700 ml, or a maximum $\dot{V}O_2$ >10 ml/kg/min. Thus, some patients could meet criteria for surgery if they had a maximum $\dot{V}O_2$ >10 ml/kg/min despite having very poor FEV_1.

Postoperative exercise capacity is well maintained after lung resectional surgery. In a study of 57 patients (47) retested 6 months after surgery, lobectomy patients had a mean decrease in FEV_1 of 8% while exercise capacity as measured by peak $\dot{V}O_2$ declined 13%. Interestingly, pneumonectomy patients in this study had a decrease in FEV_1 averaging 23% while maximum $\dot{V}O_2$ decreased by only 16%. Similar data were reported by Pelletier et al. (48) and Bolliger and colleagues (49) showing little or no change with lobectomy and a 20–25% decrease in maximum work capacity after pneumonectomy.

Abdominal Surgery

The usefulness of the lactic acidosis threshold (*LAT*) was demonstrated by Older et al. (50) in elderly patients undergoing major abdominal surgeries. In 187 patients older than 60 years, mean $\dot{V}O_2$ at the

LAT averaged 12.4 ± 2.7 ml/min/kg. If the *LAT* was <11 ml/min/kg (found in 30% of the study patients), mortality from cardiovascular complications was 18%. On the other hand, if the *LAT* was >11 ml/min/kg, the cardiovascular death rate in the postoperative period was only 0.8%. Of interest, those patients who manifested evidence of cardiac ischemia in addition to having a low lactic acidosis threshold had a 42% mortality rate.

Epstein et al. (51) compared peak $\dot{V}O_2$ as a predictor of postoperative complications with a cardiopulmonary risk index that combined pulmonary function, clinical information, and a cardiac risk index. Their index clearly separated patients who had complications from those who did not. Those patients with a peak $\dot{V}O_2$ <500 ml/m^2/min had a sixfold increase in complications compared with those with a higher peak $\dot{V}O_2$. Although both variables were predictive, a multiple logistic regression analysis did not identify peak $\dot{V}O_2$ as an independent predictor.

Analysis

There remain several questions about the use of cardiopulmonary exercise testing in preoperative evaluation. First, who are the most suitable candidates? It is unlikely that all patients need to be tested, but patients with unsuspected cardiopulmonary disease (especially cardiac) may be discovered with testing. It does appear important to offer exercise testing to older patients and those with marginal lung or cardiac function who would otherwise be excluded from major thoracic or abdominal surgery. These patients may have surprisingly good exercise capacity that may translate into surprisingly low perioperative risk. Second, there is the question about the type of exercise testing to be performed for preoperative evaluation. Measurement of peak $\dot{V}O_2$ and $\dot{V}O_2$ at the *LAT* provide objective data that can be compared with high- and low-risk populations, but how useful in comparison are more simple tests with less sophisticated measurements, such as stair-climbing or timed walking tests? (51, 52) Third, there is need for further focus on specific types of surgery in relationship to postoperative complications and cardiopulmonary exercise testing. Results of exercise testing in patients have been largely used in those undergoing thoracic (lung) and abdominal surgery. The value of exercise testing for predicting complications of other forms of surgery, such as heart or vascular surgery, or orthopedic procedures, has not been determined. Finally, there is a need for more evidence that improvement in preoperative

exercise capacity after smoking cessation, medical therapy, exercise training, or other interventions can reduce postoperative risks.

MEASURING IMPAIRMENT FOR DISABILITY EVALUATION

Impairment and Disability

In impairment and disability evaluation, exercise testing has an important role. Sometimes, the focus is on establishing causation of disease from a substance encountered in the workplace; in other cases, the process is to determine the degree of impairment.

Impairment, as used in the United States, is a measurable, objective decrease in functional capacity. Disability is an assessment of the impact of impairment on the individual and requires socioeconomic and environmental input, including factors such as age, gender, education, economic and social environment, and energy requirements of the occupation (53). A World Health Organization statement (54) defined impairment as "any loss or abnormality of psychological, physiological, or anatomical structure or function," while disability was defined as "any restriction or lack (resulting from impairment) of ability to perform an activity within the range considered normal for a human being." Physicians are asked to identify and measure impairment but, although opinions are often sought about a patient's disability, disability decisions are usually made through an administrative or legal process. Because exercise testing permits objective measurement of physiologic function, it determines impairment rather than disability.

Problems in Assessing Impairment from Resting Measures Only

In 1986, the American Thoracic Society statement on evaluation of impairment and disability secondary to respiratory disorders recommended a systematic evaluation process (53). The statement was "concerned primarily with impairments related to reduced lung function," and presented a rating system for impairment from lung disease based on vital capacity (FVC), forced expiratory volume in 1 sec (FEV$_1$), FEV$_1$/FVC, and single-breath diffusing capacity for carbon monoxide (D$_{LCO}$). It also implied that there was a well-documented relationship between measurements made at rest (e.g., FEV$_1$ and

$D_{L}CO$) and measurements made during exercise (maximum $\dot{V}O_2$ and work capacity). The authors concluded that the majority of subjects undergoing an evaluation for impairment would not require exercise testing.

This assumption can be challenged by examining whether maximum work capacity can be predicted theoretically from resting pulmonary function. Consider the relationship between FEV_1 and peak $\dot{V}O_2$. In this analysis, begin by assuming that a subject's $FEV_1 = 1.5$ L. If FEV_1 is used to predict maximum exercise minute ventilation ($\dot{V}E$) by using two reported estimates (55, 56,) ($FEV_1 \times 35$ and $FEV_1 \times 40$), the maximum $\dot{V}E$ values would range from 52.5 L/min to 60 L/min. Next, assume that dead space/tidal volume ratio (VD/VT) at maximum exercise ranges from a low of 0.15 in a normal subject to 0.40 in someone with moderate ventilation-perfusion mismatching from lung disease. Using this range, the estimated maximum alveolar ventilation ($\dot{V}A = \dot{V}E \times [1 - VD/VT]$) would span 31.5 to 51 L/min for the maximum $\dot{V}E$ values calculated from the FEV_1 values, above. Then, assuming that $PACO_2$ would be between 25 to 35 mmHg (not unusual numbers), one could estimate the extremes of $\dot{V}CO_2$ that could be present by $\dot{V}CO_2$ L/min (STPD) $= PACO_2 \times \dot{V}A$ L/min (BTPS)/863. The estimated $\dot{V}CO_2$, using these examples, ranges from 0.91 to 2.10 L/min. Finally, what is the relationship between $\dot{V}CO_2$ and $\dot{V}O_2$? $\dot{V}O_2 = \dot{V}CO_2/R$, and R at maximum exercise ranges from 0.9 to 1.2. Our hypothetical subject's maximum $\dot{V}O_2$ might be as low as 0.76 L/min or as high as 2.33 L/min for the same FEV_1 value. Therefore, while the *ventilatory capacity* of the respiratory system for ventilation may be successfully predicted from resting FEV_1 (and this, too, is open to question), the *ventilatory requirement* for a given level of work cannot be predicted from the FEV_1.

Cotes and co-workers (57) tested the hypothesis that exercise limitation could be predicted accurately from lung function impairment by using maximum $\dot{V}O_2$ as the dependent variable in a stepwise multiple regression. In this way, they determined which variables significantly affect peak $\dot{V}O_2$. A group of 157 referred men with a variety of suspected or known occupational lung disorders was studied. Each had abnormal pulmonary function, were limited during the exercise test by dyspnea, and had a maximum $\dot{V}E$ within 2 SD of the maximum $\dot{V}E$ predicted from the FEV_1. In addition, all subjects had to have a satisfactory treadmill exercise test, with the endpoint being the point at which subjects stopped

voluntarily or when their heart rate exceeded 80% of predicted value.

Results were expressed as the correlation coefficient (r) and as the fraction of total variance accounted for (r^2) by variables taken individually and stepwise with peak $\dot{V}O_2$ as the dependent variable. For single variables, r and %-variance were FVC (0.39, 15%), FEV_1 (0.45, 20%), FEV_1/FVC (0.29, 8.4%), and $D_{L}CO$ (0.50, 25%). The combination of FEV_1 and $D_{L}CO$ could account for only 29% of the variance in peak $\dot{V}O_2$. However, when FEV_1 (or FVC and FEV_1/FVC) was combined with measured $\dot{V}E$ during exercise, 54% of the variance of peak $\dot{V}O_2$ was explained. The authors of this analysis concluded that loss of exercise capacity was not accurately predicted from resting lung function indices, but the predictability of peak $\dot{V}O_2$ could be enhanced by adding the measurement of $\dot{V}E$ during submaximal exercise.

Exercise Testing and Impairment Evaluation

A number of investigators have emphasized the usefulness of integrative cardiopulmonary exercise testing for determination of impairment (57–67). Exercise testing complements clinical evaluation and adds to resting pulmonary function and roentgenographic studies. It increases diagnostic accuracy, both quantitively (measurement of work capacity, maximum $\dot{V}O_2$, and sustained work capacity) and qualitatively (identification of the cause of exercise limitation).

For example, during an approximately 3-year period, we had the opportunity to see 490 current or retired shipyard workers (62). Of these, 348 men who had complaints of exercise limitation or who were suspected of having exercise limitation were studied using 1-minute incremental cycle ergometry exercise with gas exchange measurements. A conclusion was made by the referring physician as to the likelihood of exercise limitation, if any, and the specific organ system limiting exercise, but this conclusion was based solely on non-exercise data, including chest roentgenograms, resting pulmonary function tests, resting electrocardiogram, medical history, physical examination, and smoking history (Fig. 8.9). Following the exercise test, another conclusion was made, but this time using all data acquired during the evaluation including the exercise test (Fig. 8.9).

On the initial assessment, 143 subjects were pre-

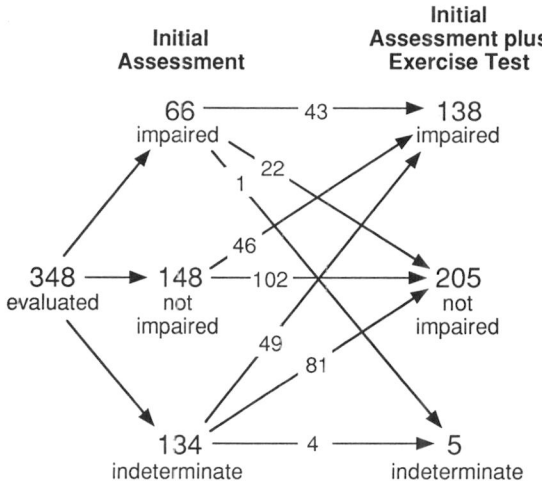

FIGURE 8.9.   The influence of cardiopulmonary exercise testing on the evaluation of work impairment; 348 patients were initially referred for suspicion of functional impairment secondary to asbestos exposure. The initial assessment was done without exercise testing but with all other clinical modalities available to the evaluating physician. This assessment concluded that 66 were impaired but no decision could be reached on 134 of the 348 patients being evaluated. In the final assessment, cardiopulmonary exercise data were added to the information available to the physician rendering the interpretation. This new information confirmed (cardiopulmonary exercise testing taken as the gold standard) impairment in 43 of the 66, with 22 going into the not impaired category and 1 into the indeterminate category. In contrast, 95 subjects were added to the impaired category, 46 from the "not impaired" category and 49 from the indeterminate category; 102 of the 148 subjects thought to be not impaired were confirmed as being not impaired. However, 81 were added to this category from the indeterminate category and 22 from the impaired category making a total of 205 subjects for whom it was thought that there was no basis on which to conclude that the patient had a physiological impairment in the ability to perform physical work. Only 4 of the 130 subjects whose impairment was uncertain before cardiopulmonary exercise testing remained in this category after the cardiopulmonary exercise test.

dicted to have normal work capacity, but 46 (31%) of these subjects turned out to have a peak $\dot{V}O_2$ below the 95% confidence limit. The accuracy of the clinical prediction of a low work capacity was similar; 66 subjects were expected to have low work capacity, and of these, only 43 (67%) were correctly categorized. Furthermore, the referring physicians judged that the work capacity of a large number of subjects could not be estimated (134 subjects). Of these, 60% had normal peak $\dot{V}O_2$ while 37% had abnormally low peak $\dot{V}O_2$. While the magnitude of reduction of peak $\dot{V}O_2$ had a significant correlation with resting pulmonary function (VC, FEV_1, $D_{L}CO$ as %-predicted), prediction of reduced work capacity from resting pulmonary function was not always helpful. Overall, 138 workers had abnormally low peak $\dot{V}O_2$: 43 were correctly predicted, 46 were in-

correctly expected to be normal, and 49 were uncertain. The sensitivity of resting pulmonary function tests, chest x-ray, and other studies for detecting low peak $\dot{V}O_2$ was only about 31%.

The cause of exercise limitation may have an effect on the accuracy of resting studies, largely because the most often used resting data are the tests of pulmonary function. However, among our 138 subjects with low peak $\dot{V}O_2$, only 25 were limited by obstructive or restrictive lung disease, whereas 95/138 (69%) had a cardiovascular cause of exercise limitation (Table 8.3). The presence of a high proportion of cardiovascular disease in this patient population is not unique; Agostoni et al. found that 37% of 120 asbestos workers had unexpected cardiac limitation rather than ventilatory limitation.

O_2 Cost of Work

In approximate terms, the oxygen cost ($\dot{V}O_2$) for office work might be about 5–7 ml/kg/min, moderate labor about 15 ml/kg/min, and strenuous labor 20–30 ml/kg/min. Some guidelines suggest, in addition, that workers could perform manual labor at a comfortable "work pace" when this was approximately 40% of peak $\dot{V}O_2$, a value interestingly close to the lactic acidosis threshold in most subjects.

Having obtained measurements of peak $\dot{V}O_2$ and $\dot{V}O_2$ at the anaerobic threshold, it might be tempting to relate these to the oxygen cost of specific activities, including specific work tasks. There are a number of sources of information about specific O_2 costs of various physical activities, both for various occupations and for specific kinds of movements, but many of these are estimates rather than actual measurements. These values should be used with caution. For given individuals whose age, weight, gender, rate of work, efficiency of movement, degree of intermittency of the work task, and other factors differ, the true metabolic cost of work ($\dot{V}O_2$) may

TABLE 8.3.   **Diagnostic Causes (%) of Reduced Work Capacity in 138 Workers with Impairment***

69% cardiovascular
41% cardiac
28% peripheral arterial or other
14% airway obstruction
4% restrictive lung disease
11% neurologic or musculoskeletal
2% obesity

* Work Capacity below the 95% confidence limits of predicted

vary greatly. For this reason, we recommend that broad estimates of metabolic cost of exercise be used rather than trying to make estimates for very specific tasks.

Analysis

A report of a working group of the European Society for Clinical Respiratory Physiology (68) concluded that equating the degree of respiratory impairment from pulmonary function tests with the degree of reduced exercise capacity was overly simplistic because of the weak correlation between the two. The best assessment about exercise capacity was obtained from a symptom-limited progressive exercise test. A proposed scale of percentage "respiratory disability" was suggested with a score ranging from 0–100%. [In this paper, "respiratory disability" refers to the estimated loss of function as determined from exercise testing rather than the way "disability" is defined by others and contrasted to "impairment."] The peak $\dot{V}O_2$, which excluded the lowest 5% of normal subjects, was taken as the point of 0% disability (using 1.64 SD below the mean predicted value). For 100% disability, the value chosen corresponded to a peak $\dot{V}O_2$ that was compatible with extremely low exercise capacity, about 0.5 L/min or about twice resting $\dot{V}O_2$ for normal sized persons. The group proposed that %-disability should be calculated as a linear function of maximum observed $\dot{V}O_2$ ranging from 0.5 L/min (100% disability) to mean predicted peak $\dot{V}O_2$ − 1.64 × SD (0% disability). They presented data from 157 men with respiratory impairment and found that, as assessed by exercise testing, 28% had no impairment; 38% had 1–19% respiratory disability; 11% had severe disability (60–79% respiratory disability); and 1% had 100% respiratory disability. Although this scheme was intended as a way of expressing impairment from lung disease, the same criteria could probably be applied to heart and other diseases.

Cardiopulmonary exercise testing is indicated when a precise measurement of work capacity (work rate, peak $\dot{V}O_2$, or $\dot{V}O_2$ at the anaerobic threshold) is required, often when symptoms or subjective exercise capacity are inconsistent with resting measurements. The ATS recommendation for exercise testing includes the potential of *underestimating* the degree of impairment in a patient with mildly to moderately reduced resting pulmonary function. Furthermore, we have evaluated patients whose claimed exercise capacity exceeded estimates based on resting pulmonary function; and, on occasion,

the cardiopulmonary exercise test confirmed that the patient's impairment was considerably *overestimated* from spirometry and D_LCO.

In selected patients, exercise testing is a valuable diagnostic tool. The greatest potential advantages may be in evaluating those with co-existing disease (heart disease, peripheral arterial disease, etc.) along with lung disease, or those with potentially confounding risk factors such as cigarette smoking. In some of these patients, exercise capacity may be limited by a mechanism other than respiratory impairment that would not be predicted from resting pulmonary function testing. In others, the sensitivity of exercise-related abnormalities of arterial blood gases, alveolar-arterial Po_2 difference, or dead space/tidal volume ratio may be useful in identifying subtle evidence of respiratory disease.

EXERCISE REHABILITATION
Physiological Basis of Exercise Rehabilitation

Endurance exercise training is commonly used to improve exercise tolerance and quality of life. It has proved useful in healthy subjects (e.g., athletes) and in a number of patient groups. It is widely conceded that an exercise training program is the most beneficial portion of rehabilitation programs. Cardiopulmonary exercise testing is uniquely suited to gauge the specific benefits of exercise training. Moreover, exercise testing serves to rule out co-existing disease processes that would contraindicate a rigorous exercise program. Cardiopulmonary exercise testing is necessary to understand the physiologic changes induced by exercise training in patients and normal subjects. The general physiological changes in response to training are described.

Skeletal Muscle

Skeletal muscles are composed of two major varieties of contractile cells (69). One type of fiber seems designed for prolonged repetitive contraction. These fibers are known as "type I," "oxidative" or "slow-twitch" fibers. The other fiber type has rapid contractile properties, but has a limited capacity for prolonged repetitive contraction, and is known as "type II," "glycolytic" or "fast-twitch." The relative proportion of these two fiber types varies from muscle group to muscle group. After an effective program of training, subpopulations of type II fibers remodel. Type IIb fibers, which have a very low capacity for oxidative metabolism remodel into type IIa fibers (70), which have a high oxidative potential—in some ways similar to type I fibers. Type I fibers undergo extensive biochemical and structural modification (69). In these fibers, the mitochondrial number and size increase. The concentrations of a number of enzymes in both the cytosol and the mitochondria increase (71). These enzymatic changes facilitate the Krebs cycle reactions and oxidative phosphorylation so that the capacity to oxidatively metabolize the end product of glycolysis (pyruvate) and fatty acids and ketone bodies is increased (69). In parallel with the increased ability to utilize oxygen, the ability to supply oxygen to the muscle cells increases. Myoglobin levels in the trained muscle are higher (72); this may contribute to the ability to transport oxygen from the muscle capillary to the site of metabolism. More importantly, muscle capillaries proliferate (73). The number of capillaries increases out of proportion to the increase in muscle fiber size so that more capillaries surround a given muscle fiber. This decreases the diffusion distance from the oxygen source (hemoglobin in the muscle capillary) to the oxygen sink (the mitochondrion in the muscle cell). Therefore, a lower capillary P_{O_2} can sustain a given level of oxygen consumption.

These structural and biochemical changes are seen only in the muscle groups involved in the training regimen (74); this is known as the principle of specificity (75). For example, walking or running does not induce changes in the arm muscles. Training on a stationary bicycle will not fully translate into improvements in running performance, as a somewhat different group of muscles are involved.

Changes in other organ systems besides the exercising muscles also occur. The cardiovascular system undergoes significant changes as a result of exercise training (75–77). The heart hypertrophies, with increases in both ventricular wall thickness and chamber size. Body composition usually changes as a result of an effective program of endurance training (78, 79). Muscle size increases and this is reflected by an increase in lean body mass. Body fat often decreases more than muscle mass increases, so that body weight falls (although changes in body weight vary).

Cardiac Output and Heart Rate

After an effective program of training, cardiac output at peak exercise is increased, though cardiac output at rest and at a given work rate is not appreciably altered. However, stroke volume is higher at rest, at any given work rate, and at peak exercise. Consequently, heart rate at rest and at a given level of exercise is distinctly lower after exercise training, though peak heart rate is unchanged. Both systolic and diastolic blood pressure tend to be lower after training, especially in the hypertensive subject.

Blood Lactate

After an effective program of endurance training, the remodeling of the exercising muscles yields both improved oxygen delivery to the mitochondria and improved mitochondrial capability for aerobic metabolism. As a result, the onset of anaerobic metabolism is delayed. At any given work rate above the pre-training anaerobic threshold, blood lactate levels are lower after exercise training (80, 81) (Fig. 8.10). Sullivan et al. (82) demonstrated that knowledge of peak $\dot{V}_{O_2}$ and anaerobic threshold allowed

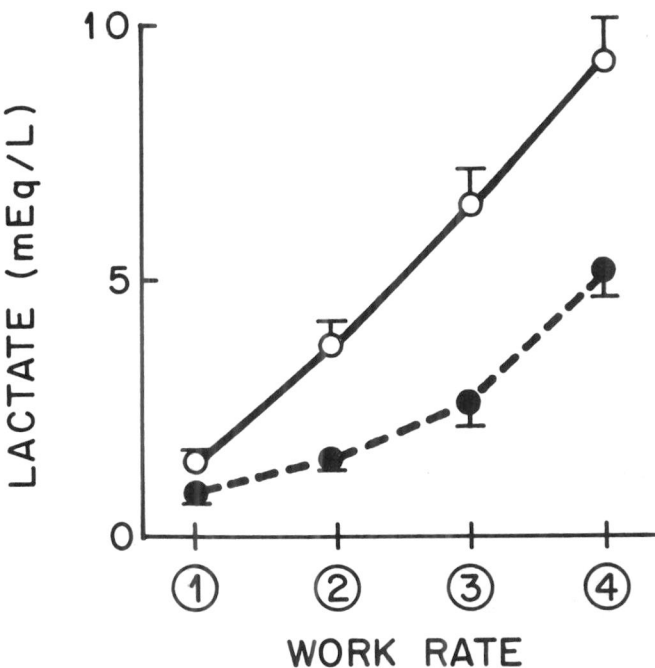

FIGURE 8.10.   Effect of endurance training on end-exercise blood lactate levels at four work rates. Values plotted are the average (± SE) responses of 10 subjects before (solid line) and after (dashed line) endurance training. Subjects exercised for 15 minutes at work rates ranging from moderate (work rate 1) to very heavy intensity (work rate 4). After training, blood lactate levels are lower in response to identical exercise tasks. Reprinted with permission from Casaburi R, Storer TW, Ben-Dov I, et al. Effect of endurance training on possible determinants of $\dot{V}_{O_2}$ during heavy exercise. J Appl Physiol 1987;62:199–207.

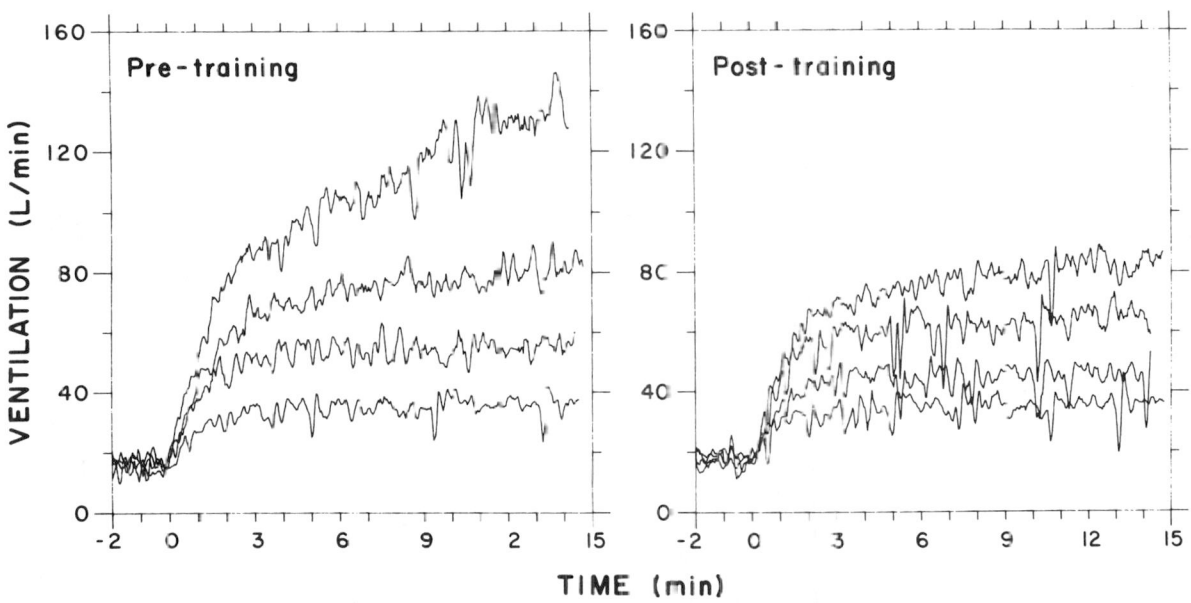

FIGURE 8.11.   Effect of endurance training on the breath-by-breath time course of ventilation following the onset of constant work rate exercise in a healthy subject. Left: pre-training responses to 95, 148, 191, and 233 watts. Right: post-training responses to identical work rates after 8 weeks of endurance training. Note the dramatic decrease in ventilation at the higher work rates after training. Reprinted with permission from Casaburi R, Storer TW, Ben-Dov I, et al. Effect of endurance training on possible determinants of $\dot{V}O_2$ during heavy exercise. J Appl Physiol 1987;62:199–207.

good prediction of an individual's blood lactate level in response to a given level of constant work rate exercise. This relationship was unaltered by training, despite appreciable increases in both peak $\dot{V}O_2$ and anaerobic threshold.

Oxygen Uptake

Endurance training increases maximal $\dot{V}O_2$, both because arteriovenous O_2 content difference widens and maximal cardiac output is higher (79). In healthy subjects, improvements on the order of 8–15% are commonly seen. During incremental exercise tests at sub-AT work rates, $\dot{V}O_2$ is not altered by training. For above-AT work rates, there is a tendency for $\dot{V}O_2$ to be lower at a given work rate after training, though in most cases the differences are difficult to appreciate (the overall $\Delta\dot{V}O_2/\Delta WR$ slope remains approximately 10 ml/min/watt). Following the onset of heavy constant work rate exercise, however, distinct differences are induced by exercise training. A decrease in the slow (phase III) rise in $\dot{V}O_2$ is seen, and this decrease is in close proportion to the decrease in blood lactate elicited by training (80). Despite this close correlation, the mechanism of the decreased oxygen requirement remains controversial (83).

Ventilation

In both the steady-state and during exercise transients, $\dot{V}E$ responds in close proportion to CO_2 output (84). After training, at a given work rate, $\dot{V}E$ is lower in proportion to the decrease in CO_2 output. Moreover, because lactic acid production is lower, the hydrogen ion stimulation of the carotid bodies is lower and less hyperventilation is present at a given heavy work rate (81). This additional decrease in ventilation means that arterial PCO_2 is higher at a given heavy work rate. Figure 8.11 shows the responses to 15 minutes of exercise at four progressively higher work rates before and after a program of endurance training. At the higher (above AT) work rates, there is a dramatically lower ventilatory response to exercise.

Other Physiological Responses

Blood catecholamine responses to a given level of heavy exercise are often dramatically lower after training (85), although the fractional reduction varies appreciably among subjects (80). Other hormonal responses are reduced as well (85, 86). The body temperature increase that occurs with exercise is ameliorated somewhat (80, 87). Finally, ratings of perceived exertion for a given work rate are generally lower (88). Whether this reduction is predominantly linked to improved physiologic function or to psychologic factors is unclear (89).

Exercise Rehabilitation in Heart Disease

The objective of exercise training is to improve exercise tolerance and quality of life. Because patients with heart disease become physically inactive as a result of reduced ability to deliver blood to the muscles of locomotion, the skeletal muscles undergo change similar to that of detraining. Therefore when cardiac function and ability to increase cardiac output improves, the changes in muscle due to inactivity will probably limit the patient's exercise performance. With this logic in mind, Itoh and Kato (90) studied the effect of short-term training after cardiac surgery for valvular heart disease and coronary artery bypass graft surgery. They used as their training work rate the anaerobic threshold rather than the level of exercise training recommended by the American College of Sports Medicine (91), which is 40 to 85% of the predicted maximum heart rate. They found the latter impractical because of the range of heart rate recommended and also because most of the patients with coronary artery bypass graft surgery received β-adrenoreceptor blockade therapy, which limits the heart rate increase. Using peak $\dot{V}O_2$, AT, $\Delta\dot{V}O_2/\Delta WR$ and the time constant for the $\dot{V}O_2$ in response to constant work rate exercise as outcome measures, they found significant improvement in aerobic function in the group of post-surgery patients who underwent exercise training, but did not find improvement in the control group of post-surgical patients who did not undergo exercise training.

Itoh and Kato (54) selected the work rate at the subject's anaerobic threshold because they regarded it as a safe and yet effective work level for exercise training. They reasoned that, at the AT, patients are able to supply the O_2 required to perform work because they do not endure a significant lactic acidosis and therefore the heart is not overstressed. The sympathetic nervous system is not excessively stimulated at this work level since only minor changes in norepinephrine and epinephrine take place at the AT (see Chapter 2). Also, patients find this training program acceptable since they are able to maintain work at the AT over a prolonged exercise period.

Using similar logic to Itoh and Kato, Dubach et al. (92) contrasted the effect of a 2-month endurance exercise training program, using a combination of walking and cycling training at a work rate comparable to that which would approximate the subject's anaerobic threshold, with no formal exercise training program. Training was started approximately 36 days after myocardial infarction. Myocardial injury was not extended by the training program, as evaluated by magnetic resonance imaging of the heart. The trained patients increased peak $\dot{V}O_2$ and lactate threshold by 26% and 39%, respectively, whereas there was no detectable improvement in the non-trained control group.

Despite the obvious importance of the question as to whether exercise training improves exercise tolerance and left ventricular function in chronic left ventricular failure, there are few studies in which objective measurements have been made, as pointed out in the review of the topic by McKelvie et al. in 1995 (93). However, the studies that have been done indicate that peak $\dot{V}O_2$ improves after an exercise training program. More recently, Belardinelli et al. (94) studied the effect of exercise training on left ventricular diastolic filling in patients with dilated cardiomyopathy, using pulsed Doppler echocardiography. They found that exercise training increased the LAT and peak $\dot{V}O_2$ in patients with dilated cardiomyopathy and impaired left ventricular relaxation. The basis of the increase in cardiac function was an improvement in peak early filling of the left ventricle.

The key physiological effect of training in the heart disease patient is the reduction in heart rate, thereby allowing more time for blood to flow through the coronary blood vessels and more time for cardiac filling. Also, because of more aerobic and less anaerobic regeneration of ATP after training, the lactic acidosis is less severe at a given level of exercise. Thus, there is less ventilatory drive and therefore less breathing stress as a result of the reduced lactic acidosis. Finally, of great importance, is a greater sense of well being in patients as they find that they are physically stronger and more active.

Exercise Rehabilitation in Chronic Obstructive Pulmonary Disease

The message of approximately 15 randomized trials and more than 30 observational studies is clear. Rehabilitative exercise training improves exercise tolerance and reduces dyspnea on exertion of patients with chronic lung disease (95). But whether these benefits are the result of the psychological or physiologic effects of an exercise program is not always clear (96). Cardiopulmonary exercise testing provides unequivocal evidence of the physiologic benefits of training in pulmonary patients. Best studied are patients with chronic obstructive pulmonary disease (COPD), but results of exercise programs in patients with cystic fibrosis (97) and asthma (98) have also been published.

Patients with COPD are often ventilatory limited, in that their exercise tolerance is limited by the level of ventilation tolerance they can sustain. This occurs both because the level of ventilation that can be sustained is low, and the level of ventilation required for a given level of exercise is elevated. The low ventilatory ceiling is related to respiratory muscle fatigue induced by high work of breathing from high expiratory airways resistance and hyperinflation-induced mechanical disadvantage of the diaphragm and chest wall muscles (99). The high ventilatory requirement for a given level of exercise is dictated by inefficient gas exchange (high V_D/V_T), hypoxic stimulation of ventilation and H^+ stimulation resulting from the production of CO_2 and lactate (100, 101). In some patients, contributing factors to the early onset of lactic acidosis include decreased oxygen delivery due to increased pulmonary vascular resistance and arterial hypoxemia. But, increasingly, abnormalities in the skeletal muscles are being suspected as limiting aerobic energy production and causing early onset of lactic acidosis. A portion of these abnormalities is likely related to severe deconditioning related to inactivity (101), but other sources (malnutrition, low anabolic hormone levels and myopathy related to corticosteroid use) may be present.

Until the present decade, it was doubted that COPD patients could gain physiological benefits from a program of exercise training (102). New strategies, chief among them the employment of exercise intensities that are a high percentage of peak exercise tolerance (103), have now demonstrated that physiologic benefits are achievable. Cardiopulmonary exercise testing shows that the increased exercise tolerance after a rigorous program of rehabilitative exercise training in COPD patients is associated with a decreased ventilatory requirement at a given level of exercise. In a group of patients with predominantly moderate COPD, training-induced reduction in ventilatory requirement was closely correlated with the reduction in blood lactate levels

(104). In a group of patients with more severe disease, the reduction in ventilatory requirement was associated with the adoption of a more efficient (slower, deeper) breathing pattern (105). Besides determining the degree (and mechanism) of improvement in exercise tolerance that occurs as a result of an exercise program, cardiopulmonary exercise testing has other well-defined uses in the context of pulmonary rehabilitation:

1. The contraindications to a rigorous exercise program can be defined.
2. The need for supplemental oxygen during exercise can be determined.
3. Exercise prescription guidelines can be developed.
4. The mechanism of exercise limitation can be clarified.

ASSESSING EFFECTIVENESS OF TREATMENT

The major role of the heart, pulmonary and peripheral circulations, lungs, and ventilatory apparatus is to support the respiration of the cells, and specifically the increased respiration of the skeletal muscles during exercise. Therefore, measurements of respiration in response to exercise should give the most direct global assessment of the function of these organ systems.

But to use cardiopulmonary exercise testing for the purpose of evaluating therapy, it is necessary for the laboratory calibration to be accurate, to use sensitive end points, and to be consistent in methodology. Based on the experience of the multicenter Vasodilator Heart Failure Trials (V-HeFT II) of the Veterans Affairs Hospitals, Cohn et al. (106) pointed out the need for well-trained technicians and careful calibration of the cardiopulmonary exercise system. Thus it was of concern that some centers were performing cardiopulmonary exercise testing without a good understanding of what constituted a good or poor test. Several centers produced results in which tests of normal subjects (controls) yielded $\Delta\dot{V}O_2/\Delta WR$ values that were either too low or too high to be physiologic. By the third year of the study, the normal control subjects at all centers had the same and proper values for $\Delta\dot{V}O_2/\Delta WR$, i.e., 10 ml/min/W. If the leaders at these centers had been trained in cardiopulmonary exercise physiology, they would have recognized immediately that their results were incorrect, rather than recognizing a

a)

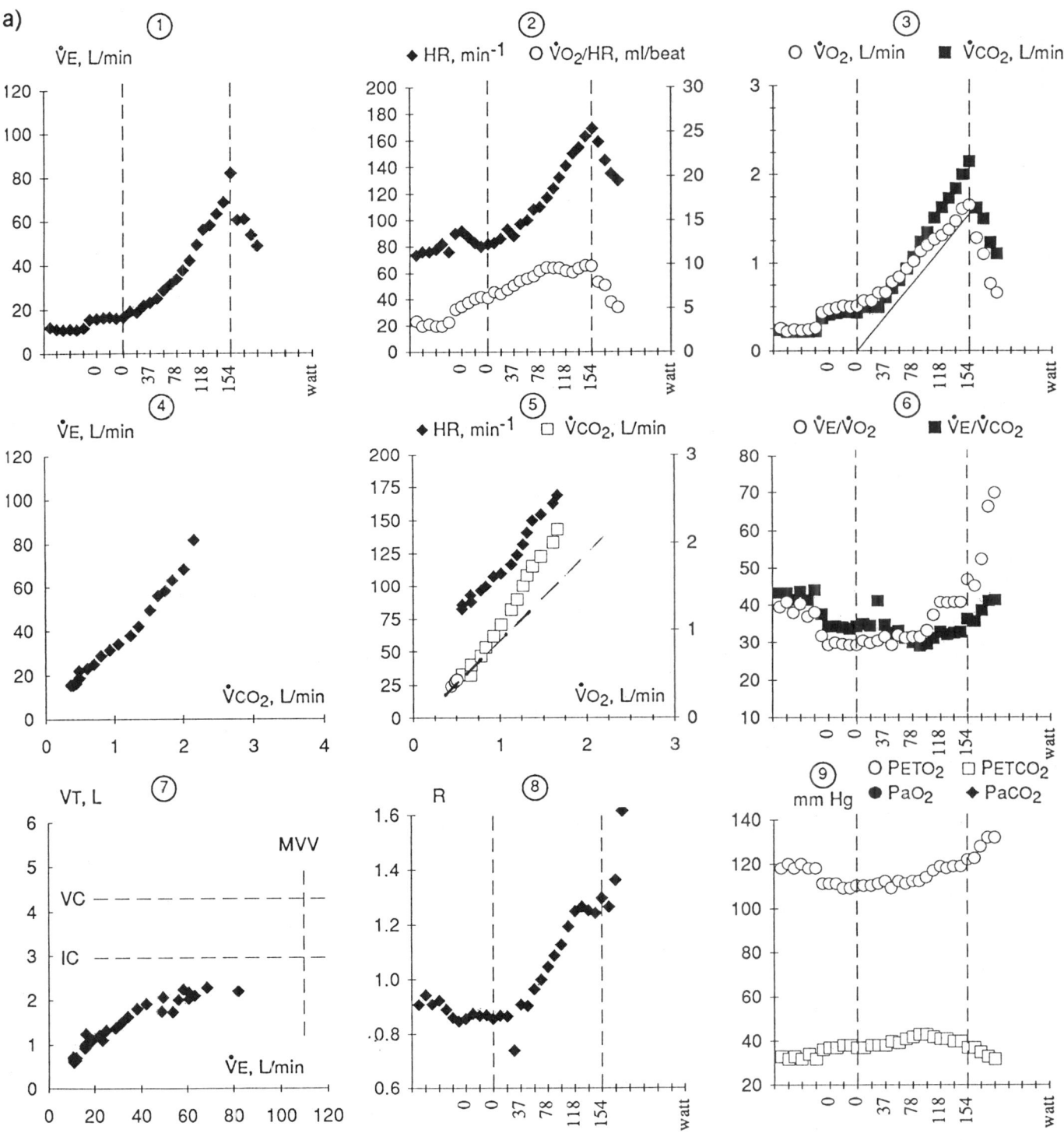

FIGURE 8.12.   Reproducibility of cardiopulmonary exercise testing in patient presented as case 81 in Chapter 9. This 29-year-old male, who noted progressive decrease in exercise tolerance over about a year, was studied by us three times over a period of 6 months to confirm a diagnosis made at the time of the first study (8.12a). While he was symptomatic during this period of evaluation, he was stable. Because of skepticism by the consulting cardiologist regarding the diagnosis of cardiomyopathy with diastolic dysfunction suggested by the first evaluation, the second study (8.12b) was done 3 months later, this time with arterial blood gas analysis (not shown). As can be seen, despite a 3-month interval between studies a and b, the peak $\dot{V}O_2$ (1.6 L/min) and AT (0.8 l/min) were

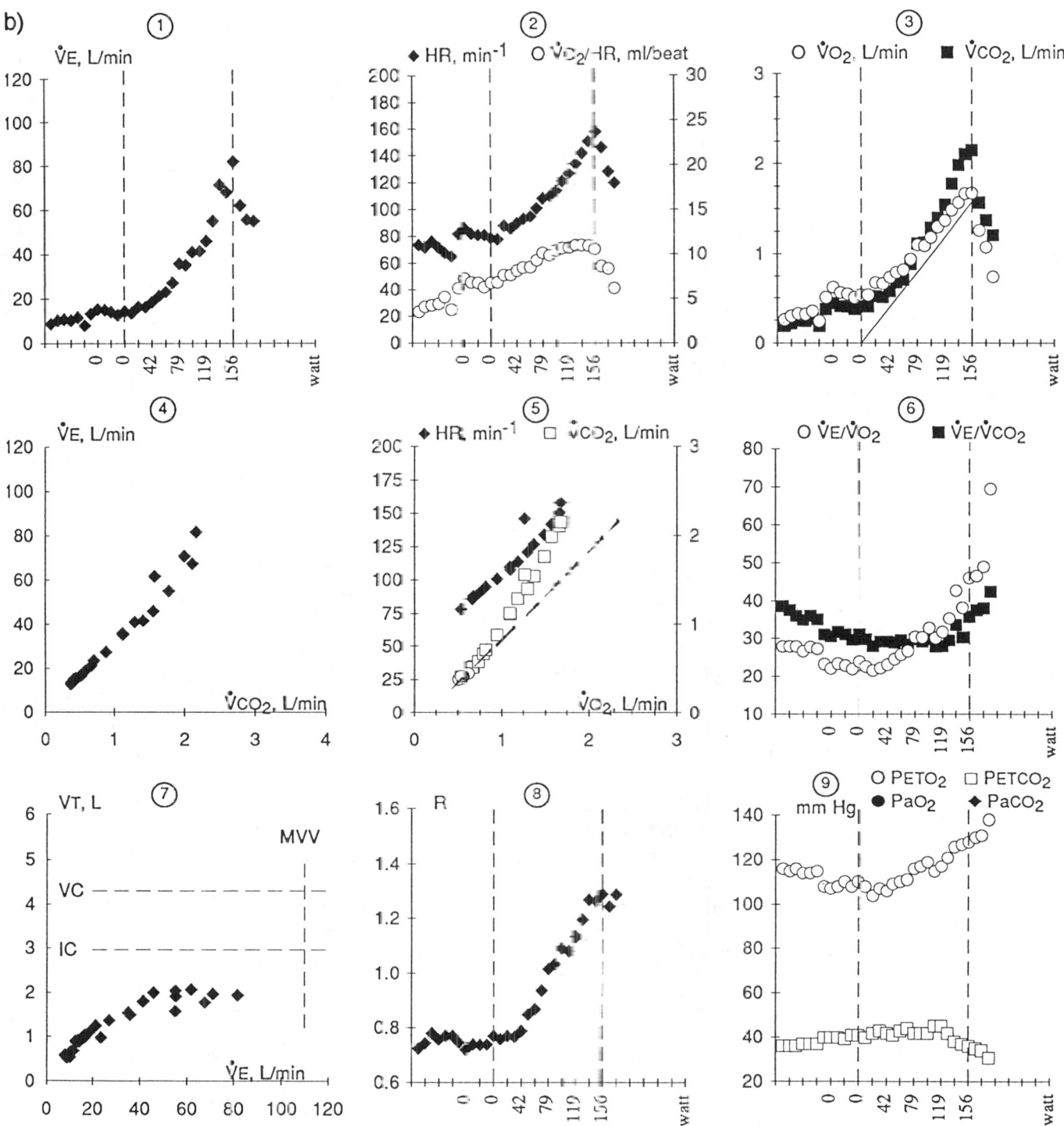

essentially the same and the graphs are almost superimposable. A third test was done 3 months after study b in another exercise laboratory at our institution, this time with right heart catheterization to confirm the low exercise stroke volume of the patient predicted from tests a and b. This third test, with cardiac output, mixed venous and femoral vein blood gases, is shown as case 81 in Chapter 9. Again, the results of the gas exchange studies of this third test are virtually superimposable on the first two, including very similar peak $\dot{V}O_2$, AT and O_2 pulse values. See case 81, Chapter 9 for the predicted normal values for this patient.

problem only when experts reviewed the collected data. Knowing that $\Delta\dot{V}O_2/\Delta WR$ should be 10 ml/min/W in all normal subjects for any increasing work rate exercise test protocol provides an internal calibration of a laboratory and an ability to detect gross errors. Despite this problem in V-Heft II, from the peak $\dot{V}O_2$ in the studies in which the patients performed exercise to work levels above their AT, they concluded that peak $\dot{V}O_2$ was a powerful predictor of the annual mortality rate.

Figure 3.2 and the cases in Chapter 9 show the consistency of the value of $\Delta\dot{V}O_2/\Delta WR$ in all normal subjects. We obtain the same exercise gas exchange measurements when studying the same subject in any of our three hospital laboratories. All give the same results despite different equipment because of the use of trained technicians and the calibration procedures used as described in Chapter 5 and the appendix. Accuracy is further validated by use of a metabolic simulator (107).

The physiological responses to exercise are reproducible in patients with relatively stable pathophysiology. Figure 8.12 shows the first and second tests done at 3-month intervals of a 29-year-old male diagnosed after the first test (Fig. 8.12a) as having a cardiomyopathy. Case 81 in Chapter 9 shows the third evaluation of this man. In the third test (case 81) a right heart and femoral vein and arterial catheterization was done for blood sampling of blood gases and lactate during cardiopulmonary exercise testing. Figure 8.12a and 8.12b show tests 1 and 2 performed on this subject, 6 and 3 months earlier, respectively, in a different laboratory in our institution. Despite the different times and different laboratories, the parameters of aerobic function (e.g., peak $\dot{V}O_2$ and AT) and the cardiovascular and ventilatory changes as related to work rate and metabolism are highly reproducible.

Use of cardiopulmonary exercise testing for assessment of treatment is further illustrated by the case shown in Figure 8.7. This figure illustrates the wealth of information obtained from a single exercise test and sequential exercise testing to evaluate efficacy of epoprostenol treatment in this patient. These studies demonstrate that at the outset of therapy, the patient was totally and critically incapacitated but that she responded to the therapy in a gratifying way. At 8 months, based on improved perfusion to ventilated lung evident from the gas exchange measurements (reduction in $\dot{V}E/\dot{V}CO_2$ and slope of $\dot{V}E$ vs. $\dot{V}CO_2$) and O_2 transport (increase in peak $\dot{V}O_2$, AT and O_2 pulse), she was taken off the lung transplantation list. She had no further

functional gain past test 5 over the succeeding 8 months. Thus she is left with abnormally low peak $\dot{V}O_2$ and O_2 pulse (60% and 70% of predicted, respectively) and high $\dot{V}E/\dot{V}CO_2$ at the AT (third panel down, Fig. 8.7), but with the earlier improvement being sustained. These objective assessments allow her and her physicians to understand her functional disability and capacity much better than without the cardiopulmonary exercise tests.

In Chapter 9, several other cases are presented in which sequential studies helped determine that therapy improved (cases 25, 28, 45, 53, 54, 57) and several in which therapy did not change the exercise pathophysiology (cases 44, 51, 60). Importantly, the cardiopulmonary exercise tests provide the physician with reproducible and objective information needed to evaluate the clinical course of the patient and the effectiveness of therapeutic interventions.

SCREENING FOR DEVELOPMENT OF DISEASE IN HIGH RISK PATIENTS

No investigative studies have been done to our knowledge that take advantage of noninvasive cardiopulmonary exercise testing to detect developing disease in those organ systems whose major function is to transport O_2 to metabolically active cells. A normal peak $\dot{V}O_2$, AT, and $\Delta\dot{V}O_2/\Delta WR$ in response to exercise are required for an individual to function normally. Because these measurements of aerobic function depend on cardiovascular function, sequential measurements of these during cardiopulmonary exercise testing are likely to be the most sensitive measurements that a physician can use to detect the abnormal deterioration of cardiovascular function with time, such as illustrated by cases 13, 19, and 82 in chapter 9. Thus periodic cardiopulmonary exercise tests might be important to perform to detect myocardial ischemia (including silent myocardial ischemia) in people with strong family histories of coronary artery disease.

Similarly, the measurement of the slope of $\dot{V}E$ vs. $\dot{V}CO_2$ and $\dot{V}E/\dot{V}CO_2$, in view of the uniformity of these measurements among different people, would likely be a sensitive noninvasive method to detect the development of pulmonary vascular disease in patients such as those with thromboembolic disease and the pulmonary vasculopathy that leads to primary pulmonary hypertension. In addition, it might be possible to detect the development of any inheritable disease of the muscles or lungs earlier than otherwise possible because of the changing pattern in exercise gas exchange that distinguishes normal from abnormal.

The intimate relationship between O_2 transport and exercise bioenergetics is clear. The normal gas exchange response to exercise is also well defined. Abnormal gas exchange responses to exercise are characteristic for disease in a specific organ system. Thus to detect disease of impaired coupling of external to cellular respiration at an early stage, and possibly prevent serious progression of the illness, a non-invasive cardiopulmonary exercise test is probably the most sensitive, most comprehensive and most cost effective single test available to patients and physicians at this time.

GRADED EXERCISE TESTING AND THE ATHLETE

Training for athletic competition, especially of the endurance kind, owes as much to the accumulated lore of the practices of previously successful athletes as to the application of training strategies based on the results of physiological experimentation. The underlying theme of the various approaches to endurance training, however, is that of stressing the "system" during training beyond the demands of the actual event. How far beyond the power demands of the event and with what patterns of work-rest repetition remains the central issue.

While many approaches will improve performance, the challenge is to determine the optimum pattern: the one that will achieve the greatest improvement in the available time. Laboratory exercise testing of the graded or incremental kind can provide a basis for establishing such a strategy, ensuring that the chosen strategy is successfully accomplished during the training session, and establishing objective criteria to support the physiological benefits of the training scheme.

This is most clearly evident in considering the extremes of event duration: sprints and marathon— and beyond. It is hard to see how knowledge of a subject's $\dot{V}O_2$ max, critical power, anaerobic threshold, etc. can possibly influence the choice of training speeds for a sprinter. Considerations of the recovery kinetics of, for example, muscle or blood lactate (which for the purposes of this discussion we will use as proxy variables for the fatigue-inducing mechanisms) might be beneficial to the choice of interval strategy in the future. Indices of peak and mean power over a short maximum-effort sprint,

such as provided by the Wingate Test (108), offer more in this regard. For example, if these indices show improvement as a result of the training program but performance at the event does not, this would suggest that the athlete's technique be the focus of attention.

For events of marathon duration or longer, the glycogen-squandering aspects of anaerobic glycolysis, and consequent increased rate of lactate production are detrimental to performance. Consequently, a knowledge of the athlete's speed at the *AT*, by an appropriate measurement or estimation technique (including perceptual correlates [109]), can serve both as a means of optimizing the rate at which the event is actually performed (110) and as a frame of reference for a strategy for training at some higher speed that will induce a given degree of lactic acidemia. That is, one that is sustained at some target value aimed at inducing a training effect: in this case to increase the threshold and hence the potential optimum performance rate.

At the intervening "middle distances," knowledge of the subject's profile of aerobic function is likely to be of considerably more importance. Although Newsholme has suggested that muscle glycogen depletion can contribute to fatigue at running events as "short" as 10,000 meters, it is likely that in these events fatigue is a result of metabolites increasing inexorably (locally within muscle [112] and/or sites within the brain [113] at a rate which causes then, or their perceptual consequences, to attain a maximal, and limiting, value at the end of the race).

The upper limit of the work rate at which both $\dot{V}O_2$ and blood lactate can be maintained at a high but constant level has been demonstrated to be the subject's critical power (114). In healthy young subjects, this occurs, on average, at a $\dot{V}O_2$ of approximately 50% of the difference between the *AT* and the peak $\dot{V}O_2$, and at a blood lactate level of approximately 4–5 mM. However, these levels vary among subjects and hence it is important to determine the specific level for a given subject rather than relying on a group mean value to guide training. These profiles will therefore establish whether the training intensity is sufficiently high for the training target and also monitor training-induced improvements. However, it is important to recognize that a particular level of blood lactate, for instance, can be attained either by a relatively low constant-load exercise bout or by work-rest repetitions involving appreciably greater work rates. This allows the recruitment pattern of muscle fibers and the metabolic and acid-base consequences of work to be proportionally manipulated for the training purpose.

Overtraining is also important to the athlete as it can lead to increased risk of infections and depressed immunologic function, in addition to decrements of performance (115). This appears to be a manifestation of prolonged high-intensity training; lower levels can boost immune function. The use of graded exercise testing to establish the upper level of beneficial training intensities and duration should provide insight into the deleterious aspects of inappropriate training.

As more is learned about the physiological mechanisms that trigger "training effects" and how the variables of intensity, duration, and recovery interact to induce the effects (116), laboratory testing will become even more useful in training prescriptions.

SUMMARY

Up until recently, cardiopulmonary exercise testing has not been applied in a general way in medicine because of the time-consuming effort to obtain the useful data. However, with the advent of automated gas analyzers, sensitive measuring devices, and computerized methods to calculate and display the massive amount of useful data that can be obtained from cardiopulmonary exercise tests, it is being recognized as a technology with growing applications. We have used it most effectively for differential diagnosis, including unique diagnoses that cannot be made objectively without cardiopulmonary exercise testing. It takes the guess-work and bias out of differential diagnosis. It also makes impairment evaluation for disability more objective. It has been a very helpful guide in both cardiac and pulmonary rehabilitation for determining both the training work rate and whether improvement in exercise performance had occurred. In recent years, cardiopulmonary exercise testing has been shown to be a more accurate predictor of severity of cardiac illness and predictor of survival time in patients with heart failure than other techniques currently used by cardiologists for grading severity of chronic heart failure. Thus it is now used to prioritize patients for heart transplantation, with peak $\dot{V}O_2$ over-riding other cardiologic measurements. Likely these same guidelines can be applied to lung transplantation in patients with primary pulmonary hypertension and lung diseases.

Cardiopulmonary exercise testing has obvious applications in determining the therapeutic effectiveness of drugs and procedures. Less clear, but obvious in application, is the use of this quantitative approach to detect disease earlier, before it is so advanced that abnormalities develop at rest and are irreversible. The increasing number of applications for which cardiopulmonary exercise testing is currently employed attests to its growing importance in medicine. It has the potential to reduce health care costs by streamlining the diagnostic approach to disease and facilitating treatment decisions.

REFERENCES

1. Higginbotham MB. Diastolic dysfunction and exercise gas exchange. In: Wasserman K, ed. Gas Exchange in Heart Disease. Armonk, NY: Futura Publishing Company, Inc., 1996;39–54.
2. Wasserman K, Zhang YY, Gitt A, Belardinelli R, Koike A, Lubarsky L, Agostini PG. Lung function and exercise gas exchange in chronic heart failure. Circulation 1997;96:2221–2227.
3. Riley M, Nugent A, Steele IC, Bell N, Trimble ER, Nicholls DP, Patterson VH. Gas exchange during exercise in McArdle's disease. J Appl Physiol 1993;75:745–754.
4. Bogaard JM, Scholte HR, Busch FM, Stam H, Versprille A. Anaerobic threshold as detected from ventilatory and metabolic exercise responses in patients with mitochondrial respiratory chain defect. In: Tavassi L, DiPrampero PE eds. Advances in Cardiology. The Anaerobic Threshold: Physiological and Clinical Significance. Basel: Karger, 1986;135–145.
5. Bogaard JM, Busch HFM, Scholte HR, Stam H, Versprille A. Exercise responses in patients with an enzyme deficiency in the mitochrondrial respiratory chain. Eur Respir J 1988;1:445–452.
6. Pardee HEB, DeGraff AG, Della Chapelle CE, Eggleston C, Kossman CE, Maynard E, Schwedel JB, Stewart HJ, Wright IS. Functional capacity classification of patients: In: Nomenclature and criteria for diagnosis of diseases of the heart and blood vessels. New York: New York Heart Association, 1953;81.
7. Matsumura N, Nishijima H, Kojima S, Hashimoto F, Minami M, Yasuda H. Determination of anaerobic threshold for assessment of functional state in patients with chronic heart failure. Circulation 1983;68:360–367.
8. Weber KT, Janicki JS. Cardiopulmonary exercise testing for evaluation of chronic cardiac failure. Am J Cardiol 1985;55:22A-31A.
9. Mudge GH, Goldstein S, Addonizio LJ, Caplan A, Mancini D, Levine TB, Ritsch ME, Stevenson LW. Task Force 3: Recipient Guidelines/Prioritization. J Am Coll Cardiol 1993;22:21–26.
10. Stelken AM, Younis LT, Jennison SH, Miller DD, Miller LW, Shaw LJ, Kargl D, Chaitman BR. Prognostic value of cardiopulmonary exercise testing using percent achieved of predicted peak oxygen uptake for patients with ischemic and dilated cardiomyopathy. J Am Coll Cardiol 1996;27:345–352.

11. Stevenson LW. Role of exercise testing in the evaluation of candidates for cardiac transplantation. In: Wasserman K ed. Exercise Gas Exchange in Heart Disease. Armonk, NY: Futura Publishing Co., 1996;271–286.

12. Mancini D, Eisen H, Kussmaul W, Mull R, Edmunds L, Wilson J. Value of peak exercise oxygen consumption for optimal timing of cardiac transplantation of ambulatory patients with heart failure. Circulation 1991;83:778–786.

13. Likoff MJ, Chandler SL. Clinical determinants of mortality in chronic congestive heart failure secondary to idiopathic dilated or to ischemic cardiomyopathy. Am J Cardiol 1987;59:634–638.

14. Stringer W, Hansen J, Wasserman K. Cardiac output estimated non-invasively from oxygen uptake ($\dot{V}O_2$) during exercise. J Appl Physiol 1997;82:908–912.

15. Sullivan MJ, Knight D, Higginbotham MB, Cobb FR. Relation between central and peripheral hemodynamics during exercise in patients with chronic heart failure. Muscle blood flow is reduced with maintenance of arterial perfusion pressure. Circulation 1989;80:769–781.

16. Agostoni PG, Wasserman K, Perego GB, Marenzi GC, Guazzi M, Assanelli E, Lauri G, Guazzi MD. Oxygen transport to muscle during exercise in chronic congestive heart failure secondary to idiopathic dilated cardiomyopathy. Am J Cardiol 1997;79:1120–4.

17. Sullivan MJ, Hawthorne MH. Exercise intolerance in patients with chronic heart failure. Prog Cardiovasc Dis 1995;38:1–22.

18. Weber KT. Cardiopulmonary exercise testing and the evaluation of systolic dysfunction. In: Wasserman K ed. Exercise Gas Exchange in Heart Disease. Armonk, NY: Futura Publishing Company, 1996;55–62.

19. Itoh H, Taniguichi K, Koike A, Doi M. Evaluation of severity of heart failure using ventilatory gas analysis. Circulation 1990;81(Suppl. II):II31-II37.

20. Koike A, Hiroe M, Adachi H, Yajima T, Nogami A, Ito H, Takamoto T, Taniguichi K, Marumo F. Anaerobic metabolism as an indicator of aerobic function during exercise in cardiac patients. J Am Coll Cardiol 1992; 20:120–126.

21. Rickenbacher PR, Trindade PT, Haywood GA, Vagelos RH, Schroeder JS, Willson K, Prikazsky L., Fowler MB. Transplant candidates with severe left ventricular dysfunction managed with medical treatment: characteristics and survival. J Am Coll Cardiol 1996;27:1192–1197.

22. Szlachic J, Massie BM, Kramer BL, Topic N, Tubau J. Correlates and prognostic indication of exercise capacity in chronic congestive heart failure. Am J Cardiol 1985; 55:1037–1042.

23. Chua TP, Ponikowski P, Harrington D, Anker SD, Webb-Peploe K, Clark AL, Poole-Wilson PA, Coats AJ. Clinical correlates and prognostic significance of the ventilatory response to exercise in chronic heart failure. J Am Coll Cardiol 1997;29:1585–1590.

24. Opasich C, Pinna GD, Bobbio M, Sisti M, Demichelis B, Febo O, Forni G, Riccardi R, Riccardi PG, Capomolla S, Cobelli F, Tavazzi L. Peak exercise oxygen consumption in chronic heart failure: toward efficient use in the individual patient. J Am Coll Cardiol 1998;29:766–775.

25. Costanzo MR, Augustine S, Bourge R, Bristow M,

O'Connell JB, Driscoll D, Rose E. Selection and treatment of candidates for heart transplantation. A statement for health professionals from the Committee on Heart Failure and Cardiac Transplantation of the Council on Clinical Cardiology, American Heart Association. Circulation 1995;92:3593–3612.

26. Mancini DM, Eisen H, Kussmaul W, Mull R, Edmunds LH Jr, Wilson JR. Value of peak exercise oxygen consumption for optimal timing of cardiac transplantation in ambulatory patients with heart failure. Circulation 1991;83:778–786.

27. Aaronson KD, Mancini DM. Is percentage of predicted maximal oxygen consumption a better predictor of survival than peak exercise oxygen consumption for patients with severe heart failure? J Heart Lung Transplant 1995;14:981–989.

28. Roul G, Moulichon ME, Bareiss P, Gries P, Sacrez J, Germain P, Messard JM, Sacrez A. Exercise peak $\dot{V}O_2$ determination in chronic heart failure: is it still of value? Eur Heart J 1994;15:495–502.

29. Osada N, Chaitman BR, Miller LW, Yip D, Cishek MB, Wolford TL, Donohue TJ. Cardiopulmonary exercise testing identifies low risk patients with heart failure and severely impaired exercise capacity considered for heart transplation. J Am Coll Cardiol 1998;31:577–582.

30. Kao W, Winkel EM, Johnson MR, Piccione W, Lichtenberg R, Costanzo MR. Role of maximal oxygen consumption in establishment of heart transplant candidacy for heart failure patients with intermediate exercise tolerance. Am J Cardiol 1997;79:1124–1127.

31. Stevenson LW, Steimle AE, Fonarow G, Kermani M, Kermani D, Hamilton MA, Moriguchi JD, Walden J, Tillisch JH, Drinkwater DC, Laks H. Improvement in exercise capacity of candidates awaiting heart transplantation. J Am Coll Cardiol 1995;25:163–170.

32. Meyers J, Gullestad L, Vagelos R, Do D, Bellin D, Ross H, Fowler MB. Clinical, hemodynamic, and cardiopulmonary exercise test determinants of survival in patients referred for evaluation of heart failure. Ann Intern Med 1998; 129:286–293.

33. Olsen GN, Weiman DS, Bolton JWR, Gass GD, Mclain WC, Schoonover GA, Hornung CA. Submaximal invasive exercise testing and quantitative lung scanning in the evaluation for tolerance of lung resection. Chest 1989;95:267–273.

34. Olsen GN. The evolving role of exercise testing prior to lung resection. Chest 1989;9:218–225.

35. Olsen GN. Preoperative physiology and lung resection (editorial). Chest 1992;101:300–301.

36. Miyoshi S, Nakahara K, Ohno K, Monden Y, Kawashima Y. Exercise tolerance in lung cancer patients: the relationship between exercise capacity and postthoracotomy hospital mortality. Ann Thor Surg 1987;44:487–490.

37. Gilbreth EM, Weisman IM. Role of exercise stress testing in preoperative evaluation of patients for lung resection. Clin Chest Med 1994;15:389–403.

38. Sue DY, Wasserman K. Impact of integrative cardiopulmonary exercise testing on clinical decision making. Chest 1991;99:981–992.

39. Wasserman K. Preoperative evaluation of cardiovascular exercise training on clinical decision making. Chest 1993;104:663–664.

40. Smith TP, Kinasewitz GT, Tucker WY, Spillers WP, George WP. Exercise capacity as a predictor of post-thoracotomy morbidity. Am Rev Respir Dis 1984; 129:730–734.

41. Bechard D, Wetstein L. Assessment of exercise oxygen consumption as preoperative criterion for lung resection. Ann Thor Surg 1987;44:344–349.

42. Bolliger CT, Jordan P, Soler M, Stulz P, Gradel E, Skarvan K, Elsasser S, Gonon M, Wyser C, Tamm M, et al. Exercise capacity as a predictor of postoperative complications in lung resection candidates. Am J Respir Crit Care Med 1995; 151:1472–1480.

43. Bolliger CT, Wyser C, Roser H, Soler M, Perruchoud AP. Lung scanning and exercise testing for the prediction of postoperative performance in lung resection candidates at increased risk for complications. Chest 1995; 108:341–348.

44. Morice RC, Peters EJ, Ryan MB, Putnam JB, Ali MK, Rith JA. Exercise testing in the evaluation of patients at high risk for complications from lung resection. Chest 1992;101:356–361.

45. Nakagawa K, Nakahara K, Miyoshi S, Kawashima Y. Oxygen transport during incremental exercise load as a predictor of operative risk in lung cancer patients. Chest 1992;101:1369–1375.

46. Pate P, Tenholder MF, Griffin JP, Eastridge CE, Weiman DS. Preoperative assessment of the high-risk patient for lung resection. Ann Thor Surg 1996;61:1494–1500.

47. Larsen KR, Svendsen UG, Milman N, Brenoe J, Petersen BN. Cardiopulmonary function at rest and during exercise after resection for bronchial carcinoma. Ann Thor Surg 1997;64:960–964.

48. Pelletier C, Lapointe L, LeBlanc P. Effects of lung resection on pulmonary function and exercise capacity. Thorax 1990;45:497–502.

49. Bolliger CT, Perruchoud AP. Functional evaluation of lung resection candidate. Eur Respir J 1998;11:198–212.

50. Older P, Smith R, Courtney P, Hone R. Preoperative evaluation of cardiac failure and ischemia in elderly patients by cardiopulmonary exercise testing. Chest 1993;104:701–704.

51. Epstein SK, Faling LJ, Daly BD, Celli BR. Predicting complications after pulmonary resection. Preoperative exercise testing vs. a multifactorial cardiopulmonary risk index. Chest 1993;104:694–700.

52. Holden DA, Rice TW, Stelmach K, Meeker DP. Exercise testing, 6-min walk, and stair climb in the evaluation of patients at high risk for pulmonary resection. Chest 1992;102:1774–1779.

53. Renzetti AD, Bleecker ER, Epler GR, Jones RN, Kanner RE, Repsher LH. Evaluation of impairment/disability secondary to respiratory disorders. Am Rev Respir Dis 1986;133:1205–1209.

54. Wood PH. Appreciating the consequences of disease: International classification of impairments, disabilities, and handicaps. Who Chronicle 1980;34:376–380.

55. Campbell SC. A comparison of the maximum volume ventilation with forced expiratory volume in one second: an assessment of subject cooperation. J Occup Med 1982;24:531–533.

56. Gandevia B, Hugh-Jones P. Terminology for measurements of ventilatory capacity. Thorax 1957;1:290–293.

57. Cotes JE, Zejda J, King B. Lung function impairment as a guide to exercise limitation in work-related lung disorders. Am Rev Respir Dis 1988;137:1089–1093.

58. Agostoni P, Smith DD, Schoene RGB, Robertson HT, Butler J. Evaluation of breathlessness in asbestos workers. Am Rev Respir Dis 1987;135:812–816.

59. Agusti AGN, Roca J, Rodriguez-Roisin R, Xaubet A, Agusti-Vidal A. Different patterns of gas exchange response to exercise in asbestos and idiopathic pulmonary fibrosis. Eur Respir J 1988;1:510–516.

60. Howard J, Mohsenifar Z, Brown HV, Koerner SK. Role of exercise testing in assessing functional respiratory impairment due to asbestos exposure. J Occup Med 1982;24:685–689.

61. Markos J, Musk AW, Finucane KE. Functional similarities of asbestosis and cryptogenic fibrosing alveolitis. Thorax 1988;43:708–714.

62. Oren A, Sue DY, Hansen JE, Torrance DJ, Wasserman K. The role of exercise testing in impairment evaluation. Am Rev Respir Dis 1987;135:230–235.

63. Pearle J. Exercise performance and functional impairment in asbestos-exposed workers. Chest 1981;80: 701–705.

64. Risk C, Epler GR, Gaensler EA. Exercise alveolar-arterial oxygen pressure difference in interstitial lung disease. Chest 1984;85:69–74.

65. Sue DY, Oren A, Hansen JE, Wasserman K. Lung function and exercise performance in smoking and non-smoking asbestos-exposed workers. Am Rev Respir Dis 1985;132:612–618.

66. Wiedemann HP, Gee JBL, Balmes JR. Exercise testing in occupational lung disease. Clin Chest Med 1984; 5:157–171.

67. Ortega F, Montemayor T, Sanchez A, Cabello F, Castillo J. Role of cardiopulmonary exercise testing and the criteria used to determine disability in patients with severe chronic obstructive pulmonary disease. Am J Respir Crit Care Med 1994;150:747–751.

68. Cotes JE. Rating respiratory disability: a report on behalf of a working group of the European Society for Clinical Respiratory Physiology. Eur Respir J 1990;3:1074–1077.

69. Saltin B, Gollnick PD. Skeletal muscle adaptability: significance for metabolism and performance. In: Handbook of Physiology. Washington D.C.: Am Physiol Soc, 1986;555.

70. Anderson P, Henriksson J. Training induced changes in the subgroups of human type II skeletal muscle fibers. Acta Physiol Scand 1977;99:123–125.

71. Holloszy JO. Adaptation of skeletal muscle to endurance exercise. Med Sci Sports 1975;7:155–164.

72. Pattengale PK, Holloszy JO. Augmentation of skeletal muscle myoglobin by a program of treadmill running. Am J Physiol 1967;213:783–785.

73. Saltin B, Henriksson J, Nygaard E, Andersen P, Jansson E. Fiber types and metabolic potentials of skeletal muscles in sedentary men and endurance runners. Ann NY Acad Sci 1977;301:3–29.

74. Henriksson J. Training induced adaptation of skeletal muscle and metabolism during submaximal exercise. J Physiol 1977;270:661–675.

75. McArdle WD, Katch FI, Pechar GS. Comparison of continuous and discontinuous treadmill and bicycle tests for max $\dot{V}O_2$. Med Sci Sports Exerc 1972;5:156–160.

76. Clausen JP, Klausen K, Rasmussen B, Trap-Jersen J. Central and peripheral circulatory changes after training of the arms and legs. Am J Physiol 1973;225:675–682.

77. Saltin B. Cardiovascular and pulmonary adaptation to physical activity. In: Exercise, Fitness, and Health. A Consensus of Current Knowledge. Champaign, IL: Human Kinetics, 1990;187.

78. Pollock ML, Miller HS, Janeway R. Effects of walking on body composition and cardiovascular function of middle-aged men. J Appl Physiol 1971;30:126–130.

79. Pollock ML, Wilmore JH. Exercise in Health and Disease. Philadelphia: Saunders, 1990.

80. Casaburi R, Storer TW, Ben-Dov I, Wasserman K. Effect of endurance training on possible determinants of $\dot{V}O_2$ during heavy exercise. J Appl Physiol 1987;62:199–207.

81. Casaburi R, Storer TW, Wasserman K. Mediation of reduced ventilatory response to exercise after endurance training. J Appl Physiol 1987;63:1533–1538.

82. Sullivan CS, Casaburi R, Storer TW, Wasserman K. Prediction of blood lactate response to constant power outputs. Eur J Appl Physiol 1995;71:349–354.

83. Poole DC, Barstow TJ, Gaesser GA, Willis WT, Whipp BJ. $\dot{V}O_2$ slow component: physiological and functional significance. Med Sci Sports Exerc 1994;26:1354–1358.

84. Casaburi R, Whipp BJ, Wasserman K, Beaver WL, Koyal SN. Ventilatory and gas exchange dynamics in response to sinusoidal work. J Appl Physiol 1977;42:300–311.

85. Winder WW, Hickson RC, Hagberg JA, Ehsani AA, McLane JA. Training-induced changes in hormonal and metabolic responses to submaximal exercise. J Appl Physiol 1979;46:766–771.

86. Sutton JR, Farrell PS, Harber VJ. Hormonal adaptation to physical activity. In: Exercise, Fitness, and Health. Champaign, IL: Human Kinetics Books, 1990;217.

87. Gisolfi C, Robinson S. Relations between physical training, acclimatization and heat tolerance. J Appl Physiol 1969;26:530–534.

88. Hill DW, Cureton KJ, Grisham SC, Collins MA. Effect of training on the rating on perceived exertion at the ventilatory threshold. Eur J Appl Physiol 1987;56:206–211.

89. Haas F, Schicchi JS, Axen K. Desensitization to dyspnea in chronic obstructive pulmonary disease. In: Casaburi R, Petty TL, eds. Principles and Practice of Pulmonary Rehabilitation. Philadelphia: Saunders, 1993;241–251.

90. Itoh H, Kato K. Short-term exercise training after cardiac surgery. In: Wasserman K, ed. Exercise Gas Exchange in Heart Disease. Armonk, NY: Futura Publishing Company, 1996;229–244.

91. ACSM's Guidelines for Exercise Testing and Prescription. Baltimore: Williams & Wilkins, 1995;151–235.

92. Dubach P, Myers J, Dziekan G, Goebbels U, Reinhart W, Vogt P, Ratti R, Muller P, Miettunen R, Buser P. Effect of exercise training on myocardial remodeling in patients with reduced left ventricular function after myocardial infarction. Circulation 1997;95:2060–2067.

93. McKelvie R, Teo KK, McCartney N, Humen D, Montague T, Yusuf S. Effects of exercise training in patients with congestive heart failure: a critical review. J Am Coll Cardiol 1995;25:789–796.

94. Belardinelli R, Georgiou D, Cianci G, Berman N, Ginzton L, Purcaro A. Exercise training improves left ventricular diastolic filling in patients with dilated cardiomyopathy. Circulation 1995;91:2775–2784.

95. Ries AL, Carlin BW, Carrieri-Kohlman V, Casaburi R, Celli BR, Emery CF, Hodgkin JE, Mahler DA, Make B. Pulmonary rehabilitation: evidence based guidelines. Chest 1997;112:1363–1396.

96. Casaburi R. Exercise training in chronic obstructive lung disease. In: Casaburi R, Petty TL, eds. Principles and Practice of Pulmonary Rehabilitation. Philadelphia: Saunders, 1993;204–224.

97. Orenstein DM, Noyes BE. Cystic fibrosis. In: Casaburi R, Petty TL, eds. Principles and Practice of Pulmonary Rehabilitation. Philadelphia: Saunders, 1993;439–458.

98. Clark CJ. The role of physical training in asthma. In: Casaburi R, Petty TL, eds. Principles and Practice of Pulmonary Rehabilitation. Philadelphia: Saunders, 1993;424–438.

99. Whipp BJ, Casaburi R. Physical activity, fitness and chronic lung disease. In: Boucher C, Shephard RJ, Stephens T, eds. Physical Activity, Fitness and Health. Champaign, IL: Human Kinetics, 1994;749–761.

100. Wasserman K, Sue DY, Moricca RB, Casaburi R. Selection criteria for exercise training in pulmonary rehabilitation. Eur J Appl Physiol 1989;2(Suppl 7):S604-S610.

101. Casaburi R. Deconditioning. In: Fishman AP, ed. Pulmonary Rehabilitation. Lung Biology in Health and Disease Series. New York: Marcel Dekker, 1996;213–230.

102. Belman MJ. Exercise training in chronic obstructive pulmonary disease. Clin Chest Med 1986;7:585–597.

103. Ries AL, Archibald CJ. Endurance exercise training at maximal targets in patients with chronic obstructive pulmonary disease. J Cardiopulm Rehabil 1987;7:594–601.

104. Casaburi R, Patessio A, Ioli F, Zanaboni S, Donner C, Wasserman K. Reductions in exercise lactic acidosis and ventilation as a result of exercise training in patients with obstructive lung disease. Am Rev Respir Dis 1991;143:9–18.

105. Casaburi R, Porszasz J, Burns MR, Carithers ER, Chang RSY, Cooper CB. Physiologic benefits of exercise training in rehabilitation of severe COPD patients. Am J Respir Crit Care Med 1997;155:1541–1551.

106. Cohn JN, Ziesche S, Johnson G, Cobb F. Use of exercise gas exchange measurements in multicenter drug studies. In: Wasserman K, ed. Exercise Gas Exchange in Heart Disease. Armonk, NY: Futura Publishing Company, Inc., 1996;245–256.

107. Huszczuk A, Whipp BJ, Wasserman K. A respiratory gas

exchange simulator for routine calibration in metabolic studies. Eur Respir J 1990;3:465–468.

108. Bar-Or O. The Wingate test. An update on methodology, reliability and validity. Sports Med 1987;4:381–394.

109. Cafarelli E. Sensory processes and endurance performance. In: Shephard RJ, Astrand PO, eds. Endurance in Sport. Oxford: Blackwell Scientific, 1992;261–269.

110. Zoladz JA, Sargeant AJ, Emmerich J, Stoklosa J, Zychowski A. Changes in acid-base status of marathon runners during incremental field test. Eur J Appl Physiol 1993; 67:71–76.

111. Newsholme EA, Blomstrand E, Ekblom B. Physical and mental fatigue: metabolic mechanisms and importance of plasma amino acids. Br Med Bull 1992;48:477–495.

112. Sargeant AJ, Beelen A. Human muscle fatigue in dynamic exercise. In: Sargeant AJ, Kernell D, eds. Neuro-

muscular Fatigue. Amsterdam: North Holland Publishers, 1992;81–92.

113. Newsholme E, Castell LM. Can amino acids influence exercise performance in athletes? In: Steinacker J, Ward SA, eds. The Physiology and Pathophysiology of Exercise Tolerance. New York: Plenum Press, 1996;269–274.

114. Poole DC, Ward SA, Gardner GW, Whipp BJ. Metabolic and respiratory profile of the upper limit for prolonged exercise in man. Ergonomics 1988;31:1265–1279.

115. Hoffman-Goetz L, Pedersen BK. Exercise and the immune system: a model of the stress response? Immunol Today 1994;15:382–387.

116. Banister EW, Morton RH, Fitz-Clarke JR. Clinical dose-response effects of exercise. In: Steinacker J, Ward SA, eds. The Physiology and Pathophysiology of Exercise Tolerance. New York: Plenum Press, 1996;297–309.

CHAPTER 9

Case Presentations

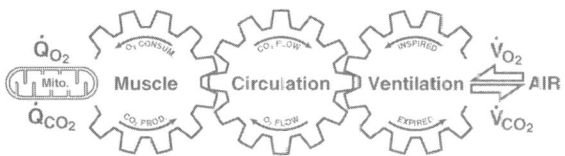

We selected the cases presented in this section because they are either representative of specific pathophysiology or they teach a unique lesson. They were not selected because they show data from especially cooperative subjects or are pretty records. In fact, these studies were done on typical patients evaluated in our clinical exercise laboratory and therefore include records that range between the best and the worst with respect to appearance. The primary goal of this chapter is to offer a systematic approach to interpretation of exercise performance. We demonstrate how measurements can be used as decision-making branchpoints for reaching an appropriate diagnosis and how to apply these measurements to a range of abnormalities that lead to exercise intolerance.

The data given in these case presentations are restricted to information needed to interpret the exercise test. Generally, two sets of resting blood gas data are included in Table 3 of each report. The first is obtained with the subject sitting on the ergometer but before breathing on the mouthpiece (i.e., without accompanying respiratory gas exchange data), and the second is obtained with the subject on the ergometer while breathing on the mouthpiece prior to exercise (i.e., with accompanying gas exchange data). Both sets of data are reported for comparison, when available.

The graphic data given with each case display data points every 30 seconds, calculated as the average of whole breath-by-breath measurements over the preceding 15- to 20-second period. The protocol is shown on panels 1, 2, 3, 6, 8, and 9 of these figures in which the abscissa is the work rate increase. After a period of rest and unloaded pedalling (0 W), the work rate is increased in equal increments each minute or in a ramp pattern. The time at which the work rate is being progressively increased begins at the left vertical dashed line, and the termination of exercise is indicated by the right vertical dashed line. Two minutes of recovery data are also plotted. In panel 3, work rate is scaled to be 1/10 of that of $\dot{V}O_2$. Thus, when the $\dot{V}O_2$ increase exactly parallels the work rate increase, $\Delta\dot{V}O_2/\Delta$ work rate = 10 ml/min/W. Interrelated ventilatory and cardiovascular variables are plotted on panels 4, 5, and 7 during rest and exercise, but not recovery. In panel 5, the mean predicted peak $\dot{V}O_2$ and maximum HR for a sedentary person of the same sex, age, and body size are marked with an "X." Moreover, plotted on panel 5 is $\dot{V}CO_2$ as a function of $\dot{V}O_2$. The dashed diagonal line through this plot has a slope of 1. Thus, when $\dot{V}CO_2$ versus $\dot{V}O_2$ increases more steeply than this line, the $\dot{V}O_2$ is above the subject's anaerobic threshold, and the break-point is the anaerobic threshold. In each case, the summary data shown in second Table are taken from the third Table (and the fourth Table, if provided) and the Figure(s).

The predicted values given for each case are the mean values taken from Chapter 6. As with any predicted values, there are normal ranges. To the best of our judgement, our interpretations take the range of normal values into account.

Eighty-three cases are presented for interpretation. Practical considerations limited our ability to provide more examples, and of course, there are many disorders of exercise performance that we have not studied directly. Because each category of disease can have perturbations that are instructive to review, we found it desirable sometimes to present more than one case example of each type of disorder. Moreover, patients frequently have more than one abnormality. Thus, we thought it important to present some of these complex cases and to provide the rationale for our conclusions regarding the dominant pathophysiology.

Of the 83 cases, the first 15 are of men and women whom we concluded were normal at the time of the initial study. They were selected to show the effect of age, gender, form of ergometry used for testing, effect of O_2 breathing, effect of β-adrenergic blockade, effect of obesity, and effect of cigarette smoking on the test results.

Cases 16 to 29 are examples of coronary artery disease, valvular heart disease, cardiomyopathies, and congenital heart disease. Other examples of heart diseases are provided in the "complex" case category described later.

Cases 30 to 35 are examples of peripheral arterial diseases. Again, some examples are included in the "complex" case category because these disorders are commonly associated with primary heart disease.

Cases 36 to 45 include several types and severity of diseases primarily associated with airflow obstruction. Other examples of obstructive airway disease can be found in the "complex" category.

Cases 46 to 58 are examples of pulmonary fibrosis or respiratory restriction of various causes or identified as idiopathic. Two cases show results before and after treatment.

Cases 59 to 64 are examples of chronic pulmonary vascular diseases of several types. Two of the major roles of exercise testing are diagnosis and the noninvasive evaluation of the effect of therapy in these disorders. Other examples of pulmonary vascular diseases are presented in the group of patients with lung diseases.

Cases 65 to 67 are examples of subjects who were classified as having made a poor effort during exercise testing. It was concluded that they did not have evidence of organic disease reducing exercise tolerance.

Examples of disorders of the respiratory "pump" are presented in cases 68 to 70. These disorders can be found in many forms, and the three cases presented are representative.

Cases 71 to 79 are among the most challenging in that these are patients with multiple abnormalities (complex cases). We have analyzed these cases with the intent of diagnosing the limiting disorder or disorders.

Case 80 is a young lady with primary pulmonary hypertension. This case highlights the abnormalities that can be used to track the progress of the patient's disorder.

Cases 81 and 82 are two men with heart disease. The first is a young man with a restrictive cardiomyopathy, the diagnosis first made by cardiopulmonary exercise testing and later documented with cardiac catheterization. The second shows a senior citizen who transitioned from normal to cardiomyopathy, thought to be based on diastolic dysfunction. Case 83 is an example of psychogenic dyspnea complicated by an impaired ability to increase cardiac output due to heavy beta-adrenergic blockade.

In a few instances, the conclusions we reached in the Case Analysis will not be obtained easily from the logical sequence suggested by the flow charts (Chapter 7). Nevertheless, we started each analysis by applying the flow chart logic. The supporting data listed under each diagnosis in the flow chart should always be used to confirm the diagnosis derived from the flow chart analysis.

This section is intended to provide examples of cardiorespiratory disorders that reduce exercise tolerance and the pathophysiology that accompanies each disorder. Cases with arterial blood gas measurements were preferred in the case selection process for inclusion in this book so that the effect of exercise on arterial blood gases can be illustrated in health and disease. Because of the variety of conditions that can interfere with the coupling of external to cellular respiration, it is not possible to include examples of all conditions that limit exercise in the case selection. Nevertheless, we hope that the principles taught by the cases selected and the preparatory chapters provide the reader with the necessary physiologic background to interpret the many pathophysiologic conditions that lead to exercise intolerance.

Case 1 Normal Man
Clinical Findings

This 55-year-old executive was referred for exercise testing because of his complaint of decreased exercise tolerance. He complained of weakness, fatigue, and some dyspnea after jogging 1 block, but he could walk 3 miles on the level without difficulty. He had become symptomatic after recovery from an ankle injury 2 years earlier and felt unable to satisfactorily improve his exercise tolerance. He did not report chest pain, syncope, palpitations, coughing, or wheezing. He had smoked half a pack of cigarettes per day for 10 years but had reduced his smoking to 3 to 4 cigarettes per week. He took no medications. Physical examination, chest roentgenograms, and resting ECG were normal.

Exercise Findings

The patient performed exercise on a cycle ergometer. He pedalled at 60 rpm without added load for 3 minutes. The work rate was then increased 20 W per minute to his symptom-limited maximum. Arterial blood was sampled every second minute, and intra-arterial blood pressure was recorded from a percutaneously placed brachial artery catheter. The patient stopped exercise because of thigh fatigue. Twelve-lead ECG recordings remained normal during exercise.

TABLE 9.1.1. Selected Respiratory Function Data

Measurement	Predicted	Measured
Age, yr		55
Sex		Male
Height, cm		182
Weight, kg	83	80
Hematocrit, %		41
VC, L	4.75	6.06
IC, L	3.17	4.16
TLC, L	7.08	8.24
FEV_1, L	3.76	4.52
FEV_1/VC, %	79	75
MVV, L/min	151	200
D_LCO, ml/mm Hg/min	28.8	28.3

TABLE 9.1.2. Selected Exercise Data

Measurement	Predicted	Measured
Peak $\dot{V}O_2$, L/min	2.47	2.53
Maximum HR, beats/min	165	176
Maximum O_2 pulse, ml/beat	15.0	14.5
$\Delta\dot{V}O_2/\Delta WR$, ml/min/W	10.3	9.8
AT, L/min	>1.07	1.2
Blood pressure, mmHg (rest, max)		144/81, 225/87
Maximum $\dot{V}E$, L/min		107
Exercise breathing reserve, L/min	>15	93
PaO_2, mmHg (rest, max ex)		98, 110
$P(A - a)O_2$, mmHg (rest, max ex)		5, 15
$P(a - ET)CO_2$, mmHg (rest, max ex)		0, −5
VD/VT (rest, heavy ex)		0.26, 0.15
HCO_3^-, mEq/L (rest, 2-min recov)		25, 12

FIGURE 9.1.1.

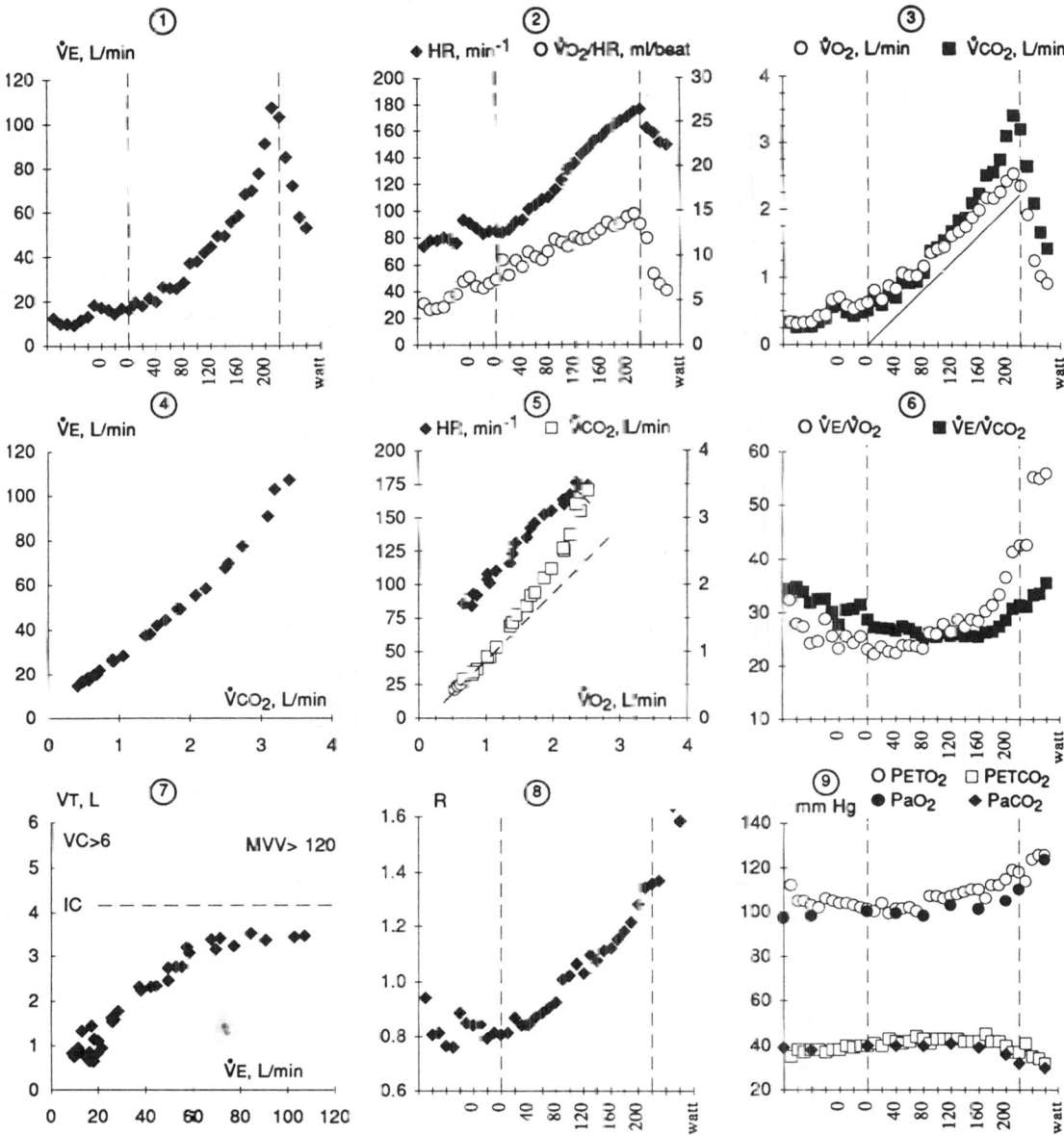

1. Vertical dashed lines in panels 1 to 3 and 6, 8, and 9 indicate the beginning and the end of increasing work period.
2. Unloaded cycling is performed for 3 minutes before the left vertical dashed line.
3. In panel 3, the diagonal line shows the increase of $\dot{V}O_2$ at a slope of 10 ml/min/W.
4. In panel 5, the diagonal dashed line has a slope of 1.

TABLE 9.1.3. Air Breathing

Time min	Work rate watts	BP mmHg	HR min⁻¹	f min⁻¹	$\dot{V}_E$ L/min BTPS	$\dot{V}_{CO_2}$ L/min STPD	$\dot{V}_{O_2}$ L/min STPD	$\dot{V}_{O_2}$/HR ml/beat	R	pH	HCO₃⁻ meq/L	Po₂ ET	Po₂ a	Po₂ (A−a)	Pco₂ ET	Pco₂ a	Pco₂ (a−ET)	$\dot{V}_E/\dot{V}_{CO_2}$	$\dot{V}_E/\dot{V}_{O_2}$	VD/VT
	Rest	153/87								7.42	25		97			39				
	Rest		74	14	12.2	0.32	0.34	4.6	0.94			112			35			34	32	
	Rest		78	13	9.8	0.25	0.31	4.0	0.81			105			38			35	28	
	Rest		78	13	9.9	0.26	0.32	4.1	0.81			105			37			34	27	
	Rest	144/81	80	11	9.2	0.26	0.34	4.3	0.76	7.42	24	103	93	5	38	38	0	32	24	0.26
	Rest		79	12	11.4	0.32	0.42	5.3	0.76			102			38			32	25	
	Rest		76	10	13.2	0.38	0.43	5.7	0.88			105			37			33	29	
	Unloaded		93	16	18.2	0.56	0.66	7.1	0.85			105			38			30	26	
	Unloaded		91	12	17.1	0.58	0.69	7.6	0.84			104			38			28	23	
	Unloaded		87	19	16.2	0.48	0.57	6.6	0.84			104			40			30	26	
	Unloaded		83	19	14.5	0.42	0.53	6.4	0.79			103			39			31	24	
	Unloaded		85	22	16.9	0.48	0.59	6.9	0.81			102			40			31	25	
	Unloaded	171/87	85	25	16.4	0.50	0.62	7.3	0.81	7.41	25	101	100	2	40	40	0	29	23	0.21
0.5	20		84	24	19.7	0.65	0.80	9.5	0.81			100			41			27	22	
1.0	20		86	28	18.1	0.58	0.67	7.8	0.87			104			40			27	23	
1.5	40		92	23	21.6	0.73	0.87	9.5	0.84			99			43			27	23	
2.0	40	183/84	93	18	19.9	0.69	0.82	8.8	0.84	7.40	24	101	99	5	42	40	−2	27	22	0.18
2.5	60		101	17	26.7	0.92	1.06	10.5	0.87			101			41			27	24	
3.0	60		104	17	26.0	0.91	1.03	9.9	0.88			102			42			27	24	
3.5	80		108	16	25.8	0.93	1.03	9.5	0.90			100			44			26	24	
4.0	80	195/81	110	16	28.4	1.07	1.16	10.5	0.92	7.38	23	103	98	9	43	40	−3	25	23	0.14
4.5	100		116	16	37.3	1.38	1.37	11.8	1.01			107			41			26	26	
5.0	100		123	17	38.1	1.44	1.41	11.5	1.02			107			43			25	26	
5.5	120		131	18	42.0	1.54	1.45	11.1	1.06			106			43			26	28	
6.0	120	207/87	135	19	44.5	1.67	1.62	12.0	1.03	7.37	23	107	103	7	43	41	−2	26	26	0.17
6.5	140		142	18	49.4	1.83	1.67	11.8	1.10			108			43			26	29	
7.0	140		146	20	49.4	1.87	1.74	11.9	1.07			109			42			26	27	
7.5	160		152	20	55.5	2.09	1.88	12.4	1.11			110			42			26	29	
8.0	160	213/90	155	19	58.3	2.23	1.99	12.8	1.12	7.35	21	110	101	13	42	39	−3	25	28	0.13
8.5	180		160	20	67.7	2.51	2.18	13.6	1.15			106			45			26	30	
9.0	180		163	22	69.5	2.55	2.16	13.3	1.18			112			42			27	31	
9.5	200		167	24	77.3	2.74	2.26	13.5	1.21			112			42			27	33	
10.0	200	225/87	170	27	90.7	3.10	2.42	14.2	1.28	7.31	18	115	105	15	40	36	−4	29	37	0.16
10.5	220		174	31	107.2	3.40	2.53	14.5	1.34			119			37			31	41	
11.0	220	216/90	176	30	102.9	3.20	2.36	13.4	1.36	7.30	15	118	110	15	37	32	−5	31	43	0.14
	Recovery		162	24	84.3	2.64	1.93	11.9	1.37			114			41			31	43	
	Recovery		158	21	71.5	2.10	1.26	8.0	1.67			124			35			33	55	
	Recovery		151	18	57.6	1.67	1.02	6.8	1.64			126			34			34	55	
	Recovery	165/75	149	19	52.7	1.44	0.91	6.1	1.58	7.22	12	126	124	5	32	30	−2	35	56	0.18

Interpretation

Comments

The results of the respiratory function studies are within normal limits (Table 9.1.1).

Analysis

Referring to flow chart 1 (Chapter 7), the peak $\dot{V}_{O_2}$ and anaerobic threshold are normal (Table 9.1.2).

See flow chart 2. The ECG and arterial blood gases (Table 9.1.3) are normal throughout exercise; the O_2-pulse at the maximum work rate is normal.

Conclusion

This is a normal man, with high level of anxiety regarding his physical status.

Case 2 Normal Athlete

Clinical Findings

This 31-year-old physiologist was a frequent marathon runner. He had no known health problems and trained several times weekly.

Exercise Findings

The subject performed exercise on a cycle ergometer. He pedalled without added load at 60 rpm for 2 minutes. The work rate was then increased 30 W every minute to his symptom-limited maximum. There were no arrhythmias, and the ECG remained normal.

TABLE 9.2.1.   Selected Respiratory Function Data

Measurement	Predicted	Measured
Age, yr		31
Sex		Male
Height, cm		182
Weight, kg	83	81
Hematocrit, %		43
VC, L	5.48	6.27
IC, L	3.65	3.56
FEV$_1$, L	4.43	4.51
FEV$_1$/VC, %	81	72
MVV, L/min	182	185

TABLE 9.2.2.   Selected Exercise Data

Measurement	Predicted	Measured
Peak $\dot{V}O_2$, L/min	3.22	4.95
Maximum HR, beats/min	189	175
Maximum O_2 pulse, ml/beat	17.0	28.3
$\Delta \dot{V}O_2/\Delta WR$, ml/min/W	10.3	11.5
AT, L/min	>1.32	2.5
Maximum $\dot{V}E$, L/min		186
Exercise breathing reserve, L/min	>15	−1

Figure 9.2.1.

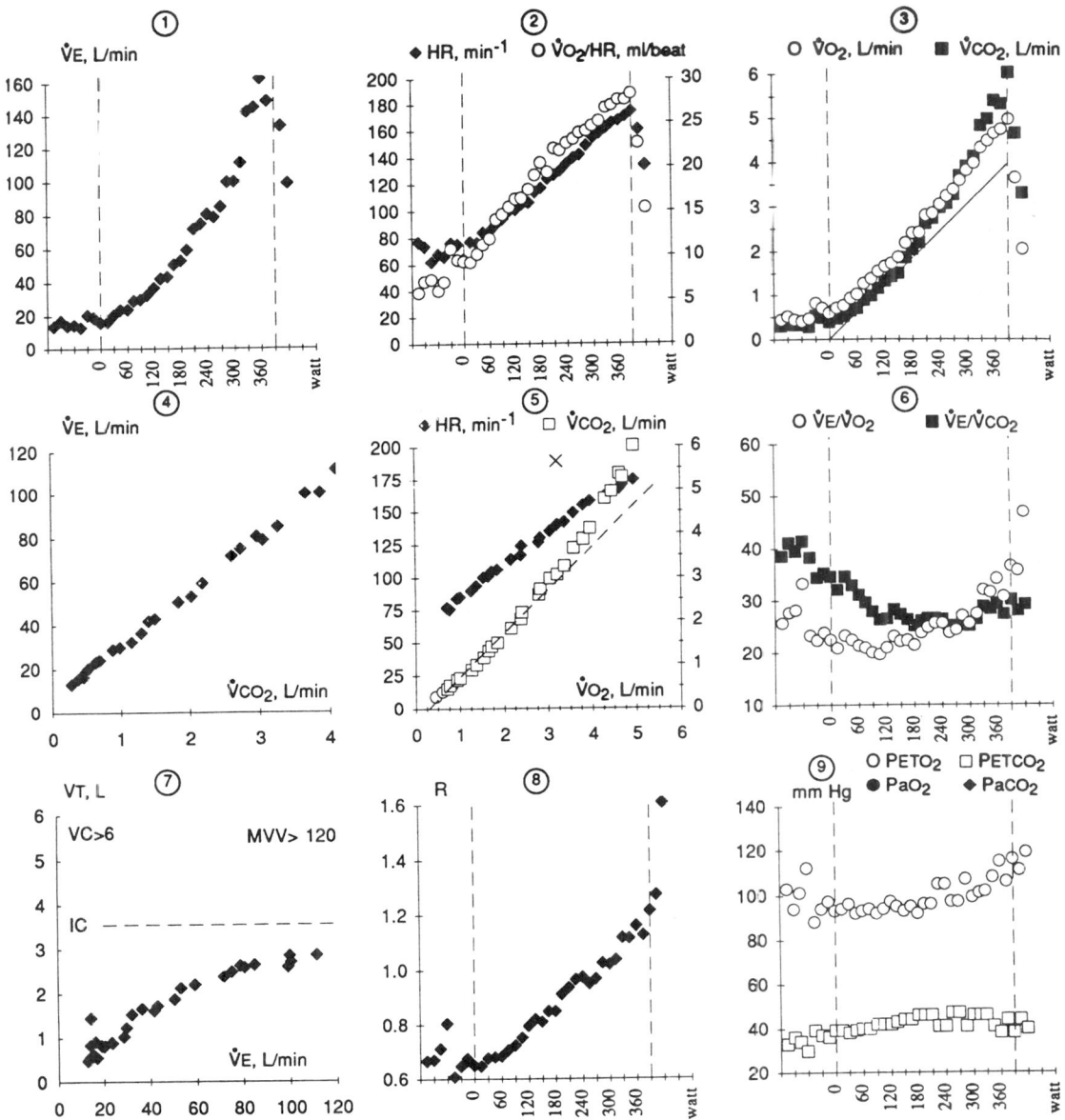

1. Vertical dashed lines in panels 1 to 3 and 6, 8, and 9 indicate the beginning and the end of increasing work period.

2. Unloaded cycling is performed for 3 minutes before the left vertical dashed line.

3. In panel 3, the diagonal line shows the increase of $\dot{V}O_2$ at a slope of 10 ml/min/W.

4. In panel 5, the diagonal dashed line has a slope of 1; the "x" in the upper right is the predicted maximum heart rate and $\dot{V}O_2$ for the subject.

TABLE 9.2.3. Air Breathing

Time min	Work rate watts	BP mmHg	HR min⁻¹	f min⁻¹	$\dot{V}_E$ L/min BTPS	$\dot{V}_{CO_2}$ L/min STPD	$\dot{V}_{O_2}$ L/min STPD	$\dot{V}_{O_2}$/HR ml/beat	R	pH	HCO₃⁻ meq/L	P_{O_2}, mmHg ET	a	(A − a)	P_{CO_2} mmHg ET	a	(a − ET)	$\dot{V}_E$/$\dot{V}_{CO_2}$	$\dot{V}_E$/$\dot{V}_{O_2}$	V_D/V_T
	Rest		77	25	13.7	0.30	0.45	5.8	0.67			103			33			39	26	
	Rest		74	31	17.0	0.35	0.52	7.0	0.67			94			36			41	28	
	Rest		62	17	14.1	0.32	0.45	7.3	0.71			101			34			40	28	
	Rest		68	10	14.5	0.33	0.41	6.0	0.80			112			30			41	33	
	Unloaded		66	27	13.0	0.28	0.46	7.0	0.61			88			39			38	23	
	Unloaded		76	25	20.4	0.53	0.82	10.8	0.65			94			37			34	22	
	Unloaded		75	23	18.9	0.48	0.71	9.5	0.68			97			36			35	24	
	Unloaded		64	26	15.7	0.39	0.60	9.4	0.65			93			39			35	22	
0.5	30		77	18	16.3	0.46	0.71	9.2	0.65			94			39			32	21	
1.0	30		76	25	20.1	0.52	0.77	10.1	0.68			96			38			35	23	
1.5	60		84	26	23.3	0.64	0.94	11.2	0.68			92			39			33	22	
2.0	60		85	27	23.8	0.69	1.01	11.9	0.68			93			40			31	21	
2.5	90		90	28	28.7	0.89	1.26	14.0	0.71			94			40			30	21	
3.0	90		94	24	29.6	0.99	1.37	14.6	0.72			92			42			28	20	
3.5	120		100	21	32.2	1.16	1.54	15.4	0.75			94			42			26	20	
4.0	120		101	22	36.5	1.31	1.65	16.3	0.79			97			42			26	21	
4.5	150		105	26	41.9	1.41	1.72	16.4	0.82			95			43			28	23	
5.0	150		106	25	43.1	1.50	1.85	17.5	0.81			93			44			27	22	
5.5	180		114	27	50.6	1.84	2.17	19.0	0.85			95			44			26	22	
6.0	180		117	25	53.2	2.03	2.39	20.4	0.85			92			46			25	21	
6.5	210		124	27	59.3	2.19	2.40	19.4	0.91			96			46			26	24	
7.0	210		127	30	71.7	2.61	2.79	22.0	0.94			96			46			26	25	
7.5	240		130	30	75.0	2.73	2.83	21.8	0.96			105			41			27	26	
8.0	240		135	31	80.6	2.97	3.05	22.6	0.97			105			41			26	26	
8.5	270		140	30	78.9	3.06	3.22	23.0	0.95			97			47			25	24	
9.0	270		142	32	85.0	3.27	3.38	23.8	0.97			97			47			25	24	
9.5	300		149	35	100.0	3.67	3.58	24.0	1.03			107			41			26	27	
10.0	300		155	37	100.4	3.83	3.80	24.5	1.02			99			46			25	26	
10.5	330		158	39	111.6	4.11	3.96	25.1	1.04			101			46			26	27	
11.0	330		162	48	142.4	4.81	4.31	26.6	1.12			102			46			29	32	
11.5	360		166	48	144.8	4.97	4.46	26.9	1.11			108			41			28	32	
12.0	360		168	53	162.6	5.38	4.64	27.3	1.16			115			38			29	34	
12.5	390		171	50	149.1	5.31	4.71	27.5	1.13			106			44			27	31	
13.0	390		175	63	186.0	6.01	4.95	28.3	1.21			116			38			30	36	
	Recovery		161	46	133.7	4.63	3.64	22.6	1.27			111			44			28	36	
	Recovery		134	38	99.1	3.29	2.05	15.3	1.60			119			40			29	47	

Interpretation

Comments

This case is presented to illustrate results of a normal, athletic subject.

Analysis

Referring to flow chart 1, the peak $\dot{V}_{O_2}$ and the anaerobic threshold are considerably above the predicted values (Table 9.2.2). The predicted values are, of course, those for a sedentary population. The results of this study demonstrate how much better an athlete can perform than the average member of the sedentary group. The exceptionally high O_2 pulse at maximum work rate reflects the large stroke volume and $C(a - \bar{v})_{O_2}$ that this subject must have. Assuming that the mixed venous O_2 saturation was as low as 20%, the O_2 pulse of 28.3 ml/beat would indicate that the subject's stroke volume must be approximately 175 ml. The normal ventilatory equivalent for O_2 and CO_2 at the anaerobic threshold (panel 6, Fig. 9.2.1) reflects the ventilation-perfusion matching of a normal subject. The maximum exercise ventilation is approximately equal to his MVV. Thus, his breathing reserve is approximately zero, a common finding in exceptionally fit people.

Conclusion

This is an exceptionally fit, normal subject.

Case 3 Normal Man: Air and Oxygen Breathing
Clinical Findings

The patient was a 59-year-old retired shipyard worker with a history of asbestos exposure and a 2-pack/day history of cigarette smoking. He had stopped working 4 years previously. He was asymptomatic at the time of this examination. Physical and laboratory examinations were normal; chest roentgenograms revealed focal pleural plaques with calcification.

Exercise Findings

After we obtained informed consent, the patient participated in a blinded-crossover exercise study on a cycle ergometer, receiving one of two humidified gas mixtures (compressed air or 100% oxygen) just prior to and during each study. He pedalled at 60 rpm without added load for 3 minutes. The work rate was then increased 15 W per minute to his symptom-limited maximum. Arterial blood was sampled every second minute, and intra-arterial blood pressure was recorded from a percutaneously placed brachial artery catheter. He rested 1 hour between the two studies and exercised to his maximum tolerance on each occasion. On both occasions, he stopped exercise because of general fatigue. Resting and exercise ECG readings were normal.

TABLE 9.3.1. Selected Respiratory Function Data

Measurement	Predicted	Measured
Age, yr		59
Sex		Male
Height, cm		155
Weight, kg	62	53
Hematocrit, %		46
VC, L	2.90	3.19
IC, L	1.94	2.12
TLC, L	4.51	4.62
FEV_1, L	2.26	2.49
FEV_1/VC, %	78	78
MVV, L/min	112	118
$D_{L}CO$, ml/mm Hg/min	19.9	20.7

TABLE 9.3.2. Selected Exercise Data

Measurement	Predicted	Air	O_2
Peak $\dot{V}CO_2$, L/min		2.03	1.93
Peak $\dot{V}O_2$, L/min	1.65	1.57	
Maximum HR, beats/min	161	192	188
Maximum O_2 pulse, ml/beat	10.2	8.2	
$\Delta\dot{V}O_2/\Delta WR$, ml/min/W	10.3	9.7	
AT, L/min	>0.73	0.8	
Blood pressure, mmHg (rest, max)		100/56, 213/88	100/63, 231/94
Maximum $\dot{V}E$, L/min		89	72
Exercise breathing reserve, L/min	>15	29	46
PaO_2, mmHg (rest, max ex)		102, 101	585, 586
$P(A - a)O_2$, mmHg (rest, max ex)		24, 25	103, 93
$P(a - ET)CO_2$, mmHg (rest, max ex)		−4, −4	1, −2
VD/VT (rest, heavy ex)		0.19, 0.27	0.37, 0.26
HCO_3^- mEq/L (rest, 2-min recov)		23, 12	19, 14

FIGURE 9.3.1.   Air breathing.

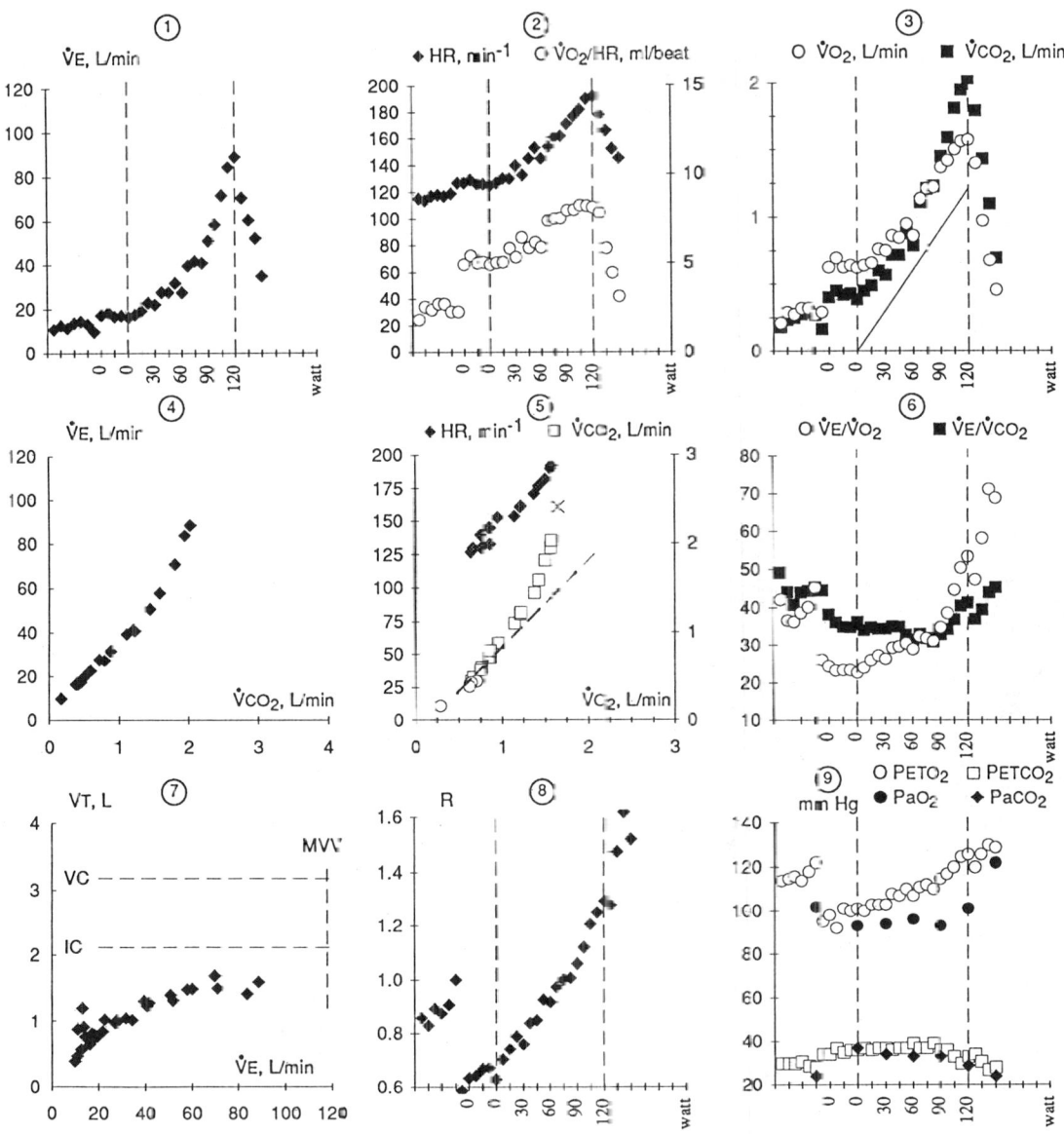

1. Vertical dashed lines in panels 1 to 3 and 6, 8, and 9 indicate the beginning and the end of increasing work period.

2. Unloaded cycling is performed for 3 minutes before the left vertical dashed line.

3. In panel 3, the diagonal line shows the increase of $\dot{V}O_2$ at a slope of 10 ml/min/W.

4. In panel 5, the diagonal dashed line has a slope of 1; the "z" in the upper right is the predicted maximum heart rate and $\dot{V}O_2$ for the subject.

FIGURE 9.3.2.   Oxygen breathing.

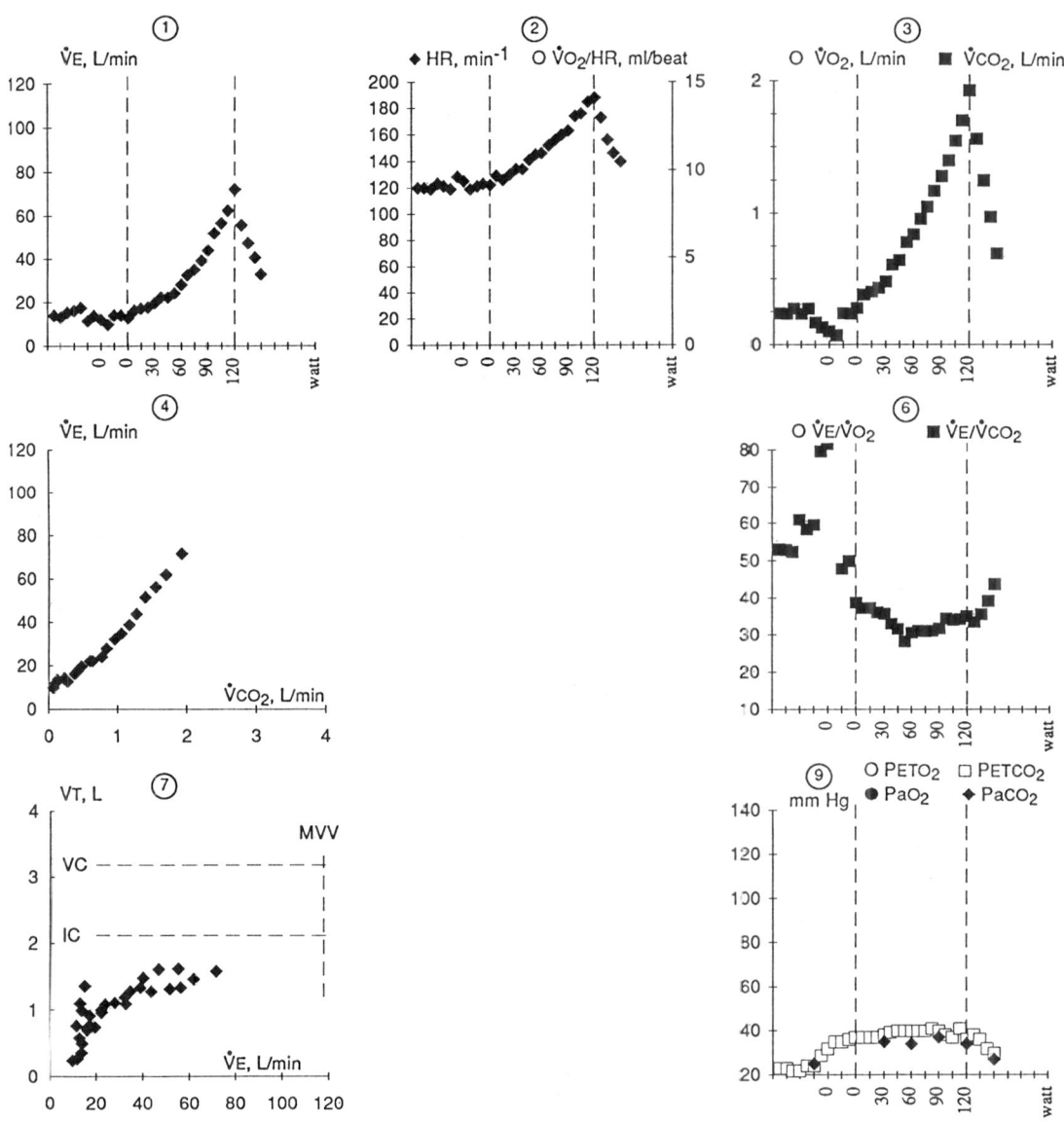

1. Vertical dashed lines in panels 1 to 3 and 6 and 9 indicate the beginning and the end of increasing work period.
2. Unloaded cycling is performed for 3 minutes before the left vertical dashed line.

TABLE 9.3.3. **Air Breathing**

Time min	Work rate watts	BP mmHg	HR min⁻¹	f min⁻¹	$\dot{V}_E$ L/min BTPS	$\dot{V}_{CO_2}$ L/min STPD	$\dot{V}_{O_2}$ L/min STPD	$\dot{V}_{O_2}$/HR ml/beat	R	pH	HCO₃ meq/L	P_{O_2}, mmHg ET	a	(A − a)	P_{CO_2}, mmHg ET	a	(a − ET)	$\dot{V}_E$/$\dot{V}_{CO_2}$	$\dot{V}_E$/$\dot{V}_{O_2}$	VD/VT
	Rest		115	23	10.8	0.18	0.21	1.8	0.86			114			30			49	42	
	Rest		114	22	12.5	0.24	0.29	2.5	0.83			115			30			44	37	
	Rest		117	13	11.3	0.25	0.28	2.4	0.89			116			30			41	36	
	Rest		118	15	13.6	0.28	0.32	2.7	0.88			114			31			44	39	
	Rest		117	19	14.5	0.29	0.32	2.7	0.91			113			29			44	40	
	Rest	100/56	119	11	13.2	0.27	0.27	2.3	1.00	7.48	18	122	102	24	28	24	−4	45	45	0.19
	Unloaded		127	25	9.7	0.17	0.29	2.3	0.59			95			34			45	26	
	Unloaded		127	21	17.1	0.40	0.63	5.0	0.63			98			34			38	24	
	Unloaded		129	23	18.2	0.45	0.70	5.4	0.64			92			37			36	23	
	Unloaded		126	23	16.7	0.42	0.63	5.0	0.67			10⁻			35			35	23	
	Unloaded		126	24	17.0	0.43	0.64	5.1	0.67			100			36			35	23	
	Unloaded	150/75	125	25	16.3	0.39	0.62	5.0	0.63	7.41	23	101	93	3	36	37	1	36	23	0.31
0.5	15		127	23	17.3	0.45	0.64	5.0	0.70			100			37			34	24	
1.0	15		130	25	19.2	0.49	0.66	5.1	0.74			103			36			35	26	
1.5	30		130	22	22.6	0.60	0.76	5.8	0.79			103			37			35	27	
2.0	30	163/75	140	26	21.9	0.57	0.75	5.4	0.76	7.40	21	103	94	14	37	34	−3	35	26	0.24
2.5	45		133	27	27.6	0.72	0.86	6.5	0.84			108			36			35	29	
3.0	45		145	28	27.6	0.72	0.85	5.9	0.85			107			37			35	30	
3.5	60		153	30	31.5	0.88	0.95	6.2	0.93			110			37			33	30	
4.0	60	194/81	145	28	27.2	0.79	0.86	5.9	0.92	7.40	20	107	96	19	39	33	−6	31	29	0.15
4.5	75		154	30	39.4	1.11	1.14	7.4	0.97			111			37			33	32	
5.0	75		161	32	41.4	1.21	1.21	7.5	1.00			112			37			32	32	
5.5	90		162	34	40.8	1.23	1.22	7.5	1.01			110			39			31	31	
6.0	90	194/75	171	36	50.8	1.45	1.37	8.0	1.06	7.39	20	115	93	25	36	33	−3	33	35	0.19
6.5	105		177	39	58.0	1.59	1.42	8.0	1.12			117			36			34	39	
7.0	105		182	47	71.0	1.81	1.50	8.2	1.21			120			33			37	45	
7.5	120		190	59	83.9	1.95	1.56	8.2	1.25			125			30			40	51	
8.0	120	213/88	192	55	88.6	2.03	1.57	8.2	1.29	7.37	16	126	101	25	33	29	−4	41	53	0.27
	Recovery		178	41	69.9	1.79	1.40	7.9	1.28			120			34			37	47	
	Recovery		166	40	60.0	1.43	0.97	5.8	1.47			126			31			40	58	
	Recovery		152	39	51.8	1.10	0.68	4.5	1.62			130			27			44	71	
	Recovery	169/63	145	34	34.6	0.70	0.46	3.2	1.52	7.33	12	129	122	11	28	24	−4	45	69	0.19

Interpretation

Comments

Resting respiratory function is normal (Table 9.3.1). The exercise test was repeated with the patient breathing O_2, as part of an experimental study. At rest, the patient acutely hyperventilated while breathing with the mouthpiece; this ceased as soon as the exercise started. The associated relative hypoventilation noted in the transition from rest to unloaded cycling (panel 9, Fig. 9.3.1) caused a simultaneous marked decrease in R (panel 8, Fig. 9.3.1).

Analysis

Referring to flow chart 1, the peak $\dot{V}_{O_2}$ is normal (Table 9.3.2 and panel 3 of Fig. 9.3.1). See flow chart 2: The ECG and arterial blood gases at peak $\dot{V}_{O_2}$ are normal (branchpoint 2.1). The subject is not obese (branchpoint 2.2). While the patient and we thought that he was volunteering for this study as a normal subject, we noted a resting tachycardia that persisted during exercise so that he went 31 beats/min higher than his maximum predicted heart rate at the peak work rate. As a consequence, he had a reduced peak O_2 pulse. Questioning the pa-

TABLE 9.3.4. Oxygen Breathing

Time min	Work rate watts	BP mmHg	HR min⁻¹	f min⁻¹	$\dot{V}_E$ L/min BTPS	$\dot{V}_{CO_2}$ L/min STPD	$\dot{V}_{O_2}$ L/min STPD	$\dfrac{\dot{V}_{O_2}}{HR}$ ml/beat	R	pH	HCO₃⁻ meq/L	P_{O_2}, mmHg ET	a	(A − a)	P_{CO_2}, mmHg ET	a	(a − ET)	$\dfrac{\dot{V}_E}{\dot{V}_{CO_2}}$	$\dfrac{\dot{V}_E}{\dot{V}_{O_2}}$	$\dfrac{V_D}{V_T}$
	Rest		120	14	13.9	0.24									23			53		
	Rest		120	12	13.2	0.23									23			53		
	Rest		119	11	15.1	0.27									22			52		
	Rest		123	22	15.9	0.23									22			61		
	Rest		121	19	17.4	0.27									24			58		
	Rest	100/63	119	15	11.4	0.17				7.49	19	585	103		24	25	1	60		0.37
	Unloaded		128	38	13.6	0.13									29			80		
	Unloaded		125	44	11.9	0.10									32			82		
	Unloaded		119	41	9.8	0.07									35			90		
	Unloaded		121	28	13.9	0.24									35			48		
	Unloaded		123	28	13.9	0.23									36			50		
	Unloaded	163/81	122	22	12.7	0.28									37			39		
0.5	15		129	23	16.1	0.38									37			37		
1.0	15		126	22	16.8	0.40									37			37		
1.5	30		130	23	17.5	0.43									37			36		
2.0	30	181/88	134	26	19.4	0.48				7.40	21	591	87		38	35	−3	36		0.28
2.5	45		134	23	22.2	0.61									39			33		
3.0	45		141	22	22.1	0.64									40			32		
3.5	60		145	22	23.9	0.78									40			28		
4.0	60	206/88	146	25	27.9	0.84				7.38	20	576	103		40	34	−6	31		0.16
4.5	75		152	27	32.3	0.96									40			31		
5.0	75		156	27	34.8	1.05									40			31		
5.5	90		160	29	39.0	1.17									41			31		
6.0	90	225/91	163	34	43.7	1.28				7.37	21	581	95		40	37	−3	32		0.25
6.5	105		174	39	51.6	1.40									38			34		
7.0	105		176	42	56.3	1.55									37			34		
7.5	120		185	42	62.0	1.70									41			34		
8.0	120	231/94	188	45	71.7	1.93				7.35	18	586	93		36	34	−2	35		0.26
	Recovery		173	34	55.3	1.56									38			34		
	Recovery		156	29	46.9	1.25									36			36		
	Recovery		146	27	40.3	0.97									32			39		
	Recovery	219/75	140	30	32.7	0.69				7.33	14	584	102		30	27	−3	44		0.25

tient about medication and examining the patient for hyperthyroidism did not provide us with a satisfactory explanation of his tachycardia. The recommendation was to restudy this subject on another occasion with request that he take no recreational drugs or medications.

The major difference between the air and O_2 breathing studies is a significantly reduced exercise ventilation in the latter when performing at the same work rate (Tables 9.3.3 and 9.3.4 and panel 1 of Figs. 9.3.1 and 9.3.2). Consistent with this is the higher Pa_{CO_2} at maximum exercise during the O_2 breathing study. Arterial oxygen tension was normal (585 mmHg) at rest and remained unchanged throughout exercise during the oxygen breathing study, demonstrating the absence of a significant right to left shunt.

Conclusion

Probably a normal subject with unexplained tachycardia. Repeat study recommended.

Case 4 Normal Woman: Air and Oxygen Breathing
Clinical Findings

This 45-year-old housewife was referred for evaluation of dyspnea. She had recently begun to increase her activity and felt that she was shorter of breath than she should be. Physical and laboratory examinations revealed no abnormalities.

Exercise Findings

The patient performed exercise on a cycle ergometer. She pedalled at 60 rpm without added load for 3 minutes. The work rate was then increased 10 W per minute to her symptom-limited maximum. Arterial blood was sampled every second minute, and intra-arterial blood pressure was recorded from a percutaneously placed brachial artery catheter. A second incremental exercise test was performed with O_2 breathing, 1½ hours after recovery from

the first, with work rate increments of 20 W per minute. She stopped exercise in each case complaining of general fatigue and shortness of breath. Resting and exercise ECGs were normal.

TABLE 9.4.1. Selected Respiratory Function Data

Measurement	Predicted	Measured
Age, yr		45
Sex		Female
Height, cm		165
Weight, kg	64	61
Hematocrit, %		40
VC, L	3.30	3.21
IC, L	2.20	1.99
FEV_1, L	2.68	2.71
FEV_1/VC, %	81	84
MVV, L/min	112	117
$D_{L}CO$, ml/mmHg/min	24.1	21.1

TABLE 9.4.2. Selected Exercise Data

Measurement	Predicted	Room Air	O_2
Peak work rate, W		130	160
Peak $\dot{V}O_2$, L/min	1.60	1.71	
Maximum HR, beats/min	175	160	155
Maximum O_2 pulse, ml/beat	9.1	10.7	
$\Delta\dot{V}O_2/\Delta WR$, ml/min/W	10.3	11.9	
AT, L/min	>0.78	0.9	
Blood pressure, mmHg (rest, max)		135/81, 194/81	106/75, 181/88
Maximum $\dot{V}E$, L/min		70	54
Exercise breathing reserve, L/min	>15	47	63
PaO_2, mmHg (rest, max ex)		105, 108	643, 552
$P(A - a)O_2$, mmHg (rest, max ex)		5, 16	33, 117
$P(a - ET)CO_2$, mmHg (rest, max ex)		−1, −6	4, −3
VD/VT (rest, heavy ex)		0.21, 0.11	0.34, 0.18
HCO_3^-, mEq/L (rest, 2-min recov)		25, 13	25, unknown

FIGURE 9.4.1.   Air breathing.

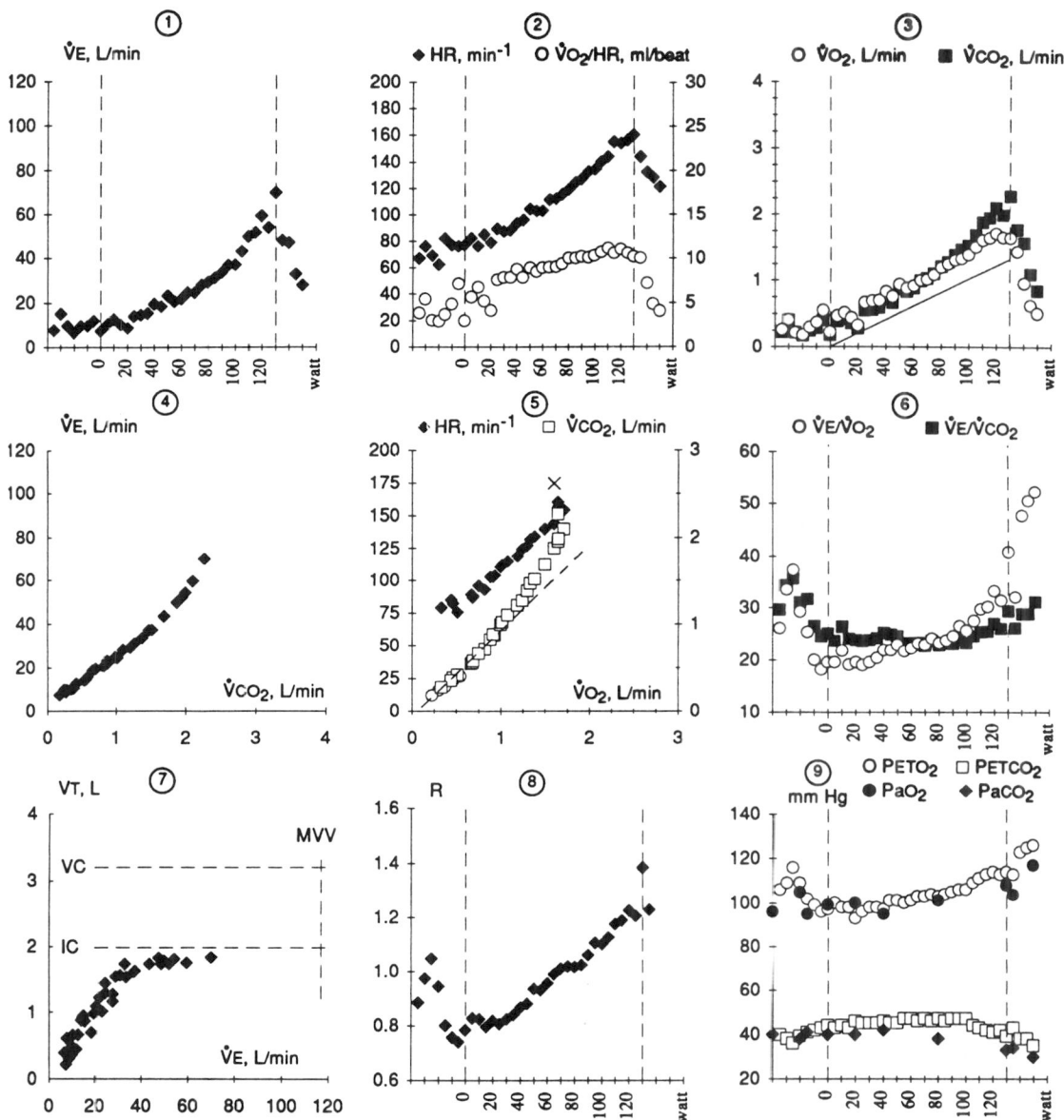

1. Vertical dashed lines in panels 1 to 3 and 6, 8, and 9 indicate the beginning and the end of increasing work period.

2. Unloaded cycling is performed for 3 minutes before the left vertical dashed line.

3. In panel 3, the diagonal line shows the increase of $\dot{V}O_2$ at a slope of 10 ml/min/w.

4. In panel 5, the diagonal dashed line has a slope of 1; the "x" in the upper right is the predicted maximum heart rate and $\dot{V}O_2$ for the subject.

FIGURE 9.4.2.   Oxygen breathing.

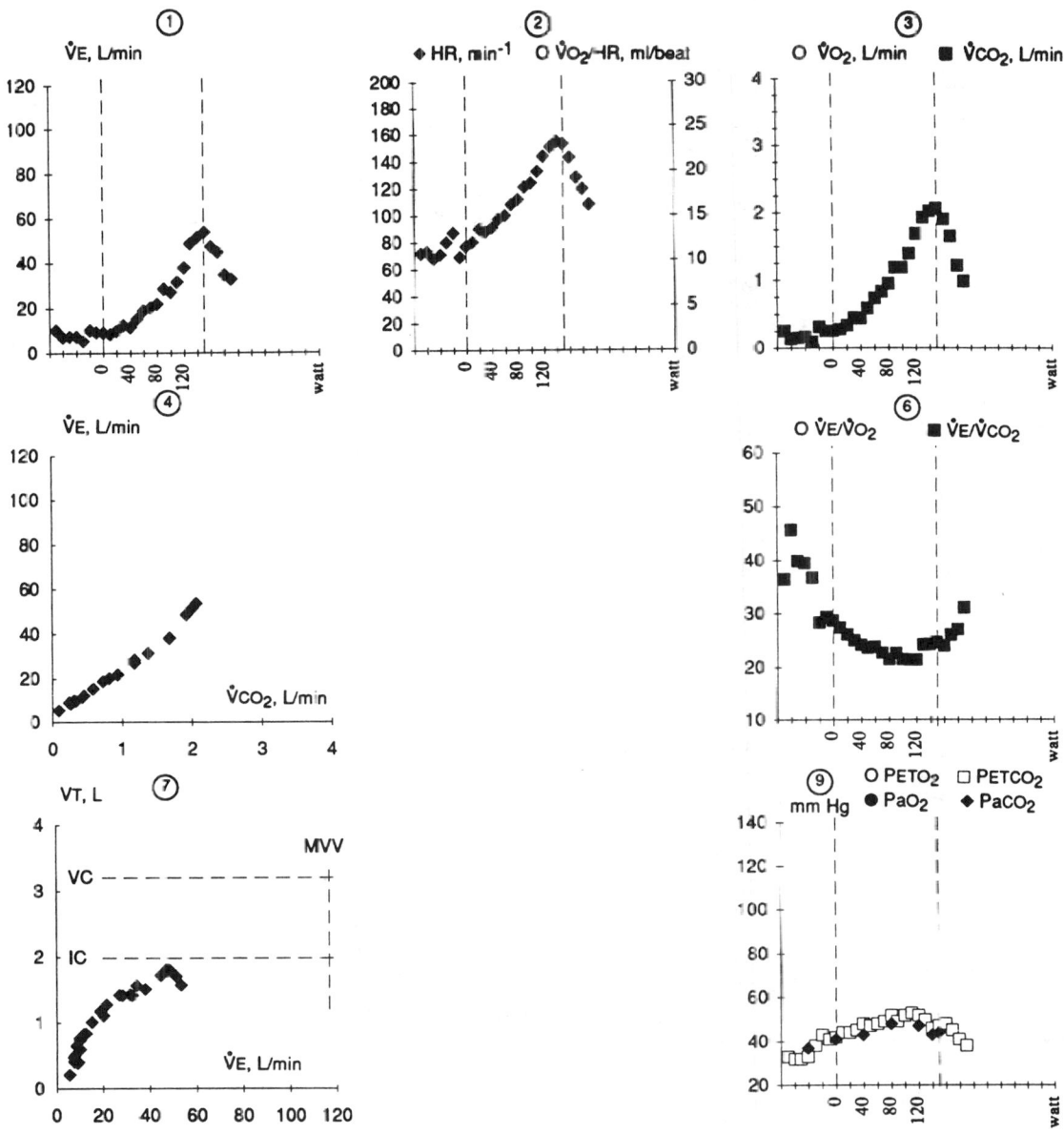

1. Vertical dashed lines in panels 1 to 3 and 6 and 9 indicate the beginning and the end of increasing work period.
2. Unloaded cycling is performed for 3 minutes before the left vertical dashed line.

TABLE 9.4.3. Air Breathing

Time min	Work rate watts	BP mmHg	HR min⁻¹	f min⁻¹	$\dot{V}_E$ L/min BTPS	$\dot{V}_{CO_2}$ L/min STPD	$\dot{V}_{O_2}$ L/min STPD	$\dot{V}_{O_2}$/HR ml/beat	R	pH	HCO_3^- meq/L	P_{O_2}, mmHg ET	a	(A−a)	P_{CO_2}, mmHg ET	a	(a−ET)	$\dot{V}_E$/$\dot{V}_{CO_2}$	$\dot{V}_E$/$\dot{V}_{O_2}$	V_D/V_T
	Rest	138–81								7.42	25		96			40				
	Rest		67	13	7.9	0.23	0.26	3.9	0.88			106			40			30	26	
	Rest		76	16	15.1	0.40	0.41	5.4	0.98			109			38			34	34	
	Rest		69	22	9.7	0.22	0.21	3.0	1.05			116			36			36	37	
	Rest	138/75	62	17	6.7	0.17	0.18	2.9	0.94	7.43	25	109	105	5	39	38	−1	31	29	0.21
	Unloaded	138/81	82	27	9.9	0.24	0.30	3.7	0.80	7.41	26	102	95	6	41	41	0	32	25	0.26
	Unloaded		77	28	9.8	0.28	0.37	4.8	0.76			99			42			27	20	
	Unloaded		76	27	12.1	0.40	0.54	7.1	0.74			96			43			25	18	
	Unloaded	144/75	77	34	7.4	0.18	0.23	3.0	0.78	7.41	25	97	99	2	44	40	−4	25	20	0.08
0.5	10		82	16	10.4	0.38	0.46	5.6	0.83			100			43			24	20	
1.0	10		76	19	12.7	0.42	0.51	6.7	0.82			98			44			26	22	
1.5	20		85	21	10.2	0.35	0.44	5.2	0.80			98			43			24	19	
2.0	20	144/75	79	29	8.9	0.27	0.33	4.2	0.82	7.41	25	93	100	3	46	40	−6	24	20	0.07
2.5	30		89	16	14.1	0.54	0.67	7.5	0.81			96			45			24	19	
3.0	30		87	16	14.7	0.56	0.68	7.8	0.82			98			45			24	20	
3.5	40		88	18	15.6	0.58	0.69	7.8	0.84			98			45			24	20	
4.0	40	144/75	93	20	19.6	0.71	0.82	8.8	0.87	7.39	25	97	95	8	46	42	−4	25	22	0.17
4.5	50		96	27	18.7	0.66	0.75	7.8	0.88			101			45			25	22	
5.0	50		104	23	23.3	0.87	0.93	8.9	0.94			101			45			25	23	
5.5	60		103	19	20.7	0.82	0.88	8.5	0.93			100			47			23	22	
6.0	60	156/75	103	18	22.0	0.88	0.92	8.9	0.96			101			47			23	22	
6.5	70		111	19	24.7	0.99	1.00	9.0	0.99			103			46			23	23	
7.0	70		112	17	24.6	1.02	1.01	9.0	1.01			103			47			23	23	
7.5	80		115	24	28.0	1.10	1.08	9.4	1.02			104			46			24	24	
8.0	80	163/75	119	19	29.3	1.21	1.19	10.0	1.02	7.37	22	103	101	11	47	38	−9	23	23	0.01
8.5	90		124	20	31.2	1.27	1.24	10.0	1.02			104			46			23	24	
9.0	90		127	22	33.7	1.38	1.30	10.2	1.06			105			47			23	24	
9.5	100		132	23	37.1	1.47	1.33	10.1	1.11			106			47			24	26	
10.0	100	175/81	134	23	37.4	1.52	1.38	10.3	1.10			106			47			23	26	
10.5	110		140	25	43.5	1.69	1.50	10.7	1.13			109			44			24	28	
11.0	110		144	28	50.0	1.88	1.60	11.1	1.18			111			43			25	30	
11.5	120		155	30	52.1	1.95	1.64	10.6	1.19			113			42			25	30	
12.0	120		154	34	59.6	2.10	1.71	11.1	1.23			114			41			27	33	
12.5	130		156	30	54.3	1.99	1.65	10.6	1.21			113			42			26	31	
13.0	130	194/81	160	38	70.0	2.27	1.64	10.3	1.38	7.31	16	114	108	16	39	33	−6	29	41	0.11
	Recovery	156/69	144	28	48.6	1.77	1.44	10.0	1.23	7.28	16	113	104	17	43	34	−9	26	32	0.03
	Recovery		132	26	47.5	1.57	0.95	7.2	1.65			123			38			29	48	
	Recovery		128	19	33.0	1.09	0.62	4.8	1.76			125			38			29	51	
	Recovery	131/63	121	22	28.0	0.84	0.50	4.1	1.68	7.26	13	126	117	13	35	30	−5	31	52	0.07

TABLE 9.4.4. Oxygen Breathing

Time min	Work rate watts	BP mmHg	HR min⁻¹	f min⁻¹	$\dot{V}_E$ L/min BTPS	$\dot{V}_{CO_2}$ L/min STPD	$\dot{V}_{O_2}$ L/min STPD	$\dot{V}_{O_2}$/HR ml/beat	R	pH	HCO₃ meq/L	P_{O_2} ET	P_{O_2} a	P_{O_2} (A-a)	P_{CO_2} ET	P_{CO_2} a	P_{CO_2} (a-ET)	$\dot{V}_E/\dot{V}_{CO_2}$	$\dot{V}_E/\dot{V}_{O_2}$	V_D/V_T
	Rest		72	14	10.3	0.25									33			36		
	Rest		73	15	7.2	0.13									32			46		
	Rest		68	18	7.5	0.15									32			40		
	Rest	106/75	71	15	7.6	0.16				7.44	25		643	33	33	37	4	40		0.34
	Unloaded		80	27	5.6	0.09									38			37		
	Unloaded		87	17	10.2	0.31									43			28		
	Unloaded		69	23	9.3	0.25									41			29		
	Unloaded	113/69	77	24	9.2	0.25				7.39	24		605	67	42	41	-1	29		0.21
0.5	20		80	13	8.5	0.27									44			27		
1.0	20		90	13	10.0	0.34									44			26		
1.5	40		88	15	12.5	0.45									45			25		
2.0	40	125/69	91	14	11.6	0.43				7.39	26		595	75	48	43	-5	24		0.15
2.5	60		97	15	15.2	0.59									47			24		
3.0	60		100	16	18.8	0.73									48			24		
3.5	80		108	18	20.1	0.82									49			23		
4.0	80	144/75	112	17	21.7	0.94				7.34	25		601	64	52	48	-4	22		0.15
4.5	100		121	20	28.3	1.18									49			23		
5.0	100		124	19	27.1	1.18									52			22		
5.5	120		133	22	31.5	1.38									53			21		
6.0	120	169/81	144	25	38.0	1.68				7.29	22		587	79	52	47	-5	21		0.13
6.5	140		151	27	48.7	1.92									50			24		
7.0	140	175/81	155	30	51.4	2.01				7.30	21		564	106	46	43	-3	24		0.17
7.5	160	181/88	153	34	53.6	2.06				7.28	20		552	117	47	44	-3	25		0.19
	Recovery		143	26	47.4	1.89									48			24		
	Recovery		128	26	44.8	1.64									45			26		
	Recovery		120	22	34.6	1.21									41			27		
	Recovery		108	23	32.5	0.98									38			31		

Interpretation

Comments

Resting respiratory function (Table 9.4.1) and ECG are normal.

Analysis

Referring to flow chart 1, the peak $\dot{V}_{O_2}$ and anaerobic threshold are normal (Table 9.4.2). See flow chart 2 for further analysis. There are no ECG abnormalities, and arterial blood gas values and V_D/V_T are normal throughout exercise (Table 9.4.3) (branchpoint 2.1). The patient is not obese (Table 9.4.1) (branchpoint 2.2). Thus, this patient has no limitation to exercise for her age and has no physiologic evidence of cardiovascular or pulmonary disease.

Pa_{O_2} is also normal during 100% O_2 breathing (Table 9.4.4), ruling out a significant right to left shunt.

Of special note is that the patient was able to exercise to a higher work rate with a slightly lower heart rate during O_2 breathing instead of air breathing. Moreover, respiratory compensation for the metabolic acidosis (decrease in Pa_{CO_2}) was less evident during the O_2 breathing study.

Conclusion

Our final assessment is that this patient was actually normal and her symptoms were the result of anxiety regarding her performance at sports.

Case 5 Normal Woman

Clinical Findings

This non-smoking occupational therapist was referred for evaluation of dyspnea. She described the sensation as the inability to take a deep breath. She also noted nervousness, dizziness, and shortness of breath while eating. She was usually active in sports, but also noted shortness of breath in these activities. Physical examination was normal except for resting tachycardia and a 2/6 systolic ejection murmur. Echocardiogram revealed a mitral valve prolapse. There were no dysrhythmias on 24-hour Holter monitoring. Chest roentgenograms, ECG, and respiratory function tests were normal, except for some reduction in expiratory flow rates attributable to reduced effort.

Exercise Findings

The patient performed exercise on a cycle ergometer. She pedalled at 60 rpm without added load for 3 minutes. The work rate was then increased 15 W per minute to her symptom-limited maximum. Arterial blood was sampled every second minute, and intra-arterial blood pressure was recorded from a percutaneously placed brachial artery catheter. She stopped pedalling at 150 W complaining of fatigue and a feeling of palpitations. She felt somewhat short of breath. There were no abnormal ST changes or arrhythmia. No wheezing or diminution of FEV_1 occurred in the post-exercise period.

TABLE 9.5.1. Selected Respiratory Function Data

Measurement	Predicted	Measured
Age, yr		24
Sex		Female
Height, cm		159
Weight, kg	61	51
Hematocrit, %		40
VC, L	3.60	3.50
IC, L	2.40	2.11
TLC, L	4.91	4.71
FEV_1, L	3.01	2.55
FEV_1/VC, %	84	73
MVV, L/min	115	118
D_LCO, ml/mm Hg/min	26.5	29.8

TABLE 9.5.2. Selected Exercise Data

Measurement	Predicted	Measured
Peak $\dot{V}O_2$, L/min	1.84	1.62
Maximum HR, beats/min	196	198
Maximum O_2 pulse, ml/beat	9.4	8.2
$\Delta\dot{V}O_2/\Delta WR$, ml/min/W	10.3	9.1
AT, L/min	>0.83	1.0
Blood pressure, mmHg (rest, max)		135/84, 177/87
Maximum $\dot{V}E$, L/min		64
Exercise breathing reserve, L/min	>15	54
PaO_2, mmHg (rest, max ex)		95, 100
$P(A - a)O_2$, mmHg (rest, max ex)		14, 17
$P(a - ET)CO_2$, mmHg (rest, max ex)		−1, −3
VD/VT (rest, heavy ex)		0.20, 0.16
HCO_3^-, mEq/L (rest, 2-min recov)		25, 15

FIGURE 9.5.1.

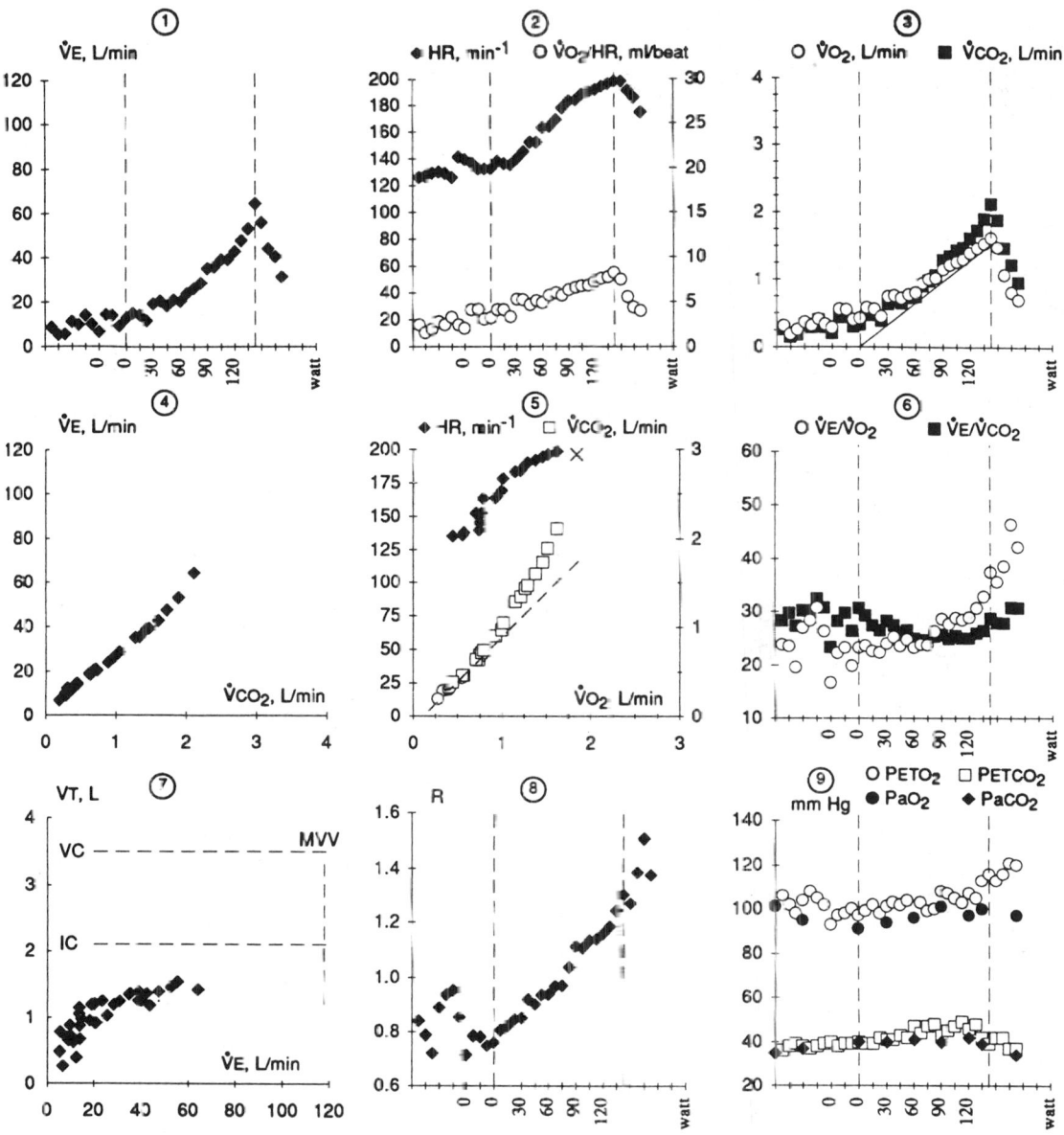

1. Vertical dashed lines in panels 1 to 3 and 6, 8, and 9 indicate the beginning and the end of increasing work period.

2. Unloaded cycling is performed for 3 minutes before the left vertical dashed line.

3. In panel 3, the diagonal line shows the increase of $\dot{V}O_2$ at a slope of 10 ml/min/w.

4. In panel 5, the diagonal dashed line has a slope of 1; the "x" in the upper right is the predicted maximum heart rate and $\dot{V}O_2$ for the subject.

TABLE 9.5.3. Air Breathing

Time min	Work rate watts	BP mmHg	HR min^{-1}	f min^{-1}	$\dot{V}_E$ L/min BTPS	$\dot{V}_{CO_2}$ L/min STPD	$\dot{V}_{O_2}$ L/min STPD	$\dot{V}_{O_2}$/HR ml/beat	R	pH	HCO$_3^-$ meq/L	P$_{O_2}$, mmHg ET	a	(a − a)	P$_{CO_2}$, mmHg ET	a	(a − ET)	$\dot{V}_E$/$\dot{V}_{CO_2}$	$\dot{V}_E$/$\dot{V}_{O_2}$	V$_D$/V$_T$
	Rest	135/84								7.47	25		101			35				
	Rest		126	12	8.4	0.26	0.31	2.5	0.84			106			36			28	24	
	Rest		127	11	5.4	0.15	0.19	1.5	0.79			102			38			30	24	
	Rest		129	7	5.5	0.18	0.25	1.9	0.72			98			39			27	20	
	Rest	144/84	130	18	11.2	0.32	0.36	2.8	0.89	7.44	25	104	95	14	38	37	−1	30	27	0.20
	Rest		129	11	9.7	0.29	0.31	2.4	0.94			108			37			30	28	
	Rest		126	13	13.7	0.39	0.41	3.3	0.95			105			38			32	31	
	Unloaded		141	14	10.1	0.29	0.34	2.4	0.85			102			39			31	26	
	Unloaded		139	25	6.8	0.20	0.28	2.0	0.71			93			40			23	17	
	Unloaded		137	21	14.2	0.44	0.56	4.1	0.79			97			38			28	22	
	Unloaded		132	12	13.8	0.43	0.55	4.2	0.78			98			39			30	23	
	Unloaded		132	14	9.1	0.30	0.40	3.0	0.75			100			39			26	20	
	Unloaded	141/81	132	32	12.5	0.32	0.42	3.2	0.76	7.42	25	97	91	9	40	40	0	31	23	0.23
0.5	15		138	15	14.7	0.46	0.57	4.1	0.81			99			39			29	24	
1.0	15		136	16	14.0	0.46	0.56	4.1	0.82			102			39			27	23	
1.5	30		135	17	11.5	0.38	0.45	3.3	0.84			98			42			26	22	
2.0	30	150/84	140	16	19.1	0.63	0.74	5.3	0.85	7.42	25	101	94	10	41	40	−1	28	24	0.22
2.5	45		145	17	20.4	0.69	0.75	5.2	0.92			103			41			27	25	
3.0	45		152	19	18.3	0.64	0.71	4.7	0.90			102			43			26	24	
3.5	60		152	23	21.0	0.72	0.77	5.1	0.94			104			42			26	25	
4.0	60	159/84	163	22	20.3	0.74	0.79	4.8	0.94	7.40	25	96	96	11	47	41	−6	25	23	0.14
4.5	75		164	19	23.8	0.90	0.93	5.7	0.97			103			44			25	24	
5.0	75		169	25	25.9	0.97	1.00	5.9	0.97			99			47			25	24	
5.5	90		178	24	28.6	1.05	1.01	5.7	1.04			100			48			25	26	
6.0	90	171/81	183	26	35.1	1.28	1.15	6.3	1.11	7.38	23	108	101	12	43	40	−3	26	29	0.15
6.5	105		184	26	35.6	1.34	1.21	6.6	1.11			107			45			25	28	
7.0	105		188	31	39.0	1.43	1.26	6.7	1.13			105			47			25	29	
7.5	120		190	28	39.1	1.47	1.29	6.8	1.14			103			49			25	28	
8.0	120	174/87	192	31	42.6	1.60	1.38	7.2	1.16	7.32	21	107	97	16	46	42	−4	25	29	0.17
8.5	135		194	34	47.6	1.73	1.46	7.5	1.18			105			48			26	31	
9.0	135	177/87	196	36	52.8	1.89	1.52	7.8	1.24	7.31	19	113	100	17	42	39	−3	26	33	0.15
9.5	150		198	45	64.2	2.11	1.62	8.2	1.30			116			39			29	37	
	Recovery		198	36	55.6	1.88	1.48	7.5	1.27			113			42			28	36	
	Recovery		191	37	43.9	1.47	1.06	5.5	1.39			116			42			28	38	
	Recovery		186	32	40.3	1.22	0.81	4.4	1.51			121			37			31	46	
	Recovery	153/78	175	25	31.2	0.95	0.69	3.9	1.38	7.27	15	120	97	26	37	34	−3	31	42	0.16

Interpretation

Comments

This young woman, who experienced occasions of dyspnea, has normal lung volumes and flow rates indicating the absence of restrictive or obstructive lung disease (Table 9.5.1). In addition, her diffusing capacity is normal. Her resting ECG is also normal.

Analysis

Referring to flow chart 1, the peak $\dot{V}_{O_2}$ and anaerobic threshold are normal (Table 9.5.2). See flow chart 2: Her ECG and O_2 pulse at maximum exercise are normal and her arterial blood gases remain normal

through exercise (branchpoint 2.1). This patient is not obese (branchpoint 2.2). This leads to the diagnosis of a normal subject with anxiety; however, she has a marked tachycardia at rest and an appropriate heart rate response to exercise. Hyperthyroidism was ruled out and the tachycardia was not a persistent observation (Holter monitoring), as might be found with vasoregulatory asthenia.

Conclusion

This is a normal young woman with anxiety; however, the sensation of palpitations was not related to a cardiac arrhythmia. The patient deserves follow-up for endocrine disorders or other conditions that might account for her symptoms.

Case 6 Normal Man

Clinical Findings

This 37-year-old shipyard machinist was evaluated because of complaints of dyspnea. He stated that he had been unable to play a full game of baseball for the last 6 years and that he gets out of breath and has to stop after climbing 3 to 4 flights on shipboard. He never smoked. He denied cough, chest pain, edema, or other symptoms. Physical, roentgenographic, and laboratory examinations were normal.

Exercise Findings

The patient performed exercise on a cycle ergometer. He pedalled at 60 rpm without added load for 3 minutes. The work rate was then increased 25 W per minute to his symptom-limited maximum. Arterial blood was sampled every second minute, and intra-arterial blood pressure was recorded from a percutaneously placed brachial artery catheter. He stopped exercise because of general fatigue. Resting and exercise ECGs were normal.

TABLE 9.6.1. Selected Respiratory Function Data

Measurement	Predicted	Measured
Age, yr		37
Sex		Male
Height, cm		157
Weight, kg	63	67
Hematocrit, %		45
VC, L	3.30	4.38
IC, L	2.20	2.80
TLC, L	4.52	5.30
FEV_1, L	2.66	3.52
FEV_1/VC, %	81	80
MVV, L/min	127	124
$D_{L}CO$, ml/mm Hg/min	22.4	29.8

TABLE 9.6.2. Selected Exercise Data

Measurement	Predicted	Measured
Maximum $\dot{V}O_2$, L/min	2.36	2.23
Maximum HR, beats/min	183	188
Maximum O_2 pulse, ml/beat	12.9	11.9
$\Delta\dot{V}O_2$/ΔWR, ml/min/W	10.3	10.4
AT, L/min	>0.99	1.1
Blood pressure, mmHg (rest, max)		125/75, 188/94
Maximum $\dot{V}E$, L/min		90
Exercise breathing reserve, L/min	>15	34
$PaCO_2$, mmHg (rest, max ex)		84, 114
$P(A - a)O_2$, mmHg (rest, max ex)		7, 2
$P(a - ET)CO_2$, mmHg (rest, max ex)		0, −4
VD/VT (rest, heavy ex)		0.31, 0.16
HCO_3^-, mEq/L (rest, 2-min recov)		24, 16

FIGURE 9.6.1.

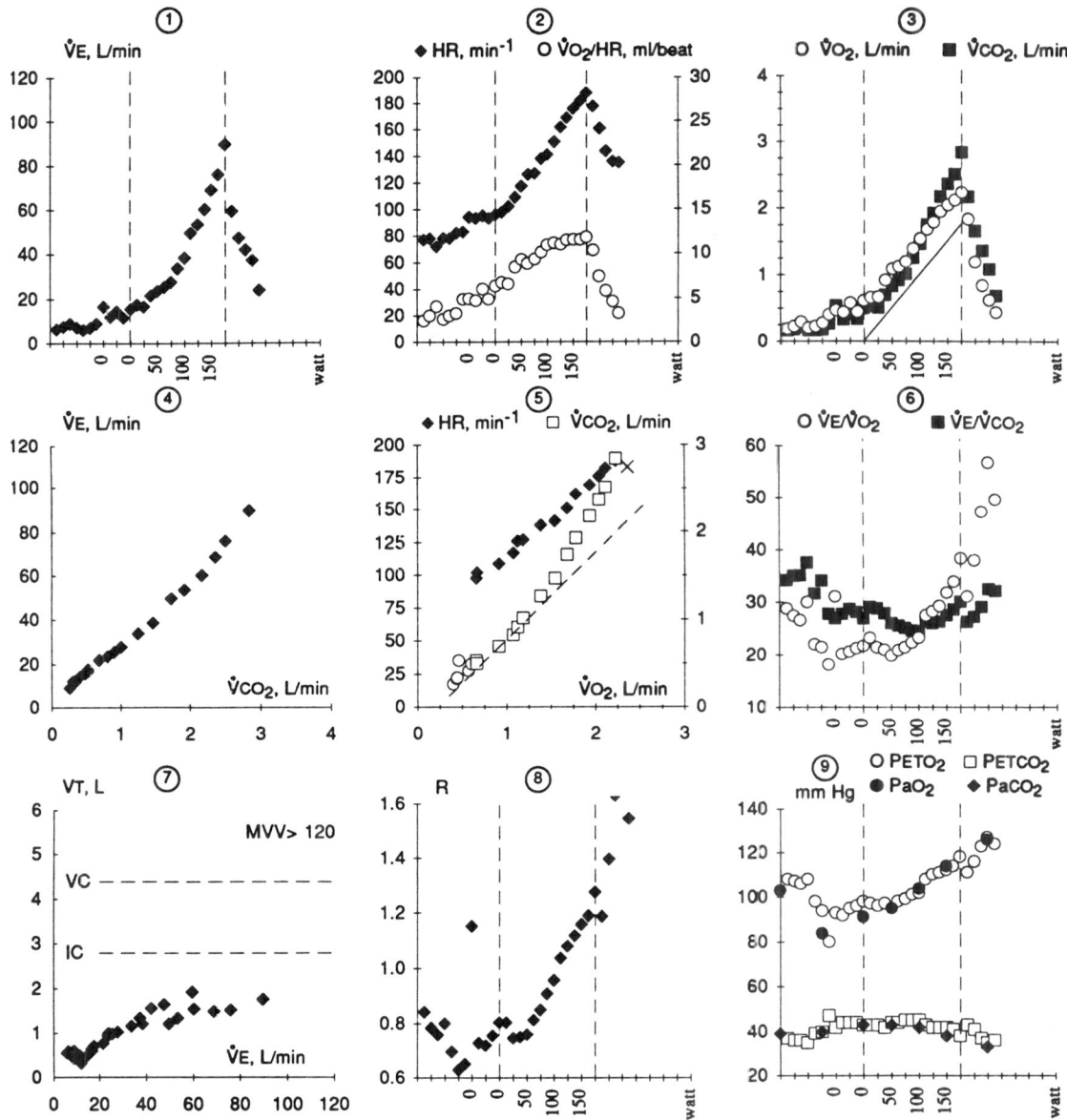

1. Vertical dashed lines in panels 1 to 3 and 6, 8, and 9 indicate the beginning and the end of increasing work period.

2. Unloaded cycling is performed for 3 minutes before the left vertical dashed line.

3. In panel 3, the diagonal line shows the increase of $\dot{V}_{O_2}$ at a slope of 10 ml/min/w.

4. In panel 5, the diagonal dashed line has a slope of 1; the "x" in the upper right is the predicted maximum heart rate and $\dot{V}_{O_2}$ for the subject.

TABLE 9.6.3. Air Breathing

Time min	Work rate watts	BP mmHg	HR min⁻¹	f min⁻¹	V̇E L/min BTPS	V̇CO₂ L/min STPD	V̇O₂ L/min STPD	V̇O₂/HR ml/beat	R	pH	HCO₃⁻ meq/L	PO₂ ET	PO₂ a	PO₂ (A−a)	PCO₂ ET	PCO₂ a	PCO₂ (a−ET)	V̇E/V̇CO₂	V̇E/V̇O₂	VD/VT
	Rest	125/75								7.41	24		103			39				
	Rest		77	11	6.4	0.16	0.19	2.5	0.84			103			37			34	29	
	Rest		78	14	7.5	0.18	0.23	2.9	0.78			107			36			35	27	
	Rest		72	15	9.0	0.22	0.29	4.0	0.76			106			36			35	27	
	Rest		78	13	7.1	0.16	0.20	2.6	0.80			108			35			37	30	
	Rest		78	11	6.0	0.16	0.23	2.9	0.70			98			39			32	22	
	Rest	125/81	82	13	6.9	0.17	0.27	3.3	0.63	7.39	24	94	84	7	40	40	0	34	21	0.31
	Unloaded		83	21	9.0	0.25	0.40	4.8	0.65			80			47			28	18	
	Unloaded		94	28	16.7	0.53	0.46	4.9	1.15			93			42			27	31	
	Unloaded		93	38	12.1	0.32	0.44	4.7	0.73			92			44			28	20	
	Unloaded		95	31	14.4	0.41	0.57	6.0	0.72			95			44			29	21	
	Unloaded		93	23	11.5	0.34	0.45	4.8	0.76			96			44			28	21	
	Unloaded	144/81	96	28	15.6	0.49	0.61	6.4	0.80	7.37	24	98	91	8	43	43	0	27	22	0.22
0.5	25		98	25	17.5	0.53	0.66	6.7	0.80			97			43			29	23	
1.0	25		102	26	16.6	0.50	0.67	6.6	0.75			96			43			29	21	
1.5	50		109	28	21.6	0.69	0.92	8.4	0.75			97			42			28	21	
2.0	50	150/81	117	25	23.5	0.82	1.08	9.2	0.76	7.38	25	95	95	1	44	43	−1	26	20	0.21
2.5	75		126	26	25.5	0.91	1.12	8.9	0.81			98			44			26	21	
3.0	75		127	27	27.7	1.01	1.19	9.4	0.85			99			45			25	21	
3.5	100		138	29	33.6	1.26	1.39	10.1	0.91			101			45			25	22	
4.0	100	181/94	141	32	38.6	1.47	1.54	10.9	0.95	7.37	24	102	104	2	45	42	−3	24	23	0.15
4.5	125		151	41	49.7	1.74	1.63	11.1	1.04			108			43			27	28	
5.0	125		162	40	53.5	1.92	1.73	11.0	1.08			110			42			26	28	
5.5	150		169	39	60.2	2.17	1.94	11.5	1.12			111			42			26	29	
6.0	150	188/94	176	46	68.8	2.36	2.04	11.6	1.16	7.37	22	112	114	2	42	38	−4	27	32	0.16
6.5	175		182	50	76.0	2.51	2.11	11.6	1.19			114			41			29	34	
7.0	175		188	51	89.7	2.84	2.23	11.9	1.27			118			38			30	38	
	Recovery		178	31	59.6	2.17	1.83	0.3	1.19			111			43			26	31	
	Recovery		161	29	47.5	1.66	1.19	7.4	1.39			116			41			27	38	
	Recovery		144	27	42.0	1.37	0.84	5.8	1.63			123			37			29	47	
	Recovery	181/100	136	28	37.5	1.08	0.62	4.6	1.74	7.30	16	127	126	2	35	33	−2	33	57	0.18
	Recovery		135	24	23.9	0.68	0.44	3.3	1.55			124			36			32	50	

Interpretation

Comments

The results of this patient's resting respiratory function studies are normal (Table 9.6.1). The resting ECG is normal.

Analysis

Referring to flow chart 1, peak V̇O₂ and the anaerobic threshold are within normal limits (Table 9.6.2). See flow chart 2: ECG, O₂ pulse at peak V̇O₂, and arterial blood gases are normal (branchpoint 2.1). The patient is not obese (branchpoint 2.2).

Conclusion

This is a normal 37-year-old man. Symptoms probably relate to anxiety and lack of fitness.

Case 7 Normal Man

Clinical Findings

This 74-year-old retired shipyard worker was referred for evaluation and exercise testing because work-up at another institution had resulted in a diagnosis of "emphysema" despite no evidence of airway obstruction. The patient had a mild, nonproductive cough, had smoked approximately 35 years, and continued to smoke. He had no other circulatory or respiratory symptoms, except for shortness of breath from climbing 2 flights of stairs but not from walking for 1 mile on the level. Physical examination was normal. Exercise testing was performed to help resolve the difference between clinical impressions.

Exercise Findings

The patient performed exercise on a cycle ergometer. He pedalled at 60 rpm without added load for 3 minutes. The work rate was then increased 15 W per minute to his symptom-limited maximum. Arterial blood was sampled every second minute, and intra-arterial blood pressure was recorded from a percutaneously placed brachial artery catheter. The patient stopped exercise because of shortness of breath. Resting and exercise ECGs were normal.

TABLE 9.7.1. Selected Respiratory Function Data

Measurement	Predicted	Measured
Age, yr		74
Sex		Male
Height, cm		169
Weight, kg	73	82
Hematocrit, %		44
VC, L	3.37	4.88
IC, L	2.25	4.12
TLC, L	5.60	6.05
FEV_1, L	2.58	3.96
FEV_1/VC, %	77	81
MVV, L/min	110	107
$D_{L}CO$, ml/mm Hg/min	21.6	24.8

TABLE 9.7.2. Selected Exercise Data

Measurement	Predicted	Measured
Peak $\dot{V}O_2$, L/min	1.74	1.95
Maximum HR, beats/min	146	132
Maximum O_2 pulse, ml/beat	11.9	14.8
$\Delta\dot{V}O_2/\Delta WR$, ml/min/W	10.3	10.6
AT, L/min	>0.78	1.4
Blood pressure, mmHg (rest, max)		150/84, 177/79
Maximum $\dot{V}E$, L/min		68
Exercise breathing reserve, L/min	>15	39
PaO_2, mmHg (rest, max ex)		97, 101
$P(A - a)O_2$, mmHg (rest, max ex)		20, 16
$P(a - ET)CO_2$, mmHg (rest, max ex)		3, 0
VD/VT (rest, heavy ex)		0.35, 0.22
HCO_3^-, mEq/L (rest, 2-min recov)		20, 15

FIGURE 9.7.1.

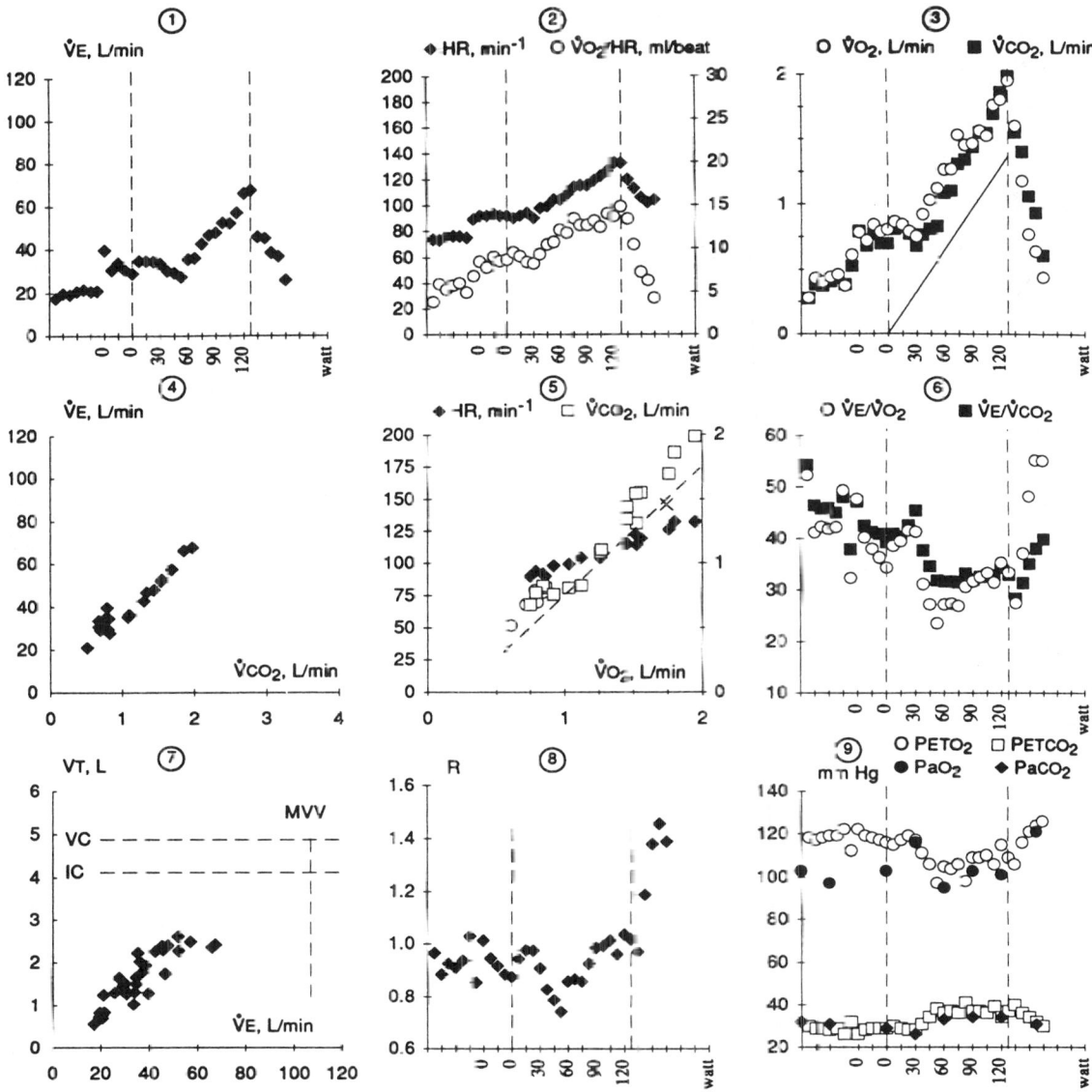

1. Vertical dashed lines in panels 1 to 3 and 6, 8, and 9 indicate the beginning and the end of increasing work period.
2. Unloaded cycling is performed for 3 minutes before the left vertical dashed line.
3. In panel 3, the diagonal line shows the increase of $\dot{V}O_2$ at a slope of 10 ml/min/w.
4. In panel 5, the diagonal dashed line has a slope of 1; the "x" in the upper right is the predicted maximum heart rate and $\dot{V}C_2$ for the subject.

TABLE 9.7.3.   Air Breathing

Time min	Work rate watts	BP mmHg	HR min⁻¹	f min⁻¹	$\dot{V}_E$ L/min BTPS	$\dot{V}_{CO_2}$ L/min STPD	$\dot{V}_{O_2}$ L/min STPD	$\dot{V}_{O_2}$/HR ml/beat	R	pH	HCO₃⁻ meq/L	PO₂ ET	PO₂ a	PO₂ (A−a)	PCO₂ ET	PCO₂ a	PCO₂ (a−ET)	$\dot{V}_E/\dot{V}_{CO_2}$	$\dot{V}_E/\dot{V}_{O_2}$	VD/VT
	Rest	150/82								7.41	20		103			32				
	Rest		74	31	17.3	0.27	0.28	3.8	0.96			118			30			54	52	
	Rest		73	24	19.7	0.38	0.43	5.9	0.88			117			29			46	41	
	Rest		76	27	19.2	0.37	0.40	5.3	0.93			118			29			46	42	
	Rest	147/84	76	27	20.7	0.40	0.44	5.8	0.91	7.42	20	119	97	20	28	31	3	46	42	0.35
	Rest		76	26	21.6	0.43	0.46	6.1	0.93			119			29			45	42	
	Rest		75	30	20.8	0.38	0.37	4.9	1.03			122			26			48	49	
	Unloaded		89	17	21.1	0.52	0.61	6.9	0.85			112			32			38	32	
	Unloaded		92	31	39.8	0.79	0.78	8.5	1.01			122			26			47	48	
	Unloaded		92	23	30.8	0.68	0.72	7.8	0.94			119			28			42	40	
	Unloaded		93	26	34.0	0.77	0.84	9.0	0.92			118			29			41	38	
	Unloaded		92	24	30.7	0.70	0.79	8.6	0.89			117			29			41	36	
	Unloaded	162/84	92	20	29.1	0.70	0.80	8.7	0.88	7.42	18	116	103	15	29	29	0	39	34	0.23
0.5	15		90	21	34.9	0.81	0.86	9.6	0.94			115			30			41	39	
1.0	15		92	21	34.8	0.82	0.84	9.1	0.98			117			29			40	39	
1.5	30		94	23	34.7	0.77	0.79	8.4	0.97			119			28			43	41	
2.0	30	159/81	90	33	33.7	0.68	0.75	8.3	0.91	7.44	17	117	116	6	28	26	−2	45	41	0.25
2.5	45		98	20	30.3	0.76	0.92	9.4	0.83			111			31			38	31	
3.0	45		99	20	29.7	0.81	1.03	10.4	0.79			106			34			35	27	
3.5	60		100	17	27.8	0.83	1.12	10.8	0.74			97			38			32	24	
4.0	60	168/84	104	16	35.6	1.08	1.26	12.1	0.86	7.37	19	105	95	18	36	33	−3	32	27	0.17
4.5	75		108	18	36.4	1.10	1.27	11.8	0.87			104			37			32	27	
5.0	75		114	19	42.8	1.31	1.53	13.4	0.86			106			36			31	27	
5.5	90		115	27	46.8	1.34	1.45	12.6	0.92			98			41			33	31	
6.0	90	186/90	115	20	47.9	1.44	1.46	12.7	0.99	7.36	19	109	103	13	37	34	−3	32	32	0.20
6.5	105		119	23	52.5	1.55	1.56	13.1	0.99			109			37			33	32	
7.0	105		122	20	52.2	1.54	1.52	12.5	1.01			110			36			33	33	
7.5	120		126	23	57.2	1.69	1.76	14.0	0.96			106			39			33	31	
8.0	120	177/79	132	28	66.1	1.86	1.80	13.6	1.03	7.33	18	115	101	16	34	34	0	34	35	0.25
8.5	135		132	28	67.5	1.98	1.95	14.8	1.02			109			37			33	33	
	Recovery		120	20	45.8	1.55	1.60	13.3	0.97			106			40			28	28	
	Recovery		113	19	45.4	1.40	1.18	10.4	1.19			116			36			31	37	
	Recovery		106	20	38.8	1.06	0.77	7.3	1.38			121			34			35	48	
	Recovery	168/78	102	21	37.1	0.93	0.64	6.3	1.45	7.31	15	124	121	6	32	31	−1	38	55	0.25
	Recovery		104	20	25.9	0.61	0.44	4.2	1.39			126			30			40	55	

Interpretation

Comments

This patient's resting respiratory function is normal (Table 9.7.1). The resting ECG is normal.

Analysis

In flow chart 1, the maximum $\dot{V}_{O_2}$ is normal. The anaerobic threshold is normal (Table 9.7.2). See flow chart 2: The ECG, O_2 pulse, arterial blood gases, and VD/VT are normal (branchpoint 2.1). The patient is not obese (branchpoint 2.2).

Conclusion

This is a normal cardiovascular and respiratory response to exercise. The patient has no evidence of abnormalities consistent with the diagnosis of "emphysema" given to the patient in a previous examination.

Case 8 Normal, with Ventilatory Chemoreflex Insensitivity

Clinical Findings

This 67-year-old retired man had worked for 30 years in the shipyards. He had never smoked. Three months previously, he was diagnosed with hypertension for which he was treated with triamterene and hydrochlorothiazide. He noted shortness of breath after climbing 2 flights of stairs and frequent mild substernal pressure not related to exertion, meals, body position, or stress. Physical, roentgenographic, laboratory, and ECG results were normal.

Exercise Findings

The patient performed exercise on a cycle ergometer. He pedalled at 60 rpm without added load for 3 minutes. The work rate was then increased 20 W per minute to his symptom-limited maximum. Arterial blood was sampled every second minute, and intra-arterial blood pressure was recorded from a percutaneously placed brachial artery catheter. He stopped exercise with shortness of breath, but without chest pain or pressure. ECG pattern remained normal.

TABLE 9.8.1. Selected Respiratory Function Data

Measurement	Predicted	Measured
Age, yr		67
Sex		Male
Height, cm		173
Weight, kg	76	80
Hematocrit, %		48
VC, L	3.82	3.86
IC, L	2.55	2.42
TLC, L	6.06	6.04
FEV_1, L	2.97	3.07
FEV_1/VC, %	78	80
MVV, L/min	124	121
D_{LCO}, ml/mm Hg/min	26.3	32.3

TABLE 9.8.2. Selected Exercise Data

Measurement	Predicted	Measured
Peak $\dot{V}O_2$, L/min	1.98	1.94
Maximum HR, beats/min	153	142
Maximum O_2 pulse, ml/beat	13.0	13.7
$\Delta\dot{V}O_2$/ΔWR, ml/min/W	10.3	9.9
AT, L/min	>0.89	1.5
Blood pressure, mmHg (rest, max)		176/92, 215/92
Maximum $\dot{V}E$, L/min		56
Exercise breathing reserve, L/min	>15	65
PaO_2, mmHg (rest, max ex)		96, 81
$P(A - a)O_2$, mmHg (rest, max ex)		8, 22
$P(a - ET)CO_2$, mmHg (rest, max ex)		1, −6
VD/VT (rest, heavy ex)		0.39, 0.26
HCO_3^-, mEq/L (rest, 2-min recov)		27, 22

FIGURE 9.8.1. Air Breathing

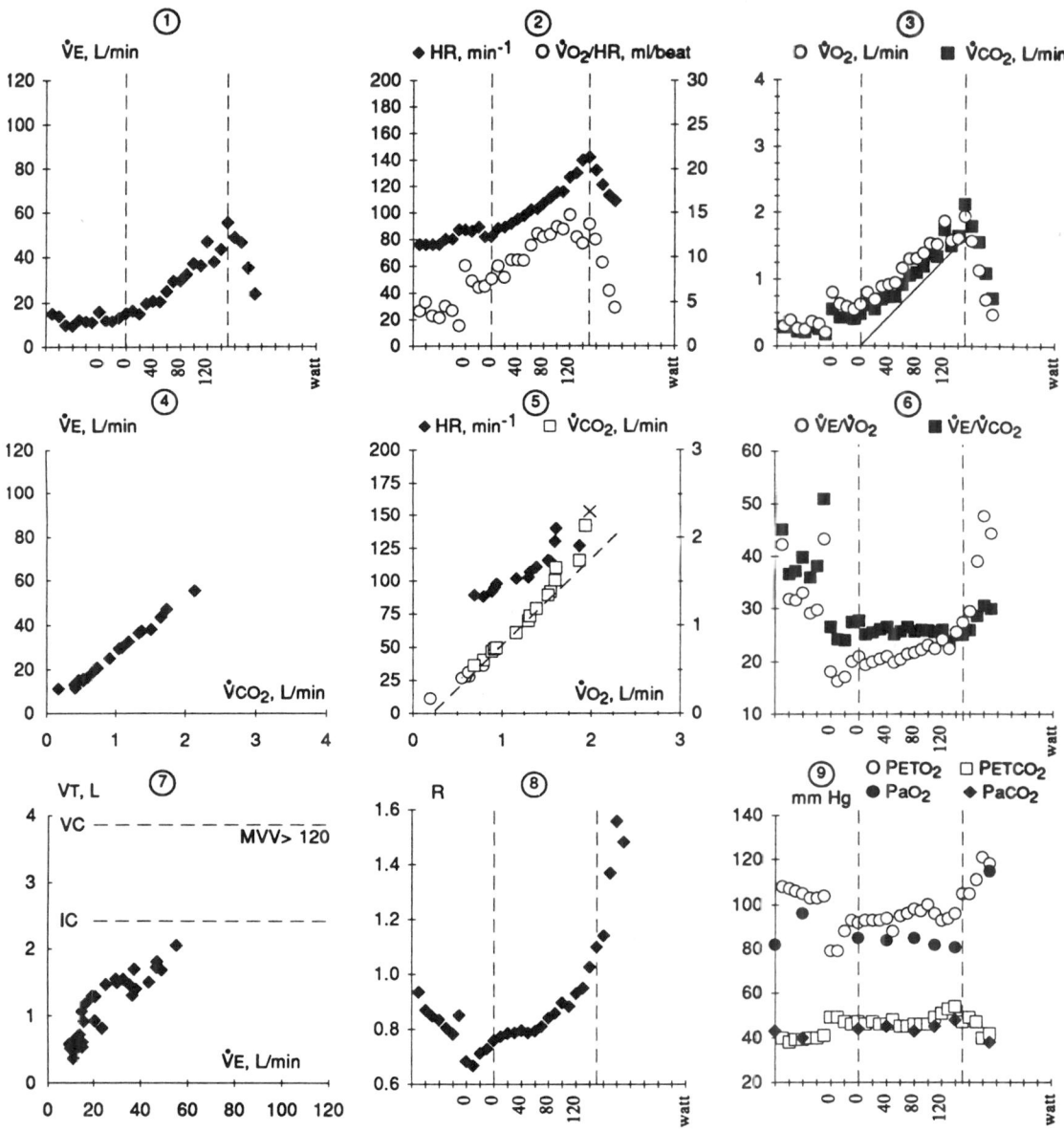

1. Vertical dashed lines in panels 1 to 3 and 6, 8, and 9 indicate the beginning and the end of increasing work period.

2. Unloaded cycling is performed for 3 minutes before the left vertical dashed line.

3. In panel 3, the diagonal line shows the increase of $\dot{V}O_2$ at a slope of 10 ml/min/w.

4. In panel 5, the diagonal dashed line has a slope of 1; the "x" in the upper right is the predicted maximum heart rate and $\dot{V}O_2$ for the subject.

TABLE 9.8.3. Air Breathing

Time min	Work rate watts	BP mmHg	HP min⁻¹	f min⁻¹	V̇E L/min BTPS	V̇CO2 L/min STPD	V̇O2 L/min STPD	V̇O2/HR ml/beat	R	pH	HCO3⁻ meq/L	PO2 ET	PO2 a	PO2 (A−a)	PCO2 ET	PCO2 a	PCO2 (a−ET)	V̇E/V̇CO2	V̇E/V̇O2	VD/VT
	Rest	176/92								7.41	27		82			43				
	Rest		76	28	15.0	0.28	0.30	3.9	0.93			108			40			45	42	
	Rest		76	19	13.7	0.33	0.38	5.0	0.87			107			38			37	32	
	Rest		76	19	9.8	0.22	0.26	3.4	0.85			106			39			37	31	
	Rest	164/92	76	16	9.3	0.20	0.24	3.2	0.83	7.43	26	105	96	8	39	40	1	40	33	0.39
	Rest		80	22	12.3	0.29	0.36	4.5	0.81			103			40			36	29	
	Rest		80	22	11.4	0.25	0.32	4.0	0.78			103			40			38	30	
	Unloaded		87	30	11.2	0.17	0.20	2.3	0.85			104			41			51	43	
	Unloaded		87	17	15.7	0.54	0.79	9.1	0.68			79			49			26	18	
	Unloaded		86	19	11.8	0.42	0.63	7.3	0.67			79			49			24	16	
	Unloaded		89	18	11.6	0.42	0.59	6.6	0.71			88			47			24	17	
	Unloaded		82	25	13.1	0.40	0.55	6.7	0.73			93			46			27	20	
	Unloaded	185/92	82	25	15.1	0.47	0.62	7.6	0.76	7.40	27	92	85	10	47	44	−3	28	21	0.25
0.5	20		88	14	16.5	0.61	0.79	9.0	0.77			93			46			25	19	
1.0	20		89	14	14.9	0.54	0.69	7.8	0.78			93			47			25	20	
1.5	40		92	15	19.5	0.70	0.89	9.7	0.79			93			46			26	20	
2.0	40	194/89	95	16	20.7	0.73	0.92	9.7	0.79	7.40	27	94	84	12	46	45	−1	26	21	0.26
2.5	60		98	22	20.5	0.74	0.94	9.6	0.79			88			48			25	20	
3.0	60		102	17	25.1	0.92	1.16	11.4	0.79			95			45			26	20	
3.5	80		103	19	29.5	1.05	1.30	12.6	0.81			96			45			27	21	
4.0	80	203/89	107	20	30.0	1.10	1.31	12.2	0.84	7.40	26	98	85	16	46	43	−3	26	22	0.21
4.5	100		111	21	32.6	1.19	1.39	12.5	0.86			97			46			26	22	
5.0	100		115	22	37.4	1.38	1.54	13.4	0.90			100			46			26	23	
5.5	120	209/89	116	28	36.6	1.34	1.52	13.1	0.88	7.38	26	96	82	18	49	45	−4	26	23	0.23
6.0	120		127	26	47.2	1.74	1.87	14.7	0.93			93			51			26	24	
6.5	140		130	27	38.1	1.51	1.59	12.2	0.95			94			53			24	23	
7.0	140	215/92	140	29	43.6	1.65	1.61	11.5	1.02	7.35	26	96	81	22	54	48	−6	25	26	0.26
7.5	160		142	27	55.5	2.13	1.94	13.7	1.10			105			47			25	27	
	Recovery		132	29	49.0	1.80	1.58	12.0	1.14			105			49	38	−4	26	29	
	Recovery		121	27	46.8	1.56	1.14	9.4	1.37			111			47			29	39	
	Recovery		113	24	35.4	1.09	0.70	6.2	1.56			121			40			31	48	
	Recovery	209/92	109	29	23.7	0.71	0.48	4.4	1.48	7.37	22	118	115	7	42			30	44	0.22

Interpretation

Comments

Results of the resting respiratory function studies are normal (Table 9.8.1). The resting ECG is normal.

Analysis

Referring to flow chart 1, the peak V̇O2 and anaerobic threshold are normal (Table 9.8.2). See flow chart 2: The exercise ECG, arterial blood gases, VD/VT, and O2 pulse at peak V̇O2 are normal (branchpoint 2.1). The patient is not obese (branchpoint 2.2). While the arterial CO2 tension is normal at rest, the increase in ventilation lagged the increase in CO2 production, causing arterial PCO2 to rise gradually during exercise (panel 9, Fig. 9.8.1 and Table 9.8.3). This is occasionally seen when the ventilatory chemoreflex is relatively insensitive to the exercise metabolic acidosis. Because the CO2 stores are increasing in the body as a consequence of the rising PaCO2, CO2 output does not rise as steeply as it otherwise might, particularly above the anaerobic threshold. Thus, V̇E/V̇CO2 at the termination of work is not increased over that at the AT (panel 6, Fig. 9.8.1) and there is no steepening in the V̇E-work rate relationship (panels 1 and 4, Fig. 9.8.1).

Conclusion

This is normal cardiovascular and respiratory function in a patient likely to have a ventilatory chemoreflex that is relatively insensitive to pH decrease.

Case 9 Exceptionally Fit Man with Mild Lung Disease

Clinical Findings

This 59-year-old worker had no complaints or history of heart or lung disease. He had sustained a gunshot wound to the right chest at age 24 that was not surgically treated. He had been exposed to asbestos 20 years previously and had smoked 1 pack of cigarettes daily for 12 years until 20 years ago. He cycled approximately 50 miles a week. Physical, roentgenographic, and ECG examinations were normal except for evidence of focal, old granulomatous disease and an old rib fracture.

Exercise Findings

The patient performed exercise on a cycle ergometer. He pedalled at 60 rpm without added load for 3 minutes. The work rate was then increased 20 W per minute to his symptom-limited maximum. Arterial blood was sampled every second minute, and intra-arterial blood pressure was recorded from a percutaneously placed brachial artery catheter. He stopped exercise because of general exhaustion. Exercise ECGs were normal.

TABLE 9.9.1. Selected Respiratory Function Data

Measurement	Predicted	Measured
Age, yr		59
Sex		Male
Height, cm		175
Weight, kg	78	93
Hematocrit, %		46
VC, L	4.21	4.34
IC, L	2.79	3.57
TLC, L	6.36	5.86
FEV_1, L	3.58	3.57
FEV_1/VC, %	80	82
MVV, L/min	137	152
D_{LCO}, ml/mm Hg/min	28.2	29.5

TABLE 9.9.2. Selected Exercise Data

Measurement	Predicted	Measured
Peak $\dot{V}O_2$, L/min	2.32	3.40
Maximum HR, beats/min	161	195
Maximum O_2 pulse, ml/beat	14.4	17.4
$\Delta\dot{V}O_2/\Delta WR$, ml/min/W	10.3	12.7
AT, L/min	>1.02	1.4
Blood pressure, mmHg (rest, max)		125/75, 200/88
Maximum $\dot{V}E$, L/min		174
Exercise breathing reserve, L/min	>15	−22
PaO_2, mmHg (rest, max ex)		120, 71
$P(A - a)O_2$, mmHg (rest, max ex)		5, 49
$P(a - ET)CO_2$, mmHg (rest, max ex)		−4, −13
VD/VT (rest, heavy ex)		0.17, 0.02
HCO_3^-, mEq/L (rest, 2-min recov)		25, 10

FIGURE 9.9.1.

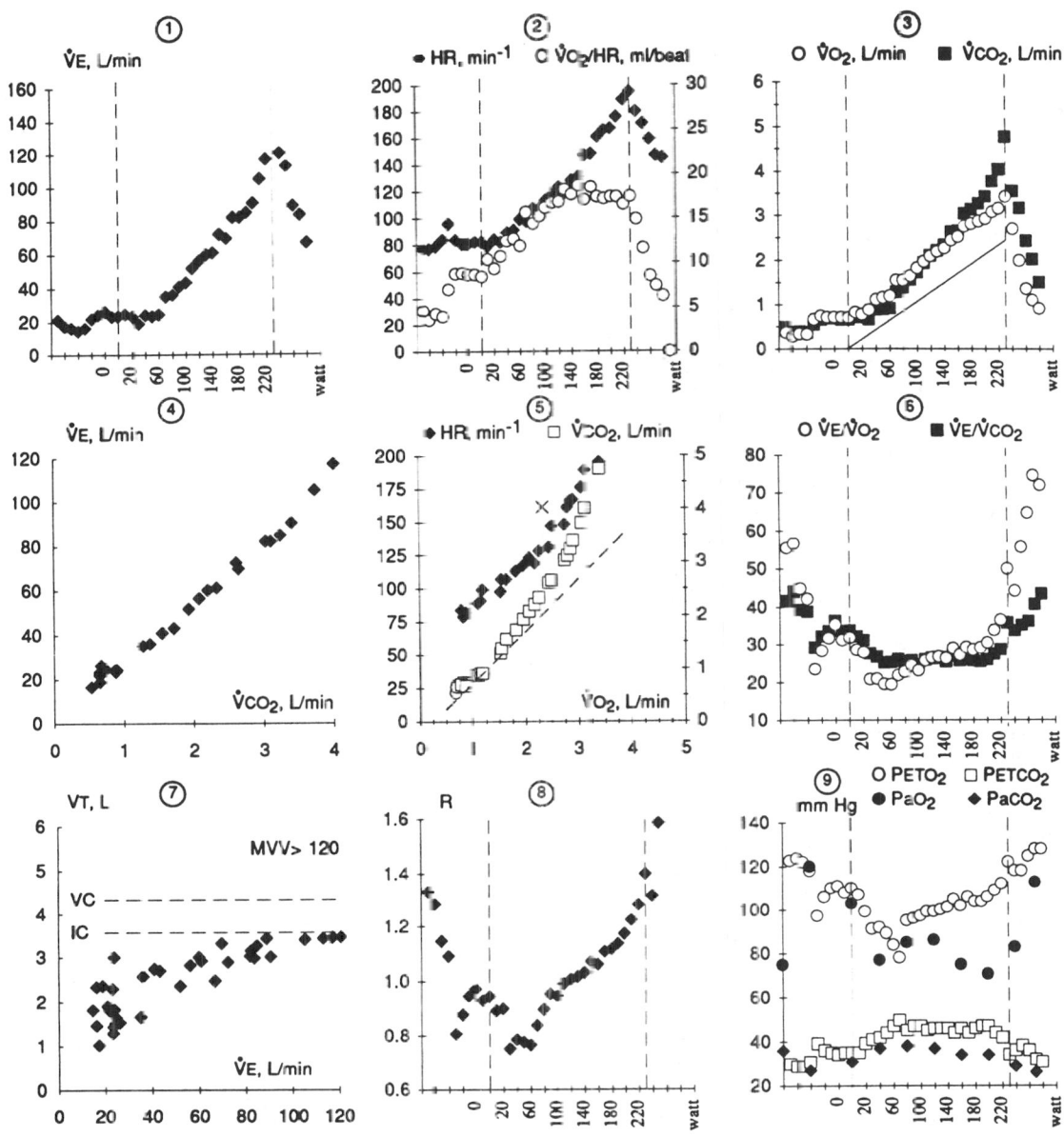

1. Vertical dashed lines in panels 1 to 3 and 6, 8, and 9 indicate the beginning and the end of increasing work period.
2. Unloaded cycling is performed for 3 minutes before the left vertical dashed line.
3. In panel 3, the diagonal line shows the increase of $\dot{V}O_2$ at a slope of 10 ml/min/w.
4. In panel 5, the diagonal dashed line has a slope of 1; the "x" in the upper right is the predicted maximum heart rate and $\dot{V}O_2$ for the subject.

Interpretation

Comments

The results of this patient's respiratory function studies are within normal limits (Table 9.9.1). The resting ECG is normal. The respiratory alkalosis at rest, while breathing on the mouthpiece, is acute, developing in anticipation of exercise. It disappears after exercise started. When starting to breathe on the mouthpiece, the patient hyperventilates to a pH of 7.52, $PaCO_2$ of 27 mmHg and PaO_2 of 120. The

TABLE 9.9.3. Air Breathing

Time min	Work rate watts	BP mmHg	HR min⁻¹	f min⁻¹	$\dot{V}_E$ L/min BTPS	$\dot{V}_{CO_2}$ L/min STPD	$\dot{V}_{O_2}$ L/min STPD	$\dot{V}_{O_2}$/HR ml/beat	R	pH	HCO₃⁻ meq/L	P_{O_2} ET	P_{O_2} a	P_{O_2} (A−a)	P_{CO_2} ET	P_{CO_2} a	P_{CO_2} (a−ET)	$\dot{V}_E/\dot{V}_{CO_2}$	$\dot{V}_E/\dot{V}_{O_2}$	V_D/V_T
	Rest	125/75								7.45	25		75			36				
	Rest		77	11	20.9	0.48	0.36	4.7	1.33			123			30			42	55	
	Rest		77	17	17.3	0.36	0.28	3.6	1.29			124			29			44	57	
	Rest		79	11	16.2	0.39	0.34	4.3	1.15			122			29			39	45	
	Rest	119/75	84	8	14.6	0.36	0.33	3.9	1.09	7.52	22	118	120	5	31	27	−4	39	42	0.17
	Unloaded		96	7	16.4	0.54	0.67	7.0	0.81			97			39			29	24	
	Unloaded		84	12	21.9	0.65	0.74	8.8	0.88			106			36			32	28	
	Unloaded		81	13	23.9	0.68	0.72	8.9	0.94			110			35			34	32	
	Unloaded		81	17	26.2	0.68	0.70	8.6	0.97			111			34			36	35	
	Unloaded		82	10	23.0	0.66	0.71	8.7	0.93			108			35			34	31	
	Unloaded	156/81	82	16	23.3	0.65	0.69	8.4	0.94	7.47	22	110	103	14	35	31	−4	34	32	0.17
0.5	20		79	15	24.7	0.73	0.82	10.4	0.89			107			35			32	29	
1.0	20		84	18	23.3	0.70	0.78	9.3	0.90			99			39			31	28	
1.5	40		82	8	13.9	0.66	0.88	10.7	0.75			91			41			28	21	
2.0	40	163/81	89	8	24.0	0.87	1.11	12.5	0.78	7.43	24	92	77	28	42	37	−5	27	21	0.13
2.5	60		91	13	23.5	0.89	1.15	12.6	0.77			89			44			25	19	
3.0	60		99	16	24.2	0.90	1.18	11.9	0.76			84			47			25	19	
3.5	80		98	21	35.2	1.28	1.53	15.6	0.84			78			50			26	22	
4.0	80	175/81	107	14	36.1	1.38	1.54	14.4	0.90	7.41	24	95	85	24	45	38	−7	25	23	0.10
4.5	100		107	15	41.1	1.55	1.63	15.2	0.95			96			47			26	24	
5.0	100		113	16	43.4	1.72	1.82	16.1	0.95			97			47			24	23	
5.5	120		117	22	52.0	1.93	1.95	16.7	0.99			99			45			26	26	
6.0	120		123	20	56.5	2.08	2.07	16.8	1.00	7.37	21	99	86	27	46	37	−9	26	26	0.11
6.5	140		119	20	60.0	2.20	2.17	18.2	1.01			100			46			27	27	
7.0	140		128	21	61.2	2.33	2.26	17.7	1.03			101			46			26	26	
7.5	160		131	25	72.5	2.61	2.44	18.6	1.07			105			44			27	29	
8.0	160	200/88	147	21	69.8	2.65	2.50	17.0	1.06	7.35	18	102	75	43	46	34	−12	26	27	0.01
8.5	180		148	27	82.1	3.03	2.74	18.5	1.11			106			44			26	29	
9.0	180		161	26	82.2	3.11	2.79	17.3	1.11			104			46			26	29	
9.5	200		166	26	85.0	3.24	2.85	17.2	1.14			104			47			26	29	
10.0	200		167	30	90.6	3.40	2.90	17.4	1.17	7.29	16	106	71	49	47	34	−13	26	30	0.02
10.5	220		176	31	105.5	3.74	3.06	17.4	1.22			109			44			28	34	
11.0	220		189	34	117.3	4.01	3.13	16.6	1.28			112			42			29	37	
11.5	240		195	55	174.5	4.75	3.40	17.4	1.40			122			34			36	50	
	Recovery	200/88	180	35	121.1	3.52	2.68	14.9	1.31	7.26	13	118	83	43	36	29	−7	34	44	0.11
	Recovery		171	33	1¯3.3	3.15	1.99	11.6	1.58			118			38			35	56	
	Recovery		159	26	89.2	2.42	1.35	8.5	1.79			125			36			36	64	
	Recovery	163/75	147	28	83.7	2.01	1.09	7.4	1.84	7.20	10	128	113	20	32	26	−6	40	75	0.17
	Recovery		145	27	67.1	1.50	0.90	6.2	1.67			128			31			43	72	
	Recovery																			

extraordinarily large increase in Pa_{O_2} when starting to breathe on the mouthpiece at rest is probably due to: 1) hypoxemia off the mouthpiece due to microatelectasis associated with obesity (a common problem in overweight subjects); and 2) the large increase in Pa_{O_2}, which accompanies acute hyperventilation, and a high R.

Analysis

Referring to flow chart 1, this patient's peak $\dot{V}_{O_2}$ and anaerobic threshold are above predicted (Table 9.9.2). Because he cycled regularly to maintain his fitness, he performed exceedingly well. See flow chart 2: The ECG and O_2 pulse (high because of fitness) at maximal exercise are normal, but the blood gases are abnormal (branchpoint 2.1). V_D/V_T and $P(a − ET)_{CO_2}$ are normal, but $P(A − a)_{O_2}$ at maximum exercise is increased and suggests the presence of mild lung disease (branchpoint 2.3).

Conclusion

This exceptionally fit man of 59 years has features of mild lung disease.

Case 10 Normal: Cycle and Treadmill

Clinical Findings

This 37-year-old hospital employee was asymptomatic and volunteered for an exercise study. He did not exercise regularly or smoke. Physical examination, chest roentgenograms and resting ECG were normal.

Exercise Findings

On 2 separate days, 1 month apart, the subject exercised to maximum tolerance using an incremental protocol, first on the cycle and second on the treadmill. He stopped on both occasions because of calf fatigue. There was no arrhythmia or abnormality in the ECG.

TABLE 9.10.1.   Selected Respiratory Function Data

Measurement	Predicted	Measured
Age, yr		37
Sex		Male
Height, cm		161
Weight, kg	66	53
Hematocrit, %		45
VC, L	3.56	3.21
IC, L	2.37	2.51
TLC, L	4.90	5.01
FEV$_1$, L	2.87	2.64
FEV$_1$/VC, %	81	82
MVV, L/min	132	107
D$_{LCO}$, ml/mm Hg/min	23.1	22.3

TABLE 9.10.2.   Selected Exercise Data

Measurement	Predicted		Measured	
	Cycle	Treadmill	Cycle	Treadmill
Peak $\dot{V}O_2$, L/min	2.21	2.45	1.37	2.07
Maximum HR, beats/min	183	183	173	183
Maximum O_2 pulse, ml/beat	12.1	13.4	10.8	11.3
$\Delta\dot{V}C_2/\Delta$WR, ml/min/W	10.3		8.4	
AT, L/min	>0.93	>1.03	1.7	1.15
Maximum $\dot{V}E$, L/min			76	85
Exercise breathing reserve, L/min	>15	>15	31	22

TABLE 9.10.3. Cycle Ergometry

Time min	Work rate watts	BP mmHg	HR min⁻¹	f min⁻¹	$\dot{V}_E$ L/min BTPS	$\dot{V}_{CO_2}$ L/min STPD	$\dot{V}_{O_2}$ L/min STPD	$\dot{V}_{O_2}$/HR ml/beat	R	pH	HCO₃⁻ meq/L	P_{O_2}, mmHg ET	a	(A − a)	P_{CO_2}, mmHg ET	a	(a − ET)	$\dot{V}_E$/$\dot{V}_{CO_2}$	$\dot{V}_E$/$\dot{V}_{O_2}$	V_D/V_T
	Rest		79	15	9.5	0.28	0.33	4.2	0.85			99			44			29	25	
	Rest		95	14	11.1	0.36	0.42	4.4	0.86			97			45			28	24	
	Rest		78	13	7.8	0.23	0.26	3.3	0.88			101			44			29	26	
	Rest		74	14	7.3	0.19	0.21	2.8	0.90			102			43			32	29	
	Unloaded		109	18	17.3	0.58	0.55	5.0	1.05			105			44			27	29	
	Unloaded		97	8	11.1	0.44	0.52	5.4	0.85			96			46			24	20	
	Unloaded		103	17	14.3	0.53	0.63	6.1	0.84			92			48			24	20	
	Unloaded		104	16	15.1	0.56	0.65	6.3	0.86			94			47			25	21	
	Unloaded		108	16	17.7	0.67	0.71	6.6	0.94			97			47			24	23	
	Unloaded		97	16	14.8	0.55	0.55	5.7	1.00			103			46			24	24	
0.5	25		107	16	16.4	0.61	0.60	5.6	1.02			104			46			25	25	
1.0	25		108	18	16.2	0.57	0.57	5.3	1.00			103			45			26	26	
1.5	50		113	18	15.8	0.58	0.64	5.7	0.91			96			47			25	22	
2.0	50		110	17	17.1	0.67	0.74	6.7	0.91			94			50			23	21	
2.5	75		122	19	22.0	0.86	0.89	7.3	0.97			99			48			24	23	
3.0	75		129	17	19.8	0.85	0.90	7.0	0.94			93			52			22	20	
3.5	100		132	21	26.4	1.07	1.04	7.9	1.03			99			50			23	24	
4.0	100		133	17	22.9	1.07	1.12	8.4	0.96			89			57			20	19	
4.5	125		143	21	31.1	1.40	1.29	9.0	1.09			97			55			21	23	
5.0	125		147	22	35.1	1.64	1.50	10.2	1.09			95			56			20	22	
5.5	150		155	26	41.4	1.82	1.52	9.8	1.20			102			53			22	26	
6.0	150		159	27	44.4	1.94	1.58	9.9	1.23			103			53			22	27	
6.5	175		168	31	53.2	2.24	1.71	10.2	1.31			107			52			23	30	
7.0	175		173	44	75.8	2.79	1.87	10.8	1.49			114			46			26	39	
	Recovery		167	34	60.1	2.31	1.67	10.0	1.38			109			50			25	34	
	Recovery		158	30	49.5	1.88	1.29	8.2	1.46			112			49			25	36	
	Recovery		146	31	48.8	1.68	0.98	6.7	1.71			118			44			27	47	
	Recovery		140	27	40.1	1.30	0.73	5.2	1.78			121			42			29	52	

FIGURE 9.10.1.   Cycle ergometry.

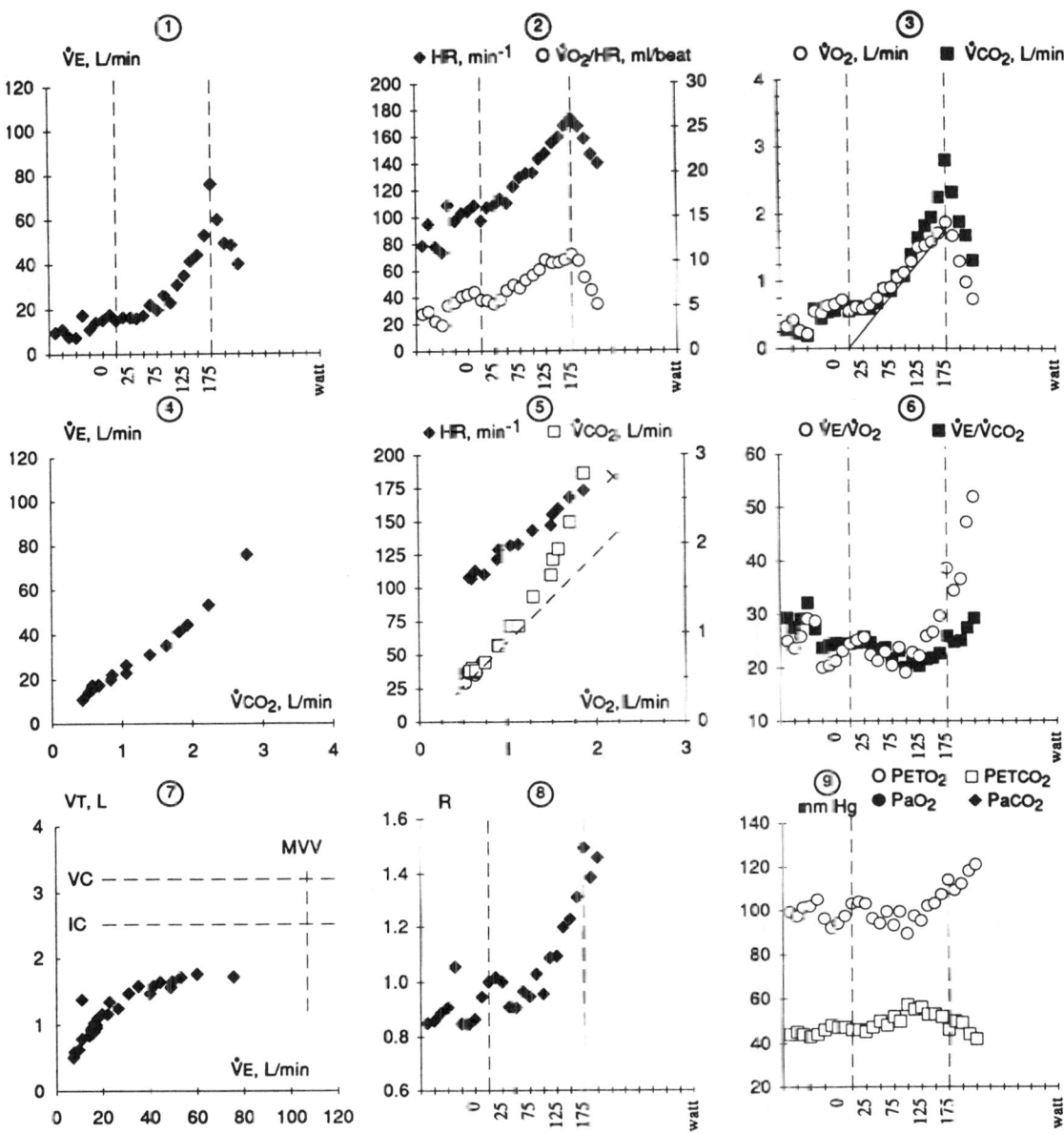

1. Vertical dashed lines in panels 1 to 3 and 6, 8, and 9 indicate the beginning and the end of increasing work period.

2. Unloaded cycling is performed for 3 minutes before the left vertical dashed line.

3. In panel 3, the diagonal line shows the increase of $\dot{V}O_2$ at a slope of 10 ml/min/w.

4. In panel 5, the diagonal dashed line has a slope of 1; the "x" in the upper right is the predicted maximum heart rate and $\dot{V}O_2$ for the subject.

FIGURE 9.10.2.   Treadmill ergometry.

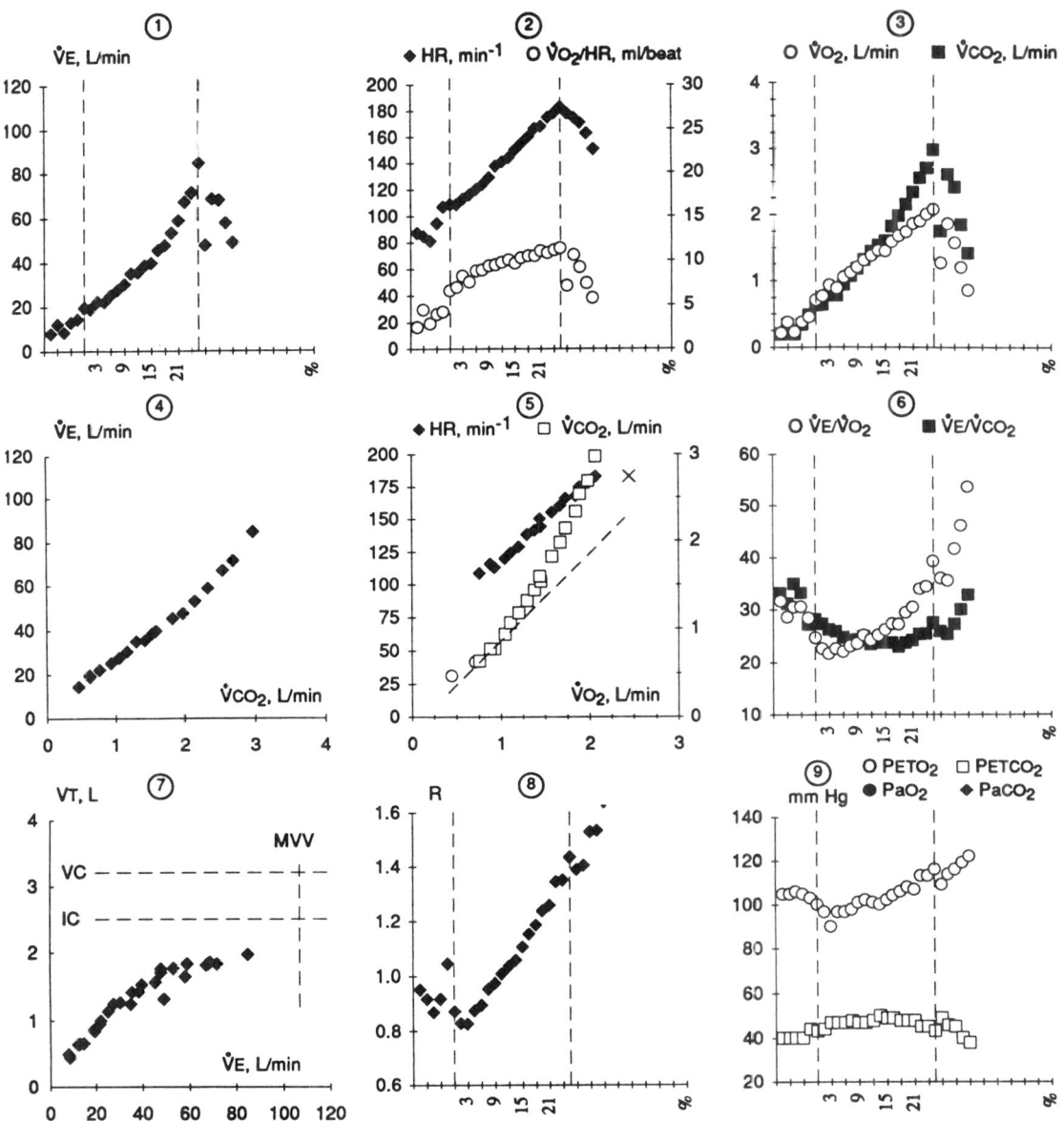

1. Vertical dashed lines in panels 1 to 3 and 6, 8, and 9 indicate the beginning and the end of increasing work period.
2. Zero grade walking is performed for 1 minute before the left vertical dashed line.
3. In panel 5, the diagonal dashed line has a slope of 1; the "x" in the upper right is the predicted maximum heart rate and $\dot{V}O_2$ for the subject.

TABLE 9.10.4.   Treadmill Ergometry

Time min	Treadmill grade, %	BP mmHg	HR min⁻¹	f min⁻¹	$\dot{V}_E$ L/min BTPS	$\dot{V}_{CO_2}$ L/min STPD	$\dot{V}_{O_2}$ L/min STPD	$\dot{V}_{O_2}$ HR ml/beat	R	pH	HCO₃ meq/L	P_{O_2}, mmHg ET	a	(A − a)	P_{CO_2}, mmHg ET	a	(a − ET)	$\dot{V}_E$ $\dot{V}_{CO_2}$	$\dot{V}_E$ $\dot{V}_{O_2}$	VD VT
	Rest		87	16	8.0	0.20	0.21	2.4	0.95			105			40			33	32	
	Rest		85	19	12.2	0.34	0.37	4.4	0.92			105			40			31	29	
	Rest		81	19	8.6	0.20	0.23	2.8	0.87			106			40			35	30	
	Rest		95	20	13.0	0.34	0.37	3.9	0.92			105			40			33	31	
	0		107	22	14.6	0.47	0.45	4.2	1.04			103			44			27	28	
	0		109	23	19.4	0.62	0.71	6.5	0.87			100			43			28	25	
0.5	3		109	22	19.1	0.63	0.76	7.0	0.83			97			44			27	23	
1.0	3		113	22	22.1	0.77	0.93	8.2	0.83			90			47			26	22	
1.5	6		116	23	21.9	0.77	0.88	7.6	0.88			97			47			26	23	
2.0	6		120	22	25.1	0.94	1.05	8.8	0.90			97			47			25	22	
2.5	9		124	22	27.5	1.06	1.11	9.0	0.95			98			48			24	23	
3.0	9		129	24	30.4	1.17	1.20	9.3	0.98			101			47			24	24	
3.5	12		138	28	35.0	1.31	1.30	9.4	1.01			102			47			25	25	
4.0	12		141	25	35.6	1.43	1.38	9.8	1.04			101			48			23	24	
4.5	15		144	27	38.6	1.53	1.45	10.1	1.06			100			50			24	25	
5.0	15		150	26	39.8	1.59	1.44	9.6	1.10			102			49			24	26	
5.5	18		155	29	45.6	1.82	1.58	10.2	1.15			104			49			24	27	
6.0	18		160	27	47.8	1.98	1.67	10.4	1.19			106			48			23	27	
6.5	21		166	30	53.3	2.14	1.73	10.4	1.24			108			48			24	29	
7.0	21		168	32	59.0	2.33	1.85	11.0	1.26			107			48			24	30	
7.5	24		175	37	67.3	2.54	1.89	10.8	1.34			113			45			25	34	
8.0	24		178	39	71.7	2.69	1.99	11.2	1.35			113			45			25	34	
8.5	27		183	43	84.9	2.97	2.07	11.3	1.43			116			43			27	39	
	Recovery		178	28	47.8	1.75	1.26	7.1	1.39			109			49			26	36	
	Recovery		175	37	68.8	2.60	1.85	10.6	1.41			114			46			25	35	
	Recovery		171	37	68.3	2.40	1.57	9.2	1.53			116			45			27	42	
	Recovery		163	35	58.1	1.84	1.20	7.4	1.53			119			40			30	46	
	Recovery		151	37	49.2	1.41	0.86	5.7	1.64			122			38			33	54	

Interpretation
Comments

The results of this subject's resting respiratory function studies are normal (Table 9.10.1). The resting ECG is normal. This study is presented to contrast the results when the same subject performed on the cycle and on the treadmill.

Analysis

Referring to flow chart 1, the peak $\dot{V}_{O_2}$ and the anaerobic threshold are normal for both cycle and treadmill exercise (Table 9.10.2). The ECG and O_2 pulse are normal at maximum work rate (branchpoint 2.1). See flow chart 2: The subject is not obese (branchpoint 2.2). The peak $\dot{V}_{O_2}$ is about 10% higher on the treadmill than on the cycle.

Conclusion

This subject shows normal exercise performance.

Case 11 Normal: Pre- and Post-β-adrenergic Blockade

Clinical Findings

This 23-year-old asthmatic student voluntarily participated in a double-blind study evaluating the effect of a β-adrenergic blocker, pindolol, on exercise-induced asthma. He had had hay fever and asthma since childhood but was otherwise in excellent health. He was taking no medications. Physical examination, chest roentgenograms, ECG, and hemogram were normal.

Exercise Findings

Two similar cycle exercise studies were performed a week apart. After baseline spirometry, 0.4 mg of pindolol or placebo was given over a 20-minute period through a venous catheter. After repeat spirometry, the subject pedalled without added resistance at 60 rpm for 3 minutes and at 60 W for an additional 3 minutes. Thereafter, the work rate was increased 20 W every minute. On each occasion the subject stopped because of fatigue. ECG pattern remained normal. Repeat spirometry in duplicate or triplicate, performed 2, 7, 12, 17, 22, and 27 minutes after exercise, did not reveal exercise-induced bronchospasm.

TABLE 9.11.1. Selected Respiratory Function Data

Measurement	Predicted	Measured
Age, yr		23
Sex		Male
Height, cm		170
Weight, kg	68	64
Hematocrit, %		45
VC, L	4.79	4.86
IC, L	3.21	3.40
TLC, L	6.46	6.72
FEV$_1$, L	4.04	3.58
FEV$_1$/VC, %	84	74
MVV, L/min	175	142
D$_L$CO, ml/mm Hg/min	33.2	32.5

TABLE 9.11.2. Selected Exercise Data

Measurement	Predicted	Placebo	Pindolol
Peak $\dot{V}O_2$, L/min	2.90	2.57	2.39
Maximum HR, beats/min	197	189	156
Maximum O$_2$ pulse, ml/beat	14.7	13.6	15.3
$\Delta\dot{V}O_2$/ΔWR, ml/min/W	10.3	10.5	9.7
AT, L/min	>1.16	1.5	1.4
Maximum $\dot{V}E$, L/min		94	85
Exercise breathing reserve, L/min	>15	48	57

FIGURE 9.11.1.   Pre-β-adrenergic blockade.

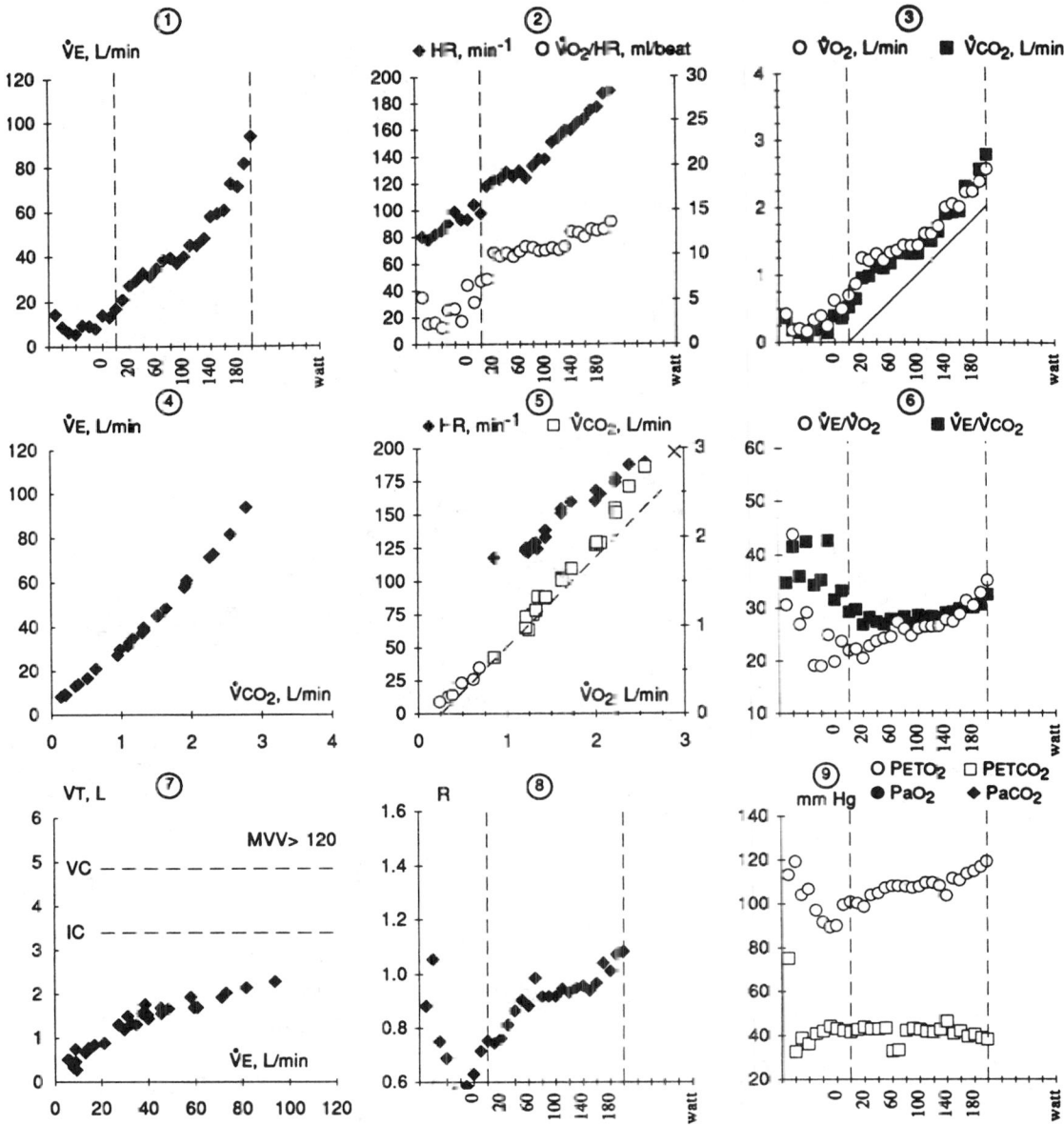

1. Vertical dashed lines in panels 1 to 3 and 6, 8, and 9 indicate the beginning and the end of increasing work period.

2. Unloaded cycling is performed for 3 minutes before the left vertical dashed line.

3. In panel 3, the diagonal line shows the increase of $\dot{V}O_2$ at a slope of 10 ml/min/w.

4. In panel 5, the diagonal dashed line has a slope of 1; the "x" in the upper right is the predicted maximum heart rate and $\dot{V}O_2$ for the subject.

FIGURE 9.11.2.   Post-β-adrenergic blockade.

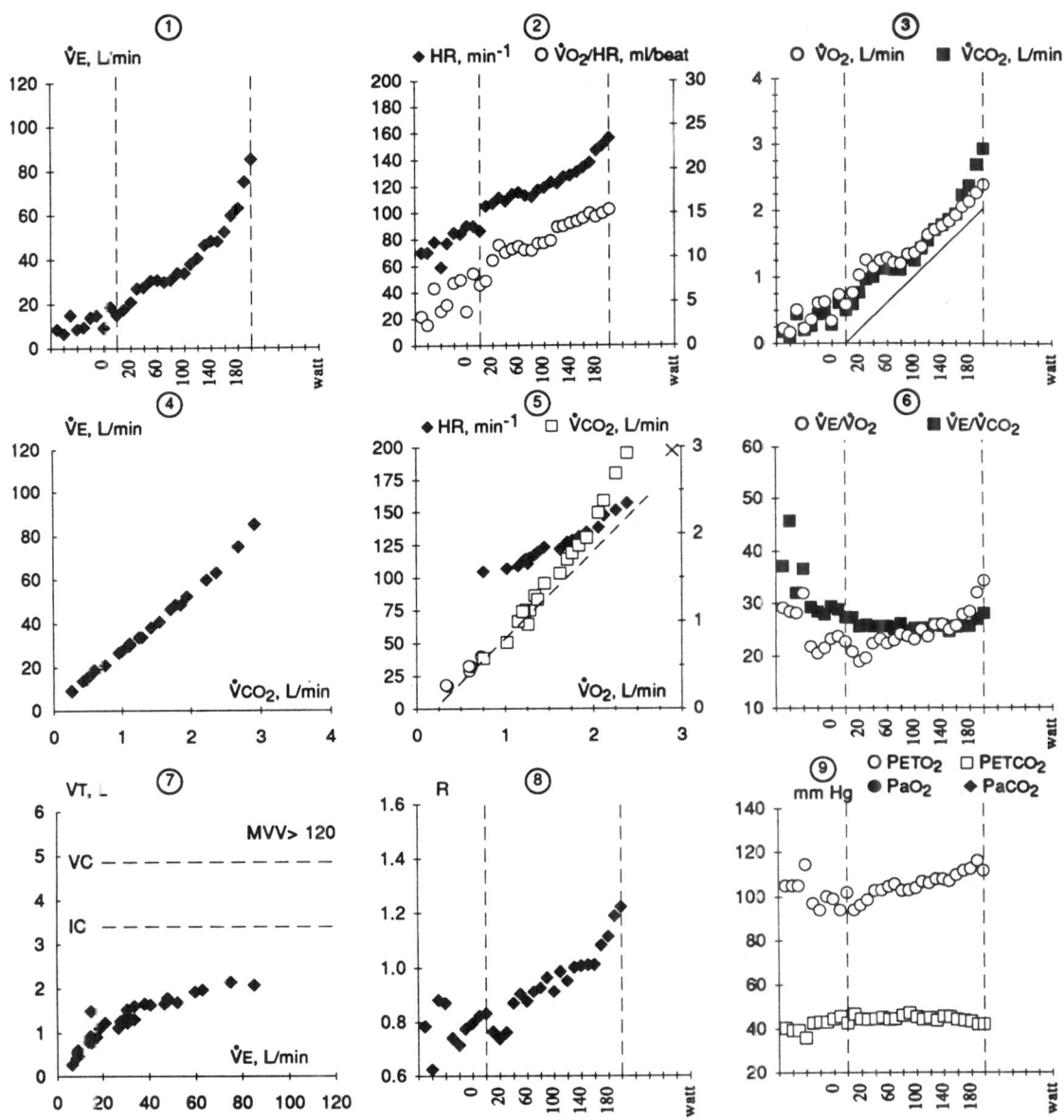

1. Vertical dashed lines in panels 1 to 3 and 6, 8, and 9 indicate the beginning and the end of increasing work period.
2. Unloaded cycling is performed for 3 minutes before the left vertical dashed line.
3. In panel 3, the diagonal line shows the increase of $\dot{V}O_2$ at a slope of 10 ml/min/w.
4. In panel 5, the diagonal dashed line has a slope of 1; the "x" in the upper right is the predicted maximum heart rate and $\dot{V}O_2$ for the subject.

TABLE 9.11.3. Pre-β-adrenergic Blockade

Time min	Work rate watts	BP mmHg	HR min⁻¹	f min⁻¹	V̇E L/min BTPS	V̇CO₂ L/min STPD	V̇O₂ L/min STPD	V̇O₂/HR ml/beat	R	pH	HCO₃ meq/L	PO₂, mmHg ET	a	(A − a)	PCO₂, mmHg ET	a	(a − ET)	V̇E/V̇CO₂	V̇E/V̇O₂	VD/VT
	Rest		80	19	14.5	0.37	0.42	5.3	0.88			113			75			35	31	
	Rest		78	12	8.9	0.19	0.18	2.3	1.06			119			32			41	44	
	Rest		82	13	6.5	0.15	0.20	2.4	0.75			104			39			36	27	
	Rest		85	11	5.6	0.11	0.16	1.9	0.69			107			36			42	29	
	Unloaded		90	34	9.4	0.19	0.34	3.8	0.56			97			41			34	19	
	Unloaded		99	20	9.1	0.21	0.39	3.9	0.54			92			42			35	19	
	Unloaded		93	25	8.1	0.14	0.24	2.6	0.58			90			44			43	25	
	Unloaded		93	20	14.0	0.39	0.62	6.7	0.63			90			43			32	20	
	Unloaded		104	20	13.3	0.35	0.49	4.7	0.71			99			42			33	24	
	Unloaded		98	20	16.9	0.52	0.69	7.0	0.75			101			41			29	22	
0.5	20		118	24	21.1	0.64	0.86	7.3	0.74			100			42			30	22	
1.0	20		122	21	27.3	0.95	1.25	0.2	0.76			99			44			27	20	
1.5	40		123	25	29.8	0.98	1.21	9.8	0.81			104			43			28	23	
2.0	40		128	25	32.9	1.12	1.30	10.2	0.86			105			43			27	24	
2.5	60		125	21	31.4	1.10	1.22	9.8	0.90			107			43			27	24	
3.0	60		129	27	34.9	1.17	1.33	10.3	0.88			108			33			28	25	
3.5	80		124	22	38.7	1.33	1.35	10.9	0.99			108			33			28	27	
4.0	80		133	26	39.7	1.32	1.44	10.8	0.92			108			42			28	26	
4.5	100		138	24	37.5	1.31	1.43	10.4	0.92			107			43			27	25	
5.0	100		138	28	40.1	1.32	1.44	10.4	0.92			108			42			29	26	
5.5	120		151	27	45.3	1.53	1.62	10.7	0.94			110			42			28	27	
6.0	120		154	29	45.4	1.51	1.62	10.5	0.93			110			41			28	27	
6.5	140		159	29	48.5	1.64	1.73	10.9	0.95			108			42			28	27	
7.0	140		160	30	58.0	1.91	2.00	12.5	0.96			104			46			29	28	
7.5	160		165	35	59.4	1.93	2.06	12.5	0.94			112			41			29	27	
8.0	160		168	36	61.0	1.94	2.01	12.0	0.97			111			42			30	29	
8.5	180		174	36	72.9	2.32	2.23	12.8	1.04			114			39			30	31	
9.0	180		177	37	71.3	2.27	2.24	12.7	1.01			115			40			30	30	
9.5	200		187	38	81.7	2.56	2.39	12.8	1.07			117			39			31	33	
10.0	200		189	41	93.8	2.78	2.57	13.6	1.08			119			38			32	35	

Interpretation

Comments

This study is presented to demonstrate the effect of β-adrenergic blockade on exercise. The lowest work rate after unloaded cycling is 60 W, followed by 1-minute increments of 20 W. This uneven increase in the work rate increment causes the upward dis- tortion in the V̇O₂-work rate slope (panel 3, Figs. 9.11.1 and 9.11.2). Results of respiratory function testing are normal at the time of study (Table 9.11.1).

Analysis

Referring to flow chart 1, the maximum aerobic capacity and AT are within normal limits on both

TABLE 9.11.4. Post-β-adrenergic Blockade

Time min	Work rate watts	BP mmHg	HR min⁻¹	ṙ min⁻¹	V̇E L/min BTPS	V̇CO₂ L/min STPD	V̇O₂ L/min STPD	V̇O₂ HR ml/beat	R	pH	HCO₃⁻ meq/L	PO₂, mmHg ET	a	(A − a)	PCO₂, mmHg ET	a	(a − ET)	V̇E V̇CO₂	V̇E V̇O₂	VD VT
	Rest		70	20	8.4	0.18	0.23	3.3	0.78			105			40			37	29	
	Rest		70	24	6.6	0.10	0.16	2.3	0.63			105			39			46	29	
	Rest		78	10	14.9	0.44	0.50	6.4	0.88			105			39			32	28	
	Rest		59	16	8.7	0.20	0.23	3.9	0.87			114			36			37	32	
	Unloaded		77	20	9.3	0.26	0.35	4.5	0.74			97			42			29	22	
	Unloaded		85	17	13.7	0.43	0.60	7.1	0.72			94			43			29	20	
	Unloaded		84	16	14.7	0.48	0.62	7.4	0.77			100			43			28	22	
	Unloaded		90	15	9.2	0.27	0.34	3.8	0.79			99			44			29	23	
	Unloaded		90	17	18.7	0.60	0.73	8.1	0.82			94			46			29	24	
	Unloaded		86	19	15.0	0.49	0.59	6.9	0.83			102			42			27	23	
0.5	20		105	19	17.4	0.58	0.76	7.2	0.76			94			47			27	21	
1.0	20		107	17	20.9	0.76	1.03	9.6	0.74			96			44			26	19	
1.5	40		111	24	26.8	0.96	1.26	11.4	0.76			99			44			26	20	
2.0	40		109	22	27.5	1.00	1.15	10.6	0.87			103			45			26	22	
2.5	60		114	20	30.4	1.12	1.24	10.9	0.90			103			45			26	23	
3.0	60		115	25	30.7	1.12	1.28	11.1	0.88			104			44			26	22	
3.5	80		113	23	29.9	1.11	1.22	10.8	0.91			106			44			25	23	
4.0	80		112	22	30.7	1.11	1.20	10.7	0.93			103			46			26	24	
4.5	100		117	21	33.6	1.29	1.34	11.5	0.96			103			47			25	24	
5.0	100		119	26	33.7	1.25	1.37	11.5	0.91			104			45			25	23	
5.5	120		123	23	38.0	1.43	1.45	11.8	0.99			107			44			25	25	
6.0	120		122	25	40.6	1.55	1.63	13.4	0.95			106			45			25	24	
6.5	140		127	28	46.5	1.71	1.71	13.5	1.00			108			44			26	26	
7.0	140		128	28	48.2	1.78	1.77	13.8	1.01			108			46			26	26	
7.5	160		131	27	48.1	1.86	1.84	14.0	1.01			107			45			25	25	
8.0	160		134	31	52.2	1.95	1.93	14.4	1.01			110			44			25	26	
8.5	180		138	31	59.8	2.23	2.06	14.9	1.08			111			44			26	28	
9.0	180		147	32	63.1	2.37	2.13	14.5	1.11			112			43			25	28	
9.5	200		151	35	75.1	2.69	2.26	15.0	1.19			116			42			27	32	
10.0	200		156	41	85.2	2.92	2.39	15.3	1.22			111			42			28	34	

pre- and post-β-adrenergic blockade exercise tests (Table 9.11.2). See flow chart 2: The ECG and O₂ pulse at maximum work rate are normal (branch-point 2.1). The large reduction in maximum HR, with slight reduction in peak V̇O₂ and increase in maximum O₂ pulse, is typical of the effect of β-adrenergic blockade. The chronotropic effect of the β-blockade increases the time for ventricular filling and results in a larger O₂ pulse at the same work rate.

Conclusion

This study is normal with demonstration of heart rate slowing and the slight decrease in peak V̇O₂ following β-adrenergic blockade.

Case 12 Normal: Immediate Effects of Cigarette Smoking

Clinical Findings

This 27-year-old subject was one of several men who volunteered for a study to investigate the effect of recent cigarette smoking on cardiovascular and respiratory function during exercise. The subject was apparently in excellent general health, but had smoked cigarettes for 10 years. Physical examination, chest roentgenogram, and ECG were normal.

Exercise Findings

Two similar exercise studies were performed 6 days apart on a cycle ergometer. In the 5 hours before the first study, the subject smoked 15 medium tar cigarettes. In the second study, the subject was under observation for 5 hours without smoking. He breathed oxygen for the first 3 of those 5 hours to reduce the carboxyhemoglobin in his blood. On both occasions he pedalled without added load at 60 rpm for 3 minutes. The work rate was then increased 25 W every minute to his symptom-limited maximum. On both occasions, the subject stopped exercise because of fatigue. ECG remained normal. Carboxyhemoglobin levels were 6.1% at the start of the first study and 1.5% at the start of the second study.

TABLE 9.12.1. Selected Respiratory Function Data

Measurement	Predicted	With Prior Smoking	Without Smoking
Age, yr		27	
Sex		Male	
Height, cm		168	
Weight, kg	69	83	
Hematocrit, %		47	47
VC, L	4.65	4.18	4.20
IC, L	3.10	3.43	3.43
TLC, L	6.19	6.26	6.68
FEV_1, L	3.79	3.57	3.55
FEV_1/VC, %	81	85	85
MVV, L/min	168	149	163
$D_{L}CO$, ml/mm Hg/min	31.2	34.7	37.4

TABLE 9.12.2. Selected Exercise Data

Measurement	Predicted	With Prior Smoking	Without Prior Smoking
Peak $\dot{V}O_2$, L/min	2.99	2.55	2.73
Maximum HR, beats/min	193	178	182
Maximum O_2 pulse, ml/beat	15.5	14.3	15.0
$\Delta\dot{V}O_2/\Delta WR$, ml/min/W	10.3	9.0	9.9
AT, L/min	>1.23	1.1	1.25
Blood pressure, mmHg (rest, max)		138/84, 183/110	132/84, 186/105
Maximum $\dot{V}E$, L/min		110	121
Exercise breathing reserve, L/min	>15	39	42
PaO_2, mmHg (rest, max ex)		102, 103	109, 106
$P(A - a)O_2$, mmHg (rest, max ex)		5, 19	−1, 16
$P(a - ET)CO_2$, mmHg (rest, max ex)		−1, −3	−2, −3
VD/VT (rest, heavy ex)		0.37, 0.13	0.27, 0.20
HCO_3^-, mEq/L (rest, 2-min recov)		25, 14	26, 15

FIGURE 9.12.1.   With prior smoking.

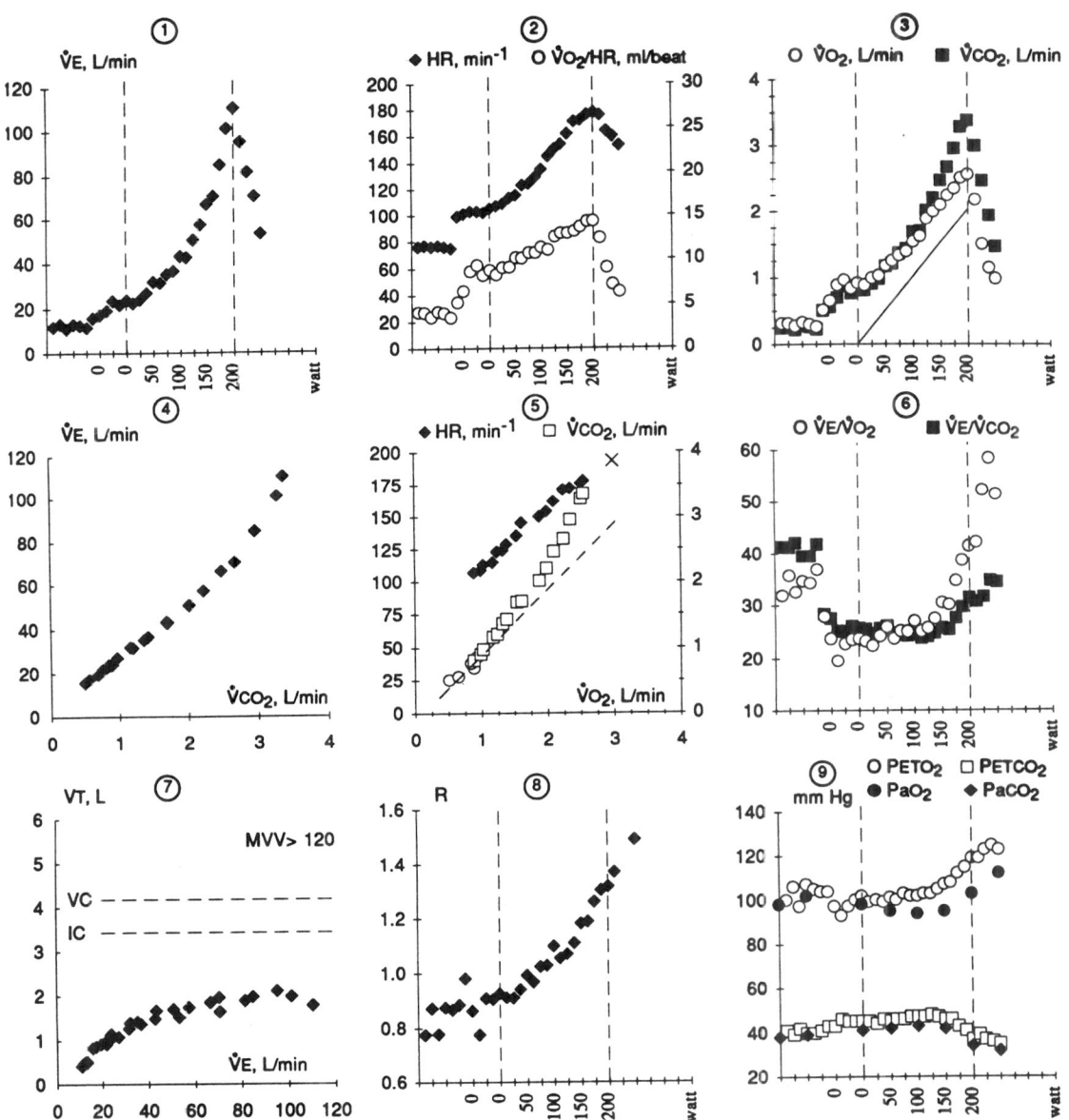

1. Vertical dashed lines in panels 1 to 3 and 6, 8, and 9 indicate the beginning and the end of increasing work period.

2. Unloaded cycling is performed for 3 minutes before the left vertical dashed line.

3. In panel 3, the diagonal line shows the increase of $\dot{V}O_2$ at a slope of 10 ml/min/w.

4. In panel 5, the diagonal dashed line has a slope of 1; the "x" in the upper right is the predicted maximum heart rate and $\dot{V}O_2$ for the subject.

FIGURE 9.12.2.   Without prior smoking.

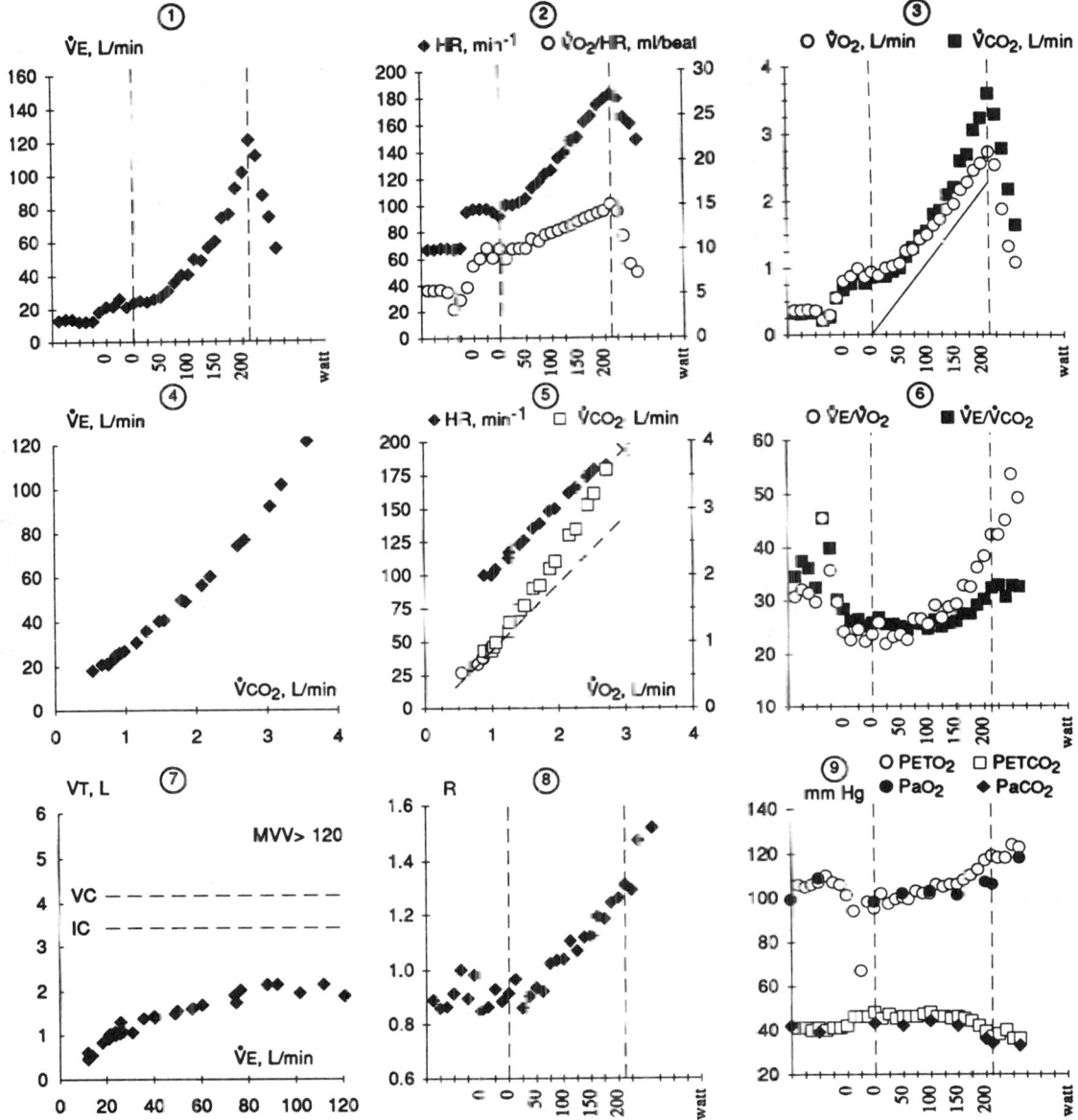

1. Vertical dashed lines in panels 1 to 3 and 6, 8, and 9 indicate the beginning and the end of increasing work period.
2. Unloaded cycling is performed for 3 minutes before the left vertical dashed line.
3. In panel 3, the diagonal line shows the increase of $\dot{V}O_2$ at a slope of 10 ml/min/w.
4. In panel 5, the diagonal dashed line has a slope of 1; the "x" in the upper right is the predicted maximum heart rate and $\dot{V}O_2$ for the subject.

TABLE 9.12.3. With Prior Smoking

Time min	Work rate watts	BP mmHg	HR min^{-1}	f min^{-1}	$\dot{V}_E$ L/min BTPS	$\dot{V}_{CO_2}$ L/min STPD	$\dot{V}_{O_2}$ L/min STPD	$\dot{V}_{O_2}$/HR ml/beat	R	pH	HCO$_3^-$ meq/L	Po$_2$, mmHg ET	a	(A − a)	Pco$_2$, mmHg ET	a	(a − ET)	$\dot{V}_E/\dot{V}_{CO_2}$	$\dot{V}_E/\dot{V}_{O_2}$	V_D/V_T
	Rest	138/84								7.42	24		98			38				
	Rest		76	26	12.1	0.24	0.31	4.1	0.77			100			41			41	32	
	Rest		77	27	13.4	0.27	0.31	4.0	0.87			106			39			41	36	
	Rest		76	27	11.1	0.21	0.27	3.6	0.78			97			42			42	33	
	Rest	138/84	77	25	13.2	0.28	0.32	4.2	0.88	7.42	25	107	102	5	40	39	−1	40	35	0.37
	Rest		76	25	12.4	0.26	0.30	3.9	0.87			105			40			40	34	
	Rest		75	25	11.7	0.23	0.26	3.5	0.88			104			41			42	37	
	Unloaded		99	19	15.8	0.50	0.51	5.2	0.98			104			43			28	28	
	Unloaded		101	20	17.1	0.56	0.65	6.4	0.86			97			43			28	24	
	Unloaded		103	21	19.2	0.69	0.89	8.6	0.78			93			46			25	20	
	Unloaded		103	21	23.6	0.87	0.96	9.3	0.91			97			45			25	23	
	Unloaded		102	24	21.8	0.76	0.84	8.2	0.90			100			45			26	24	
	Unloaded	156/96	105	23	23.8	0.85	0.92	8.8	0.92	7.39	24	102	98	8	45	41	−4	26	24	0.17
0.5	25		107	22	22.5	0.81	0.89	8.3	0.91			99			45			25	23	
1.0	25		109	21	24.0	0.90	0.99	9.1	0.91			100			44			25	22	
1.5	50		113	25	27.0	0.97	1.03	9.1	0.94			99			46			26	24	
2.0	50	165/93	115	23	32.1	1.16	1.17	10.2	0.99	7.38	24	101	95	13	45	42	−3	26	26	0.20
2.5	75		123	25	31.6	1.20	1.24	10.1	0.97			100			46			25	24	
3.0	75		124	25	35.4	1.36	1.33	10.7	1.02			103			46			24	25	
3.5	100		129	27	36.8	1.42	1.38	10.7	1.03			102			47			24	25	
4.0	100	177/96	135	26	43.4	1.68	1.53	11.3	1.10	7.36	24	102	94	16	47	43	−4	25	27	0.17
4.5	125		145	29	43.0	1.70	1.61	11.1	1.06			103			47			24	25	
5.0	125		150	30	50.8	2.01	1.88	12.5	1.07			103			48			24	26	
5.5	150		154	33	57.5	2.21	1.99	12.9	1.11			105			47			25	27	
6.0	150	177/99	162	36	66.6	2.47	2.09	12.9	1.18	7.33	22	107	95	18	46	42	−4	26	30	0.19
6.5	175		171	36	70.4	2.66	2.24	13.1	1.19			108			46			25	30	
7.0	175		172	43	84.8	2.95	2.34	13.6	1.26			112			43			28	35	
7.5	200		176	51	101.2	3.27	2.51	14.3	1.30			115			41			30	39	
8.0	200		178	62	110.6	3.36	2.55	14.3	1.32	7.32	17	119	103	19	37	34	−3	31	41	0.18
	Recovery		176	45	95.2	2.99	2.18	12.4	1.37			119			39			31	42	
	Recovery		164	43	81.4	2.46	1.49	9.1	1.65			123			37			32	52	
	Recovery		160	43	70.6	1.93	1.15	7.2	1.68			125			36			35	58	
	Recovery	165/84	153	35	53.3	1.46	0.98	6.4	1.49	7.27	14	123	112	14	35	32	−3	34	51	0.21

Interpretation

Comments

This study is presented because it illustrates small but significant effects of short-term cigarette smoking on the peak $\dot{V}_{O_2}$ and the anaerobic threshold. It also illustrates the reproducibility of the cardiac and gas exchange responses to exercise performed on different days, and the effects of obesity.

Results of resting respiratory function studies are normal (Table 9.12.1). The resting ECG is normal.

Analysis

Referring to flow chart 1, the peak $\dot{V}_{O_2}$ is reduced with prior smoking as compared with the non-smoking study and borderline normal. However, it was clearly normal without prior smoking (Table

TABLE 9.12.4. Without Prior Smoking

Time min	Work rate watts	BP mmHg	HR min⁻¹	f min⁻¹	$\dot{V}_E$ L/min BTPS	$\dot{V}_{CO_2}$ L/min STPD	$\dot{V}_{O_2}$ L/min STPD	$\dot{V}_{O_2}$/HR ml/beat	R	pH	HCO₃⁻ meq/L	PO₂ mmHg ET	a	(A−a)	PCO₂ mmHg ET	a	(a−ET)	$\dot{V}_E/\dot{V}_{CO_2}$	$\dot{V}_E/\dot{V}_{O_2}$	VD/VT
	Rest	129/84								7.40	26		99			42				
	Rest		67	24	13.1	0.32	0.36	5.4	0.89			106			41			35	31	
	Rest		67	26	13.8	0.31	0.36	5.4	0.86			105			41			37	32	
	Rest		68	26	13.8	0.32	0.37	5.4	0.86			106			40			36	31	
	Rest	132/84	68	20	12.1	0.32	0.35	5.1	0.91	7.43	25	107	109	−1	41	39	−2	33	30	0.27
	Rest		67	27	12.3	0.22	0.22	3.3	1.00			110			40			45	45	
	Rest		68	25	12.5	0.26	0.29	4.3	0.90			107			41			40	36	
	Unloaded		95	22	18.2	0.54	0.55	5.8	0.98			106			41			30	30	
	Unloaded		97	23	21.0	0.67	0.79	8.1	0.85			101			42			28	24	
	Unloaded		97	21	21.4	0.75	0.87	9.0	0.86			94			46			26	23	
	Unloaded		97	20	26.0	0.92	0.99	10.2	0.93			67			46			26	25	
	Unloaded		95	21	21.0	0.76	0.86	9.1	0.88			98			46			25	22	
	Unloaded	141/87	92	22	23.8	0.85	0.93	10.1	0.91	7.39	26	95	98	6	48	43	−5	26	24	0.20
0.5	25		100	24	25.0	0.86	0.89	8.9	0.97			102			45			27	26	
1.0	25		100	24	24.0	0.86	1.00	10.0	0.86			97			47			26	22	
1.5	50		102	25	25.9	0.93	1.03	10.1	0.90			99			45			26	23	
2.0	50	153/90	105	25	27.0	0.99	1.06	10.1	0.93	7.39	25	100	102	4	46	42	−4	25	23	0.17
2.5	75		113	29	30.9	1.16	1.26	11.2	0.92			99			46			25	23	
3.0	75		117	26	35.8	1.30	1.27	10.9	1.02			103			46			26	26	
3.5	100		123	28	40.3	1.48	1.43	11.6	1.03			102			47			26	27	
4.0	100	168/93	126	29	40.6	1.55	1.49	11.8	1.04	7.37	25	102	103	4	48	44	−4	25	26	0.19
4.5	125		135	32	50.0	1.80	1.63	12.1	1.10			106			46			26	29	
5.0	125		139	33	49.0	1.85	1.73	12.4	1.07			105			46			25	27	
5.5	150		148	35	56.6	2.09	1.87	12.6	1.12			106			45			26	29	
6.0	150	177/99	150	36	60.4	2.20	1.96	13.1	1.12	7.36	23	106	101	11	46	42	−4	26	29	0.20
6.5	175		162	39	74.3	2.59	2.17	13.4	1.19			108			45			27	33	
7.0	175		166	38	76.8	2.69	2.27	13.7	1.19			110			44			27	32	
7.5	200		174	43	92.2	3.05	2.45	14.1	1.24			113			42			29	36	
8.0	200	186/105	179	52	101.8	3.22	2.55	14.2	1.26	7.35	20	117	107	13	39	36	−3	30	38	0.20
8.5	225		182	64	121.0	3.58	2.73	15.0	1.31	7.32	17	119	106	16	37	34	−3	32	42	0.20
	Recovery		179	52	111.9	3.28	2.54	14.2	1.29			118			38			33	42	
	Recovery		165	41	88.0	2.77	1.88	11.4	1.47			118			40			31	45	
	Recovery		160	43	74.9	2.18	1.33	8.3	1.64			124			36			33	54	
	Recovery	162/90	148	35	56.1	1.64	1.08	7.3	1.52	7.26	15	123	118	8	36	33	−3	32	49	0.18

9.12.2). The anaerobic threshold is reduced after smoking but is normal without prior smoking (Table 9.12.2). See flow chart 2: The subject is 20% overweight (branchpoint 2.2). This obese subject's $\dot{V}_{O_2}$ during unloaded cycling is approximately 0.95 L/min (Table 9.12.3 and panel 3 of Figs. 9.12.1 and 9.12.2).

Indices other than peak $\dot{V}_{O_2}$ and AT that might reflect the effect of the increased carboxyhemoglobin during exercise are the O_2 pulse and $\Delta\dot{V}_{O_2}/\Delta WR$. These are both reduced after cigarette smoking (Table 9.12.2). Although the indices of ventilation–perfusion matching are normal at maximum exercise in this and most normal subjects, they tend to become abnormal immediately after smoking (1).

Conclusion

Cigarette smoking and obesity have affected exercise performance in an otherwise normal subject.

Reference

1. Hirsch GL, Sue DY, Wasserman K, et al. Immediate effects of cigarette smoking on cardiorespiratory responses to exercise. J Appl Physiol 1985;58:1975–1981.

Case 13 Cardiologic Misdiagnoses in a Man at Ages 65 and 72

Clinical Findings

At age 65, this self-employed male executive had cardiopulmonary exercise testing to evaluate dyspnea that had occurred while he was hiking with a group of young men at an altitude of 10,000 ft (3 km). He had been an avid hiker but had noted a decreased ability to hike at high altitudes in the last 3 to 4 years. He was referred by his private physician to a cardiologist, who gave him an extensive cardiologic work-up, including treadmill exercise tests (without gas exchange measurements), gated cardiac wall motion studies, echocardiogram, and a coronary angiogram. The results of these were negative. He was told that he probably had heart failure secondary to a cardiomyopathy and was prescribed an ACE inhibitor. The patient believed that the drug did not help him but caused untoward side effects. The results of the cardiopulmonary exercise tests done at Harbor-UCLA reported below show that this man did not have heart failure and, in fact, had above normal parameters of aerobic function which depend on matched cardiac function.

Seven years later, he still liked to hike but he no longer did it at high altitude. Because he found exercise fatigue and that he was not able to maintain the pace of his female companion, he went to a cardiologist who gave him an extensive cardiologic work-up including an exercise study without gas exchange measurements. During the exercise test, he developed ST segment depression in the left precordial leads which became more marked as exercise progressed, and had a run of 3 PVCs at a heart rate of 171, his maximum. The cardiologist concluded that the patient had "excellent exercise tolerance" and discounted the ECG changes as a "false positive EKG response" based on normal echocardiographic studies. The PA systolic pressure was estimated to be 70–75 during exercise. Because of the pulmonary hypertension, the patient was referred to a pulmonologist. $\dot{V}/\dot{Q}$ scans were read as low probability of pulmonary embolus. This patient was referred by the pulmonologist to Harbor-UCLA for evaluation because of fatigue with exercise and a diagnosis of pulmonary hypertension, based on the interpretation of echocardiographic studies, which he felt could not be attributed to lung disease.

Exercise Findings

Age 65: The patient performed exercise on a cycle ergometer while he breathed room air and a second time breathing 15% O_2 (equivalent to 8000-ft altitude). On both occasions, he pedalled at 60 rpm without an added load for 3 minutes. The work rate was then increased 20 W per minute to tolerance. Arterial blood was sampled every second minute, and intra-arterial pressure was recorded from a percutaneously placed brachial artery catheter. The patient stopped exercise because of fatigue and shortness of breath on both occasions. No ECG abnormalities were noted at rest or during exercise.

Age 72: The air-breathing exercise study was repeated, using exactly the same protocol as that used in the initial evaluation at age 65, including arterial blood sampling and pressure measurements. The ST segment was depressed in AVF by 1½ mm at a heart rate of 125. By a heart rate of 137, the ST segment was depressed by 2 mm in standard lead III, AVF and V5 with smaller depression in V4 and V6. He had no ectopic beats or chest pain.

TABLE 9.13.1. Selected Respiratory Function Data, Age 65

Measurement	Predicted	Measured
Age, yr		65
Sex		Male
Height, cm		183
Weight, kg	83	83
Hematocrit, %		44
VC, L	4.60	4.70
IC, L	3.06	3.70
FEV$_1$, L	3.45	3.47
FEV$_1$/VC, %	75	74
MVV, L/min	142	129
D$_L$CO, ml/mm Hg/min	28.0	28.6

TABLE 9.13.2. Selected Exercise Data, Age 65

Measurement	Predicted (Room air)	Measured Air	Measured 15% O_2
Peak $\dot{V}O_2$, L/min	2.21	2.69	2.19
Maximum HR, beats/min	155	175	172
Maximum O_2 pulse, ml/beat	14.3	15.9	12.9
$\Delta\dot{V}O_2/\Delta WR$, ml/min/W	10.3	10.3	7.8
AT, L/min	>0.99	1.9	1.2
Blood pressure, mmHg (rest, max ex)		132/72, 210/90	114/66, 198/96
Maximum $\dot{V}E$, L/min		115	108
Exercise breathing reserves, L/min	>15	14	21
PaO_2, mmHg (rest, max ex)		113, 106	77, 52
$P(A - a)O_2$ mmHg (rest, max ex)		−1, 16	0, 27
$P(a - ET)CO_2$, mmHg (rest, max ex)		1, −3	2, 0
VD/VT (rest, max ex)		0.25, 0.21	0.36, 0.19
HCO_3^-, mEq/L (rest, 2-min recovery)		21, 15	21, 17

TABLE 9.13.3. Room Air, Age 65

Time min	Work rate watts	BP mmHg	HR min⁻¹	f min⁻¹	$\dot{V}E$ L/min BTPS	$\dot{V}CO_2$ L/min STPD	$\dot{V}O_2$ L/min STPD	$\dot{V}O_2$/HR ml/beat	R	pH	HCO_3^- meq/L	PO_2 ET	a	(A − a)	PCO_2 ET	a	(a − ET)	$\dot{V}E/\dot{V}CO_2$	$\dot{V}E/\dot{V}O_2$	VD/VT
	Rest		68	24	15.6	0.33	0.31	4.6	1.06			119			30			41	44	
	Rest		68	16	17.5	0.40	0.33	4.9	1.21			119			30			40	49	
	Rest		77	17	14.4	0.31	0.27	3.5	1.15			118			31			42	48	
	Rest		83	22	17.8	0.39	0.33	4.0	1.18			114			32			41	48	
	Unloaded		83	19	19.9	0.53	0.55	6.6	0.96			113			33			35	33	
	Unloaded		80	21	21.3	0.53	0.49	6.1	1.08			115			32			37	40	
	Unloaded		80	19	19.9	0.55	0.52	6.5	1.06			111			34			33	35	
	Unloaded		76	19	21.2	0.58	0.63	8.3	0.92			112			33			34	31	
	Unloaded		75	19	21.0	0.55	0.58	7.7	0.95			113			33			35	33	
	Unloaded	135/72	81	23	19.8	0.52	0.58	7.2	0.90	7.40	21	110	113	−1	34	35	1	34	31	0.25
0.5	20		81	18	24.5	0.67	0.65	8.0	1.03			109			34			34	35	
1.0	20		85	20	22.8	0.63	0.71	8.4	0.89			111			34			33	30	
1.5	40		87	21	27.1	0.81	0.85	9.8	0.95			105			33			31	30	
2.0	40	144/75	88	19	25.1	0.75	0.79	9.0	0.95	7.40	21	111	120	−6	36	35	−1	31	30	0.20
2.5	60		98	19	28.0	0.81	0.87	8.9	0.93			112			34			33	30	
3.0	60		100	20	29.4	0.91	1.10	11.0	0.83			107			35			30	25	
3.5	80		99	21	33.7	1.04	1.24	12.5	0.84			108			36			31	26	
4.0	80	144/75	112	21	34.5	1.07	1.23	11.0	0.87	7.40	21	108	106	5	36	35	−1	31	27	0.18
4.5	100		110	23	33.3	1.20	1.39	12.6	0.86			109			36			26	23	
5.0	100	162/84	113	23	42.6	1.33	1.50	13.3	0.89	7.40	22	110	109	1	35	36	1	31	27	0.21
5.5	120		120	25	45.6	1.43	1.57	13.1	0.91			109			36			30	28	
6.0	120	168/84	124	24	49.6	1.57	1.69	13.6	0.93	7.40	23	110	107	4	36	37	1	30	28	0.22
6.5	140		130	24	51.2	1.67	1.84	14.2	0.91			108			37			29	27	
7.0	140		135	27	59.8	1.81	1.99	14.7	0.91			111			36			32	29	
7.5	160		140	29	61.2	1.87	2.03	14.5	0.92			109			38			31	29	
8.0	160	174/84	149	32	66.7	2.14	2.18	14.6	0.98	7.40	21	113	107	7	36	35	−1	30	29	0.17
8.5	180		152	27	64.3	2.12	2.14	14.1	0.99			108			39			29	29	
9.0	180		154	31	73.7	2.45	2.45	15.9	1.00			112			37			29	29	
9.5	200		160	33	78.7	2.61	2.54	15.9	1.03			110			38			29	30	
10.0	200	207/84	172	36	91.8	2.91	2.60	15.1	1.12	7.40	21	117	100	18	35	35	0	30	34	0.19
10.5	220		175	42	102.1	3.09	2.69	15.4	1.15			118			34			32	37	
11.0	220	210/90	174	49	115.3	3.25	2.69	15.5	1.21	7.40	20	121	106	15	32	33	1	34	41	0.23
	Recovery		162	34	92.9	2.94	2.24	13.8	1.31	7.30	16	119	107	16	36	33	−3	31	40	0.14
	Recovery		154	36	87.3	2.44	1.58	10.3	1.54			125			32			35	53	
	Recovery		140	29	62.8	1.73	1.07	7.6	1.62			127			32			35	56	
	Recovery		125	24	49.1	1.39	0.89	7.1	1.56	7.30	15	125	132	−4	33	31	−2	34	53	0.17

FIGURE 9.13.1.   Room air, Age 65.

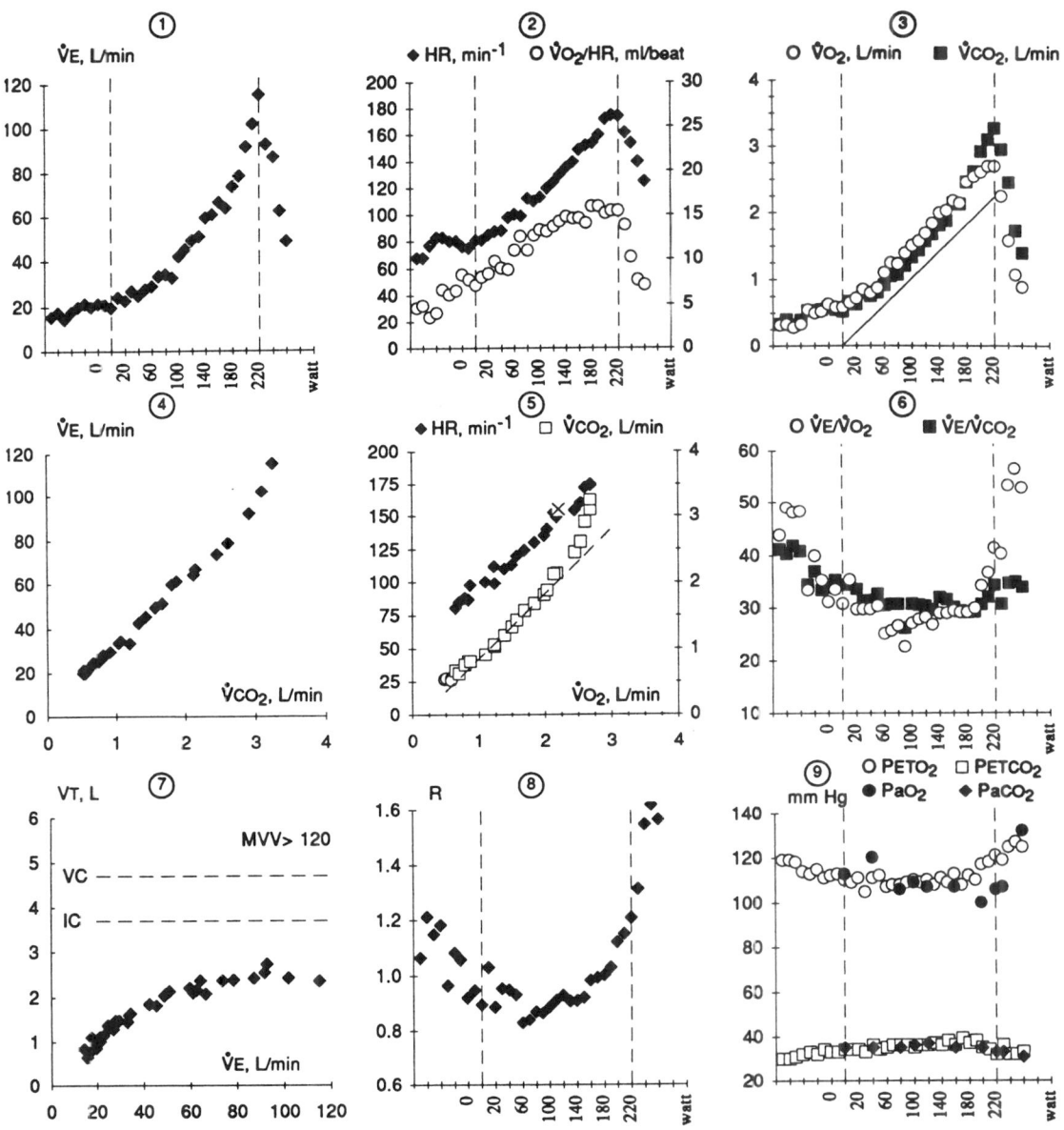

1. Vertical dashed lines in panels 1 to 3 and 6, 8, and 9 indicate the beginning and the end of increasing work period. Unloaded cycling is performed for 3 minutes before the left vertical dashed line.

2. Unloaded cycling is performed for 3 minutes before the left vertical dashed line.

3. In panel 3, the diagonal line shows the increase of $\dot{V}O_2$ at a slope of 10 ml/min/w.

4. In panel 5, the diagonal dashed line has a slope of 1; the "x" in the upper right is the predicted maximum heart rate and $\dot{V}O_2$ for the subject.

FIGURE 9.13.2.   15% oxygen. Age 65.

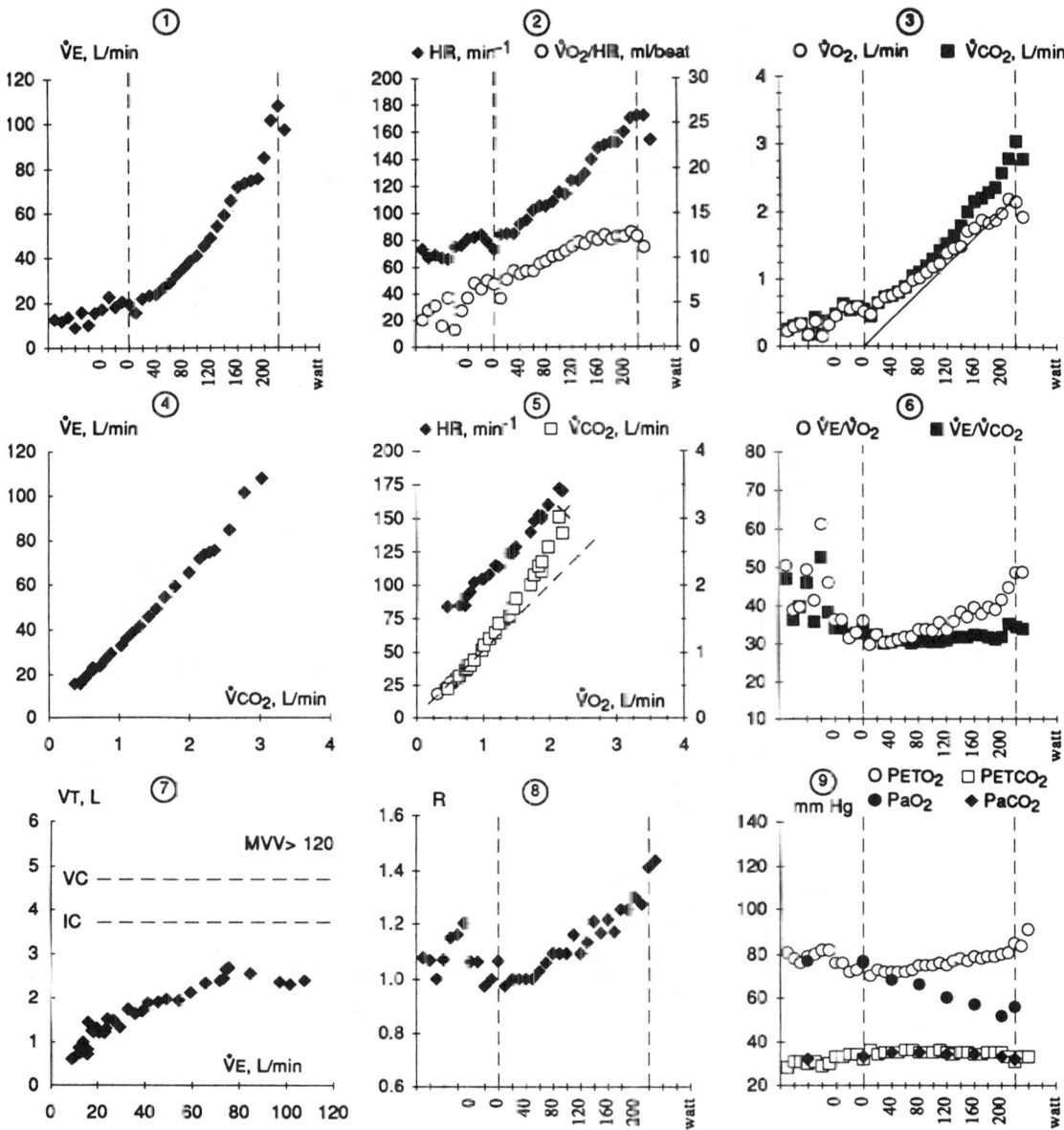

1. Vertical dashed lines in panels 1 to 3 and 6, 8, and 9 indicate the beginning and the end of increasing work period.

2. Unloaded cycling is performed for 3 minutes before the left vertical dashed line.

3. In panel 3, the diagonal line shows the increase of $\dot{V}O_2$ at a slope of 10 ml/min/w.

4. In panel 5, the diagonal dashed line has a slope of 1; the "x" in the upper right is the predicted maximum heart rate and $\dot{V}O_2$ for the subject.

TABLE 9.13.4. 15% Oxygen, Age 65

Time min	Work rate watts	BP mmHg	HR min⁻¹	f min⁻¹	$\dot{V}_E$ L/min BTPS	$\dot{V}_{CO_2}$ L/min STPD	$\dot{V}_{O_2}$ L/min STPD	$\dot{V}_{O_2}$/HR ml/beat	R	pH	HCO₃⁻ meq/L	PO₂ ET	PO₂ a	PO₂ (A − a)	PCO₂ ET	PCO₂ a	PCO₂ (a − ET)	$\dot{V}_E$/$\dot{V}_{CO_2}$	$\dot{V}_E$/$\dot{V}_{O_2}$	VD/VT
	Rest		73	17	12.7	0.24	0.22	3.0	1.08			81			28			47	51	
	Rest		67	14	12.1	0.30	0.28	4.2	1.07			78			31			36	39	
	Rest		69	14	13.9	0.32	0.32	4.6	1.00			76			31			40	40	
	Rest	114/56	67	15	9.1	0.17	0.16	2.4	1.07	7.44	21	79	77	0	30	32	2	46	49	0.36
	Rest		66	11	16.0	0.42	0.37	5.5	1.15			80			31			36	41	
	Rest		75	16	10.3	0.17	0.15	2.0	1.16			82			29			53	61	
	Unloaded		76	19	15.8	0.37	0.31	4.0	1.20			82			30			38	46	
	Unloaded		81	14	17.5	0.48	0.45	5.6	1.07			76			33			34	36	
	Unloaded		82	19	23.1	0.63	0.59	7.2	1.07			76			33			34	36	
	Unloaded		84	15	18.4	0.53	0.54	6.5	0.97			72			34			32	31	
	Unloaded		79	17	20.8	0.59	0.59	7.5	1.00			73			34			33	33	
	Unloaded	132/36	73	15	19.8	0.55	0.51	7.1	1.07	7.39	20	77	76	0	32	33	1	34	36	0.21
0.5	20		84	22	15.7	0.45	0.46	5.5	0.97			70			36			31	30	
1.0	20		85	18	22.2	0.64	0.64	7.5	1.00			73			34			32	32	
1.5	40		85	18	23.6	0.73	0.73	8.6	1.00			72			35			30	30	
2.0	40	114/60	92	16	24.2	0.75	0.75	8.1	1.00	7.41	22	72	68	4	35	35	0	30	30	0.18
2.5	60		95	18	26.8	0.81	0.81	8.5	1.00			72			35			31	31	
3.0	60		102	22	29.4	0.89	0.86	8.5	1.03			72			36			31	32	
3.5	80		105	19	33.0	1.04	0.98	9.3	1.06			73			36			30	32	
4.0	80	144/66	105	22	36.0	1.11	1.01	9.7	1.10	7.42	22	75	66	9	35	35	0	31	34	0.19
4.5	100		108	23	38.9	1.20	1.10	10.1	1.10			75			35			31	34	
5.0	100		115	22	41.5	1.30	1.19	10.3	1.10			75			35			30	33	
5.5	120		114	24	45.7	1.43	1.23	10.8	1.16			76			36			31	36	
6.0	120	144/66	124	25	49.2	1.53	1.40	11.3	1.10	7.42	22	75	60	15	35	34	−1	31	34	0.17
6.5	140		124	28	54.5	1.65	1.45	11.7	1.14			77			34			32	36	
7.0	140		129	28	59.4	1.80	1.49	11.5	1.21			78			35			32	38	
7.5	160		140	28	65.7	2.00	1.71	12.2	1.17			77			35			32	37	
8.0	160	174/73	148	30	72.0	2.15	1.77	11.9	1.22	7.41	21	79	57	21	34	34	0	32	39	0.21
8.5	180		150	30	73.6	2.21	1.88	12.5	1.17			78			34			32	38	
9.0	180		152	28	74.6	2.29	1.83	12.0	1.25			79			35			32	39	
9.5	200		152	28	75.6	2.36	1.88	12.4	1.25			79			35			31	39	
10.0	200	195/34	160	33	84.8	2.57	1.98	12.4	1.30	7.38	19	80	52	28	35	33	−2	32	41	0.17
10.5	220		170	44	101.6	2.78	2.19	12.9	1.27			81			33			35	45	
11.0	220	198/96	172	45	107.9	3.03	2.15	12.5	1.41	7.33	17	85	56	27	31	32	1	34	49	0.21
	Recovery		172	41	97.3	2.77	1.93	11.2	1.44			84			33			34	49	
	Recovery		154									91			33					

TABLE 9.13.5. Selected Respiratory Function Data, Age 72

Measurement	Predicted	Measured
Age, yr		72
Sex		Male
Height, cm		184
Weight, kg	83	84
Hematocrit, %		47
VC, L	4.61	4.39
IC, L	3.08	3.82
FEV₁, L	3.29	2.94
FEV₁/VC, %	75	68
MVV, L/min	134	130
D$_L$CO, ml/mm Hg/min	27.0	19.2

TABLE 9.13.6. Selected Exercise Data, Age 72

Measurement	Predicted	Measured
Peak $\dot{V}_{O_2}$, L/min	2.02	1.99
Maximum HR, beats/min	148	152
Maximum O₂ pulse, ml/beat	13.6	13.1
Δ$\dot{V}_{O_2}$/ΔWR, ml/min/W	10.3	8.6
AT, L/min	>0.95	1.4
Blood pressure, mmHg (rest, max)		110/60, 200/75
Maximum $\dot{V}_E$, L/min		85
Exercise breathing reserve, L/min	>15	46
Pa$_{O_2}$, mmHg (rest, max ex)		102, 105
P(A − a)$_{O_2}$, mmHg (rest, max ex)		15, 21
P(a − ET)CO₂, mmHg (rest, max ex)		5, −2
VD/VT (rest, heavy ex)		0.53, 0.18
HCO₃⁻, mEq/L (rest, 2 min recov)		24, 20

FIGURE 9.13.3.   Room air, Age 72.

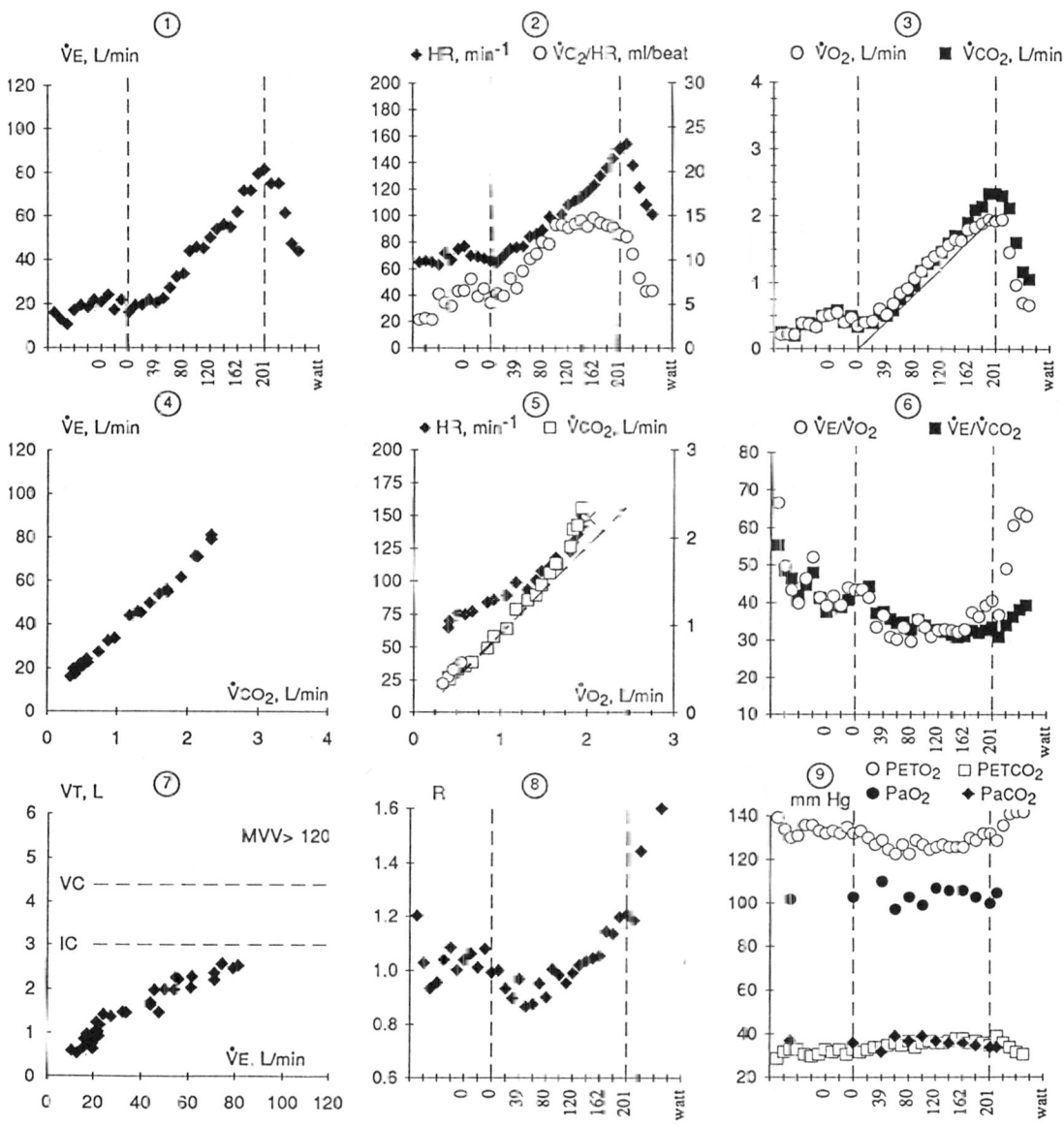

1. Vertical dashed lines in panels 1 to 3 and 6, 8, and 9 indicate the beginning and the end of increasing work period.

2. Unloaded cycling is performed for 3 minutes before the left vertical dashed line.

3. In panel 3, the diagonal line shows the increase of $\dot{V}O_2$ at a slope of 10 ml/min/w.

4. In panel 5, the diagonal dashed line has a slope of 1; the "x" in the upper right is the predicted maximum heart rate and $\dot{V}O_2$ for the subject.

TABLE 9.13.7.　Room Air; Age 72

Time min	Work rate watts	BP mmHg	HR min⁻¹	f min⁻¹	V̇E L/min BTPS	V̇CO2 L/min STPD	V̇O2 L/min STPD	V̇O2/HR ml/beat	R	pH	HCO3⁻ meq/L	PO2, mmHg ET	a	(A − a)	PCO2, mmHg ET	a	(a − ET)	V̇E/V̇CO2	V̇E/V̇O2	VD/VT
	Rest		65	24	15.9	0.26	0.21	3.3	1.20			139			29			55	67	
	Rest		65	24	12.9	0.23	0.22	3.4	1.03			134			32			48	50	
	Rest	110/60	65	18	10.6	0.20	0.21	3.3	0.93	7.42	24	130	102	9	33	37	4	46	43	0.43
	Rest		63	21	17.1	0.37	0.39	6.2	0.96			131			33			42	40	
	Rest		72	26	19.3	0.39	0.37	5.2	1.04			136			31			45	46	
	Rest		67	23	18.4	0.35	0.32	4.8	1.08			136			30			48	52	
	Unloaded		75	24	22.0	0.49	0.49	6.5	1.00			132			31			41	41	
	Unloaded		77	17	21.1	0.53	0.51	6.6	1.04			133			33			38	39	
	Unloaded		70	17	24.2	0.58	0.55	7.8	1.06			132			32			39	42	
	Unloaded		69	18	17.3	0.41	0.41	5.9	1.01			133			33			39	39	
	Unloaded		68	21	21.8	0.50	0.46	6.8	1.08			132			31			41	44	
	Unloaded	130/65	66	19	16.2	0.34	0.34	5.2	0.99	7.40	22	135	103	11	33	36	3	44	43	0.41
0.5	7		65	25	19.4	0.40	0.40	6.2	1.00			133			32			43	44	
1.0	18		70	31	19.6	0.39	0.42	6.0	0.93			130			33			44	41	
1.5	29		75	22	21.7	0.54	0.60	8.0	0.90			127			34			37	33	
2.0	39	105/40	76	20	20.5	0.50	0.52	6.8	0.97	7.47	23	129	110	7	34	32	−2	38	37	0.27
2.5	50		77	19	22.5	0.59	0.68	8.8	0.87			125			35			36	31	
3.0	62	105/40	84	20	27.4	0.75	0.85	10.2	0.88	7.41	24	123	97	10	36	39	3	35	30	0.34
3.5	71		86	22	32.4	0.88	0.92	10.7	0.95			127			35			35	33	
4.0	80	120/50	89	23	33.7	0.97	1.07	12.0	0.90	7.42	24	123	103	7	37	37	0	33	30	0.28
4.5	90		99	26	43.9	1.18	1.18	11.9	1.01			129			34			36	36	
5.0	100	115/40	94	23	45.7	1.29	1.31	13.9	0.98	7.41	24	127	99	12	36	39	3	34	34	0.34
5.5	109		101	23	45.5	1.35	1.41	13.9	0.96			125			37			33	31	
6.0	120	135/50	108	25	50.0	1.46	1.47	13.6	0.99	7.43	24	126	107	6	36	37	1	33	33	0.28
6.5	129		111	27	53.9	1.60	1.57	14.1	1.02			127			36			32	33	
7.0	141	145/55	114	25	55.8	1.70	1.65	14.4	1.03	7.42	23	126	106	9	37	36	−1	32	33	0.23
7.5	149		118	24	54.7	1.71	1.63	13.8	1.04			126			38			31	32	
8.0	162	150/55	123	27	61.7	1.91	1.81	14.7	1.05	7.40	22	126	106	9	38	36	−2	31	33	0.23
8.5	169		130	30	71.3	2.10	1.84	14.2	1.14			130			36			33	38	
9.0	177	175/65	136	32	71.2	2.14	1.89	13.9	1.14	7.40	21	129	103	15	37	35	−2	32	36	0.22
9.5	192		143	32	79.1	2.34	1.95	13.7	1.20			132			36			33	39	
10.0	201	180/65	150	32	81.1	2.34	1.94	12.9	1.21	7.40	21	132	100	21	35	34	−1	34	41	0.24
	Recovery		154	29	74.5	2.31	1.95	12.7	1.18	7.39	20	129	105	15	39	34	−5	31	37	0.18
	Recovery		138	29	74.7	2.13	1.47	10.7	1.44			136			36			34	49	
	Recovery		121	30	61.2	1.62	0.97	8.0	1.67			141			34			36	61	
	Recovery		108	32	47.3	1.17	0.70	6.5	1.66			142			32			38	64	
	Recovery		101	27	44.1	1.07	0.67	6.6	1.60			142			31			40	63	

Interpretation

Comments

Resting respiratory function studies were normal.

Analysis

Age 65: Referring to flow chart 1, peak V̇O2 and the anaerobic threshold are both normal, well above predicted values for sedentary men. Proceeding to flow chart 2 through branchpoints 2.1 and 2.2, it is apparent that the patient is an exceptionally fit man. The low breathing reserve is compatible with good motivation. While the patient was breathing 15%

O2, peak V̇O2 and the anaerobic threshold decreased. ΔV̇O2/ΔWR and exercise tolerance decreased somewhat; these decreases are expected because all of these measurements are O2 transport dependent.

Age 72: The patient's predicted V̇O2 had decreased by 0.2 L/min but his actual V̇O2 had decreased by 0.7 L/min. Referring to flow chart 1, his peak V̇O2 is still within normal limits (branchpoint 1.1). Referring to flow chart 2, his ECG is abnormal (branchpoint 2.1). His VD/VT, P(A − a)O2 and P(a − ET)CO2 are normal (branchpoint 2.3) indicating that the patient probably has early cardiovascular disease, but does not have functionally significant lung or pulmonary vascular disease. Because there were important changes in O_2 transport such as decreasing slope of the $\dot{V}O_2$-work rate relationship, O_2 pulse becoming constant at a lower than predicted value, and the steepening of the heart rate response to increasing $\dot{V}O_2$ (panel 5 of Fig. 9.13.3) above the heart rate at which the ST segments begin to decrease, it should be concluded that the ECG changes did reflect functionally important myocardial ischemia. This patient probably developed significant myocardial ischemia with exercise at a $\dot{V}O_2$ of about 1.4 L/min and a heart rate of about 110 beats/min (heart rate at which heart rate-$\dot{V}O_2$ relationship starts to become more steep and O_2 pulse becomes constant). Because systemic $C(a - \bar{v})O_2$ increases with increasing $\dot{V}O_2$, the constant O_2 pulse could be interpreted as indicating that the stroke volume starts to decrease above the work rate at which the O_2 pulse becomes constant. The decreasing stroke volume is the likely cause of the non-linear steepening of the heart rate-$\dot{V}O_2$ relationship (Fig. 9.13.3, panel 5) as peak $\dot{V}O_2$ is approached. The heart rate-$\dot{V}O_2$ plot at age 72 contrasts with the same plot at age 65.

Conclusion

Age 65: This man had excellent cardiovascular function with no evidence to support the diagnosis of cardiomyopathy. His symptoms were most likely due to the decrease in cardiovascular function associated with aging while he tries to continue his physical feats of earlier years.

Age 72: This man decreased his aerobic function considerably more rapidly than predicted despite maintaining an exercise schedule. At this time, he has physiologic and ECG evidence of myocardial ischemia during exercise above a $\dot{V}O_2$ of 1.4 L/min and heart rate of 110 beats/min. He did not have significant pulmonary vascular disease as evidenced by the blood gas and V_D/V_T data during exercise and the normal $\dot{V}E/\dot{V}CO_2$ at the AT.

Two different cardiologists misdiagnosed this patient because they did not have the benefit of exercise gas exchange measurements. At age 65, the patient was given the diagnosis of heart failure and accordingly treated, when he in fact had better than normal cardiac function as evidenced by his ability to transport more than the predicted amount of O_2 to the tissues. At age 72, he was told that he had "excellent exercise tolerance" and also that he had pulmonary vascular disease (not compatible conclusions), and that he did not have myocardial ischemia. The cardiopulmonary exercise test showed that his overall cardiovascular function was average for sedentary men of his age and size, that he had myocardial ischemia at submaximal exercise, both electrocardiographically and functionally, and that he did not have significant pulmonary vascular disease.

Case 14 Obesity, Hypertension, and Cigarette Smoking

Clinical Findings

This 53-year-old former mechanic had retired because of medical disability 3 years previously with symptoms of vertigo, nausea, and ataxia and a diagnosis of vestibular neuronitis. He had no other complaints except for some shortness of breath when bicycling uphill. He had 30 years of cigarette smoking and claimed to be smoking one-half pack per day. Hypertension, diagnosed 14 years ago, was being treated with methyldopa. Chest roentgenograms were normal except for symmetric pleural thickening considered to represent extrapleural fat.

Exercise Findings

The patient performed exercise on a cycle ergometer. He pedalled at 60 rpm without added load for 3 minutes. The work rate was then increased 15 W per minute to his symptom-limited maximum. Arterial blood was sampled every second minute, and intra-arterial blood pressure was recorded from a percutaneously placed brachial artery catheter. Resting and exercise ECGs were normal. Resting carboxyhemoglobin was 7.4%. The patient stopped exercise complaining of leg fatigue.

TABLE 9.14.1. Selected Respiratory Function Data

Measurement	Predicted	Measured
Age, yr		53
Sex		Male
Height, cm		171
Weight, kg	74	104
Hematocrit, %		51
VC, L	4.15	4.00
IC, L	2.77	3.64
TLC, L	6.15	5.69
FEV_1, L	3.28	3.25
FEV_1/VC, %	79	81
MVV, L/min	140	126
D_LCO, ml/mm Hg/min	28.8	29.8

TABLE 9.14.2. Selected Exercise Data

Measurement	Predicted	Measured
Peak $\dot{V}O_2$, L/min	2.48	2.45
Maximum HR, beats/min	167	168
Maximum O_2 pulse, ml/beat	14.9	15.6
$\Delta\dot{V}O_2 I/\Delta WR$, ml/min/W	10.3	10.4
AT, L/min	>1.07	1.45
Blood pressure, mmHg (rest, max)		160/90, 274/137
Maximum $\dot{V}E$, L/min		116
Exercise breathing reserve, L/min	>15	10
PaO_2, mmHg (rest, max ex)		81, 85
$P(A - a)O_2$, mmHg (rest, max ex)		26, 37
$P(a - ET)CO_2$, mmHg (rest, max ex)		1, −7
VD/VT (rest, heavy ex)		0.31, 0.23
HCO_3^-, mEq/L (rest, 2-min recov)		24, 14

FIGURE 9.14.1.

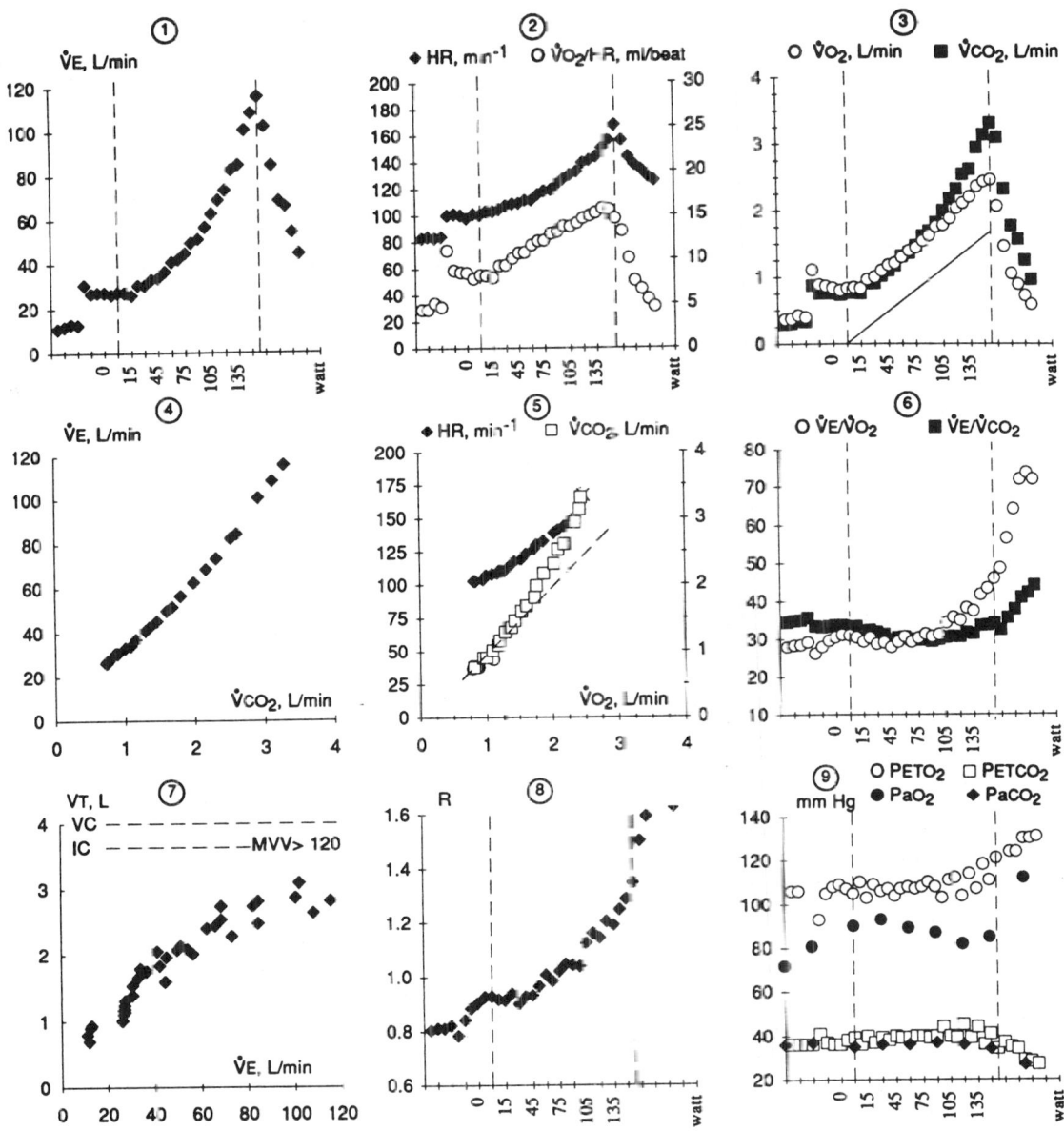

1. Vertical dashed lines in panels 1 to 3 and 6, 8, and 9 indicate the beginning and the end of increasing work period.

2. Unloaded cycling is performed for 3 minutes before the left vertical dashed line.

3. In panel 3, the diagonal line shows the increase of $\dot{V}O_2$ at a slope of 10 ml/min/w.

4. In panel 5, the diagonal dashed line has a slope of 1; the "x" in the upper right is the predicted maximum heart rate and $\dot{V}O_2$ for the subject.

TABLE 9.14.3.

Time min	Work rate watts	BP mmHg	HR min⁻¹	f min⁻¹	$\dot{V}_E$ L/min BTPS	$\dot{V}_{CO_2}$ L/min STPD	$\dot{V}_{O_2}$ L/min STPD	$\dot{V}_{O_2}$/HR ml/beat	R	pH	HCO_3^- meq/L	P_{O_2} ET	P_{O_2} a	P_{O_2} (A−a)	P_{CO_2} ET	P_{CO_2} a	P_{CO_2} (a−ET)	$\dot{V}_E/\dot{V}_{CO_2}$	$\dot{V}_E/\dot{V}_{O_2}$	V_D/V_T
	Rest	160/100								7.44	24		72		36					
	Rest		83	14	11.2	0.29	0.36	4.3	0.81			106			36			35	28	
	Rest		84	17	11.9	0.30	0.37	4.4	0.81			106			36			35	28	
	Rest		83	14	13.1	0.34	0.42	5.1	0.81			167			36			35	28	
	Rest	160/90	84	14	12.6	0.32	0.39	4.6	0.82	7.43	24	168	81	26	36	37	1	36	29	0.31
	Unloaded		100	20	30.8	0.87	1.11	11.1	0.78			93			41			33	26	
	Unloaded		101	23	26.9	0.75	0.89	8.8	0.84			105			37			33	28	
	Unloaded		100	22	27.3	0.76	0.86	8.6	0.88			108			36			33	30	
	Unloaded		98	23	27.3	0.75	0.83	8.5	0.90			109			36			34	31	
	Unloaded		101	24	26.6	0.73	0.79	7.8	0.92			107			38			34	31	
	Unloaded	200/110	100	24	27.4	0.76	0.82	8.2	0.93	7.43	23	105	90	23	39	35	−4	33	31	0.24
0.5	15		103	21	27.5	0.77	0.84	8.2	0.92			110			36			33	31	
1.0	15		103	26	26.3	0.75	0.82	8.0	0.91			103			40			32	29	
1.5	30		104	20	30.8	0.90	0.96	9.2	0.94			109			37			32	30	
2.0	30	200/110	107	22	30.6	0.90	1.00	9.3	0.90	7.43	23	106	93	18	39	36	−3	32	29	0.23
2.5	45		108	20	33.3	1.01	1.09	10.1	0.93			107			38			31	29	
3.0	45		109	19	34.0	1.09	1.17	10.7	0.93			104			40			30	28	
3.5	60		111	21	36.9	1.16	1.20	10.8	0.97			107			39			30	29	
4.0	60		111	20	41.2	1.30	1.29	11.6	1.01	7.42	23	108	89	25	39	36	−3	30	31	0.20
4.5	75		115	23	42.4	1.36	1.38	12.0	0.99			107			40			30	29	
5.0	75		118	23	45.2	1.46	1.43	12.1	1.02			108			40			30	30	
5.5	90		119	24	49.9	1.60	1.53	12.9	1.05			110			39			30	31	
6.0	90	215/106	123	24	51.4	1.68	1.61	13.1	1.04	7.39	22	108	87	27	40	37	−3	29	31	0.20
6.5	105		127	28	56.6	1.81	1.74	13.7	1.04			103			44			30	31	
7.0	105		130	26	62.6	1.99	1.77	13.6	1.12			111			40			30	34	
7.5	120		133	27	68.8	2.17	1.87	14.1	1.16			112			39			31	36	
8.0	120		139	32	73.3	2.32	2.03	14.6	1.14	7.38	21	104	82	36	45	36	−9	30	35	0.20
8.5	135		141	30	82.4	2.53	2.10	14.9	1.20			114			39			32	38	
9.0	135		144	34	84.5	2.61	2.19	15.2	1.19			107			44			31	37	
9.5	150		150	35	100.8	2.93	2.35	15.7	1.25			118			36			33	42	
10.0	150	274/137	156	41	108.4	3.13	2.43	15.6	1.29	7.37	19	111	85	37	41	34	−7	34	43	0.23
10.5	165		168	41	115.8	3.30	2.45	14.6	1.35			121			34			34	46	
	Recovery		156	33	102.3	3.08	2.05	13.1	1.50			1			37			32	49	
	Recovery		144	30	84.5	2.31	1.45	10.1	1.59			124			35			35	57	
	Recovery		138	25	68.7	1.76	1.04	7.5	1.69			124			34			38	64	
	Recovery	210/100	134	27	66.1	1.56	0.89	6.6	1.75	7.32	14	130	112	20	29	27	−2	41	72	0.21
	Recovery		129	26	54.4	1.24	0.71	5.5	1.75			130			28			42	74	
	Recovery		126	28	44.7	0.96	0.59	4.7	1.63			131			27			44	72	

Interpretation

Comments

Results of this patient's resting respiratory function studies are normal except for a low ERV/IC ratio consistent with obesity (Table 9.14.1). The resting ECG is normal. The patient is 30 kg overweight (Table 9.14.1); his resting carboxyhemoglobin of 7.4% suggests recent cigarette smoking.

Analysis

Referring to flow chart 1, peak $\dot{V}_{O_2}$ and anaerobic threshold are within normal limits (Table 9.14.2).

See flow chart 2: The ECG, arterial blood gases, and O_2 pulse at peak $\dot{V}_{O_2}$ are normal (branchpoint 2.1). The patient is 30 kg overweight (branchpoint 2.2). Supporting the diagnosis of obesity as the cause of this patient's shortness of breath is his high oxygen cost for unloaded cycling ($\dot{V}_{O_2}$ = 0.9 L/min), and low breathing reserve at the maximum work rate (Table 9.14.2).

Conclusion

Obesity has contributed to dyspnea in an otherwise normal, cigarette-smoking hypertensive patient.

Case 15 Extreme Obesity

Clinical Findings

This 45-year-old man was referred for an exercise study to evaluate his capacity for work as a security guard. Because of his obesity, his employer believed that he was unable to perform his duties, which could include running up stairs and chasing after thieves. The evaluee denied any exercise limitation and is not taking any medications. He does not smoke or drink alcoholic beverages. Resting ECG was normal.

Exercise Findings

The patient performed exercise on a treadmill because this was believed to best simulate the tasks he might be called on to perform. He walked on the level at 3 miles per hour (4.8 km per hour) for 3 minutes, after which the grade was increased 2 degrees per minute to tolerance. Heart rate and rhythm were continuously monitored. Blood pressure was measured by sphygmomanometry and oxygen saturation by ear oximetry. Multiple-lead ECGs were taken during rest, exercise, and recovery. The patient appeared to give an excellent effort and stopped exercise because of fatigue; he denied chest pain or dyspnea during or after the study. No ectopy or abnormal ECG changes occurred during or after exercise.

TABLE 9.15.1. Selected Respiratory Function Data

Measurement	Predicted	Measured
Age, yr		45
Sex		Male
Height, cm		168
Weight, kg	72	157
Hematocrit, %		47
VC, L	4.11	3.67
C, L	2.74	3.63
FEV$_1$, L	3.31	3.19
FEV$_1$/VC, %	81	87
MVV, L/min	132	140

TABLE 9.15.2. Selected Exercise Data

Measurement	Predicted	Measured
Peak $\dot{V}O_2$, L/min	3.28	4.14
Maximum HR, beats/min	175	191
Maximum O$_2$ pulse, ml/beat	18.7	21.8
AT, L/min	>1.39	3.25
Blood pressure, mmHg (rest, max)		160/90, 225/100
Maximum $\dot{V}E$, L/min		128
Exercise breathing reserve, L/min	>15	12

FIGURE 9.15.1.

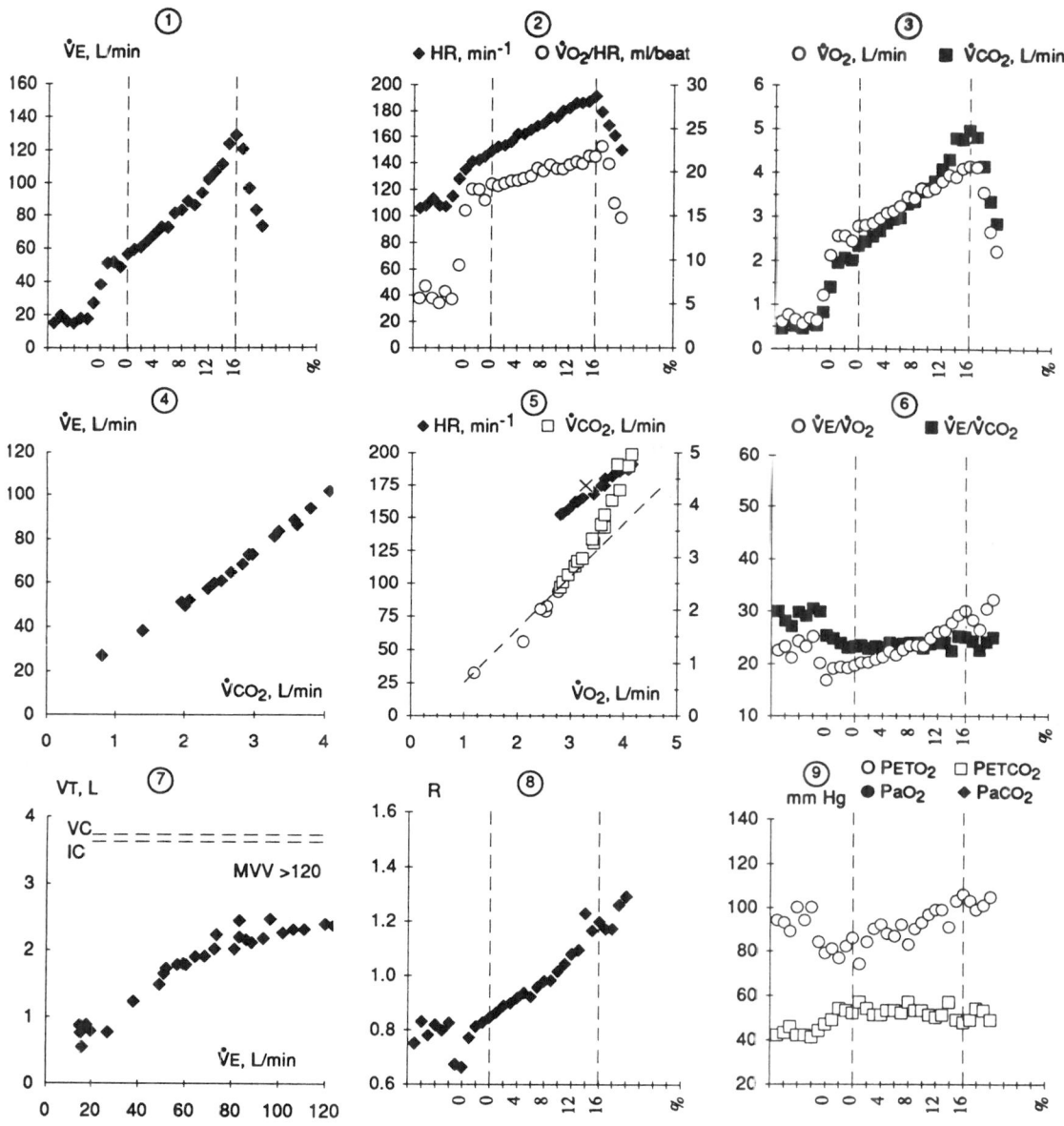

1. Vertical dashed lines in panels 1 to 3 and 6, 8, and 9 indicate the beginning and the end of increasing work period.

2. Zero grade walking is performed for 3 minutes before the left vertical dashed line.

3. In panel 5, the diagonal dashed line has a slope of 1; the "x" in the upper right is the predicted maximum heart rate and $\dot{V}O_2$ for the subject.

TABLE 9.15.3. Air Breathing

Time min	Treadmill grade, %	BP mmHg	HR min⁻¹	f min⁻¹	$\dot{V}_E$ L/min BTPS	$\dot{V}_{CO_2}$ L/min STPD	$\dot{V}_{O_2}$ L/min STPD	$\dot{V}_{O_2}$/HP ml/beat	R	pH	HCO₃⁻ meq/L	P$_{O_2}$, mmHg ET	a	(A−a)	P$_{CO_2}$, mmHg ET	a	(a−ET)	$\dot{V}_E$/$\dot{V}_{CO_2}$	$\dot{V}_E$/$\dot{V}_{O_2}$	V$_D$/V$_T$
	Rest	160/90																		
	Rest		106	20	15.2	0.45	0.60	5.7	0.75			94			42			30	23	
	Rest		108	25	19.8	0.63	0.76	7.0	0.83			93			43			28	23	
	Rest		113	29	16.0	0.50	0.64	5.7	0.78			89			46			27	21	
	Rest	150/100	108	17	14.8	0.45	0.55	5.1	0.82			100			42			30	24	
	Rest		107	20	17.7	0.55	0.69	6.4	0.80			94			42			29	23	
	Rest		115	20	17.5	0.52	0.63	5.5	0.83			100			41			30	25	
0.5	0		128	35	27.1	0.81	1.20	9.4	0.68			84			44			30	20	
1.0	0		135	31	38.1	1.40	2.11	15.6	0.66			79			47			25	17	
1.5	0		141	31	51.1	1.96	2.54	18.0	0.77			81			49			25	19	
2.0	0		142	30	52.0	2.07	2.55	18.0	0.81			77			54			24	19	
2.5	0		145	33	49.2	2.01	2.43	16.8	0.83			82			53			23	19	
3.0	0	210/100	149	32	57.0	2.34	2.77	18.6	0.84			86			52			23	20	
3.5	2		152	33	59.5	2.42	2.80	18.4	0.86			74			57			23	20	
4.0	2		153	34	60.6	2.53	2.85	18.6	0.89			84			54			23	20	
4.5	4		156	34	64.6	2.66	2.96	19.0	0.90			90			51			23	21	
5.0	4	210/90	162	36	68.6	2.83	3.08	19.0	0.92			92			51			23	21	
5.5	6		162	36	72.7	2.92	3.12	19.3	0.94			88			53			24	22	
6.0	6		165	36	72.8	2.97	3.22	19.5	0.92			87			53			23	22	
6.5	8		168	40	81.1	3.28	3.43	20.4	0.96			92			52			24	23	
7.0	8	210/90	170	38	83.4	3.34	3.41	20.1	0.98			83			57			24	24	
7.5	10		175	42	88.7	3.56	3.63	20.7	0.98			90			53			24	23	
8.0	10		175	40	86.3	3.61	3.56	20.3	1.01			93			53			23	23	
8.5	12		180	43	93.6	3.79	3.64	20.2	1.04			97			51			24	25	
9.0	12	220/90	182	45	101.8	4.07	3.78	20.8	1.08			99			50			24	26	
9.5	14		186	46	106.3	4.28	3.92	21.1	1.09			99			51			24	26	
10.0	14		186	48	111.0	4.77	3.38	20.9	1.23			91			57			22	28	
10.5	16		187	52	123.5	4.75	4.08	21.8	1.16			103			49			25	29	
11.0	16	225/100	191	53	128.4	4.96	4.14	21.7	1.20			106			48			25	30	
	Recovery		179	50	120.1	4.80	4.10	22.9	1.17			103			49			24	28	
	Recovery	200/80	169	39	96.4	4.13	3.53	20.9	1.17			99			54			23	26	
	Recovery		161	34	83.2	3.34	2.65	16.5	1.26			101			53			24	30	
	Recovery	180/80	150	33	73.6	2.85	2.21	14.7	1.29			105			49			25	32	

Interpretation

Comments

Resting lung studies are typical of extreme obesity.

Analysis

Referring to flow chart 1, peak $\dot{V}_{O_2}$ and the anaerobic threshold are high normal as predicted from height. Through branchpoints 1.1 in this flow chart and branchpoints 2.1 and 2.2 in flow chart 2, the diagnosis of obesity is confirmed. The breathing reserve is low at maximal exercise. The metabolic cost ($\dot{V}_{C_2}$) of walking at zero grade at 3 miles per hour is seen to be 2.5 L/min, which is much higher than would be seen in an individual of normal weight. The anaerobic threshold is reached at a grade of 6 to 8%, and $\dot{V}_{O_2}$max is reached at a 16% grade. These are roughly the tasks that would correspond to the anaerobic threshold and $\dot{V}_{O_2}$max in a subject of normal weight (albeit at a much lower $\dot{V}_{O_2}$ cost).

Conclusion

Except for systolic hypertension, no evidence of cardiopulmonary disease was found. There is a fit thin person hiding in this obese man! Despite his fitness, obesity has added a significant burden to his ability to perform an exercise task as well as a normal weight person of equal fitness.

Case 16 Coronary Artery Disease

Clinical Findings

This 58-year-old man had been exposed to asbestos, sandblasting, and 35 years of cigarettes. On questioning, he admitted to a grinding chest pain, originating in the midback and radiating around the left chest into the substernal area. The pain, brought on when walking on cold days and relieved in a few minutes by rest, had not previously been treated or diagnosed. He denied shortness of breath. A physical examination revealed no evidence of peripheral vascular disease, heart murmurs, or abnormal heart sounds. The resting 12-lead ECG was within normal limits.

Exercise Findings

The patient performed exercise on a cycle ergometer. He pedalled at 60 rpm without added load for 3 minutes. The work rate was then increased 20 W per minute to his symptom-limited maximum. Arterial blood was sampled every second minute, and intra-arterial blood pressure was recorded from a percutaneously placed brachial artery catheter. The patient stopped exercise because of interscapular pain and right anterior chest pain. The ECG showed a 2-mm ST segment depression in leads 2, 3, AVF, and V3 through V6 during exercise but returned to normal after 9 minutes of recovery. The chest pain resolved within 1 minute of cessation of exercise.

TABLE 9.16.1. Selected Respiratory Function Data

Measurement	Predicted	Measured
Age, yr		58
Sex		Male
Height, cm		173
Weight, kg	76	82
Hematocrit, %		41
VC, L	4.09	4.04
IC, L	2.73	3.39
TLC, L	6.20	5.93
FEV_1, L	3.21	3.43
FEV_1/VC, %	79	85
MVV, L/min	135	155
$D_{L}CO$, ml/mm Hg/min	25.5	25.9

TABLE 9.16.2. Selected Exercise Data

Measurement	Predicted	Measured
Peak $\dot{V}O_2$, L/min	2.25	1.47
Maximum HR, beats/min	162	146
Maximum O_2 pulse, ml/beat	13.9	10.3
$\Delta\dot{V}O_2/\Delta WR$, ml/min/W	10.3	7.2
AT, L/min	>0.99	1.0
Blood pressure, mmHg (rest, max)		174/81, 222/99
Maximum $\dot{V}E$, L/min		75
Exercise breathing reserve, L/min	>15	80
PaO_2, mmHg (rest, max ex)		87, 115
$P(A - a)O_2$, mmHg (rest, max ex)		18, 10
$P(a - ET)CO_2$, mmHg (rest, max ex)		−3, −6
VD/VT (rest, heavy ex)		0.21, 0.12
HCO_3^-, mEq/L (rest, 2-min recov)		22, 16

FIGURE 9.16.1.

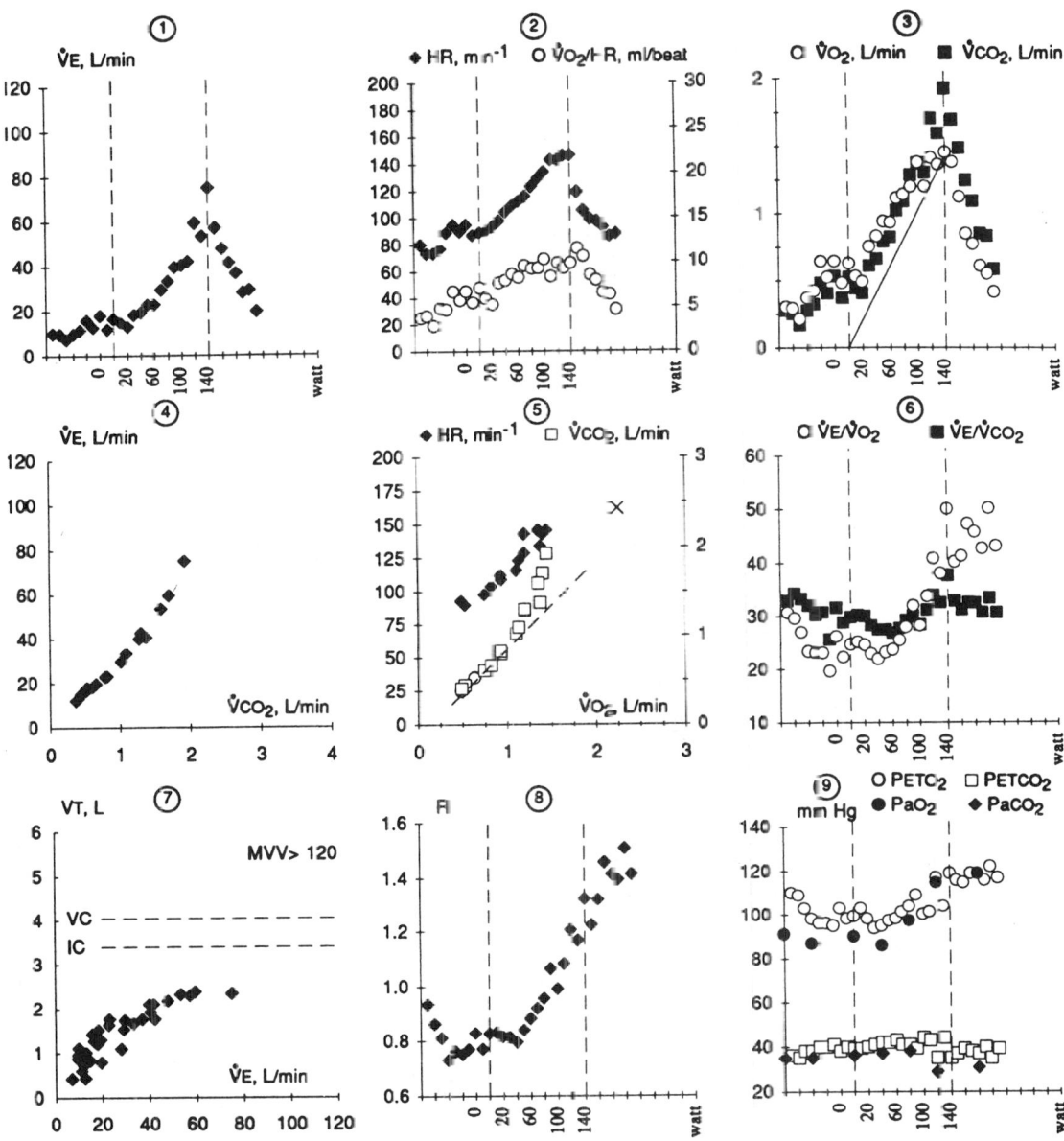

1. Vertical dashed lines in panels 1 to 3 and 6, 8, and 9 indicate the beginning and the end of increasing work period.

2. Unloaded cycling is performed for 3 minutes before the left vertical dashed line.

3. In panel 3, the diagonal line shows the increase of $\dot{V}O_2$ at a slope of 10 ml/min/w.

4. In panel 5, the diagonal dashed line has a slope of 1; the "x" in the upper right is the predicted maximum heart rate and $\dot{V}O_2$ for the subject.

TABLE 9.16.3. Air Breathing

Time min	Work rate watts	BP mmHg	HR min⁻¹	f min⁻¹	$\dot{V}E$ L/min ETPS	$\dot{V}CO_2$ L/min STPD	$\dot{V}O_2$ L/min STPD	$\dot{V}O_2$/HR ml/beat	R	pH	HCO₃⁻ meq/L	PO_2, mmHg ET	a	(A − a)	PCO_2, mmHg ET	a	(a − ET)	$\dot{V}E$/$\dot{V}CO_2$	$\dot{V}E$/$\dot{V}O_2$	VD/VT
	Rest									7.42	22		91			35				
	Rest		80	9	10.0	0.28	0.30	3.8	0.93			110			36			33	31	
	Rest		74	11	9.5	0.25	0.29	3.9	0.86			109			35			34	30	
	Rest		74	17	7.1	0.17	0.21	2.8	0.81			103			38			33	27	
	Rest		77	10	9.5	0.27	0.37	4.8	0.73	7.41	22	98	87	18	38	35	−3	32	23	0.21
	Rest		89	19	11.3	0.32	0.42	4.7	0.76			96			40			30	23	
	Rest		95	11	15.7	0.48	0.64	6.7	0.75			96			40			31	23	
	Unloaded		90	30	12.8	0.40	0.52	5.8	0.77			95			41			26	20	
	Unloaded		95	15	18.0	0.53	0.64	6.7	0.83			103			38			32	26	
	Unloaded		87	17	12.1	0.37	0.48	5.5	0.77			98			40			29	22	
	Unloaded	174/81	89	13	16.6	0.52	0.63	7.1	0.83	7.41	22	99	90	18	39	36	−3	30	25	0.18
0.5	20		90	18	14.8	0.44	0.53	5.9	0.83			103			39			30	25	
1.0	20		93	13	13.1	0.40	0.49	5.3	0.82			98			40			30	24	
1.5	40		98	12	18.2	0.61	0.75	7.7	0.81			94			41			28	23	
2.0	40	192/84	104	15	19.4	0.66	0.83	8.0	0.80	7.40	23	95	86	19	42	37	−5	27	22	0.14
2.5	60		109	14	22.9	0.79	0.94	8.6	0.84			97			42			27	23	
3.0	60		112	13	23.0	0.82	0.93	8.3	0.88			98			43			27	24	
3.5	80		116	17	29.6	1.02	1.11	9.6	0.92			101			41			28	25	
4.0	80	204/90	123	20	33.4	1.09	1.14	9.3	0.96	7.39	23	104	97	14	41	38	−3	29	28	0.21
4.5	100		129	19	39.9	1.28	1.20	9.3	1.07			109			39			30	32	
5.0	100		134	21	40.5	1.37	1.38	10.3	0.99			100			44			28	28	
5.5	120		143	24	42.4	1.30	1.20	8.4	1.08			101			43			31	34	
6.0	120	222/99	143	25	59.6	1.70	1.41	9.9	1.21	7.42	18	117	115	10	35	29	−6	34	41	0.12
6.5	140		146	23	53.6	1.59	1.36	9.3	1.17			104			44			32	38	
7.0	140		146	32	75.1	1.92	1.45	9.9	1.32			119			35			38	50	
	Recovery	210/72	119	25	57.4	1.69	1.38	11.6	1.22			116			37			33	40	
	Recovery		105	22	48.0	1.48	1.12	10.7	1.32			115			39			31	41	
	Recovery		99	20	41.9	1.24	0.85	8.6	1.46			119			38			32	47	
	Recovery		97	21	37.0	1.09	0.77	7.9	1.42	7.34	16	119	119	7	37	31	−6	32	46	0.13
	Recovery		93	26	28.2	0.85	0.61	6.6	1.39			116			40			31	43	
	Recovery		86	19	29.2	0.83	0.55	6.4	1.51			122			35			33	50	
	Recovery		88	25	19.8	0.58	0.41	4.7	1.41			117			39			30	43	

Interpretation

Comments

Resting respiratory function is normal (Table 9.16.1).

Analysis

In flow chart 1, the peak $\dot{V}O_2$ is reduced, whereas the anaerobic threshold is normal (Table 9.16.2), which directs us through branchpoints 1.1, 1.2, and 1.3 to flow chart 3. The breathing reserve (branchpoint 3.1) is high while the ECG (branchpoint 3.3) is abnormal, directing us to "myocardial ischemia."

The patient's chest pain and low $\Delta\dot{V}O_2/\Delta WR$ are confirmatory; even more significant are the plateau in $\dot{V}O_2$ and O_2 pulse concurrently with the onset of abnormal ST segment changes. The rise in O_2 pulse after heavy exercise ceased is evidence for recovery of stroke volume from ischemia-induced left ventricular dysfunction. None of these abnormalities would have been evident if exercise had been terminated at a pulse rate below 140 beats per minute.

Conclusion

Myocardial ischemia secondary to coronary artery disease.

Case 17 Coronary Artery Disease

Clinical Findings

This 61-year-old retired shipyard worker complained of breathing difficulties that he could not quantify or describe well. He denied shortness of breath but stated that he stopped using stairs because of a "peculiar feeling in his chest." He also complained of a stabbing substernal and right flank pain not associated with exertion or stress and neck pain, associated with movement of the head attributed to degenerative cervical spine arthritis. He had never smoked cigarettes. Examination revealed psoriasis and normal blood pressure, heart sounds, and peripheral pulses. He had bilateral pleural plaques on chest roentgenograms. He also had ECG findings suggestive of left ventricular hypertrophy.

Exercise Findings

The patient performed exercise on a cycle ergometer. He pedalled at 60 rpm without added load for 3 minutes. The work rate was then increased 20 W per minute to his symptom-limited maximum. Arterial blood was sampled every second minute, and intra-arterial blood pressure was recorded from a percutaneously placed brachial artery catheter. The patient stopped exercise because of shortness of breath and tired thighs. He denied chest pain. The ECG developed slight ST segment depression in leads 2, 3, AVF, V5, and V6 at 120 W of exercise (HR 150) that gradually became more prominent with a maximum ST depression of 5 mm at the cessation of exercise (180 W). A rare, unifocal, premature ventricular contraction was noted. The ECG returned to baseline after 14 minutes of recovery.

TABLE 9.17.1.   Selected Respiratory Function Data

Measurement	Predicted	Measured
Age, yr		61
Sex		Male
Height, cm		176
Weight, kg	78	70
Hematocrit, %		39
VC, L	4.23	3.95
IC, L	2.82	2.60
TLC, L	6.47	6.01
FEV_1, L	3.32	3.25
FEV_1/VC, %	78	82
MVV, L/min	137	121
D_LCO, ml/mm Hg/min	25.5	33.3

TABLE 9.17.2.   Selected Exercise Data

Measurement	Predicted	Measured
Peak $\dot{V}O_2$, L/min	2.08	1.90
Maximum HR, beats/min	159	180
Maximum O_2 pulse, ml/beat	13.1	10.6
$\Delta\dot{V}O_2/\Delta WR$, ml/min/W	10.3	7.5
AT, L/min	>0.91	1.1
Blood pressure, mmHg (rest, max)		144/75, 246/108
Maximum $\dot{V}E$, L/min		86
Exercise breathing reserve, L/min	>15	35
PaO_2, mmHg (rest, max ex)		87, 103
$P(A - a)O_2$, mmHg (rest, max ex)		5, 15
$P(a - ET)CO_2$, mmHg (rest, max ex)		2, −1
VD/VT (rest, heavy ex)		0.48, 0.24
HCO_3^-, mEq/L (rest, 2-min recov)		26, 20

FIGURE 9.17.1.

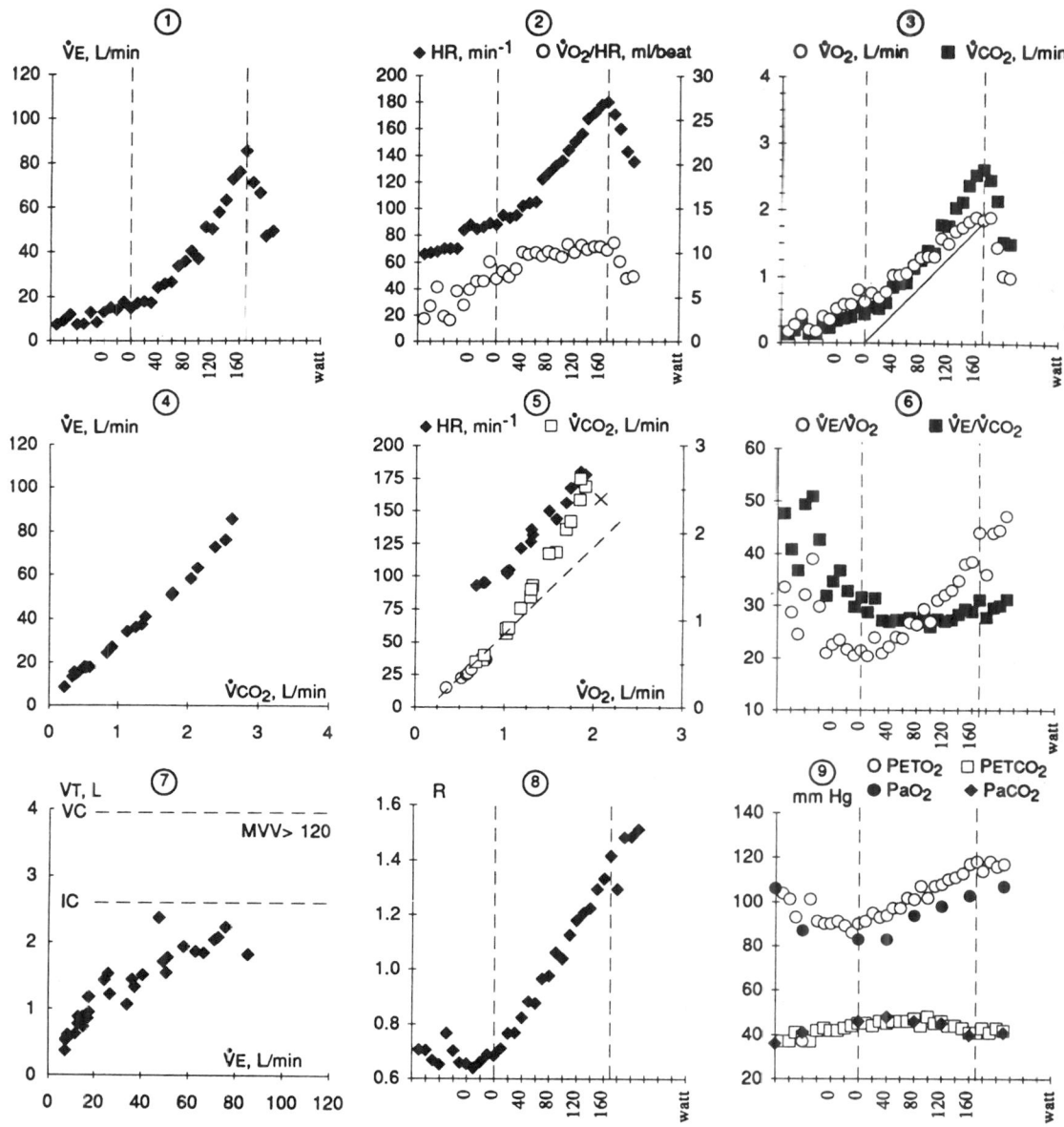

1. Vertical dashed lines in panels 1 to 3 and 6, 8, and 9 indicate the beginning and the end of increasing work period.

2. Unloaded cycling is performed for 3 minutes before the left vertical dashed line.

3. In panel 3, the diagonal line shows the increase of $\dot{V}O_2$ at a slope of 10 ml/min/w.

4. In panel 5, the diagonal dashed line has a slope of 1; the "x" in the upper right is the predicted maximum heart rate and $\dot{V}O_2$ for the subject.

TABLE 9.17.3.

Time min	Work rate watts	BP mmHg	HR min⁻¹	f min⁻¹	$\dot{V}_E$ L/min BTPS	$\dot{V}_{CO_2}$ L/min STPD	$\dot{V}_{O_2}$ L/min STPD	$\dot{V}_{O_2}$/HR ml/beat	R	pH	HCO₃ meq/L	Po₂, mmHg ET	a	(A−a)	Pco₂, mmHg ET	a	(a−ET)	$\dot{V}_E$/$\dot{V}_{CO_2}$	$\dot{V}_E$/$\dot{V}_{O_2}$	VD/VT
	Rest	144/75								7.43	26		106			36				
	Rest		66	20	7.4	0.12	0.17	2.3	0.71			104			37			48	34	
	Rest		67	16	9.1	0.19	0.27	4.0	0.73			101			37			41	29	
	Rest		68	19	11.9	0.28	0.42	6.2	0.67			98			41			37	24	
	Rest	150/75	70	14	7.6	0.13	0.20	2.9	0.65	7.44	27	97	97	5	39	41	2	49	32	0.48
	Rest		70	15	7.9	0.13	0.17	2.4	0.76			101			37			51	39	
	Rest		70	15	13.2	0.28	0.40	5.7	0.70			91			42			43	30	
	Unloaded		84	14	8.5	0.23	0.35	4.2	0.66			90			43			32	21	
	Unloaded		88	17	13.2	0.34	0.52	5.9	0.65			90			42			35	23	
	Unloaded		85	21	15.4	0.37	0.58	6.8	0.64			91			42			37	23	
	Unloaded		86	17	14.2	0.39	0.59	6.9	0.66			89			43			33	22	
	Unloaded		89	15	17.7	0.55	0.80	9.0	0.69			86			44			30	21	
	Unloaded	171/78	88	17	15.0	0.43	0.63	7.2	0.68	7.4	29	90	83	4	45	46	1	32	22	0.37
0.5	20		95	20	17.2	0.54	0.76	8.0	0.71			91			45			29	20	
1.0	20		93	19	17.9	0.52	0.68	7.3	0.76			95			44			31	24	
1.5	40		95	15	17.6	0.60	0.78	8.2	0.77			93			46			27	21	
2.0	40	192/78	102	17	24.3	0.85	1.03	10.1	0.83	7.40	29	94	83	11	45	48	3	27	22	0.31
2.5	60		104	17	26.0	0.90	1.02	9.8	0.88			97			46			27	24	
3.0	60		105	22	26.9	0.92	1.05	10.0	0.88			97			46			27	24	
3.5	80		122	32	34.2	1.14	1.18	9.7	0.97			102			46			28	27	
4.0	80	216/87	127	25	36.1	1.26	1.29	10.2	0.98	7.40	28	101	94	9	47	43	−1	27	26	0.29
4.5	100		132	27	40.8	1.39	1.31	9.9	1.06			107			44			28	29	
5.0	100		136	28	37.4	1.35	1.30	9.6	1.04			102			48			26	27	
5.5	120		144	29	51.4	1.78	1.58	11.0	1.13			107			45			27	31	
6.0	120	231/96	150	33	50.8	1.77	1.50	10.0	1.18	7.39	27	108	98	12	46	45	−1	27	32	0.28
6.5	140		156	30	58.1	2.04	1.69	10.8	1.21			110			44			27	33	
7.0	140		168	34	63.3	2.13	1.74	10.4	1.22			111			44			28	35	
7.5	160		172	35	72.8	2.38	1.84	10.7	1.29			113			43			29	38	
8.0	160	234/99	178	34	76.0	2.53	1.90	10.7	1.33	7.39	24	117	103	15	41	40	−1	29	38	0.24
8.5	180	246/108	180	47	85.5	2.62	1.85	10.3	1.42			113			41			31	44	
	Recovery		171	35	71.3	2.43	1.90	11.1	1.29			114			43			28	36	
	Recovery		160	36	66.6	2.15	1.45	9.1	1.48			113			41			30	44	
	Recovery		143	20	47.5	1.53	1.03	7.2	1.49			116			43			30	44	
	Recovery	192/78	135	29	49.6	1.51	1.00	7.4	1.51	7.30	20	117	107	13	42	41	−1	31	47	0.31

Interpretation

Comments

Resting respiratory function (Table 9.17.1) and ECG are normal.

Analysis

Referring to flow chart 1, the peak $\dot{V}_{O_2}$ and anaerobic threshold are normal (Table 9.17.2), which directs us through branchpoint 1.1 to flow chart 2. The ECG is abnormal and the O_2 pulse is reduced, reaching a plateau for the last 5 minutes of incremental exercise (panel 2, Fig 9.17.1) (branchpoint 2.1). The indices of ventilation-perfusion matching are normal (branchpoint 2.3). The low O_2 pulse, steep heart rate-$\dot{V}_{O_2}$ relationship and reduced $\Delta\dot{V}_{O_2}/\Delta WR$ indicate that the ST segment changes are functionally significant, i.e., consistent with coronary artery disease.

Conclusion

Silent myocardial ischemia.

Case 18 Small Vessel Coronary Artery Disease

Clinical Findings

This 47-year-old asymptomatic man was referred for cardiopulmonary exercise testing because of a strong family history of coronary artery disease and the finding of coronary artery calcification on an ultrafast CT cardiac scan. Physical examination, chest roentgenograms, and resting ECGs were normal.

Exercise Findings

The patient performed exercise on a cycle ergometer. He pedalled at 60 rpm without an added load for 3 minutes. The work rate was then increased 25 W per minute to tolerance. Heart rate and rhythm were continuously monitored; 12-lead ECGs were obtained during rest, exercise, and recovery. Blood pressure was measured with a sphygmomanometer and oxygen saturation with an ear oximeter. The patient appeared to give an excellent effort and stopped exercise because of leg fatigue. He denied chest pain during or after the study. The ECGs showed progressive down-sloping ST segment depression in leads II, III, AVF, and V3 to V6 after 150 W of exercise and reached approximately 3 mm in leads II and V4 at the cessation of exercise. These changes resolved by 5 minutes of recovery. No ectopy was present.

TABLE 9.18.1. Selected Respiratory Function Data

Measurement	Predicted	Measured
Age, yr		47
Sex		Male
Height, cm		175
Weight, kg	78	64
Hematocrit, %		42
VC, L	4.78	5.04
IC, L	3.19	3.70
FEV$_1$, L	3.91	4.03
FEV$_1$/VC, %	81	80
MVV, L/min	153	180

TABLE 9.18.2. Selected Exercise Data

Measurement	Predicted	Measured
Peak $\dot{V}O_2$, L/min	2.35	1.88
Maximum HR, beats/min	173	181
Maximum O$_2$ pulse, ml/beat	13.6	10.4
$\Delta \dot{V}O_2/\Delta WR$, ml/min/W	10.3	6.4
AT, L/min	>1.01	1.3
Blood pressure, mmHg (rest, max)		125/82, 160/90
Maximum $\dot{V}E$, L/min		78
Exercise breathing reserve, L/min	>15	102
O$_2$ saturation, oximeter (rest, max)		99, 95

FIGURE 9.18.1.

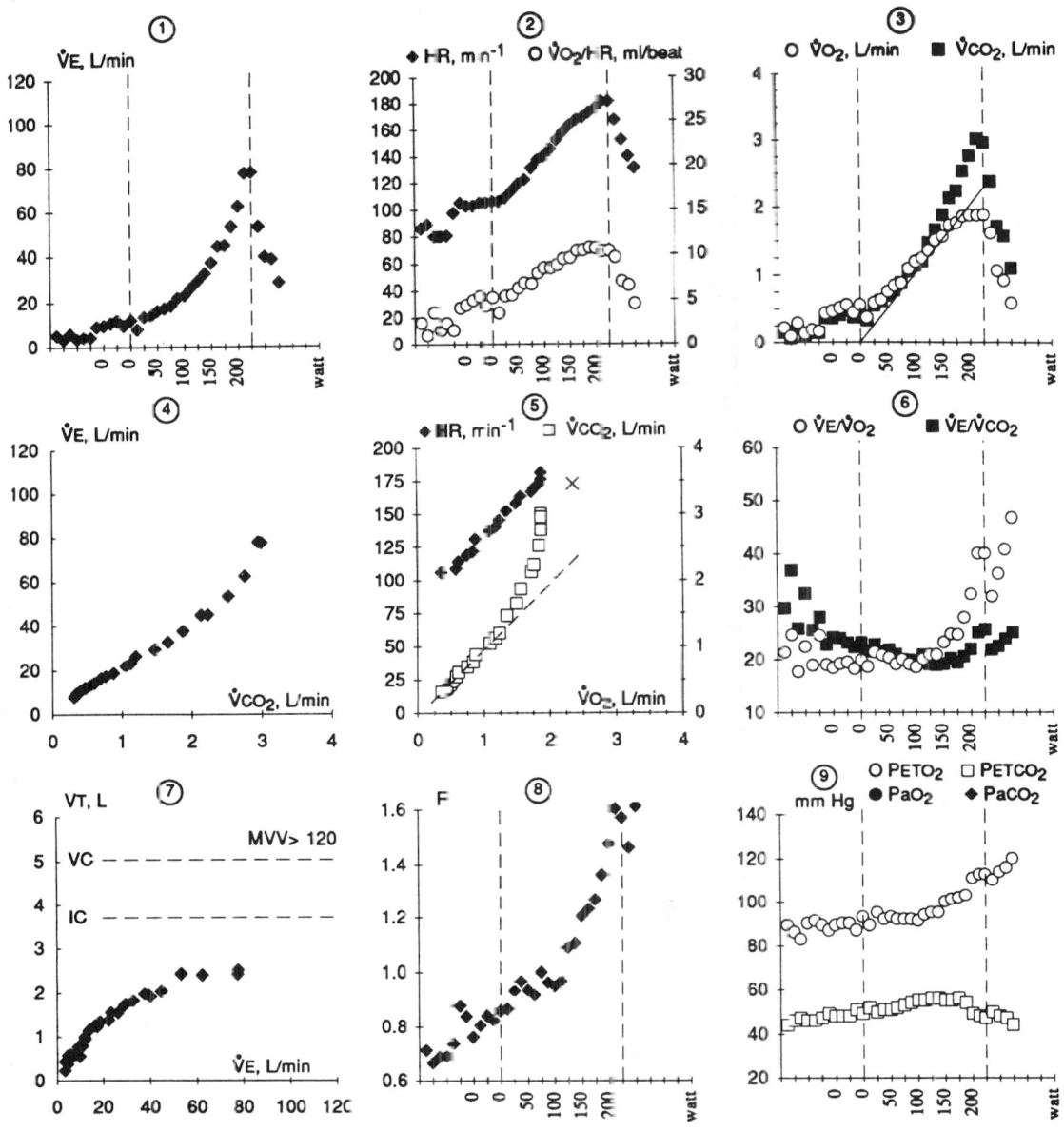

1. Vertical dashed lines in panels 1 to 3 and 6, 8, and 9 indicate the beginning and the end of increasing work period.

2. Unloaded cycling is performed for 3 minutes before the left vertical dashed line.

3. In panel 3, the diagonal line shows the increase of $\dot{V}O_2$ at a slope of 10 ml/min/w.

4. In panel 5, the diagonal dashed line has a slope of 1; the "x" in the upper right is the predicted maximum heart rate and $\dot{V}O_2$ for the subject.

TABLE 9.18.3. Air Breathing

Time min	Work rate watts	BP mmHg	HR min⁻¹	f min⁻¹	V̇E L/min BTPS	V̇CO₂ L/min STPD	V̇O₂ L/min STPD	V̇O₂/HR ml/beat	R	pH	HCO₃⁻ meq/L	PO₂, mmHg ET	a	(A−a)	PCO₂, mmHg ET	a	(a−ET)	V̇E/V̇CO₂	V̇E/V̇O₂	VD/VT
	Rest	125/82																		
	Rest		86	11	5.4	0.15	0.21	2.4	0.71			89			44			30	21	
	Rest		89	14	3.4	0.06	0.09	1.0	0.67			86			46			37	25	
	Rest		80	10	6.0	0.20	0.29	3.6	0.69			83			47			26	18	
	Rest	110/60	80	8	3.6	0.09	0.13	1.6	0.69			90			46			32	22	
	Rest		81	12	4.6	0.14	0.19	2.3	0.74			91			46			26	19	
	Rest		98	8	4.6	0.14	0.16	1.6	0.88			89			47			28	25	
	Unloaded		105	12	9.2	0.36	0.43	4.1	0.84			87			49			23	19	
	Unloaded		103	12	9.5	0.35	0.46	4.5	0.76			89			48			24	18	
	Unloaded		103	14	11.0	0.41	0.51	5.0	0.80			90			48			24	19	
	Unloaded		105	12	11.9	0.47	0.56	5.3	0.84			90			48			23	19	
	Unloaded		105	17	9.7	0.37	0.45	4.3	0.82			87			51			22	18	
	Unloaded	120/82	106	13	12.2	0.48	0.56	5.3	0.86			93			49			23	20	
0.5	25		106	13	8.0	0.32	0.37	3.5	0.86			89			52			22	19	
1.0	25		109	12	13.6	0.55	0.59	5.4	0.93			95			50			23	21	
1.5	50		114	12	14.1	0.61	0.63	5.5	0.97			92			51			21	21	
2.0	50	130/90	119	13	16.3	0.70	0.75	6.3	0.93			93			51			22	20	
2.5	75		122	14	17.3	0.77	0.84	6.9	0.92			92			52			21	19	
3.0	75		131	14	18.7	0.88	0.88	6.7	1.00			92			53			20	20	
3.5	100		137	16	22.2	1.05	1.09	8.0	0.96			92			54			20	19	
4.0	100	130/90	140	15	23.3	1.13	1.19	8.5	0.95			91			55			19	19	
4.5	125		145	17	26.3	1.20	1.24	8.6	0.97			94			55			21	20	
5.0	125		152	17	29.5	1.47	1.35	8.9	1.09			95			56			19	21	
5.5	150		158	18	32.8	1.66	1.50	9.5	1.11			95			56			19	21	
6.0	150	145/90	163	19	37.7	1.88	1.56	9.6	1.21			100			55			19	23	
6.5	175		167	22	44.8	2.13	1.73	10.4	1.23			101			55			20	25	
7.0	175		169	22	45.1	2.23	1.76	10.4	1.27			102			56			19	25	
7.5	200		173	22	53.4	2.52	1.85	10.7	1.36			103			54			20	28	
8.0	200	160/90	176	26	62.5	2.76	1.87	10.6	1.48			111			49			22	32	
8.5	225		181	32	77.5	3.00	1.87	10.3	1.60			113			48			25	40	
9.0	225		181	31	77.8	2.95	1.88	10.4	1.57			113			47			25	40	
	Recovery		167	22	53.4	2.37	1.62	9.7	1.46			110			50			22	32	
	Recovery		152	21	40.2	1.71	1.06	7.0	1.61			114			48			22	36	
	Recovery		140	20	39.1	1.57	0.92	6.6	1.71			116			47			24	41	
	Recovery	160/75	131	17	28.9	1.10	0.59	4.5	1.86			120			44			25	47	

Interpretation

Comments

Normal spirometry.

Analysis

Referring to flow chart 1, peak $\dot{V}O_2$ is reduced, but the anaerobic threshold is within normal limits (Table 9.18.2). Proceeding next to flow chart 3, the high breathing reserve (branchpoint 3.1) and abnormal ECG that developed during exercise (branchpoint 3.3) lead us to the diagnosis of myocardial ischemia. The low O_2 pulse and the failure of $\dot{V}O_2$ and the O_2 pulse to rise appropriately for the last 2½ minutes of exercise indicate that an O_2 delivery problem developed at that time. The constant O_2 pulse indicates that the product of the arterial-mixed venous O_2 content difference and stroke volume reached its maximum value prematurely. The constant value might reflect a decreasing stroke volume while arteriovenous difference increased.

Conclusion

The combination of O_2 delivery abnormalities (which imply a failure of cardiac output to increase appropriately for the work rate) and ECG findings consistent with myocardial ischemia suggest that the patient had functionally important coronary artery disease. Follow-up coronary angiograms showed diffuse distal coronary artery disease.

Case 19 Coronary Artery Disease Developed Over a 3-year Interval

Clinical Findings

This 57-year-old male asbestos worker was evaluated at 3-year intervals. At the time of his first evaluation he had a several-year history of diabetes mellitus treated with insulin injections, hypertension treated with hydrochlorothiazide, obesity, arthritis of the hip, and moderate exertional dyspnea. He had never smoked tobacco. Examination at that time revealed moderate obesity and minimal pleural thickening on his chest roentgenograms. The respiratory function and exercise study data of that evaluation are shown in Tables 9.19.1 to 9.19.3 and Figure 9.19.1. When evaluated 3 years later (Tables 9.19.4 to 9.19.6 and Figure 9.19.2), he had developed left-sided "gas" pains at the left sternal border, associated with exercise, which were being treated with cimetidine.

Exercise Findings

On both occasions, the patient performed exercise on a cycle ergometer. He pedalled at 60 rpm without an added load for 2 or 3 minutes. The work rate was then increased 20 W per minute to tolerance. On the first occasion, arterial blood was sampled every second minute and intra-arterial pressure was recorded from a percutaneously placed brachial artery catheter. The patient was well motivated and cooperative and stopped exercise because of thigh pain, without chest or abdominal pain. No ECG abnormalities were noted at rest, but during high work levels, 1- to 2-mm J-point depression with upsloping ST segments was seen in a few leads.

On the second exercise test, the patient stopped exercise because of calf fatigue and an inability to maintain his cycling frequency. During the last 1 to 2 minutes of exercise he noted left parasternal non-radiating "gas" pain which subsided within 3 minutes of recovery. He denied shortness of breath. The resting ECG was entirely normal; however, at 120 W, 1.5 mm of ST segment depression was seen in leads II, III, AVF, V3 and V4; at 140 W, 2.5- to 3-mm ST segment depression was seen in the same leads plus V5 and V6. The ECG returned to normal by 3 minutes after exercise.

TABLE 9.19.1.   Selected Respiratory Function Data: First Study

Measurement	Predicted	Measured
Age, yr		57
Sex		Male
Height, cm		171
Weight, kg	74	96
Hematocrit, %		46
VC, L	3.99	4.25
IC, L	2.66	3.37
TLC, L	6.03	6.00
FEV$_1$, L	3.14	3.52
FEV$_1$/VC, %	79	83
MVV, L/min	134	135
D$_L$CO, ml/mm Hg/min	26.4	36.4

TABLE 9.19.2.   Selected Exercise Data: First Study

Measurement	Predicted	Measured
Peak $\dot{V}O_2$, L/min	2.32	2.20
Maximum HR, beats/min	163	148
Maximum O$_2$ pulse, ml/beat	14.2	14.9
$\Delta\dot{V}O_2/\Delta WR$, ml/min/W	10.3	10.3
AT, L/min	>1.02	1.2
Blood pressure, mmHg (rest, max ex)		156/94, 250/113
Maximum $\dot{V}E$, L/min		143
Exercise breathing reserves, L/min	>15	−8
PaO$_2$, mmHg (rest, max ex)		100, 129
P(A − a)O$_2$ mmHg (rest, max ex)		10, 3
P(a − ET)CO$_2$, mmHg (rest, max ex)		−4, −2
VD/VT (rest, max ex)		0.16, 0.19
HCO$_3^-$ mEq/L (rest, 2-min recovery)		24, 15

FIGURE 9.19.1. First Study.

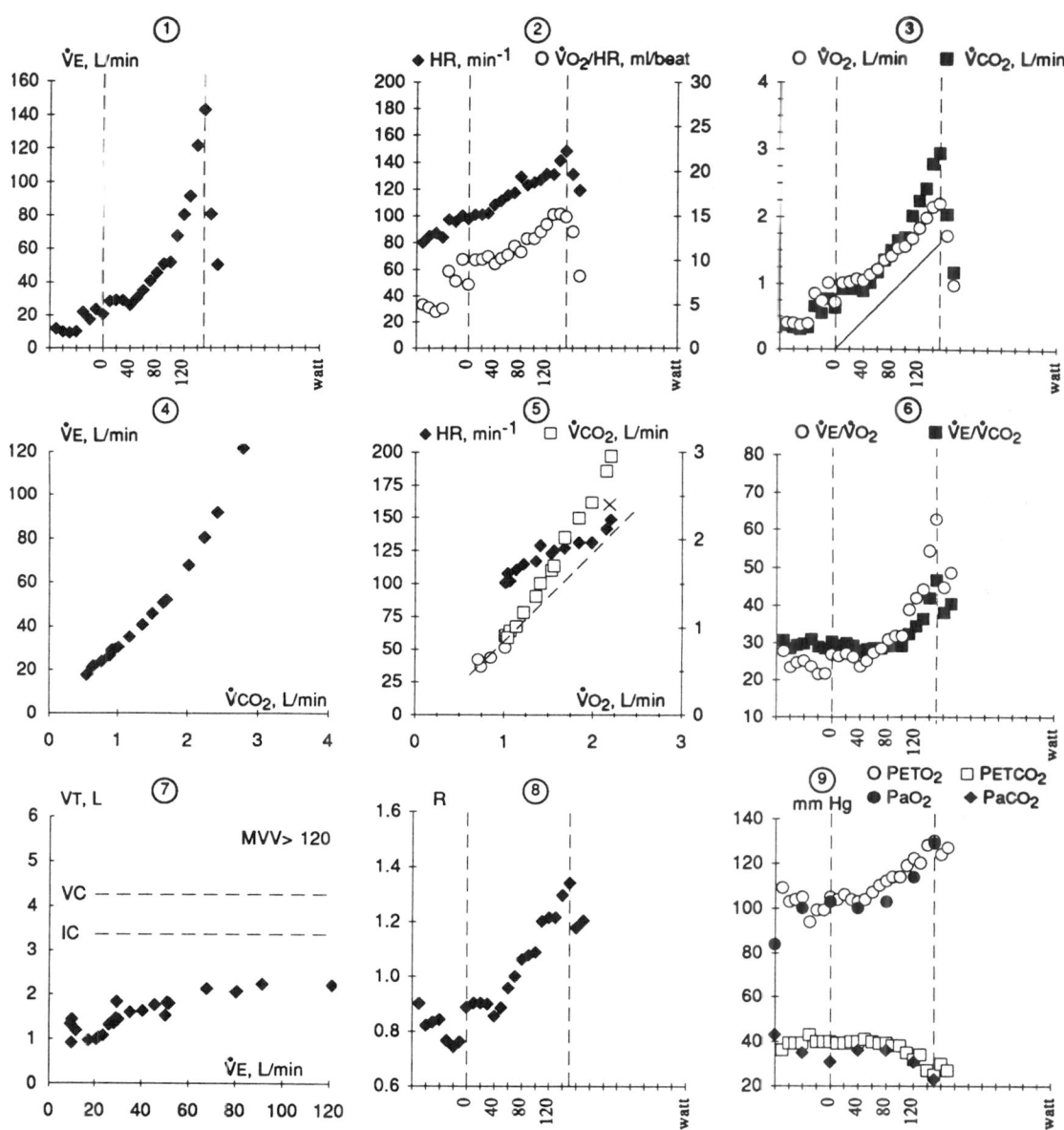

1. Vertical dashed lines in panels 1 to 3 and 6, 8, and 9 indicate the beginning and the end of increasing work period.

2. Unloaded cycling is performed for 3 minutes before the left vertical dashed line.

3. In panel 3, the diagonal line shows the increase of $\dot{V}O_2$ at a slope of 10 ml/min/w.

4. In panel 5, the diagonal dashed line has a slope of 1; the "x" in the upper right is the predicted maximum heart rate and $\dot{V}O_2$ for the subject.

FIGURE 9.19.2.   Second Study.

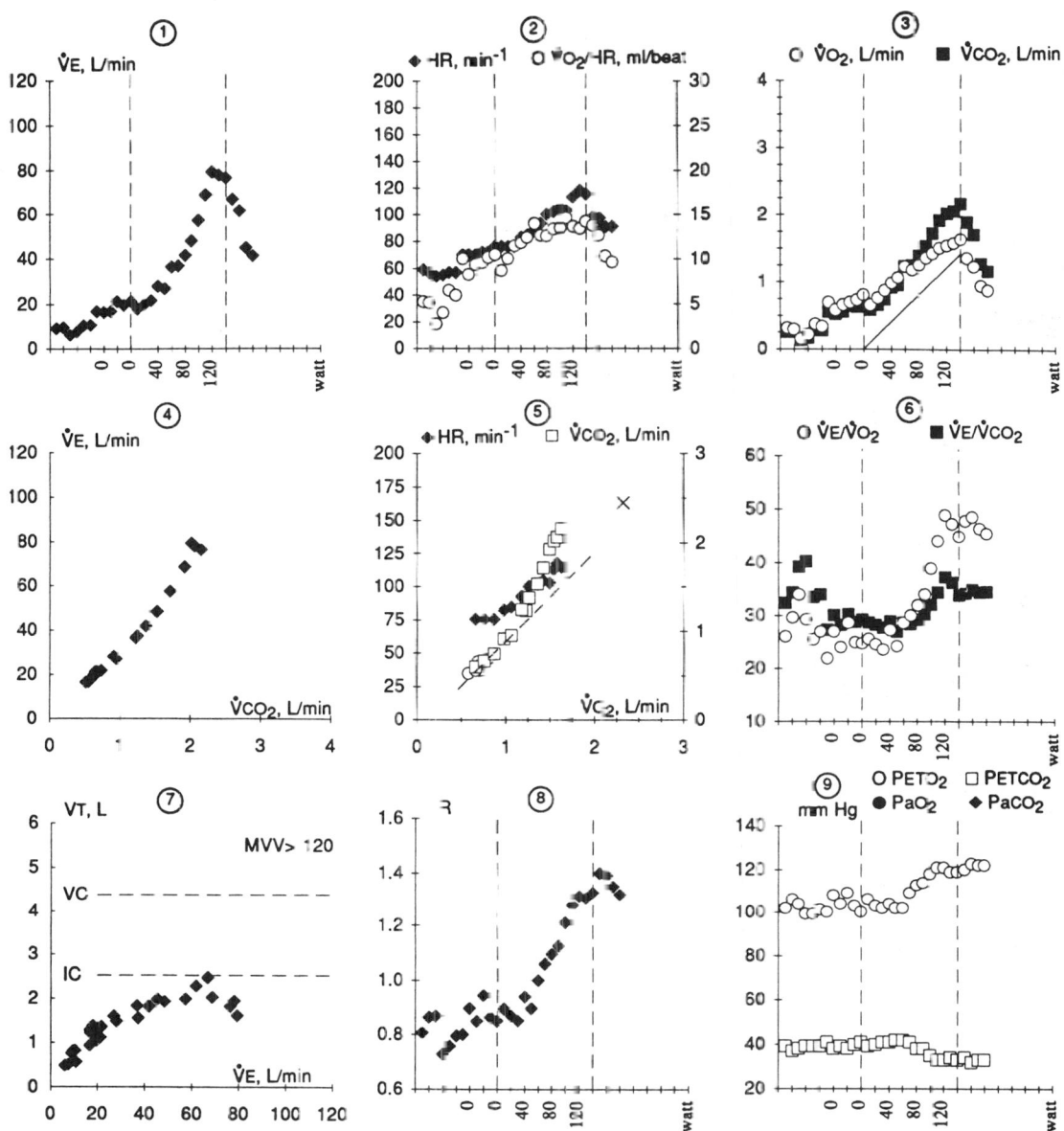

1. Vertical dashed lines in panels 1 to 3 and 6, 8, and 9 indicate the beginning and the end of increasing work period.

2. Unloaded cycling is performed for 3 minutes before the left vertical dashed line.

3. In panel 3, the diagonal line shows the increase of $\dot{V}O_2$ at a slope of 10 ml/min/w.

4. In panel 5, the diagonal dashed line has a slope of 1; the "×" in the upper right is the predicted maximum heart rate and $\dot{V}O_2$ for the subject.

TABLE 9.19.3. First Study

Time min	Work rate watts	BP mmHg	HR min⁻¹	f min⁻¹	V̇E L/min BTPS	V̇CO₂ L/min STPD	V̇O₂ L/min STPD	V̇O₂/HR ml/beat	R	pH	HCO₃⁻ meq/L	PO₂ ET	PO₂ a	PO₂ (A−a)	PCO₂ ET	PCO₂ a	PCO₂ (a−ET)	V̇E/V̇CO₂	V̇E/V̇O₂	VD/VT
	Rest	156/94								7.37	24		84			43				
	Rest		80	10	11.9	0.36	0.40	5.0	0.90			109			36			31	28	
	Rest		85	11	10.0	0.32	0.39	4.6	0.82			103			39			28	23	
	Rest		87	7	9.4	0.30	0.36	4.1	0.83			104			39			29	24	
	Rest	175/100	84	7	10.1	0.32	0.38	4.5	0.84	7.40	21	105	100	10	39	35	−4	30	25	0.16
	Unloaded		97	21	21.8	0.65	0.85	8.8	0.76			94			43			31	24	
	Unloaded		96	18	17.4	0.55	0.74	7.7	0.74			99			40			29	21	
	Unloaded		100	22	23.7	0.77	1.01	10.1	0.76			99			40			28	22	
	Unloaded	206/113	98	21	20.8	0.63	0.71	7.2	0.89	7.41	19	105	103	13	40	31	−9	30	27	0.07
0.5	20		101	21	28.3	0.91	1.01	10.0	0.90			104			39			29	26	
1.0	20		101	20	29.2	0.92	1.02	10.1	0.90			106			39			30	27	
1.5	40		102	16	29.4	0.96	1.07	10.5	0.90			104			40			29	26	
2.0	40	219/106	108	20	26.3	0.89	1.04	9.6	0.86	7.39	21	103	100	9	40	36	−4	28	24	0.12
2.5	60		111	21	30.3	1.01	1.14	10.3	0.89			104			41			28	25	
3.0	60		115	22	35.2	1.17	1.22	10.6	0.96			107			40			28	27	
3.5	80		117	25	40.7	1.36	1.36	11.6	1.00			110			39			28	28	
4.0	80	238/106	129	26	45.7	1.50	1.41	10.9	1.06	7.39	21	112	103	13	39	36	−3	29	31	0.16
4.5	100		123	28	50.9	1.65	1.53	12.4	1.08			114			38			29	32	
5.0	100		125	29	51.9	1.70	1.56	12.5	1.09			114			38			29	32	
5.5	120		127	32	67.8	2.02	1.68	13.2	1.20			119			35			32	39	
6.0	120	250/113	131	39	80.3	2.24	1.84	14.0	1.22	7.41	19	122	114	9	32	31	−1	34	42	0.18
6.5	140		131	41	91.5	2.42	1.99	15.2	1.22			120			34			36	44	
7.0	140		141	55	121.3	2.79	2.15	15.2	1.30			128			27			42	54	
7.5	160	235/110	148	59	142.8	2.95	2.20	14.9	1.34	7.42	15	130	129	3	25	23	−2	47	63	0.19
	Recovery		131	39	80.8	2.04	1.73	13.2	1.18			124			30			38	45	
	Recovery		119	33	50.4	1.18	0.98	8.2	1.20			127			27			40	49	

TABLE 9.19.4. Selected Respiratory Function Data: Second Study

Measurement	Predicted	Measured
Age, yr		60
Sex		Male
Height, cm		171
Weight, kg	74	87
VC, L	3.92	4.38
IC, L	2.61	2.53
TLC, L	6.11	5.87
FEV₁, L	3.06	3.59
FEV₁/VC, %	78	81
MVV, L/min	132	158
D$_{L}$CO, ml/mm Hg/min	26.4	31.8

TABLE 9.19.5. Selected Exercise Data: Second Study

Measurement	Predicted	Measured
Peak V̇O₂, L/min	2.19	1.63
Maximum HR, beats/min	160	118
Maximum O₂ pulse, ml/beat	13.7	14.2
ΔV̇O₂/ΔWR, ml/min/W	10.3	6.8
AT, L/min	>0.96	1.05
Blood pressure, mmHg (rest, max ex)		140/80, 210/100
Maximum V̇E, L/min		79
Exercise breathing reserve, L/min	>15	79

TABLE 9.19.6. Second Study

Time min	Work rate watts	BP mmHg	HR min^{-1}	f min^{-1}	$\dot{V}E$ L/min BTPS	$\dot{V}CO_2$ L/min STPD	$\dot{V}O_2$ L/min STPD	$\dot{V}O_2$/HR ml/beat	R	pH	HCO_3^- meq/L	PO_2 ET	PO_2 a	PO_2 (a–a)	PCO_2 ET	PCO_2 a	PCO_2 (a–ET)	$\dot{V}E/\dot{V}CO_2$	$\dot{V}E/\dot{V}O_2$	VD/VT
Rest		140/80																		
Rest			69	12	9.1	0.25	0.31	5.3	0.81			102			39			32	26	
Rest		140/90	67	12	9.6	0.25	0.29	5.1	0.86			106			37			34	30	
Rest			64	13	6.2	0.13	0.15	2.3	0.87			104			38			39	34	
Rest		140/90	55	15	7.7	0.16	0.22	4.0	0.73			99			39			40	29	
Rest			57	13	10.5	0.28	0.37	6.5	0.76			99			39			34	25	
Rest			57	19	10.8	0.27	0.34	6.0	0.79			101			39			34	27	
	Unloaded		70	18	16.8	0.56	0.70	10.0	0.80			100			41			27	22	
	Unloaded		70	13	16.7	0.52	0.58	8.3	0.90			108			38			30	27	
	Unloaded		70	14	17.0	0.56	0.66	9.4	0.85			104			39			28	24	
	Unloaded		72	19	21.3	0.65	0.69	9.6	0.94			109			38			30	29	
	Unloaded		72	19	19.8	0.63	0.73	10.1	0.86			103			40			29	25	
	Unloaded	145/90	76	16	21.2	0.68	0.80	10.5	0.85			100			41			29	25	
0.5	20		76	13	18.0	0.59	0.66	8.7	0.89			106			39			29	26	
1.0	20		76	15	19.9	0.66	0.76	10.0	0.87			103			40			28	25	
1.5	40		76	16	21.8	0.74	0.87	11.4	0.85			102			41			28	23	
2.0	40	180/90	83	19	28.2	0.92	0.98	11.8	0.94			104			41			29	27	
2.5	60		85	17	27.1	0.95	1.06	12.5	0.90			102			42			27	24	
3.0	60		88	20	36.8	1.23	1.23	14.0	1.00			102			42			29	29	
3.5	80		93	24	37.4	1.25	1.18	12.7	1.06			109			41			28	30	
4.0	80	195/85	100	23	42.1	1.38	1.26	12.6	1.10			113			38			29	32	
4.5	100		102	25	48.4	1.53	1.36	13.3	1.13			114			38			30	34	
5.0	100		105	29	57.6	1.72	1.42	13.5	1.21			118			35			32	39	
5.5	120		103	34	68.8	1.92	1.50	14.6	1.28			121			33			34	44	
6.0	120	210/100	113	49	79.3	2.02	1.54	13.6	1.31			121			33			37	49	
6.5	140		118	40	78.0	2.06	1.58	13.4	1.30			119			34			36	47	
7.0	140		115	42	76.5	2.16	1.63	14.2	1.33			119			33			34	45	
	Recovery		98	27	66.8	1.89	1.35	13.8	1.40			120			34			34	48	
	Recovery	210/90	97	27	61.9	1.71	1.23	12.7	1.39			123			32			35	48	
	Recovery		91	23	45.5	1.27	0.94	10.3	1.35			122			33			34	46	
	Recovery	180/90	91	23	41.9	1.16	0.88	9.7	1.32			122			33			34	45	

Interpretation

Comments

Resting respiratory function studies and arterial blood gases and pH were normal at both evaluations.

Analysis

Referring to flow chart 1, in the first study all findings were normal with the exception of a negative breathing reserve, which we interpret as indicating the patient's sensitive ventilatory response to the exercise-induced metabolic acidosis with precise pH regulation. To maintain this normal pH, he lowered his $PaCO_2$ from 35 to 23 mmHg over a 3½-minute period. He had no evidence of pulmonary or cardiovascular dysfunction.

In the second study, 3 years later, the peak $\dot{V}O_2$ was reduced while the anaerobic threshold, al-though lower than that of the earlier study, remained normal (Table 9.19.5). Referring to flow chart 6, the breathing reserve was normal (branchpoint 3.1). The ECG during the second exercise study was clearly abnormal, leading to the diagnosis of myocardial ischemia. The low $\Delta \dot{V}O_2/\Delta WR$ and flat O_2 pulse during the period of increasing work rate are supportive of this diagnosis.

Conclusion

This patient, with several risk factors for coronary artery disease, had an initially normal cardiovascular response to incremental exercise. Three years later, his O_2 flow became clearly abnormal during incremental exercise. At about the same time, he developed ECG abnormalities and chest pain. The ECG changes, symptoms, and the gas exchange abnormalities establish the diagnosis of myocardial ischemia.

Case 20 Myocardial Ischemia with Mild Interstitial and Obstructive Airway Disease
Clinical Findings

This 54-year-old man was referred by a government agency for cardiopulmonary exercise testing because of his work exposure to asbestos of 15 years. He no longer smoked but had a 30-year history of cigarette smoking. He denied dyspnea, cough, chest pain, weight change, or ankle edema. He got little exercise and felt numbness in his legs after 20 minutes of walking. He had borderline hypertension and an elevated serum cholesterol. There were crackles at the left lung base, and a chest roentgenogram showed linear scarring in that area. Heart sounds and the resting ECGs were normal.

Exercise Findings

The patient performed exercise on a cycle ergometer. He pedalled at 60 rpm without an added load for 3 minutes. The work rate was then increased 15 W per minute to tolerance. Heart rate and rhythm were continuously monitored; 12-lead ECGs were obtained during rest, exercise, and recovery. Blood pressure was measured with a sphygmomanometer and arterial oxygen saturation was estimated with an ear oximeter. The patient appeared to give a good effort and stopped exercise because of leg fatigue; he denied chest pain or dyspnea during or after the study. Significant ST segment depression in leads II, III, aVF, and V3 to V6 was noted beginning at the 120-W work rate with a maximum of 2.5-mm depression at end-exercise. The ST-segment abnormalities resolved after 9 minutes of recovery. No ectopy was present. Saturation as estimated by oximetry remained normal.

TABLE 9.20.1. Selected Respiratory Function Data

Measurement	Predicted	Measured
Age, yr		54
Sex		Male
Height, cm		191
Weight, kg	90	98
Hematocrit, %		47
VC, L	5.36	4.79
IC, L	3.58	3.78
FEV$_1$, L	4.25	3.05
FEV$_1$/VC, %	79	64
MVV, L/min	164	126
D$_L$CO, ml/mm Hg/min	29.5	27.7

TABLE 9.20.2. Selected Exercise Data

Measurement	Predicted	Measured
Peak $\dot{V}O_2$, L/min	2.81	2.09
Maximum HR, beats/min	166	142
Maximum O$_2$ pulse, ml/beat	16.9	14.8
$\Delta\dot{V}O_2/\Delta$WR, ml/min/W	10.3	8.9
AT, L/min	>1.21	1.4
Blood pressure, mmHg (rest, max)		154/90, 198/78
Maximum $\dot{V}E$, L/min		72
Exercise breathing reserve, L/min	>15	54

TABLE 9.20.3. Air Breathing

Time min	Work rate watts	BP mmHg	HR min⁻¹	f min⁻¹	$\dot{V}_E$ L/min BTPS	$\dot{V}_{CO_2}$ L/min STPD	$\dot{V}_{O_2}$ L/min STPD	$\dot{V}_{O_2}$/HR ml/beat	R	pH	HCO₃⁻ meq/L	P_{O_2} ET	P_{O_2} a	P_{O_2} (A–a)	P_{CO_2} ET	P_{CO_2} a	P_{CO_2} (a–ET)	$\dot{V}_E/\dot{V}_{CO_2}$	$\dot{V}_E/\dot{V}_{O_2}$	V_D/V_T
	Rest	154/90																		
	Rest		77	5	16.6	0.45	0.53	6.9	0.85			106			35			36	31	
	Rest		78	10	14.9	0.44	0.50	6.4	0.88			112			33			32	28	
	Rest		80	6	12.4	0.37	0.43	5.4	0.86			109			34			32	28	
	Rest	150/96	79	5	9.9	0.32	0.40	5.1	0.80			107			34			30	24	
	Rest		77	9	13.5	0.38	0.48	6.2	0.79			107			34			34	27	
	Rest		79	10	9.4	0.27	0.32	4.1	0.84			107			35			32	27	
	Unloaded		83	16	18.1	0.52	0.70	8.4	0.74			102			36			32	24	
	Unloaded		82	13	16.4	0.50	0.64	7.8	0.78			104			36			31	24	
	Unloaded		84	14	18.5	0.58	0.74	8.8	0.78			103			37			30	23	
	Unloaded		86	15	16.7	0.52	0.66	7.7	0.79			100			39			30	23	
	Unloaded		88	13	21.0	0.67	0.80	9.1	0.84			104			37			30	25	
	Unloaded	148/88	85	13	26.1	0.82	0.93	10.9	0.88			105			37			30	27	
0.5	15		87	15	22.6	0.74	0.85	9.8	0.87			103			39			29	25	
1.0	15		87	15	24.7	0.77	0.88	10.1	0.88			107			37			30	27	
1.5	30		88	12	19.9	0.65	0.75	8.5	0.87			106			37			29	25	
2.0	30	152/90	90	16	27.5	0.85	0.93	10.9	0.87			107			36			31	27	
2.5	45		92	12	22.5	0.74	0.86	9.3	0.86			100			41			29	25	
3.0	45		94	13	28.3	0.94	1.06	11.3	0.89			105			39			29	26	
3.5	60		98	16	30.9	1.02	1.17	11.9	0.87			105			39			29	25	
4.0	60	148/84	98	16	33.9	1.12	1.25	12.8	0.90			104			39			29	26	
4.5	75		99	15	35.6	1.21	1.34	13.5	0.90			103			41			28	26	
5.0	75		103	17	37.7	1.27	1.36	13.2	0.93			105			40			29	27	
5.5	90		102	18	38.3	1.31	1.39	13.6	0.94			105			41			28	26	
6.0	90	178/86	108	18	43.4	1.49	1.54	14.3	0.97			105			41			28	27	
6.5	105		112	21	49.4	1.62	1.57	14.0	1.03			110			39			29	30	
7.0	105		109	20	49.6	1.71	1.71	15.7	1.00			103			44			28	28	
7.5	120		115	22	55.1	1.83	1.69	14.7	1.08			110			40			29	31	
8.0	120	170/88	120	23	51.4	1.79	1.72	14.3	1.04			108			41			28	29	
8.5	135		128	24	60.8	2.04	1.87	14.6	1.09			111			39			29	31	
9.0	135		132	25	64.8	2.15	1.95	14.8	1.10			110			41			29	32	
9.5	150		139	27	64.4	2.17	1.98	14.2	1.10			108			43			29	31	
10.0	150	198/78	142	30	71.9	2.34	2.09	14.7	1.12			113			39			30	33	
	Recovery		137	23	68.4	2.33	2.02	14.7	1.15			113			40			29	33	
	Recovery		122	23	55.4	1.95	1.52	12.5	1.28			114			42			27	35	
	Recovery		119	22	60.1	2.02	1.29	10.8	1.57			119			40			29	45	
	Recovery		127	20	58.5	1.81	1.04	8.2	1.74			124			37			31	55	

Interpretation

Comments

Resting studies showed a mild obstructive ventilatory defect.

Analysis

Referring to flow chart 1, peak $\dot{V}_{O_2}$ is mildly decreased, but the anaerobic threshold is normal. Proceeding next to flow chart 3, the high breathing reserve (branchpoint 3.1) and abnormal exercise ECG (branchpoint 3.3) lead to the diagnosis of myocardial ischemia, although the patient had no chest pain or distress. The $\Delta\dot{V}_{O_2}/\Delta WR$ is within normal limits, but the plateau in the O_2 pulse for the last 4 minutes of exercise suggests the inability to further increase stroke volume and the arterio-venous O_2 difference or that stroke volume is decreasing as arterio-venous O_2 difference is increasing. This is coincident with the onset of abnormal ECG findings and is further supported by a slowing of $\dot{V}_{O_2}$ increase as work rate is increased.

FIGURE 9.20.1.

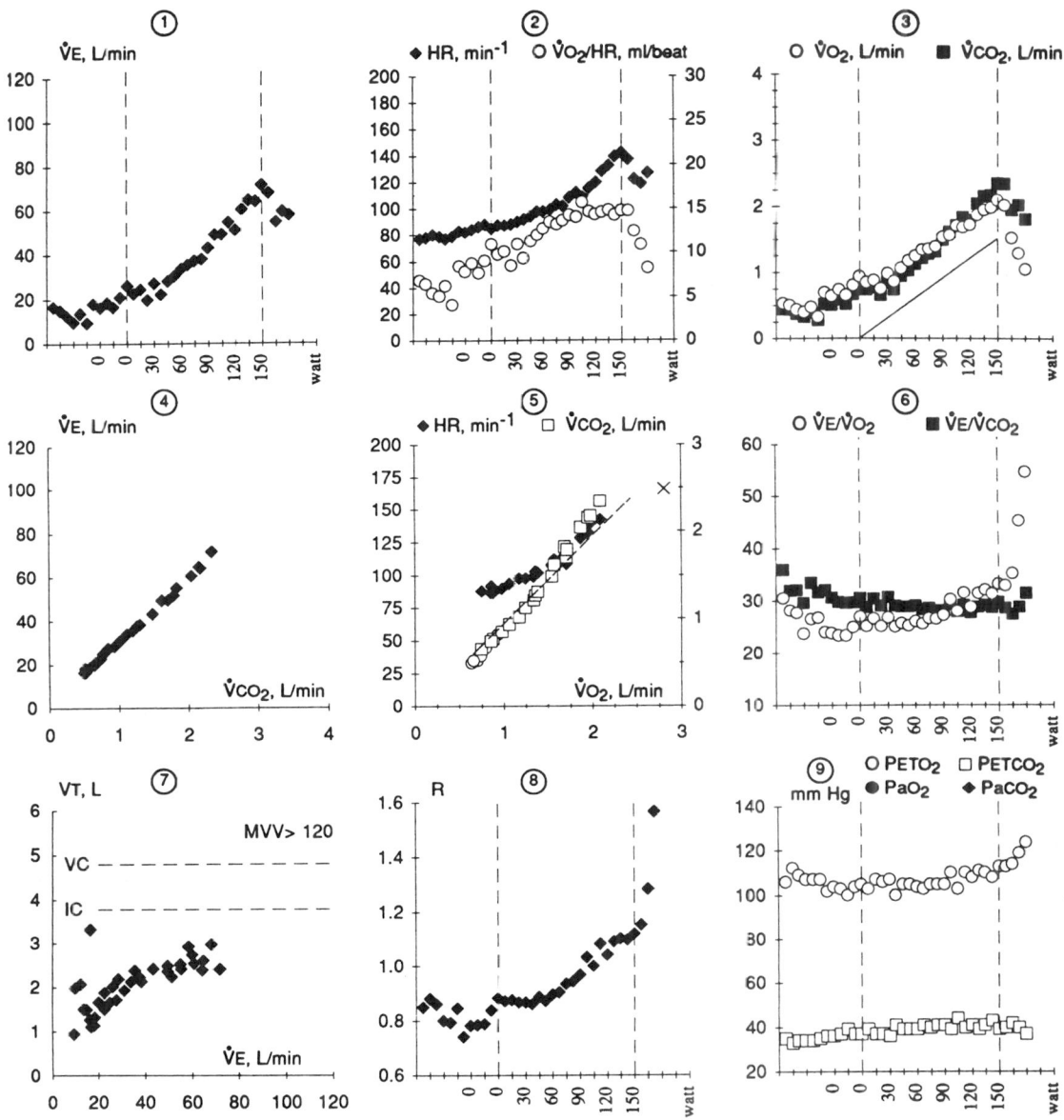

1. Vertical dashed lines in panels 1 to 3 and 6, 8, and 9 indicate the beginning and the end of increasing work period.
2. Unloaded cycling is performed for 3 minutes before the left vertical dashed line.
3. In panel 3, the diagonal line shows the increase of $\dot{V}O_2$ at a slope of 10 ml/min/w.
4. In panel 5, the diagonal dashed line has a slope of 1; the "x" in the upper right is the predicted maximum heart rate and $\dot{V}O_2$ for the subject.

Conclusion

The patient has evidence of myocardial ischemia associated with concurrent evidence of myocardial dysfunction. This is most likely due to coronary artery disease. The normal ventilatory equivalents indicate essentially normal ventilation-perfusion matching despite the mild obstructive and interstitial lung disease. The patient was referred to his private internist for further diagnostic and therapeutic evaluation of his cardiac disease.

Case 21 Silent Myocardial Ischemia, Systemic Hypertension, and Mild Interstitial Lung Disease

Clinical Findings

This 65-year-old man was referred for evaluation. He had retired from work in the shipyard 5 years previously. He had noted slight dyspnea on exertion beginning 6 years prior to evaluation but could still climb 2 flights of stairs without shortness of breath. He had smoked half a pack of cigarettes a day between the ages 24 and 40. He denied cough, sputum production, or wheezing. He had recently become short of breath on a fishing trip at high altitude. At age 25, he was discharged from the Army because of a "cardiac murmur," but this was not noted on later examinations. There was no history of rheumatic fever or congestive heart failure. He took no medications. Physical examination was normal except for bilateral arcus senilis. Chest roentgenograms revealed bilateral pleural plaques and possible bibasilar interstitial disease.

Exercise Findings

The patient performed exercise on a cycle ergometer. He pedalled at 60 rpm without added load for 3 minutes. The work rate was then increased 20 W per minute. Blood was sampled every second minute, and intra-arterial blood pressure was recorded from a percutaneously placed brachial artery catheter. Resting ECG showed deep Q waves in leads 2, 3, and AVF compatible with an old inferior infarction. During exercise, occasional single ventricular premature contractions were noted. At 120 watts the ST segments were depressed 2 mm in V4 through V6 and then 4 mm before exercise was stopped at 160 W. The ST segments became isoelectric within 5 minutes of recovery. The patient experienced leg fatigue but denied any chest pain or discomfort.

TABLE 9.21.1. Selected Respiratory Function Data

Measurement	Predicted	Measured
Age, yr		65
Sex		Male
Height, cm		174
Weight, kg	77	65
Hematocrit, %		45
VC, L	3.97	3.58
IC, L	2.64	2.24
TLC, L	6.21	6.68
FEV, L	3.09	2.60
FEV/VC, %	78	73
MVV, L/min	128	117
D_{LCO}, ml/mm Hg/min	25.6	21.7

TABLE 9.21.2. Selected Exercise Data

Measurement	Predicted	Measured
Peak $\dot{V}O_2$, L/min	1.88	1.41
Maximum HR, beats/min	155	176
Maximum O_2 pulse, ml/beat	12.1	8.0
$\Delta\dot{V}O_2/\Delta WR$, ml/min/W	10.3	7.3
AT, L/min	>0.84	1.05
Blood pressure, mmHg (rest, max)		189/108, 234/126
Maximum $\dot{V}E$, L/min		74
Exercise breathing reserve, L/min	>15	43
PaO_2 mmHg (rest, max ex)		93, 89
$P(A - a)O_2$, mmHg (rest, max ex)		15, 35
$P(a - ET)CO_2$, mmHg (rest, max ex)		3, 1
V_D/V_T (rest, heavy ex)		0.32, 0.37

FIGURE 9.21.1.

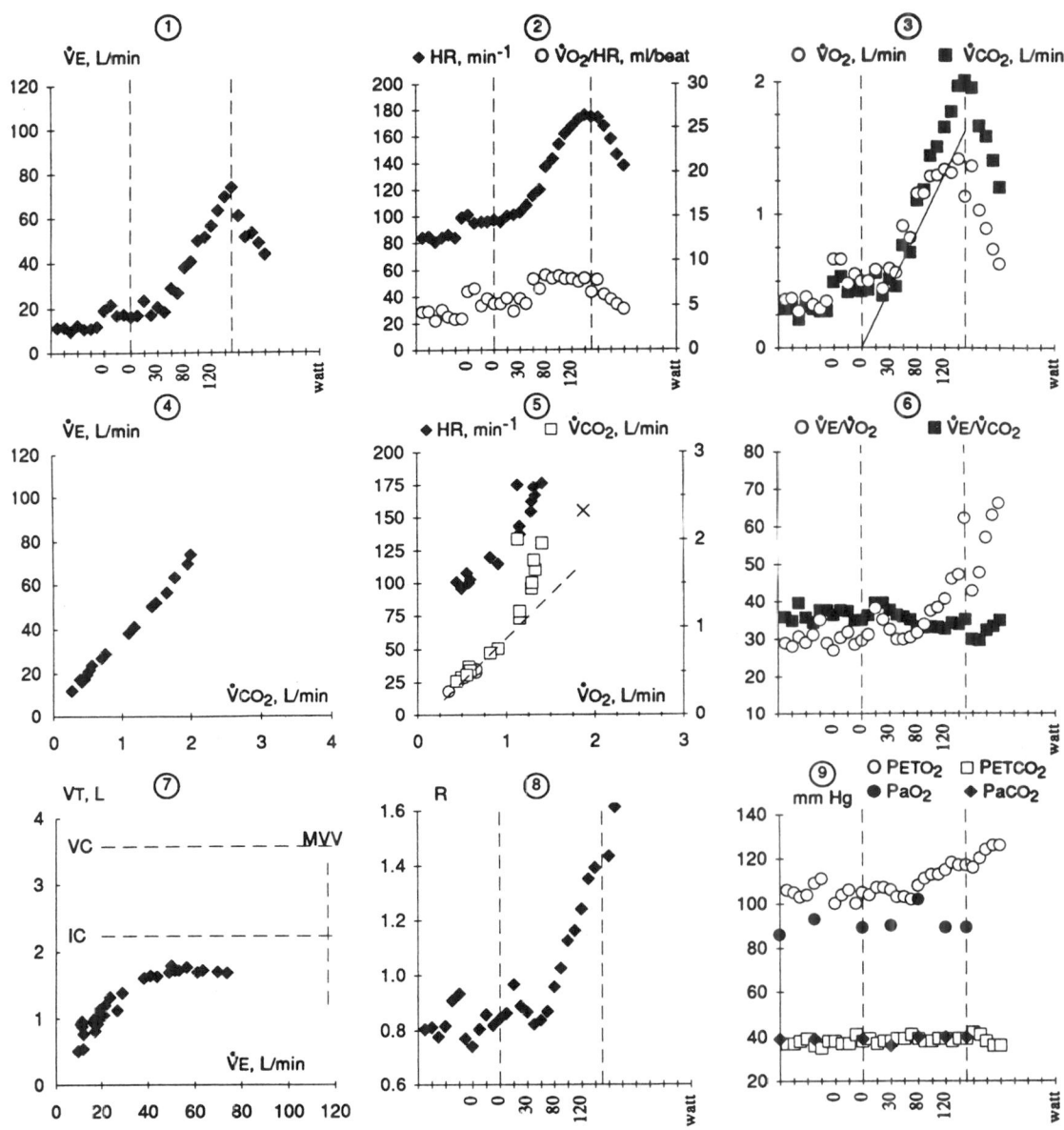

1. Vertical dashed lines in panels 1 to 3 and 6, 8, and 9 indicate the beginning and the end of increasing work period.

2. Unloaded cycling is performed for 3 minutes before the left vertical dashed line.

3. In panel 3, the diagonal line shows the increase of $\dot{V}O_2$ at a slope of 10 ml/min/w.

4. In panel 5, the diagonal dashed line has a slope of 1; the "x" in the upper right is the predicted maximum heart rate and $\dot{V}O_2$ for the subject.

Interpretation

Comments

Results of the resting respiratory function studies are within normal limits (Table 9.21.1). The resting ECG is abnormal and suggests that the patient had an inferior wall myocardial infarction in the past.

Analysis

Referring to flow chart 1, the peak $\dot{V}O_2$ is reduced but the anaerobic threshold is within normal limits (Table 9.21.2). See flow chart 3: The breathing reserve is high (branchpoint 3.1). The ECG became abnormal as the maximum work rate was approached (branchpoint 3.3). While

TABLE 9.21.3. Air Breathing

Time min	Work rate watts	BP mmHg	HR min⁻¹	f min⁻¹	V̇E L/min BTPS	V̇CO₂ L/min STPD	V̇O₂ L/min STPD	V̇O₂/HR ml/beat	R	pH	HCO₃⁻ meq/L	Po₂ ET	Po₂ a	Po₂ (A−a)	Pco₂ ET	Pco₂ a	Pco₂ (a−ET)	V̇E/V̇CO₂	V̇E/V̇O₂	VD/VT
	Rest	189/108								7.44	26		86			39				
	Rest		84	12	11.4	0.29	0.36	4.3	0.81			106			37			36	29	
	Rest		85	13	11.5	0.30	0.37	4.4	0.81			105			37			35	28	
	Rest		81	19	9.9	0.21	0.27	3.3	0.78			103			38			39	31	
	Rest		84	16	12.4	0.31	0.38	4.5	0.82			104			39			36	29	
	Rest	192/114	86	12	11.0	0.29	0.32	3.7	0.91	7.44	26	109	93	15	36	39	3	34	31	0.32
	Rest		84	12	11.2	0.27	0.29	3.5	0.93			111			35			38	35	
	Unloaded		99	22	12.0	0.27	0.35	3.5	0.77			103			38			38	29	
	Unloaded		101	17	19.2	0.49	0.66	6.5	0.74			100			38			36	27	
	Unloaded		95	18	21.5	0.53	0.66	6.9	0.80			104			37			38	30	
	Unloaded		93	18	16.8	0.41	0.48	5.0	0.85			106			37			37	32	
	Unloaded		96	19	17.3	0.45	0.55	5.7	0.82			100			41			35	29	
	Unloaded	213/120	97	17	16.2	0.42	0.50	5.2	0.84	7.43	25	105	89	16	38	39	1	35	30	0.34
0.5	20		96	17	17.0	0.43	0.50	5.2	0.86			104			39			36	31	
1.0	20		100	18	23.6	0.56	0.58	5.8	0.97			107			37			39	38	
1.5	30		101	21	17.2	0.39	0.44	4.4	0.89			107			38			40	35	
2.0	30	210/114	103	20	20.9	0.51	0.59	5.7	0.86	7.50	28	106	90	20	38	36	−2	38	33	0.33
2.5	60		108	20	18.4	0.46	0.56	5.2	0.82			103			39			36	30	
3.0	60		115	21	29.0	0.73	0.91	7.9	0.84			103			39			36	30	
3.5	80		120	24	26.9	0.71	0.82	6.8	0.87			102			41			35	30	
4.0	80	219/117	137	24	38.3	1.10	1.15	8.4	0.96	7.36	22	108	102	7	39	40	1	33	32	0.33
4.5	100		143	25	41.0	1.13	1.15	8.0	1.03			111			38			33	34	
5.0	100		154	28	50.1	1.44	1.28	8.3	1.13			113			38			33	37	
5.5	120		162	30	51.8	1.50	1.29	8.0	1.16			113			39			33	38	
6.0	120	234/126	167	32	56.6	1.65	1.33	8.0	1.24	7.35	22	115	89	27	39	40	1	33	41	0.32
6.5	140		173	37	63.5	1.77	1.31	7.6	1.35			113			38			34	46	
7.0	140		176	41	69.8	1.96	1.41	8.0	1.39			117			39			34	47	
7.5	160	234/126	178	44	73.9	2.00	1.13	6.5	1.77	7.35	22	117	89	35	39	40	1	35	62	0.37
	Recovery		174	36	61.1	1.95	1.36	7.8	1.43			116			42			30	43	
	Recovery		168	30	51.6	1.66	1.03	6.1	1.61			120			41			30	48	
	Recovery		158	31	53.3	1.58	0.89	5.6	1.78			124			38			32	57	
	Recovery	220/120	146	29	49.0	1.40	0.74	5.1	1.89			126			36			33	63	
	Recovery		138	27	44.0	1.20	0.63	4.6	1.90			126			36			35	66	

the patient did not experience chest pain, the diagnosis of myocardial ischemia is supported by the marked change in slope in V̇O₂ in response to increasing work rate (panel 3, Fig. 9.21.1) and a reduced ΔV̇O₂/ΔWR. The very marked increase in R starting at 80 W (Table 9.21.3 and panel 8, Fig. 9.21.1) reflects the development of a significant metabolic acidosis as the anaerobic threshold is exceeded. The steepening heart rate response with increasing oxygen uptake (panel 5, Fig. 9.21.1) and the failure of O₂ pulse to increase at a low work rate (panel 2, Fig. 9.21.1) reflect a low stroke volume and a maximal C(a − v̄)O₂ being reached at a relatively low work rate.

This patient has significant systemic hypertension. We cannot therefore exclude the possibility that the myocardial ischemia and impaired cardiac function demonstrated here are due, in part, to ab-

normally increased myocardial work and coronary artery disease.

There is evidence of ventilation-perfusion mismatching (high VD/VT and positive P(a − ET)CO₂). These abnormal findings might be due to the abnormalities that develop in the lungs in response to chronic heart failure (due to an ischemic cardiomyopathy) as described in Chapter 4. The normal resting respiratory function suggests that the decrease in perfusion of ventilated lung reflected by these blood gas abnormalities is unlikely to be due to primary lung disease.

Conclusion

Myocardial ischemia with reduced exercise performance secondary to coronary artery disease and systemic hypertension.

Case 22 Ischemic Cardiomyopathy

Clinical Findings

This 65-year-old man had sustained an acute myocardial infarction 6 years ago. Since then he had required one to two nitroglycerin tablets per day and propranolol for "stable angina." He had had 30 years of asbestos exposure in the shipyards and had smoked for 23 years. He could walk 2 to 3 miles before becoming dyspneic and admitted to a scantily productive morning cough. Resting ECG was normal. An exercise study was performed to evaluate the relative contributions of his pulmonary and cardiac illnesses.

Exercise Findings

The patient performed exercise on a cycle ergometer. He pedalled at 60 rpm without added load for 3 minutes. The work rate was then increased 10 W per minute. Arterial blood was sampled every second minute, and intra-arterial blood pressure was recorded from a percutaneously placed brachial artery catheter. The incremental cycle exercise test was terminated at 70 W because of moderate substernal chest pain and the development of 3 mm of ST segment depression in leads 2, 3, and AVF, and occasional premature ventricular beats. These abnormalities resolved promptly after termination of exercise.

TABLE 9.22.1. Selected Respiratory Function Data

Measurement	Predicted	Measured
Age, yr		65
Sex		Male
Height, cm		167
Weight, kg	71	55
Hematocrit, %		41
VC, L	3.54	3.42
IC, L	2.36	1.81
TLC, L	5.57	6.16
FEV_1, L	2.75	2.33
FEV_1/VC, %	78	68
MVV, L/min	120	101
$D_L CO$, ml/mm Hg/min	22.6	26.4

TABLE 9.22.2. Selected Exercise Data

Measurement	Predicted	Measured
Peak $\dot{V}O_2$, L/min	1.68	1.01
Maximum HR, beats/min	155	152
Maximum O_2 pulse, ml/beat	10.8	7.3
$\Delta\dot{V}O_2/\Delta WR$, ml/min/W	10.3	5.7
AT, L/min	>0.74	0.9
Blood pressure, mmHg (rest, max)		165/87, 159/84
Maximum $\dot{V}E$, L/min		39
Exercise breathing reserve, L/min	>15	62
PaO_2, mmHg (rest, max ex)		94, 95
P(A − a)O_2, mmHg (rest, max ex)		13, 18
P(a − ET)CO_2, mmHg (rest, max ex)		4, 2
VD/VT (rest, heavy ex)		0.40, 0.29
HCO_3^-, mEq/L (rest, 2-min recov)		27, 23

FIGURE 9.22.1.

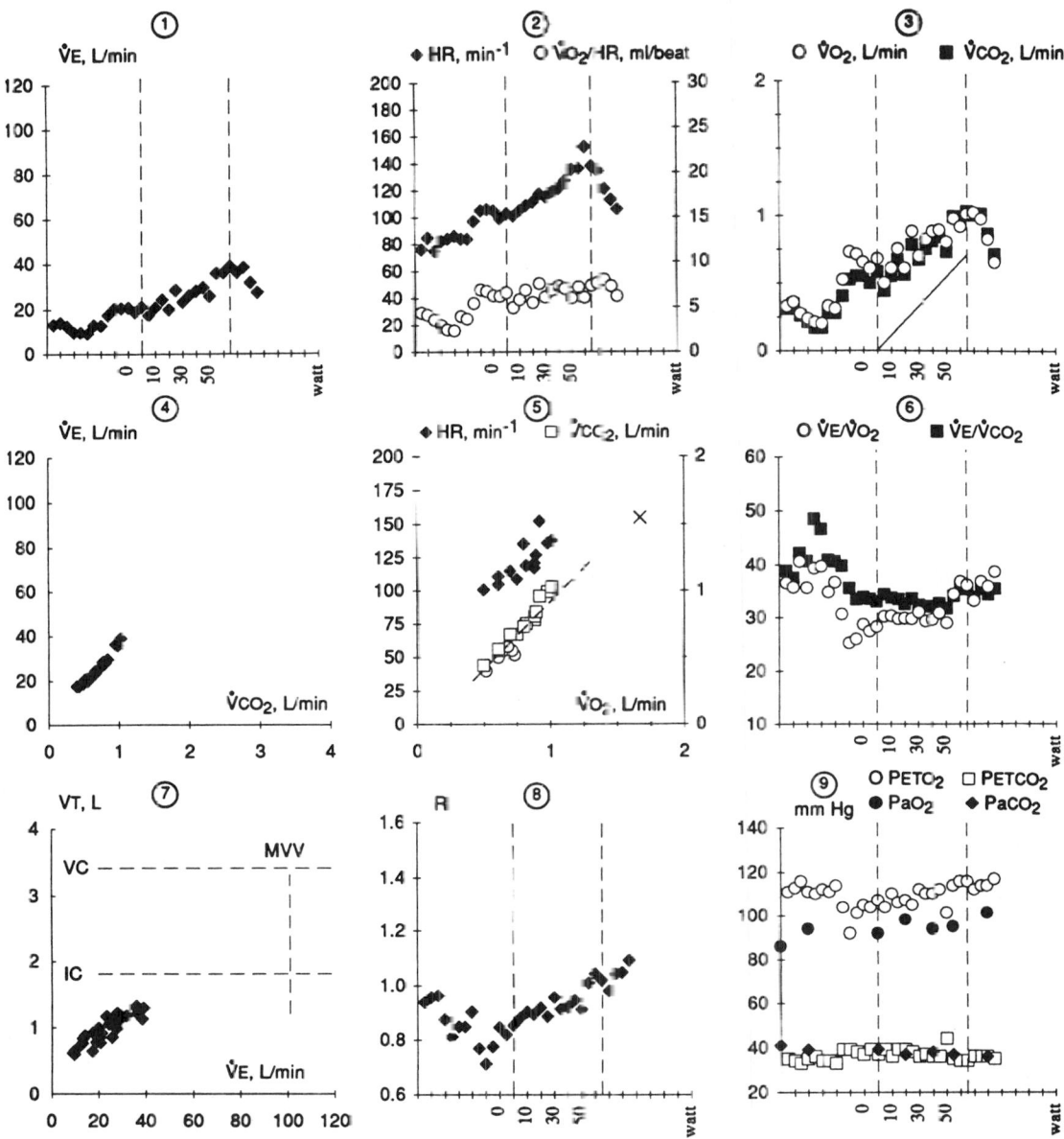

1. Vertical dashed lines in panels 1 to 3 and 6, 8, and 9 indicate the beginning and the end of increasing work period.

2. Unloaded cycling is performed for 3 minutes before the left vertical dashed line.

3. In panel 3, the diagonal line shows the increase of $\dot{V}O_2$ at a slope of 10 ml/min/w.

4. In panel 5, the diagonal dashed line has a slope of 1; the "x" in the upper right is the predicted maximum heart rate and $\dot{V}O_2$ for the subject.

TABLE 9.22.3. Air Breathing

Time min	Work rate watts	BP mmHg	HR min⁻¹	f min⁻¹	$\dot{V}_E$ L/min BTPS	$\dot{V}_{CO_2}$ L/min STPD	$\dot{V}_{O_2}$ L/min STPD	$\dot{V}_{O_2}$/HR ml/beat	R	pH	HCO₃⁻ meq/L	P$_{O_2}$ ET	P$_{O_2}$ a	P$_{O_2}$ (A−a)	P$_{CO_2}$ ET	P$_{CO_2}$ a	P$_{CO_2}$ (a−ET)	$\dot{V}_E$/$\dot{V}_{CO_2}$	$\dot{V}_E$/$\dot{V}_{O_2}$	V$_D$/V$_T$
	Rest	165/87								7.43	27		86			41				
	Rest		76	16	13.4	0.31	0.33	4.3	0.94			111			35			39	36	
	Rest		85	16	14.1	0.34	0.36	4.2	0.96			113			34			37	36	
	Rest		75	17	12.4	0.26	0.27	3.6	0.96			116			33			42	41	
	Rest		82	15	9.8	0.21	0.24	2.9	0.88	7.44	26	111	94	13	35	39	4	41	36	0.40
	Rest	156/84	84	16	9.6	0.17	0.21	2.5	0.81			110			36			48	39	
	Rest		86	15	9.2	0.17	0.20	2.3	0.85			112			34			47	40	
	Rest		84	17	12.9	0.28	0.33	3.9	0.85			111			34			41	35	
	Rest		84	17	12.8	0.28	0.31	3.7	0.90			114			33			41	37	
	Unloaded		97	19	17.5	0.40	0.52	5.4	0.77			104			39			40	31	
	Unloaded		105	22	20.3	0.52	0.73	7.0	0.71			92			39			35	25	
	Unloaded		106	24	20.4	0.55	0.71	6.7	0.77			101			38			33	26	
	Unloaded		105	23	20.6	0.55	0.65	6.2	0.85			105			37			34	29	
	Unloaded		99	24	18.8	0.50	0.61	6.2	0.82			104			39			34	27	
	Unloaded	162/84	103	23	21.1	0.58	0.68	6.6	0.85	7.44	26	107	92	14	37	39	2	33	28	0.30
0.5	10		101	27	17.4	0.44	0.50	5.0	0.88			104			39			34	30	
1.0	10		105	27	20.8	0.55	0.61	5.8	0.90			110			36			34	30	
1.5	20		109	23	24.3	0.67	0.75	6.9	0.89			106			39			33	30	
2.0	20	165/87	111	20	19.9	0.56	0.61	5.5	0.92	7.45	25	107	98	12	39	37	−2	33	30	0.26
2.5	30		117	26	28.4	0.78	0.88	7.5	0.89			105			38			34	30	
3.0	30		115	20	23.3	0.67	0.70	6.1	0.96			112			36			32	31	
3.5	40		119	23	26.0	0.75	0.82	6.9	0.91			110			37			32	29	
4.0	40	156/84	121	23	27.9	0.81	0.88	7.3	0.92	7.44	25	110	94	15	36	38	2	32	29	0.27
4.5	50		127	25	29.5	0.84	0.89	7.0	0.94			112			36			33	31	
5.0	50		135	30	25.7	0.73	0.80	5.9	0.91			101			44			32	29	
5.5	60	162/84	136	27	35.9	0.99	0.98	7.2	1.01	7.44	25	114	5	18	35	37	2	34	34	0.29
6.0	60		152	28	36.2	0.96	0.92	6.1	1.04			116			34			35	37	
6.5	70	159/84	138	30	38.9	1.03	1.01	7.3	1.02			116			34			35	36	
	Recovery		134	30	36.3	1.00	1.02	7.6	0.98			112			36			34	33	0.28
	Recovery		121	34	38.5	1.01	0.97	8.0	1.04			114			36			35	37	
	Recovery	162/84	113	27	31.7	0.86	0.82	7.3	1.05	7.43	23	114	101	14	36	36	0	34	36	
	Recovery		106	28	27.5	0.71	0.65	6.1	1.09			117			35			35	39	

Interpretation

Comments

The resting respiratory function studies indicate that the patient has mild airflow obstruction (Table 9.22.1). The resting ECG is normal.

Analysis

Referring to flow chart 1, the peak $\dot{V}_{O_2}$ is reduced and the anaerobic threshold is normal (Table 9.22.2). See flow chart 3: The breathing reserve is high (branchpoint 3.1), while the exercise ECG (branchpoint 3.3) was clearly abnormal. The chest pain, low $\Delta\dot{V}_{O_2}/\Delta WR$ and low O$_2$ pulse that fails to rise during exercise all add support to the primary diagnosis of myocardial ischemia. The high breathing reserve and normal indices of ventilation-perfusion matching indicate that the lungs and pulmonary circulation are functioning normally. In contrast, the cardiovascular response to exercise is abnormal.

Conclusion

Reduced exercise performance secondary to ischemic cardiomyopathy with mild airflow obstruction.

Case 23 Cardiomyopathy

Clinical Findings

This 41-year-old former brickworker, woodworker, sandblaster, and security guard had been placed on disability for a back injury 9 years ago. Hypertension had been diagnosed 6 years ago. He had started complaining of dyspnea and a productive cough 3 years ago. He had been diagnosed as having "probable pulmonary asbestosis" and "asthmatic bronchitis" 2 years ago. He denied smoking but had had repeated hospitalizations for alcoholism. He was being treated with propranolol, hydrochlorothiazide, oxtriphylline, and potassium supplementation. Auscultation of the heart and lungs were normal, as were posteroanterior, lateral, and oblique chest roentgenograms.

Exercise Findings

The patient performed exercise on a cycle ergometer. He pedalled at 60 rpm without added load for 3 minutes. The work rate was then increased 20 W per minute to his symptom limited maximum. Arterial blood was sampled every second minute, and intra-arterial blood pressure was recorded from a percutaneously placed brachial artery catheter. Resting ECG was normal. He stopped exercise with complaints of shortness of breath, a feeling that he was "going to faint," and leg "tiredness." One PVC occurred during exercise, but exercise and recovery ECG were otherwise normal.

TABLE 9.23.1. Selected Respiratory Function Data

Measurement	Predicted	Measured
Age, yr		41
Sex		Male
Height, cm		170
Weight, kg	74	78
Hematocrit, %		44
VC, _	3.95	4.00
IC, L	2.63	3.30
TLC, L	5.58	5.28
FEV$_1$, L	3.16	3.43
FEV$_1$/VC, %	80	86
MVV, L/min	137	118
D$_{CO}$, ml/mm Hg/min	25.8	24.7

TABLE 9.23.2. Selected Exercise Data

Measurement	Predicted	Measured
Peak $\dot{V}O_2$, L/min	2.64	1.75
Maximum HR, beats/min	179	150
Maximum O$_2$ pulse, ml/beat	14.7	11.7
$\Delta\dot{V}O_2/\Delta WR$, ml/min/W	10.3	8.3
AT, L/min	>1.11	0.85
Blood pressure, mmHg (rest, max)		132/87, 204/108
Maximum $\dot{V}E$, L/min		78
Exercise breathing reserve, L/min	>15	40
PaCO$_2$, mmHg (rest, max ex)		87, 117
P(A − a)O$_2$, mmHg (rest, max ex)		4, 3
P(a − ET)CO$_2$, mmHg (rest, max ex)		2, −2
VD/VT (rest, heavy ex)		0.36, 0.23
HCO$_3^-$, mEq/L (rest, 2-min recov)		27, 18

FIGURE 9.23.1.

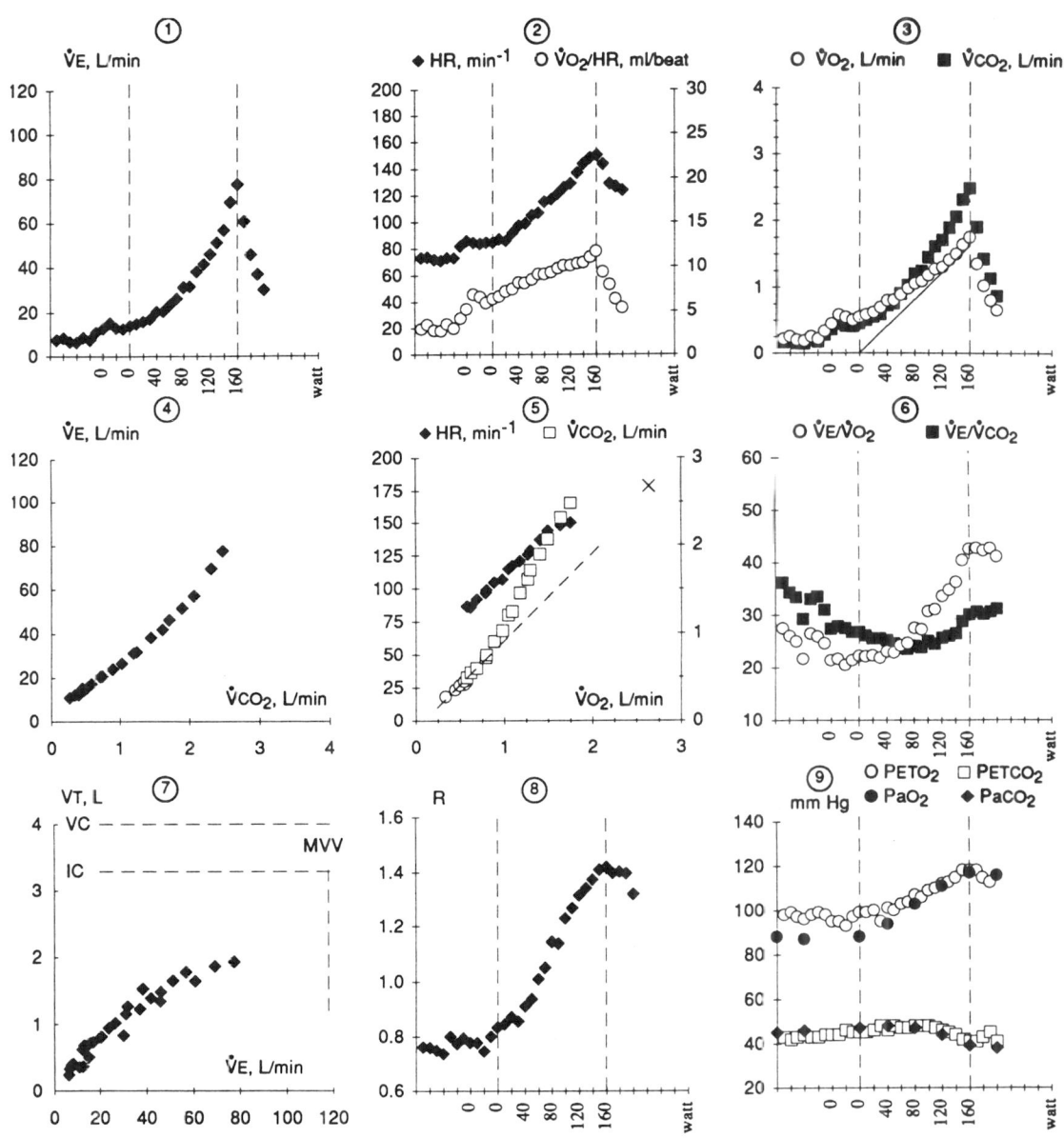

1. Vertical dashed lines in panels 1 to 3 and 6, 8, and 9 indicate the beginning and the end of increasing work period.
2. Unloaded cycling is performed for 3 minutes before the left vertical dashed line.
3. In panel 3, the diagonal line shows the increase of $\dot{V}_{O_2}$ at a slope of 10 ml/min/w.
4. In panel 5, the diagonal dashed line has a slope of 1; the "x" in the upper right is the predicted maximum heart rate and $\dot{V}_{O_2}$ for the subject.

Interpretation

Comments

Resting pulmonary function (Table 9.23.1) and ECG are normal.

Analysis

Referring to flow chart 1, the peak $\dot{V}_{O_2}$ and anaerobic threshold are reduced (Table 9.23.2). See flow chart 4: The breathing reserve is normal (branchpoint 4.1) and the ventilatory equivalent at the anaerobic

TABLE 9.23.3. Air Breathing

Time min	Work rate watts	BP mmHg	HR min⁻¹	f min⁻¹	V̇E L/min BTPS	V̇CO₂ L/min STPD	V̇O₂ L/min STPD	V̇O₂/HR ml/beat	R	pH	HCO₃⁻ meq/L	PO₂, mmHg ET	a	(A−a)	PCO₂, mmHg ET	a	(a−ET)	V̇E/V̇CO₂	V̇E/V̇O₂	VD/VT
	Rest	132/87								7.39	27		88			45				
	Rest		73	19	7.4	0.16	0.21	2.9	0.76			98			43			36	28	
	Rest		74	21	8.3	0.19	0.25	3.4	0.76			99			42			34	26	
	Rest		72	20	6.7	0.15	0.20	2.8	0.75			97			43			33	25	
	Rest	126/84	71	17	6.4	0.14	0.19	2.7	0.74	7.39	27	96	87	4	44	46	2	35	26	0.36
	Rest		73	21	8.4	0.20	0.25	3.4	0.80			98			43			33	26	
	Rest		73	20	7.4	0.17	0.22	3.0	0.77			99			43			34	26	
	Unloaded		82	31	11.0	0.27	0.34	4.1	0.79			98			44			31	25	
	Unloaded		86	34	12.5	0.35	0.45	5.2	0.78			95			44			27	21	
	Unloaded		85	30	15.1	0.45	0.58	6.8	0.78			95			44			28	22	
	Unloaded		84	19	12.9	0.41	0.55	6.5	0.75			93			46			28	21	
	Unloaded		85	20	12.4	0.40	0.50	5.9	0.80			97			45			27	21	
	Unloaded	138/84	85	21	13.8	0.45	0.54	6.4	0.83	7 37	27	99	88	8	45	47	2	27	22	0.27
0.5	20		87	21	14.6	0.49	0.58	6.7	0.84			99			45			26	22	
1.0	20		86	22	15.7	0.54	0.62	7.2	0.87			100			46			26	22	
1.5	40		92	23	17.0	0.59	0.69	7.5	0.86			95			48			26	22	
2.0	40	147/90	97	25	20.3	0.72	0.79	8.1	0.91	7.38	28	101	94	4	46	48	2	25	23	0.26
2.5	60		99	25	20.5	0.75	0.80	8.1	0.94			100			48			25	23	
3.0	60		105	25	23.6	0.90	0.89	8.5	1.01			103			47			24	24	
3.5	80		107	26	26.4	1.03	0.98	9.2	1.05			104			47			23	25	
4.0	80	159/90	115	27	31.2	1.20	1.05	9.1	1.14	7.36	26	107	103	5	48	47	−1	24	28	0.22
4.5	100		117	25	31.7	1.24	1.09	9.3	1.14			106			48			24	27	
5.0	100		121	25	38.3	1.45	1.18	9.8	1.23			109			48			25	31	
5.5	120		126	30	41.9	1.61	1.27	10.1	1.27			110			47			24	31	
6.0	120	192/105	129	31	46.2	1.71	1.30	10.1	1.32	7.35	24	112	111	3	46	44	−2	25	34	0.22
6.5	140		137	31	51.5	1.89	1.41	10.3	1.34			113			45			26	35	
7.0	140		144	32	57.0	2.06	1.50	10.4	1.37			115			44			26	36	
7.5	160		148	37	69.3	2.31	1.64	11.1	1.41			113			42			29	40	
8.0	160	204/108	150	40	77.6	2.48	1.75	11.7	1.42	7.34	21	113	117	3	41	39	−2	30	42	0.25
	Recovery		144	37	61.0	1.90	1.36	9.4	1.40			118			41			30	43	
	Recovery		129	34	45.8	1.43	1.02	7.9	1.40			115			43			30	42	
	Recovery		127	30	37.0	1.13	0.81	6.4	1.40			113			45			30	43	
	Recovery	150/78	124	36	30.1	0.87	0.66	5.3	1.32	7.28	18	116	116	3	41	38	−3	31	41	0.24

threshold (branchpoint 4.3) and the indices of venti-lation-perfusion matching are normal. These find-ings indicate that this patient does not have an abnormal pulmonary circulation, but does have a non-pulmonary O₂ flow problem. Because the he-matocrit is normal (branchpoint 4.4), this is most likely due to cardiovascular disease. The exercise ECG is essentially normal throughout exercise. His $\Delta \dot{V}O_2/\Delta WR$ is low and he has a low but rising O₂ pulse at maximum work rate (panel 2 of Fig. 9.23.1). The patient's blood pressure response to exercise and heart rate reserve are normal (Table 9.23.2), and the patient did not have leg pain with exercise, making peripheral arterial disease unlikely. Because

propranolol, itself, one of this patient's medications, ordinarily gives a high O₂ pulse during exercise, the finding of a low O₂ pulse at maximum exercise supports the diagnosis of primary heart disease. (Pulmonary vascular disease is already ruled out.)

Conclusion

This patient is a 41-year-old chronic alcoholic with cardiovascular limitation. Pulmonary vascular, pe-ripheral arterial, and coronary artery disease were shown to be unlikely causes of the limitation. Two-dimensional echocardiography with exercise sup-ported the diagnosis of cardiomyopathy.

Case 24 Cardiomyopathy, Hypertrophic Type

Clinical Findings

This 65-year-old female real estate broker was referred for evaluation of exertional dyspnea of 1 year's duration. She noted dyspnea without chest pain when walking half a block on the level or climbing less than one flight of stairs. She denied asthma but had smoked cigarettes until 6 years previously. She had been treated 2 decades ago for hyperthyroidism. Work-up elsewhere revealed mild airway obstruction, hypertension, and normal thyroid status. Cardiac catheterization showed 40% stenosis of one coronary artery; echocardiogram was interpreted as normal; and a wall motion study showed a left ventricular ejection fraction of 72%, decreasing slightly during exercise. Medications were clonidine, triamterene, and hydrochlorothiazide. Examination was normal except for systemic hypertension, mild obesity, and a variable systolic murmur at the third left interspace near the sternum. Resting ECG showed left ventricular hypertrophy.

Exercise Findings

The patient performed cycle ergometer exercise on two occasions. During the first study, the murmur was loud, her O_2 pulse decreased as exercise progressed, and she was more hypertensive and became symptomatic with minimal exercise. Two weeks later she returned for the second study shortly after taking clonidine. She had less hypertension and a barely audible systolic murmur. She pedalled at 60 rpm without added load for 3 minutes. The work rate was then increased 10 W per minute to her symptom-limited maximum. Arterial blood was sampled every second minute, and intra-arterial blood pressure recorded from a percutaneously placed brachial artery catheter. The patient stopped exercise because of overall fatigue and shortness of breath. Less than 1 mm of downsloping ST segment depression developed in leads 1, AVL, and V6, while an increasing number of atrial and ventricular premature contractions developed near the end of exercise. A recording of brachial artery pressure is shown.

TABLE 9.24.1. Selected Respiratory Function Data

Measurement	Predicted	Measured
Age, yr		65
Sex		Female
Height, cm		164
Weight, kg	64	69
Hematocrit, %		40
VC, L	2.86	2.78
IC, L	1.91	2.30
TLC, L	4.93	5.45
FEV$_1$, L	2.26	1.88
FEV$_1$/VC, %	79	67
MVV, L/min	85	67
D$_L$CO, ml/mm Hg/min	21.0	19.3

TABLE 9.24.2. Selected Exercise Data

Measurement	Predicted	First Study	Second Study
Peak $\dot{V}O_2$, L/min	1.28	0.88	1.15
Maximum HR, beats/min	155	142	148
Maximum O_2 pulse, ml/beat	8.3	5.8	7.8
$\Delta\dot{V}O_2/\Delta WR$, ml/min/W	10.3		6.3
AT, L/min	>0.63	Indeterminate	1.0
Blood pressure, mmHg (rest, max)		168/80, 243/102	159/69, 240/79
Maximum $\dot{V}E$, L/min		54	65
Exercise breathing reserve, L/min	>15	13	2
Pao$_2$, mmHg (rest, max ex)			84, 109
P(A − a)o$_2$, mmHg (rest, max ex)			20, 16
P(a − ET)co$_2$, mmHg (rest, max ex)			5, 2
VD/VT (rest, heavy ex)			0.35, 0.32
HCO$_3^-$, mEq/L (rest, 2-min recov)			26, 22

FIGURE 9.24.1.   Second study.

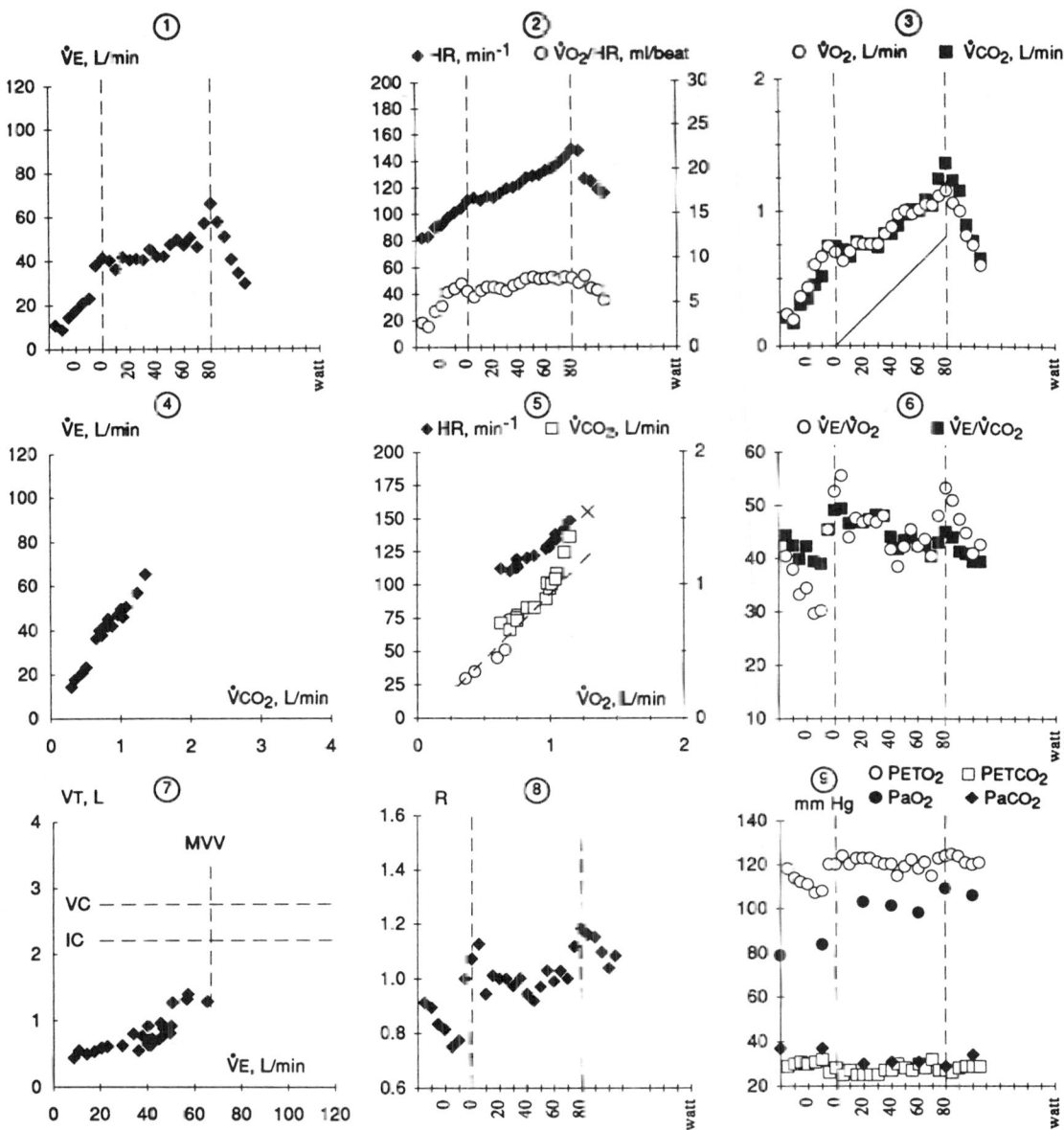

1. Vertical dashed lines in panels 1 to 3 and 6, 8, and 9 indicate the beginning and the end of increasing work period.

2. Unloaded cycling is performed for 3 minutes before the left vertical dashed line.

3. In panel 3, the diagonal line shows the increase of $\dot{V}O_2$ at a slope of 10 ml/min/w.

4. In panel 5, the diagonal dashed line has a slope of 1; the "x" in the upper right is the predicted maximum heart rate and $\dot{V}O_2$ for the subject.

TABLE 9.24.3. Second Study

Time min	Work rate watts	BP mmHg	HR min⁻¹	f min⁻¹	$\dot{V}_E$ L/min BTPS	$\dot{V}_{CO_2}$ L/min STPD	$\dot{V}_{O_2}$ L/min STPD	$\dot{V}_{O_2}$/HR ml/beat	R	pH	HCO₃⁻ meq/L	P_{O_2} ET	P_{O_2} a	P_{O_2} (A−a)	P_{CO_2} ET	P_{CO_2} a	P_{CO_2} (a−ET)	$\dot{V}_E$/$\dot{V}_{CO_2}$	$\dot{V}_E$/$\dot{V}_{O_2}$	V_D/V_T
	Rest	159/69								7.46	26		79			37				
	Rest		82	20	11.0	0.21	0.23	2.8	0.91			118			29			44	40	
	Rest		83	20	8.9	0.17	0.19	2.3	0.89			114			30			42	38	
	Unloaded		90	29	14.4	0.30	0.36	4.0	0.83			112			31			40	33	
	Unloaded		92	33	17.6	0.35	0.43	4.7	0.81			111			30			42	34	
	Unloaded		97	35	20.7	0.45	0.60	6.2	0.75			107			31			39	30	
	Unloaded	184/75	101	38	23.1	0.51	0.66	6.5	0.77	7.47	26	108	84	20	32	37	5	39	30	0.35
	Unloaded		104	49	37.8	0.74	0.74	7.1	1.00			120			26			45	45	
	Unloaded		110	58	41.2	0.74	0.69	6.3	1.07			120			28			49	53	
0.5	10		112	60	40.1	0.71	0.63	5.6	1.13			124			25			49	56	
1.0	10		110	66	36.3	0.66	0.70	6.4	0.94			120			27			47	44	
1.5	20		113	66	41.7	0.77	0.76	6.7	1.01			123			25			47	47	
2.0	20	201/90	112	63	40.4	0.75	0.75	6.7	1.00	7.52	24	123	103	17	25	30	5	47	47	0.33
2.5	30		115	65	40.9	0.75	0.75	6.5	1.00			123			25			47	47	
3.0	30		119	62	40.4	0.73	0.75	6.3	0.97			121			25			48	47	
3.5	40		120	63	45.1	0.83	0.83	6.9	1.00			120			27			48	48	
4.0	40	193/73	122	64	42.0	0.83	0.88	7.2	0.94	7.51	24	120	101	17	27	31	4	44	42	0.32
4.5	50		127	58	42.1	0.89	0.97	7.6	0.92			115			30			42	38	
5.0	50		128	60	47.1	0.97	1.00	7.8	0.97			119			28			43	42	
5.5	60		129	61	49.7	1.01	0.98	7.6	1.03			122			27			44	45	
6.0	60	220/73	132	53	47.0	1.00	1.01	7.7	0.99	7.49	23	118	98	21	30	31	1	42	42	0.31
6.5	60		134	55	50.4	1.08	1.05	7.8	1.03			121			28			42	44	
7.0	70		138	48	46.0	1.04	1.04	7.5	1.00			115			32			40	40	
7.5	80		142	43	56.8	1.24	1.11	7.8	1.12			123			27			43	48	
8.0	80	240/79	148	51	65.5	1.36	1.15	7.8	1.18	7.49	22	124	109	16	27	29	2	45	53	0.32
	Recovery		147	41	57.4	1.23	1.06	7.2	1.16			125			26			44	51	
	Recovery		126	40	50.8	1.15	1.00	7.9	1.15			124			28			41	47	
	Recovery		124	44	40.4	0.90	0.82	6.6	1.10			121			29			41	45	
	Recovery	261/92	118	43	34.3	0.78	0.75	6.4	1.04	7.42	22	120	106	11	29	34	5	39	41	0.32
	Recovery		115	47	29.5	0.65	0.60	5.2	1.08			121			29			39	43	

Interpretation

Comments

The results of the resting respiratory function studies are compatible with mild airflow obstruction. A resting ECG is normal except for left ventricular hypertrophy. Her left ventricular ejection fraction at rest is 72%.

Analysis

Referring to flow chart 1, in the first study the peak $\dot{V}_{O_2}$ is reduced and the anaerobic threshold is indeterminate. In the second study, the peak $\dot{V}_{O_2}$ and anaerobic threshold are normal (Table 9.24.2). If we use flow chart 2, because of the abnormal blood gases, we go to the right sides of branchpoint 2.1 and branchpoint 2.3 we arrive at the diagnoses of "lung or pulmonary vascular disease." Because the cardiovascular abnormalities are more striking than the evidence for ventilation-perfusion mismatching or for obstructive lung disease, we should refer to flow chart 5. Addressing the question of branchpoint 5.1, V_D/V_T and P(a − ET)$_{CO_2}$ are mildly abnormal, but P(A − a)$_{O_2}$ is normal (Tables 9.24.2, 9.24.3). Taking the abnormal branch of branchpoint 5.1, we address the question of the breathing reserve (branchpoint 5.3). In this patient, it is normal in the first study and slightly reduced, primarily because of hyperventilation that she developed during exercise. Because of the normal heart rate reserve and the absence of respiratory acidosis at maximal exercise, we must examine the other side of branchpoint 5.1.

In this study the prominent disorders are a low $\Delta\dot{V}_{O_2}$/ΔWR and a low O_2 pulse that does not in-

FIGURE 9.24.2. Four tracings of ECG (upper) and brachial artery blood pressure (lower) during and immediately after cycle ergometer exercise: (1) unloaded pedalling; (2) 30 W; (3) 80W; and (4) early recovery. Each tracing is 4 seconds in duration. Note premature contractions at unloaded pedalling and early recovery and their effect on the contour of the following pulse.

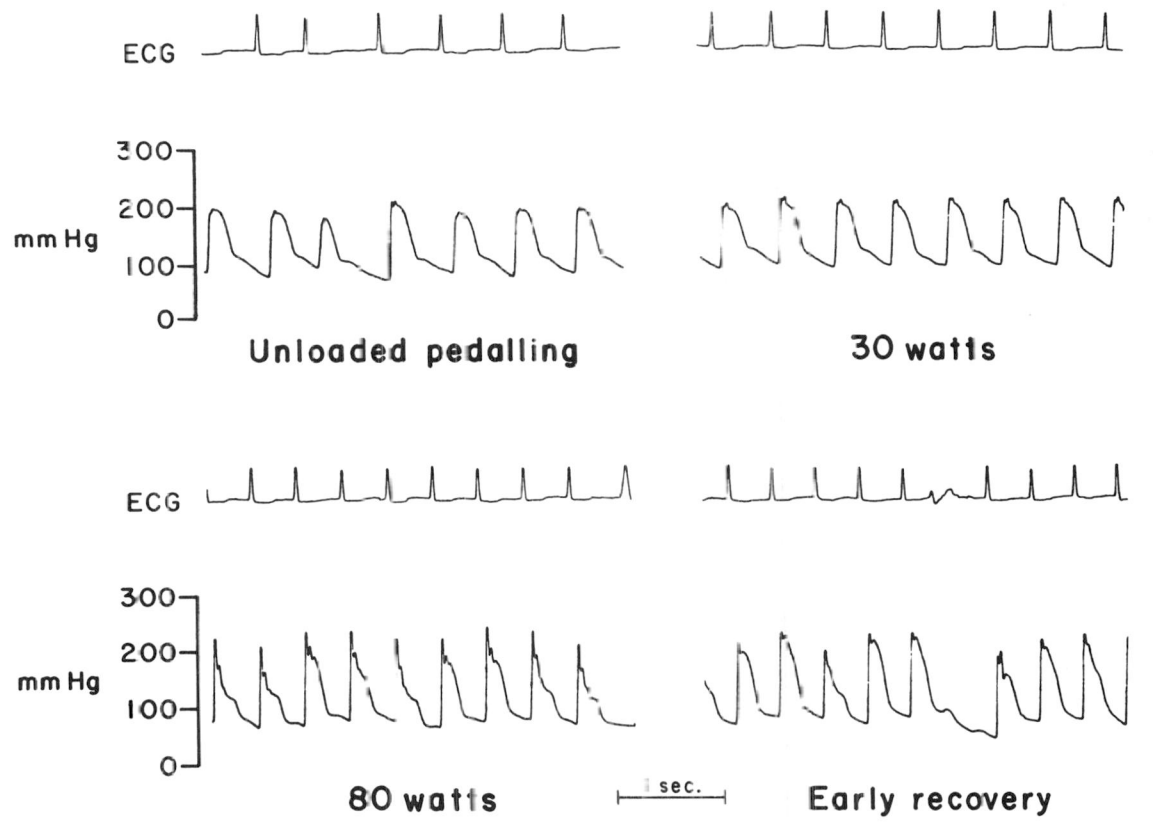

crease with increasing work rate (Table 9.24.2 and panel 2 of Fig. 9.24.1). Therefore, it seems more likely that this patient has a cardiovascular defect. Taking the left sides of branchpoint 5.1, 5.2, and 5.4, we should conclude that this patient has myocardial ischemia or a heart disease which prevents the normal increase in cardiac output with work rate increase, as the cause of the exercise limitation. To support this diagnosis are the observations that the $\dot{V}O_2$ does not rise normally in response to increasing work rate (panel 3, Fig. 9.24.1A), the O_2 pulse is flat (panel 2, Fig. 9.24.1), and heart rate becomes steeper with increasing $\dot{V}O_2$ (panel 5, Fig. 9.24.1). During her more symptomatic test (not shown here), not only was her limitation greater, but her O_2 pulse actually decreased with increasing work rate.

The directly recorded arterial pressures are un-usual and provide a clue to her cardiac diagnosis. The upstrokes in arterial pressure during systole are steep and abruptly stop increasing. Thus, the pressure wave takes on a spike and dome pattern. This pattern becomes more prominent with increasing work rate and remains so during early recovery (Fig. 9.24.2), characteristic of idiopathic hypertrophic cardiomyopathy. Premature ventricular contractions in recovery were followed by heart beats with a reduced, rather than increased, systolic and pulse pressure, a finding also characteristic of this disorder.

Conclusion

Reduced exercise tolerance secondary to hypertrophic cardiomyopathy.

Case 25 Chronic Heart Failure: Before and After Therapy

Clinical Findings

This 64-year-old retired man had recurrent episodic shortness of breath for 11 years, initially diagnosed as "asthma," and hypertension. He had recently been hospitalized repeatedly for congestive heart failure without evidence of prior myocardial infarction or valvular heart disease. He had been a cigarette smoker and was being treated with digoxin, furosemide, hydralazine, KCl, prednisone, ranitidine, occasional albuterol, and diazepam. Examination revealed a heavy-set man without peripheral edema, or abnormal physical findings on examination of the chest. Chest roentgenograms showed cardiomegaly and Kerley B lines; resting ECG showed left atrial enlargement and probable left ventricular hypertrophy. Exercise studies were performed after stabilization and every several weeks during 3 months of a drug study. The patient had progressive improvement; the first and final exercise tests of this period are presented.

Exercise Findings

On both occasions, the patient performed exercise on a cycle ergometer. He pedalled at 60 rpm without an added load for 3 minutes. The work rate was then increased in a ramp fashion 10 W per minute to tolerance. Blood pressure was measured with a sphygmomanometer. On both occasions, the patient was well motivated and cooperative and stopped exercise because of generalized fatigue. The patient had no chest pain, arrhythmia, or abnormal ST-T wave changes.

TABLE 9.25.1. Selected Respiratory Function Data

Measurement	Predicted	Measured
Age, yr		64
Sex		Male
Height, cm		170
Weight, kg	73	82
VC, L	3.65	2.70 (2.80*)
IC, L	2.43	1.92
TLC, L	5.95	4.33
FEV$_1$, L	2.92	2.01 (2.30*)
FEV$_1$/VC, %	80	74
MVV, L/min, indirect	117	80 (92*)
D$_L$CO, ml/mm Hg/min	23.4	22
Hematocrit		44

*After 4 breaths of aerosolized albuterol.

TABLE 9.25.2. Selected Exercise Data

Measurement	Predicted	First Study	Final Study
Peak V̇O$_2$, L/min	2.03	0.91	1.34
Maximum HR, beats/min	156	131	160
Maximum O$_2$ pulse, ml/beat	13.0	7.0	9.0
ΔV̇O$_2$/ΔWR, ml/min/W	10.3	8.0	9.2
AT, L/min	>0.89	0.6	1.0
Blood pressure, mmHg (rest, max ex)		112/95, 139/88	139/88, 204/104
Maximum V̇E, L/min		44	55
Exercise breathing reserve, L/min	>15	36	25

FIGURE 9.25.1.   First study.

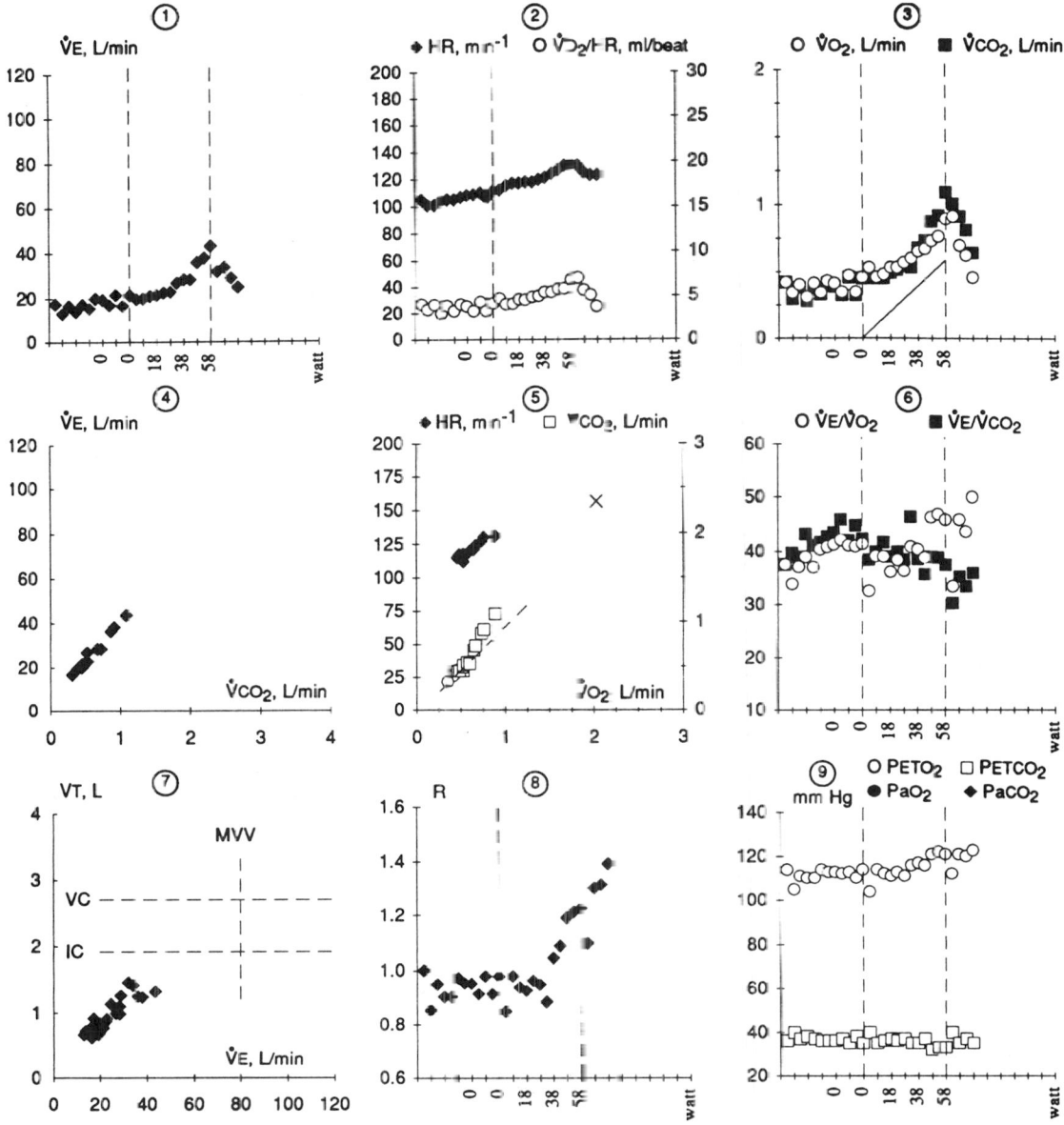

1. Vertical dashed lines in panels 1 to 3 and 6, 8, and 9 indicate the beginning and the end of increasing work period.

2. Unloaded cycling is performed for 3 minutes before the left vertical dashed line.

3. In panel 3, the diagonal line shows the increase of $\dot{V}O_2$ at a slope of 10 ml/min/w.

4. In panel 5, the diagonal dashed line has a slope of 1; the "x" in the upper right is the predicted maximum heart rate and $\dot{V}O_2$ for the subject.

TABLE 9.25.3. First Study

Time min	Work rate watts	BP mmHg	HR min⁻¹	f min⁻¹	V̇E L/min BTPS	V̇CO₂ L/min STPD	V̇O₂ L/min STPD	V̇O₂/HR ml/beat	R	pH	HCO₃⁻ meq/L	PO₂, mmHg ET	a	(A−a)	PCO₂, mmHg ET	a	(a−ET)	V̇E/V̇CO₂	V̇E/V̇O₂	VD/VT
	Rest	112/95	105	19	17.4	0.42	0.42	4.0	1.00			114			36			38	38	
	Rest		101	20	13.2	0.29	0.34	3.4	0.85			105			40			40	34	
	Rest		101	21	16.6	0.38	0.40	4.0	0.95			111			37			39	37	
	Rest		104	19	13.7	0.28	0.31	3.0	0.90			110			38			43	39	
	Rest		105	24	17.2	0.37	0.41	3.9	0.90			110			37			41	37	
	Rest		105	22	15.6	0.33	0.34	3.2	0.97			114			36			42	40	
	Unloaded		107	28	19.9	0.41	0.43	4.0	0.95			113			36			43	41	
	Unloaded		108	29	19.4	0.39	0.41	3.8	0.95			113			36			43	41	
	Unloaded		109	26	16.9	0.32	0.35	3.2	0.91			112			37			46	42	
	Unloaded		110	26	21.5	0.46	0.47	4.3	0.98			113			35			42	41	
	Unloaded		106	27	16.6	0.32	0.35	3.3	0.91			110			38			45	41	
	Unloaded		111	28	21.4	0.45	0.46	4.1	0.98			114			35			42	41	
0.5	3		112	29	19.7	0.45	0.53	4.7	0.85			104			40			38	33	
1.0	8		115	24	20.0	0.45	0.46	4.0	0.98			114			35			40	39	
1.5	13		117	28	21.1	0.45	0.48	4.1	0.94			112			36			42	39	
2.0	18		117	25	21.2	0.49	0.53	4.5	0.92			111			37			39	36	
2.5	23		118	26	22.5	0.51	0.53	4.5	0.96			113			36			40	38	
3.0	28		118	25	22.8	0.54	0.57	4.8	0.95			111			37			38	36	
3.5	33		120	27	26.8	0.53	0.60	5.0	0.88			116			35			46	41	
4.0	38		121	26	28.4	0.68	0.65	5.4	1.05			117			35			39	40	
4.5	43		124	29	28.4	0.73	0.67	5.4	1.09			116			37			36	39	
5.0	48		127	29	36.2	0.87	0.73	5.7	1.19			121			32			39	46	
5.5	53		130	31	38.2	0.92	0.76	5.8	1.21			122			33			39	47	
6.0	58	139/88	131	33	43.5	1.09	0.89	6.8	1.22			121			33			37	46	
	Recovery		130	22	32.1	1.00	0.91	7.0	1.10			112			40			30	33	
	Recovery		125	24	34.0	0.91	0.70	5.6	1.30			121			35			35	46	
	Recovery		123	23	29.0	0.81	0.62	5.0	1.31			120			37			33	44	
	Recovery		123	22	24.8	0.64	0.46	3.7	1.39			123			35			36	50	

Interpretation

Comments

Initial resting respiratory function studies showed respiratory restriction and mild airway obstruction with some response to inhaled albuterol. The resting respiratory function tests were not repeated 3 months later.

Analysis

Referring to flow chart 1 (first study), the patient has a reduced peak V̇O₂ and anaerobic threshold (Table 9.25.2 and Fig. 9.25.1) referring us to flow chart 4. Referring to flow chart 4, the breathing reserve is high (branchpoint 4.1), and the V̇E/V̇CO₂ at AT is also high (branchpoint 4.3), suggesting an abnormal pulmonary circulation. Because the vital

FIGURE 9.25.2.   Final study.

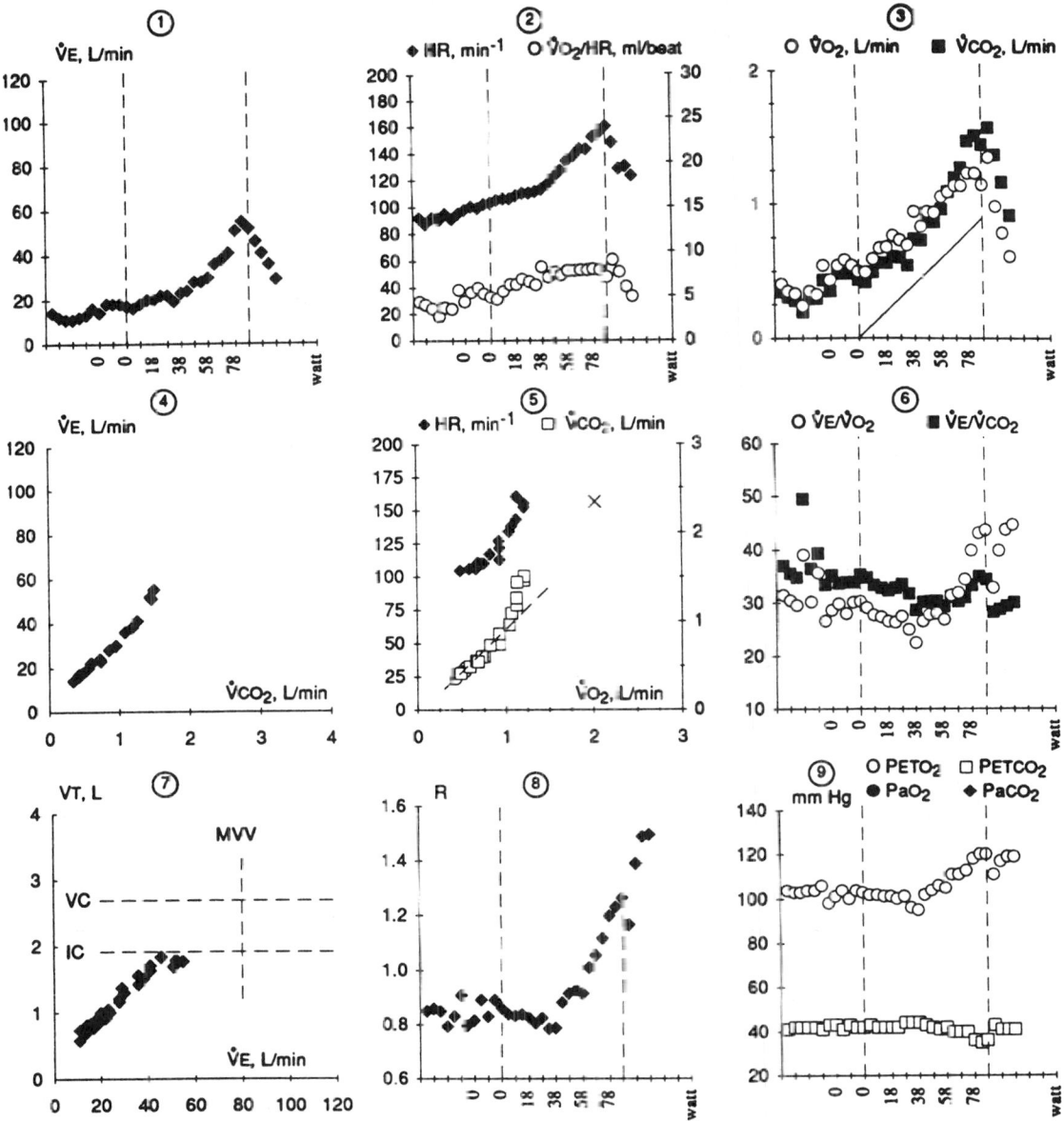

1. Vertical dashed lines in panels 1 to 3 and 6, 8, and 9 indicate the beginning and the end of increasing work period.
2. Unloaded cycling is performed for 3 minutes before the left vertical dashed line.
3. In panel 3, the diagonal line shows the increase of $\dot{V}O_2$ at a slope of 10 ml/min/w.
4. In panel 5, the diagonal dashed line has a slope of 1; the "x" in the upper right is the predicted maximum heart rate and $\dot{V}O_2$ for the subject.

TABLE 9.25.4. Final Study

Time min	Work rate watts	BP mmHg	HR min⁻¹	f min⁻¹	$\dot{V}_E$ L/min BTPS	$\dot{V}_{CO_2}$ L/min STPD	$\dot{V}_{O_2}$ L/min STPD	$\dot{V}_{O_2}$/HR ml/beat	R	pH	HCO₃⁻ meq/L	P_{O_2}, mmHg ET	a	(A − a)	P_{CO_2}, mmHg ET	a	(a − ET)	$\dot{V}_E$/$\dot{V}_{CO_2}$	$\dot{V}_E$/$\dot{V}_{O_2}$	V_D/V_T
	Rest	139/88	92	17	14.0	0.34	0.40	4.3	0.85			104			41			37	31	
	Rest		87	16	12.0	0.30	0.35	4.0	0.86			103			42			35	30	
	Rest		92	15	11.0	0.28	0.33	3.6	0.85			103			42			35	29	
	Rest		90	19	11.0	0.19	0.24	2.7	0.79			104			42			49	39	
	Rest		95	17	12.0	0.29	0.35	3.7	0.83			104			42			36	30	
	Rest		91	19	13.0	0.29	0.32	3.5	0.91			106			41			39	36	
	Unloaded		95	19	16.0	0.43	0.54	5.7	0.80			98			43			33	27	
	Unloaded		98	20	14.0	0.35	0.43	4.4	0.81			101			43			35	29	
	Unloaded		100	22	18.0	0.48	0.54	5.4	0.89			104			41			34	30	
	Unloaded		99	21	18.0	0.48	0.58	5.9	0.83			100			43			34	28	
	Unloaded		102	21	18.0	0.48	0.54	5.3	0.89			104			42			34	30	
	Unloaded		103	22	17.0	0.43	0.50	4.9	0.86			103			42			35	30	
0.5	3		105	21	16.0	0.41	0.49	4.7	0.84			102			43			35	29	
1.0	8		106	20	18.0	0.49	0.59	5.6	0.83			102			42			33	28	
1.5	13		106	20	20.0	0.56	0.67	6.3	0.84			101			42			33	27	
2.0	18		108	23	20.0	0.56	0.68	6.3	0.82			101			42			32	27	
2.5	23		110	24	22.0	0.61	0.76	6.9	0.80			100			42			33	26	
3.0	28		110	23	22.0	0.60	0.73	6.6	0.82			101			44			33	27	
3.5	33		111	22	19.0	0.54	0.69	6.2	0.78			96			44			32	25	
4.0	38		113	22	23.0	0.74	0.94	8.3	0.79			95			44			29	22	
4.5	43		117	24	24.0	0.73	0.83	7.1	0.88			102			43			30	26	
5.0	48		122	24	28.0	0.86	0.94	7.7	0.91			104			42			30	28	
5.5	53		127	23	28.0	0.86	0.93	7.3	0.92			106			41			30	28	
6.0	58		134	23	30.0	0.96	1.05	7.8	0.91			105			42			29	27	
6.5	63		138	25	36.0	1.09	1.08	7.8	1.01			111			40			31	31	
7.0	68		143	25	38.0	1.19	1.13	7.9	1.05			111			40			30	32	
7.5	73		143	25	41.0	1.26	1.13	7.9	1.12			113			40			31	34	
8.0	78		152	30	51.0	1.46	1.22	8.0	1.20			118			36			33	40	
8.5	83		155	31	55.0	1.50	1.22	7.9	1.23			120			35			35	43	
9.0	88	204/104	160	29	52.0	1.44	1.14	7.1	1.26			120			36			34	43	
	Recovery		148	25	46.0	1.56	1.34	9.1	1.16			111			43			28	33	
	Recovery		128	24	41.0	1.36	0.98	7.7	1.39			117			41			29	40	
	Recovery		130	23	36.0	1.16	0.78	6.0	1.49			119			41			29	44	
	Recovery		123	21	29.0	0.91	0.61	5.0	1.49			119			41			30	45	

capacity is low (branchpoint 4.5), we are directed to consider moderate to severe left ventricular failure. The patient has physiologic features of this problem including low O_2 pulse and low $\Delta\dot{V}_{O_2}/\Delta WR$. The reduced and slowly increasing O_2 pulse during exercise and the increase when exercise stopped are consistent with left ventricular dysfunction.

Three months after treatment including afterload reduction (Table 9.25.4 and Fig. 9.25.2), the maximum work rate, peak $\dot{V}_{O_2}$, maximum O_2 pulse, an- aerobic threshold, and $\Delta\dot{V}_{O_2}/\Delta WR$ findings are considerably improved.

Conclusion

This study is presented to show the findings of severe left ventricular dysfunction, as may be seen with cardiomyopathy of any cause, and the improvement in the functional abnormalities with effective therapy.

Case 26 Cardiomyopathy with Oscillatory Function

Clinical Findings

This 35-year-old former truck driver with idiopathic cardiomyopathy underwent exercise testing as part of his evaluation for a study using new pharmaceutical agents. He had developed loss of energy and shortness of breath over the past 3 years and had been hospitalized twice for "pneumonia." He used alcohol occasionally but denied use of tobacco or other oral or intravenous drugs. He had no history of angina, hypertension, rheumatic fever, or edema. An endocardial biopsy 2 years previously was non-diagnostic. The patient was taking 40 mg furosemide, 0.25 mg digoxin, and 60 mg isosorbide daily. Resting heart rate was 104 and blood pressure 122/86. On physical examination there was cardicmegaly, an audible S-3, and fine basilar rales, but no peripheral edema. Chest roentgenograms were normal except for left ventricular enlargement. Resting ECG revealed sinus rhythm, left ventricular hypertrophy, and diffuse ST-T wave depression, more marked in the anterolateral leads.

Exercise Findings

The patient performed exercise on a cycle ergometer. After 2 minutes of rest, he pedalled at 60 rpm without added load for 3 minutes. The work rate was then increased in ramp pattern 15 W per minute

to his symptom-limited maximum. Arm blood pressure was measured with a sphygmomanometer. Exercise was stopped because of lightheadedness. No further ECG abnormalities were noted.

TABLE 9.26.1. Selected Respiratory Function Data

Measurement	Predicted	Measured
Age, yr		35
Sex		Male
Height, cm		178
Weight, kg	80	82
Hematocrit, %		45
VC, L	5.23	4.72
IC, L	3.47	3.10
FEV$_1$, L	4.29	3.78
FEV$_1$/VC, %	82	80
MVV, L/min	172	148

TABLE 9.26.2. Selected Exercise Data

Measurement	Predicted	Measured
Peak $\dot{V}O_2$, L/min	3.02	1.71
Maximum HR, beats/min	185	157
Maximum O$_2$ pulse, ml/beat	16.3	10.9
$\Delta\dot{V}O_2$/ΔWR, ml/min/W	10.3	10.8
AT, L/min	>1.27	1.0
Maximum $\dot{V}E$, L/min		81
Exercise breathing reserve, L/min	>15	67

FIGURE 9.26.1.

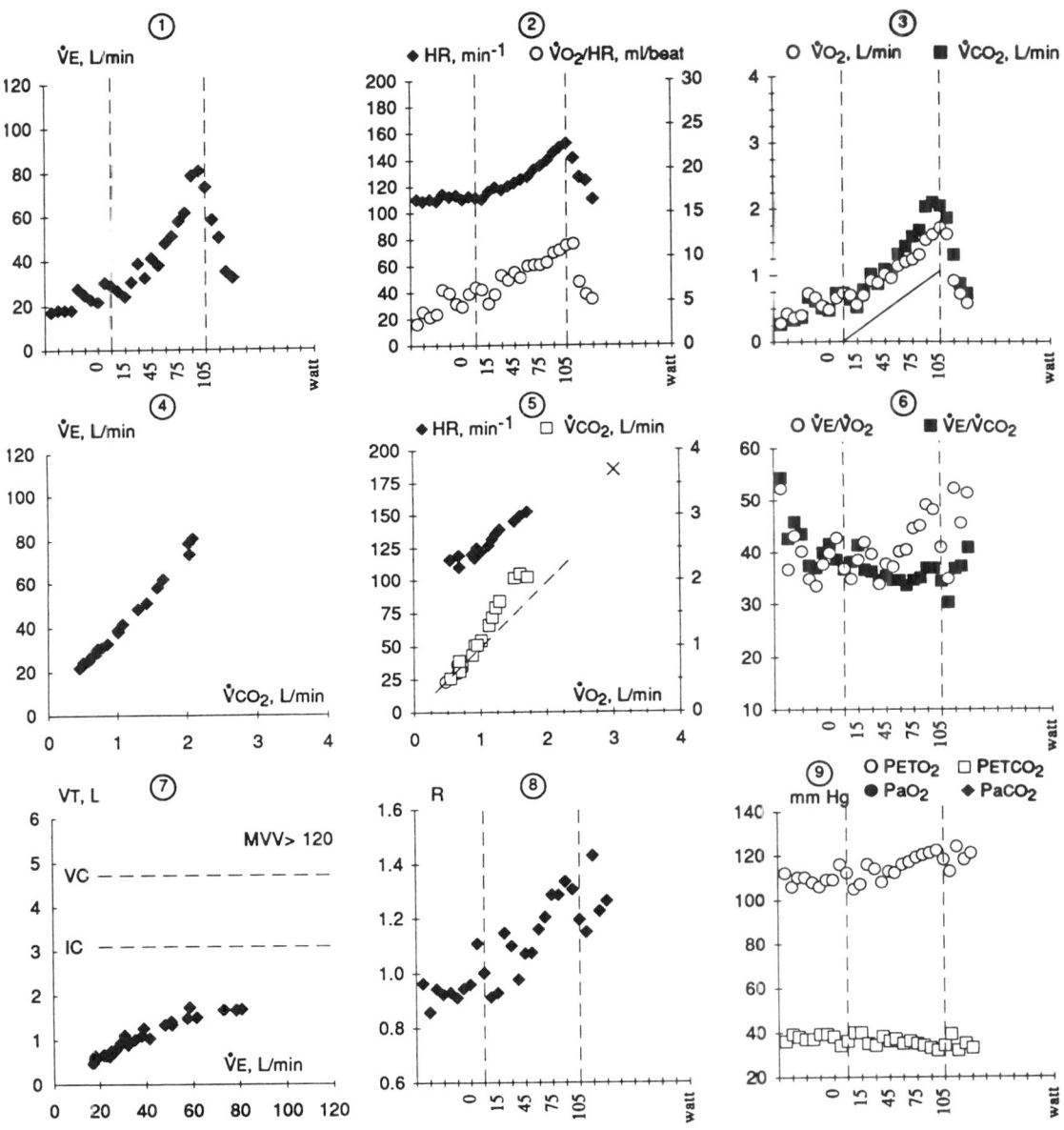

1. Vertical dashed lines in panels 1 to 3 and 6, 8, and 9 indicate the beginning and the end of increasing work period.
2. Unloaded cycling is performed for 3 minutes before the left vertical dashed line.
3. In panel 3, the diagonal line shows the increase of $\dot{V}O_2$ at a slope of 10 ml/min/w.
4. In panel 5, the diagonal dashed line has a slope of 1; the "x" in the upper right is the predicted maximum heart rate and $\dot{V}O_2$ for the subject.

TABLE 9.26.3. Air Breathing

Time min	Work rate watts	BP mmHg	HR min⁻¹	f min⁻¹	$\dot{V}_E$ L/min BTPS	$\dot{V}_{CO_2}$ L/min STPD	$\dot{V}_{O_2}$ L/min STPD	$\dot{V}_{O_2}$/HR ml/beat	R	pH	HCO₃ meq/L	P$_{O_2}$, mmHg ET	a	(A − a)	P$_{CO_2}$, mmHg ET	a	(a − ET)	$\dot{V}_E$/$\dot{V}_{CO_2}$	$\dot{V}_E$/$\dot{V}_{O_2}$	V$_D$/V$_T$
	Rest	119/81																		
	Rest		110	36	17.2	0.26	0.27	2.5	0.96			112			36			54	52	
	Rest		109	30	17.9	0.36	0.42	3.9	0.86			106			39			43	37	
	Rest		110	33	17.9	0.33	0.35	3.2	0.94			110			38			46	43	
	Rest		109	28	18.0	0.36	0.39	3.6	0.92			110			37			43	40	
	Unloaded		114	33	27.8	0.67	0.72	6.3	0.93			108			37			37	35	
	Unloaded		112	33	24.9	0.60	0.66	5.9	0.91			106			39			37	33	
	Unloaded		113	34	22.8	0.50	0.53	4.7	0.94			109			39			40	38	
	Unloaded		110	32	21.8	0.46	0.48	4.4	0.96			109			38			41	40	
	Unloaded		112	31	30.3	0.72	0.65	5.8	1.11			113			34			38	43	
	Unloaded		111	31	29.0	0.72	0.72	6.5	1.00			112			36			37	37	
0.5	7.5	122/87	110	35	26.9	0.63	0.69	6.3	0.91			105			40			38	35	
1.0	15		116	38	24.3	0.61	0.55	4.7	0.93			107			40			41	38	
1.5	22.5		119	28	30.8	0.78	0.68	5.7	1.15			116			35			36	42	
2.0	30		117	31	39.0	1.01	0.92	7.9	1.10			114			34			36	40	
2.5	37.5	140/92	120	34	32.5	0.86	0.88	7.3	0.98			108			38			34	34	
3.0	45		122	40	41.4	1.08	1.01	8.3	1.07			113			36			35	38	
3.5	52.5		125	35	38.1	1.02	0.95	7.6	1.07			112			37			34	37	
4.0	60		127	36	48.2	1.31	1.13	8.9	1.13			116			35			34	40	
4.5	67	154/85	132	38	51.1	1.43	1.19	9.0	1.20			117			36			33	40	
5.0	75		135	39	57.8	1.53	1.23	9.1	1.28			119			35			34	44	
5.5	82		190	41	61.8	1.67	1.30	9.4	1.28			120			34			35	45	
6.0	90		145	47	78.7	2.03	1.52	10.5	1.34			121			33			37	49	
6.5	97	156/87	149	48	80.9	2.09	1.60	10.7	1.31			122			32			37	48	
7.0	105		152	44	73.4	2.04	1.71	11.3	1.19			118			34			34	41	
	Recovery	144/83	141	34	58.7	1.85	1.61	11.4	1.15			113			39			30	35	
	Recovery		127	36	50.7	1.30	0.91	7.2	1.43			124			32			37	52	
	Recovery		124	35	35.2	0.87	0.71	5.7	1.23			118			35			37	45	
	Recovery		110	36	32.3	0.72	0.57	5.2	1.26			121			33			41	51	
		137/85																			

Interpretation

Comments

This patient has an idiopathic cardiomyopathy, New York Heart Association Class II. Respiratory function is normal. An oscillatory pattern of change in $\dot{V}_{O_2}$, $\dot{V}_{CO_2}$, and $\dot{V}_E$ is seen during exercise testing in some patients with cardiomyopathy and is well illustrated in this patient in Figure 9.26.2, which uses an 8-second rolling average of the breath-by-breath values.

Analysis

Referring to flow chart 1, the peak $\dot{V}_{O_2}$ and anaerobic threshold are reduced (Table 9.26.2). Go to flow chart 4. The breathing reserve is normal (branch-point 4.1), whereas the ventilatory equivalents are high at the anaerobic threshold (branchpoint 4.3). The rightward direction takes us to the diagnostic box "abnormal pulmonary circulation." The vital capacity is low normal (branchpoint 4.5). We do not have blood gases to help distinguish between moderate to severe left ventricular function (right branch) and pulmonary vascular disease (left branch), but the periodic (oscillatory) breathing pattern brought out during low level exercise makes the former more likely. A number of studies have described an increase in V$_D$/V$_T$ and an increased ventilatory requirement depending on the severity of left ventricular failure. The phenomenon and possible mechanism is addressed by Wasserman et al (1).

Finally, we should consider in this analysis the most striking finding, i.e., the oscillatory pattern of the $\dot{V}_{O_2}$, $\dot{V}_{CO_2}$ depicted in Figure 9.26.2, and the

FIGURE 9.26.2.   Tracings of $\dot{V}O_2$ (left) and $\dot{V}CO_2$ (right) using an 8-second rolling average of breath-by-breath data during 2 minutes of rest, 3 minutes of unloaded pedalling, 7 minutes of ramp (incremental) exercise, and 2 minutes of recovery. The vertical dashed lines indicate the onset and end of exercise. Although oscillations can be seen throughout this 14-minute period, they are most marked during mild and moderate exercise. It is thought that the increased catecholamine response that occurs with heavy exercise obliterates the changing vasomotor tone from the central nervous system (Traube-Hering's waves in blood pressure) (1). When the data are plotted with less temporal resolution, i.e., every half minute, the oscillations become indistinct.

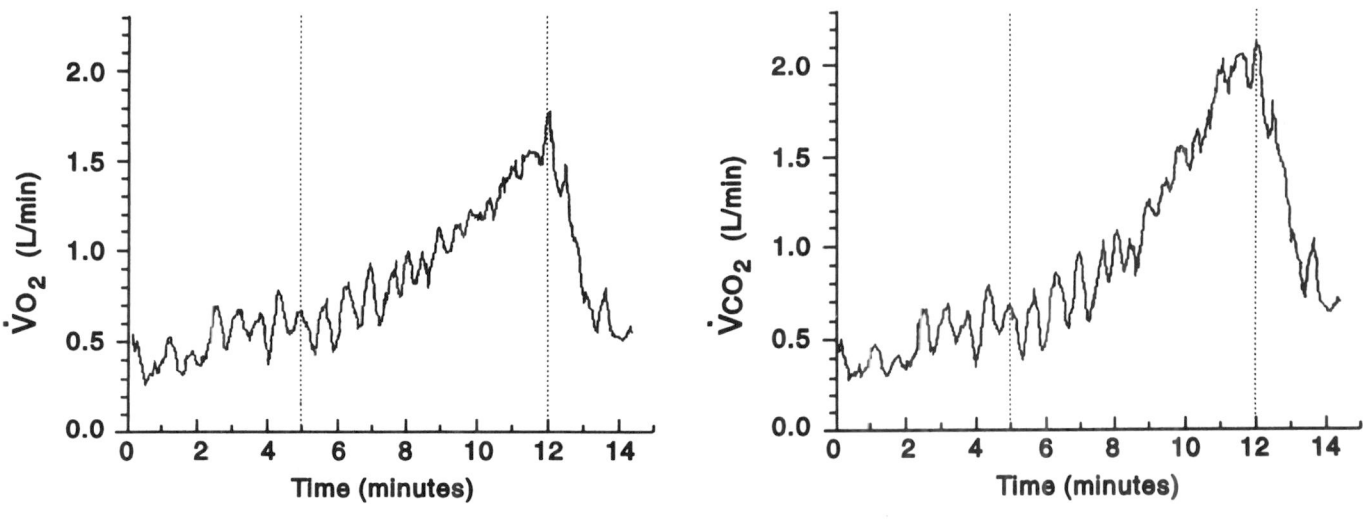

accompanying oscillatory pattern of $\dot{V}E$ and R, which are not displayed here. The oscillations have a period of about 40 seconds from peak to peak and are greatest for mild to moderate exercise. This phenomenon is typical for some patients with congestive heart failure and appears to be from cyclic changes in cardiac output rather than secondary to cyclic changes in ventilation (2).

Conclusion

This patient is presented to illustrate the oscillatory pattern in O_2 uptake and other accompanying pa-

rameters that frequently occur in patients with congestive heart failure, especially during mild to moderate exercise.

Reference

1. Wasserman K, Zhang Y-Y, Gitt A, et al. Lung function and exercise gas exchange in chronic heart failure. Circulation 1997; 96:2221–2227.
2. Ben-Dov I, Sietsema KE, Casaburi R, et al. Evidence that circulatory oscillations accompany ventilatory oscillations during exercise in patients with heart failure. Am Rev Respir Dis 1992; 145:776–781.

Case 27 Mitral Insufficiency
Clinical Findings

This 43-year-old female electronics assembler had rheumatic fever at age 10. In the last 6 months she developed increasing dyspnea and orthopnea, with intermittent atrial fibrillation and pleural effusion, requiring repeated hospitalizations. There was no evidence of mitral stenosis or coronary artery disease on catheterization, angiography, or echocardiography. At the time of exercise study, she had a sinus rhythm, findings of mitral regurgitation with left atrial and left ventricular enlargement, but no pleural effusion or dependent edema. Her medications were digoxin, furosemide, and potassium chloride.

Exercise Findings

The patient performed exercise on a cycle ergometer. She pedalled at 60 rpm without added load for 3 minutes. The work rate was then increased 5 W per minute to her symptom-limited maximum. She stopped cycling because of general fatigue. There were no ST segment changes or arrhythmia.

TABLE 9.27.1. Selected Respiratory Function Data

Measurement	Predicted	Measured
Age, yr		43
Sex		Female
Height, cm		160
Weight, kg	61	56
Hematocrit, %		40
VC, L	2.88	2.03
IC, L	1.92	1.49
TLC, L	4.33	3.32
FEV$_1$, L	2.36	1.81
FEV$_1$/VC, %	82	89
MVV, L/min	90	90
D$_L$CO, ml/mm Hg/min	21.7	23.5

TABLE 9.27.2. Selected Exercise Data

Measurement	Predicted	Measured
Peak V̇o$_2$, L/min	1.57	0.79
Maximum HR, beats/min	177	186
Maximum O$_2$ pulse, ml/beat	8.9	4.2
ΔV̇o$_2$/ΔWR, ml/min/W	10.3	5.6
AT, L/min	>0.74	0.65
Maximum V̇E, L/min		31
Exercise breathing reserve, L/min	>15	59

Figure 9.27.1.

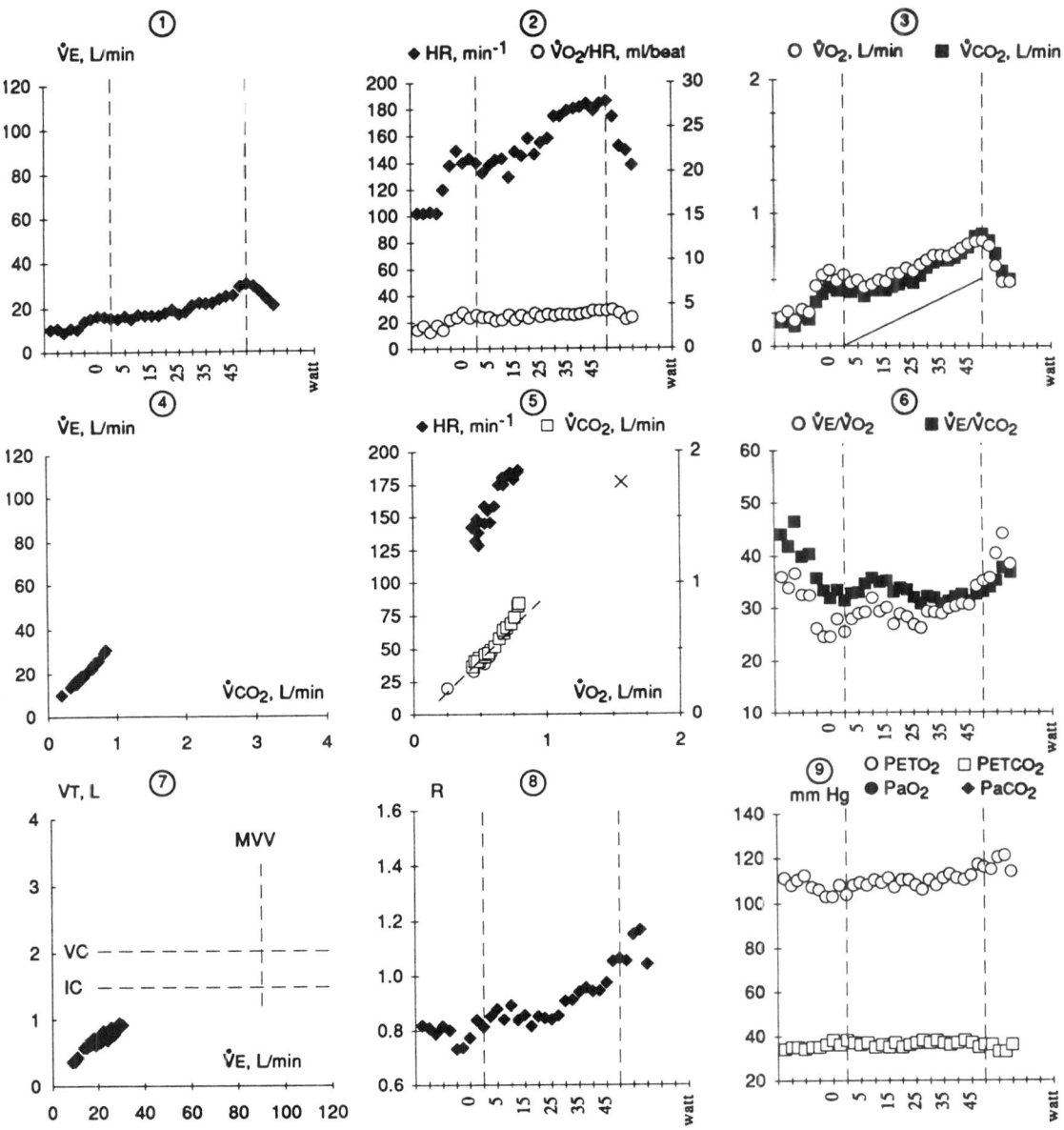

1. Vertical dashed lines in panels 1 to 3 and 6, 8, and 9 indicate the beginning and the end of increasing work period.

2. Unloaded cycling is performed for 3 minutes before the left vertical dashed line.

3. In panel 3, the diagonal line shows the increase of $\dot{V}O_2$ at a slope of 10 ml/min/w.

4. In panel 5, the diagonal dashed line has a slope of 1; the "x" in the upper right is the predicted maximum heart rate and $\dot{V}O_2$ for the subject.

TABLE 9.27.3. Air Breathing

Time min	Work rate watts	BP mmHg	HR min⁻¹	f min⁻¹	$\dot{V}_E$ L/min BTPS	$\dot{V}_{CO_2}$ L/min STPD	$\dot{V}_{O_2}$ L/min STPD	$\dfrac{\dot{V}_{O_2}}{HR}$ ml/beat	R	pH	HCO₃ meq/L	P_{O_2}, mmHg ET	a	(A − a)	P_{CO_2}, mmHg ET	a	(a − ET)	$\dfrac{\dot{V}_E}{\dot{V}_{CO_2}}$	$\dfrac{\dot{V}_E}{\dot{V}_{O_2}}$	$\dfrac{V_D}{V_T}$
	Rest		102	27	10.2	0.18	0.22	2.2	0.82			111			34			44	36	
	Rest		102	26	11.0	0.21	0.26	2.5	0.81			108			35			42	34	
	Rest		103	24	9.0	0.15	0.19	1.8	0.79			110			35			46	37	
	Rest		102	25	10.9	0.22	0.27	2.6	0.81			112			34			40	33	
	Unloaded		120	25	10.2	0.20	0.25	2.1	0.80			107			35			40	32	
	Unloaded		138	24	13.8	0.33	0.45	3.3	0.73			106			35			36	26	
	Unloaded		149	25	15.1	0.39	0.53	3.6	0.74			103			36			33	24	
	Unloaded		140	26	16.2	0.44	0.57	4.1	0.77			103			38			32	25	
	Unloaded		143	26	15.9	0.41	0.49	3.4	0.84			108			36			33	28	
	Unloaded		140	24	15.5	0.43	0.53	3.8	0.81			104			38			31	25	
0.5	5		132	25	15.2	0.40	0.47	3.6	0.85			108			37			33	28	
1.0	5		138	26	16.4	0.43	0.49	3.6	0.83			109			36			33	29	
1.5	10		142	26	15.0	0.37	0.44	3.1	0.84			108			37			35	29	
2.0	10		143	27	16.9	0.41	0.46	3.2	0.89			110			35			36	32	
2.5	15		129	27	16.6	0.41	0.49	3.8	0.84			109			36			35	29	
3.0	15		148	26	16.6	0.41	0.48	3.2	0.85			111			35			35	30	
3.5	20		145	26	16.7	0.44	0.54	3.7	0.81			107			37			33	27	
4.0	20		158	27	17.8	0.43	0.54	3.4	0.85			110			35			34	29	
4.5	25		146	31	19.0	0.43	0.58	4.0	0.84			110			36			33	28	
5.0	25		155	25	17.1	0.47	0.56	3.6	0.84			108			37			32	27	
5.5	30		158	25	18.1	0.52	0.61	3.9	0.85			106			38			31	26	
6.0	30		175	28	21.0	0.58	0.64	3.7	0.91			110			37			32	29	
6.5	35		175	29	22.2	0.62	0.68	3.9	0.91			108			38			32	29	
7.0	35		179	27	21.9	0.64	0.68	3.8	0.94			111			37			31	29	
7.5	40		180	27	22.3	0.64	0.67	3.7	0.96			113			36			31	30	
8.0	40		181	30	23.7	0.66	0.70	3.9	0.94			111			37			32	30	
8.5	45		184	30	24.9	0.69	0.73	4.0	0.95			110			38			32	31	
9.0	45		179	29	25.6	0.74	0.76	4.2	0.97			112			37			31	30	
9.5	50		184	31	29.2	0.82	0.78	4.2	1.05			117			35			32	34	
10.0	50		186	33	30.5	0.84	0.79	4.2	1.06			113			36			33	35	
	Recovery		174	33	29.6	0.79	0.75	4.3	1.05			115			36			34	36	
	Recovery		152	35	27.2	0.69	0.60	3.9	1.15			120			33			35	40	
	Recovery		149	35	24.1	0.56	0.48	3.2	1.17			121			33			38	44	
	Recovery		138	32	21.1	0.50	0.48	3.5	1.04			114			36			37	38	

Interpretation

Comments

Respiratory function at rest is compatible with a restrictive defect but the diffusing capacity (D_LCO) is normal (Table 9.27.1).

Analysis

Referring to flow chart 1, the peak $\dot{V}_{O_2}$ and anaerobic threshold are low (Table 9.27.2). See flow chart 4. The breathing reserve is high (branchpoint 4.1). The ventilatory equivalent for CO_2 is slightly elevated at the anaerobic threshold (branchpoint 4.3). Therefore we are led to consider an abnormal pulmonary circulation. The vital capacity is reduced (branchpoint 4.5) leading us to the diagnosis of left ventricular failure, undoubtedly due to the valvular heart disease. The striking finding is the low and flat O_2 pulse throughout exercise (panel 2, Fig. 9 27.1) and

steep heart rate-$\dot{V}_{O_2}$ relationship (panel 5, Fig. 9.27.1), low heart rate reserve and low $\Delta\dot{V}_{O_2}/\Delta WR$, all findings confirming the diagnosis of heart disease. The low and unchanging O_2 pulse suggests that the patient's effective stroke volume is very low and the arterial-mixed venous O_2 difference is maximized at a low work rate. Note that if the $\dot{V}_E/\dot{V}_{CO_2}$ at the AT were normal (branchpoint 4.3) we would have been led to the same diagnosis of heart disease through branchpoint 4.6. The difference reflects on the extent to which the pulmonary circulation has been affected by the left-sided heart failure.

Conclusion

Valvular heart disease, as suggested by the patient's history, has caused marked exercise intolerance because of an inadequate cardiac output response to exercise (heart failure).

Case 28 Mitral Stenosis: Pre- and Post-β-adrenergic Blockade

Clinical Findings

This 57-year-old former receptionist had had rheumatic fever at age 16. She had had orthopnea during pregnancy at age 24. She was otherwise well except for gradually increasing dyspnea of 6 years' duration and exertional dull substernal aching radiating to the jaw and left arm of 3 months' duration. Examination revealed a grade II pre-systolic murmur and an opening snap. The mitral valve area was mildly decreased and the left atrium was moderately dilated. Coronary arteriography was normal. The second exercise study was performed 17 months after the first while the patient was receiving propranolol 3 times daily. At that time she complained of increasing dyspnea, even at rest, associated with light-headedness, sweating, numbness of the fingers, and perioral tingling.

Exercise Findings

On both occasions the patient exercised on a cycle ergometer to her symptom-limited maximum. She pedalled at 60 rpm without added load for 3 minutes. During the first test the work rate was increased 10 W per minute, and during the second test (17 months later), it was increased 5 W per minute. Arterial blood was sampled every second minute, and intra-arterial blood pressure was recorded from a percutaneously placed brachial artery catheter. Resting ECGs showed left atrial enlargement and sinus rhythm; there were no abnormal ST segment changes, nor arrhythmia during exercise. She stopped exercise in both studies complaining of leg fatigue, not dyspnea or chest pain.

TABLE 9.28.1. Selected Respiratory Function Data

Measurement	Predicted	Before Blockade	After Blockade
Age, yr		57	59
Sex		Female	
Height, cm		166	
Weight, kg	65	67	
Hematocrit, %		40	
Vc, L	3.10	3.16	2.73
IC, L	2.07	2.26	2.19
TLC, L	5.15	5.01	4.62
FEV$_1$, L	2.48	2.58	2.26
FEV$_1$/Vc, %	80	82	83
MVV, L/min	93	96	81
D$_L$CO, ml/mmHg/min	21.9	20.3	18.7

TABLE 9.28.2. Selected Exercise Data

Measurement	Predicted	Before Blockade	After Blockade
Peak $\dot{V}O_2$, L/min	1.42	0.74	0.91
Maximum HR, beats/min	162	120	108
Maximum O$_2$ pulse, ml/beat	8.7	6.2	8.4
$\Delta\dot{V}O_2/\Delta WR$, ml/min/W	10.3	Indeterminate	7.4
AT, L/min	>0.70	Indeterminate	Indeterminate
Blood pressure, mmHg (rest, max)		128/62, 164/83	153/72, 168/78
Maximum $\dot{V}E$, L/min		43	47
Exercise breathing reserve, L/min	>15	53	34
PaO$_2$, mmHg (rest, max ex)		97, 125	87, 122
P(A − a)O$_2$, mmHg (rest, max ex)		10, 2	11, 5
P(a − ET)CO$_2$, mmHg (rest, max ex)		0, −1	3, −1
VD/VT (rest, heavy ex)		0.26, 0.25	0.28, 0.19
HCO$_3^-$, mEq/L (rest, 2-min recov)		24, 18	24, 18

FIGURE 9.28.1.   Pre-β-adrenergic blockade.

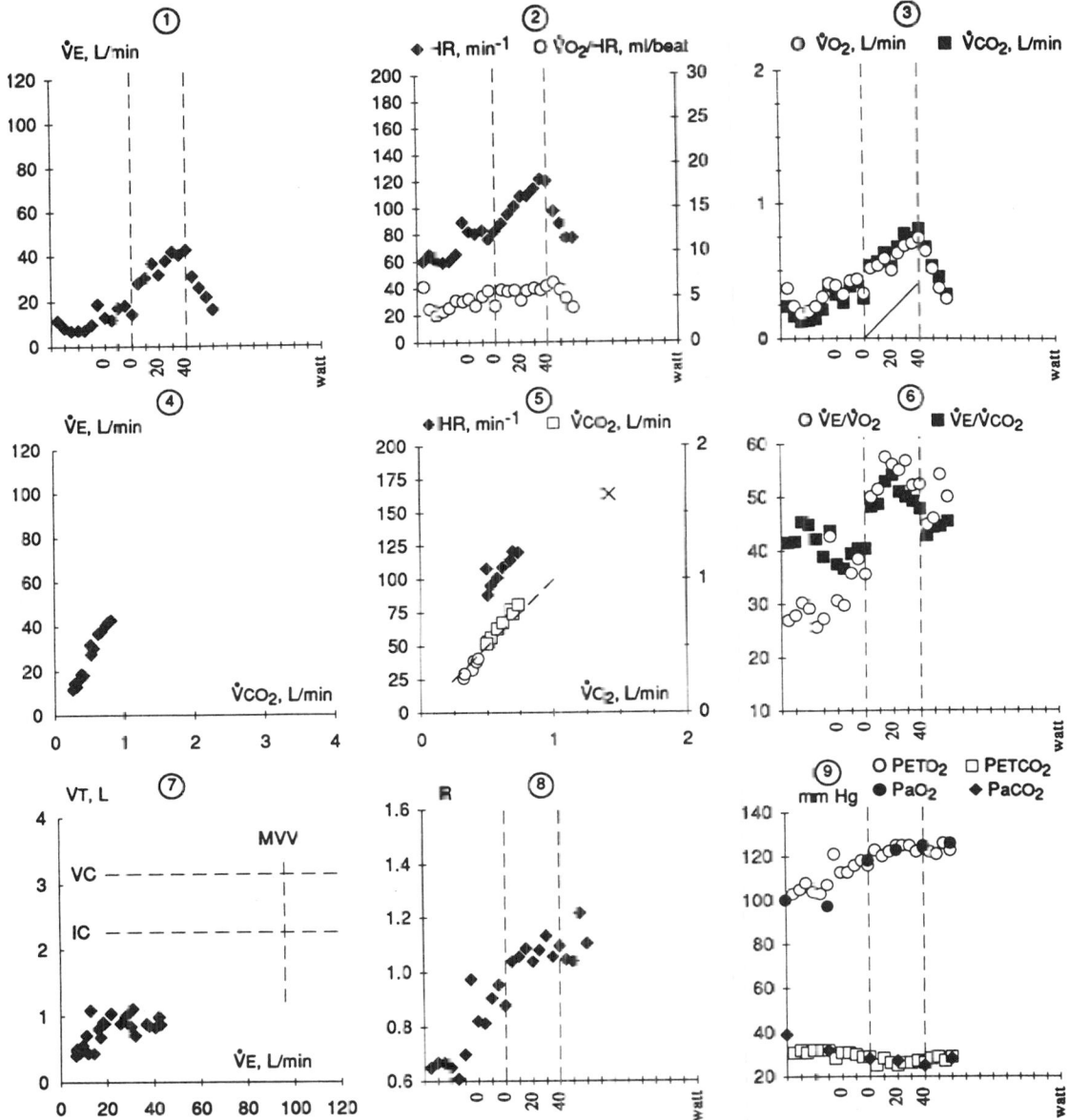

1. Vertical dashed lines in panels 1 to 3 and 6, 8, and 9 indicate the beginning and the end of increasing work period.

2. Unloaded cycling is performed for 3 minutes before the left vertical dashed line.

3. In panel 3, the diagonal line shows the increase of $\dot{V}C_2$ at a slope of 10 ml/min/w.

4. In panel 5, the diagonal dashed line has a slope of 1; the "≃" in the upper right is the predicted maximum heart rate and $\dot{V}O_2$ for the subject.

TABLE 9.28.3. Pre-β-adrenergic Blockade

Time min	Work rate watts	BP mmHg	HR min⁻¹	f min⁻¹	V̇E L/min BTPS	V̇CO₂ L/min STPD	V̇O₂ L/min STPD	V̇O₂/HR ml/beat	R	pH	HCO₃ meq/L	PO₂ ET	PO₂ a	PO₂ (A-a)	PCO₂ ET	PCO₂ a	PCO₂ (a-ET)	V̇E/V̇CO₂	V̇E/V̇O₂	VD/VT
	Rest	128/62								7.40	24		100			39				
	Rest		60	16	11.3	0.24	0.37	6.2	0.65			103			31			41	27	
	Rest		65	18	8.2	0.16	0.24	3.7	0.67			105			32			42	28	
	Rest		60	17	6.9	0.12	0.18	3.0	0.67			108			31			45	30	
	Rest		59	15	7.1	0.13	0.20	3.4	0.65			104			32			45	29	
	Rest		60	14	7.1	0.14	0.23	3.8	0.61			103			32			42	26	
	Rest	140/77	65	17	9.6	0.21	0.30	4.6	0.70	7.43	21	107	97	10	32	32	0	39	27	0.26
	Unloaded		89	21	18.8	0.39	0.40	4.5	0.98			121			28			44	43	
	Unloaded		82	12	13.0	0.32	0.39	4.8	0.82			113			31			37	31	
	Unloaded		80	27	11.8	0.26	0.32	4.0	0.81			113			31			37	30	
	Unloaded		83	25	17.1	0.38	0.42	5.1	0.90			116			30			39	36	
	Unloaded		76	20	18.2	0.41	0.43	5.7	0.95			118			29			40	38	
	Unloaded	146/80	82	33	14.5	0.29	0.33	4.0	0.88	7.47	20	116	118	1	29	28	-1	40	35	0.19
0.5	10		88	28	27.9	0.53	0.51	5.8	1.04			123			25			48	50	
1.0	10		95	36	30.3	0.56	0.53	5.6	1.06			120			28			49	51	
1.5	20		101	42	36.9	0.63	0.58	5.7	1.09			122			26			53	57	
2.0	20	152/80	108	45	31.9	0.52	0.50	4.6	1.04	7.50	21	125	123	1	25	27	2	54	56	0.36
2.5	30		109	44	37.8	0.67	0.62	5.7	1.08			125			26			51	55	
3.0	30		114	43	42.2	0.77	0.68	6.0	1.13			125			26			50	57	
3.5	40		121	49	40.6	0.74	0.70	5.8	1.06			122			27			49	52	
4.0	40	164/83	120	49	42.9	0.81	0.74	6.2	1.09	7.49	19	124	125	2	26	25	-1	48	52	0.25
	Recovery		97	28	31.0	0.67	0.64	6.6	1.05			122			28			43	45	
	Recovery		88	29	25.9	0.53	0.51	5.8	1.04			121			29			44	46	
	Recovery		77	21	21.8	0.45	0.37	4.8	1.22			126			27			44	54	
	Recovery	149/71	77	20	16.2	0.32	0.29	3.8	1.10	7.42	18	123	126	-2	29	28	-1	45	50	0.29

Interpretation

Comments

Resting pulmonary function is normal on both occasions of study (Table 9.28.1). The ECG is normal except for evidence of left atrial enlargement. This case is presented because it illustrates the abnormalities of mitral stenosis and changes in O_2 pulse with propranolol. Moreover, it is presented because the development of respiratory alkalosis during exercise is unusual.

Analysis

During exercise, the peak $\dot{V}O_2$ is decreased and the anaerobic threshold is indeterminate (Table 9.28.2).

See flow chart 5. The indices of distribution of ventilation relative to perfusion are normal at maximum exercise, making lung disease and pulmonary vascular disease unlikely diagnoses (branchpoint 5.1). The heart rate reserve was high in the pre-β-adrenergic blocked state leading us to branchpoint 5.5. We only had enough data to calculate $\Delta\dot{V}O_2/\Delta WR$ from the post-β-adrenergic blocked state and it was low, taking us to branchpoint 5.8. The arterial pressure response to exercise was not high leading us to the diagnosis of left ventricular failure. Consistent with heart disease as the primary diagnosis is the low O_2 pulse that fails to rise as the work rate increases.

Commonly, an anticipatory respiratory alkalosis occurs at rest, but disappears with the start of exer-

FIGURE 9.28.2.   Post-β-adrenergic blockade.

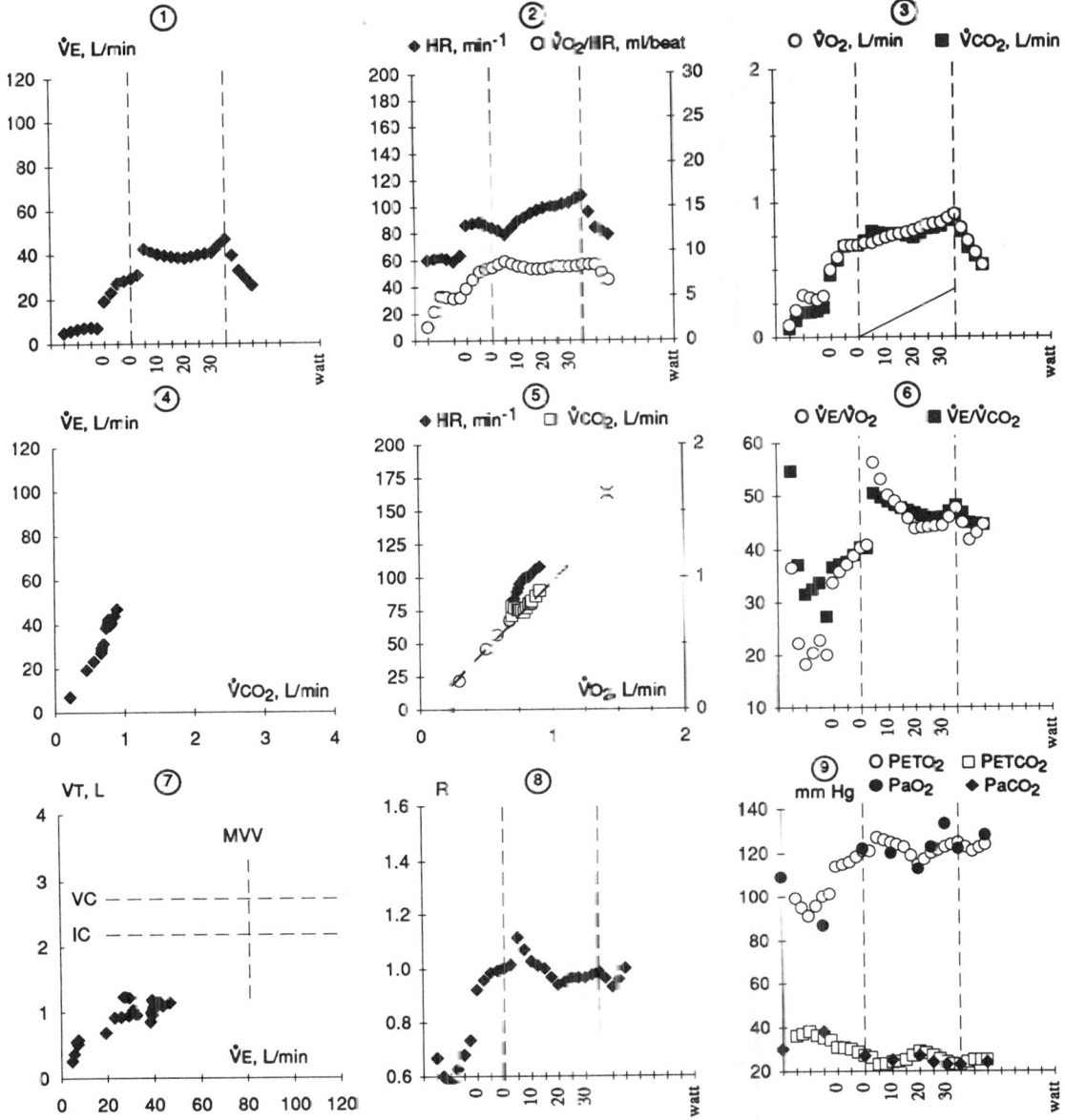

1. Vertical dashed lines in panels 1 to 3 and 6, 8 and 9 indicate the beginning and the end of increasing work period.

2. Unloaded cycling is performed for 3 minutes before the left vertical dashed line.

3. In panel 3, the diagonal line shows the increase of $\dot{V}O_2$ at a slope of 10 ml/min/w.

4. In panel 5, the diagonal dashed line has a slope of 1; the "x" in the upper right is the predicted maximum heart rate and $\dot{V}O_2$ for the subject.

TABLE 9.28.4. Post-β-adrenergic Blockade

Time min	Work rate watts	BP mmHg	HR min⁻¹	f min⁻¹	$\dot{V}_E$ L/min BTPS	$\dot{V}_{CO_2}$ L/min STPD	$\dot{V}_{O_2}$ L/min STPD	$\dot{V}_{O_2}$/HR ml/beat	R	pH	HCO_3^- meq/L	P_{O_2} ET	P_{O_2} a	P_{O_2} (A−a)	P_{CO_2} ET	P_{CO_2} a	P_{CO_2} (a−ET)	$\dot{V}_E/\dot{V}_{CO_2}$	$\dot{V}_E/\dot{V}_{O_2}$	V_D/V_T
	Rest	153/72								7.48	22		109			30				
	Rest																			
	Rest		60	19	4.9	0.06	0.09	1.5	0.67			99			36			55	37	
	Rest		61	16	5.8	0.12	0.20	3.3	0.60			95			37			37	22	
	Rest		62	12	6.7	0.18	0.31	5.0	0.58			91			38			32	18	
	Rest		61	13	7.1	0.19	0.30	4.8	0.63			96			37			32	20	
	Rest	159/72	59	13	7.5	0.19	0.28	4.7	0.68	7.41	24	100	87	11	35	38	3	34	23	0.28
	Unloaded		63	14	7.2	0.22	0.30	4.8	0.73			101			34			27	20	
	Unloaded		86	28	19.2	0.46	0.50	5.8	0.92			114			31			37	34	
	Unloaded		87	25	23.2	0.57	0.59	6.8	0.96			115			31			37	36	
	Unloaded		88	22	27.1	0.67	0.68	7.7	0.99			116			30			38	37	
	Unloaded		86	23	28.3	0.68	0.68	7.9	0.99			119			29			39	39	
	Unloaded	162/78	84	24	29.4	0.68	0.68	8.1	1.00	7.50	21	121	122	1	27	27	0	40	40	0.19
0.5	5		82	30	31.1	0.71	0.70	8.5	1.01			121			26			40	41	
1.0	5		79	37	42.5	0.78	0.70	8.9	1.11			127			23			50	56	
1.5	10		84	36	41.3	0.77	0.72	8.6	1.07			126			24			50	53	
2.0	10	168/78	89	35	40.1	0.76	0.74	8.3	1.03	7.52	20	125	120	6	24	25	1	49	50	0.27
2.5	15		92	34	39.6	0.76	0.75	8.2	1.01			124			25			48	49	
3.0	15		95	33	39.1	0.76	0.76	8.0	1.00			123			25			48	48	
3.5	20		97	39	38.8	0.75	0.78	8.0	0.97			119			27			47	46	
4.0	20	171/81	99	45	38.4	0.74	0.79	8.0	0.94	7.49	20	115	113	9	29	27	−2	47	44	0.28
4.5	25		100	41	39.1	0.77	0.81	8.1	0.95			113			28			46	44	
5.0	25	168/78	100	37	39.8	0.80	0.83	8.3	0.96	7.51	19	120	123	2	27	24	−3	46	44	0.20
5.5	30		102	38	40.4	0.81	0.84	8.2	0.96			122			26			46	44	
6.0	30	168/78	103	38	40.9	0.82	0.85	8.3	0.96	7.51	18	123	133	−7	24	23	−1	46	44	0.17
6.5	35		106	40	43.9	0.86	0.88	8.3	0.98			124			24			47	46	
7.0	35	168/78	108	41	46.8	0.90	0.91	8.4	0.99	7.50	18	125	122	5	23	23	0	48	48	0.20
	Recovery		96	38	39.7	0.78	0.81	8.4	0.96			123			24			47	45	
	Recovery		84	34	32.5	0.66	0.71	8.5	0.93			121			25			45	42	
	Recovery		82	31	29.3	0.60	0.62	7.6	0.96			123			25			45	43	
	Recovery	156/72	79	28	26.0	0.53	0.53	6.7	1.00	7.49	18	124	128	−2	25	24	−1	45	45	0.18

cise. The respiratory alkalosis in response to exercise as observed in this patient on both study occasions is unusual and probably abnormal.

In the post-propranolol study (Fig. 9.28.2), after an initial elevation, $\dot{V}_E$ remains relatively unchanged (panel 1, Fig. 9.28.2) while R remains high (panel 8, Fig. 9.28.2) and Pa_{CO_2} falls further as work rate is increased (panel 9, Fig. 9.28.2 and Table 9.28.4). The further hyperventilation of the arterial blood (decrease in Pa_{CO_2}) without an increase in $\dot{V}_E$ probably results from an inordinately small pulmonary blood flow increase in response to increasing work rate. This also accounts for the shallow $\dot{V}_{O_2}$ response as work rate is increased (panel 3, Fig. 9.28.2) and the low flat O_2-pulse response (panel 2, Fig. 9.28.2).

Conclusion

Exercise response to exercise reflecting left-sided heart failure due to mitral stenosis, with and without β-adrenergic blockade. A rare occurrence of exercise-induced respiratory alkalosis is presented.

Case 29 Congenital Heart Disease

Clinical Findings

This 18-year-young woman was referred to evaluate exercise dyspnea. She had a known history of dextrocardia and had had a pulmonic valve replacement as a child. Pulmonary hypertension and pulmonic valve insufficiency were recently diagnosed. She had had dyspnea from climbing less than one flight of stairs. She had smoked cigarettes for 1 year. Examination revealed normal breath sounds and a grade II diastolic murmur over the upper sternum.

Exercise Findings

Exercise studies with the patient breathing room air and 100% O_2 were performed in the same morning on a cycle ergometer with an intermediate rest period. On both occasions, arterial blood was sampled every second minute and intra-arterial pressure was recorded from a percutaneously placed brachial artery catheter. The patient pedalled at 60 rpm without an added load for 3 minutes. The work rate was then increased in a ramp of 7 W per minute to tolerance. The patient was cooperative, appeared to

give good efforts, and stopped exercise on both occasions because of dyspnea. Resting and repeated ECGs during exercise (taken with reversed limb and right chest leads) did not reveal arrhythmias or evidence of myocardial ischemia. Arterial saturation by ear oximetry fell from 97% at rest to 87% at maximal exercise, but direct arterial blood gas measurements did not support this change.

TABLE 9.29.1.   Selected Respiratory Function Data

Measurement	Predicted	Measured
Age yr		18
Sex		Female
Height, cm		160
Weight, kg	61	49
Hematocrit, %		39
VC, _	3.38	2.20
IC, L	2.25	1.61
TLC, L	4.31	3.62
FEV_1, L	2.97	1.91
FEV_1/VC, %	88	87
MVV L/min		
Direct	118	58
Indirect	119	76
$D_{L}CO$ ml/mm Hg/min	25.1	12.6

TABLE 9.29.2.   Selected Exercise Data

Measurement	Predicted	Room Air	Oxygen
Peak $\dot{V}O_2$, L/min	1.93	0.76	
Maximum HR, beats/min	202	111	113
Maximum O_2 pulse, ml/beat	9.6	6.8	
$\Delta \dot{V}O_2/\Delta WR$, ml/min/W	10.3	6.3	
AT, L/min	>0.87	<0.65	
Work rate, max, W		<35	35
Blood pressure, mmHg (rest, max ex)		96/60, 126/66	102/60, 114/66
Maximum $\dot{V}E$, L/min		47	38
Exercise breathing reserve, L/min			
Using direct MVV	>15	11	20
Using indirect MVV	>15	19	38
O_2 saturation, oximeter (rest, max ex)		97, 87	
PaO_2, mmHg (rest, max ex)		75, 81	479, 532
$P(A - a)O_2$, mmHg (rest, max ex)		40, 42	203, 150
$P(a - ET)CO_2$, mmHg (rest, max ex)		5, 6	3, 4
VD/VT (rest, max ex)		0.31, 0.37	0.35, 0.35
HCO_3^-, mEq/L (rest, recovery)		20, 19	21, 20

FIGURE 9.29.1.   Air breathing.

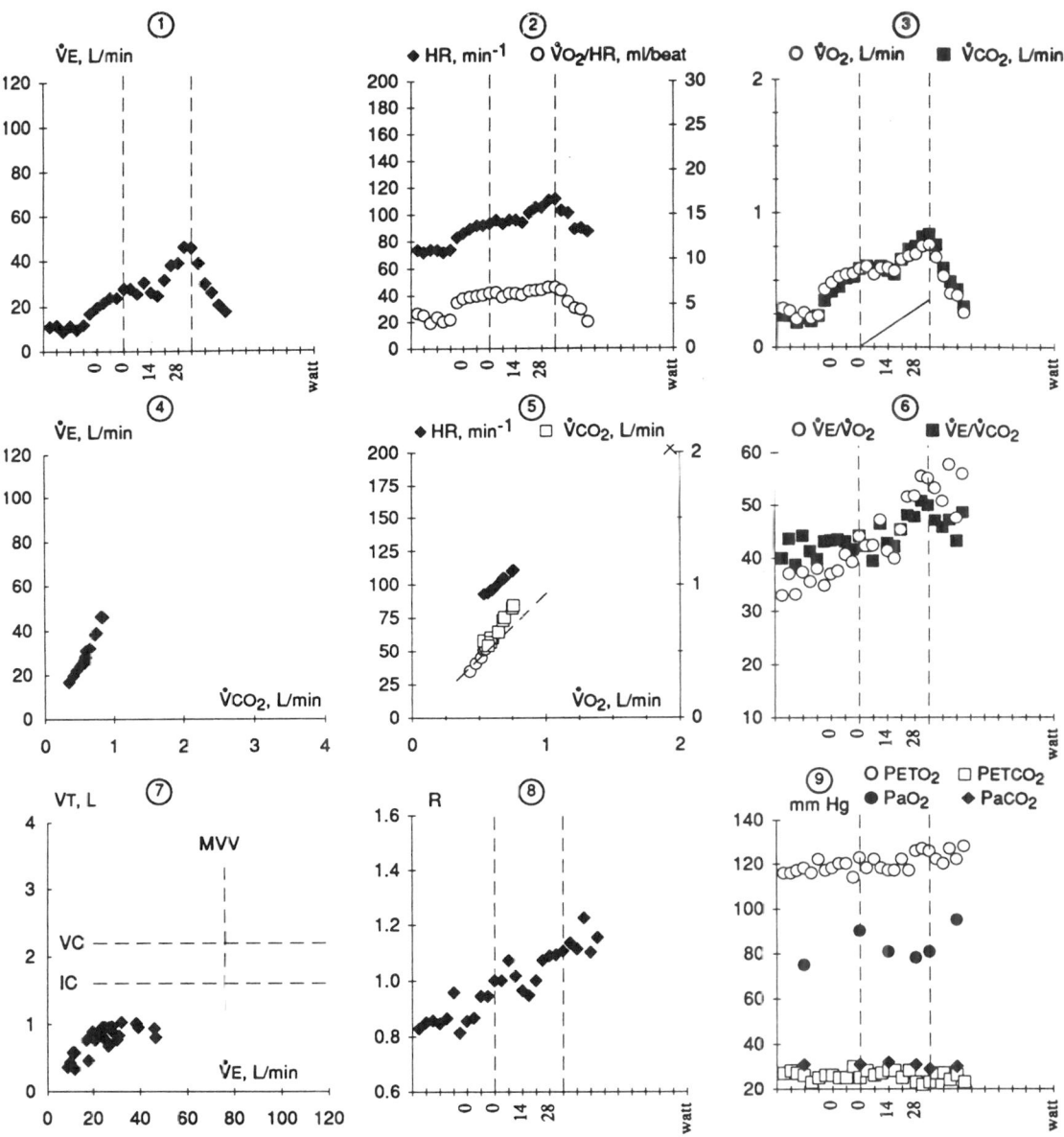

1. Vertical dashed lines in panels 1 to 3 and 6, 8, and 9 indicate the beginning and the end of increasing work period.

2. Unloaded cycling is performed for 3 minutes before the left vertical dashed line.

3. In panel 3, the diagonal line shows the increase of $\dot{V}O_2$ at a slope of 10 ml/min/w.

4. In panel 5, the diagonal dashed line has a slope of 1; the "x" in the upper right is the predicted maximum heart rate and $\dot{V}O_2$ for the subject.

FIGURE 9.29.2. Oxygen breathing.

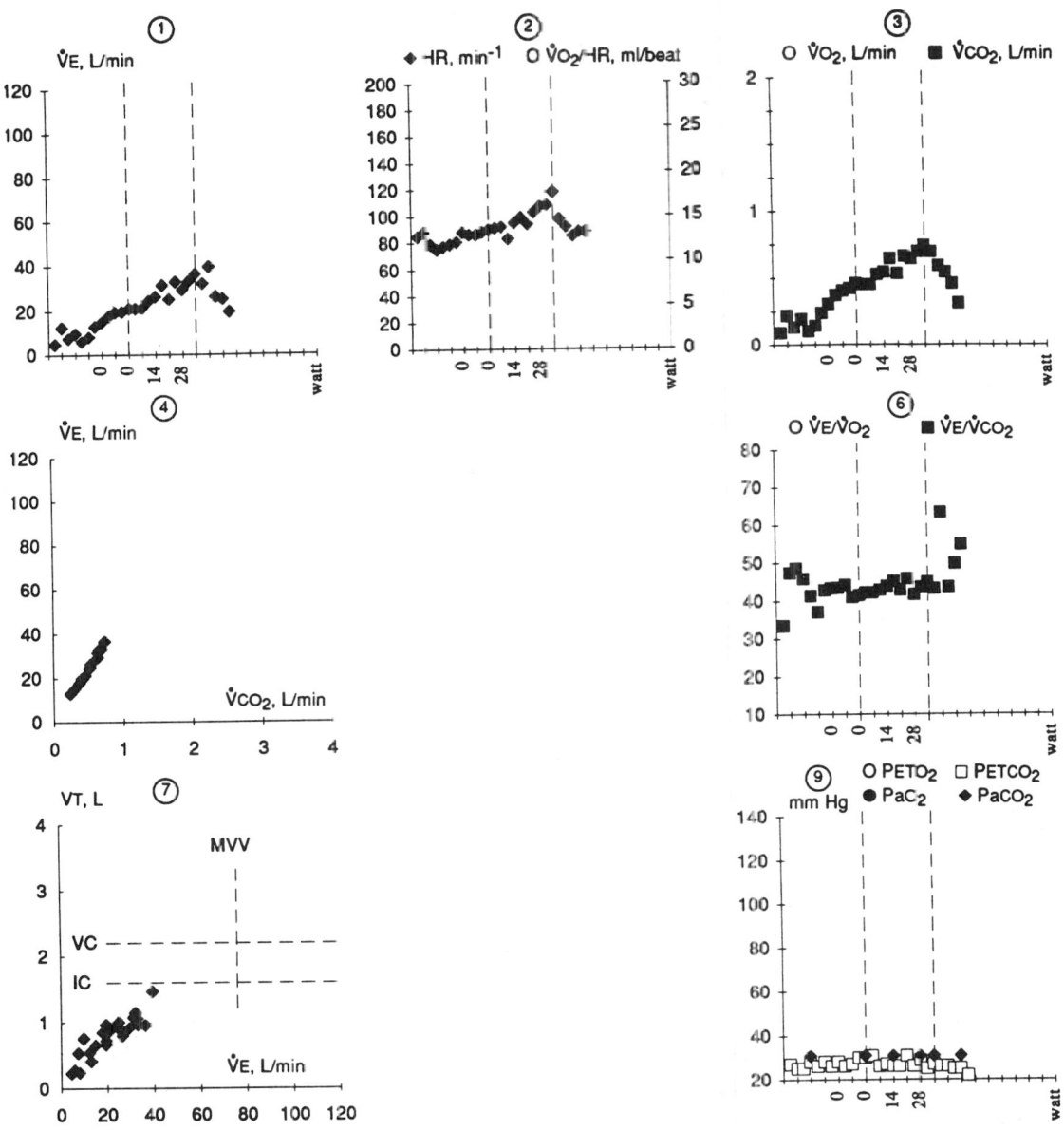

1. Vertical dashed lines in panels 1 to 3 and 6 and 9 indicate the beginning and the end of increasing work period.
2. Unloaded cycling is performed for 3 minutes before the left vertical dashed line.

TABLE 9.29.3. Air Breathing

Time min	Work rate watts	BP mmHg	HR min⁻¹	f min⁻¹	$\dot{V}_E$ L/min BTPS	$\dot{V}_{CO_2}$ L/min STPD	$\dot{V}_{O_2}$ L/min STPD	$\dot{V}_{O_2}$/HR ml/beat	R	pH	HCO₃⁻ meq/L	PO₂, mmHg ET	a	(A−a)	PCO₂, mmHg ET	a	(a−ET)	$\dot{V}_E$/$\dot{V}_{CO_2}$	$\dot{V}_E$/$\dot{V}_{O_2}$	VD/VT
	Rest		74	19	11.2	0.24	0.29	3.9	0.83			116			27			40	33	
	Rest		72	20	11.7	0.23	0.27	3.8	0.85			116			28			43	37	
	Rest		74	24	9.0	0.18	0.21	2.8	0.86			117			27			39	33	
	Rest	96/60	74	20	11.4	0.22	0.26	3.5	0.85	7.43	20	118	75	40	26	31	5	44	37	0.31
	Rest		72	22	9.7	0.19	0.22	3.1	0.86			116			23			41	36	
	Rest		74	35	12.1	0.23	0.24	3.2	0.96			122			25			40	38	
	Unloaded		83	22	16.9	0.35	0.43	5.2	0.81			117			26			43	35	
	Unloaded		86	22	19.6	0.41	0.48	5.6	0.85			118			26			43	37	
	Unloaded		89	27	21.8	0.45	0.52	5.8	0.87			120			25			43	38	
	Unloaded		92	25	24.0	0.51	0.54	5.9	0.94			120			25			43	41	
	Unloaded		92	29	24.0	0.52	0.55	6.0	0.95			114			30			41	39	
	Unloaded	102/66	93	29	28.0	0.58	0.58	6.2	1.00	7.46	22	123	90	29	25	31	6	44	44	0.34
0.5	4		96	31	27.9	0.60	0.60	6.3	1.00			118			28			42	42	
1.0	7		93	34	25.7	0.58	0.54	5.8	1.07			122			26			39	42	
1.5	11		96	37	30.9	0.60	0.59	6.1	1.02			118			27			46	47	
2.0	14	114/66	96	28	26.7	0.57	0.59	6.1	0.97	7.43	21	117	81	36	28	32	4	43	41	0.34
2.5	18		94	26	24.9	0.54	0.57	6.1	0.95			117			28			42	40	
3.0	21		101	31	32.0	0.65	0.65	6.4	1.00			122			25			45	45	
3.5	25		105	38	38.3	0.73	0.68	6.5	1.07			117			28			48	52	
4.0	28	126/66	105	41	39.2	0.75	0.69	6.6	1.09	7.43	20	126	78	43	23	31	8	48	52	0.38
4.5	32		110	57	46.5	0.82	0.75	6.8	1.09			127			22			51	56	
5.0	35		111	49	46.1	0.84	0.76	6.8	1.11	7.45	20	126	81	42	23	29	6	50	55	0.37
	Recovery		103	41	39.2	0.76	0.67	6.5	1.13			122			27			47	53	
	Recovery		101	39	30.2	0.59	0.53	5.2	1.11			120			27			46	51	
	Recovery		89	39	26.4	0.49	0.40	4.5	1.23			127			24			47	58	
	Recovery	108/60	90	27	20.8	0.43	0.39	4.3	1.10	7.41	19	122	95	27	26	30	4	43	47	0.29
	Recovery		87	38	17.8	0.30	0.26	3.0	1.15			128			23			49	56	

Interpretation

Comments

This is a patient with known congenital heart disease, previously surgically repaired, with recent deterioration, and mild restrictive lung disease. The arterial oxyhemoglobin saturation did not fall during the brief exercise period when directly measured, but ear oximetry saturation declined 10% during the same time.

Analysis

Referring to flow chart 1, in the room air study the peak $\dot{V}_{O_2}$ was reduced while the anaerobic threshold was also low (Table 9.29.2). This directs us to flow chart 4. Using the indirect MVV measurement, the breathing reserve is normal (branchpoint 4.1). This leads us to branchpoint 4.3 in which we address the $\dot{V}_E/\dot{V}_{CO_2}$ at the AT, which is elevated. This leads us to abnormal pulmonary circulation taking us to branchpoint 4.5. The vital capacity is reduced leading us to the diagnosis of moderate to severe left-sided heart failure. However the differential feature between the left ventricular failure disorder and pulmonary vascular disease based on the reduced vital capacity might be incorrect because her prior surgery, rather than moderate severe heart failure, might have accounted for the reduction. Addressing the diagnosis through flow chart 5, the VD/VT, $P(A − a)_{O_2}$, and $P(a − ET)_{CO_2}$ are abnormal (branchpoint 5.1), whereas the breathing reserve is normal (branchpoint 5.3). Evidence of a reduced cardiac output response and of a reduced $\Delta\dot{V}_{O_2}/\Delta WR$ is indicative of a circulatory limitation. O_2 breathing

TABLE 9.29.4.   Oxygen Breathing

Time min	Work rate watts	BP mmHg	HR min⁻¹	f min⁻¹	$\dot{V}E$ L/min BTPS	$\dot{V}CO_2$ L/min STPD	$\dot{V}O_2$ L/min STPD	$\dfrac{\dot{V}O_2}{HR}$ ml/beat	R	pH	HCO₃ meq/L	PO₂, mmHg ET	a	(A−a)	PCO₂, mmHg ET	a	(a−ET)	$\dfrac{\dot{V}E}{\dot{V}CO_2}$	$\dfrac{\dot{V}E}{\dot{V}O_2}$	$\dfrac{VD}{VT}$
	Rest		85	20	4.7	0.09									27			33		
	Rest		88	23	12.4	0.22									25			47		
	Rest		79	14	7.5	0.13									25			49		
	Rest	102/60	75	13	9.8	0.19				7.45	21		479	203	28	31	3	46		0.35
	Rest		77	22	6.0	0.10									26			41		
	Rest		79	33	8.0	0.14									28			37		
	Unloaded		81	31	12.9	0.24									26			43		
	Unloaded		88	23	14.9	0.30									28			43		
	Unloaded		86	21	17.8	0.37									26			43		
	Unloaded		86	20	19.4	0.40									27			44		
	Unloaded		88	27	19.5	0.42									30			41		
	Unloaded	114/66	90	23	21.0	0.46				7.42	20		533	49	30	31	1	41		0.30
0.5	4		91	24	21.0	0.45									31			42		
1.0	7		92	24	21.0	0.45									26			42		
1.5	11		83	26	24.4	0.52									27			43		
2.0	14	120/72	95	33	26.4	0.54				7.44	21		536	46	26	31	5	44		0.32
2.5	18		99	29	31.3	0.64									26			45		
3.0	21		94	28	25.1	0.53									31			43		
3.5	25		103	31	32.8	0.66									26			46		
4.0	28	114/72	107	32	29.4	0.64				7.42	20		534	148	29	31	2	42		0.30
4.5	32		108	34	33.0	0.69									25			44		
5.0	35	114/66	118	38	36.4	0.74				7.43	20		532	150	27	31	4	45		0.35
	Recovery		98	28	32.1	0.69									26			43		
	Recovery		92	27	39.6	0.59									26			63		
	Recovery		85	30	26.1	0.54									25			44		
	Recovery	90/48	88	25	25.0	0.46				7.42	20		543	139	25	31	6	50		0.40
	Recovery		88	29	19.4	0.31									22			55		

provided no benefit to the patient with respect to work capacity or the ventilatory response. Neither the breathing frequency nor the VT/IC is abnormally high on either test. The high heart rate reserve suggests chronotropic insufficiency. The high PaO_2 during O_2 breathing excludes a significant right to left shunt. The tight control of pH, and failure to recruit new pulmonary blood vessels during exercise, reflected in the increase in ventilatory equivalent for CO_2 during exercise, i.e., decrease in gas exchange efficiency (panel 6), might account for this patient's dyspnea.

Conclusion

This patient demonstrates a severe cardiovascular limitation to exercise, secondary to congenital heart disease, subjectively experienced as dyspnea For some reason, the patient regulates her $PaCO_2$ at a low level (has a low set-point), thereby requiring a high ventilation to eliminate the metabolic CO_2 of exercise (see the high $\dot{V}E/\dot{V}CO_2$ at the anaerobic threshold in panel 6 of Fig. 9.29.1). This high ventilatory requirement is likely the main factor stimulating dyspnea and limiting exercise tolerance.

As is not uncommonly seen in patients with cardiovascular limitation to exercise, the ear oximeter values were falsely decreased at maximal exercise, probably because of inadequate cardiac output and reduced perfusion of the ear lobe (1).

Reference

1. Hansen JE, Casaburi R. Validity of ear oximetry in clinical exercise testing. Chest 1987;91:333–337.

Case 30 Peripheral Arterial Disease

Clinical Findings

This 65-year-old cigarette-smoking man was evaluated as part of a research study looking for coronary artery calcification. He had been overweight and a known diabetic for approximately 6 years. He had continued to lead an active life, but had been limited in his speed of walking for approximately 5 years, with pain in his thighs and calves, especially on the right side. He had had some cough and sputum production for a decade. He denied chest pain, shortness of breath, wheezing, edema, or skin problems. Pulses could not be palpated in the legs except for a faint right femoral artery pulse. The patient had no edema; skin warmth and color were good. The coronary arteries were free of calcification.

Exercise Findings

The patient performed exercise on a cycle ergometer. He pedalled at 60 rpm without an added load for 3 minutes. The work rate was then increased 15 W per minute to tolerance. Heart rate and rhythm were continuously monitored; 12-lead ECGs were obtained during rest, exercise, and recovery. Blood pressure was measured with a sphygmomanometer every minute. The patient appeared to give an excellent effort and stopped exercise because of bilateral thigh and calf pain. He denied chest pain or discomfort during or after the study. The ECGs showed occasional premature ventricular contractions both at rest and during exercise, but were otherwise normal. No abnormal ST segments or T waves were noted before, during, or after exercise.

TABLE 9.30.1 Selected Respiratory Function Data

Measurement	Predicted	Measured
Age, yr		65
Sex		Male
Height, cm		170
Weight, kg	74	88
Hematocrit, %		42
VC, L	3.43	3.65
IC, L	2.44	3.20
FEV$_1$, L	2.74	2.48
FEV$_1$/VC, %	79	68
MVV, L/min	110	92

TABLE 9.30.2 Selected Exercise Data

Measurement	Predicted	Measured
Peak $\dot{V}O_2$, L/min	2.04	1.06
Maximum HR, beats/min	155	135
Maximum O$_2$ pulse, ml/beat	13.2	7.9
$\Delta\dot{V}O_2/\Delta WR$, ml/min/W	10.3	6.9
AT, L/min	>0.95	0.8
Blood pressure, mmHg (rest, max)		164/88, 278/110
Maximum $\dot{V}E$, L/min		33
Exercise breathing reserve, L/min	>15	59

FIGURE 9.30.1.

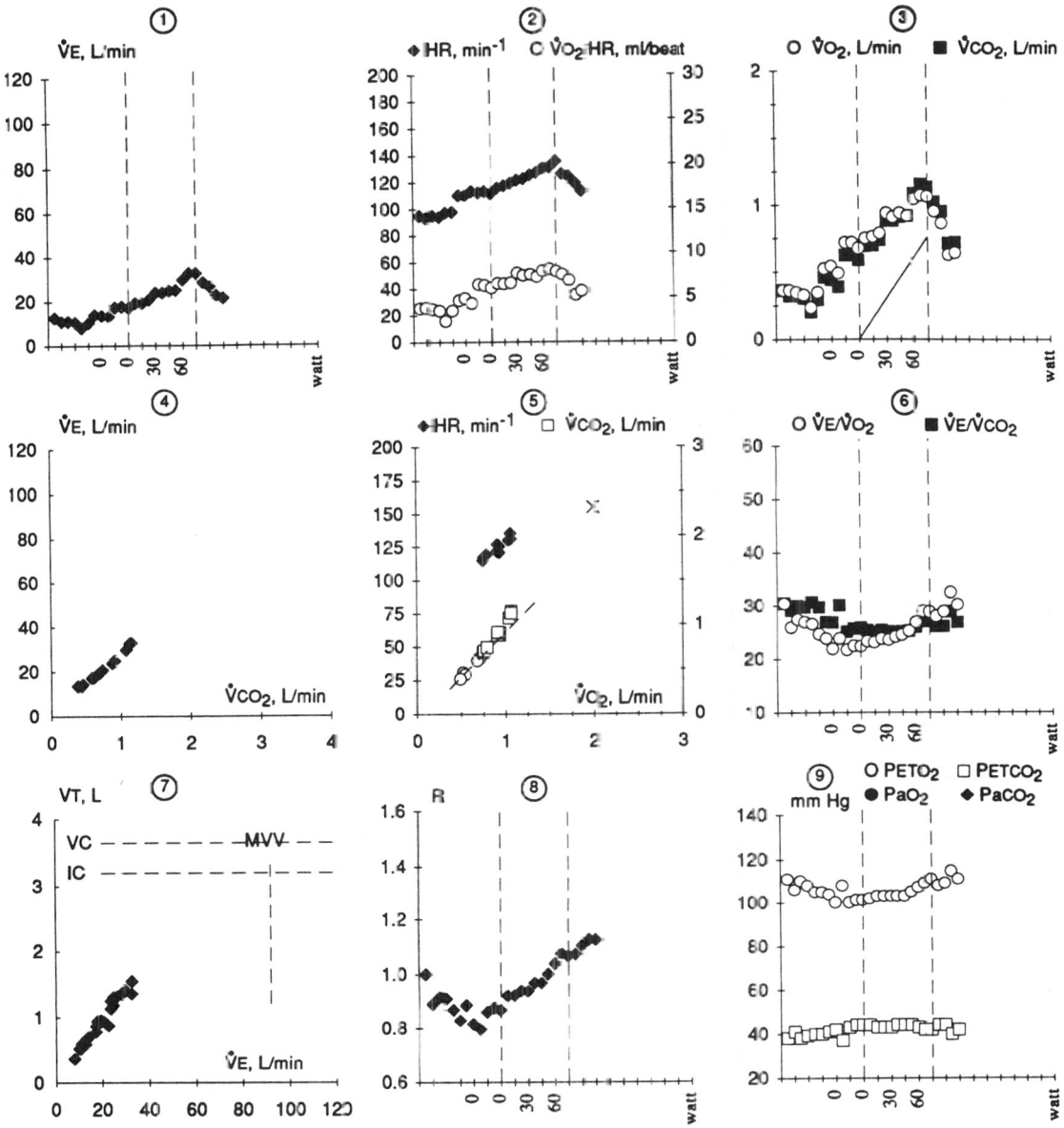

1. Vertical dashed lines in panels 1 to 3 and 6, 8, and 9 indicate the beginning and the end of increasing work period.
2. Unloaded cycling is performed for 3 minutes before the left vertical dashed line.
3. In panel 3, the diagonal line shows the increase of $\dot{V}O_2$ at a slope of 10 ml/min/w.
4. In panel 5, the diagonal dashed line has a slope of 1; the ">" in the upper right is the predicted maximum heart rate and $\dot{V}O_2$ for the subject.

TABLE 9.30.3. Air Breathing

Time min	Work rate watts	BP mmHg	HR min⁻¹	f min⁻¹	$\dot{V}_E$ L/min BTPS	$\dot{V}_{CO_2}$ L/min STPD	$\dot{V}_{O_2}$ L/min STPD	$\dot{V}_{O_2}$/HR ml/beat	R	pH	HCO_3^- meq/L	P_{O_2}, mmHg ET	a	(A − a)	P_{CO_2}, mmHg ET	a	(a − ET)	$\dot{V}_E/\dot{V}_{CO_2}$	$\dot{V}_E/\dot{V}_{O_2}$	V_D/V_T
	Rest	164/88										111								
	Rest		95	22	12.8	0.36	0.36	3.8	1.00			106			38			30	30	
	Rest	188/80	93	21	11.1	0.32	0.36	3.9	0.89			110			41			29	26	
	Rest		95	19	11.2	0.32	0.35	3.7	0.91			108			38			30	27	
	Rest	218/80	94	20	10.6	0.30	0.33	3.5	0.91			105			39			30	27	
	Rest		97	22	8.0	0.20	0.23	2.4	0.87			105			40			31	27	
	Rest	198/82	98	20	10.3	0.29	0.35	3.6	0.83						40			30	25	
	Unloaded		110	20	14.1	0.46	0.52	4.7	0.88			104			41			27	24	
	Unloaded	214/100	110	20	13.5	0.44	0.54	4.9	0.81			100			42			27	22	
	Unloaded		113	20	13.4	0.39	0.49	4.3	0.80			108			37			30	24	
	Unloaded	238/96	112	20	17.3	0.62	0.72	6.4	0.86			100			43			25	22	
	Unloaded		113	19	17.8	0.63	0.72	6.4	0.88			101			44			26	22	
	Unloaded	254/90	111	22	17.1	0.59	0.68	6.1	0.87			101			44			26	22	
0.5	7.5		115	20	19.2	0.69	0.75	6.5	0.92			102			44			25	23	
1.0	15	255/100	117	20	19.2	0.70	0.76	6.5	0.92			103			43			25	23	
1.5	22.5		119	22	20.6	0.74	0.79	6.6	0.94			103			43			25	24	
2.0	30	245/114	121	19	23.7	0.88	0.94	7.8	0.94			103			43			25	23	
2.5	37.5		122	21	23.7	0.88	0.91	7.5	0.97			103			44			25	24	
3.0	45	252/110	125	21	24.7	0.91	0.94	7.5	0.97			103			44			25	24	
3.5	52.5		127	19	24.8	0.92	0.92	7.2	1.00			105			44			25	25	
4.0	60	256/114	130	21	29.7	1.08	1.04	8.0	1.04			107			43			26	27	
4.5	67.5		131	21	32.7	1.15	1.07	8.2	1.07			109			42			27	29	
5.0	75	278/110	135	24	32.6	1.13	1.06	7.9	1.07			111			42			27	29	
	Recovery		126	21	28.4	1.02	0.95	7.5	1.07			108			44			26	28	
	Recovery	268/90	124	20	26.5	0.95	0.86	6.9	1.10			109			44			26	29	
	Recovery		119	26	22.6	0.71	0.63	5.3	1.13			115			40			29	32	
	Recovery	241/86	113	23	21.2	0.72	0.64	5.7	1.13			111			42			27	30	

Interpretation

Comments

The patient has mild, asymptomatic airways obstruction, diabetes mellitus, obesity, and clinical evidence of peripheral arterial disease without heart disease.

Analysis

Referring to flow chart 1, peak $\dot{V}_{O_2}$ and the anaerobic threshold are reduced (Table 9.30.2). Proceeding next to flow chart 4, the high breathing reserve (branchpoint 4.1) and normal $\dot{V}_E/\dot{V}_{CO_2}$ at the anaerobic threshold (branchpoint 4.3) lead us to "O_2 flow problem of non-pulmonary origin." The normal hematocrit (branchpoint 4.4) indicates a cardiovascular disorder with a low non-changing O_2 pulse (branchpoint 4.6). The findings of exercise-induced systemic hypertension, leg pain, low $\Delta\dot{V}_{O_2}/\Delta WR$, and high heart rate reserve all support the diagnosis of peripheral arterial disease. The absence of ECG changes of myocardial ischemia suggests that the coronary vessels are relatively uninvolved.

Conclusion

The exercise-induced hypertension is especially typical of peripheral arterial disease. In addition, the increase in $\dot{V}_{CO_2}$ with work rate is reduced similar to the $\dot{V}_{O_2}$-work rate relationship in contrast to primary heart disease or disease of the pulmonary circulation. Perhaps this is because the leg blood flow contributes in a relatively small way to the total systemic circulation and the reduction in $\dot{V}_{O_2}$ would result in a reduction in aerobic CO_2 production. Although many patients with peripheral arterial disease are limited by associated coronary artery disease, this does not seem to be true for this man.

Case 31 Peripheral Arterial Disease with Pulmonary Vascular and Obstructive Airway Disease

Clinical Findings

This 69-year-old retired shipyard worker had been a heavy cigarette smoker until 5 years before. For more than a decade he had noted excessive shortness of breath on climbing one flight of stairs. For the last several years his activity had been limited by cramps in the calves after walking approximately 100 yards; they were relieved by rest. He took no medication. Examination revealed a left cataract and reduced arterial pulsations in the legs, but no rales, wheezing, or edema. Chest x-ray studies showed pleural thickening on the right, an elevated left leaf of the diaphragm, and normal heart size.

Exercise Findings

The patient performed exercise on a cycle ergometer. He pedalled at 60 rpm without added load for 3 minutes. The work rate was then increased 10 W per minute to his symptom-limited maximum. Blood was sampled every second minute, and intra-arterial blood pressure was recorded from a percutaneously placed brachial artery catheter. The patient stopped exercise because of pain in both calves. He developed frequent premature ventricular contractions and hypertension during exercise that resolved during recovery. Resting, exercise, and recovery ECG tracings were otherwise normal.

TABLE 9.31.1. Selected Respiratory Function Data

Measurement	Predicted	Measured
Age, yr		69
Sex		Male
Height, cm		165
Weight, kg	70	76
Hematocrit, %		40
VC, L	3.68	3.25
IC, L	2.45	2.69
TLC, L	6.11	6.05
FEV, L	2.87	1.92
FEV/VC, %	73	59
MVV, L/min	113	87
$D_{L}CO$, ml/mm Hg/min	21.8	17.5

TABLE 9.31.2. Selected Exercise Data

Measurement	Predicted	Measured
Peak $\dot{V}O_2$, L/min	1.78	0.83
Maximum HR, beats/min	151	115
Maximum O_2 pulse, ml/beat	11.8	7.2
$\Delta\dot{V}O_2/\Delta WR$, ml/min/W	10.3	5.2
AT, L/min	>0.80	not reached
Blood pressure, mmHg (rest, max)		198/84, 264/120
Maximum $\dot{V}E$, L/min		30
Exercise breathing reserve, L/min	>15	57
Pao_2, mmHg (rest, max ex)		87, 80
P(A − a)O_2, mmHg (rest, max ex)		11, 28
P(a − ET)CO_2, mmHg (rest, max ex)		5, 1
V_D/V_T (rest, heavy ex)		0.47, 0.38
HCO_3, mEq/L (rest, 2-min recov)		24, 23

FIGURE 9.31.1.

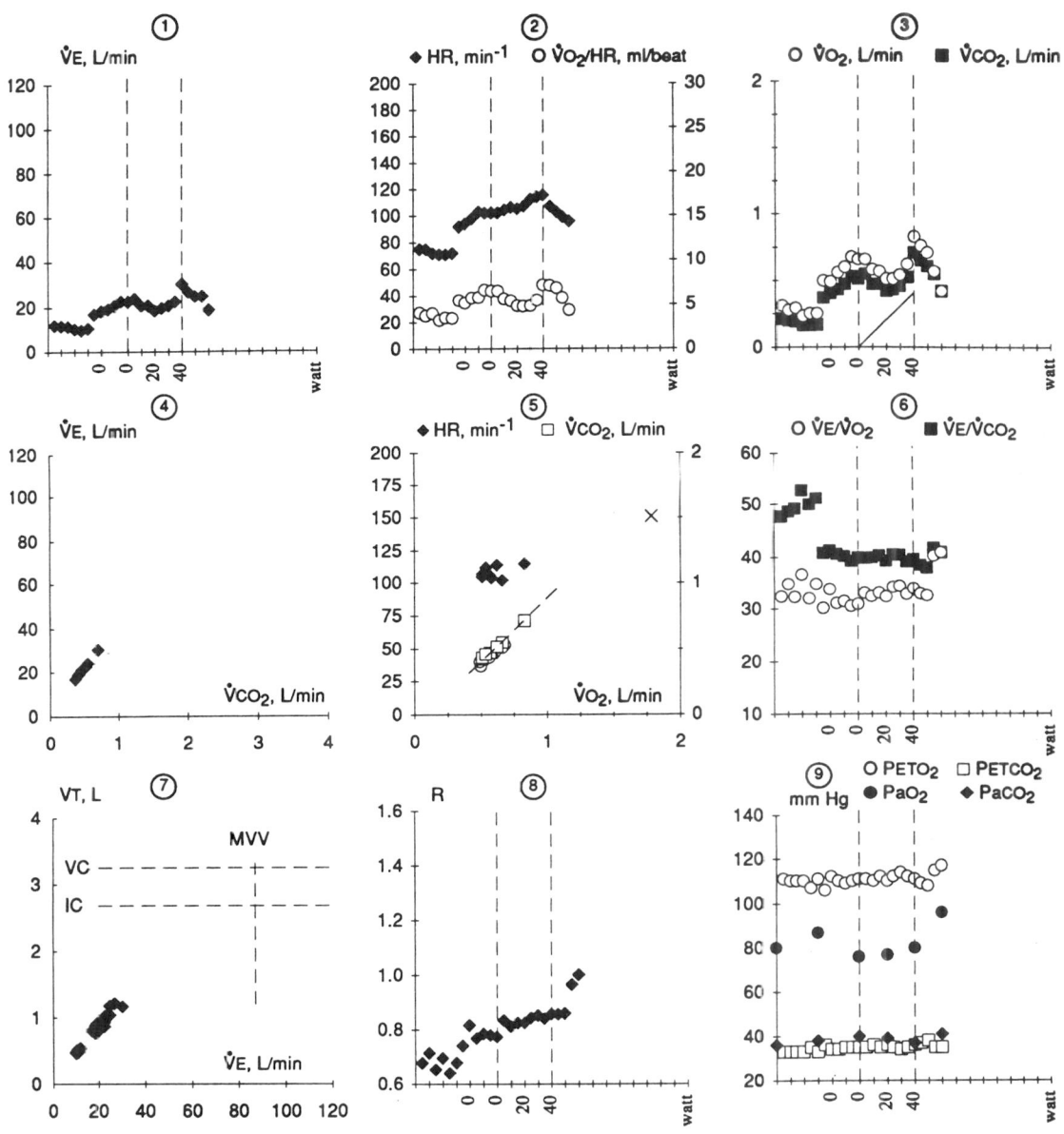

1. Vertical dashed lines in panels 1 to 3 and 6, 8, and 9 indicate the beginning and the end of increasing work period.
2. Unloaded cycling is performed for 3 minutes before the left vertical dashed line.
3. In panel 3, the diagonal line shows the increase of $\dot{V}O_2$ at a slope of 10 ml/min/w.
4. In panel 5, the diagonal dashed line has a slope of 1; the "x" in the upper right is the predicted maximum heart rate and $\dot{V}O_2$ for the subject.

Interpretation

Comments

Resting respiratory function studies show the patient to have moderate airflow obstruction (Table 9.31.1). The resting electrocardiogram is normal.

Analysis

Referring to flow chart 1, the peak $\dot{V}O_2$ is reduced while the anaerobic threshold was not measurable (Table 9.31.2). The latter is not unexpected for peripheral arterial disease because of the difficulty for the muscle lactic acidosis to be reflected systemically

TABLE 9.31.3. Air Breathing

Time min	Work rate watts	BP mmHg	HR min^{-1}	f min^{-1}	$\dot{V}_E$ L/min BTPS	$\dot{V}_{CO_2}$ L/min STPD	$\dot{V}_{O_2}$ L/min STPD	$\dot{V}_{O_2}$/HR ml/beat	R	pH	HCO$_3$ meq/L	PO$_2$, mmHg ET	a	(A−a)	PCO$_2$, mmHg ET	a	(a−ET)	$\dot{V}_E$/$\dot{V}_{CO_2}$	$\dot{V}_E$/$\dot{V}_{O_2}$	V_D/V_T
	Rest	210/84								7.43	23	80			36					
	Rest		75	22	11.9	0.21	0.31	4.1	0.63			111			33			48	32	
	Rest		75	22	11.6	0.20	0.28	3.7	0.71			110			33			49	35	
	Rest		72	23	11.3	0.19	0.29	4.0	0.66			110			33			49	32	
	Rest		71	22	10.3	0.16	0.23	3.2	0.70			110			33			53	37	
	Rest		71	20	9.7	0.16	0.25	3.5	0.64			107			33			50	32	
	Rest	198/84	72	20	10.4	0.17	0.25	3.5	0.68	7.41	24	111	87	11	33	38	5	51	35	0.47
	Unloaded		92	21	16.9	0.37	0.50	5.4	0.74			106			36			41	30	
	Unloaded		94	21	18.3	0.40	0.49	5.2	0.82			112			34			41	34	
	Unloaded		98	21	19.2	0.43	0.56	5.7	0.77			110			34			41	31	
	Unloaded		103	22	20.7	0.47	0.60	5.8	0.78			109			35			40	31	
	Unloaded		102	22	22.6	0.53	0.68	6.7	0.78			110			35			39	30	
	Unloaded	246/93	102	24	22.4	0.51	0.66	6.5	0.77	7.40	24	111	76	25	35	40	5	40	31	0.42
0.5	10		102	23	23.8	0.55	0.66	6.5	0.83			111			35			40	3	
1.0	10		104	23	20.7	0.47	0.58	5.6	0.81			110			36			40	32	
1.5	20		106	24	20.9	0.47	0.57	5.4	0.82			112			35			40	33	
2.0	20	252/114	105	24	18.5	0.42	0.51	4.9	0.82	7.40	24	110	77	27	36	39	3	39	32	0.39
2.5	30		107	25	19.5	0.43	0.51	4.8	0.84			112			35			40	34	
3.0	40		112	25	20.7	0.46	0.54	4.8	0.85			114			34			40	34	
3.5	40		114	26	22.5	0.52	0.62	5.4	0.84			112			35			39	33	
4.0	40	264/120	115	26	30.3	0.71	0.83	7.2	0.86	7.40	23	111	80	28	36	37	1	40	34	0.38
	Recovery		107	22	26.8	0.65	0.76	7.1	0.86			109			37			38	33	
	Recovery		103	21	24.8	0.61	0.71	6.9	0.86			108			38			38	32	
	Recovery		99	24	24.9	0.55	0.57	5.8	0.96			115			35			42	40	
	Recovery	210/96	96	21	18.9	0.42	0.42	4.4	1.00	7.37	23	117	96	13	35	41	6	41	41	0.44

as discussed in Case 30. Therefore, we consider the anaerobic threshold to be indeterminate and use flow chart 5. While the maximum work rate performed is quite low, the maximum exercise V_D/V_T is high, and $P(a - ET)CO_2$ and $P(A - a)O_2$ are at the borderline of abnormality (branchpoint 5.1). The breathing reserve is high (branchpoint 5.3). This suggests that the disease process is either that of pulmonary vascular or left ventricular failure. However, neither diagnosis fits very well with the measurements shown in the two supporting boxes. The failure to develop a systemic metabolic acidosis, the high heart rate reserve and the systemic hypertension are particularly incompatible with either diagnosis and suggests that this patient has a mixed disorder, with neither of the two choices derived by the flow chart being the dominant limiting disorder. Returning to branchpoint 5.1 and taking the normal branch, we continue through branchpoints 5.2, and 5.5 and finally reach branchpoint 5.8. The patient has systemic hypertension, reduced arterial pulses

in the legs and lower extremity pain with exercise suggesting that peripheral arterial disease is the diagnosis limiting exercise performance. Supporting this is the very low $\Delta\dot{V}_{O_2}$/ΔWR (branchpoint 5.8) and the failure to develop a systemic metabolic acidosis. ($\dot{V}_{O_2}$ and $\dot{V}_{CO_2}$ could increase only slightly above that required for unloaded cycling.)

Conclusion

Both peripheral and pulmonary vascular disease are present, with the former being the primary limiting disorder. The exercise-induced arrhythmia also suggests the presence of myocardial ischemia, perhaps from the high cardiac afterload induced by systemic hypertension. The poor perfusion of the exercising muscles probably prevented the cellular metabolic acidosis from being reflected in the arterial blood. Note that while this patient has moderate airflow obstruction, it does not appear to be important in this patient's exercise limitation.

Case 32 Heart Failure Dominant Mixed Cardiovascular Disease in an Anemic Smoker

Clinical Findings

This 54-year-old male bartender was referred for preoperative study to evaluate his exercise capacity. He occasionally had calf pain at rest and always after walking one block. He had smoked at least 60 pack years but denied cardiac or respiratory symptoms. The left iliac and superficial femoral arteries were demonstrated to be obstructed on angiography. He was moderately anemic (hematocrit = 34) with occult blood in the stool.

Exercise Findings

The patient performed exercise on a cycle ergometer. He pedalled at 60 rpm without added load for 3 minutes. The work rate was then increased 15 W per minute to his symptom-limited maximum. Blood was sampled every second minute, and intra-arterial blood pressure was recorded from a percutaneously placed brachial artery catheter. Resting and exercise ECGs were normal. He stopped exercise because of severe leg pain, which was more prominent on the left. Carboxyhemoglobin was 5.6% in his resting arterial blood.

TABLE 9.32.1. Selected Respiratory Function Data

Measurement	Predicted	Measured
Age, yr		59
Sex		Male
Height, cm		168
Weight, kg	72	60
Hematocrit, %		34
VC, L	3.94	3.84
IC, L	2.63	3.64
TLC, L	5.86	7.16
FEV_1, L	3.12	3.07
FEV_1/VC, %	79	80
MVV, L/min	136	110
$D_{L}CO$, ml/mm Hg/min	23.0	22.9

TABLE 9.32.2. Selected Exercise Data

Measurement	Predicted	Measured
Peak $\dot{V}O_2$, L/min	1.90	0.82
Maximum HR, beats/min	161	141
Maximum O_2 pulse, ml/beat	11.8	5.8
$\Delta\dot{V}O_2/\Delta WR$, ml/min/W	10.3	6.2
AT, L/min	>0.84	0.7
Blood pressure, mmHg (rest, max)		168/72, 255/114
Maximum $\dot{V}E$, L/min		60
Exercise breathing reserve, L/min	>15	50
PaO_2, mmHg (rest, max ex)		94, 117
$P(A - a)O_2$, mmHg (rest, max ex)		20, 11
$P(a - ET)CO_2$, mmHg (rest, max ex)		3, 2
VD/VT (rest, heavy ex)		0.45, 0.38
HCO_3^-, mEq/L (rest, 2-min recov)		20, 16

FIGURE 9.32.1.

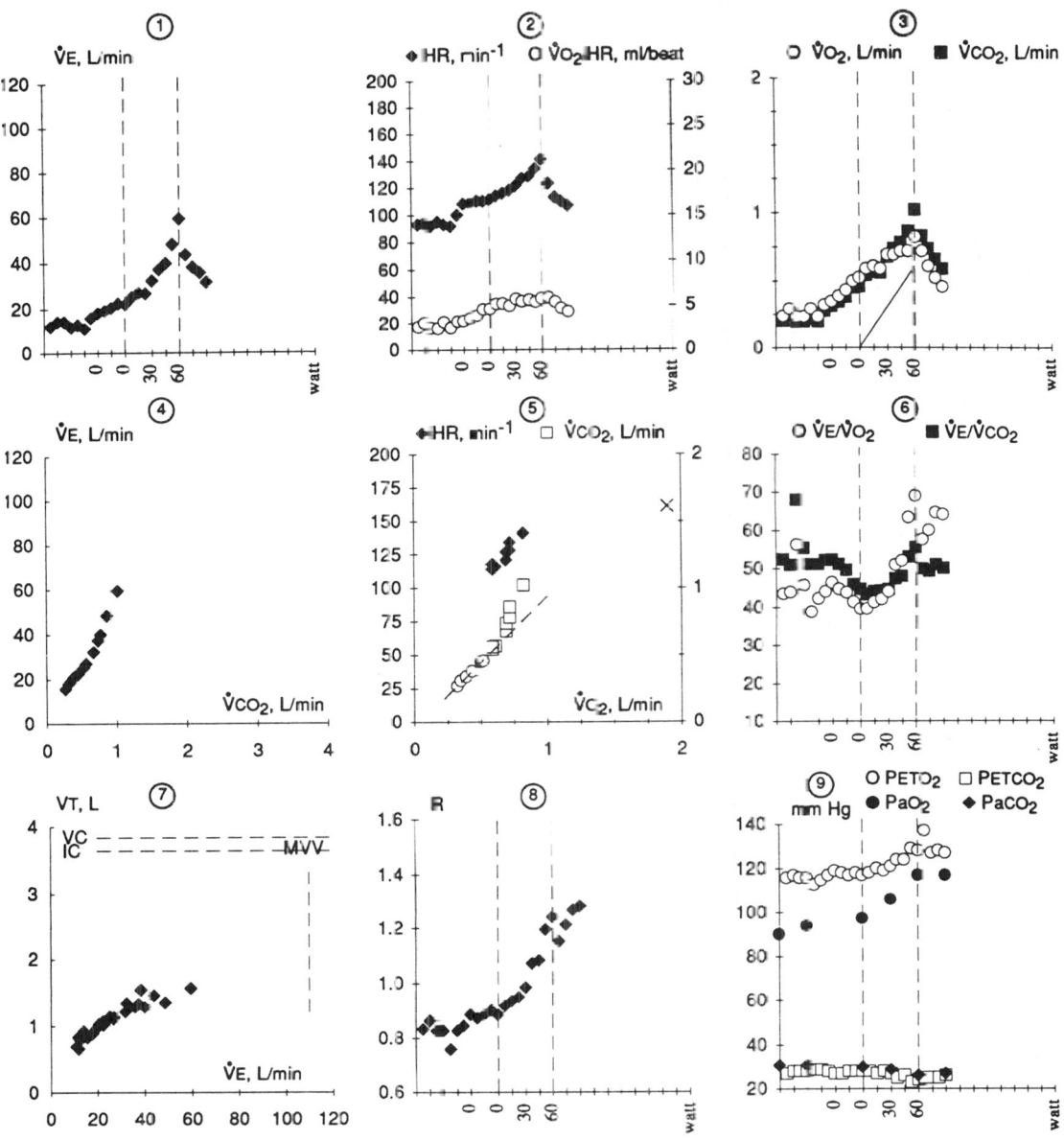

1. Vertical dashed lines in panels 1 to 3 and 6, 3, and 9 indicate the beginning and the end of increasing work period.

2. Unloaded cycling is performed for 3 minutes before the left vertical dashed line.

3. In panel 3, the diagonal line shows the increase of $\dot{V}O_2$ at a slope of 10 ml/min/w.

4. In panel 5, the diagonal dashed line has a slope of 1; the "×" in the upper right is the predicted maximum heart rate and $\dot{V}O_2$ for the subject.

TABLE 9.32.3. Air Breathing

Time min	Work rate watts	BP mmHg	HR min⁻¹	f min⁻¹	$\dot{V}_E$ L/min BTPS	$\dot{V}_{CO_2}$ L/min STPD	$\dot{V}_{O_2}$ L/min STPD	$\dot{V}_{O_2}$/HR ml/beat	R	pH	HCO₃⁻ meq/L	P_{O_2}, mmHg ET	a	(A − a)	P_{CO_2}, mmHg ET	a	(a − ET)	$\dfrac{\dot{V}_E}{\dot{V}_{CO_2}}$	$\dfrac{\dot{V}_E}{\dot{V}_{O_2}}$	$\dfrac{V_D}{V_T}$
	Rest	168/72								7.43	20		90			31				
	Rest		93	18	12.0	0.20	0.24	2.6	0.83			116			27			52	44	
	Rest		94	15	14.0	0.25	0.29	3.1	0.86			117			28			51	44	
	Rest		92	16	14.3	0.19	0.23	2.5	0.83			116			28			68	56	
	Rest	168/72	95	14	11.7	0.19	0.23	2.4	0.83	7.42	20	116	94	20	28	31	3	55	46	0.45
	Rest		93	16	12.6	0.22	0.29	3.1	0.76			113			29			51	39	
	Rest		92	16	11.1	0.19	0.23	2.5	0.83			115			29			51	42	
	Unloaded		100	19	15.7	0.27	0.32	3.2	0.84			117			28			52	44	
	Unloaded		108	20	17.9	0.31	0.35	3.2	0.89			119			27			52	46	
	Unloaded		109	20	19.1	0.34	0.39	3.6	0.87			118			27			51	45	
	Unloaded		110	20	20.5	0.38	0.43	3.9	0.88			117			28			49	44	
	Unloaded		110	22	22.5	0.45	0.50	4.5	0.90			118			28			46	41	
	Unloaded	231/93	111	21	22.3	0.46	0.52	4.7	0.88	7.43	20	117	97	20	28	30	2	45	39	0.33
0.5	15		114	22	25.2	0.54	0.59	5.2	0.92			118			28			43	40	
1.0	15		116	24	27.1	0.57	0.61	5.3	0.93			120			27			44	41	
1.5	30		118	24	26.8	0.56	0.59	5.0	0.95			119			28			44	42	
2.0	30	245/102	121	24	32.3	0.68	0.69	5.7	0.99	7.43	19	121	106	15	27	29	2	45	44	0.31
2.5	45		127	28	37.4	0.74	0.69	5.4	1.07			124			25			47	51	
3.0	45		128	31	40.1	0.78	0.72	5.6	1.08			124			26			48	52	
3.5	60		134	36	48.6	0.86	0.72	5.4	1.19			129			23			53	63	
4.0	60	255/114	141	38	59.7	1.02	0.82	5.8	1.24	7.44	17	128	117	11	24	26	2	55	69	0.38
	Recovery		123	30	43.9	0.83	0.72	5.9	1.15			137			25			50	57	
	Recovery		113	25	38.6	0.74	0.61	5.4	1.21			127			25			49	60	
	Recovery		110	28	35.9	0.66	0.52	4.7	1.27			128			25			51	64	
	Recovery	258/102	107	26	31.7	0.59	0.46	4.3	1.28	7.39	16	127	117	11	26	27	1	50	64	0.34

Interpretation

Comments

The resting respiratory function is normal, including the diffusing capacity (Table 9.32.1).

Analysis

Referring to flow chart 1, peak $\dot{V}_{O_2}$ and anaerobic threshold are reduced during exercise testing (Table 9.32.2). See flow chart 4 for further analysis. The breathing reserve is high (branchpoint 4.1). This patient has a combination of abnormalities that fit the major diagnoses leading from both branches of branchpoint 4.3. Mildly elevated values of V_D/V_T and $P(a − {\scriptstyle ET})_{CO_2}$, and normal $P(A − a)_{O_2}$ and Pa_{O_2} at maximal exercise suggest the reduced perfusion to ventilated lung seen in moderate to severe heart failure (right branch of branchpoint 4.5). The abnormality in V_D/V_T with normal $P(A − a)_{O_2}$, low $\Delta\dot{V}_{O_2}/$

ΔWR, and low and flat O_2-pulse, are the abnormalities seen with moderate to severe left-sided heart failure. The patient's anemia and carboxyhemoglobinemia may contribute to the abnormality in peripheral oxygenation. The steep heart rate versus $\dot{V}_{O_2}$ relationship and low O_2 pulse noted with increasing work rate is consistent with either a cardiac abnormality, anemia, or a combination of both disorders.

Conclusion

Although the patient has ischemic peripheral arterial disease as documented by angiography, and reflected by his leg pain in response to exercise, the flat O_2 pulse pattern as work rate is increased, the manifestation of a systemic lactic acidosis and the steep heart rate response to exercise suggest that heart failure with anemia, and carboxyhemoglobinemia are dominant factors in the patient's pathophysiology.

Case 33 Hypertensive Cardiovascular Disease and Carboxyhemoglobinemia

Clinical Findings

This 46-year-old current shipyard worker was referred for evaluation of shortness of breath. He complained of chronic cough and sputum production of 8 to 10 years' duration. He dated the shortness of breath to a hospitalization for a leg fracture 6 years before. He had previously abused alcohol and smoked. Physical examination revealed a smooth liver edge 5 cm below the right costal margin without other evidence of liver disease. There were no physical signs of cardiovascular or pulmonary disease. Chest roentgenogram showed small bilateral pleural plaques. ECG showed a left anterior hemiblock.

Exercise Findings

The patient performed exercise on a cycle ergometer. He pedalled at 60 rpm without added load for 3 minutes. The work rate was then increased 20 W per minute to his symptom-limited maximum. Arterial blood was sampled every second minute, and intra-arterial blood pressure was recorded from a percutaneously placed brachial artery catheter. He stopped exercise complaining of shortness of breath and exhaustion. Carboxyhemoglobin level was 7.5% at the start of exercise, suggesting that the patient had recently smoked. There was no chest pain or abnormal ECG changes.

TABLE 9.33.1.   Selected Respiratory Function Data

Measurement	Predicted	Measured
Age, yr		46
Sex		Male
Height, cm		161
Weight, kg	67	70
Hematocrit, %		43
VC, L	3.32	3.23
IC, –	2.22	2.24
TLC, L	4.77	4.77
FEV_1, L	2.65	2.62
FEV_1/VC, %	80	81
MVV, L/min	122	104
D_{CO}, ml/mm Hg/min	22.3	22.1

TABLE 9.33.2.   Selected Exercise Data

Measurement	Predicted	Measured
Peak $\dot{V}O_2$, L/min	2.26	1.17
Maximum HR, beats/min	174	149
Maximum O_2 pulse, ml/beat	13.0	8.1
$\Delta\dot{V}O_2/\Delta WR$, m/min/W	10.3	7.6
AT, L/min	>0.97	0.9
Blood pressure, mmHg (rest, max)		168/108, 228/126
Maximum $\dot{V}E$, L/min		45
Exercise breathing reserve, L/min	>15	59
PaO_2, mmHg (rest, max ex)		93, 101
$P(A - a)O_2$, mmHg (rest, max ex)		12, 21
$P(a - ET)CO_2$, mmHg (rest, max ex)		0, −2
$\dot{V}D/\dot{V}T$ (rest, heavy ex)		0.25, 0.19
HCO_3, mEq/L (rest, 2-min recov)		23, 18

FIGURE 9.33.1.

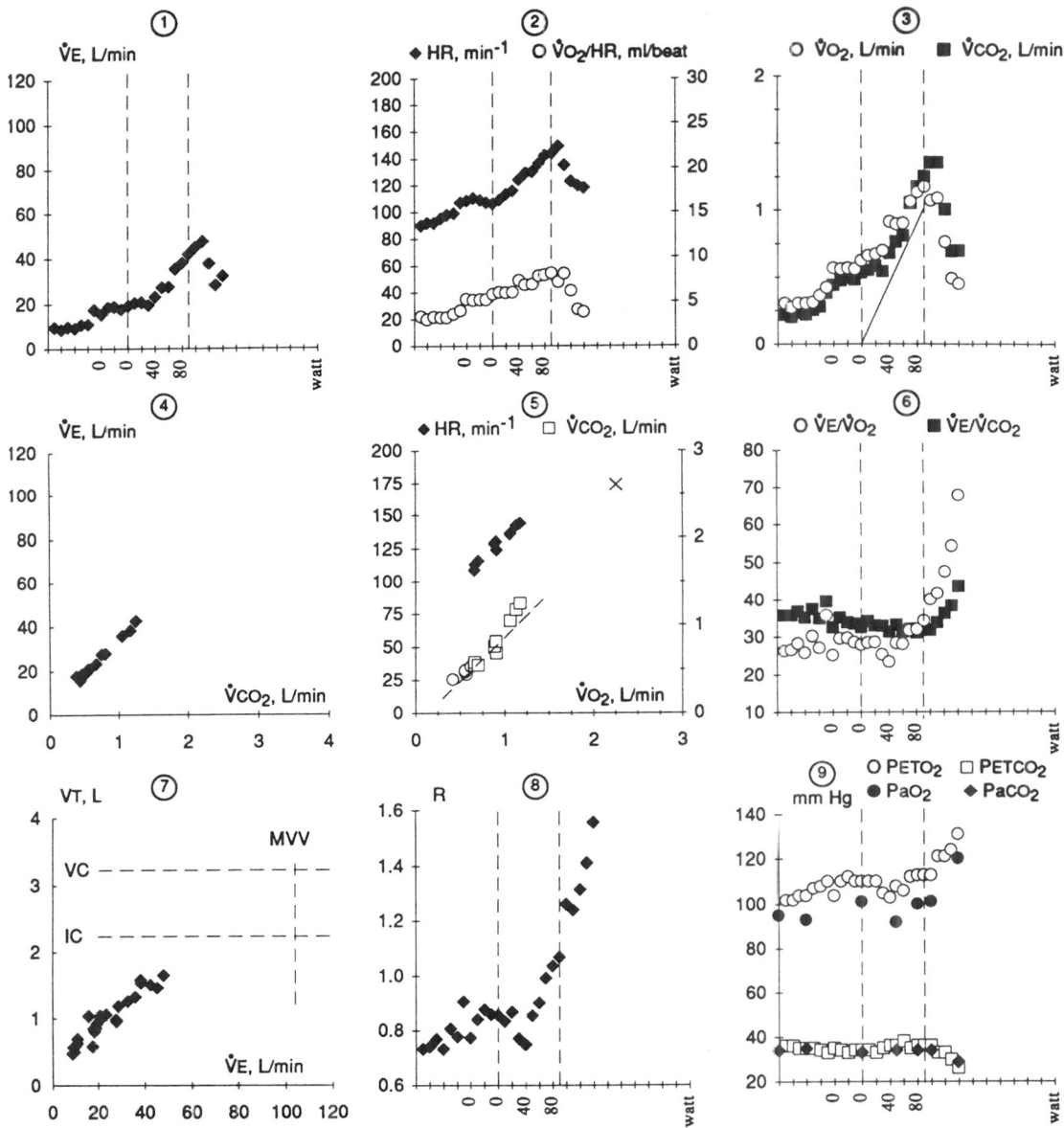

1. Vertical dashed lines in panels 1 to 3 and 6, 8, and 9 indicate the beginning and the end of increasing work period.

2. Unloaded cycling is performed for 3 minutes before the left vertical dashed line.

3. In panel 3, the diagonal line shows the increase of $\dot{V}O_2$ at a slope of 10 ml/min/w.

4. In panel 5, the diagonal dashed line has a slope of 1; the "x" in the upper right is the predicted maximum heart rate and $\dot{V}O_2$ for the subject.

TABLE 9.33.3.   Air Breathing

Time min	Work rate watts	BP mmHg	HR min⁻¹	f min⁻¹	V̇E L/min BTPS	V̇CO₂ L/min STPD	V̇O₂ L/min STPD	V̇O₂/HR ml/beat	R	pH	HCO₃ meq/L	PO₂ ET	PO₂ a	PO₂ (A−a)	PCO₂ ET	PCO₂ a	PCO₂ (a−ET)	V̇E/V̇CO₂	V̇E/V̇O₂	VD/VT
	Rest	168/108								7.44	23		95			34				
	Rest		90	19	9.5	0.22	0.30	3.3	0.73			102			36			36	26	
	Rest		92	18	8.7	0.20	0.27	2.9	0.74			102			36			36	27	
	Rest		92	17	9.9	0.23	0.30	3.3	0.77			104			35			37	28	
	Rest	168/108	95	16	9.1	0.22	0.30	3.2	0.73	7.4	22	104	93	12	35	35	0	35	26	0.25
	Rest		98	17	10.8	0.25	0.31	3.2	0.81			107			35			37	30	
	Rest		99	16	11.1	0.28	0.36	3.6	0.78			108			34			35	27	
	Unloaded		107	30	17.6	0.38	0.42	3.9	0.90			110			33			40	36	
	Unloaded		108	15	15.6	0.44	0.57	5.3	0.77			104			35			33	25	
	Unloaded		110	23	18.5	0.47	0.56	5.1	0.84			110			34			35	30	
	Unloaded		109	22	18.8	0.50	0.57	5.2	0.88			112			33			34	30	
	Unloaded		107	21	17.8	0.48	0.56	5.2	0.86			110			34			33	29	
	Unloaded	186/111	106	21	19.1	0.53	0.62	5.8	0.85	7.45	23	110	101	12	34	33	−1	33	28	0.18
0.5	20		109	21	20.5	0.55	0.66	6.1	0.83			110			34			34	28	
1.0	20		113	20	20.8	0.58	0.67	5.9	0.87			110			33			33	29	
1.5	40		116	21	19.5	0.54	0.70	6.0	0.77			105			35			33	25	
2.0	40		124	22	23.2	0.63	0.91	7.3	0.75			103			36			31	23	
2.5	60	204/120	129	28	27.5	0.76	0.89	6.9	0.85	7.43	22	108	92	19	36	34	−2	33	28	0.21
3.0	60		130	29	27.8	0.81	0.90	6.9	0.90			106			38			31	28	
3.5	80		136	27	35.8	1.05	1.06	7.8	0.99			112			35			32	32	
4.0	80	225/123	142	25	38.3	1.17	1.13	8.0	1.04	7.41	21	113	100	17	36	34	−2	31	32	0.17
4.5	100		144	28	42.4	1.25	1.17	8.1	1.07			113			36			32	34	
	Recovery	228/126	149	31	45.3	1.35	1.07	7.2	1.26	7.40	21	113	101	21	36	34	−2	32	40	0.19
	Recovery		135	29	47.9	1.35	1.09	8.1	1.24			121			33			34	42	
	Recovery		123	24	38.1	1.00	0.76	6.2	1.32			121			33			36	47	
	Recovery		120	24	28.5	0.69	0.49	4.1	1.41			124			30			38	54	
	Recovery	183/111	118	26	32.7	0.70	0.45	3.8	1.56	7.41	18	131	120	9	26	29	3	44	68	0.30

Interpretation

Comments

Respiratory function at rest is normal (Table 9.33.1). Resting ECG is consistent with a left anterior hemiblock.

Analysis

Referring to flow chart 1, the peak V̇O₂ and anaerobic threshold are reduced during exercise (Table 9.33.2). See flow chart 4: The breathing reserve is high (Table 9.33.2) (branchpoint 4.1). The ventilatory equivalent for CO₂ at the anaerobic threshold is normal (see Fig. 9.33.1), and the indices of distribution of ventilation relative to perfusion are normal (branchpoint 4.3), supporting the diagnosis of an O₂ flow problem of non-pulmonary origin. The hematocrit is normal (branchpoint 4.4). The maximum O₂ pulse is re-

duced but increasing (branchpoint 4.6) supporting a diagnosis of peripheral arterial pathophysiology. Confirmatory are a high heart rate reserve, hypertension and a shallow ΔV̇O₂/ΔWR. The patient did not experience chest pain and his ECG remained normal throughout the exercise test.

Conclusion

The patient evidently has exercise intolerance secondary to cardiovascular disease. This is possibly secondary to combined peripheral arterial disease secondary to essential hypertension and failure of the heart to respond adequately to the increased after-load; however, the reduced O₂ capacity of the blood and shift to the left of the oxyhemoglobin dissociation curve, caused by the elevated carboxyhemoglobin concentration, may also contribute to the patient's circulatory dysfunction.

Case 34 Patent Ductus Arteriosus

Clinical Findings

This 25-year-old man recently developed exertional dyspnea. He was found to have a patent ductus arteriosus. Cardiac angiography demonstrated normal coronary arteries, a left ventricular ejection fraction of 56%, a large flow from the aorta through the patent ductus to the pulmonary artery, and normal pulmonary artery pressures at rest. The surgeon desired a pre-operative cycle ergometer study with a pulmonary artery catheter in place to assess pulmonary artery pressures during exercise. The patient was sent to the exercise laboratory with a right radial artery catheter and pulmonary artery catheter placed via the right subclavian vein. Resting 12-lead ECGs showed left atrial enlargement and left ventricular hypertrophy.

Exercise Findings

The patient performed exercise on a cycle ergometer. He pedalled at 60 rpm without an added load for 3 minutes. The work rate was then increased 15 W per minute to tolerance. Intra-arterial pressures were recorded continuously except when blood was simultaneously sampled every 2 minutes from the systemic and pulmonary arterial catheters. The patient stopped exercise because of calf and thigh fatigue. The patient had no chest pain and no further ECG abnormalities.

TABLE 9.34.1. Selected Respiratory Function Data

Measurement	Predicted	Measured
Age, yr		25
Sex		Male
Height, cm		170
Weight, kg	74	56
Hemoglobin, g/100 ml		14.6
VC, L	4.39	4.27
IC, L	2.93	2.42
TLC, L	5.81	6.62
FEV_1, L	3.57	3.62
FEV_1/VC, %	81	85
MVV, L/min	156	158
D_LCO, ml/mm Hg/min	29.6	35.6

TABLE 9.34.2. Selected Exercise Data

Measurement	Predicted	Measured
Peak $\dot{V}O_2$, L/min	2.68	1.68
Maximum HR, beats/min	195	166
Maximum O_2 pulse, ml/beat	13.7	10.1
$\Delta\dot{V}O_2/\Delta WR$, ml/min/W	10.3	8.2
AT, L/min	>1.09	1.0
Systemic blood pressure, mmHg (rest, max)		154/70, 228/105
Pulmonary artery pressure, mmHg (rest, max)		20/10, 30/15
Maximum $\dot{V}E$, L/min		54
Exercise breathing reserve, L/min	>15	104
PaO_2, mmHg (rest, max ex)		103, 95
$P(A - a)O_2$, mmHg (rest, max ex)		6, 17
$P(a - ET)CO_2$, mmHg (rest, max ex)		0, −3
VD/VT (rest, max ex)		0.39, 0.20
HCO_3^-, mEq/L (rest, 2-min recov)		25, 18

FIGURE 9.34.1.

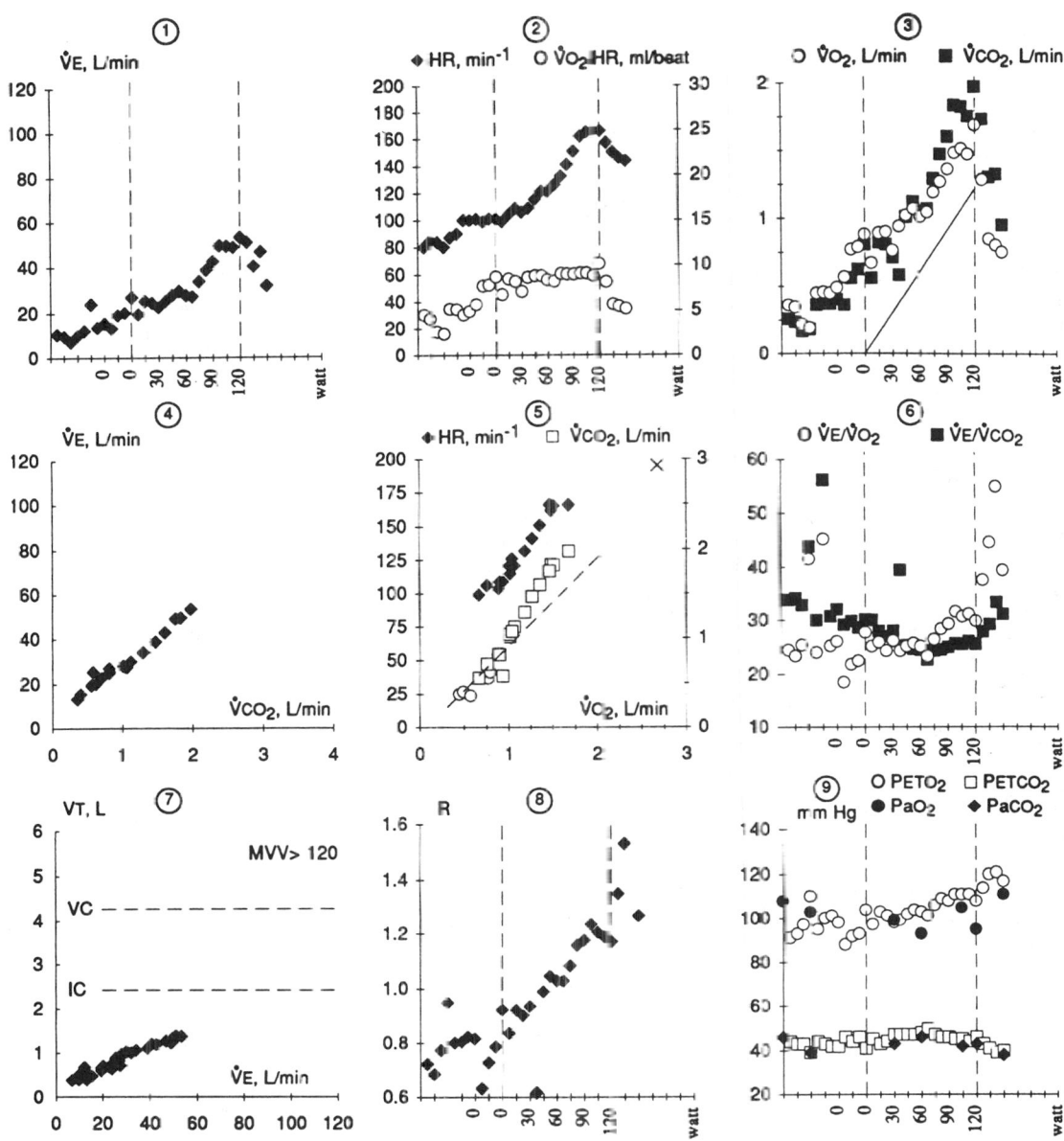

1. Vertical dashed lines in panels 1 to 3 and 6, 8, and 9 indicate the beginning and the end of increasing work period.
2. Unloaded cycling is performed for 3 minutes before the left vertical dashed line.
3. In panel 3, the diagonal line shows the increase of $\dot{V}O_2$ at a slope of 10 ml/min/w.
4. In panel 5, the diagonal dashed line has a slope of 1; the ">" in the upper right is the predicted maximum heart rate and $\dot{V}O_2$ for the subject.

Interpretation

Comments

Resting respiratory function studies were normal with a high normal $D_{L}CO$ suggestive of an increase in pulmonary capillary blood volume. For the level of $\dot{V}O_2$, the left ventricular output at rest and exercise, as calculated from the Fick equation, was considerably elevated. The exercise systemic blood pressure was high, but the pulmonary artery pressure was normal. The breathing reserve was high and gas exchange measures were normal.

TABLE 9.34.3. Air Breathing

Time min	Work rate watts	BP mmHg	HR min⁻¹	f min⁻¹	$\dot{V}_E$ L/min ETPS	$\dot{V}_{CO_2}$ L/min STPD	$\dot{V}_{O_2}$ L/min STPD	$\dot{V}_{O_2}$/HR ml/beat	R	pH	HCO₃⁻ meq/L	PO₂, mmHg ET	a	(A − a)	PCO₂, mmHg ET	a	(a − ET)	$\dot{V}_E$/$\dot{V}_{CO_2}$	$\dot{V}_E$/$\dot{V}_{O_2}$	VD/VT
	Rest	154/69								7.32	23		108			46				
	Rest		80	20	10.5	0.26	0.36	4.5	0.72			91			44			34	24	
	Rest		85	19	9.8	0.24	0.35	4.1	0.69			93			43			34	23	
	Rest		84	18	7.1	0.17	0.22	2.6	0.77			97			43			33	25	
	Rest		80	25	10.0	0.18	0.19	2.4	0.95	7.42	25	110	103	6	39	39	0	44	41	0.39
	Rest	180/87	87	18	12.3	0.36	0.45	5.2	0.80			95			44			30	24	
	Rest		90	37	23.9	0.37	0.46	5.1	0.80			100			43			56	45	
	Unloaded		100	25	13.5	0.37	0.45	4.5	0.82			101			42			31	25	
	Unloaded		100	32	15.5	0.40	0.49	4.9	0.82			98			42			32	26	
	Unloaded		101	33	13.3	0.36	0.57	5.6	0.63			88			46			29	18	
	Unloaded		99	29	19.2	0.56	0.77	7.8	0.73			92			44			30	22	
	Unloaded		101	29	20.2	0.62	0.79	7.8	0.78			93			46			29	22	
	Unloaded		101	33	27.1	0.81	0.88	8.7	0.92			104			41			30	28	
0.5	15		99	32	19.5	0.56	0.67	6.8	0.84			97			45			30	25	
1.0	15		104	29	25.4	0.82	0.89	8.6	0.92			103			43			28	26	
1.5	30		109	33	24.7	0.81	0.90	8.3	0.90			101			44			27	24	
2.0	30	222/102	106	33	22.7	0.71	0.76	7.2	0.93	7.39	26	98	99	6	47	43	−4	28	26	0.25
2.5	45		109	30	25.4	0.58	0.94	8.6	0.62			99			47			39	24	
3.0	45		115	29	28.0	1.01	1.02	8.9	0.99			102			47			25	25	
3.5	60		121	29	30.0	1.12	1.07	8.8	1.05			104			47			25	26	
4.0	60	231/96	121	30	27.9	1.04	1.01	8.3	1.03	7.35	25	103	93	12	48	46	−2	24	25	0.21
4.5	75		126	38	27.4	1.07	1.04	8.3	1.03			101			50			23	23	
5.0	75		132	32	34.1	1.29	1.19	9.0	1.08			106			47			24	26	
5.5	90		141	35	38.9	1.47	1.27	9.0	1.16			109			46			24	28	
6.0	90		151	36	42.8	1.60	1.36	9.0	1.18			108			46			25	29	
6.5	105		162	37	49.8	1.83	1.48	9.1	1.24			111			45			25	32	
7.0	105	246/108	165	40	49.6	1.82	1.51	9.2	1.21	7.34	22	111	105	9	45	42	−3	25	31	0.18
7.5	120		166	40	49.0	1.75	1.47	8.9	1.19			111			44			26	31	
8.0	120	228/105	166	39	53.5	1.97	1.68	10.1	1.17	7.30	21	108	95	17	46	43	−3	25	30	0.20
	Recovery		157	37	51.1	1.73	1.28	8.2	1.35			114			43			28	37	
	Recovery		150	34	40.8	1.30	0.85	5.7	1.53			120			41			29	45	
	Recovery		146	37	47.0	1.32	0.80	5.5	1.65			121			39			33	55	
	Recovery	171/90	144	32	32.2	0.95	0.75	5.2	1.27	7.29	18	117	111	7	40	38	−2	31	39	0.25

Analysis

Referring to flow chart 1, peak $\dot{V}_{O_2}$ and the anaerobic threshold are decreased. If one goes next to flow chart 4, the high breathing reserve (branchpoint 4.1), normal $\dot{V}_E/\dot{V}_{CO_2}$ (branchpoint 4.3), normal hematocrit (branchpoint 4.4), and low, unchanging O_2 pulse (branchpoint 4.6) lead us to the diagnosis of heart disease. The ECG does not show evidence of myocardial ischemia, but the low $\Delta\dot{V}_{O_2}/\Delta WR$ and steep HR versus $\dot{V}_{O_2}$ response confirm the presence of cardiovascular dysfunction.

Conclusion

The patient's large left to right shunt through the patent ductus arteriosus requires an increased left ventricular output to support the peripheral O_2 requirements. Thus, while the left ventricular output is high, the recirculation of part of it through the lungs deprives the peripheral tissues of the O_2 they need. Thus the pathophysiology is similar to left ventricular failure with a low anaerobic threshold and peak $\dot{V}_{O_2}$. In addition, the noninvasively measured low and relatively unchanging O_2 pulse throughout incremental exercise indicates that the patient reached a maximum product of stroke volume and arterial-mixed venous O_2 difference early in the exercise study. Presumably, by removing the pulmonary steal of systemic blood flow by closing the ductus, these abnormalities would be corrected. Following surgical correction of the patent ductus arteriosus, the patient's dyspnea and exercise tolerance improved considerably.

Case 35 Vasoregulatory Asthenia

Clinical Findings

This 31-year-old woman was referred for exercise testing because of the insidious and progressive fatigability of 10 months' duration. She had formerly been active as a homemaker, had worked frequent 12-hour shifts as an ICU nurse, and had done 2 to 3 hours of vigorous exercise daily. At this time, she recognized dyspnea on walking two blocks and often experienced rapid, forceful palpitations with exertion or emotion. Her sleep requirements had increased markedly and she had gained 17 pounds in weight. She frequently woke from sleep diaphoretic and with palpitations, but did not snore. She had had hypertension only during her two pregnancies. She did not smoke or use drugs. Work-up elsewhere revealed a normal physical examination, chest roentgenograms, ECG, spirometry, echocardiograms, ejection fraction, resting blood gases, and thyroid function. Exercise studies elsewhere, including cardiac catheterization, showed tachycardia, normal ear oximetry, normal right- and left-sided arterial pressures, and a high mixed venous PO_2 during exercise. Examination here revealed a healthy-looking, animated woman with resting tachycardia and normal peripheral pulses. The oxyhemoglobin dissociation curve was normal, as assessed by measuring the P_{50}.

Exercise Findings

The patient performed exercise on a cycle ergometer. She pedalled at 60 rpm without an added load for 3 minutes. The work rate was then increased 15 W per minute to tolerance. Heart rate and rhythm were continuously monitored; 12-lead ECGs were obtained during rest, exercise, and recovery. Blood pressure was measured with a sphygmomanometer and oxygen saturation with an ear oximeter. The patient appeared to give an excellent effort and stopped exercise because of generalized and thigh fatigue. She denied chest pain during or after the study. No arrhythmias or ischemic changes were noted on ECGs.

TABLE 9.35.1.   Selected Respiratory Function Data

Measurement	Predicted	Measured
Age, yr		31
Sex		Female
Height, cm		167
Weight, kg	66	63
Hematocrit, %		40
VC, L	3.75	4.81
IC, L	2.50	3.34
TLC, L	5.51	6.64
FEV$_1$, L	3.08	4.27
FEV$_1$/VC, %	82	89
MVV, L/min	116	146
D$_L$CO, ml/mm Hg/min	27.7	28.8

TABLE 9.35.2.   Selected Exercise Data

Measurement	Predicted	Measured
Peak $\dot{V}O_2$, L/min	1.88	1.73
Maximum HR, beats/min	189	195
Maximum O_2 pulse, ml/beat	10.1	8.9
$\Delta\dot{V}O_2/\Delta WR$, ml/min/W	10.3	10.3
AT L/min	>0.86	0.8
Blood pressure, mmHg (rest, max)		155/90, 155/90
Maximum $\dot{V}E$, L/min		67
Exercise breathing reserve, L/min	>15	79
O_2 saturation, oximeter (rest, max)		99,100

FIGURE 9.35.1.

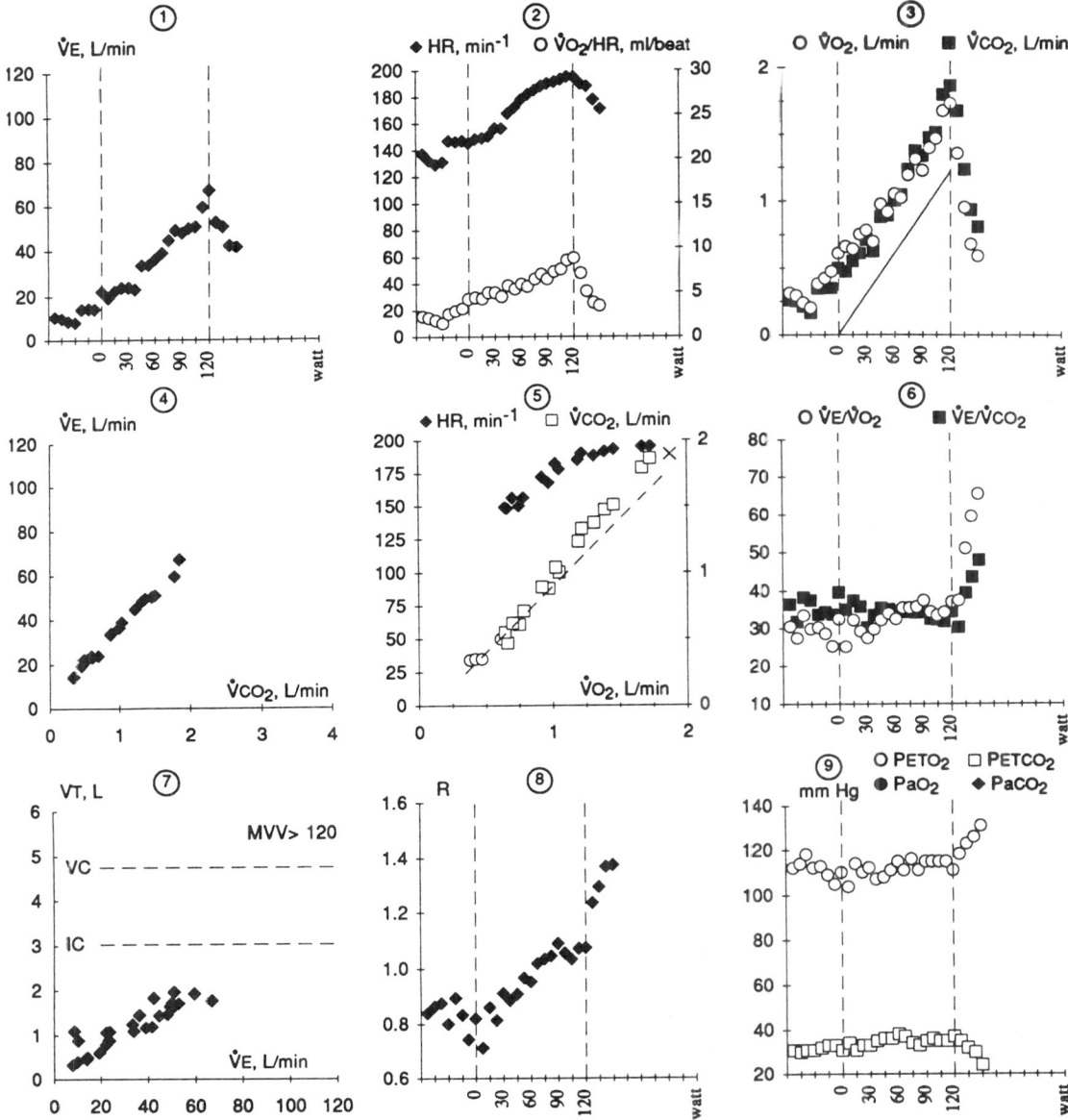

1. Vertical dashed lines in panels 1 to 3 and 6, 8, and 9 indicate the beginning and the end of increasing work period.

2. Unloaded cycling is performed for 3 minutes before the left vertical dashed line.

3. In panel 3, the diagonal line shows the increase of $\dot{V}O_2$ at a slope of 10 ml/min/w.

4. In panel 5, the diagonal dashed line has a slope of 1; the "x" in the upper right is the predicted maximum heart rate and $\dot{V}O_2$ for the subject.

TABLE 9.35.3. Air Breathing

Time min	Work rate watts	BP mmHg	HP min⁻¹	f min⁻¹	V̇E L/min BTPS	V̇CO₂ L/min STPD	V̇O₂ L/min STPD	V̇O₂/HR ml/beat	R	pH	HCO₃ meq/L	PO₂, mmHg ET	ē	(A − a)	PCO₂, mmHg ET	a	(a − ET)	V̇E/V̇CO₂	V̇E/V̇O₂	VD/VT
	Rest	115/90	137	12	10.5	0.26	0.31	2.3	0.84			112			31			36	31	
	Rest		132	25	10.1	0.25	0.29	2.2	0.88			114			30			32	28	
	Rest		129	8	8.7	0.21	0.24	1.9	0.85			118			31			38	33	
	Rest		131	25	8.1	0.16	0.20	1.5	0.80			112			31			37	30	
	Unloaded		147	31	14.1	0.34	0.38	2.6	0.89			113			32			34	30	
	Unloaded		146	29	14.5	0.35	0.42	2.9	0.83			109			33			34	29	
	Unloaded		147	28	14.2	0.35	0.47	3.2	0.74			105			33			34	25	
	Unloaded	140/95	145	28	22.1	0.50	0.61	4.2	0.82			110			31			39	32	
0.5	15		148	32	19.2	0.47	0.66	4.5	0.71			104			34			35	25	
1.0	15		149	21	22.3	0.55	0.64	4.3	0.86			114			31			37	32	
1.5	30		150	22	23.7	0.61	0.75	5.0	0.81			113			33			36	29	
2.0	30		156	27	23.7	0.71	0.78	5.0	0.91			112			33			30	27	
2.5	45		156	26	23.0	0.62	0.70	4.5	0.89			107			35			34	30	
3.0	45		168	27	33.4	0.88	0.97	5.8	0.91			108			36			35	32	
3.5	60		172	31	33.8	0.89	0.92	5.3	0.97			111			36			35	34	
4.0	60	155/90	178	25	36.3	1.00	1.05	5.9	0.95			115			38			34	33	
4.5	75		182	33	38.9	1.04	1.02	5.6	1.02			111			37			35	35	
5.0	75		185	31	44.7	1.23	1.19	6.4	1.03			116			34			34	35	
5.5	90		188	30	49.2	1.37	1.31	7.0	1.05			111			33			34	36	
6.0	90		190	33	48.2	1.33	1.22	6.4	1.09			115			35			34	37	
6.5	105		191	29	50.1	1.47	1.39	7.3	1.06			115			36			32	34	
7.0	105		193	26	51.0	1.51	1.46	7.6	1.03			115			35			32	33	
7.5	120		195	31	59.7	1.79	1.67	8.6	1.07			115			35			32	34	
8.0	120		195	38	67.1	1.86	1.73	8.9	1.08			111			37			34	37	
	Recovery		190	31	53.0	1.67	1.35	7.1	1.24			118			35			30	37	
	Recovery		188	31	50.9	1.23	0.95	5.1	1.29			123			32			39	51	
	Recovery		178	23	42.3	0.93	0.68	3.8	1.37			126			30			43	59	
	Recovery	125/60	171	35	41.6	0.81	0.59	3.5	1.37			131			24			48	65	

Interpretation

Comments

Resting respiratory function studies were better than average.

Analysis

Referring to flow chart 1, the peak V̇C₂ is normal for a sedentary person (which this patient is not), but the anaerobic threshold is low (Table 9.35.2). We are directed through branchpoints 1.1, 1.2, and 1.3 to flow chart 4. The breathing reserve was high (branchpoint 4.1). The V̇E/V̇CO₂ at the anaerobic threshold is borderline elevated, but the PETCO₂ is reduced suggesting hyperventilation. If we take the normal branch for V̇E/V̇CO₂ at AT, we go to the diagnosis labelled "O₂ flow problem of non-pulmonary origin." We are moderately confident that the patient does not have appreciable widening of the P(A − a)O₂ because of the normal ear oximetry. The hematocrit is normal (branchpoint 4.4). The O₂ pulse is not low and nonchanging (branchpoint 4.6), leading us to the diagnosis of "peripheral arterial disease." This does not fit this patient well, considering her resting tachycardia, negative heart rate reserve, absence of hypertension, and good peripheral pulses. Exploring further, she does not fit the diagnosis of "anemia" or "heart disease," but she does have a steep HR versus V̇O₂ and a low heart rate reserve. Knowing from prior studies that she did not have a low mixed venous PO₂ during heavy exercise, we can presume that the exercising muscles have difficulty extracting oxygen from their capillaries. These findings fit the diagnosis of vasoregulatory asthenia (1–3), which appears to be characterized by an inability to vasodilate the exercising muscle vascular beds and to vasoconstrict non-exercising organs. This may represent a specific defect in the autonomic nervous system.

Conclusion

The patient's findings were consistent with vaso-regulatory asthenia, but follow-up evaluation was recommended. The patient was placed on a physical training program with some objective and subjective improvement in exercise tolerance, but there was no improvement with β-adrenergic blockade. As the pathophysiologic mechanisms underlying vasoregulatory asthenia are unclear, a subsequent exercise test was performed in which serial venous blood samples were drawn. Blood lactate levels were markedly increased during exercise (reaching a peak of 8.2 mEq/L), ruling out McArdle's syndrome (4) as the cause of her exercise intolerance. Other muscle disorders (e.g., electron transport chain defects) were not excluded, however (5, 6). This disorder may be due to autonomic dysfunction of the peripheral circulation (1–3).

References

1. Holmgren A, Jonsson B, Levander M, et al. Low physical work capacity in suspected heart cases due to inadequate adjustment of peripheral blood flow (vasoregulatory asthenia). Acta Med Scand 1957;158:413–436.
2. Holmgren A, Jonsson B, Levander M, et al. Physical training of patients with vasoregulatory asthenia. Acta Med Scand 1957;158:437–446.
3. Gillum RF, Teichholz LE, Herman MV, et al. The idiopathic hyperkinetic heart syndrome: clinical course and long-term prognosis. Am Heart J 1981;102:728–734.
4. McArdle B. Myopathy due to a defect in muscle glycogen breakdown. Clin Sci 1951;10:13–18.
5. Carroll JE, Hagberg JH, Brooke MH, et al. Bicycle ergometry and gas exchange measurements in neuromuscular diseases. Arch Neurol 1979;36:457–461.
6. DiMauro S, Bonilla E, Zevina M, et al. Mitochondrial myopathies. Ann Neurol 1985;17:521–538.

Case 36 Chronic Bronchitis, Mild, with Normal Exercise Performance

Clinical Findings

This 55-year-old shipyard worker complained of dyspnea after walking up one flight of stairs or a few blocks on a level surface. He had had morning cough several months of each year and had noted occasional retrosternal pain unrelated to exertion or emotional upset. He had 35 pack years of smoking until stopping 12 years ago. He exercised regularly. The physical examination was normal except for mild obesity. Chest x-ray studies showed bilateral pleural thickening in the mid lung zones and old granulomatous disease in the right upper lobe. Resting ECG was normal.

Exercise Findings

The patient performed exercise on a cycle ergometer. He first pedalled at 60 rpm, without added load, for 3 minutes. The work rate was then increased 20 W per minute to his symptom-limited maximum. Arterial blood was sampled every second minute and intra-arterial blood pressure was recorded from a percutaneously placed brachial artery catheter. The patient stopped exercise because of "exhaustion." ECG remained normal throughout exercise.

TABLE 9.36.1. Selected Respiratory Function Data

Measurement	Predicted	Measured
Age, yr		54
Sex		Male
Height, cm		174
Weight, kg	77	88
Hematocrit, %		45
VC, L	4.28	3.59
IC, L	2.86	3.12
TLC, L	6.38	6.15
FEV_1, L	3.39	2.40
FEV_1/VC, %	79	67
MVV, L/min	142	112
D_{CO}, ml/mm Hg/min	28.8	29.8

TABLE 9.36.2. Selected Exercise Data

Measurement	Predicted	Measured
Peak $\dot{V}O_2$, L/min	2.42	2.66
Maximum HR, beats/min	136	169
Maximum O_2 pulse, ml/beat	14.6	15.7
$\Delta \dot{V}O_2/\Delta WR$, ml/min/W	10.3	9.9
AT, L/min	>1.04	1.3
Blood pressure, mmHg (rest, max)		144/93, 225/117
Maximum $\dot{V}E$, L/min		86
Exercise breathing reserve, L/min	>15	26
PO_2, mmHg (rest, max ex)		81, 92
$P(a - a)O_2$, mmHg (rest, max ex)		18, 21
$P(a - ET)CO_2$, mmHg (rest, max ex)		5, −3
VD/VT (rest, heavy ex)		0.41, 0.23
HCO_3^-, mEq/L (rest, 2-min recov)		26, 16

Figure 9.36.1.

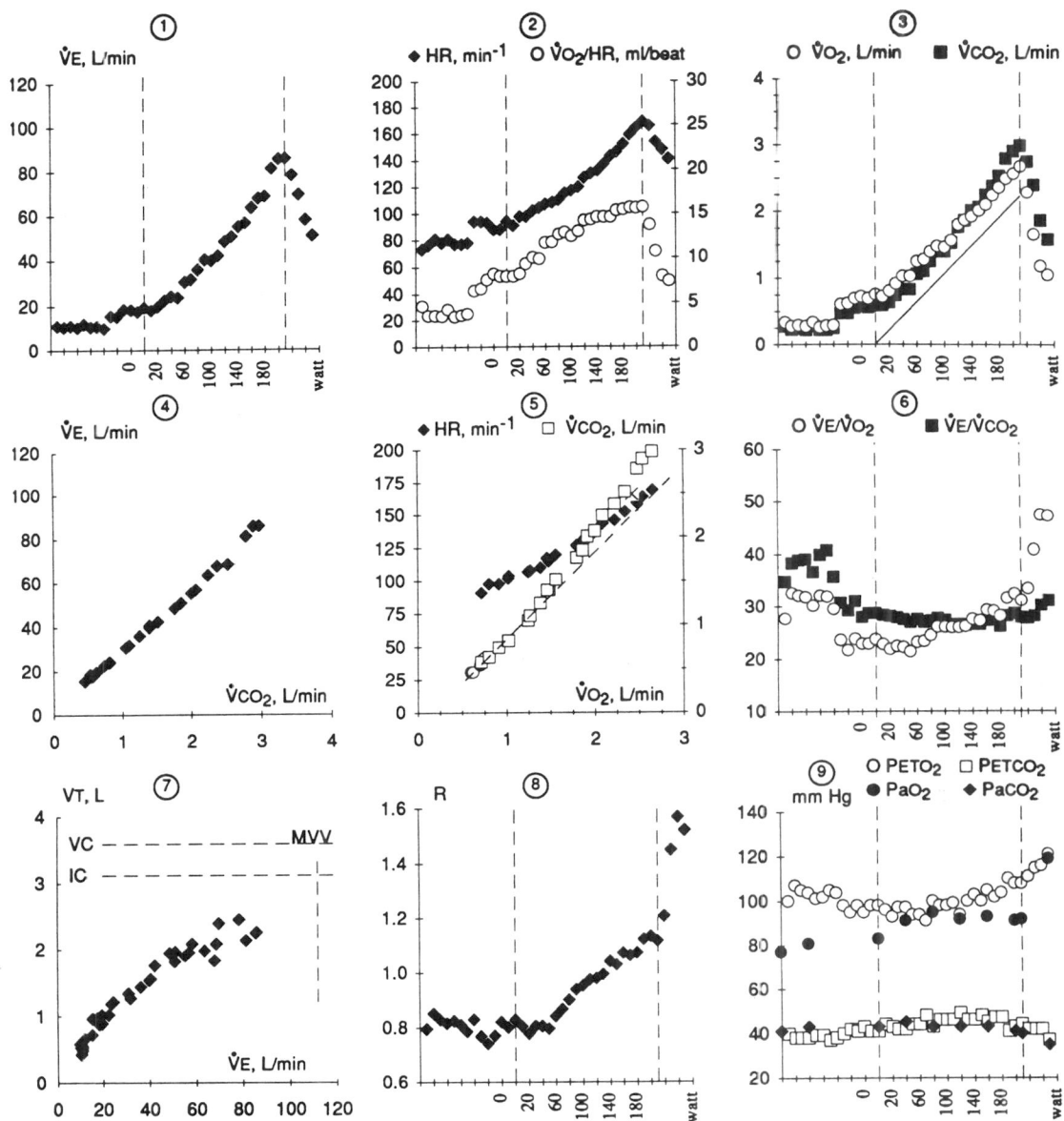

1. Vertical dashed lines in panels 1 to 3 and 6, 8, and 9 indicate the beginning and the end of increasing work period.

2. Unloaded cycling is performed for 3 minutes before the left vertical dashed line.

3. In panel 3, the diagonal line shows the increase of $\dot{V}O_2$ at a slope of 10 ml/min/w.

4. In panel 5, the diagonal dashed line has a slope of 1; the "x" in the upper right is the predicted maximum heart rate and $\dot{V}O_2$ for the subject.

TABLE 9.36.3. Air Breathing

Time min	Work rate watts	BP mmHg	HR min⁻¹	f min⁻¹	V̇E L/min BTPS	V̇CO₂ L/min STPD	V̇O₂ L/min STPD	V̇O₂/HR ml/beat	R	pH	HCO₃⁻ meq/L	PO₂ ET	PO₂ a	PO₂ (a−a)	PCO₂ ET	PCO₂ a	PCO₂ (a−ET)	V̇E/V̇CO₂	V̇E/V̇O₂	VD/VT
	Rest	141/93								7.43	26		77			41				
	Rest		73	20	11.1	0.27	0.34	4.7	0.79			100			40			35	28	
	Rest		73	20	10.5	0.23	0.27	3.6	0.85			107			38			38	33	
	Rest		81	21	11.1	0.24	0.29	3.6	0.83			105			38			39	32	
	Rest	144/90	73	19	10.2	0.22	0.27	3.5	0.81	7.40	26	104	91	18	38	43	5	39	32	0.41
	Rest		81	18	11.8	0.28	0.34	4.2	0.82			101			39			37	30	
	Rest		77	24	10.4	0.21	0.26	3.4	0.81			102			39			40	32	
	Rest		77	22	10.8	0.22	0.28	3.6	0.79			105			37			41	32	
	Rest		78	17	10.0	0.24	0.29	3.7	0.83			104			38			36	30	
	Unloaded		94	16	15.5	0.46	0.60	6.4	0.77			98			40			31	24	
	Unloaded		94	21	15.2	0.46	0.62	6.6	0.74			95			42			29	22	
	Unloaded		93	21	18.5	0.54	0.70	7.5	0.77			98			41			31	24	
	Unloaded		88	20	18.2	0.59	0.72	8.2	0.82			95			43			28	23	
	Unloaded		88	18	17.6	0.56	0.70	8.0	0.80			98			41			29	23	
	Unloaded	162/99	94	19	19.4	0.62	0.75	8.0	0.83	7.39	26	98	83	17	41	43	2	29	24	0.28
0.5	20		91	19	18.0	0.58	0.72	7.9	0.81			96			44			28	23	
1.0	20		98	22	19.6	0.63	0.81	8.3	0.78			93			43			28	22	
1.5	40		98	22	22.5	0.74	0.92	9.4	0.80			97			42			28	22	
2.0	40	174/96	102	20	24.3	0.82	1.02	10.0	0.80	7.37	26	97	91	5	42	45	3	28	22	0.28
2.5	60		104	20	23.8	0.82	1.03	9.9	0.80			94			44			27	21	
3.0	60		107	23	30.9	1.05	1.25	11.7	0.84			94			44			28	23	
3.5	80		108	25	31.8	1.10	1.27	11.8	0.87			91			48			27	23	
4.0	80	174/93	110	25	36.1	1.25	1.39	12.6	0.90	7.37	24	100	95	8	43	43	0	27	24	0.25
4.5	100		115	26	40.6	1.39	1.48	12.9	0.94			98			46			28	26	
5.0	100		117	26	40.1	1.39	1.46	12.5	0.95			98			46			27	26	
5.5	120		120	24	42.4	1.52	1.56	13.0	0.97			99			46			27	26	
6.0	120	204/99	127	25	48.7	1.76	1.80	14.2	0.98	7.36	24	94	92	14	49	43	−6	26	26	0.23
6.5	140		130	28	51.0	1.85	1.86	14.3	0.99			100			46			26	26	
7.0	140		132	29	55.4	2.00	1.92	14.5	1.04			103			46			26	28	
7.5	160		137	29	56.9	2.06	2.00	14.6	1.03			100			48			26	27	
8.0	160	210/105	143	32	63.7	2.24	2.09	14.6	1.07	7.35	23	105	93	16	45	43	−2	27	29	0.25
8.5	180		146	37	67.9	2.37	2.23	15.3	1.06			102			47			27	29	
9.0	180		152	33	68.8	2.52	2.35	15.5	1.07			104			47			26	28	
9.5	200		159	38	81.4	2.78	2.48	15.6	1.12			110			41			28	32	
10.0	200	228/114	164	38	85.7	2.89	2.55	15.5	1.13	7.33	21	108	91	22	43	41	−2	29	32	0.25
10.5	220	225/117	169	38	86.0	2.97	2.66	15.7	1.12	7.31	20	108	92	21	44	40	−4	28	31	0.22
	Recovery		166	32	78.5	2.74	2.27	13.7	1.21			111			42			28	33	
	Recovery		154	29	69.7	2.39	1.65	10.7	1.45			115			42			28	41	
	Recovery		148	28	58.3	1.85	1.18	8.0	1.57			116			42			30	47	
	Recovery	183/96	141	26	51.2	1.58	1.04	7.4	1.52	7.27	16	121	119	5	37	35	−2	31	47	0.20

Interpretation
Comments

Resting respiratory function is compatible with mild airflow obstruction (Table 9.36.1). The resting ECG is normal.

Analysis

Referring to flow chart 1, the peak oxygen uptake and anaerobic threshold are normal (Table 9.36.2). See flow chart 2: Arterial blood gases and ECG at peak V̇O₂ are normal (branchpoint 2.1). The patient is about 14% overweight (branchpoint 2.2). This is not a serious obesity problem but does contribute toward the additional metabolic cost of work. The patient also has mild airflow obstruction, however, causing a characteristic obstructive pattern at high exercise levels.

Conclusion

This study illustrates normal exercise performance in a mildly obese man with airflow obstruction.

Case 37 Chronic Bronchitis and Obesity

Clinical Findings

This 69-year-old former shipyard worker had first noted dyspnea on exertion 16 years earlier, later accompanied by cough, sputum production, and frequent wheezing. He had been receiving bronchodilators and antibiotics intermittently for 16 years. Physical examination revealed obesity, bilaterally decreased breath sounds, and some expiratory wheezes. There was no evidence of cardiovascular disease. Chest x-ray study revealed moderate pleural thickening bilaterally and scattered parenchymal calcifications compatible with inactive granulomatous disease. The heart was not enlarged. ECG was compatible with left atrial enlargement and left ventricular hypertrophy. He admitted to a 15 pack year history of cigarette smoking.

Exercise Findings

The patient performed exercise on a cycle ergometer. He first pedalled at 60 rpm, without added load, for 3 minutes. The work rate was then increased 10 W per minute to his symptom-limited maximum. Arterial blood was sampled every second minute, and intra-arterial blood pressure was recorded from a percutaneously placed brachial artery catheter. The patient stopped exercising complaining of shortness of breath and chest tightness. There were no ST segment changes or arrhythmia.

TABLE 9.37.1. Selected Respiratory Function Data

Measurement	Predicted	Measured
Age, yr		69
Sex		Male
Height, cm		166
Weight, kg	70	98
Hematocrit, %		45
VC, L	3.31	2.91 (2.15*)
IC, L	2.21	2.35 (1.89*)
TLC, L	5.38	7.32
FEV_1, L	2.55	1.47 (1.30*)
FEV_1/VC, %	77	51 (60*)
MVV, L/min	112	56 (44*)
$D_{L}CO$, ml/mm Hg/min	22.6	26.0

* On day of exercise study.

TABLE 9.37.2. Selected Exercise Data

Measurement	Predicted	Measured
Peak $\dot{V}O_2$, L/min	1.93	1.50
Maximum HR, beats/min	151	125
Maximum O_2 pulse, ml/beat	12.8	12.0
$\Delta\dot{V}O_2/\Delta WR$, ml/min/W	10.3	10.4
AT, L/min	>0.87	1.35
Blood pressure, mmHg (rest, max)		142/72, 234/99
Maximum $\dot{V}E$, L/min		55
Exercise breathing reserve, L/min	>15	1
PaO_2, mmHg (rest, max ex)		73, 92
$P(A - a)O_2$, mmHg (rest, max ex)		32, 17
$P(a - ET)CO_2$, mmHg (rest, max ex)		6, 1
VD/VT (rest, heavy ex)		0.40, 0.35
HCO_3^-, mEq/L (rest, 2-min recov)		26, 22

TABLE 9.37.3. Air Breathing

Time min	Work rate watts	BP mmHg	HR min⁻¹	f min⁻¹	V̇E L/min BTPS	V̇CO₂ L/min STPD	V̇O₂ L/min STPD	V̇O₂/HR ml/beat	R	pH	HCO₃⁻ meq/L	PO₂ ET	PO₂ a	PO₂ (A−a)	PCO₂ ET	PCO₂ a	PCO₂ (a−ET)	V̇E/V̇CO₂	V̇E/V̇O₂	VD/VT
	Rest	142/72								7.40	26		75			43				
	Rest		78	24	12.4	0.27	0.35	4.5	0.77			103			36			38	30	
	Rest		76	18	10.7	0.27	0.36	4.7	0.75			100			39			34	25	
	Rest		79	24	11.4	0.23	0.30	3.8	0.77			100			38			41	31	
	Rest	156/81	77	21	12.8	0.27	0.31	4.0	0.87	7.42	25	110	73	32	34	40	6	41	36	0.41
	Rest		79	21	13.3	0.30	0.35	4.4	0.86			109			34			38	33	
	Rest		80	22	12.9	0.24	0.28	3.5	0.86			110			34			46	39	
	Unloaded		90	36	18.0	0.29	0.38	4.2	0.76			107			34			52	39	
	Unloaded		98	50	28.0	0.53	0.66	6.7	0.80			108			34			45	36	
	Unloaded		98	56	29.5	0.57	0.65	6.6	0.85			101			40			43	38	
	Unloaded		101	43	31.8	0.79	0.89	8.8	0.89			99			42			36	32	
	Unloaded		104	49	29.1	0.69	0.77	7.4	0.90			107			38			36	32	
	Unloaded	198/93	105	47	34.6	0.76	0.85	8.1	0.89	7.40	26	106	82	22	39	42	3	40	36	0.43
0.5	10		102	55	41.2	0.90	0.96	9.4	0.94			110			36			41	38	
1.0	10		103	53	37.6	0.85	0.93	9.0	0.97			107			38			39	36	
1.5	20		105	58	46.3	0.98	0.99	9.4	0.99			114			34			42	42	
2.0	20	204/87	107	47	34.5	0.82	0.91	8.5	0.90	7.37	26	106	84	17	40	45	5	37	34	0.43
2.5	30		108	40	36.6	0.94	1.05	9.7	0.90			104			40			35	32	
3.0	30		109	50	39.8	0.95	1.05	9.6	0.90			105			39			37	34	
3.5	40		109	45	40.1	1.02	1.16	10.6	0.88			106			38			36	31	
4.0	40	207/87	110	46	42.2	1.11	1.28	11.6	0.87	7.38	24	106	80	23	38	42	4	34	30	0.37
4.5	50		113	47	42.1	1.09	1.23	10.9	0.89			105			39			35	31	
5.0	50		114	44	38.7	1.02	1.16	10.2	0.88			103			41			34	30	
5.5	60		117	45	47.1	1.25	1.39	11.9	0.91			107			39			34	31	
6.0	60	219/90	120	54	48.3	1.24	1.34	11.2	0.93	7.36	23	107	87	22	39	39	0	35	33	0.34
6.5	70		124	49	53.0	1.33	1.45	11.7	0.95			108			39			35	34	
7.0	70	234/99	125	50	55.0	1.43	1.50	12.0	0.95	7.37	22	110	92	17	38	39	1	35	34	0.35
	Recovery		128	59	51.3	1.50	1.51	11.8	0.99			109			38			31	31	
	Recovery		117	41	47.1	1.30	1.30	11.1	1.00			112			37			34	34	
	Recovery		117	52	48.5	1.20	1.22	10.4	0.98			112			36			37	36	
	Recovery		110	51	45.1	0.93	0.94	8.5	1.04			113			36			42	43	
	Recovery	204/84	107	42	31.0	0.61	0.56	5.2	1.09	7.37	22	115	95	19	36	39	3	45	49	0.45

Interpretation

Comments

Respiratory function studies indicate that this patient has a moderate obstructive defect (Table 9.37.1). The ECG is interpreted to demonstrate left ventricular hypertrophy and left atrial enlargement.

Analysis

Referring to flow chart 1, peak V̇O₂ is low and anaerobic threshold is normal. See flow chart 3: The breathing reserve is low (branchpoint 3.1) suggesting that lung disease accounts for this patient's reduced exercise performance. Supporting this is

the finding that the indices of ventilation-perfusion matching (VD/VT, P(A − a)O₂ and P(a − ET)CO₂) are abnormal and the heart rate reserve is high.

The actual maximum work rate performed by the patient is quite low, despite a mildly reduced peak V̇O₂, because the patient has an exceptionally high oxygen cost for unloaded cycling (V̇O₂ = .85 L/min). This is most likely due to his obesity (added metabolic cost of moving his lower extremities). The fall in P(A − a)O₂ and rise in PaO₂, when changing activity from rest to exercise, suggest that the resting hypoxemia in this patient is attributable to obesity-related basilar micro-atelectasis at rest that disappears with the increased ventilation accompanying exercise.

The elevated dead space fraction of the tidal vol-

FIGURE 9.37.1.

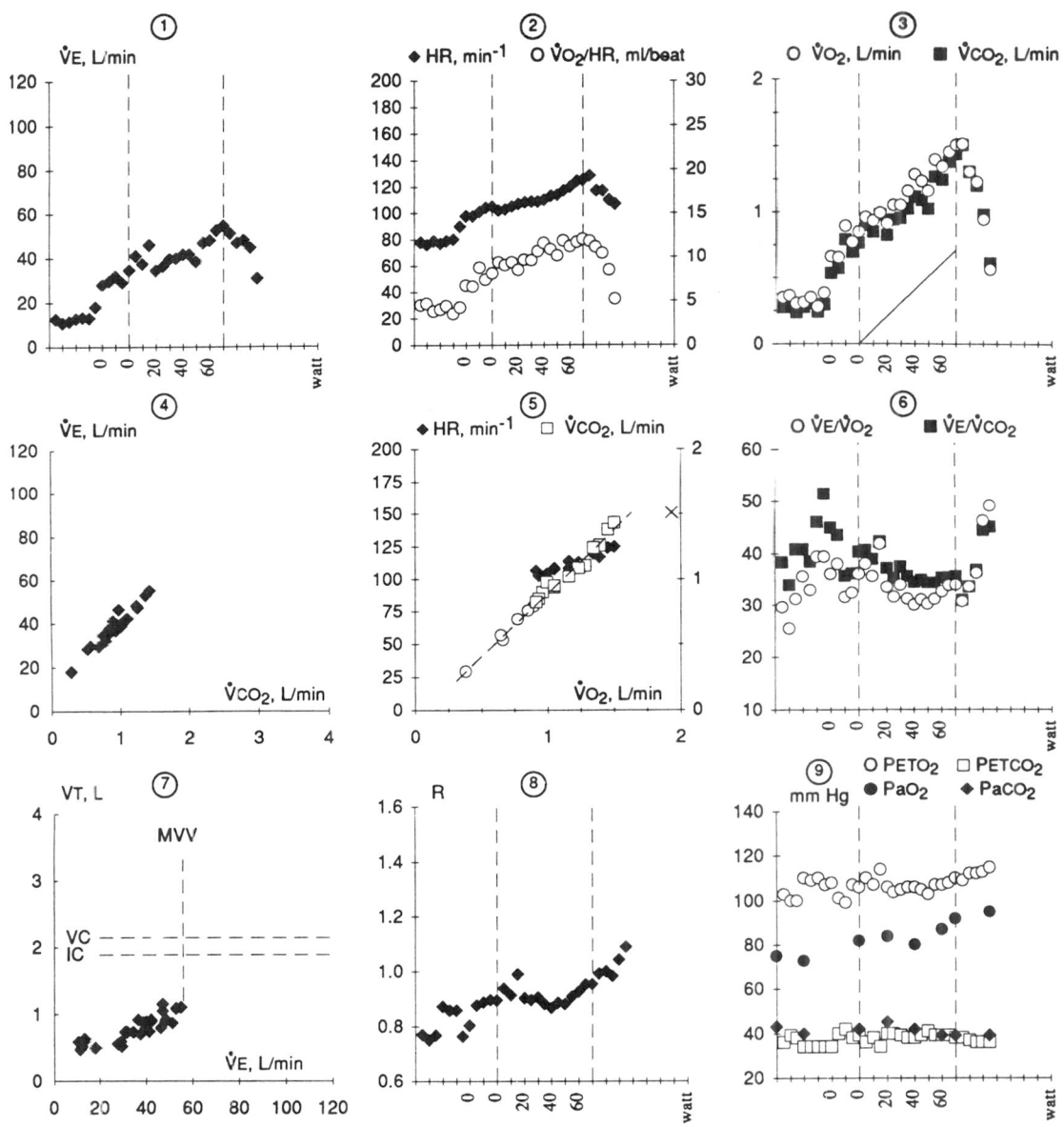

1. Vertical dashed lines in panels 1 to 3 and 6, 8, and 9 indicate the beginning and the end of increasing work period.
2. Unloaded cycling is performed for 3 minutes before the left vertical dashed line.
3. In panel 3, the diagonal line shows the increase of $\dot{V}O_2$ at a slope of 10 ml/min/w.
4. In panel 5, the diagonal dashed line has a slope of 1; the "x" in the upper right is the predicted maximum heart rate and $\dot{V}O_2$ for the subject.

ume (V_D/V_T) and high metabolic cost of exercise caused by obesity, combined with mechanical limitation to breathe due to obstructive lung disease are all potential contributors to exertional dyspnea. Evidence against primary heart disease causing this patient's symptom is the absence of myocardial ischemia on the 12-lead ECG, the high heart rate reserve at maximum exercise, the normal anaerobic threshold, and the normal $\Delta\dot{V}O_2/\Delta WR$.

Conclusion

Exertional dyspnea is secondary to moderate obstructive lung disease and obesity.

Case 38 Chronic Bronchitis, Cigarette Smoking, and Obesity

Clinical Findings

This 50-year-old shipyard worker was referred for evaluation. He had a 65 pack year history of smoking and had complained of shortness of breath and frequent chest colds with cough and sputum production for the last 7 years. He had been told that he had borderline hypertension but took no medications for this or his pulmonary symptoms. Examination was normal except for obesity, blood pressure of 140/100, and expiratory wheezes on forced expiration. Chest roentgenograms showed focal pleural plaques.

Exercise Findings

The patient performed exercise on a cycle ergometer. He pedalled at 60 rpm without added load for 3 minutes. The work rate was then increased 20 W per minute to his symptom-limited maximum. Arterial blood was sampled every second minute, and intra-arterial blood pressure was recorded from a percutaneously placed brachial artery catheter. Resting carboxyhemoglobin level was 9.4%. He stopped exercise complaining of shortness of breath. After exercise, while sitting quietly on the cycle, he became lightheaded and hypotensive. He was put in the supine position and his legs elevated; this provided immediate relief of his lightheadedness and return of his systemic blood pressure to pre-exercise levels. Resting, exercise, and recovery ECGs showed no abnormalities.

TABLE 9.38.1. Selected Respiratory Function Data

Measurement	Predicted	Before Bronchodilator	After Bronchodilator
Age, yr		50	
Sex		Male	
Height, cm		174	
Weight, kg	77	113	
Hematocrit, %		45	
VC, L	4.40	3.95	4.36
IC L	2.94	3.30	3.75
TLC, L	6.44	6.08	
FEV$_1$, L	3.49		
FEV$_1$/VC, %	79	2.53	2.96
MVV L/min	147	64	
		96	101
D$_{CO}$ ml/mm Hg/min	28.6	30.6	

TABLE 9.38.2. Selected Exercise Data

Measurement	Predicted	Measured
Peak $\dot{V}O_2$, L/min	2.68	1.84
Maximum HR, beats/min	170	131
Maximum O$_2$ pulse, ml/beat	15.8	14.3
$\Delta\dot{V}O_2/\Delta$WR, ml/min/W	10.3	10.2
AT, L/min	>1.15	1.0
Blood pressure, mmHg (rest, max)		131/88, 206/106
Maximum $\dot{V}E$, L/min		93
Exercise breathing reserve, L/min	>15	3
PaO_2, mmHg (rest, max ex)		73, 97
P(a − a)O_2, mmHg (rest, max ex)		34, 23
P(a − ET)CO_2, mmHg (rest, max ex)		7, 2
$\dot{V}D/\dot{V}T$ (rest, heavy ex)		0.41, 0.31

FIGURE 9.38.1.

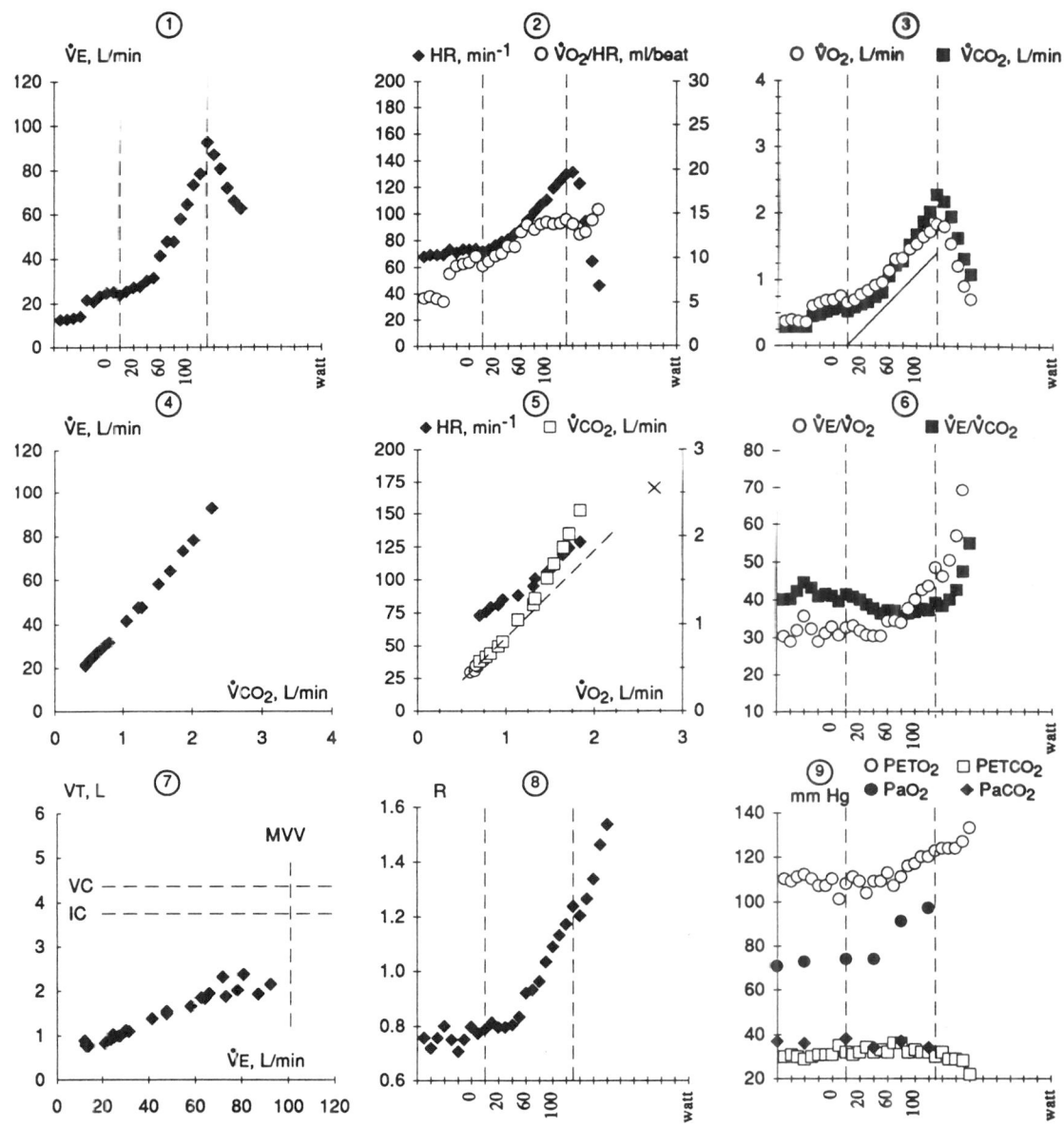

1. Vertical dashed lines in panels 1 to 3 and 6, 8, and 9 indicate the beginning and the end of increasing work period.
2. Unloaded cycling is performed for 3 minutes before the left vertical dashed line.
3. In panel 3, the diagonal line shows the increase of $\dot{V}_{O_2}$ at a slope of 10 ml/min/w.
4. In panel 5, the diagonal dashed line has a slope of 1; the "x" in the upper right is the predicted maximum heart rate and $\dot{V}_{O_2}$ for the subject.

Interpretation
Comments

Resting respiratory function studies reveal mild airflow obstruction that improves following treatment with an aerosolized bronchodilator (Table 9.38.1). The patient is 36 kg overweight. His resting carboxy-hemoglobin is 9.4% (normal < 2.0%). The patient's resting ECG is normal. This case is also presented because of the orthostasis that the patient developed when stopping exercise; this phenomenon is occasionally observed when heavy, upright exercise is abruptly terminated. To avoid this, we usually ask the patient who exercised hard to continue very

TABLE 9.38.3. Air Breathing

Time min	Work rate watts	BP mmHg	HR min^{-1}	f min^{-1}	V̇E L/min BTPS	V̇CO₂ L/min STPD	V̇O₂ L/min STPD	V̇O₂/HR ml/beat	R	pH	HCO₃ meq/L	PO₂ mmHg ET	a	(A−a)	PCO₂ mmHg ET	a	(a−ET)	V̇E/V̇CO₂	V̇E/V̇O₂	VD/VT
	Rest	131/88								7.41	23	71			37					
	Rest		68	14	12.4	0.28	0.37	5.4	0.76			110			30			40	30	
	Rest		68	16	12.6	0.28	0.39	5.7	0.72			109			31			40	29	
	Rest		69	17	13.3	0.28	0.37	5.4	0.76			111			30			42	32	
	Rest	138/88	69	18	14.0	0.28	0.35	5.1	0.80	7.38	21	112	73	34	29	36	7	45	36	0.41
	Unloaded		73	25	21.5	0.45	0.60	8.2	0.75			110			30			43	32	
	Unloaded		71	25	20.9	0.46	0.65	9.2	0.71			107			31			41	29	
	Unloaded		73	25	23.3	0.51	0.68	9.3	0.75			107			31			42	31	
	Unloaded		73	24	24.6	0.55	0.69	9.5	0.80			110			31			41	33	
	Unloaded		74	26	25.2	0.58	0.75	10.1	0.77			101			35			40	31	
	Unloaded	150/88	72	26	23.7	0.51	0.66	9.2	0.78	7.39	23	108	74	30	32	38	6	41	33	0.41
0.5	20		73	26	25.4	0.57	0.70	9.3	0.81			111			31			41	33	
1.0	20		76	27	27.0	0.62	0.78	10.3	0.79			109			32			40	32	
1.5	40		79	28	27.8	0.66	0.83	10.5	0.80			104			34			39	31	
2.0	40	156/88	81	27	30.2	0.74	0.92	11.4	0.80	7.42	22	109	74	35	32	34	2	38	30	0.30
2.5	60		85	29	31.6	0.80	0.96	11.3	0.83			109			33			36	30	
3.0	60		83	29	41.5	1.05	1.14	13.0	0.92			113			32			37	34	
3.5	80		95	32	47.8	1.22	1.31	13.8	0.93			107			36			37	34	
4.0	80	169/94	101	31	47.8	1.28	1.33	13.2	0.96	7.36	21	111	91	21	36	37	1	35	34	0.32
4.5	100		106	35	58.1	1.52	1.47	13.9	1.03			116			32			36	38	
5.0	100		110	35	64.4	1.68	1.54	14.0	1.09			117			33			37	40	
5.5	120		119	39	73.3	1.87	1.65	13.9	1.13			120			32			37	42	
6.0	120	200/100	124	39	78.3	2.02	1.72	13.9	1.17	7.35	18	120	97	23	32	34	2	37	44	0.30
6.5	140		129	43	92.6	2.28	1.84	14.3	1.24			123			30			39	48	
	Recovery		131	45	87.3	2.18	1.81	13.8	1.20			124			32			38	46	
	Recovery	131/72	122	34	80.9	1.96	1.55	12.7	1.26			124			29			40	50	
	Recovery	113/63	94	31	71.9	1.63	1.22	13.0	1.34			124			29			42	57	
	Recovery	88/44	64	34	66.1	1.33	0.91	14.2	1.46			127			28			48	69	
	Recovery	75/31	46	34	62.7	1.09	0.71	15.4	1.54			133			22			55	84	

light exercise (unloading cycle or slow walking) after completing the maximum work rate.

Analysis

Referring to flow chart 1, the peak V̇O₂ and anaerobic threshold are reduced (Table 9.38.2), which directs us through branchpoints 1.1, 1.2, and 1.3 to flow chart 4. The breathing reserve is low (branchpoint 4.1) and the VD/VT is high (branchpoint 4.2). The diagnosis of "lung disease with impaired peripheral oxygenation" is reached. The patient does have a positive P(a − ET)CO₂ and obstructive airway disease and probably a significant component of pulmonary vascular dysfunction which contributes to the low AT. The resting oxyhemoglobin saturation is reduced because of carboxyhemoglobinemia and a low PaO₂. The latter improves with the deeper breathing of exercise when due to obesity. The heart rate reserve is also high, consistent with ventilatory limitation to exercise. Both the obesity and cigarette smoking add to the degree of dysfunction caused by the obstructive airway disease

The development of a metabolic acidosis at a low V̇O₂ (i.e., a low AT) also contributed to the exercise limitation, because it stimulated ventilation at all work rates above the AT, evidenced by the steep rise in V̇E/V̇O₂ in panel 6 of Fig. 9.38.1. This response is in contrast to that seen in cases 37, 40, and 42, where the V̇E/V̇O₂ does not rise as steeply towards the end of exercise and where a circulatory-induced metabolic acidosis did not contribute to a low breathing reserve and ventilatory limitation. Sedentary life style and the carboxyhemoglobinemia from cigarette smoking contribute to the low AT. Thus this patient has reversible elements to his illness.

Conclusion

Mild airflow obstruction, obesity, and cigarette smoking all contribute to ventilatory limitation to exercise.

Case 39 Emphysema with Mild Airway Obstruction

Clinical Findings

This 50-year-old male long-term smoker was referred for cardiopulmonary exercise testing for evaluation of his exertional dyspnea. He became symptomatic after walking one block. He had mild obstructive lung disease of long duration consistent with emphysema. His only current medication was a frequently used inhaled β-agonist. The study was done to determine whether his exercise limitation was due to his lung disease.

Exercise Findings

The patient performed exercise on a cycle ergometer. He pedalled at 60 rpm without an added load for 3 minutes. The work rate was then increased 15 W per minute to tolerance. Heart rate and rhythm were continuously monitored; 12-lead ECGs were obtained during rest, exercise, and recovery. Blood pressure was measured with a sphygmomanometer and oxygen saturation with an ear oximeter. The patient appeared to give an excellent effort and stopped exercise because of shortness of breath. He denied chest pain during or after the study. Resting, exercise, and recovery ECGs were not remarkable except for occasional multifocal premature ventricular contractions during exercise and recovery.

TABLE 9.39.1. Selected Respiratory Function Data

Measurement	Predicted	Measured
Age, yr		50
Sex		Male
Height, cm		168
Weight, kg	72	66
Hematocrit, %		46
VC, L	4.06	4.10
IC, L	2.71	3.30
TLC, L	5.92	7.07
FEV_1, L	3.22	2.57
FEV_1/VC, %	79	63
MVV, L/min	141	91
D_LCO, ml/mm Hg/min	25.4	14.7

TABLE 9.39.2. Selected Exercise Data

Measurement	Predicted	Measured
Peak $\dot{V}O_2$, L/min	2.22	1.39
Maximum HR, beats/min	170	126
Maximum O_2 pulse, ml/beat	13.1	11.0
$\Delta\dot{V}O_2$/ΔWR, ml/min/W	10.3	7.3
AT, L/min	>0.95	0.9
Blood pressure, mmHg (rest, max)		120/80, 160/100
Maximum $\dot{V}E$, L/min		89
Exercise breathing reserve, L/min	>15	2
O_2 saturation (oximeter) (rest, max)		93, 88

FIGURE 9.39.1.

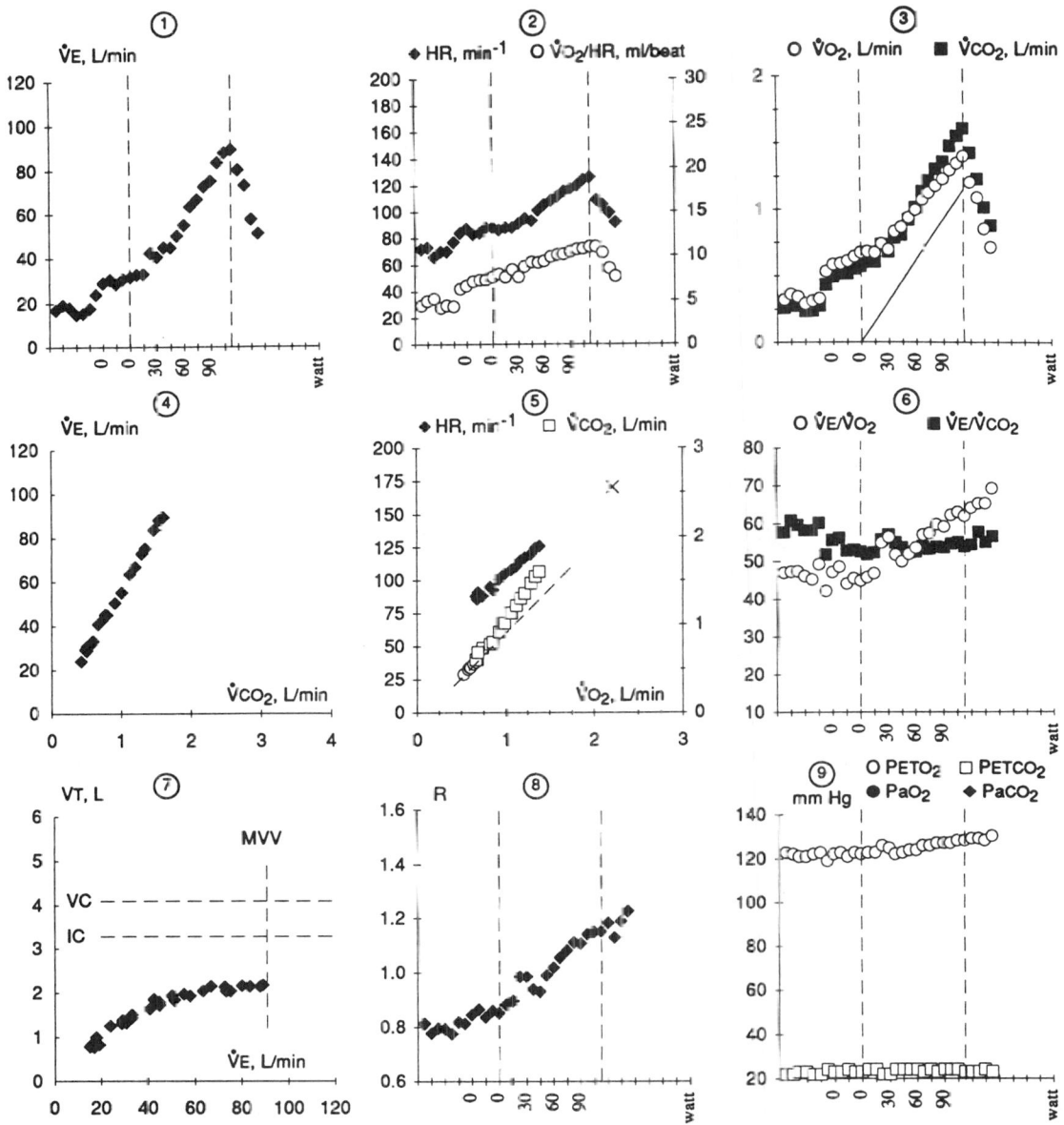

1. Vertical dashed lines in panels 1 to 3 and 6, 8, and 9 indicate the beginning and the end of increasing work period.

2. Unloaded cycling is performed for 3 minutes before the left vertical dashed line.

3. In panel 3, the diagonal line shows the increase of $\dot{V}O_2$ at a slope of 10 ml/min/w.

4. In panel 5, the diagonal dashed line has a slope of 1; the "x" in the upper right is the predicted maximum heart rate and $\dot{V}O_2$ for the subject.

TABLE 9.39.3. Air Breathing

Time min	Work rate watts	BP mmHg	HR min⁻¹	f min⁻¹	$\dot{V}_E$ L/min BTPS	$\dot{V}_{CO_2}$ L/min STPD	$\dot{V}_{O_2}$ L/min STPD	$\dot{V}_{O_2}$/HR ml/beat	R	pH	HCO₃⁻ meq/L	P_{O_2}, mmHg ET	a	(A − a)	P_{CO_2}, mmHg ET	a	(a − ET)	$\dot{V}_E$/$\dot{V}_{CO_2}$	$\dot{V}_E$/$\dot{V}_{O_2}$	V_D/V_T
	Rest	120/80																		
	Rest		72	22	16.9	0.26	0.32	4.4	0.81			123			22			58	47	
	Rest		73	23	19.0	0.28	0.36	4.9	0.78			122			22			61	47	
	Rest		66	21	17.9	0.27	0.34	5.2	0.79			121			23			60	47	
	Rest	120/80	70	19	15.0	0.23	0.29	4.1	0.79			121			23			58	46	
	Rest		70	19	15.6	0.24	0.31	4.4	0.77			122			22			58	45	
	Rest		77	18	17.8	0.27	0.33	4.3	0.82			123			22			60	49	
	Unloaded		84	19	23.9	0.43	0.53	6.3	0.81			119			24			52	42	
	Unloaded		87	21	29.1	0.49	0.58	6.7	0.84			122			23			56	47	
	Unloaded		83	23	30.6	0.51	0.59	7.1	0.86			123			23			56	49	
	Unloaded		84	22	28.8	0.51	0.61	7.3	0.84			121			24			53	44	
	Unloaded		88	23	31.1	0.55	0.64	7.3	0.86			123			23			53	46	
	Unloaded	140/90	88	22	31.9	0.57	0.67	7.6	0.85			122			23			53	25	
0.5	8		86	23	33.0	0.60	0.68	7.9	0.88			123			24			52	46	
1.0	15		88	22	33.2	0.60	0.67	7.6	0.90			123			24			52	47	
1.5	23		88	23	42.5	0.73	0.74	8.4	0.99			126			22			56	55	
2.0	30	140/90	91	25	40.9	0.68	0.69	7.6	0.99			125			22			57	56	
2.5	38		95	26	45.0	0.78	0.83	8.7	0.94			122			24			55	52	
3.0	45		93	25	44.9	0.80	0.86	9.2	0.93			123			24			53	50	
3.5	53		101	26	50.3	0.92	0.93	9.2	0.99			124			24			52	52	
4.0	60	150/92	105	28	55.3	1.01	0.99	9.4	1.02			124			24			52	53	
4.5	68		108	31	63.5	1.13	1.07	9.9	1.06			126			23			54	57	
5.0	75		111	31	66.8	1.21	1.12	10.1	1.08			126			24			53	57	
5.5	83		115	34	72.7	1.30	1.17	10.2	1.11			127			23			54	60	
6.0	90	160/100	117	37	75.2	1.35	1.22	10.4	1.11			127			24			53	59	
6.5	98		120	39	83.5	1.47	1.29	10.8	1.14			127			24			55	62	
7.0	105		124	41	87.9	1.54	1.34	10.8	1.15			128			24			55	63	
7.5	113		126	41	89.3	1.60	1.39	11.0	1.15			128			23			54	62	
	Recovery		109	37	80.1	1.42	1.20	11.0	1.18			129			23			54	64	
	Recovery	140/90	105	36	73.4	1.22	1.08	10.3	1.13			129			23			58	65	
	Recovery		99	30	57.9	1.01	0.85	8.6	1.19			128			24			55	65	
	Recovery	140/80	92	28	51.5	0.87	0.71	7.7	1.23			130			23			56	69	

Interpretation

Comments

Resting respiratory function studies showed mild obstruction, an insignificant bronchodilator response to inhaled β-agonist, and a moderately reduced $D_{L}CO$.

Analysis

Referring to flow chart 1, peak $\dot{V}_{O_2}$ and the anaerobic threshold are low (Table 9.39.2). Going next to flow chart 4, the breathing reserve (branchpoint 4.1) is very low, consistent with exercise limitation from lung disease. Although blood gases are not available, the very high ventilatory equivalents, without a high R to support acute hyperventilation, indicate increased dead space ventilation (branchpoint 4.2). The high $\dot{V}_E$/$\dot{V}_{CO_2}$ at the AT indicates that the patient requires an inordinately high ventilatory response to exercise. The high heart rate reserve is also consistent with ventilation limiting exercise. The low $\Delta\dot{V}_{O_2}$/ΔWR might be due to pulmonary vascular disease secondary to the patient's obstructive lung disease or reduced venous return during exercise resulting from high intrapleural pressure consequent to air trapping and hyperinflation.

Conclusion

This patient has mild to moderate obstructive lung disease with ventilatory limitation to exercise due to the increased ventilatory requirements secondary to ventilation-perfusion mismatching and low AT.

Case 40 Emphysema, Severe
Clinical Findings

This 65-year-old man had a long history of asbestos exposure and heavy cigarette smoking. He was being treated with aminophylline, inhaled bronchodilators, and home oxygen therapy. He was also receiving chlorothiazide for treatment of hypertension. He had stopped smoking 12 years previously. Resting ECG suggested left atrial enlargement. The question was raised with respect to the role of the patient's circulatory disease in his ventilatory impairment.

Exercise Findings

The patient performed exercise on a cycle ergometer. He first pedalled at 60 rpm, without added load, for 3 minutes. The work rate was then increased 10 W per minute to his symptom-limited maximum. Blood was sampled every second minute and intra-arterial blood pressure was recorded from a brachial artery catheter. There were no abnormal ST segment changes at rest or during exercise. He stopped exercise complaining of shortness of breath.

TABLE 9.40.1. Selected Respiratory Function Data

Measurement	Predicted	Measured
Age, yr		65
Sex		Male
Height, cm		170
Weight, kg	74	99
Hematocrit, %		53
VC, L	3.72	2.17
IC L	2.48	1.31
TLC, L	5.85	8.22
FEV_1, L	2.89	0.56
FEV_1/VC, %	78	26
MVV L/min	123	31
D_LCO ml/mm Hg/min	25.1	13.2

TABLE 9.40.2. Selected Exercise Data

Measurement	Predicted	Measured
Peak $\dot{V}O_2$, L/min	2.11	0.90
Maximum HR, beats/min	155	129
Maximum O_2 pulse, ml/beat	13.6	7.0
$\Delta\dot{V}O_2$/ΔWR, ml/min/W	10.3	8.9
AT, L/min	>0.93	not reached
Blood pressure, mmHg (rest, max)		175/94, 256/138
Maximum $\dot{V}E$, L/min		28
Exercise breathing reserve, L/min	>15	3
PaO_2, mmHg (rest, max ex)		56, 46
$P(A - a)O_2$, mmHg (rest, max ex)		39, 48
$P(a - ET)CO_2$, mmHg (rest, max ex)		4, 6
VD/VT (rest, heavy ex)		0.40, 0.41
HCO_3^-, mEq/L (rest, 2-min recov)		28, 27

FIGURE 9.40.1.

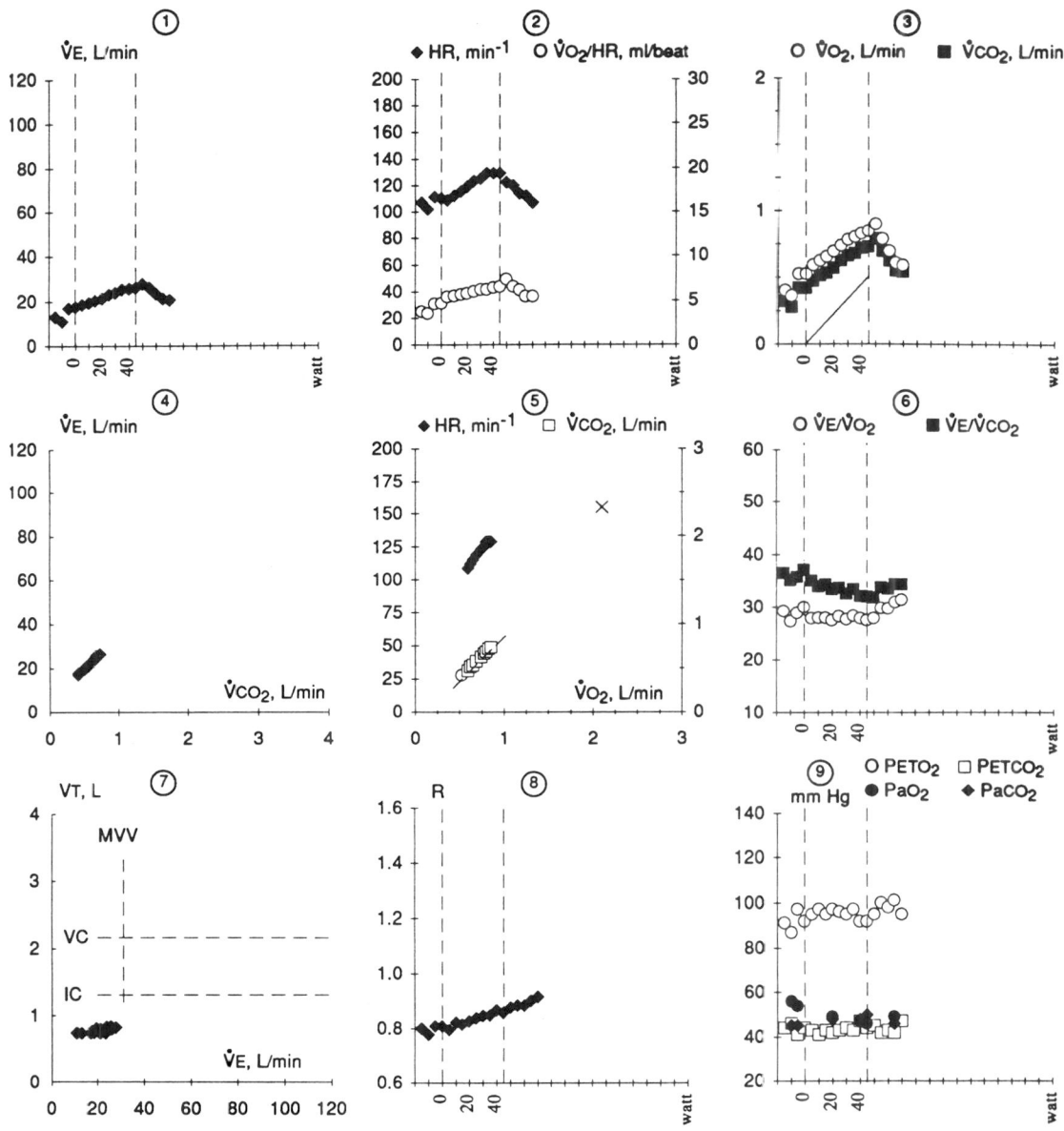

1. Vertical dashed lines in panels 1 to 3 and 6, 8, and 9 indicate the beginning and the end of increasing work period.
2. Unloaded cycling is performed for 3 minutes before the left vertical dashed line.
3. In panel 3, the diagonal line shows the increase of $\dot{V}O_2$ at a slope of 10 ml/min/w.
4. In panel 5, the diagonal dashed line has a slope of 1; the "x" in the upper right is the predicted maximum heart rate and $\dot{V}O_2$ for the subject.

TABLE 9.40.3. Air Breathing

Time min	Work rate watts	BP mmHg	HR min⁻¹	f min⁻¹	V̇E L/min BTPS	V̇CO₂ L/min STPD	V̇O₂ L/min STPD	V̇O₂/HR ml/beat	R	pH	HCO₃⁻ meq/L	PO₂, mmHg ET	ᾱ	(A − a)	PCO₂, mmHg ET	a	(a − ET)	V̇E/V̇CO₂	V̇E/V̇O₂	VD/VT
	Rest	175/94																		
	Rest		107	18	13.2	0.32	0.40	3.7	0.80			91			44			36	29	
	Rest	175/94	102	15	11.1	0.28	0.36	3.5	0.78	7.4	28	87	56	39	46	45		35	27	0.40
	Unloaded	194/100	111	23	17.0	0.42	0.52	4.7	0.81	7.4	28	97	54	43	41	45	4	36	29	0.41
	Unloaded		110	23	17.5	0.42	0.52	4.7	0.81			92			44			37	30	
0.5	10		109	25	18.6	0.47	0.59	5.4	0.80			95			43			35	28	
1.0	10		112	24	19.4	0.51	0.62	5.5	0.82			97			41			34	28	
1.5	20		115	27	20.5	0.53	0.65	5.7	0.82			95			43			34	28	
2.0	20	225/113	119	27	21.3	0.57	0.69	5.8	0.83	7.40	29	97	49	45	42	48	6	33	28	0.41
2.5	30		123	30	23.4	0.62	0.74	6.0	0.84			96			43			34	28	
3.0	30		125	29	24.0	0.66	0.78	6.2	0.85			95			44			33	28	
3.5	40		129	32	25.4	0.68	0.80	6.2	0.85			97			43			33	28	
4.0	40	250/131	129	31	25.8	0.72	0.83	6.4	0.87	7.37	27	92	47	49	47	48	1	32	28	0.40
4.5	50	256/138	129	33	26.2	0.73	0.85	6.6	0.86	7.37	28	92	46	48	44	50	6	32	28	0.41
	Recovery		122	34	28.0	0.79	0.90	7.4	0.88			95			45			32	28	
	Recovery		120	32	26.3	0.70	0.79	6.6	0.89			100			42			34	30	
	Recovery		114	32	23.5	0.62	0.70	6.1	0.89			93			43			34	30	
	Recovery	194/94	112	29	21.3	0.55	0.61	5.4	0.90	7.38	27	101	49	51	42	46	4	34	31	0.40
	Recovery		107	27	20.8	0.54	0.59	5.5	0.92			95			47			34	31	

Interpretation

Comments

This patient clearly has evidence of very severe obstructive lung disease (Table 9.40.1). His resting ECG suggests left atrial enlargement.

Analysis

Referring to flow chart 1, the peak V̇O₂ is reduced while the anaerobic threshold is not reached, but is above lower limits of normal (Table 9.40.2), which directs us through branchpoints 1.1, 1.2, and 1.3 to flow chart 3. The breathing reserve is low (branchpoint 3.1), and there is the confirmatory evidence for ventilation-perfusion mismatching (increased VD/VT, P(A − a)O₂, P(a − ET)CO₂). While there is no breathing reserve at maximal exercise there is a large heart rate reserve. The maximal ventilatory frequency is less than 50 (branchpoint 3.2), typical of obstructive lung disease. The mild respiratory acidosis during exercise is consistent with a diagnosis of ventilatory limitation.

Conclusion

The patient, while having ECG evidence of left atrial enlargement and significant systemic hypertension during exercise, clearly is limited by his obstructive lung disease and not by cardiac dysfunction. The presence of a high heart rate reserve and the absence of a ventilatory reserve, along with the development of a mild respiratory acidosis at this patient's maximum V̇O₂, support the conclusion that he has ventilatory limitation. Circulatory limitation was not severe enough to cause a metabolic acidosis over the low range of work rates the patient was able to tolerate (only one meq/L decrease in HCO₃⁻). Thus, lactic acidosis did not contribute to ventilatory drive.

Case 41 Emphysema with Pulmonary Vascular Disease

Clinical Findings

This 61-year-old man with bullous emphysema and right middle lobe scarring on chest x-ray was referred for evaluation regarding the need for oxygen supplementation. The patient had a 35 pack year history of cigarette smoking. He had not sought medical care until 4 months previously when he was hospitalized for pneumonia, severe dyspnea, and hemoptysis. Bronchoscopy, transbronchial biopsy, cytology, and mycobacterial studies were negative. Resting ECG showed poor R-wave progression.

Exercise Findings

The patient performed exercise on a cycle ergometer. He pedalled at 60 rpm without an added load for 3 minutes. The work rate was then increased 10 W per minute to tolerance. Arterial blood was sampled every second minute and intra-arterial pressure was recorded from a percutaneously placed brachial artery catheter. The patient stopped exercise because of leg fatigue. The patient had no chest pain or further ECG abnormalities.

TABLE 9.41.1. Selected Respiratory Function Data

Measurement	Predicted	Measured
Age, yr		61
Sex		Male
Height, cm		173
Weight, kg	76	63
Hematocrit, %		45
VC, L	4.00	4.37
IC, L	2.67	2.62
TLC, L	6.15	9.11
FEV_1, L	3.13	2.11
FEV_1/VC, %	78	48
MVV, L/min	131	87
$D_{L}CO$, ml/mm Hg/min	26.0	8.4

TABLE 9.41.2. Selected Exercise Data

Measurement	Predicted	Measured
Peak $\dot{V}O_2$, L/min	1.95	1.25
Maximum HR, beats/min	159	149
Maximum O_2 pulse, ml/beat	12.3	8.4
$\Delta\dot{V}O_2/\Delta WR$, ml/min/W	10.3	8.5
AT, L/min	>0.86	0.7
Blood pressure, mmHg (rest, max)		127/75, 190/96
Maximum $\dot{V}E$, L/min		85
Exercise breathing reserve, L/min	>15	2
PaO_2, mmHg (rest, max ex)		83, 72
P(A − a)O_2, mmHg (rest, max ex)		32, 52
P(a − ET)CO_2, mmHg (rest, max ex)		4, 8
VD/VT (rest, max ex)		0.28, 0.41
HCO_3^-, mEq/L (rest, 2-min recov)		22, 13

TABLE 9.41.3. Air Breathing

Time min	Work rate watts	BP mmHg	HR min⁻¹	f min⁻¹	V̇E L/min BTPS	V̇CO₂ L/min STPD	V̇O₂ L/min STPD	V̇O₂/HR ml/beat	R	pH	HCO₃ meq/L	PO₂, mmHg ET	a	(A−a)	PCO₂, mmHg ET	a	(a−ET)	V̇E/V̇CO₂	V̇E/V̇O₂	VD/VT
	Rest	129/75								7.44	22		86			33				
	Rest		77	15	13.9	0.30	0.28	3.6	1.07			122			30			42	45	
	Rest		75	13	10.8	0.23	0.23	3.1	1.00			121			31			42	42	
	Rest		76	14	9.9	0.21	0.21	2.8	1.00			118			32			41	41	
	Rest	129/75	75	15	10.8	0.27	0.26	3.5	1.04	7.44	22	118	83	32	32	36	4	35	37	0.28
	Rest		74	12	10.4	0.22	0.20	2.7	1.10			123			29			43	47	
	Rest		75	11	10.4	0.25	0.24	3.2	1.04			120			31			38	39	
	Unloaded		83	20	17.8	0.40	0.38	4.6	1.05			117			32			40	42	
	Unloaded	138/41	86	19	18.6	0.43	0.41	4.8	1.05	7.41	22	121	91	25	30	35	5	40	41	0.34
	Unloaded		89	16	19.6	0.48	0.46	5.2	1.04			120			30			38	40	
	Unloaded		94	17	21.2	0.52	0.51	5.4	1.02			120			31			38	39	
	Unloaded		94	18	24.4	0.59	0.57	6.1	1.04			121			30			39	40	
	Unloaded	168/90	95	18	25.0	0.62	0.59	6.2	1.05	7.40	21	121	78	38	30	35	5	38	40	0.33
0.5	10		97	17	25.3	0.64	0.59	6.1	1.08			120			31			37	40	
1.0	10	168/90	98	20	29.0	0.71	0.65	6.6	1.09	7.41	22	122	77	40	29	35	6	38	42	0.34
1.5	20		101	22	28.5	0.70	0.64	6.3	1.09			119			32			38	42	
2.0	20	174/90	102	21	32.5	0.78	0.70	6.9	1.11	7.40	21	123	74	45	29	34	5	39	44	0.34
2.5	30		104	24	28.9	0.73	0.67	6.4	1.09			120			32			37	40	
3.0	30	174/40	110	21	40.1	0.96	0.83	7.5	1.16	7.40	21	124	71	48	28	35	7	40	46	0.37
3.5	40		115	20	38.7	0.97	0.84	7.3	1.15			122			30			38	44	
4.0	40	180/90	119	23	44.4	1.08	0.92	7.7	1.17	7.39	20	123	71	49	29	34	5	39	46	0.34
4.5	50		123	22	47.7	1.13	0.95	7.7	1.22			125			28			40	48	
5.0	50	182/88	126	25	51.7	1.22	0.97	7.7	1.26	7.38	19	125	70	52	28	33	5	41	51	0.34
5.5	60		130	25	56.9	1.35	1.05	8.1	1.29			126			28			41	52	
6.0	60	189/93	132	26	58.7	1.40	1.08	8.2	1.30	7.36	18	125	72	51	29	33	4	40	52	0.34
6.5	70		138	26	62.3	1.47	1.12	8.1	1.31			127			28			41	54	
7.0	70	190/90	140	31	68.1	1.54	1.14	8.1	1.35	7.32	17	128	72	51	27	34	7	43	57	0.39
7.5	80		144	32	71.4	1.62	1.19	8.3	1.36			127			28			42	58	
8.0	80	190/96	149	38	80.2	1.73	1.24	8.3	1.40	7.32	17	129	72	52	26	34	8	44	62	0.41
8.5	90		148	39	85.2	1.80	1.25	8.4	1.44			129			26			45	66	
	Recovery		141	27	66.6	1.49	1.07	7.6	1.39			123			26			43	60	
	Recovery		140	26	63.3	1.38	0.90	6.4	1.53			130			26			44	68	
	Recovery		133	22	54.5	1.19	0.74	5.6	1.61			131			26			44	71	
	Recovery	174/87	126	22	51.3	1.07	0.65	5.2	1.65	7.26	13	132	115	14	25	30	5	46	76	0.36
	Recovery		120	24	45.5	0.88	0.54	4.5	1.63			133			24			49	80	

Interpretation

Comments

Resting studies showed a moderate obstructive ventilatory defect, increased total lung capacity, and low $D_{L}CO$. The ECG showed poor R-wave progression.

Analysis

Referring to flow chart 1, peak $\dot{V}O_2$ and anaerobic threshold are decreased. Proceeding next to flow chart 4, the low breathing reserve (branchpoint 4.1) and high VD/VT (branchpoint 4.2) are consistent with "lung disease with impaired peripheral oxygenation." The high VT/IC and low breathing reserve support ventilatory limitation, although ventilatory drive is increased because of the low work rate metabolic acidosis and the high VD/VT. Although the patient stated that he stopped exercise because of leg fatigue, his low breathing reserve indicated that he also had ventilatory limitation. The abnormal gas exchange (high ventilatory equivalents, high VD/VT, and positive $P(a - ET)CO_2$) with exercise are consistent with the presence of underperfusion of ventilated lung consistent with pulmonary vascular disease presumably secondary to obstructive lung disease. The severity of the metabolic acidosis (decrease in HCO_3^- from 22 to 13 mEq/L) is consistent with the low anaerobic threshold and suggests poor O_2 flow to the exercising muscle, most likely because the patient's pulmonary vascular disease limited his ability to increase cardiac output.

FIGURE 9.41.1.

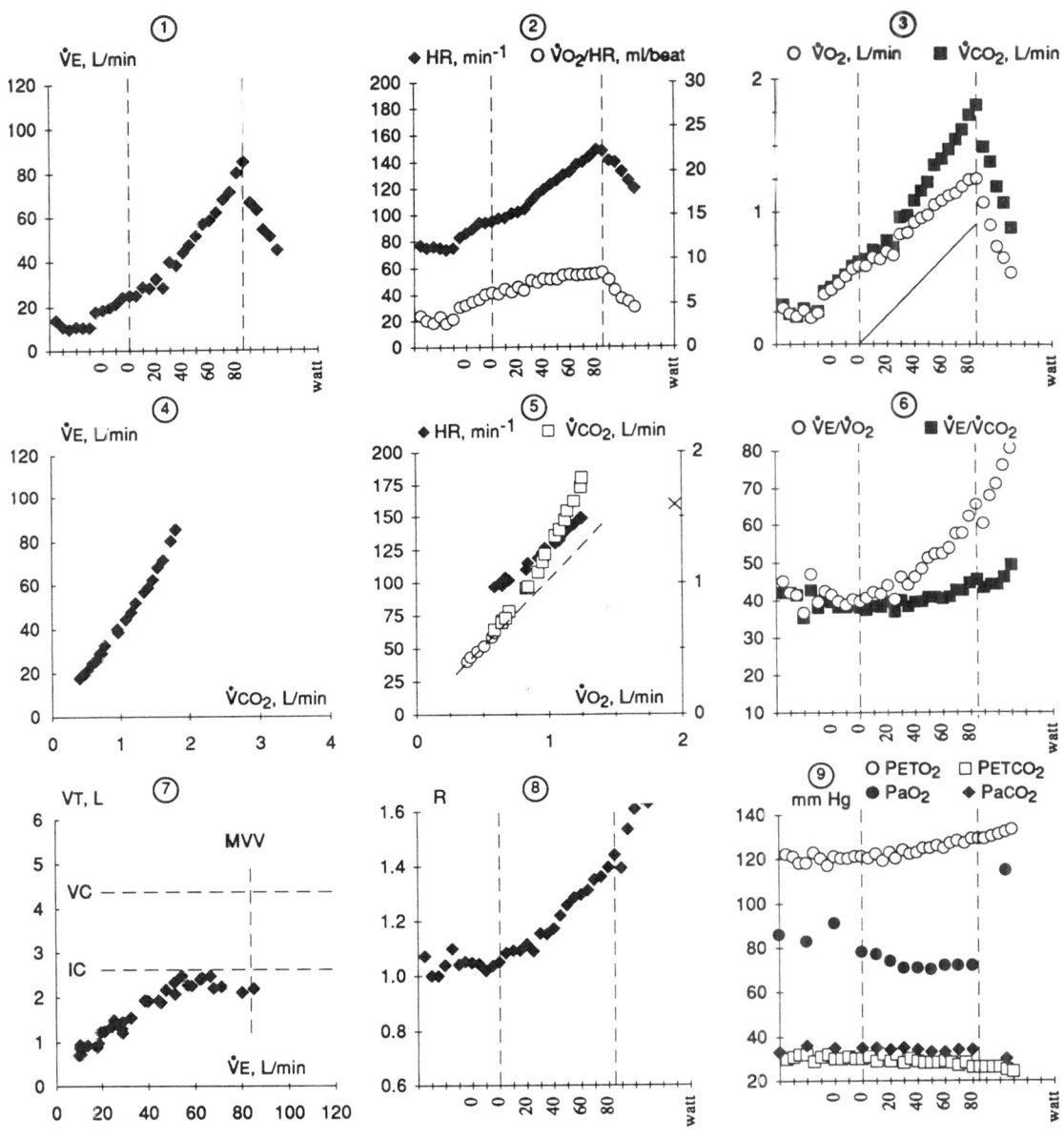

1. Vertical dashed lines in panels 1 to 3 and 6, 8, and 9 indicate the beginning and the end of increasing work period.
2. Unloaded cycling is performed for 3 minutes before the left vertical dashed line.
3. In panel 3, the diagonal line shows the increase of $\dot{V}O_2$ at a slope of 10 ml/min/w.
4. In panel 5, the diagonal dashed line has a slope of 1; the "x" in the upper right is the predicted maximum heart rate and $\dot{V}O_2$ for the subject.

Conclusion

This patient has physiologic evidence of pulmonary vascular disease, secondary to obvious obstructive lung disease. The mild degree of hypoxemia does not qualify for O_2 supplementation under current federal funding guidelines, but dyspnea may well be less with O_2 supplementation. This is an example of lung disease causing secondary cardiovascular disease, which in turn results in a high ventilatory requirement as compensation for the exercise-induced lactic acidosis. This makes the patient more exercise limited than predicted from his moderate defect in spirometry.

Case 42 Emphysema and Bronchitis, Severe: Air and Oxygen Breathing

Clinical Findings

This 62-year-old retired accountant had a long history of heavy cigarette smoking but had stopped 4 years previously. He had a chronic cough and shortness of breath. He had gradually increased his activity by physical training and rode his bicycle many miles daily. There was no history of heart failure. He took oral theophylline but no other medications. He participated in a study evaluating the effects of oxygen supplementation.

Exercise Findings

The patient performed exercise on a cycle ergometer. He pedalled at 60 rpm without added load for 3 minutes while breathing humidified compressed air. The work rate was then increased 10 W per minute to his symptom-limited maximum. Blood was sampled every second minute, and intra-arterial blood pressure was recorded from a percutaneously placed brachial artery catheter. He stopped exercise complaining of shortness of breath. Following 30 minutes of rest, he was given humidified 100% O_2 to breathe while the exercise study was repeated. He again stopped exercise complaining of shortness of breath. The 12-lead ECG showed no ST segment changes or arrhythmia. His maximum heart rate increased by 25 beats/minute and maximum work rate by 40 W.

TABLE 9.42.1. Selected Respiratory Function Data

Measurement	Predicted	Measured
Age, yr		62
Sex		Male
Height, cm		173
Weight, kg	76	78
Hematocrit, %		51
VC, L	4.30	1.67
IC, L	2.87	1.22
TLC, L	6.87	8.30
FEV_1, _	3.40	0.54
FEV_1/VC, %	79	32
MVV, L/min	131	32
D_{CO}, ml/mm Hg/min	30.9	18.5

TABLE 9.42.2. Selected Exercise Data

Measurement	Predicted	Room Air	100% O_2
Maximum WR, W		80	120
Peak $\dot{V}O_2$, L/min	2.11	0.96	
Maximum HR, beats/min	158	140	165
Maximum O_2 pulse, ml/beat	13.4	6.9	
$\Delta\dot{V}O_2/\Delta WR$, ml/min/W	10.3	8.3	
AT, L/min	>0.93	not reached	
Blood pressure, mmHg (rest, max)		169/106, 250/125	144/94, 234/119
Maximum $\dot{V}E$, L/min		32	40
Exercise breathing reserve, L/min	>15	0	−8
PaO_2, mmHg (rest, max ex)		78, 53	587, 583
$P(A - a)O_2$, mmHg (rest, max ex)		21, 51	77, 66
$P(a - ET)CO_2$, mmHg (rest, max ex)		6, 5	8, 3
VD/VT (rest, heavy ex)		0.42, 0.38	0.48, 0.37
HCO_3^-, mEq/L (rest, 2-min recov)		25, 24	27, 22

FIGURE 9.42.1.   Air Breathing.

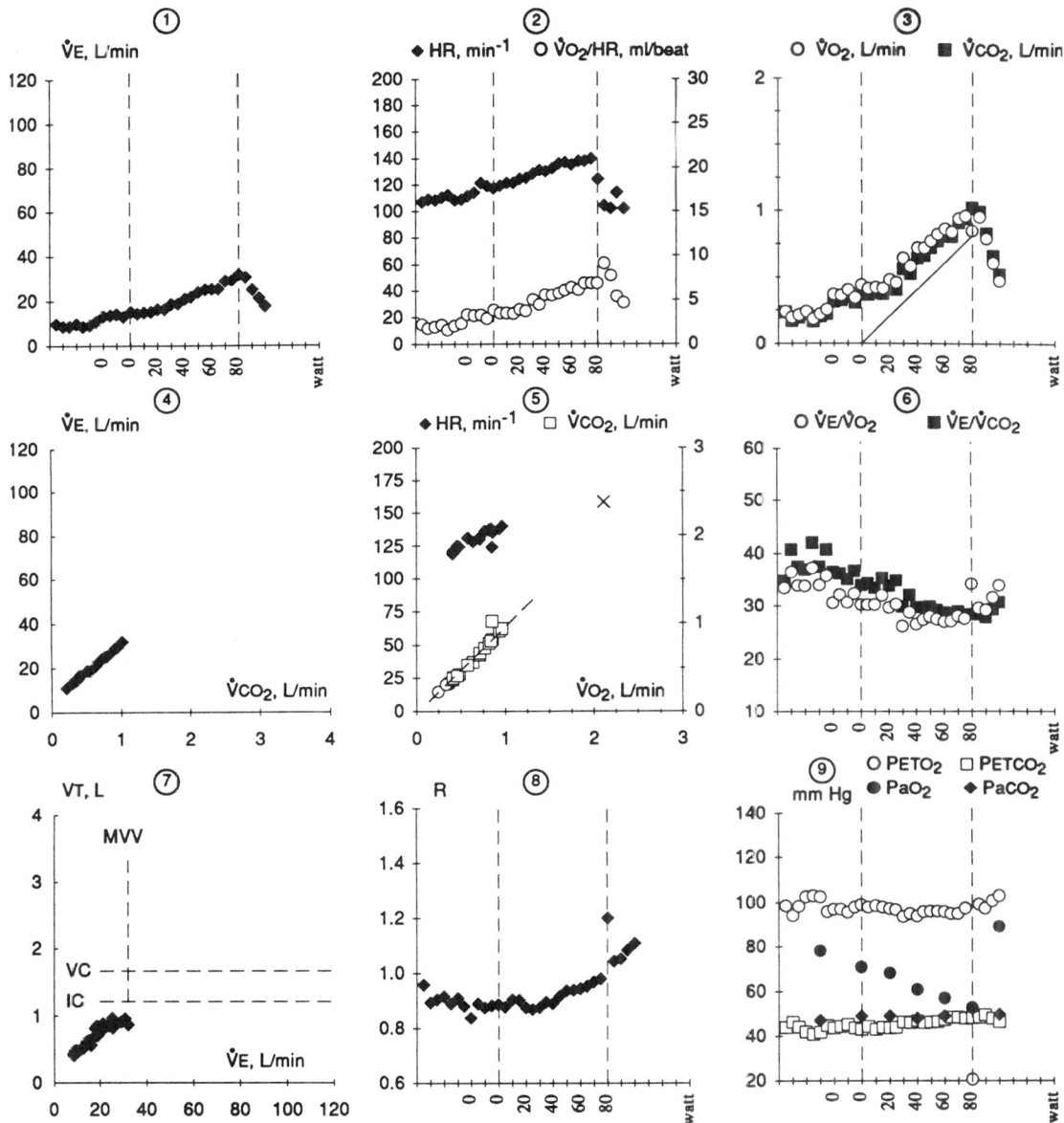

1. Vertical dashed lines in panels 1 to 3 and 6, 8, and 9 indicate the beginning and the end of increasing work period.

2. Unloaded cycling is performed for 3 minutes before the left vertical dashed line.

3. In panel 3, the diagonal line shows the increase of $\dot{V}O_2$ at a slope of 10 ml/min/w.

4. In panel 5, the diagonal dashed line has a slope of 1; the "x" in the upper right is the predicted maximum heart rate and $\dot{V}O_2$ for the subject.

TABLE 9.42.3.   Air Breathing

Time min	Work rate watts	BP mmHg	HR min⁻¹	f min⁻¹	$\dot{V}_E$ L/min BTPS	$\dot{V}_{CO_2}$ L/min STPD	$\dot{V}_{O_2}$ L/min STPD	$\frac{V_{O_2}}{HR}$ ml/beat	R	pH	HCO₃ meq/L	P_{O_2}, mmHg ET	a	(A − a)	P_{CO_2}, mmHg ET	a	(a − ET)	$\frac{\dot{V}_E}{\dot{V}_{CO_2}}$	$\frac{\dot{V}_E}{\dot{V}_{O_2}}$	$\frac{V_D}{V_T}$
	Rest		107	20	9.7	0.23	0.24	2.2	0.96			99			44			35	33	
	Rest		109	21	8.7	0.17	0.19	1.7	0.89			94			46			41	36	
	Rest		108	20	8.8	0.19	0.21	1.9	0.90			98			44			37	34	
	Rest		110	20	9.8	0.22	0.24	2.2	0.92			102			42			37	34	
	Rest		112	20	8.4	0.16	0.18	1.6	0.89			103			41			42	37	
	Rest	169/106	108	19	9.1	0.20	0.22	2.0	0.91	7.35	25	102	78	21	42	47	6	37	34	0.42
	Unloaded		109	23	10.9	0.22	0.25	2.3	0.88			96			45			41	36	
	Unloaded		111	25	13.4	0.31	0.37	3.3	0.84			97			44			36	30	
	Unloaded		114	24	13.6	0.32	0.36	3.2	0.89			97			44			36	32	
	Unloaded		121	23	14.2	0.35	0.40	3.3	0.88			96			45			35	31	
	Unloaded		119	25	13.1	0.30	0.34	2.9	0.88			98			44			37	32	
	Unloaded	181/100	117	24	15.3	0.39	0.44	3.8	0.89	7.35	27	99	71	25	43	49	6	34	30	0.42
0.5	10		119	24	14.4	0.36	0.41	3.4	0.88			98			44			34	30	
1.0	10		121	25	14.8	0.38	0.42	3.5	0.90			99			43			33	30	
1.5	20		121	24	15.1	0.37	0.41	3.4	0.90			98			44			35	32	
2.0	20	187/106	124	25	16.3	0.42	0.48	3.9	0.88	7.35	27	97	68	27	44	49	6	34	30	0.42
2.5	30		125	29	16.4	0.40	0.46	3.7	0.87			97			44			35	30	
3.0	30		128	22	18.6	0.56	0.64	5.0	0.88	7.35	27	94			46			30	26	
3.5	40		131	27	18.9	0.52	0.58	4.4	0.90			95			46			32	29	
4.0	40	213/113	130	24	21.1	0.64	0.72	5.5	0.89	7.35	26	94	61	36	47	48	1	30	26	0.36
4.5	50		132	27	21.9	0.66	0.72	5.5	0.92			96			46			30	27	
5.0	50		136	28	23.9	0.72	0.77	5.7	0.94			96			46			30	28	
5.5	60		137	30	25.0	0.77	0.82	6.0	0.94			96			47			29	27	
6.0	60	225/119	135	28	25.6	0.81	0.86	6.4	0.94	7.35	27	96	57	42	48	49	1	29	27	0.35
6.5	70		138	31	25.4	0.80	0.84	6.1	0.95			95			49			28	27	
7.0	70		138	32	29.0	0.91	0.94	6.8	0.97			95			48			29	28	
7.5	80		140	32	29.2	0.94	0.96	6.9	0.98			98			48			28	28	
8.0	80	250/125	124	37	32.1	1.02	0.85	6.9	1.20	7.32	27	101	53	51	48	53	5	28	34	0.38
	Recovery		104	32	30.7	0.99	0.95	9.1	1.04			99			48			28	29	
	Recovery		102	26	25.2	0.83	0.79	7.7	1.05			98			50			28	29	
	Recovery		114	24	21.3	0.66	0.61	5.4	1.08			101			48			29	32	
	Recovery		102	22	17.8	0.52	0.47	4.6	1.11	7.30	24	103	89	15	47	50	3	31	34	0.39

Interpretation

Comments

Resting respiratory function studies indicate that this patient has severe obstructive lung disease (Table 9.42.1); he also had significant systemic hypertension at rest.

Analysis

Referring to flow chart 1, peak $\dot{V}_{O_2}$ is moderately severely reduced and the anaerobic threshold is not reached (Table 9.42.2). We could satisfactorily use flow chart 3, but we use flow chart 5 because it is more detailed. The indices of ventilation-perfusion mismatching (V_D/V_T, $P(a - ET)_{CO_2}$ and $P(A - a)_{O_2}$) are abnormal (branchpoint 5.1). The breathing reserve is zero (branchpoint 5.3) indicating that the patient's exercise limitation is a result of lung disease. The breathing frequency (f) is less than 50 at the maximum work rate (branchpoint 5.7) consistent with the diagnosis of lung disease of the obstructive type. Other abnormal findings are an obstructive expiratory flow pattern (not shown), arterial oxygen tension, and $P(A - a)_{O_2}$ normal at rest but abnormal with exercise, a high heart rate reserve, and a respiratory acidosis at the maximum $\dot{V}_{O_2}$ (Table 9.42.3).

As a result of breathing 100% O_2, the patient was able to increase his maximal work rate by 40 W and the maximum heart rate by 25 beats per minute (i.e., from 140 during air breathing to 165 during 100% oxygen breathing). These results demonstrate that the increased heart rate reserve, during the air breathing test, results from his ventilatory limitation. Moreover, the maximum exercise ventilation

FIGURE 9.42.2.   Oxygen Breathing.

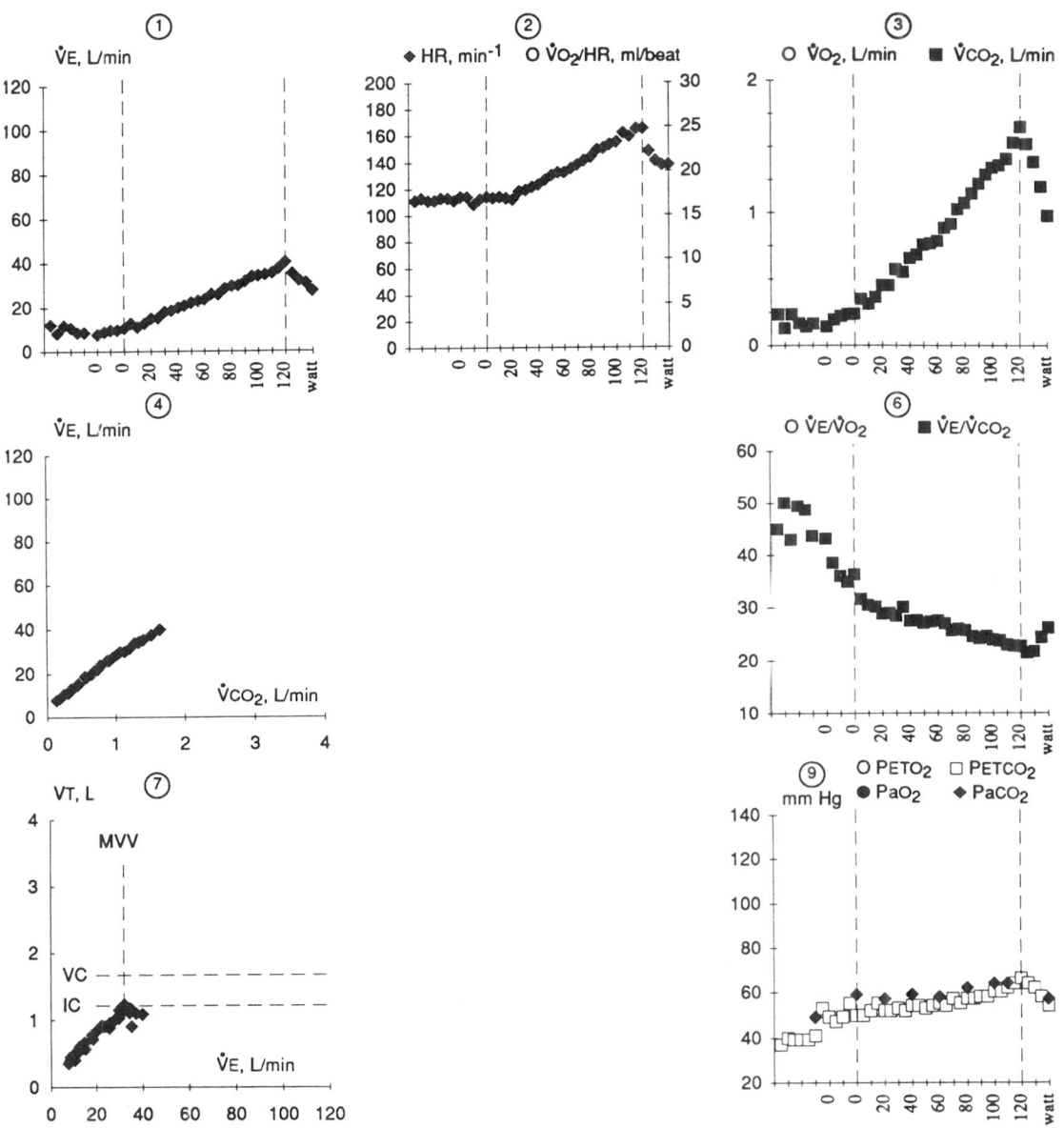

1. Vertical dashed lines in panels 1 to 3 and 6 and 9 indicate the beginning and the end of increasing work period.
2. Unloaded cycling is performed for 3 minutes before the left vertical dashed line.

TABLE 9.42.4. Oxygen Breathing

Time min	Work rate watts	BP mmHg	HR min⁻¹	f min⁻¹	V̇E L/min BTPS	V̇CO₂ L/min STPD	V̇O₂ L/min STPD	V̇O₂/HR ml/beat	F	pH	HCO₃ meq/L	PO₂ ET	PO₂ a	PO₂ (A−a)	PCO₂ ET	PCO₂ a	PCO₂ (a−ET)	V̇E/V̇CO₂	V̇E/V̇O₂	VD/VT
	Rest		111	23	12.3	0.23									37			45		
	Rest		113	21	8.3	0.13									40			50		
	Rest		111	23	11.8	0.23									39			43		
	Rest		111	26	10.6	0.17									39			49		
	Rest		113	22	8.7	0.14									39			49		
	Rest	144/94	113	19	8.6	0.16				7.35	27		587	77	41	49	8	44		0.48
	Unloaded		111	11											53					
	Unloaded		114	22	7.9	0.14									49			43		
	Unloaded		114	20	9.0	0.19									47			38		
	Unloaded		108	20	9.6	0.22									49			36		
	Unloaded		112	22	9.9	0.23									55			35		
	Unloaded	181/106	114	21	10.5	0.24				7.29	28		537	67	50	59	9	36		0.50
0.5	10		113	21	12.8	0.35									50			31		
1.0	10		114	21	11.2	0.31									52			30		
1.5	20		113	21	12.6	0.36									55			30		
2.0	20	194/106	112	22	14.8	0.45				7.30	28		584	72	52	57	5	29		0.41
2.5	30		118	27	15.3	0.45									52			29		
3.0	30		119	23	18.1	0.57									53			28		
3.5	40		121	26	18.7	0.55									52			30		
4.0	40	200/106	123	24	19.9	0.65				7.29	28		580	74	54	59	5	27		0.42
4.5	50		127	24	20.8	0.38									54			28		
5.0	50		130	24	22.2	0.75									53			27		
5.5	60		132	25	22.8	0.76									54			27		
6.0	60	206/100	132	26	23.6	0.78				7.29	27		595	60	55	58	3	27		0.41
6.5	70		135	27	25.9	0.38									54			27		
7.0	70		138	29	25.8	0.91									57			26		
7.5	80		141	28	28.7	1.02									55			26		
8.0	80	213/106	144	29	29.8	1.07				7.27	28		601	50	57	62	5	26		0.42
8.5	90		149	26	30.0	1.14									57			24		
9.0	90		150	28	31.5	1.21									58			24		
9.5	100		153	30	33.8	1.28									58			24		
10.0	100	231/106	155	29	34.2	1.33				7.24	27		606	43	60	64	4	24		0.40
10.5	110		162	31	34.5	1.35									60			24		
11.0	110	234/119	159	39	35.4	1.40				7.23	26		583	66	62	64	2	23		0.37
11.5	120		165	34	37.3	1.52									64			23		
12.0	120		165	37	40.1	1.64									66			23		
	Recovery		148	30	35.0	1.51									64			21		
	Recovery		141	26	32.1	1.38									62			22		
	Recovery		138	26	31.1	1.19									58			24		
	Recovery	214/100	138	28	27.6	0.97				7.21	22		587	69	54	57	3	26		0.38

increases during oxygen breathing at the maximum work rate from 32 L/min, the value of his resting MVV, to 40 L/min.

The increased work rate achieved during O₂ breathing is primarily the result of depression in the ventilatory response to exercise. Consequently, the patient develops a more significant respiratory and metabolic acidoses as compared to the air breathing test (increase in $PaCO_2$ of 6 mmHg above rest during air breathing, as compared to 15 mmHg for oxygen breathing). PaO_2 remains above 580 mmHg when breathing oxygen, indicating that no significant right to left shunt develops during exercise. Bicarbonate does not decrease in either study until 2 minutes after the exercise is terminated, because of the increase in $PaCO_2$ during exercise, but which decreases in recovery.

Conclusion

Exercise performance is limited by severe obstructive lung disease. Oxygen breathing results in an increased work capacity, despite a normal resting PaO_2.

Case 43 Lung Cancer and Chronic Bronchitis: Preoperative Evaluation

Clinical Findings

This 62-year-old man with a long history of chronic obstructive pulmonary disease was referred for exercise testing to assess operative risk because of the finding of a malignant pulmonary nodule. The patient had quit smoking approximately 3 months before and was being treated aggressively with bronchodilator therapy including oral corticosteroids. He had no known history of cardiovascular disease and stated he could walk 2 miles.

Exercise Findings

The patient performed exercise on a cycle ergometer. He pedalled at 60 rpm without an added load for 3 minutes. The work rate was then increased 10 W per minute to tolerance. Heart rate and rhythm were continuously monitored and ECGs were repeatedly obtained. Blood pressure was measured with a sphygmomanometer and arterial saturation estimated with an ear oximeter. The patient gave an excellent effort and stopped exercise because of shortness of breath and leg fatigue. Resting and exercise ECGs and oximetry were normal.

TABLE 9.43.1.   Selected Respiratory Function Data

Measurement	Predicted	Measured
Age, yr		62
Sex		Male
Height, cm		170
Weight, kg	74	68
Hematocrit, %		49
VC, L	3.35	2.76
IC, L	2.23	2.07
TLC, L	5.20	5.46
FEV_1, L	2.62	1.28
FEV_1/VC, %	78	46
MVV, L/min	113	62
$D_{L}CO$, ml/mm Hg/min	22.9	20.2

TABLE 9.43.2.   Selected Exercise Data

Measurement	Predicted	Measured
Peak $\dot{V}O_2$, L/min	1.98	1.22
Maximum HR, beats/min	158	175
Maximum O_2 pulse, ml/beat	12.5	7.1
$\Delta\dot{V}O_2$/ΔWR, ml/min/W	10.3	6.7
AT, L/min	>0.87	0.6
Blood pressure, mmHg (rest, max)		130/80, 220/110
Maximum $\dot{V}E$, L/min		48
Exercise breathing reserve, L/min	>15	14
O_2 saturation, oximeter (rest, max)		96, 96

FIGURE 9.43.1.

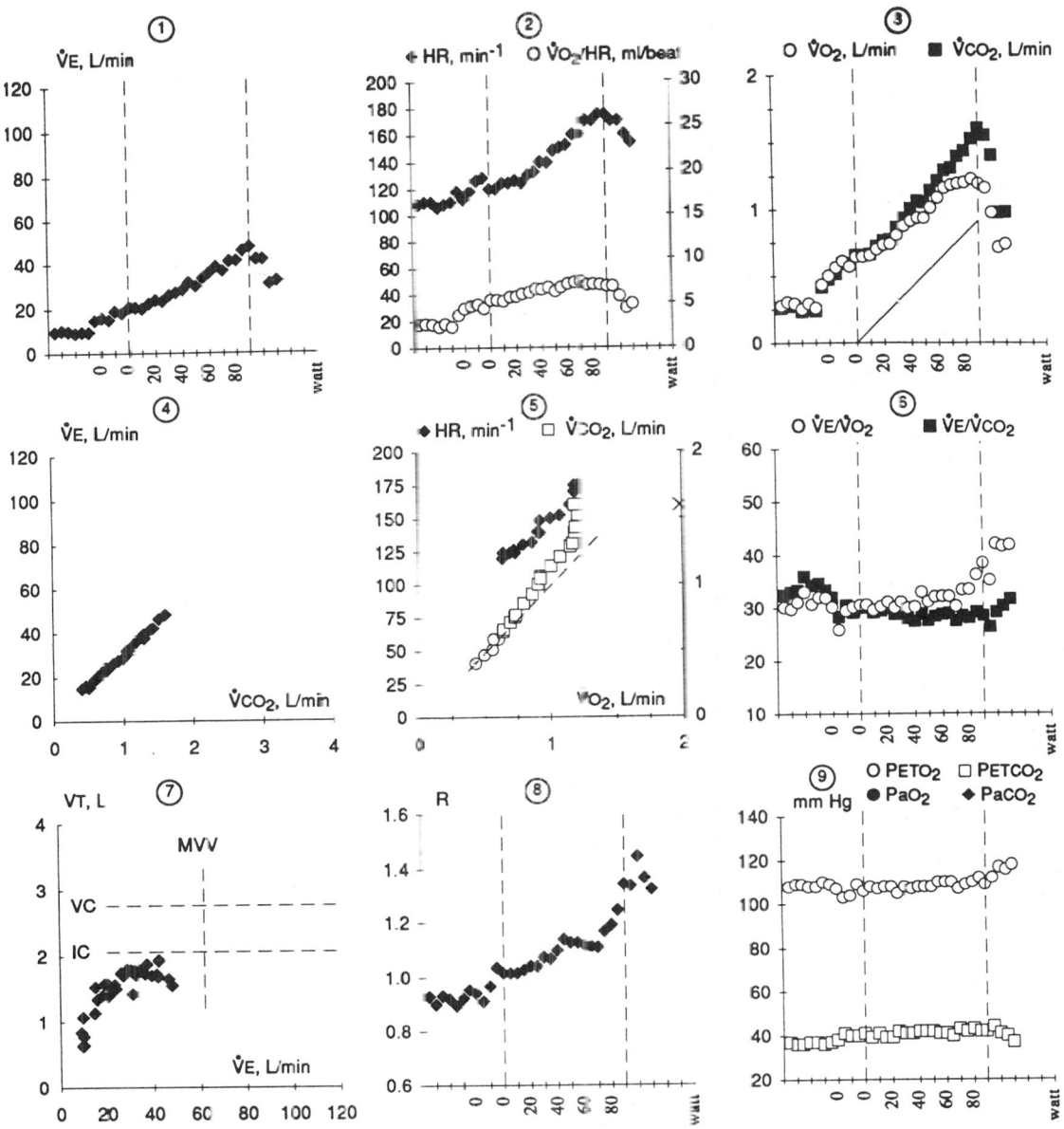

1. Vertical dashed lines in panels 1 to 3 and 6, 8, and 9 indicate the beginning and the end of increasing work period.

2. Unloaded cycling is performed for 3 minutes before the left vertical dashed line.

3. In panel 3, the diagonal line shows the increase of $\dot{V}O_2$ at a slope of 10 ml/min/w.

4. In panel 5, the diagonal dashed line has a slope of 1; the "x" in the upper right is the predicted maximum heart rate and $\dot{V}O_2$ for the subject.

Interpretation

Comments

Resting studies showed a moderately severe obstructive ventilatory defect. The anaerobic threshold is low. During unloaded pedalling, the R rose over 1.0 and persisted thereafter, evidence of excess CO_2 production because of lactic acid buffering at a low $\dot{V}O_2$.

Analysis

The most distinctive abnormalities are the exercise tachycardia, low and early plateau of the $\dot{V}O_2$ and

TABLE 9.43.3. Air Breathing

Time min	Work rate watts	BP mmHg	HR min⁻¹	f min⁻¹	V̇E L/min BTPS	V̇CO₂ L/min STPD	V̇O₂ L/min STPD	V̇O₂/HR ml/beat	R	pH	HCO₃⁻ meq/L	PO₂ mmHg ET	a	(A−a)	PCO₂ mmHg ET	a	(a−ET)	V̇E/V̇CO₂	V̇E/V̇O₂	VD/VT
	Rest	130/80																		
	Rest		108	15	9.7	0.26	0.28	2.6	0.93			108			37			32	30	
	Rest		110	16	10.3	0.27	0.30	2.7	0.90			109			36			33	30	
	Rest		110	13	10.1	0.27	0.29	2.6	0.93			109			36			33	31	
	Rest	130/80	106	11	9.2	0.23	0.25	2.4	0.92			108			37			36	33	
	Rest		108	9	9.7	0.26	0.29	2.7	0.90			108			37			34	31	
	Rest		110	15	9.6	0.24	0.26	2.4	0.92			110			36			35	32	
	Unloaded		118	13	14.8	0.41	0.43	3.6	0.95			109			37			33	32	
	Unloaded		112	12	16.1	0.47	0.50	4.5	0.94			107			38			32	30	
	Unloaded		118	10	15.3	0.51	0.56	4.7	0.91			103			41			28	26	
	Unloaded		126	12	19.0	0.59	0.61	4.8	0.97			104			40			30	29	
	Unloaded		128	13	18.3	0.59	0.57	4.5	1.04			109			40			29	30	
	Unloaded	140/80	120	13	20.6	0.65	0.64	5.3	1.02			106			41			30	30	
0.5	10		120												39			30	31	
1.0	10	150/90	124	15	20.9	0.65	0.64	5.3	1.02			108			41			29	30	
1.5	20		124	13	20.3	0.66	0.65	5.2	1.02			107			39			29	30	
2.0	20		126	15	22.5	0.72	0.70	5.6	1.03			108			39			30	31	
				16	24.1	0.76	0.73	5.8	1.04			108								
2.5	30		124	15	23.5	0.77	0.74	6.0	1.04			105			42			29	30	
3.0	30		130	15	26.2	0.86	0.80	6.2	1.08			108			41			29	31	
3.5	40		132	16	27.4	0.93	0.87	6.6	1.07			107			41			28	30	
4.0	40	150/90	140	16	28.8	1.00	0.91	6.5	1.10			108			42			27	30	
4.5	50		139	18	32.1	1.06	0.93	6.7	1.14			108			42			29	33	
5.0	50		148	17	30.4	1.05	0.93	6.3	1.13			108			42			28	31	
5.5	60		150	19	34.0	1.14	1.01	6.7	1.13			110			41			28	32	
6.0	60	200/100	152	21	36.5	1.21	1.08	7.1	1.12			110			41			29	32	
6.5	70		160	23	39.3	1.29	1.16	7.3	1.11			110			40			29	32	
7.0	70		160	20	37.5	1.31	1.18	7.4	1.11			107			43			27	30	
7.5	80		170	24	41.6	1.39	1.19	7.0	1.17			109			42			28	33	
8.0	80	200/100	170	25	42.2	1.43	1.20	7.1	1.19			110			43			28	33	
8.5	90		175	28	46.5	1.52	1.22	7.0	1.25			112			42			29	36	
9.0	90		175	31	48.2	1.60	1.19	6.8	1.34			109			42			28	38	
	Recovery		170	22	42.6	1.55	1.16	6.8	1.34			112			44			26	35	
	Recovery		170	22	42.5	1.40	0.97	5.7	1.44			117			41			29	42	
	Recovery		160	22	31.3	0.97	0.71	4.4	1.37			116			40			30	41	
	Recovery	220/110	154	19	32.6	0.98	0.74	4.8	1.32			118			37			32	42	

the O₂ pulse, and the low $\Delta\dot{V}O_2/\Delta WR$. Peak $\dot{V}O_2$ and the anaerobic threshold are decreased (Table 9.43.2) leading us to flow chart 4. The breathing reserve is borderline low (branchpoint 4.1). We do not have arterial blood gas measurements to address the question of VD/VT (branchpoint 4.2), but the $\dot{V}E/\dot{V}CO_2$ at the anaerobic threshold is normal suggesting that the VD/VT is within normal limits. The high ratio of tidal volume to inspiratory capacity and the borderline breathing reserve are compatible with obstructive lung disease. We know from panels 2, 3, 5, and 8 of the exercise test that the patient has a significant circulatory problem. Because of the normal VD/VT, the circulatory problem is not due to disease of the pulmonary circulation. Also, because of the large release of buffer CO₂ during exercise the circulatory problem is not due to peripheral

arterial disease. The steep heart rate response, low flat O₂ pulse response to exercise, low plateau in $\dot{V}O_2$ at maximal work rate, low AT and reduced $\Delta\dot{V}O_2/\Delta WR$ are all consistent with primary heart disease such as left ventricular failure limiting exercise performance.

Conclusion

The patient's $\dot{V}O_2$max of 18 ml/min/kg is associated with an intermediate risk for morbidity and mortality for lung resection. Values below 15 ml/min/kg indicate a higher risk. Unfortunately, the patient was found to have an enlarged axillary lymph node with metastatic malignant cells a few days later and was no longer a potential operative candidate.

Case 44 Bullous Emphysema: Pre- and Post-bullectomy

Clinical Findings

This 50-year-old computer technician had retired approximately 10 years prior to initial evaluation because of progressive dyspnea. He denied cough, sputum production, wheezing, or chest pain. There was no family history of lung disease. Chest x-ray studies showed large bullous lesions in the right mid and upper lung fields. Flow rates did not improve following four breaths of nebulized isoproterenol. Perfusion scan demonstrated no perfusion in the right mid and upper hemithorax or at the left apex. α-1-Antitrypsin levels were normal. One month after the first exercise test, the patient's right upper lobe and portions of the right middle lobe were resected. The resected lung showed bullous and centriacinar emphysema with patchy atelectasis; a small squamous cell scar carcinoma was found in the upper lobe. He continued to smoke heavily.

Exercise Findings

Preoperatively, the patient performed exercise on a cycle ergometer breathing room air, and following a 90-minute rest, breathing 100% oxygen. Three months postoperatively, only an air breathing study was performed. On each occasion, he pedaled at 60 rpm, on an unloaded cycle, for 2, 3, or 4 minutes.

The work rate was then increased 20 W every minute. Arterial blood was sampled every second minute, and intra-arterial blood pressure was recorded from a percutaneous brachial artery catheter. Resting ECGs were normal. Preoperatively, the patient stopped exercise because of dyspnea without an exercise-induced abnormality in the ECG. He stopped during the postoperative test because of dyspnea and pressure-like right-sided chest pain. There were multifocal, back-to-back, and salvos of premature ventricular contractions at the end of exercise and for 2 minutes of recovery without abnormal ST segment changes.

TABLE 9.44.1.   Selected Respiratory Function Data

Measurement	Predicted	Preoperative	Postoperative
Age, yr		50	
Sex		Male	
Height, cm		170	
Weight, kg	74	71	
Hematocrit, %		46	
VC, L	3.89	3.01	3.57
IC, L	2.59	2.03	2.46
TLC, L	5.69	7.05	5.56
FEV_1, L	3.09	1.93	2.44
FEV_1/VC, %	79	64	68
MVV, L/min	131	90	110
D_{LCO} ml/mm Hg/min	26.5	10.0	13.0

TABLE 9.44.2.   Selected Exercise Data

Measurement	Predicted	Preoperative	Postoperative
Peak $\dot{V}O_2$, L/min	2.32	0.99	1.06
Maximum HR, beats/min	170	144	144
Maximum O_2 pulse, ml/beat	13.7	7.5	7.9
$\Delta\dot{V}O_2/\Delta WR$, ml/min/W	10.3	5.1	5.8
AT, L/min	>1.00	0.6	0.75
Blood pressure, mmHg (rest, max)		144/90, 187/100	144/88, 238/94
Maximum $\dot{V}E$, L/min		84	80
Exercise breathing reserve, L/min	>15	6	30
PaO_2, mmHg (rest, max ex)		67, 54	74, 74
$P(A-a)O_2$, mmHg (rest, max ex)		47, 72	34, 52
$P(a-ET)CO_2$, mmHg (rest, max ex)		4, 8	4, 3
VD/VT (rest, heavy ex)		0.39, 0.47	0.41, 0.40
HCO_3^-, mEq/L (rest, 2-min recov)		21, 14	21, 14

TABLE 9.44.3. Pre-bullectomy Study

Time min	Work rate watts	BP mmHg	HR min⁻¹	f min⁻¹	V̇E L/min BTPS	V̇CO₂ L/min STPD	V̇O₂ L/min STPD	V̇O₂/HR ml/beat	R	pH	HCO₃⁻ meq/L	PO₂, mmHg ET	a	(A−a)	PCO₂, mmHg ET	a	(a−ET)	V̇E/V̇CO₂	V̇E/V̇O₂	VD/VT
	Rest									7.41	21		63			34				
	Rest		69	21	9.7	0.12	0.14	2.0	0.86			120			25			66	57	
	Rest		69	17	10.3	0.16	0.20	2.9	0.80			117			26			55	44	
	Rest		70	15	8.5	0.14	0.18	2.6	0.78			115			27			52	40	
	Rest		70	19	10.7	0.18	0.22	3.1	0.82			117			27			50	41	
	Rest		70	14	10.0	0.18	0.21	3.0	0.86			119			26			49	42	
	Rest	144/90	69	15	10.1	0.17	0.21	3.0	0.81	7.41	19	119	67	47	26	30	4	52	42	0.39
	Unloaded		76	31	29.2	0.45	0.49	6.4	0.92			124			23			59	54	
	Unloaded		80	32	30.5	0.48	0.52	6.5	0.92			125			23			58	53	
	Unloaded		80	32	31.4	0.50	0.52	6.5	0.96			125			23			57	55	
	Unloaded		84	29	28.3	0.47	0.50	6.0	0.94			124			24			55	52	
	Unloaded		88	33	29.8	0.46	0.48	5.5	0.96			124			24			59	56	
	Unloaded	156/90	87	28	28.9	0.48	0.51	5.9	0.94	7.41	18	125	62	58	24	29	5	55	52	0.42
0.5	20		91	32	32.6	0.53	0.57	6.3	0.93			125			24			56	52	
1.0	20		93	30	32.8	0.55	0.57	6.1	0.96			125			24			55	53	
1.5	40		93	32	35.0	0.57	0.59	6.3	0.97			124			24			57	55	
2.0	40	162/94	96	32	37.4	0.62	0.62	6.5	1.00	7.40	17	125	59	63	24	28	4	56	56	0.42
2.5	60		100	35	42.9	0.70	0.68	6.8	1.03			156			24			57	59	
3.0	60		104	40	50.8	0.80	0.76	7.3	1.05			156			24			59	62	
3.5	80		111	43	57.5	0.91	0.82	7.4	1.11			159			22			59	66	
4.0	80	181/96	116	45	62.7	1.00	0.87	7.5	1.15	7.40	18	159	51	72	22	30	8	59	68	0.48
4.5	100		120	58	77.3	1.13	0.95	7.9	1.19			131			20			64	76	
5.0	100		132	60	84.2	1.20	0.97	7.3	1.24			132			20			66	82	
5.5	120	187/100	144	57	78.6	1.19	0.99	6.9	1.20	7.39	17	133	54	72	20	28	8	62	75	0.47
	Recovery		138	55	76.5	1.23	1.01	7.3	1.22			132			21			58	71	
	Recovery		132	47	70.3	1.12	0.92	7.0	1.22			132			20			59	72	
	Recovery		120	44	66.2	1.08	0.83	6.9	1.30			133			20			58	75	
	Recovery	196/99	109	40	56.5	0.92	0.64	5.9	1.44	7.31	14	133	66	62	21	29	8	58	83	0.46

TABLE 9.44.4. Post-bullectomy Study

Time min	Work rate watts	BP mmHg	HR min⁻¹	f min⁻¹	V̇E L/min BTPS	V̇CO₂ L/min STPD	V̇O₂ L/min STPD	V̇O₂/HR ml/beat	R	pH	HCO₃⁻ meq/L	PO₂, mmHg ET	a	(A−a)	PCO₂, mmHg ET	a	(a−ET)	V̇E/V̇CO₂	V̇E/V̇O₂	VD/VT
	Rest	150/94								7.44	21		76			32				
	Rest		74	15	10.6	0.19	0.25	3.4	0.76			112			30			49	37	
	Rest	144/88	77	16	12.1	0.23	0.30	3.9	0.77	7.42	22	112	74	34	30	34		47	36	0.41
	Unloaded		94	21	23.3	0.46	0.57	6.1	0.81			111			30			47	38	
	Unloaded		93	19	22.0	0.45	0.54	5.8	0.83			113			30			45	38	
	Unloaded		91	19	21.9	0.46	0.56	6.2	0.82			115			29			44	36	
	Unloaded	163/88	92	19	22.2	0.47	0.49	5.3	0.96	7.42	21		68	48	31	33	2	44	42	0.37
0.5	20		103	22	24.2	0.49	0.58	5.6	0.84			116			29			46	39	
1.0	20		95	20	24.3	0.51	0.61	6.4	0.84			114			30			44	37	
1.5	40		99	21	28.3	0.60	0.69	7.0	0.87			114			30			44	38	
2.0	40	175/94	100	26	33.7	0.69	0.75	7.5	0.92	7.42	21	117	64	51	29	33	4	46	42	0.40
2.5	60		107	28	40.1	0.83	0.81	7.6	1.02			120			28			45	47	
3.0	60		112	32	47.2	0.98	0.88	7.9	1.11			121			28			45	51	
3.5	80		119	36	54.9	1.10	0.94	7.9	1.17			120			30			47	55	
4.0	80	225/94	130	42	62.4	1.25	1.03	7.9	1.21	7.39	20	123	66	55	28	34	6	47	57	0.43
4.5	100		134	44	69.9	1.40	1.06	7.9	1.32			125			28			47	62	
5.0	100	238/94	138	48	75.7	1.48	1.06	7.7	1.40	7.35	17	126	74	52	28	31	3	48	68	0.40
5.5	120		144	57	79.5	1.52	1.06	7.4	1.43			128			26			49	70	
	Recovery		144	45	74.5	1.49	1.00	6.9	1.49			129			26			47	71	
	Recovery		132	39	69.8	1.41	1.00	7.6	1.41			128			27			47	66	
	Recovery		114	36	63.5	1.26	0.85	7.5	1.48			130			26			48	71	
	Recovery	231/100	102	31	53.2	1.01	0.65	6.4	1.55	7.31	14	131	88	41	25	29	4	50	78	0.39

FIGURE 9.44.1.   Pre-bullectomy study.

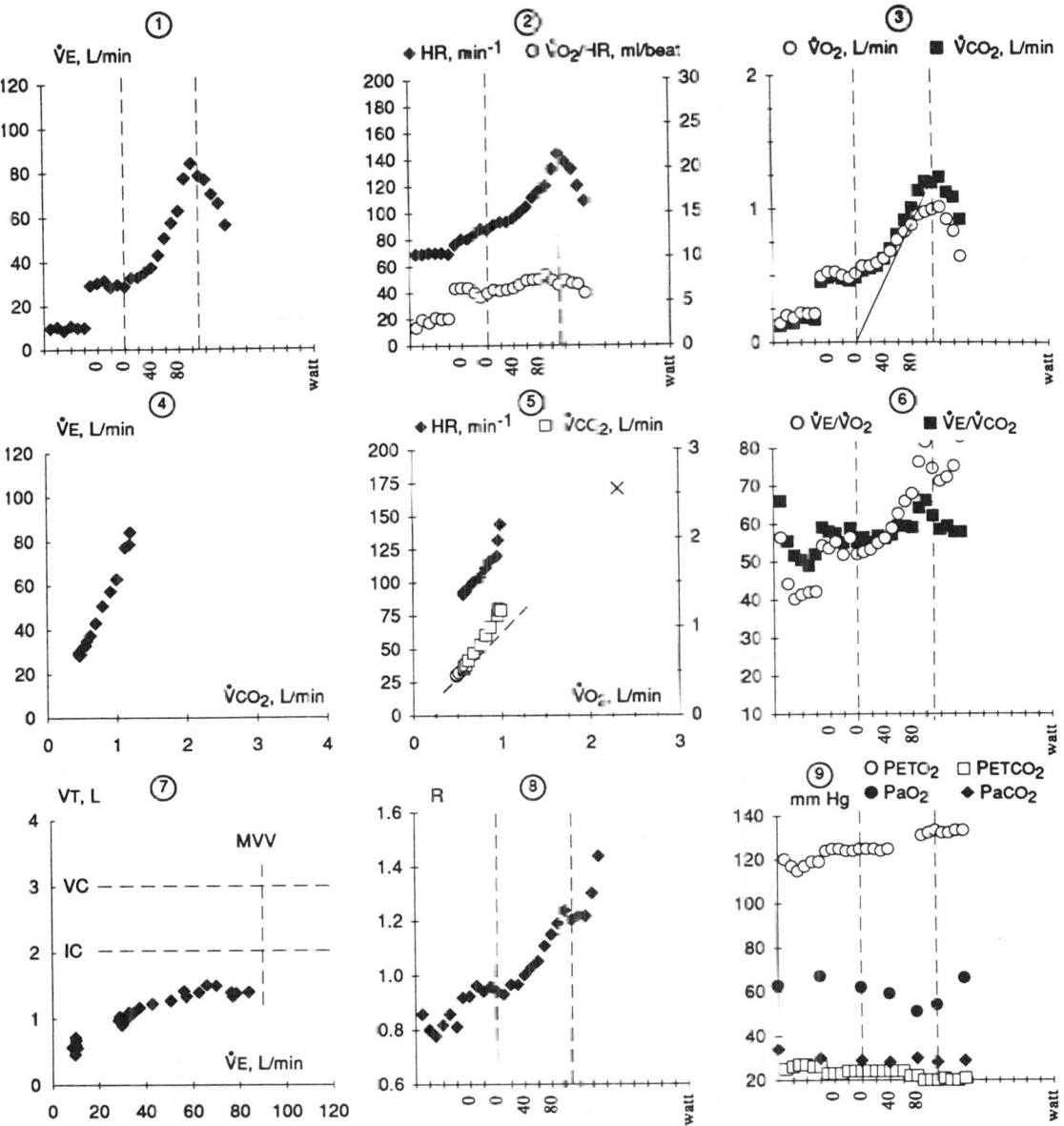

1. Vertical dashed lines in panels 1 to 3 and 6, 8, and 9 indicate the beginning and the end of increasing work period.
2. Unloaded cycling is performed for 3 minutes before the left vertical dashed line.
3. In panel 3, the diagonal line shows the increase of $\dot{V}O_2$ at a slope of 10 ml/min/w.
4. In panel 5, the diagonal dashed line has a slope of 1; the "x" in the upper right is the predicted maximum heart rate and $\dot{V}O_2$ for the subject.

FIGURE 9.44.2.   Post-bullectomy study.

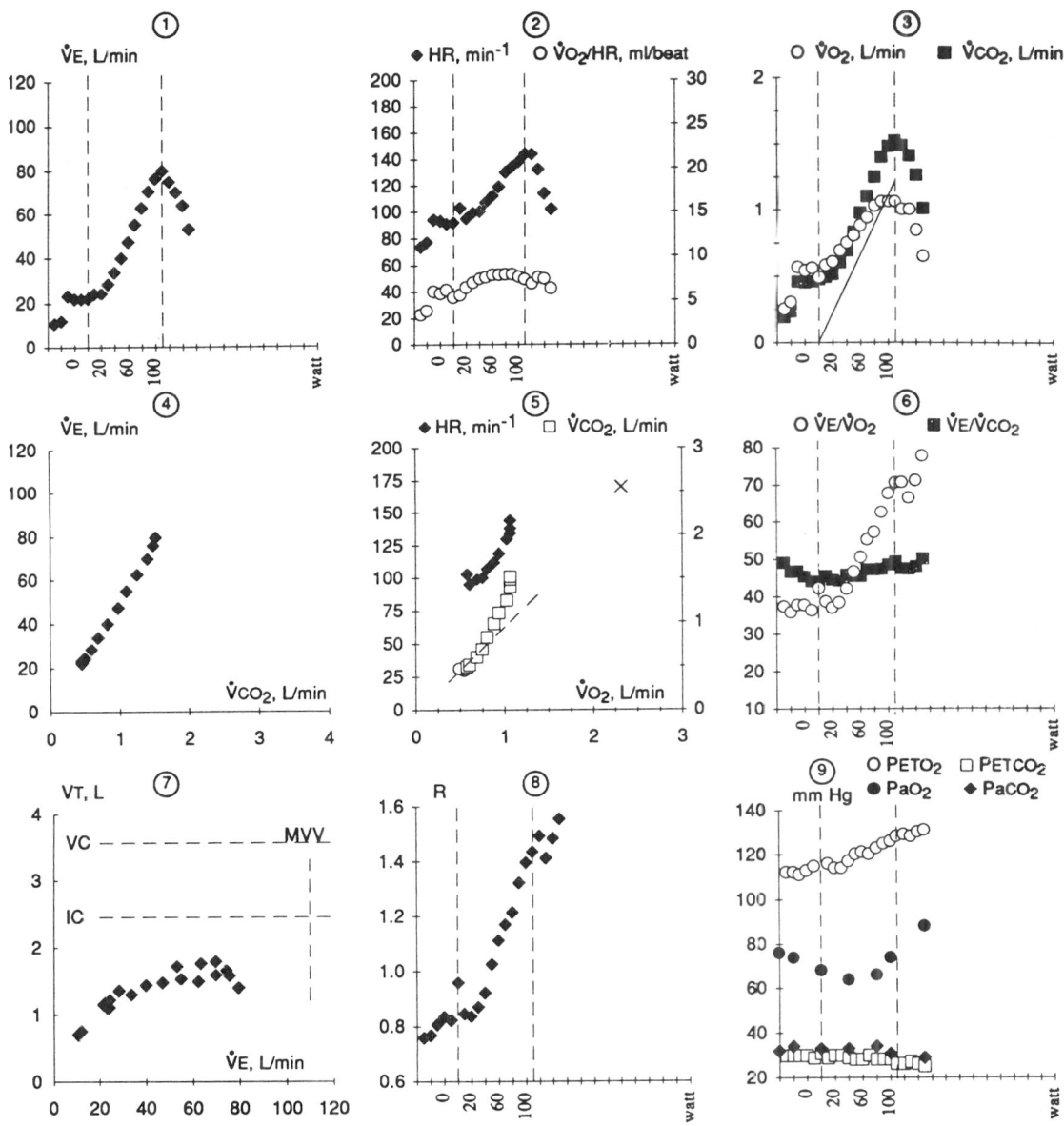

1. Vertical dashed lines in panels 1 to 3 and 6, 8, and 9 indicate the beginning and the end of increasing work period.
2. Unloaded cycling is performed for 3 minutes before the left vertical dashed line.
3. In panel 3, the diagonal line shows the increase of $\dot{V}O_2$ at a slope of 10 ml/min/w.
4. In panel 5, the diagonal dashed line has a slope of 1; the "x" in the upper right is the predicted maximum heart rate and $\dot{V}O_2$ for the subject.

Interpretation

Comments

Resting respiratory function studies show moderate obstructive lung disease with marked reduction in diffusing capacity ($D_L CO$). Following a bullectomy, the vital capacity increased, and the residual volume decreased with improvement in expiratory flow (Table 9.44.1). Although the diffusing capacity is slightly improved, it is still disproportionately reduced compared to the flow rate impairment. For example, postoperatively the MVV is 84% of predicted, whereas the diffusing capacity measurement is 50% of predicted. Exercise tolerance, surprisingly, is only slightly improved postoperatively.

Analysis

Referring to flow chart 1, the peak $\dot{V}c_2$ and anaerobic threshold are significantly reduced pre- and postoperatively (Table 9.44.2). See flow chart 4: Preoperatively the exercise breathing reserve is low, but postoperatively the breathing reserve is normal (branchpoint 4.1). Taking the low breathing reserve branch directed by the preoperative study, VD/VT is high, consistent with lung disease with impaired peripheral oxygenation (branchpoint 4.2). The confirmatory abnormalities noted in that diagnostic box are found in Table 9.44.3.

Post-bullectomy, we must take the normal breathing reserve branch at branchpoint 4.1. The ventilatory equivalent for CO_2 at the AT is high and the indices of ventilation-perfusion mismatching are abnormal, supporting the diagnosis of an abnormal pulmonary circulation (branchpoint 4.5). The vital capacity is normal suggesting that the abnormality in the pulmonary circulation is due to pulmonary vascular disease. This is supported by a low resting $D_L CO$. There is no abrupt reduction in PaO_2, postoperatively, as might be expected with a right to left shunt. This was confirmed by a repeat exercise test with the patient breathing 100% oxygen (not shown). Referring to the diagnostic box under abnormal pulmonary circulation, confirmatory observations are: 1) a steep heart rate response to the increase in $\dot{V}O_2$, becoming steeper as the peak $\dot{V}O_2$ is approached (panel 5); 2) a low O_2 pulse with a flat contour as work rate is increased (panel 2); and 3) a decreasing $\Delta\dot{V}O_2/\Delta WR$ as work rate is increased (panel 3) for both the pre- (Fig. 9.44.1) and postoperative (Fig. 9.44.2) studies. All these findings are consistent with an oxygen flow problem of the type seen with functionally important pulmonary vascular disease. Bullectomy did not improve the abnormalities in O_2 flow although it improved the ventilatory mechanics. Despite improvement in respiratory mechanics, post-operatively, exercise performance did not improve significantly. Pulmonary vascular disease was the predominant factor limiting exercise pre-operatively. The ectopy noted during exercise, after bullectomy, might be secondary to the development of critically important pulmonary hypertension.

Conclusion

The patient has bullous emphysema. Pulmonary vascular occlusive disease limited exercise performance, after bullectomy.

Case 45 Obstructive Airway Disease: Before and After Rehabilitation

Clinical Findings

This 69-year-old man with known chronic obstructive lung disease was evaluated before and after a pulmonary rehabilitation program of 2 months' duration, which featured (among other components) a program of cycle ergometer exercise. The patient exercised for 45 minutes per day, 3 days per week on a stationery bicycle at exercise intensities approaching his maximum tolerance. Resting respiratory and exercise testing data for both occasions are shown. The patient had recently stopped smoking, though he had a 51-year history of cigarette smoking. His medications included theophylline and inhaled apha-agonist and anticholinergic agents.

Exercise Findings

The patient performed exercise on a cycle ergometer before and after a 2-month training period. He pedalled at 60 rpm without an added load for 3 minutes. The work rate was then increased 5 W per minute to tolerance. Heart rate and rhythm were continuously monitored; 12-lead ECGs were obtained during rest, exercise, and recovery. Every 2 minutes, blood pressure was measured by a sphygmomanometer, and a sample of blood was drawn from a venous catheter placed in the back of the hand. Blood samples were assayed for blood lactate concentration. The patient was well motivated and cooperative and stopped exercise on both occasions because of dyspnea. No ECG abnormalities at rest or during exercise were noted.

TABLE 9.45.1. Selected Respiratory Function Data

Measurement	Predicted	Measured	
Age, yr		69	
Sex		Male	
Height, cm		170	
Weight, kg	60	74	
Hematocrit, %		40	
		Before	After*
VC, L	3.60	1.99	2.19
IC, L	2.40	1.50	1.65
FEV$_1$, L	2.78	0.99	1.11
FEV$_1$/VC, %	77	50	51
MVV, indirect, L/min	111	40	44
D$_L$CO, ml/mm Hg/min	22.4	10.6	12.7

* After training.

TABLE 9.45.2. Selected Exercise Data

Measurement	Predicted	Before	After
Peak V̇o$_2$, L/min	1.67	0.90	1.0
Maximum HR, beats/min	151	136	140
Work rate, max, W		30	50
Maximum O$_2$ pulse, ml/beat	11.1	6.6	7.6
ΔV̇o$_2$/ΔWR, ml/min/W	10.3		8.2
AT, L/min	>0.75	0.75	Indeterminate*
Maximum V̇E, L/min		40	42
Exercise breathing reserve, L/min, using indirect MVV	>15	0	2
Peak lactate, mEq/L		3.0	2.3

*Apparently, because of the small increase in lactate after training, a breakpoint in the V-slope plot (panel 5) is not observed.

FIGURE 9.45.1.   Before training.

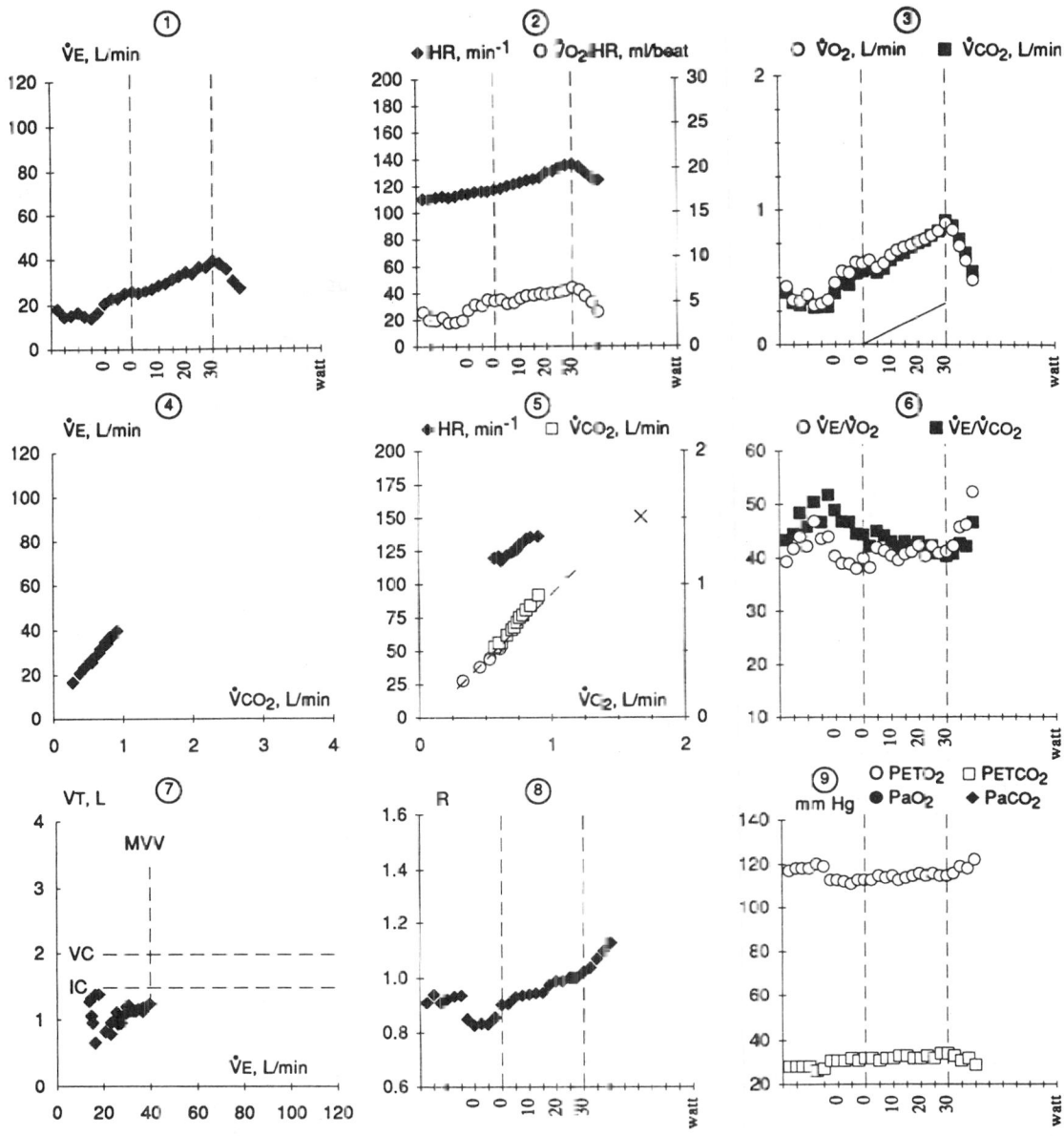

1. Vertical dashed lines in panels 1 to 3 and 6, 8, and 9 indicate the beginning and the end of increasing work period.
2. Unloaded cycling is performed for 3 minutes before the left vertical dashed line.
3. In panel 3, the diagonal line shows the increase of $\dot{V}O_2$ at a slope of 10 ml/min/w.
4. In panel 5, the diagonal dashed line has a slope of 1; the "x" in the upper right is the predicted maximum heart rate and $\dot{V}O_2$ for the subject.

TABLE 9.45.3. Before Training

Time min	Work rate watts	BP mmHg	HR min⁻¹	f̄ min⁻¹	V̇E L/min BTPS	V̇CO₂ L/min STPD	V̇O₂ L/min STPD	V̇O₂/HR ml/beat	R	pH	HCO₃⁻ meq/L	PO₂, mmHg ET	a	(A−a)	PCO₂, mmHg ET	a	(a−ET)	V̇E/V̇CO₂	V̇E/V̇O₂	VD/VT
	Rest		110	13	18.0	0.39	0.43	3.9	0.91			117			28			43	39	
	Rest		110	11	14.7	0.31	0.33	3.0	0.94			118			28			44	42	
	Rest		111	16	15.4	0.29	0.32	2.9	0.91			118			28			48	44	
	Rest		112	12	16.6	0.34	0.37	3.3	0.92			118			28			46	42	
	Rest		111	14	14.8	0.27	0.29	2.6	0.93			120			26			50	47	
	Rest		112	11	14.0	0.28	0.30	2.7	0.93			119			27			47	44	
	Unloaded		114	25	16.6	0.28	0.33	2.9	0.85			113			31			52	44	
	Unloaded		114	25	20.7	0.38	0.46	4.0	0.83			113			31			49	40	
	Unloaded		115	24	23.1	0.45	0.54	4.7	0.83			112			31			47	39	
	Unloaded		116	29	23.0	0.44	0.53	4.6	0.83			111			32			47	39	
	Unloaded		116	25	25.2	0.52	0.61	5.3	0.85			113			31			44	38	
	Unloaded		117	25	26.0	0.54	0.60	5.1	0.90			113			32			44	40	
0.5	5		118	23	25.6	0.56	0.62	5.3	0.90			113			32			42	38	
1.0	5		120	28	26.2	0.53	0.57	4.8	0.93			115			31			45	42	
1.5	10		121	27	27.0	0.56	0.60	5.0	0.93			114			32			44	41	
2.0	10		122	27	28.9	0.62	0.66	5.4	0.94			115			32			43	40	
2.5	15		124	25	29.8	0.66	0.70	5.6	0.94			113			33			42	40	
3.0	15		125	28	31.6	0.68	0.72	5.8	0.94			114			33			43	41	
3.5	20		126	29	32.8	0.72	0.74	5.9	0.97			115			32			42	41	
4.0	20		130	30	34.7	0.75	0.76	5.8	0.99			116			32			43	42	
4.5	25		131	30	33.9	0.77	0.78	6.0	0.99			115			33			41	40	
5.0	25		134	33	36.9	0.81	0.81	6.0	1.00			116			32			42	42	
5.5	30		135	31	36.9	0.84	0.84	6.2	1.00			115			34			41	41	
6.0	30		136	32	39.7	0.92	0.90	6.6	1.02			115			34			40	41	
	Recovery		134	32	38.5	0.88	0.85	6.3	1.04			116			33			41	42	
	Recovery		130	31	35.9	0.78	0.73	5.6	1.07			119			31			43	46	
	Recovery		126	25	30.7	0.68	0.62	4.9	1.10			118			32			42	46	
	Recovery		124	29	27.6	0.54	0.48	3.9	1.13			122			29			47	52	

Interpretation

Comments

This case shows the effects of a training program on resting respiratory function, work capacity, and peak V̇O₂. Resting studies show moderate obstructive lung disease, with severe loss of effective pulmonary capillary bed.

Analysis

Referring to flow chart 1, on the initial study the peak V̇O₂ was low, whereas the anaerobic threshold was at the lower limits of normal (Table 9.45.2). Regardless of which flow chart is used, we would arrive at the diagnosis of obstructive lung disease for both studies. Using flow chart 3 for the first study, we would go through branchpoints 3.1 and 3.2 to that diagnosis. Using flow chart 4, the low breathing reserve (branchpoint 4.1) and presumed high VD/VT because of the high V̇E/V̇CO₂ (branchpoint 4.2) lead us to the diagnosis of "lung disease with impaired peripheral oxygenation." If we had used flow chart 5.1, we would have arrived at the diagnosis of obstructive lung disease through branchpoints 5.1, 5.3, and 5.7.

Conclusion

Comparing the studies performed before and after pulmonary rehabilitation, it is apparent that this patient's exercise tolerance has improved appreciably. This can be explained only in part by the small improvement in airways obstruction. Insight into the cause of the improvement can be gained by comparing the physiologic responses at identical work rates in the two studies (Table 9.45.5).

FIGURE 9.45.2.   After training.

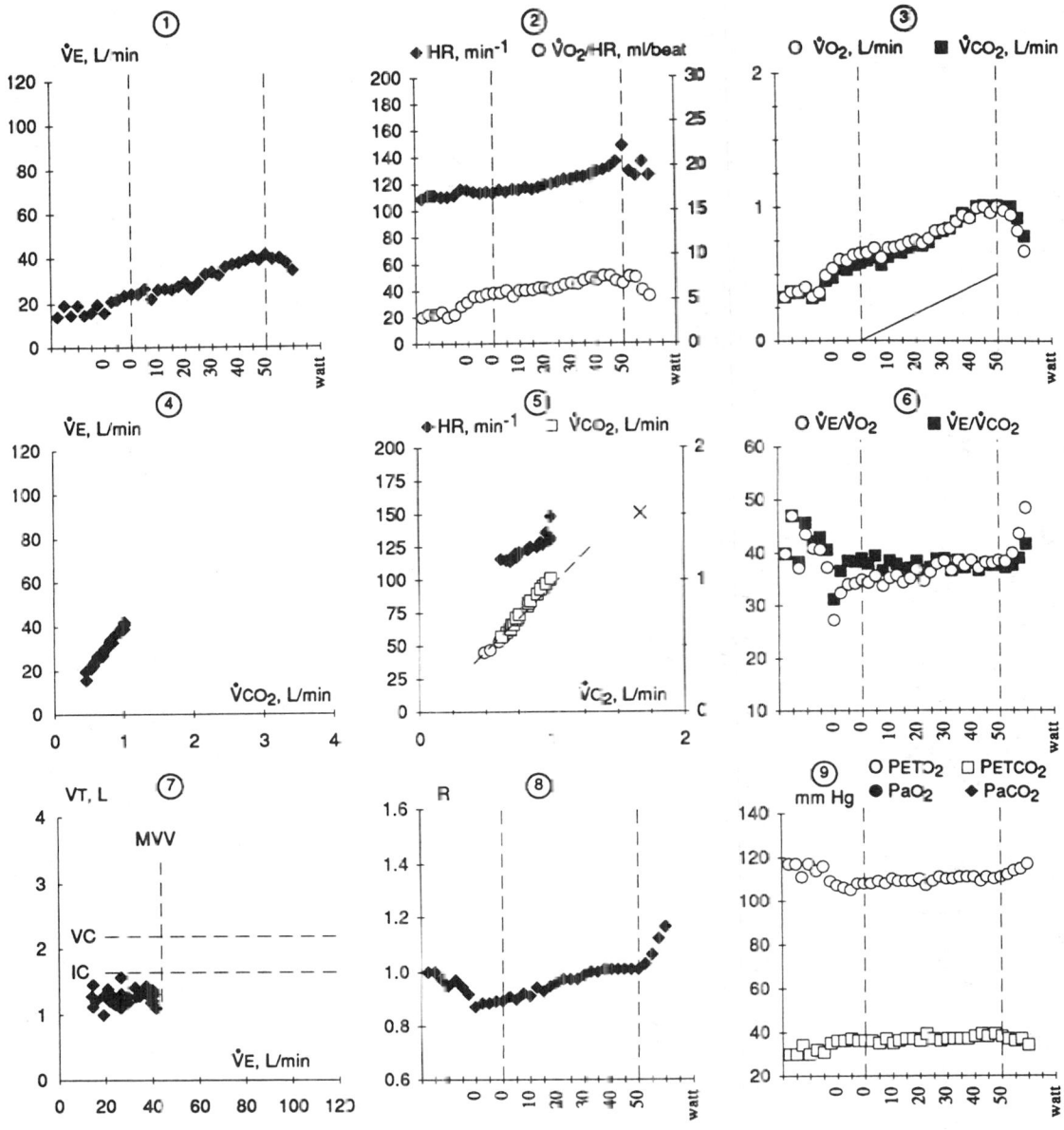

1. Vertical dashed lines in panels 1 to 3 and 6, 8, and 9 indicate the beginning and the end of increasing work period.

2. Unloaded cycling is performed for 3 minutes before the left vertical dashed line.

3. In panel 3, the diagonal line shows the increase of $\dot{V}O_2$ at a slope of 10 ml/min/w.

4. In panel 5, the diagonal dashed line has a slope of 1; the "$\times$" in the upper right is the predicted maximum heart rate and $\dot{V}O_2$ for the subject.

TABLE 9.45.4. After Training

Time min	Work rate watts	BP mmHg	HR min⁻¹	f min⁻¹	$\dot{V}_E$ L/min BTPS	$\dot{V}_{CO_2}$ L/min STPD	$\dot{V}_{O_2}$ L/min STPD	$\dfrac{\dot{V}_{O_2}}{HR}$ ml/beat	R	pH	HCO₃⁻ meq/L	PO₂, mmHg ET	a	(A−a)	PCO₂, mmHg ET	a	(a−ET)	$\dfrac{V_E}{\dot{V}_{CO_2}}$	$\dfrac{\dot{V}_E}{\dot{V}_{O_2}}$	$\dfrac{V_D}{V_T}$
	Rest		109	11	14.1	0.33	0.33	3.0	1.00			117			30			40	40	
	Rest		111	19	19.0	0.37	0.37	3.3	1.00			117			30			47	47	
	Rest		111	10	14.6	0.36	0.37	3.3	0.97			111			34			38	37	
	Rest		110	19	19.0	0.38	0.40	3.6	0.95			117			30			46	43	
	Rest		110	13	14.6	0.32	0.33	3.0	0.97			114			32			42	41	
	Rest		111	13	15.7	0.34	0.36	3.2	0.94			116			31			43	41	
	Unloaded		116	15	19.5	0.45	0.49	4.2	0.92			109			35			41	37	
	Unloaded		115	13	15.8	0.47	0.54	4.7	0.87			107			36			31	27	
	Unloaded		114	15	21.0	0.54	0.61	5.4	0.89			106			36			37	32	
	Unloaded		113	18	21.9	0.53	0.60	5.3	0.88			105			37			38	34	
	Unloaded		114	20	23.5	0.57	0.64	5.6	0.89			108			36			38	34	
	Unloaded		113	21	24.4	0.58	0.65	5.8	0.89			108			36			39	35	
0.5	5		115	20	24.4	0.60	0.66	5.7	0.91			108			36			38	34	
1.0	5		114	24	26.5	0.62	0.69	6.1	0.90			109			35			39	35	
1.5	10		116	17	22.3	0.57	0.62	5.3	0.92			108			37			37	34	
2.0	10		115	23	26.2	0.63	0.69	6.0	0.91			110			35			38	35	
2.5	15		117	20	26.6	0.66	0.70	6.0	0.94			109			36			38	36	
3.0	15		116	21	26.1	0.66	0.71	6.1	0.93			109			37			37	34	
3.5	20		117	22	27.8	0.70	0.74	6.3	0.95			109			37			37	35	
4.0	20		119	25	29.7	0.72	0.75	6.3	0.96			110			36			38	37	
4.5	25		120	17	26.7	0.71	0.73	6.1	0.97			107			39			36	35	
5.0	25		121	23	29.5	0.74	0.76	6.3	0.97			109			37			37	36	
5.5	30		123	26	33.2	0.80	0.82	6.7	0.98			111			36			39	38	
6.0	30		123	26	34.0	0.82	0.83	6.7	0.99			110			37			39	38	
6.5	35		125	23	32.6	0.84	0.84	6.7	1.00			110			37			36	36	
7.0	35		125	26	36.4	0.89	0.89	7.1	1.00			111			37			38	38	
7.5	40		127	26	37.4	0.95	0.94	7.4	1.01			111			37			37	37	
8.0	40		129	29	37.8	0.93	0.92	7.1	1.01			111			38			38	38	
8.5	45		130	29	39.0	1.00	0.99	7.6	1.01			109			39			37	37	
9.0	45		132	31	40.8	1.01	1.00	7.6	1.01			111			38			38	38	
9.5	50		136	33	39.3	0.97	0.96	7.1	1.01			110			39			38	38	
10.0	50		148	38	41.7	1.01	1.00	6.8	1.01			111			38			38	38	
	Recovery		129	33	39.9	1.00	0.97	7.5	1.03			112			37			37	38	
	Recovery		126	29	40.0	1.00	0.94	7.5	1.06			114			36			38	40	
	Recovery		136	29	38.2	0.92	0.82	6.0	1.12			115			37			39	44	
	Recovery		126	27	34.7	0.78	0.67	5.3	1.16			117			34			42	48	

TABLE 9.45.5. Selected Comparisons

	Responses to 30 Watts	
	Before Rehabilitation	After Rehabilitation
$\dot{V}_E$, L/min	40	34
$\dot{V}_{O_2}$, L/min	0.9	0.83
$\dot{V}_{CO_2}$, L/min	0.92	0.82
Heart rate, beats/min	136	123
Lactate, mEq/L	3.0	1.7

The reduction in lactate at a given work rate is characteristic of a physiologic training effect. This is also reflected in a lower $\dot{V}_{CO_2}$ (less CO_2 release from HCO_3^- buffering). The reduction in $\dot{V}_E$ and improved exercise tolerance are likely due to the reduced acid stimulus to breathing, reduced CO_2 production and improved ventilation-perfusion relationships (reduced V_D/V_T) reflected in a reduced ventilatory requirement for O_2 and CO_2.

Case 46 Early Asbestosis and Chronic Bronchitis

Clinical Findings

This 48-year-old shipyard worker denied having breathing difficulties and could climb 3 to 4 flights of stairs before noting shortness of breath. He had been treated for pneumonia 14 years before and for a pleural effusion 12 years ago. Two years previously, a benign "calcified mass" attached to a left lower rib had been removed. He had smoked a pack of cigarettes daily for 25 years and had a morning cough with small amounts of yellow sputum. No deformity, rhonchi, rales, or clubbing were noted on physical examination. Chest roentgenograms, including computerized tomographic views, showed bilateral pleural plaques and marked coarse parenchymal scarring at both bases.

Exercise Findings

The patient performed exercise on a cycle ergometer. He pedalled at 60 rpm without added load for 3 minutes. The work rate was then increased 20 W per minute to his symptom-limited maximum. Arterial blood was sampled every second minute, and intra-arterial blood pressure was recorded from a percutaneously placed brachial artery catheter. The patient stopped exercise because of chest discomfort. Resting and exercise ECG were normal. Carboxyhemoglobin was 8.3%.

TABLE 9.46.1. Selected Respiratory Function Data

Measurement	Predicted	Measured
Age, yr		48
Sex		Male
Height, cm		180
Weight, kg	82	97
Hematocrit, %		49
VC, L	4.87	4.84 (5.04*)
IC, L	3.25	3.12
TLC, L	7.06	7.12
FEV$_1$, L	3.88	3.23 (3.59*)
FEV$_1$/VC, %	80	67
MVV, L/min	158	183
D$_L$CO, ml/mm Hg/min	31.8	20.0

*After 4 breaths of aerosolized isoproterenol

TABLE 9.46.2. Selected Exercise Data

Measurement	Predicted	Measured
Peak $\dot{V}O_2$, L/min	2.77	2.37
Maximum HR, beats/min	172	149
Maximum O$_2$ pulse, ml/beat	16.1	15.9
$\Delta\dot{V}O_2/\Delta$WR, ml/min/W	10.3	10.3
AT, L/min	>1.19	1.3
Blood pressure mmHg (rest, max)		120/81, 213/84
Maximum $\dot{V}E$, L/min		98
Exercise breathing reserve, L/min	>15	85
PaO$_2$, mmHg (rest, max ex)		96, 72
P(A − a)O$_2$, mmHg (rest, max ex)		17, 47
P(a − ET)CO$_2$, mmHg (rest, max ex)		3, 1
VD/VT (rest, heavy ex)		0.41, 0.29
HCO$_3^-$, mEq/L (rest, 2-min recov)		25, 18

TABLE 9.46.3. Air Breathing

Time min	Work rate watts	BP mmHg	HR min⁻¹	f min⁻¹	$\dot{V}_E$ L/min BTPS	$\dot{V}_{CO_2}$ L/min STPD	$\dot{V}_{O_2}$ L/min STPD	$\dot{V}_{O_2}$/HR ml/beat	R	pH	HCO₃⁻ meq/L	PO₂, mmHg ET	a	(A−a)	PCO₂, mmHg ET	a	(a−ET)	$\dot{V}_E/\dot{V}_{CO_2}$	$\dot{V}_E/\dot{V}_{O_2}$	VD/VT
	Rest	120/81								7.43	25		90			38				
	Rest		60	15	9.6	0.19	0.22	3.7	0.86			111			34			44	38	
	Rest		62	14	22.6	0.54	0.64	10.3	0.84			104			36			40	33	
	Rest		66	18	18.0	0.37	0.38	5.8	0.97			117			31			45	43	
	Rest	120/78	60	18	17.3	0.35	0.38	6.3	0.92	7.45	24	114	96	17	32	35	3	45	42	0.41
	Rest		64	14	12.1	0.24	0.25	3.9	0.96			115			31			46	44	
	Rest		58	17	16.8	0.34	0.39	6.7	0.87			108			35			45	39	
	Unloaded		67	15	18.7	0.45	0.54	8.1	0.83			111			33			39	32	
	Unloaded		69	14	20.7	0.52	0.63	9.1	0.83			106			34			38	31	
	Unloaded		67	22	19.4	0.46	0.59	8.8	0.78			108			34			38	30	
	Unloaded		65	17	21.5	0.58	0.77	11.8	0.75			101			37			35	26	
	Unloaded		66	16	22.7	0.58	0.71	10.8	0.82			108			34			37	30	
	Unloaded	120/72	67	17	16.3	0.43	0.57	8.5	0.75	7.43	25	103	85	17	37	38	1	35	26	0.31
0.5	20		73	16	24.1	0.65	0.81	11.1	0.80			105			36			35	28	
1.0	20		76	14	20.4	0.69	0.78	10.3	0.88			103			37			28	25	
1.5	40		77	13	22.2	0.66	0.88	11.4	0.75			97			40			32	24	
2.0	40	129/72	84	20	22.1	0.65	0.88	10.5	0.74	7.42	25	97	81	18	41	40	−1	31	23	0.29
2.5	60		89	15	30.4	0.90	1.15	12.9	0.78			98			40			32	25	
3.0	60		91	13	23.3	0.74	0.95	10.4	0.78			91			44			30	23	
3.5	80		93	17	32.1	1.02	1.23	13.2	0.83			102			40			30	25	
4.0	80	150/75	98	21	37.7	1.16	1.34	13.7	0.87	7.39	24	101	77	27	41	41	0	31	27	0.30
4.5	100		103	18	39.4	1.26	1.41	13.7	0.89			102			41			30	27	
5.0	100		105	21	47.8	1.48	1.55	14.8	0.95			107			39			31	30	
5.5	120		106	20	47.2	1.53	1.58	14.9	0.97			107			40			30	29	
6.0	120	174/75	114	25	47.9	1.56	1.61	14.1	0.97	7.38	24	104	73	35	42	41	−1	29	28	0.27
6.5	140		124	27	61.6	1.92	1.83	14.8	1.05			110			33			31	32	
7.0	140		126	29	70.1	2.18	2.04	16.2	1.07			109			41			31	33	
7.5	160		132	31	75.6	2.25	2.01	15.2	1.12			115			36			32	36	
8.0	160	204/78	138	34	83.6	2.43	2.14	15.5	1.14	7.37	22	116	74	42	36	38	2	33	38	0.31
8.5	180		145	34	88.6	2.63	2.23	15.4	1.18			116			36			33	38	
9.0	180	213/84	149	10	97.6	2.86	2.37	15.9	1.21	7.36	20	119	72	47	37	36	−1	34	41	0.29
	Recovery		141	35	91.4	2.67	2.11	15.0	1.27			120			35			33	42	
	Recovery		122	35	84.5	2.26	1.59	13.0	1.42			124			33			36	51	
	Recovery		111	29	63.1	1.74	1.20	10.8	1.45			125			32			38	55	
	Recovery	213/72	106	23	51.2	1.32	0.96	9.1	1.38	7.33	18	123	99	24	32	34	2	37	51	0.31

Interpretation

Comments

The results of the resting respiratory function studies indicate that this patient has mild, reversible airflow obstruction and a moderate reduction in diffusing capacity (Table 9.46.1). His resting and exercise ECGs are normal. The man is a cigarette smoker with a high carboxyhemoglobin level in his blood.

Analysis

Referring to flow chart 1, the peak $\dot{V}_{O_2}$ and anaerobic threshold are at the lower limits of normal (Table 9.46.2). (See flow chart 2.) Even though these values are within the normal range and the ECG at the maximum work rate is normal, certain measurements become abnormal during exercise, indicating that the patient has ventilation-perfusion mismatching (branchpoint 2.3). These include mild arterial hypoxemia and a significant progressive increase in P(A − a)O₂ as work rate is increased. Moreover, P(a − ET)CO₂ is increased at the peak $\dot{V}_{O_2}$, and VD/VT are borderline normal.

Conclusion

Ventilation-perfusion mismatching during exercise in an asymptomatic, 48-year-old man, with maximum exercise performance at the lower limit of

FIGURE 9.46.1.

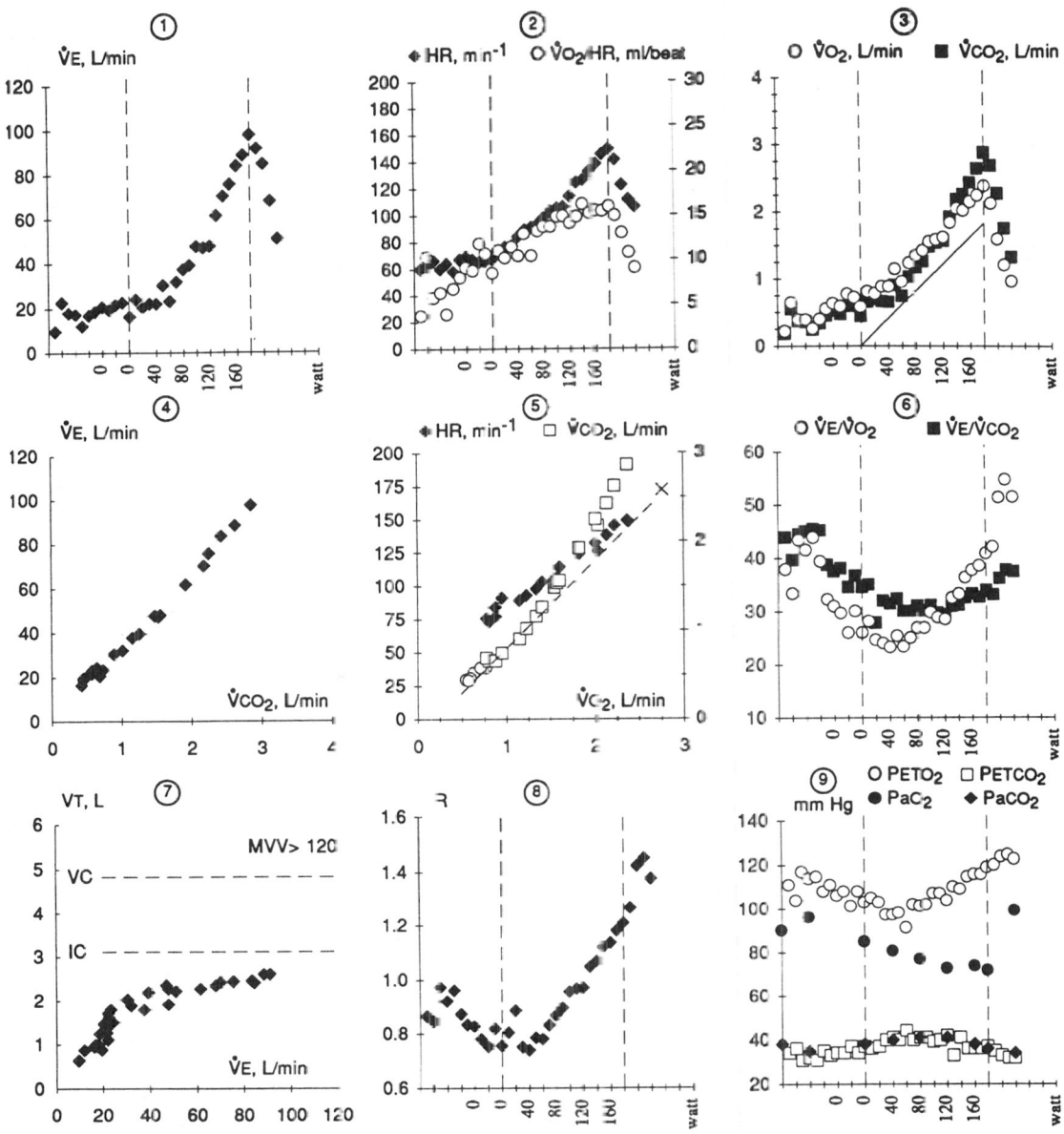

1. Vertical dashed lines in panels 1 to 3 and 6, 8, and 9 indicate the beginning and the end of increasing work period.

2. Unloaded cycling is performed for 3 minutes before the left vertical dashed line.

3. In panel 3, the diagonal line shows the increase of $\dot{V}C_2$ at a slope of 10 ml/min/w.

4. In panel 5, the diagonal dashed line has a slope of 1; the "X" in the upper right is the predicted maximum heart rate and $\dot{V}O_2$ for the subject.

normal. Putting this together with the history of a pleural effusion 12 years previously, pleural plaques, and pulmonary fibrosis evident on chest x-ray studies, the strong possibility exists that this patient is evidencing early features of pulmonary asbestosis.

The persistent cigarette smoking (high level of blood carboxyhemoglobin) in this asbestos-exposed worker provides a major neoplastic threat. It also makes him a high-risk candidate for heart disease and emphysema.

Case 47 Asbestosis, Mild

Clinical Findings

This 55-year-old male shipyard worker with a long history of asbestos and former cigarette exposure complained of shortness of breath only after climbing three to four flights of stairs and a daily cough productive of scant, yellow-tinged sputum. He denied any other symptoms or illnesses. No rales were noted on examination. Chest x-ray revealed minimal, but definite, fibrosis, typical of asbestosis. Exercise testing was requested to ascertain whether physiologic abnormalities were associated with the asbestosis.

Exercise Findings

The patient performed exercise on a cycle ergometer. He pedalled at 60 rpm without an added load for 3 minutes. The work rate was then increased 10 W per minute to tolerance. Arterial blood was sampled every second minute, and intra-arterial pressure was recorded from a percutaneously placed brachial artery catheter. The patient stopped exercise because of shortness of breath. The ECG showed nonspecific T-wave abnormalities and occasional ventricular premature contractions at rest and during exercise.

TABLE 9.47.1. Selected Respiratory Function Data

Measurement	Predicted	Measured
Age, yr		55
Sex		Male
Height, cm		181
Weight, kg	82	84
Hematocrit, %		45
VC, L	4.24	3.50
IC, L	2.83	2.26
TLC, L	6.32	5.15
FEV_1, L	3.35	2.94
FEV_1/VC, %	79	84
MVV, L/min	135	107
$D_{L}CO$, ml/mm Hg/min	27.3	22.7

TABLE 9.47.2. Selected Exercise Data

Measurement	Predicted	Measured
Peak $\dot{V}O_2$, L/min	2.50	2.03
Maximum HR, beats/min	165	154
Maximum O_2 pulse, ml/beat	15.1	13.2
$\Delta\dot{V}O_2/\Delta WR$, ml/min/W	10.3	8.7
AT, L/min	>1.08	1.3
Blood pressure, mmHg (rest, max)		156/90, 216/99
Maximum $\dot{V}E$, L/min		93
Exercise breathing reserve, L/min	>15	14
PaO_2 mmHg (rest, max ex)		88, 99
$P(A - a)O_2$ mmHg (rest, max ex)		14, 21
$P(a - ET)CO_2$, mmHg (rest, max ex)		3, −2
VD/VT (rest, max ex)		0.37, 0.30
HCO_3^-, mEq/L (rest, 2-min recov)		25, 20

FIGURE 9.47.1.

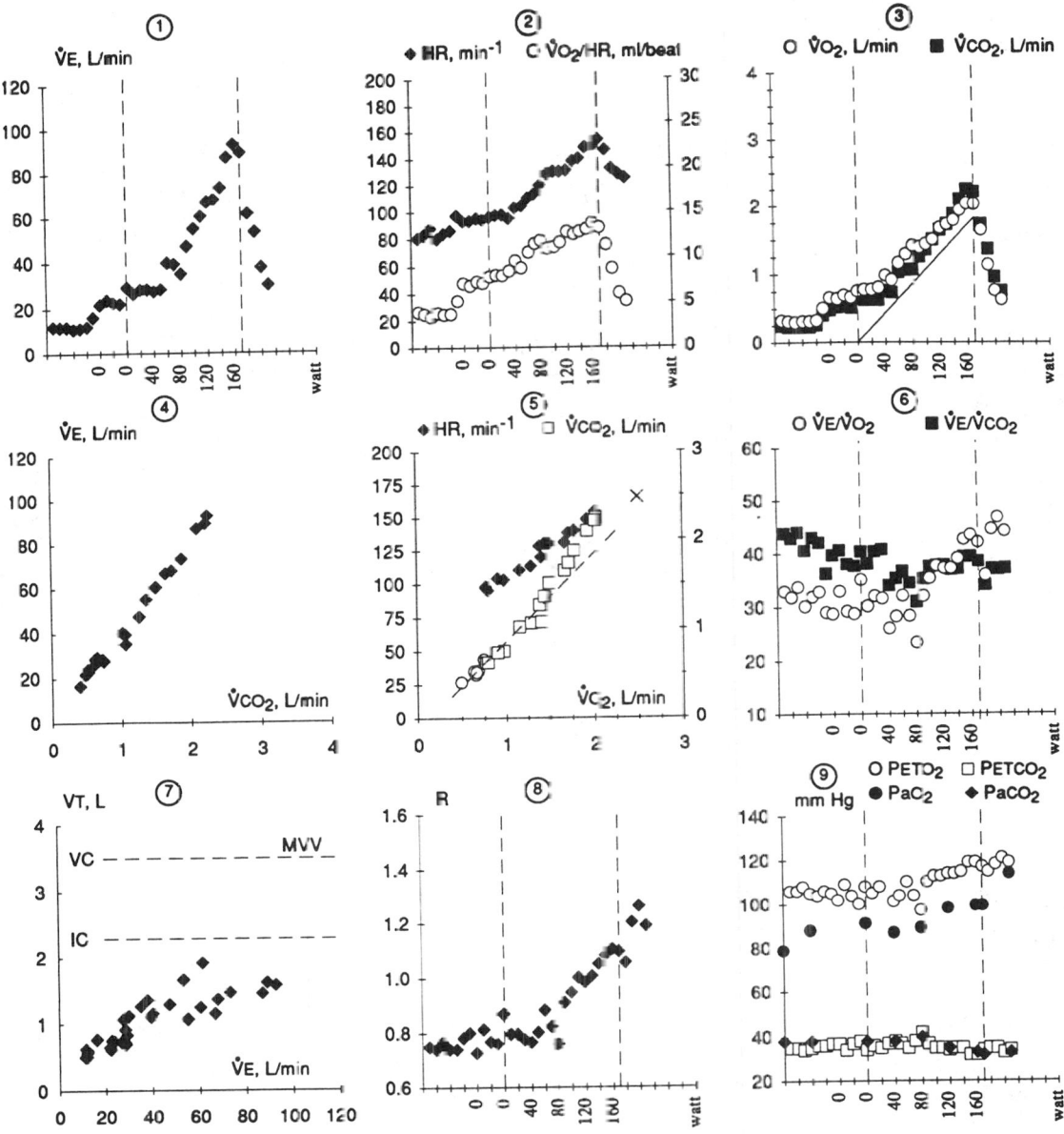

1. Vertical dashed lines in panels 1 to 3 and 6, 8. and 9 indicate the beginning and the end of increasing work period

2. Unloaded cycling is performed for 3 minutes before the left vertical dashed line.

3. In panel 3, the diagonal line shows the increase of $\dot{V}O_2$ at a slope of 10 ml/min/w.

4. In panel 5, the diagonal dashed line has a slope of 1; the "x" in the upper right is the predicted maximum heart rate and $\dot{V}O_2$ for the subject.

TABLE 9.47.3. Air Breathing

Time min	Work rate watts	BP mmHg	HR min⁻¹	f min⁻¹	V̇E L/min BTPS	V̇CO₂ L/min STPD	V̇O₂ L/min STPD	V̇O₂/HR ml/beat	R	pH	HCO₃⁻ meq/L	PO₂ ET	PO₂ a	PO₂ (A−a)	PCO₂ ET	PCO₂ a	PCO₂ (a−ET)	V̇E/V̇CO₂	V̇E/V̇O₂	VD/VT
	Rest	156/90								7.43	25		79			38				
	Rest		81	21	12.3	0.24	0.32	4.0	0.75			106			35			44	33	
	Rest		83	23	11.8	0.23	0.31	3.7	0.74			106			35			43	32	
	Rest		88	21	11.9	0.23	0.30	3.4	0.77			108			34			44	34	
	Rest	162/96	80	22	11.2	0.23	0.31	3.9	0.74	7.42	24	105	88	14	35	38	3	41	30	0.37
	Rest		84	18	11.4	0.23	0.31	3.7	0.74			104			36			43	32	
	Rest		86	20	12.2	0.25	0.32	3.7	0.78			106			36			42	33	
	Unloaded		97	21	16.3	0.40	0.50	5.2	0.80			105			37			36	29	
	Unloaded		93	33	21.8	0.48	0.66	7.1	0.73			102			37			40	29	
	Unloaded		93	32	23.8	0.52	0.64	6.9	0.81			109			34			41	33	
	Unloaded		95	30	22.7	0.53	0.69	7.3	0.77			104			37			38	29	
	Unloaded		94	36	22.3	0.51	0.67	7.1	0.76			100			38			38	29	
	Unloaded	192/96	96	35	29.2	0.65	0.75	7.8	0.87	7.43	25	108	91	16	34	38	4	40	35	0.39
0.5	20		97	36	26.6	0.62	0.78	8.0	0.79			105			36			38	30	
1.0	20		98	39	28.3	0.62	0.78	8.0	0.79			108			35			40	32	
1.5	40		95	41	28.7	0.62	0.80	8.4	0.78			204			37			41	32	
2.0	40	192/90	103	26	27.7	0.75	0.98	9.5	0.77	7.43	25	101	87	16	38	38	0	34	26	0.31
2.5	60		104	31	28.3	0.73	0.91	8.8	0.80			104			37			35	28	
3.0	60		110	35	40.2	1.02	1.16	10.5	0.88			110			35			36	32	
3.5	80		113	36	39.6	1.06	1.29	11.4	0.82			104			38			34	28	
4.0	80	198/93	120	28	35.4	1.07	1.41	11.8	0.76	7.41	25	97	89	11	42	40	−2	31	23	0.28
4.5	100		128	37	47.4	1.26	1.39	10.9	0.91			110			37			35	32	
5.0	100		130	52	55.2	1.36	1.44	11.1	0.94			113			35			37	35	
5.5	120		130	49	60.6	1.50	1.50	11.5	1.00			113			35			38	38	
6.0	120	201/93	131	58	66.8	1.64	1.67	12.7	0.98	7.43	23	114	98	16	34	35	1	38	37	0.32
6.5	140		138	50	68.0	1.73	1.72	12.5	1.01			114			35			37	37	
7.0	140		140	50	73.4	1.87	1.78	12.7	1.05			115			35			37	39	
7.5	160		148	60	87.0	2.09	1.93	13.0	1.08			119			32			39	42	
8.0	160	198/99	149	59	92.9	2.24	2.03	13.6	1.10	7.43	22	119	99	20	32	33	1	39	43	0.32
8.5	180	216/99	154	55	89.3	2.21	2.02	13.1	1.09	7.42	20	117	99	21	34	32	−2	38	42	0.28
	Recovery		146	32	61.5	1.73	1.64	11.2	1.05			115			35			34	36	
	Recovery		132	32	53.4	1.37	1.14	8.6	1.20			118			35			37	44	
	Recovery		128	28	37.8	0.96	0.76	5.9	1.26			121			33			37	47	
	Recovery	189/93	125	27	30.1	0.75	0.63	5.0	1.19	7.39	20	119	114	7	34	33	−1	37	44	0.27

Interpretation

Comments

Resting pulmonary function studies showed a mild restrictive defect with parallel loss of pulmonary capillary bed.

Analysis

Referring to flow chart 1, peak V̇O₂ is decreased, but the anaerobic threshold is normal. See flow chart 3. At branchpoint 3.1, the breathing reserve is borderline low. The VD/VT is borderline normal, but the P(A − a)O₂ and P(a − ET)CO₂ are normal. At branchpoint 3.2, the patient has a high breathing frequency, typical of restrictive lung disease. If we had used flow chart 2, we would have arrived (through branchpoints 2.1 and 2.3) at the diagnosis of lung disease.

Conclusion

This patient with asbestosis shows mild abnormalities both at rest and with exercise. There is evidence of mild restrictive lung disease at rest. Exercise testing reveals a slightly low peak V̇O₂. The high breathing frequency suggests ventilatory limitation; however, the disease at the time of testing has resulted in minimal physiologic impairments.

Case 48 Restrictive Lung Disease (Asbestosis)

Clinical Findings

This 67-year-old woman was referred for exercise testing. She had been exposed to asbestos for 3 years while working in a shipyard, approximately 40 years earlier. She had never smoked. Three years prior to this evaluation she noted fatigability, clubbing of fingernails, and shortness of breath. She was unable to climb a flight of stairs or walk rapidly on the level. A transbronchial lung biopsy at that time was reported as showing "fibrosis." Her symptoms improved markedly on 80 mg prednisone, but this medication was stopped after 1 year because of concern for its side effects. Five months prior to this evaluation she was started on oxygen therapy but corticosteroids were not restarted. Examination revealed a thin woman with fine inspiratory rales in the lateral and inferior lung fields that did not clear with coughing. There was dramatic digital clubbing. Chest roentgenograms showed extensive pulmonary infiltrates, compatible with interstitial pulmonary fibrosis. There was also a small patch of pleural calcification on the left. Resting ECG was normal.

Exercise Findings

The patient performed exercise on a cycle ergometer. She pedalled at 60 rpm without added load for 3 minutes. The work rate was then increased 5 W per minute to her symptom-limited maximum. Arterial blood was sampled every second minute, and intra-arterial blood pressure was recorded from a percutaneously placed brachial artery catheter. The patient stopped exercising because of dyspnea. She developed some premature atrial contractions during exercise but ECG otherwise was not remarkable.

TABLE 9.48.1. Selected Respiratory Function Data

Measurement	Predicted	Measured
Age, yr		67
Sex		Female
Height, cm		163
Weight, kg	63	48
Hematocrit, %		38
VC, L	2.77	1.51
IC, L	1.85	0.70
TLC, L	4.82	2.65
FEV_1, L	2.19	1.24
FEV_1/VC, %	79	82
MVV, L/min	82	33
D_{CO}, ml/mm Hg/min	22.3	6.4

TABLE 9.48.2. Selected Exercise Data

Measurement	Predicted	Measured
Peak $\dot{V}O_2$, L/min	1.12	0.42
Maximum HR, beat/min	153	108
Maximum O_2 pulse, ml/beat	7.3	4.1
AT, L/min	>0.56	Indeterminate
Blood pressure, mmHg (rest, max)		122/74, 140/80
Maximum $\dot{V}E$, L/min		29
Exercise breathing reserve, L/min	>15	4
PaO_2, mmHg (rest, max ex)		58, 46
$P(A - a)O_2$, mmHg (rest, max ex)		41, 64
$P(a - ET)CO_2$, mmHg (rest, max ex)		8, 10
VD/VT (rest, heavy ex)		0.56, 0.55
HCO_3^-, mEq/L (rest, 2-min recov)		25, 24

FIGURE 9.48.1.

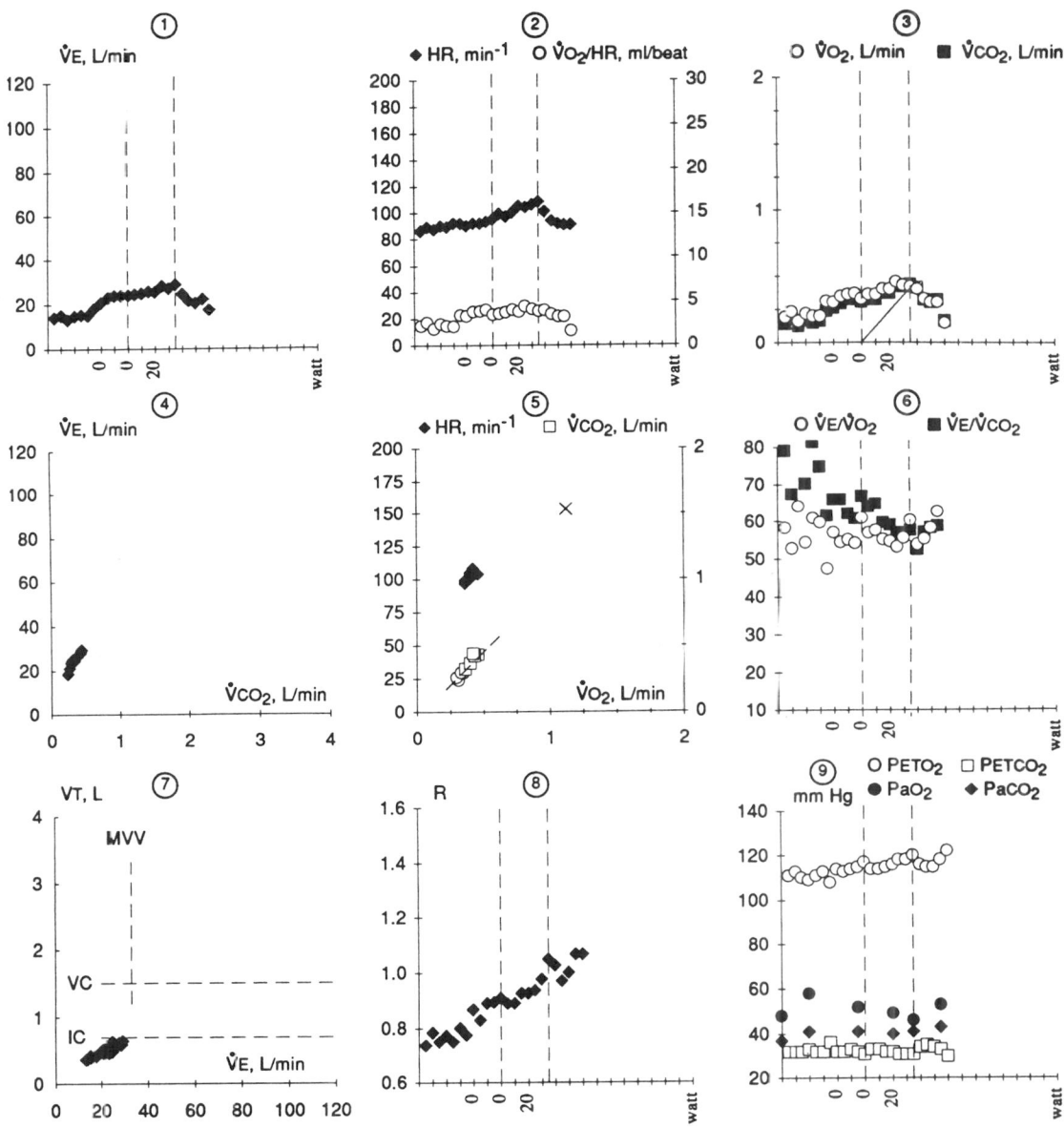

1. Vertical dashed lines in panels 1 to 3 and 6, 8, and 9 indicate the beginning and the end of increasing work period.

2. Unloaded cycling is performed for 3 minutes before the left vertical dashed line.

3. In panel 3, the diagonal line shows the increase of $\dot{V}O_2$ at a slope of 10 ml/min/w.

4. In panel 5, the diagonal dashed line has a slope of 1; the "x" in the upper right is the predicted maximum heart rate and $\dot{V}O_2$ for the subject.

TABLE 9.48.3.

Time min	Work rate watts	BP mmHg	HR min⁻¹	f min⁻¹	V̇E L/min BTPS	V̇CO₂ L/min STPD	V̇O₂ L/min STPD	V̇O₂/HR ml/beat	R	pH	HCO₃ meq/L	PO₂, mmHg ET	a	(A − a)	PCO₂, mmHg ET	a	(a − ET)	V̇E V̇CO₂	V̇E V̇O₂	VD VT
	Rest	122/74								7.44	25		48			37				
	Rest		86	38	14.3	0.14	0.19	2.2	0.74			111			32			79	58	
	Rest		89	36	15.2	0.13	0.23	2.6	0.78			113			32			67	53	
	Rest		87	37	13.4	0.12	0.16	1.8	0.75			110			32			85	64	
	Rest	119/71	90	36	15.0	0.17	0.22	2.4	0.77	7.40	25	109	58	41	33	41	8	70	54	0.56
	Rest		89	39	15.5	0.15	0.20	2.2	0.75			111			32			81	61	
	Rest		92	37	15.1	0.16	0.20	2.2	0.80			113			32			75	60	
	Unloaded		92	42	18.3	0.24	0.31	3.4	0.77			108			36			61	48	
	Unloaded		90	46	21.0	0.26	0.30	3.3	0.87			114			32			66	57	
	Unloaded		92	51	23.4	0.29	0.35	3.8	0.83			113			32			66	54	
	Unloaded		92	49	24.0	0.32	0.36	3.9	0.89			114			33			62	55	
	Unloaded	126/71	93	48	24.1	0.33	0.37	4.0	0.89	7.41	26	115	52	53	32	41	9	61	54	0.54
	Unloaded		95	50	24.3	0.30	0.33	3.5	0.91			117			31			67	61	
0.5	10		99	50	24.7	0.32	0.36	3.6	0.89			114			33			64	57	
1.0	10		97	51	25.0	0.32	0.36	3.7	0.89			114			33			65	57	
1.5	20		100	47	26.0	0.37	0.40	4.0	0.93			115			32			59	55	
2.0	20	137/74	105	47	25.8	0.37	0.40	3.8	0.93	7.41	25	116	49	58	32	40	8	59	55	0.54
2.5	30		104	49	28.6	0.43	0.46	4.4	0.93			113			31			57	53	
3.0	30		106	45	27.6	0.42	0.43	4.1	0.98			113			31			57	55	
3.5	40	140/80	108	45	29.1	0.44	0.42	3.9	1.05	7.39	24	120	46	64	31	41	10	57	60	0.55
	Recovery		101	39	24.8	0.41	0.40	4.0	1.03			116			34			52	54	
	Recovery		94	41	21.7	0.32	0.33	3.5	0.97			115			35			57	55	
	Recovery		92	40	20.8	0.30	0.30	3.3	1.00			115			34			58	58	
	Recovery	134/68	91	43	22.4	0.32	0.30	3.3	1.07	7.36	24	118	53	56	33	43	10	59	62	0.55
	Recovery		91	43	17.8	0.16	0.15	1.6	1.07			122			30			88	94	

Interpretation

Comments

Results of the respiratory function studies indicate that this patient has a moderately severe restrictive defect with a marked reduction in diffusing capacity (Table 9.48.1). The ECG is normal.

Analysis

Referring to flow chart 1, the peak V̇O₂ is markedly reduced and the anaerobic threshold is indeterminate (Table 9.48.2). See flow chart 5: VD/VT, P(a − ET)CO₂, and P(A − a)O₂ during exercise are markedly abnormal (branchpoint 5.1). The breathing reserve is low (branchpoint 5.3). The breathing frequency is high at rest and is maintained at a high level of approximately 50 breaths per minute through the incremental exercise period (branchpoint 5.7). The maximum ventilation achieved is approximately the patient's maximum ability to breathe. The foregoing findings lead to the diagnosis of restrictive lung disease. Supporting this diagnosis is the progressive decrease in PaO₂ and increase in P(A − a)O₂ at each work rate performed (Table 9.48.3 and panel 9, Fig. 9.48.1). An additional measurement consistent with restrictive lung disease is the high tidal volume/inspiratory capacity ratio (panel 7, Fig. 9.48.1). An O₂ flow limitation is demonstrated by the small rise in V̇O₂ with increasing work rate and the failure of O₂ pulse to rise (panels 3 and 2, respectively, in Fig. 9.48.1) as work rate is increased.

Conclusion

Severe exercise intolerance with marked ventilation-perfusion mismatching in a patient with restrictive lung disease.

Case 49 Idiopathic Interstitial Lung Disease

Clinical Findings

This 45-year-old woman had developed dyspnea, diffuse pulmonary infiltrates, and hypoxemia 6 months previously and was treated with oral corticosteroids without lung biopsy or specific diagnosis. She was no longer receiving medication but still had dyspnea after walking three blocks. She had never smoked and had no known exposure to known toxins except that she worked in a pet shop and sprayed bleach on cages to clean them. She had no other significant illnesses. She was evaluated to determine the pathophysiology of her dyspnea.

Exercise Findings

The patient performed exercise on a cycle ergometer. She pedalled at 60 rpm without an added load for 3 minutes. The work rate was then increased 5 W per minute to her symptom-limited maximum. Arterial blood was sampled every second minute, and intra-arterial blood pressure was recorded from a percutaneously placed brachial artery catheter. Resting and exercise ECGs were normal. The patient stopped exercise because of leg fatigue. By ear oximetry, the O_2 saturation was 96% at rest and 93% at peak exercise.

TABLE 9.49.1. Selected Respiratory Function Data

Measurement	Predicted	Measured
Age, yr		45
Sex		Female
Height, cm		152
Weight, kg	56	51
Hematocrit, %		49
VC, L	2.92	1.81
IC, L	1.95	1.23
TLC, L	4.29	3.62
FEV_1, L	2.41	1.42
FEV_1/VC, %	83	78
MVV, L/min	92	56
$D_{L}CO$, ml/mm Hg/min	22.7	4.3

TABLE 9.49.2. Selected Exercise Data

Measurement	Predicted	Measured
Peak $\dot{V}O_2$, L/min	1.44	0.88
Maximum HR, beats/min	174	174
Maximum O_2 pulse, ml/beat	8.3	5.1
$\Delta\dot{V}O_2/\Delta WR$, ml/min/W	10.3	8.7
AT, L/min	>0.69	0.65
Blood pressure, mmHg (rest, max ex)		150/90, 183/99
Maximum $\dot{V}E$, L/min		56
Exercise breathing reserve, L/min	>15	0
PaO_2, mmHg (rest, max ex)		93, 74
$P(A - a)O_2$ mmHg (rest, max ex)		24, 50
$P(a - ET)CO_2$, mmHg (rest, max ex)		1, 5
VD/VT (rest, max ex)		0.31, 0.38
HCO_3^-, mEq/L (rest, recov)		23, 17

FIGURE 9.49.1.

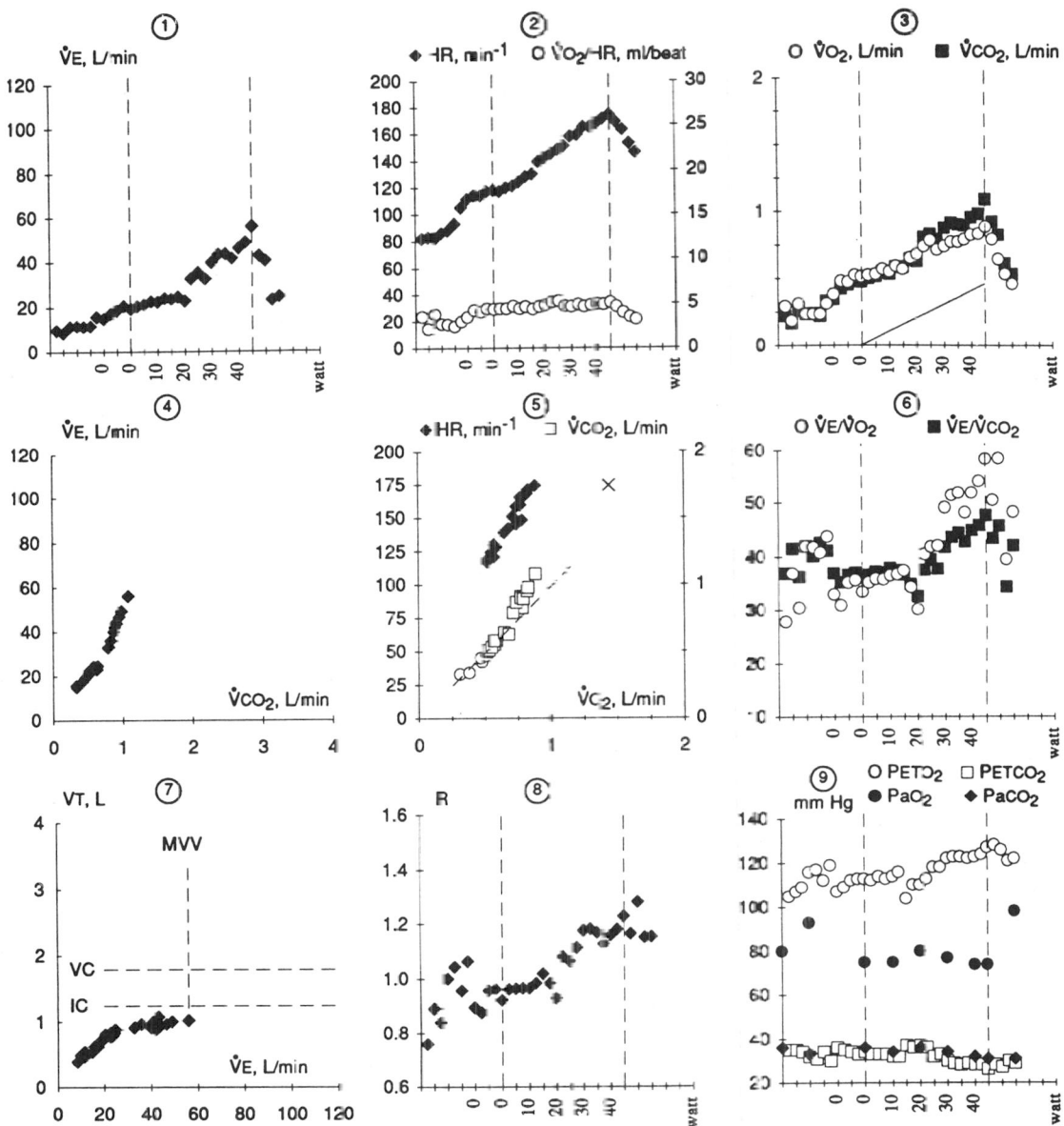

1. Vertical dashed lines in panels 1 to 3 and 6, 8, and 9 indicate the beginning and the end of increasing work period.

2. Unloaded cycling is performed for 3 minutes before the left vertical dashed line.

3. In panel 3, the diagonal line shows the increase of $\dot{V}O_2$ at a slope of 10 ml/min/w.

4. In panel 5, the diagonal dashed line has a slope of 1; the "x" in the upper right is the predicted maximum heart rate and $\dot{V}O_2$ for the subject.

Interpretation

Comments

This case is presented to show the effects of severe pulmonary vascular disease accompanying interstitial lung disease. The resting respiratory studies show extremely severe D_{LCO} reduction despite only mild to moderate restriction and normal resting PaO_2.

Analysis

Referring to flow chart 1, the patient had a low peak $\dot{V}O_2$ and anaerobic threshold (Table 9.49.2). In flow chart 4, the patient had a negligible breathing re-

TABLE 9.49.3. Air Breathing

Time min	Work rate watts	BP mmHg	HR min⁻¹	f min⁻¹	$\dot{V}_E$ L/min BTPS	$\dot{V}_{CO_2}$ L/min STPD	$\dot{V}_{O_2}$ L/min STPD	$\dot{V}_{O_2}$/HR ml/beat	R	pH	HCO₃⁻ meq/L	ET	a	(A − a)	ET	a	(a − ET)	$\dot{V}_E$/$\dot{V}_{CO_2}$	$\dot{V}_E$/$\dot{V}_{O_2}$	VD/VT
													PO₂, mmHg			PCO₂, mmHg				
	Rest	150/84								7.42	23	80			36					
	Rest		82	20	9.8	0.22	0.29	3.5	0.76			105			35			37	28	
	Rest		83	22	8.5	0.16	0.18	2.2	0.89			107			35			41	37	
	Rest		82	22	11.3	0.26	0.31	3.8	0.84			109			34			36	30	
	Rest	150/90	86	23	11.6	0.23	0.23	2.7	1.00	7.45	23	116	93	24	32	33	1	42	42	0.31
	Rest		88	21	11.4	0.24	0.23	2.6	1.04			117			31			40	42	
	Rest		93	25	11.5	0.22	0.23	2.5	0.96			112			34			43	41	
	Unloaded		105	25	15.7	0.33	0.31	3.0	1.06			119			30			41	44	
	Unloaded		111	28	14.9	0.34	0.38	3.4	0.89			107			36			37	33	
	Unloaded		114	28	17.2	0.42	0.48	4.2	0.88			109			35			35	31	
	Unloaded		114	26	18.7	0.45	0.47	4.1	0.96			112			34			37	35	
	Unloaded		117	26	20.7	0.50	0.52	4.4	0.96			113			33			37	36	
	Unloaded	177/96	118	27	19.3	0.47	0.51	4.3	0.92	7.41	22	113	75	37	34	36	2	36	33	0.30
0.5	5		117	25	20.4	0.50	0.52	4.4	0.96			112			33			37	35	
1.0	5		120	27	21.3	0.51	0.53	4.4	0.96			114			33			37	36	
1.5	10		121	27	22.6	0.55	0.57	4.7	0.96			113			33			37	36	
2.0	10	177/96	124	29	22.5	0.53	0.55	4.4	0.96	7.41	21	114	75	40	32	34	2	38	36	0.29
2.5	15		128	29	24.1	0.58	0.59	4.6	0.98			116			32			37	37	
3.0	15		130	30	23.8	0.58	0.57	4.4	1.02			104			37			37	37	
3.5	20		139	28	24.6	0.64	0.65	4.7	0.98			110			36			35	34	
4.0	20	180/99	142	28	22.8	0.63	0.68	4.8	0.93	7.39	21	110	80	32	37	36	−1	32	30	0.23
4.5	25		145	36	33.0	0.80	0.74	5.1	1.08			113			36			37	40	
5.0	25		148	37	35.8	0.83	0.78	5.3	1.06			118			32			39	42	
5.5	30		151	36	32.8	0.79	0.71	4.7	1.11			118			33			38	42	
6.0	30	180/96	158	44	40.0	0.87	0.74	4.7	1.18	7.39	20	122	77	43	30	34	4	42	49	0.35
6.5	35		159	47	43.6	0.91	0.77	4.8	1.18			123			29			44	51	
7.0	35		165	46	43.8	0.90	0.77	4.7	1.17			123			28			44	52	
7.5	40		165	43	42.1	0.89	0.79	4.8	1.13			122			29			43	48	
8.0	40	180/96	168	43	46.6	0.95	0.82	4.9	1.16	7.39	19	123	74	47	28	32	4	45	52	0.36
8.5	45		171	49	49.0	0.98	0.83	4.9	1.18			124			28			46	54	
9.0	45	183/99	174	55	56.0	1.08	0.88	5.1	1.23	7.38	18	127	74	50	26	31	5	48	58	0.38
	Recovery		169	40	43.2	0.92	0.79	4.7	1.16			128			28			43	50	
	Recovery		163	41	40.9	0.82	0.64	3.9	1.28			126			27			46	58	
	Recovery		153	30	23.4	0.61	0.53	3.5	1.15			121			30			34	39	
	Recovery	165/90	146	28	24.6	0.53	0.46	3.2	1.15	7.35	17	122	98	24	29	31	2	42	48	0.30

serve (branchpoint 4.1) and a high VD/VT (branchpoint 4.2) leading to a tentative diagnosis of "lung disease with impaired peripheral oxygenation." She had confirmatory findings of a high VT/IC, low oximeter saturation, high breathing frequency, positive $P(a − ET)CO_2$, wide and increasing $P(A − a)O_2$, and a steep HR versus $\dot{V}O_2$ relationship. The $\Delta\dot{V}O_2/\Delta WR$ is within normal limits, but the low and unchanging O_2 pulse is striking (panels 2 and 5 of Fig. 9.49.1). The decrease in O_2 saturation is small and gradual (branchpoint 4.5), making the development of a right to left shunt during exercise unlikely.

Conclusion

Although the patient has ventilatory limitation, she also has evidence of severe pulmonary vascular disease with decreased pulmonary blood flow evidenced by the steep heart rate response and the persistently low O_2 pulse. The pulmonary blood flow is so slow that there apparently is adequate time for near equilibration of pulmonary capillary PO_2 with alveolar gas even at peak exercise, the lowest exercise PaO_2 being 74.

Case 50 Mixed Connective Tissue Disease with Interstitial and Pulmonary Vascular Disease

Clinical Findings

This 38-year-old man with known mixed connective tissue disease and restrictive lung disease of 3 years' duration was referred for evaluation to determine his level of disability. He had had a productive cough for 3 years and had been dyspneic for over 2 years. He had never smoked, but had been exposed to multiple chemical agents in a rubber factory. His current medications were prednisone, theophylline, and cimetidine.

Exercise Findings

The patient performed exercise on a cycle ergometer. He pedalled at 60 rpm without an added load for 3 minutes. The work rate was then increased 15 W per minute to his symptom-limited maximum. Arterial blood was sampled every second minute and intra-arterial blood pressure was recorded from a percutaneously passed brachial artery catheter. Resting ECG was normal except for occasional premature ectopic beats. The frequency of these increased during exercise to a maximum of 12 per minute. No ST or T wave abnormalities occurred. Exercise was stopped because the patient seemed unsteady and indicated that he was lightheaded. These symptoms cleared in a few minutes. He also indicated that he was out of breath, but did not identify this as the cause of stopping.

TABLE 9.50.1.   Selected Respiratory Function Data

Measurement	Predicted	Measured
Age, yr		38
Sex		Male
Height, cm		188
Weight, kg	83	88
Hematocrit, %		43
VC, L	5.09	2.28
IC, L	3.39	1.36
TLC, L	7.14	3.43
FEV_1, L	4.09	1.99
FEV_1/VC, %	81	87
MVV, L/min		
Direct	163	107
Indirect	164	80
D_{CO}, ml/mm Hg/min	32.7	10.7

TABLE 9.50.2.   Selected Exercise Data

Measurement	Predicted	Measured
Peak $\dot{V}O_2$, L/min	3.21	1.07
Maximum HR, beats/min	182	128
Maximum O_2 pulse, ml/beat	17.6	8.4
$\Delta\dot{V}O_2/\Delta WR$, ml/min/W	>10.3	7.3
AT, L/min	>1.35	<0.9
Blood pressure, mmHg (rest, max ex)		141/90, 222/102
Maximum $\dot{V}E$, L/min		76
Exercise breathing reserve, L/min		
Using direct MVV	>15	31
Using indirect MVV	>15	4
PaO_2, mmHg (rest, max ex)		79, 63
$P(A - a)O_2$, mmHg (rest, max ex)		16, 58
$P(a - ET)CO_2$, mmHg (rest, max ex)		5, 9
V_D/V_T (rest, max ex)		0.46, 0.48
HCO_3^-, mEq/L (rest, recov)		25, 20

FIGURE 9.50.1.

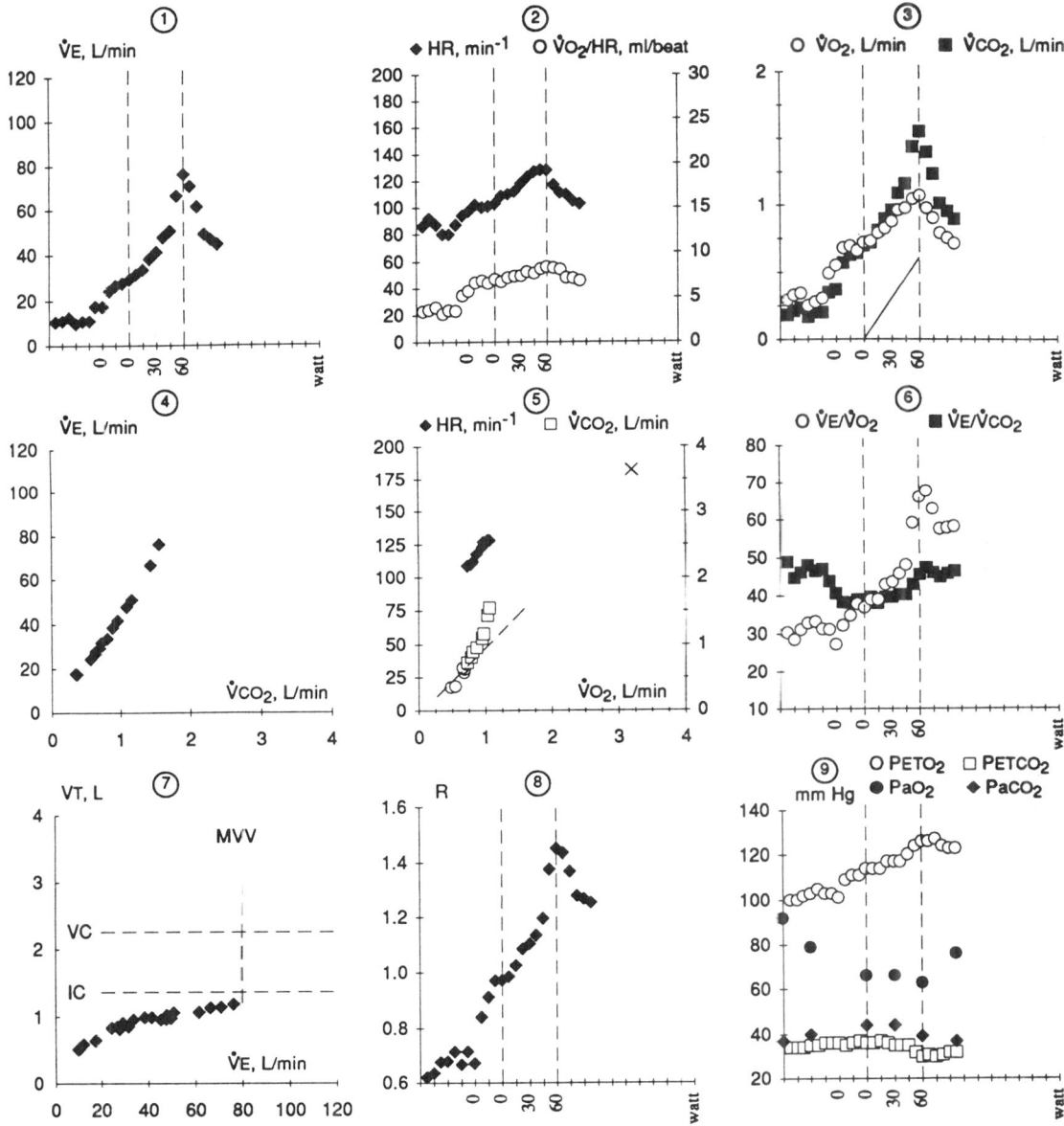

1. Vertical dashed lines in panels 1 to 3 and 6, 8, and 9 indicate the beginning and the end of increasing work period.
2. Unloaded cycling is performed for 3 minutes before the left vertical dashed line.
3. In panel 3, the diagonal line shows the increase of $\dot{V}O_2$ at a slope of 10 ml/min/w.
4. In panel 5, the diagonal dashed line has a slope of 1; the "x" in the upper right is the predicted maximum heart rate and $\dot{V}O_2$ for the subject.

TABLE 9.50.3.   Air Breathing

Time min	Work rate watts	BP mmHg	HR min⁻¹	f min⁻¹	$\dot{V}_E$ L/min BTPS	$\dot{V}_{CO_2}$ L/min STPD	$\dot{V}_{O_2}$ L/min STPD	$\dot{V}_{O_2}$/HR ml/beat	R	pH	HCO₃ meq/L	P$_{O_2}$ ET	P$_{O_2}$ a	P$_{O_2}$ (A−a)	P$_{CO_2}$ ET	P$_{CO_2}$ a	P$_{CO_2}$ (a−ET)	$\dot{V}_E$/$\dot{V}_{CO_2}$	$\dot{V}_E$/$\dot{V}_{O_2}$	VD/VT
	Rest	141/90								7.45	25		92			37				
	Rest		86	20	10.5	0.18	0.29	3.4	0.62			100			34			49	30	
	Rest		92	20	11.1	0.21	0.33	3.6	0.64			100			34			45	28	
	Rest		87	21	12.4	0.23	0.34	3.9	0.65			102			34			46	31	
	Rest	156/96	80	19	9.8	0.17	0.25	3.1	0.65	7.41	25	103	79	16	35	40	5	48	33	0.46
	Rest		80	20	11.0	0.20	0.28	3.5	0.71			105			35			47	33	
	Rest		87	20	11.1	0.20	0.30	3.4	0.67			103			36			47	31	
	Unloaded		94	27	17.6	0.35	0.49	5.2	0.71			103			36			44	31	
	Unloaded		97	27	17.3	0.37	0.55	5.7	0.67			101			36			41	27	
	Unloaded		102	29	24.3	0.57	0.68	6.7	0.84			109			35			38	32	
	Unloaded		100	31	26.6	0.63	0.69	6.9	0.91			111			36			38	35	
	Unloaded		101	34	27.8	0.64	0.66	6.5	0.97			111			37			39	38	
	Unloaded	192/99	103	32	29.2	0.70	0.72	7.0	0.97	7.38	26	114	66	39	36	44	8	38	37	0.44
0.5	15		109	37	31.6	0.72	0.73	6.7	0.98			114			36			40	39	
1.0	15		110	35	33.7	0.81	0.79	7.2	1.03			114			37			38	39	
1.5	30		112	39	38.5	0.85	0.82	7.3	1.03			117			36			40	43	
2.0	30	204/102	118	42	41.5	0.96	0.87	7.4	1.11	7.38	26	117	63	43	35	44	9	40	44	0.46
2.5	45		123	47	47.8	1.09	0.96	7.8	1.14			117			35			40	46	
3.0	45		127	48	50.8	1.16	0.97	7.6	1.23			120			35			40	48	
3.5	60		128	59	66.5	1.43	1.04	8.1	1.33			124			32			43	59	
4.0	60	222/102	128	64	76.1	1.55	1.07	8.4	1.45	7.38	23	126	63	58	30	33	9	46	66	0.48
	Recovery		117	62	70.9	1.39	0.97	8.3	1.43			126			31			47	68	
	Recovery		111	58	61.5	1.23	0.90	8.1	1.37			127			30			46	63	
	Recovery		110	51	49.7	1.01	0.79	7.2	1.23			124			31			45	57	
	Recovery		105	49	47.5	0.95	0.75	7.1	1.27			123			32			46	58	
	Recovery	180/88	103	47	45.2	0.89	0.71	6.9	1.25	7.35	20	123	76	43	32	37	5	46	58	0.45

Interpretation

Comments

This patient shows the effect of severe interstitial lung disease on the cardiac output response to exercise, presumably because of increased pulmonary vascular resistance. The resting respiratory function studies show severe restriction with severe loss of available pulmonary capillary bed and mild hypoxemia.

Analysis

Referring to flow chart 1, the patient had a low peak $\dot{V}_{O_2}$ and an extremely low anaerobic threshold (Table 9.50.2). In flow chart 4, the patient had a low breathing reserve using the indirect MVV (branchpoint 4.1). At branchpoint 4.2 we are directed to "lung disease with impaired peripheral oxygenation" by the finding of a high VD/VT. Confirmatory findings of ventilatory limitation to exercise are the high breathing frequency (64) and high VT/IC. Espe-

cially impressive are the small increases in $\dot{V}_{O_2}$ and O_2 pulse as compared to predicted, the arrhythmia, and the lightheadedness, all indicating difficulty in perfusion and/or oxygenation of the myocardium and brain as peak exercise is reached. (If we had decided that the breathing reserve were normal (branchpoint 4.1) we would also have been directed through branchpoint 4.3 with high ventilatory equivalents to "abnormal pulmonary circulation".

Conclusion

This patient demonstrates significant gas exchange, ventilatory, and cardiovascular defects, all because of his severe interstitial lung disease. Although he has no evidence of intrinsic heart disease, he has severe impairment in his ability to increase cardiac output (pulmonary blood flow). The increased CO_2 production secondary to his metabolic acidosis and the high ventilatory requirement because of his increased VD/VT combine to create an unusually large ventilatory requirement in a patient with reduced ventilatory capacity.

Case 51 Interstitial Lung Disease

Clinical Findings

This 20-year-old man with a history of exposure to crop dusting was found after extensive work-up and open lung biopsy to have an interstitial pneumonitis with mica deposits. The patient noted severe dyspnea with walking one block or climbing two flights of stairs. He denies cough, wheezing, orthopnea, chest pain, syncope, peripheral edema, or cyanosis. He was being re-evaluated following institution of daily prednisone.

Exercise Findings

The patient performed exercise on a cycle ergometer. He pedalled at 60 rpm without an added load for 3 minutes. The work rate was then increased 10 W per minute to tolerance. Arterial blood was sampled every second minute and intra-arterial pressure was recorded from a percutaneously placed brachial artery catheter. The patient was well motivated and cooperative and stopped exercise because of fatigue and shortness of breath. No ECG abnormalities occurred at rest or during exercise, but the patient developed a significant pulsus paradoxus (blood pressure variations with breathing).

TABLE 9.51.1. Selected Respiratory Function Data

Measurement	Predicted	Measured
Age, yr		20
Sex		Male
Height, cm		160
Weight, kg	66	48
Hematocrit, %		51
VC, L	3.52	1.21
IC, L	2.37	0.74
FEV$_1$, L	2.99	1.21
FEV$_1$/VC, %	85	97
MVV, L/min	125	51

TABLE 9.51.2. Selected Exercise Data

Measurement	Predicted	Measured
Peak $\dot{V}O_2$, L/min	2.46	0.74
Maximum HR, beats/min	200	182
Maximum O$_2$ pulse, ml/beat	12.3	4.1
$\Delta\dot{V}O_2/\Delta WR$, ml/min/W	10.3	4.2
AT, L/min	>0.98	<0.55
Blood pressure, mmHg (rest, max ex)		118/81, 165–126/102–63
Maximum $\dot{V}E$, L/min		47
Exercise breathing reserve, L/min	>15	4
Pao$_2$, mmHg (rest, max ex)		73, 85
P(A − a)o$_2$, mmHg (rest, max ex)		15, 36
P(a − ET)co$_2$, mmHg (rest, max ex)		3, 4
Vd/Vt (rest, max ex)		0.37, 0.36
HCO$_3^-$, mEq/L (rest, 2-min recov)		28, 14

FIGURE 9.51.1.

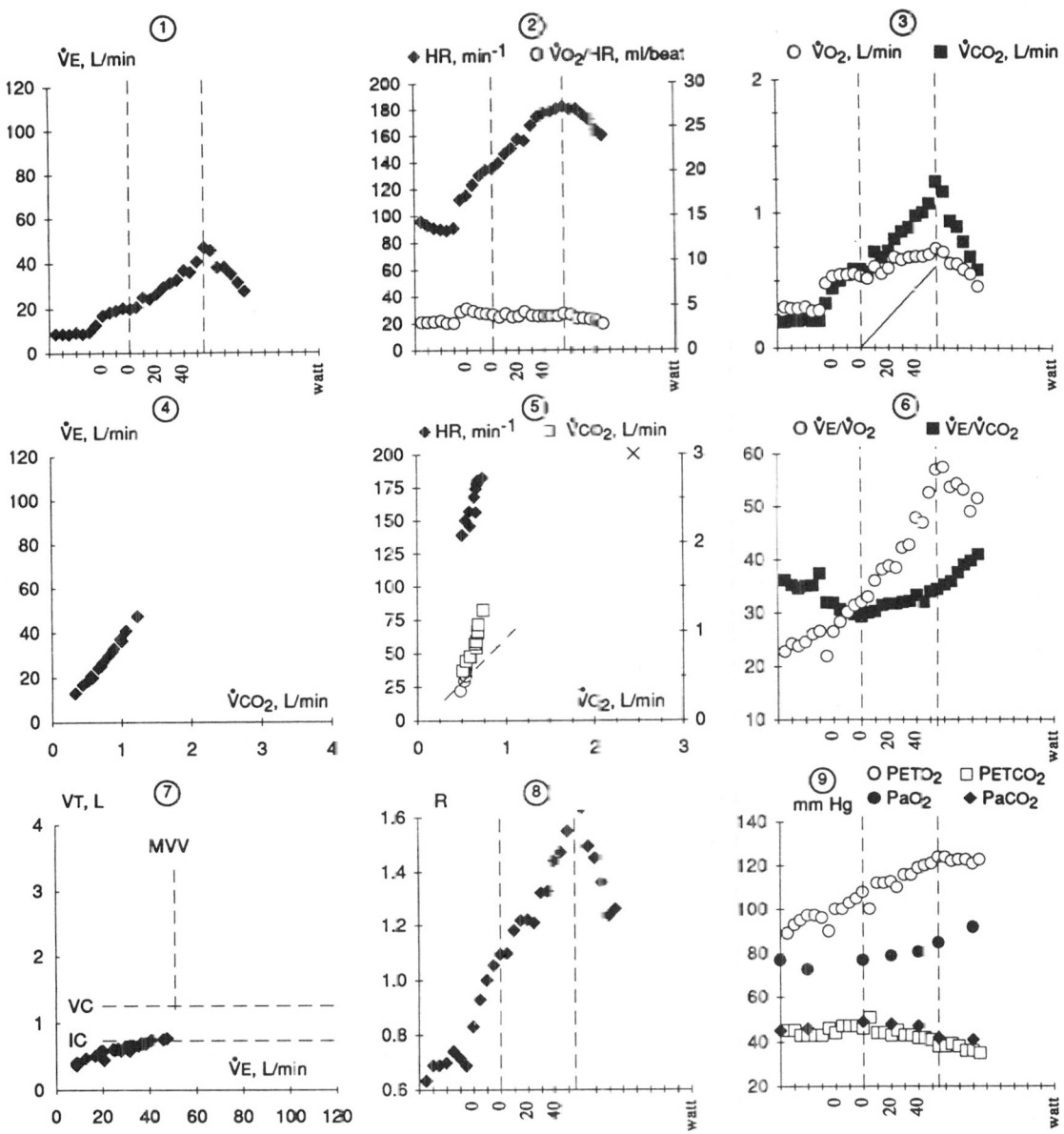

1. Vertical dashed lines in panels 1 to 3 and 6, 8, and 9 indicate the beginning and the end of increasing work period.
2. Unloaded cycling is performed for 3 minutes before the left vertical dashed line.
3. In panel 3, the diagonal line shows the increase of $\dot{V}O_2$ at a slope of 10 ml/min/w.
4. In panel 5, the diagonal dashed line has a slope of 1; the "×" in the upper right is the predicted maximum heart rate and $\dot{V}O_2$ for the subject

Interpretation

Comments

Resting respiratory function studies showed severe restrictive lung disease. Arterial blood gases revealed a chronic, compensated respiratory acidosis with mild hypoxemia.

Analysis

Referring to flow chart 1, peak $\dot{V}O_2$ and the anaerobic threshold are both markedly reduced. Proceeding to flow chart 4 through branchpoints 4.1 and 4.2, we come to lung disease with impaired peripheral oxygenation. We are instructed to look at the pulmonary vascular disease box to confirm the diagno-

TABLE 9.51.3. Air Breathing

Time min	Work rate watts	BP mmHg	HR min⁻¹	f min⁻¹	$\dot{V}_E$ L/min BTPS	$\dot{V}_{CO_2}$ L/min STPD	$\dot{V}_{O_2}$ L/min STPD	$\dot{V}_{O_2}$/HR ml/beat	R	pH	HCO_3^- meq/L	P_{O_2} ET	a	(A−a)	P_{CO_2} ET	a	(a−ET)	$\dot{V}_E/\dot{V}_{CO_2}$	$\dot{V}_E/\dot{V}_{O_2}$	V_D/V_T
	Rest	96/68								7.40	27		77			45				
	Rest		96	24	8.9	0.19	0.30	3.1	0.63			89			45			36	23	
	Rest		93	23	9.0	0.20	0.29	3.1	0.69			93			45			35	24	
	Rest		91	21	8.7	0.20	0.29	3.2	0.69			95			43			35	24	
	Rest	118/81	90	23	9.3	0.21	0.30	3.3	0.70	7.40	28	97	73	15	43	46	3	35	24	0.37
	Rest		89	22	8.9	0.20	0.27	3.0	0.74			97			43			35	26	
	Rest		91	24	9.5	0.20	0.28	3.1	0.71			96			43			37	27	
	Unloaded		112	27	12.8	0.33	0.48	4.3	0.69			90			46			32	22	
	Unloaded		115	33	16.8	0.44	0.53	4.6	0.83			100			44			32	26	
	Unloaded		123	34	18.2	0.50	0.54	4.4	0.93			100			47			31	28	
	Unloaded		130	33	19.0	0.54	0.54	4.2	1.00			103			47			30	30	
	Unloaded		134	35	20.2	0.58	0.55	4.1	1.05			105			47			30	31	
	Unloaded	147/93	135	34	19.9	0.58	0.53	3.9	1.09	7.35	27	108	77	27	46	49	3	29	32	0.34
0.5	10		139	46	20.7	0.56	0.51	3.7	1.10			100			51			30	33	
1.0	10		146	42	25.1	0.71	0.60	4.1	1.18			112			44			30	36	
1.5	20		150	40	24.4	0.67	0.55	3.7	1.22			112			44			31	38	
2.0	20	156/96	157	43	26.5	0.72	0.59	3.8	1.22	7.33	25	113	79	30	43	48	5	32	39	0.37
2.5	30		156	46	29.6	0.81	0.67	4.3	1.21			110			45			32	38	
3.0	30		168	48	31.5	0.86	0.65	3.9	1.32			116			43			32	42	
3.5	40		174	50	32.9	0.89	0.67	3.9	1.33			116			43			32	43	
4.0	40	156/90	177	54	37.1	0.98	0.68	3.8	1.44	7.28	22	119	81	33	42	47	5	33	48	0.39
4.5	50		178	52	36.3	1.00	0.68	3.8	1.47			120			42			32	47	
5.0	50		180	55	40.9	1.07	0.69	3.8	1.55			121			41			34	53	
5.5	60	65–126/102–6	182	61	47.3	1.23	0.74	4.1	1.66	7.23	17	124	85	36	38	42	4	34	57	0.36
	Recovery		180	61	45.9	1.16	0.71	3.9	1.63			124			38			35	57	
	Recovery		180	55	38.4	0.94	0.63	3.5	1.49			122			39			36	54	
	Recovery		176	56	38.4	0.90	0.62	3.5	1.45			123			38			37	54	
	Recovery		172	54	35.4	0.79	0.58	3.4	1.36			123			36			39	53	
	Recovery	136/69	164	54	31.5	0.68	0.55	3.4	1.24	7.15	14	121	92	23	36	41	5	40	49	0.40
	Recovery		160	47	27.7	0.58	0.46	2.9	1.26			123			35			41	52	

sis with other physiological measurements. The high breathing frequency, high ratio of tidal volume to inspiratory capacity (panel 7 of Fig 9.51.1), and the low breathing reserve are all typical of severe restrictive lung disease. The elevated V_D/V_T and positive $P(a − ET)CO_2$ indicate inadequate perfusion of ventilated air spaces. The lack of severe hypoxemia is at first puzzling; the extremely low O_2 pulse and low anaerobic threshold tell us that stroke volume must be extremely low. On reflection, it seems likely that the right ventricle has not hypertrophied in response to the increased pulmonary vascular resistance caused by the underlying lung disease. Thus, the cardiac output is relatively fixed, as indicated by the failure of $\dot{V}_{O_2}$ to increase despite the increasing work rate. Because cardiac output does not increase, residence time in the pulmonary capillary remains unchanged. This allows the same equilibration time for the red cells to be exposed to the alveolar gas during exercise as at rest. The striking increase in $\dot{V}_{CO_2}$ is in contrast to $\dot{V}_{O_2}$. This is explained by the severe metabolic (lactic) acidosis that the patient develops as a result of the failure of cardiac output to increase in response to exercise (arterial HCO_3^- decreases 14 meq/L in 8 minutes).

Conclusion

This is a young man with extremely severe restrictive lung disease and secondary pulmonary vascular disease with high dead space ventilation, extremely low stroke volume and cardiac output, but without significant hypoxemia.

Case 52 Sarcoidosis
Clinical Findings

This 39-year-old woman was referred for follow-up exercise testing with complaints of mild shortness of breath of 1 year's duration and diminished exercise tolerance of 18 months' duration. One year previously, following an episode of hepatitis of undetermined origin, she was found to have an enlarging right lower lung field cystic lesion. Noninvasive preoperative exercise testing at that time suggested cardiovascular limitation. During thoracic surgery, pulmonary artery pressure was normal. The resected lesion contained non-caseating granulomata compatible with sarcoidosis. No organisms were seen or cultured. The patient had never smoked cigarettes and took no medications. Her exercise test was repeated with an intra-arterial catheter.

Exercise Findings

The patient performed exercise on a cycle ergometer. She pedalled at 60 rpm without an added load for 3 minutes. The work rate was then increased 15 W per minute to tolerance. Arterial blood was sampled every second minute, and intra-arterial pressure was recorded from a percutaneously placed brachial artery catheter. The patient stopped exercise because of lightheadedness and shortness of breath. No ECG abnormalities occurred at rest or during exercise.

TABLE 9.52.1. Selected Respiratory Function Data

Measurement	Predicted	Measured
Age, yr		39
Sex		Female
Height, cm		162
Weight, kg	63	68
Hematocrit, %		41
VC, L	3.38	2.89
IC, L	2.25	1.80
TLC, L	5.84	4.34
FEV$_1$, L	2.75	2.40
FEV$_1$/VC, %	81	88
MVV, L/min	105	98
D$_L$CO, ml/mm Hg/min	24.2	17.9

TABLE 9.52.2. Selected Exercise Data

Measurement	Predicted	Measured
Peak $\dot{V}O_2$, L/min	1.70	1.12
Maximum HR, beats/min	181	173
Maximum O_2 pulse, ml/beat	9.4	6.5
$\Delta\dot{V}O_2/\Delta WR$, ml/min/W	10.3	7.3
AT, L/min	>0.81	<0.65
Blood pressure, mmHg (rest, max)		146/88, 189/105
Maximum $\dot{V}E$, L/min		55
Exercise breathing reserve, L/min	>15	43
PaO$_2$, mmHg (rest, max ex)		104, 119
P(A − a)O$_2$, mmHg (rest, max ex)		7, 7
P(a − ET)CO$_2$, mmHg (rest, max ex)		0, −4
VD/VT (rest, max ex)		0.30, 0.19
HCO$_3$, mEq/L (rest, 2-min recov)		22, 13

FIGURE 9.52.1.

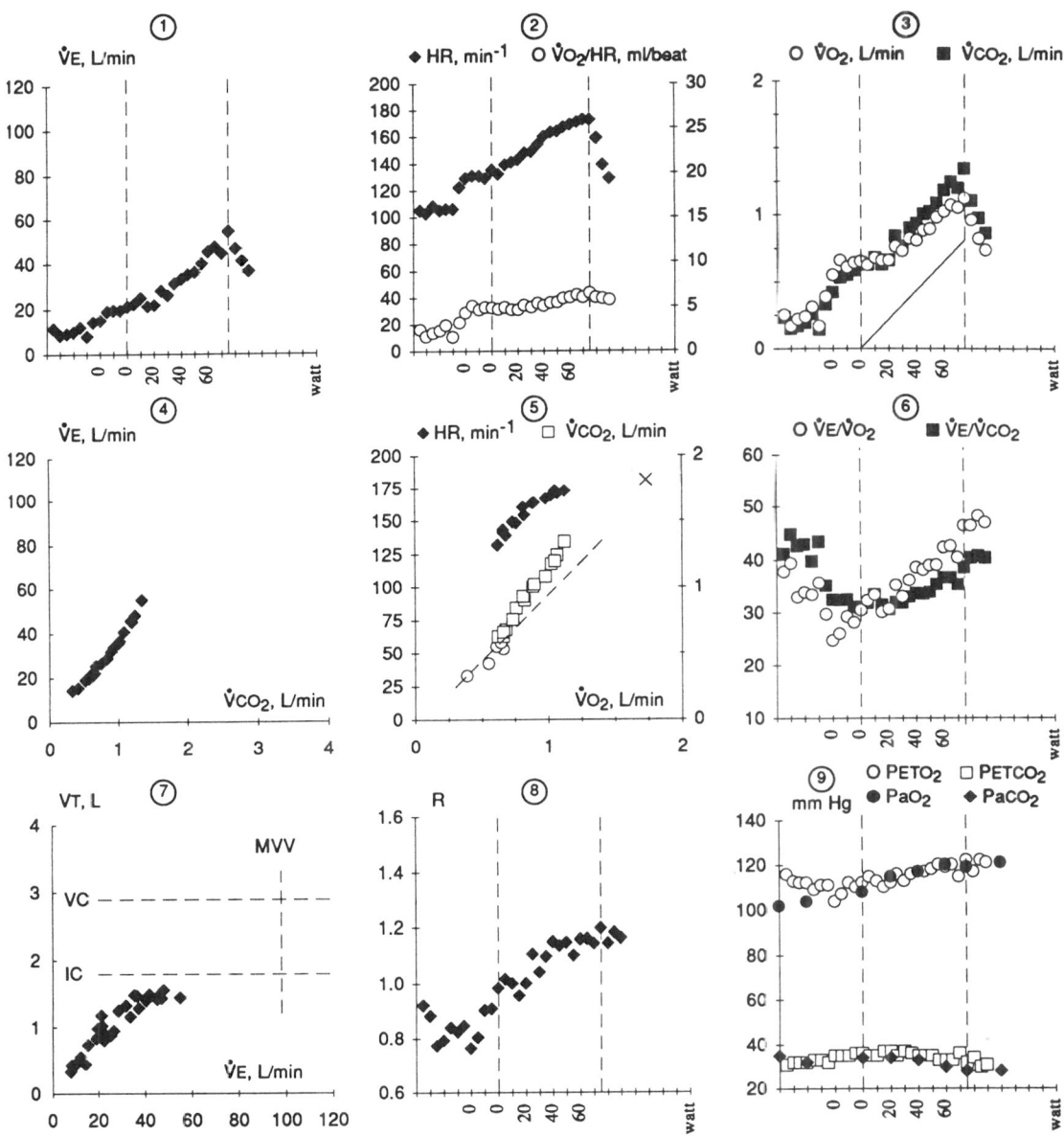

1. Vertical dashed lines in panels 1 to 3 and 6, 8, and 9 indicate the beginning and the end of increasing work period.

2. Unloaded cycling is performed for 3 minutes before the left vertical dashed line.

3. In panel 3, the diagonal line shows the increase of $\dot{V}O_2$ at a slope of 10 ml/min/w.

4. In panel 5, the diagonal dashed line has a slope of 1; the "x" in the upper right is the predicted maximum heart rate and $\dot{V}O_2$ for the subject.

TABLE 9.52.3.   Air Breathing

Time min	Work rate watts	BP mmHg	HR min⁻¹	f min⁻¹	$\dot{V}_E$ L/min BTPS	$\dot{V}_{CO_2}$ L/min STPD	$\dot{V}_{O_2}$ L/min STPD	$\frac{\dot{V}_{O_2}}{HR}$ ml/beat	R	pH	HCO₃ meq/L	P$_{O_2}$, mmHg ET	a	(A−a)	P$_{CO_2}$, mmHg ET	a	(a−ET)	$\dot{V}_E/\dot{V}_{CO_2}$	$\dot{V}_E/\dot{V}_{O_2}$	V_D/V_T
	Rest	156/90								7.41	22	102			35					
	Rest		105	23	11.4	0.23	0.25	2.4	0.92			116			31			41	38	
	Rest		103	20	8.4	0.15	0.17	1.7	0.88			113			32			45	39	
	Rest		103	23	9.2	0.17	0.22	2.0	0.77			112			32			43	33	
	Rest	146/88	105	23	10.1	0.19	0.24	2.3	0.79	7.43	21	112	104	7	32	32	0	43	34	0.30
	Rest		103	22	12.2	0.26	0.31	2.9	0.84			109			33			40	33	
	Rest		103	24	8.1	0.14	0.17	1.6	0.82			111			33			43	36	
	Unloaded		122	33	14.4	0.33	0.39	3.2	0.85			111			32			35	30	
	Unloaded		129	21	15.4	0.42	0.55	4.3	0.76			104			35			32	25	
	Unloaded		131	23	19.1	0.53	0.66	5.0	0.80			107			35			32	26	
	Unloaded		131	23	19.8	0.55	0.61	4.7	0.90			112			35			32	29	
	Unloaded		129	20	19.7	0.58	0.64	5.0	0.91			110			36			31	28	
	Unloaded	165/99	135	18	21.3	0.64	0.65	4.8	0.98	7.39	20	112	108	8	36	34	−2	31	30	0.17
0.5	10		132	28	22.4	0.63	0.62	4.7	1.02			115			35			32	32	
1.0	10		139	29	25.2	0.68	0.68	4.9	1.00			113			35			33	33	
1.5	20		141	21	21.6	0.63	0.66	4.7	0.95			110			37			31	30	
2.0	20	168/97	143	24	22.2	0.66	0.66	4.6	1.00	7.38	20	112	115	1	37	34	−3	31	31	0.15
2.5	30		148	23	28.7	0.84	0.76	5.1	1.11			116			35			32	35	
3.0	30		149	28	26.5	0.76	0.73	4.9	1.04			113			37			32	33	
3.5	40		154	24	31.7	0.90	0.82	5.3	1.10			116			36			33	36	
4.0	40	189/105	160	29	33.7	0.93	0.81	5.1	1.15	7.37	19	117	117	3	35	33	−2	34	39	0.21
4.5	50		163	24	35.6	1.00	0.88	5.4	1.14			117			35			34	38	
5.0	50		164	25	36.7	1.02	0.89	5.4	1.15			118			35			34	39	
5.5	60		167	29	40.7	1.08	0.98	5.9	1.10			120			33			35	39	
6.0	60	189/105	169	31	45.8	1.18	1.02	6.0	1.16	7.35	16	119	120	3	33	30	−3	37	42	0.20
6.5	70		171	31	48.1	1.24	1.07	6.3	1.16			120			33			37	42	
7.0	70		173	32	45.2	1.20	1.05	6.1	1.14			115			36			35	40	
7.5	80	189/105	173	38	55.0	1.34	1.12	6.5	1.20	7.32	14	122	119	7	32	28	−4	39	46	0.19
	Recovery		159	33	47.2	1.10	0.96	6.0	1.15			117			34			40	46	
	Recovery	118/60	139	28	41.8	0.97	0.82	5.9	1.18			122			30			41	48	
	Recovery		129	29	37.2	0.85	0.74	5.7	1.16			121			31			40	47	
										7.27	13	121			28					

Interpretation

Comments

The resting respiratory function studies were similar to her pre-lung resection values and showed mild restrictive lung disease. The resting blood gases reveal a mild compensated respiratory alkalosis or metabolic acidosis.

Analysis

Referring to flow chart 1, peak $\dot{V}_{O_2}$ and the anaerobic threshold are both decreased, sending us through branchpoint 1.3 to flow chart 4. The breathing reserve is high (branchpoint 4.1). The mildly elevated ventilatory equivalents can be accounted for by the low Pa_{CO_2}. The normal V_D/V_T, $P(a - ET)_{CO_2}$ and $P(A - a)_{O_2}$ (branchpoint 4.3) indicate uniform ventilation-perfusion ratios, and an O_2 flow problem of non-pulmonary origin. The hematocrit is normal (branchpoint 4.4). The maximum O_2 pulse is extremely low and increases minimally as work rate is increased. Thus the choice is peripheral arterial disease or heart disease. Because the patient did not have symptoms of claudication and the CO_2 output from HCO_3^- buffering of lactic acid is high, the cause of the O_2 flow problem must be due to heart failure. The ECG was normal. These findings are compatible with a cardiomyopathy possibly secondary to sarcoidosis.

Conclusion

The patient exercised maximally and developed a significant lactic acidosis. Pulmonary disease does not explain her low peak $\dot{V}_{O_2}$. The results are best explained by left-sided heart failure, presumably due to Sarcoidosis involvement of the myocardium.

Case 53 Sarcoidosis, Severe: Air and Oxygen Breathing

Clinical Findings

This 29-year-old man with a 6-year history of sarcoidosis was referred for evaluation of the pathophysiology of his worsening dyspnea. He was on continuous O_2 supplementation and beclomethasone diproprionate (Vanceril) inhaler, but he was not currently taking systemic corticosteroids. His weight was stable. He had smoked cigarettes for only 1 year.

Exercise Findings

The patient performed exercise on a cycle ergometer while he breathed room air. The test was repeated while he was breathing 100% O_2. On both occasions, he pedalled at 60 rpm without an added load for 3 minutes. The work rate was then increased 10 W per minute to tolerance. Arterial blood was sampled every second minute, and intra-arterial pressure was recorded from a percutaneously placed brachial artery catheter. The patient stopped exercise because of shortness of breath while breathing room air and because of leg fatigue while breathing O_2. The resting ECG showed right axis deviation and inverted T waves anteriorly. The T waves became upright during exercise. No arrhythmias were noted.

TABLE 9.53.1. Selected Respiratory Function Data

Measurement	Predicted	Measured
Age, yr		29
Sex		Male
Height, cm		171
Weight, kg	73	58
Hematocrit, %		45
VC, L	4.28	3.11
IC, L	2.85	1.59
TLC, L	5.82	4.78
FEV_1, L	3.46	2.27
FEV_1/VC, %	81	73
MVV, L/min	138	91
$D_{L}CO$, ml/mm Hg/min	29.9	6.9

TABLE 9.53.2. Selected Exercise Data

Measurement	Predicted	Measured Air	Measured 100% O_2
Maximum work rate, W		40	70
Peak $\dot{V}O_2$, L/min	2.64	0.8	
Maximum HR, beats/min	191	149	150
Maximum O_2 pulse, ml/beat	13.6	5.7	
AT, L/min	>1.08	0.7	
Blood pressure, mmHg (rest, max ex)		114/72, 135/78	111/69, 141/87
Maximum $\dot{V}E$, L/min		64	70
Exercise breathing reserve, L/min	>15	27	21
PaO_2, mmHg (rest, max ex)		42, 35	585, 605
$P(A - a)O_2$ mmHg (rest, max ex)		52, 74	84, 57
$P(a - ET)CO_2$, mmHg (rest, max ex)		16, 22	19, 28
VD/VT (rest, max ex)		0.57, 0.67	0.63, 0.71
HCO_3^-, mEq/L (rest, 2-min recov)		27, 24	25, 24

FIGURE 9.53.1.   Air breathing.

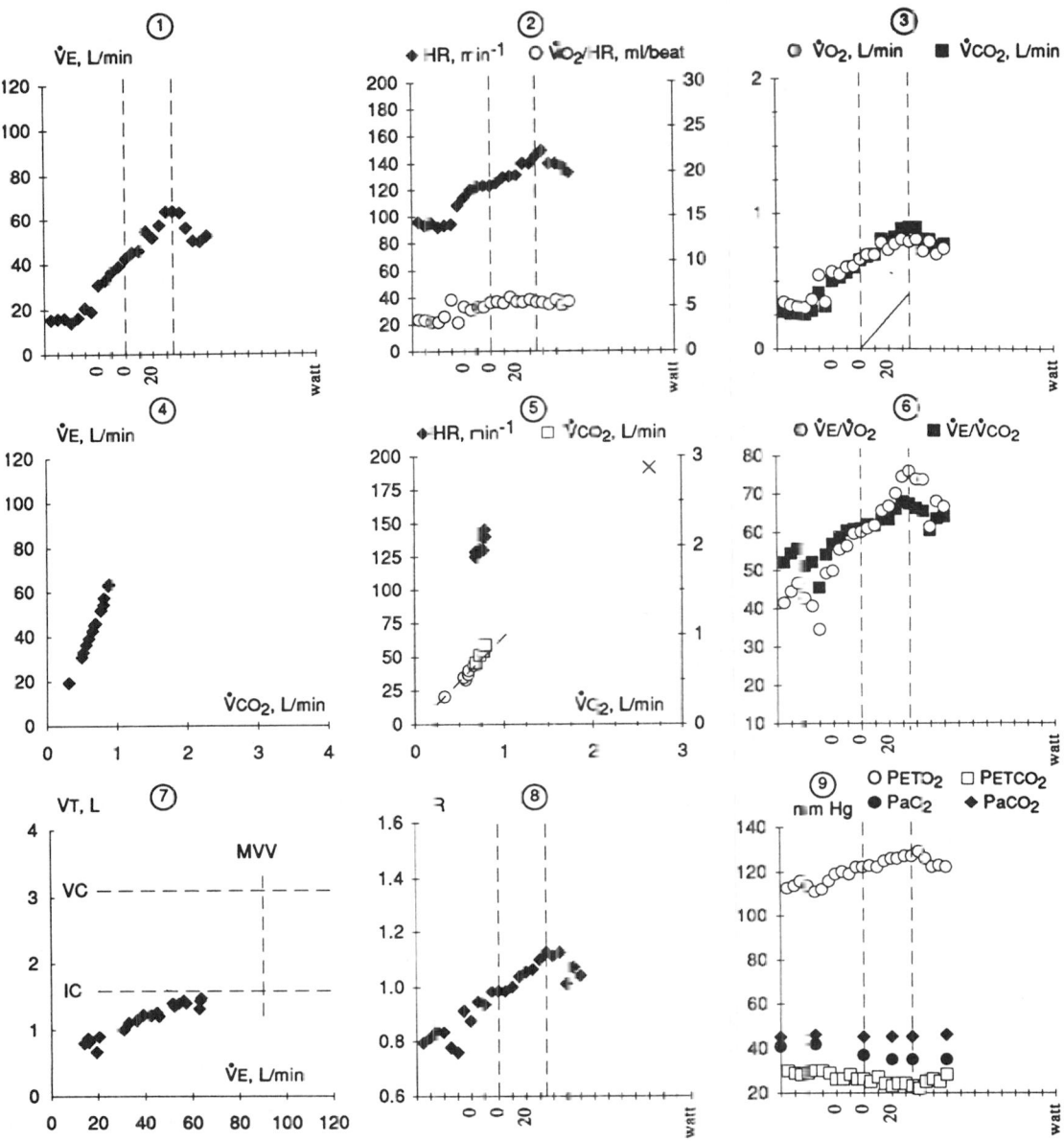

1. Vertical dashed lines in panels 1 to 3 and 6, 8, and 9 indicate the beginning and the end of increasing work period.

2. Unloaded cycling is performed for 3 minutes before the left vertical dashed line.

3. In panel 3, the diagonal line shows the increase of $\dot{V}O_2$ at a slope of 10 ml/min·w.

4. In panel 5, the diagonal dashed line has a slope of 1; the "×" in the upper right is the predicted maximum heart rate and $\dot{V}O_2$ for the subject.

FIGURE 9.53.2.   Oxygen breathing.

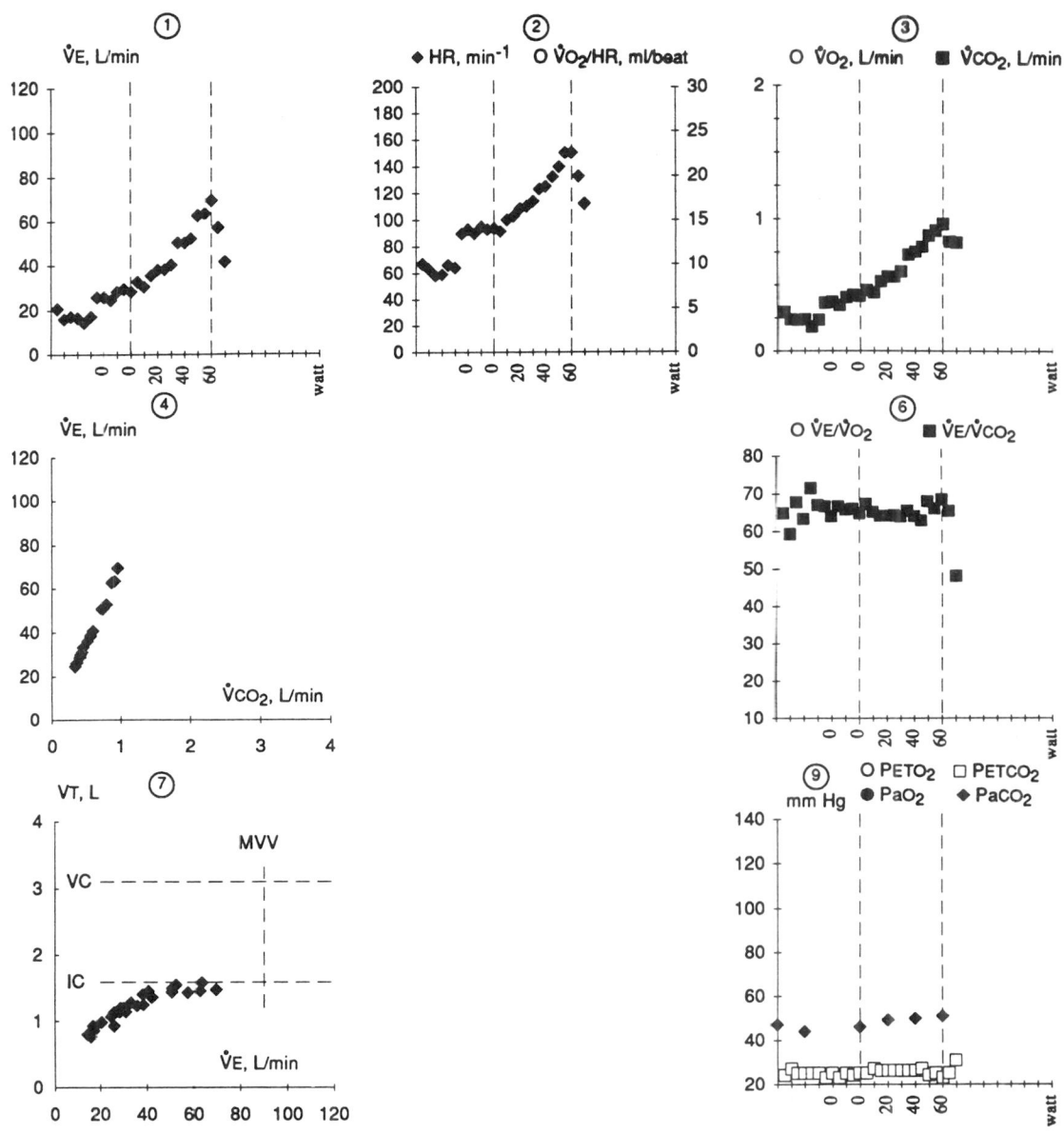

1. Vertical dashed lines in panels 1 to 3 and 6 and 9 indicate the beginning and the end of increasing work period.
2. Unloaded cycling is performed for 3 minutes before the left vertical dashed line.

TABLE 9.53.3. Air Breathing

Time min	Work rate watts	BP mmHg	HR min⁻¹	f min⁻¹	$\dot{V}_E$ L/min BTPS	$\dot{V}_{CO_2}$ L/min STPD	$\dot{V}_{O_2}$ L/min STPD	$\dot{V}_{O_2}$/HR ml/beat	R	pH	HCO₃⁻ meq/L	ET	P_{O_2}, mmHg a	(A − a)	ET	P_{CO_2}, mmHg a	(a − ET)	$\dfrac{\dot{V}_E}{\dot{V}_{CO_2}}$	$\dfrac{\dot{V}_E}{\dot{V}_{O_2}}$	$\dfrac{V_D}{V_T}$
	Rest	111/66								7.39	27		41			45				
	Rest		93	18	15.6	0.27	0.34	3.5	0.79			113			30			52	41	
	Rest		93	19	15.8	0.26	0.32	3.4	0.81			114			29			55	44	
	Rest		95	19	16.1	0.26	0.31	3.3	0.84			116			28			56	47	
	Rest		92	18	14.3	0.25	0.30	3.3	0.83			114			29			51	43	
	Rest	114/72	93	20	16.3	0.28	0.36	3.9	0.79	7.38	27	111	42	52	30	46	16	52	41	0.57
	Rest		94	23	20.6	0.41	0.54	5.7	0.79			112			30			45	35	
	Unloaded		103	29	19.2	0.31	0.34	3.1	0.91			115			29			54	49	
	Unloaded		114	31	31.0	0.50	0.57	5.0	0.88			119			26			57	50	
	Unloaded		120	30	33.0	0.52	0.55	4.6	0.95			120			26			59	55	
	Unloaded		122	32	36.5	0.56	0.60	4.9	0.93			119			28			60	56	
	Unloaded		123	32	39.1	0.60	0.61	5.0	0.93			122			26			61	60	
	Unloaded	116/72	123	35	42.5	0.65	0.66	5.4	0.93	7.38	26	122	37	67	26	45	19	61	60	0.64
0.5	10		125	36	45.1	0.68	0.69	5.5	0.99			123			25			62	61	
1.0	10		129	38	45.8	0.69	0.69	5.3	1.00			122			27			62	62	
1.5	20		130	39	54.4	0.81	0.78	6.0	1.04			125			24			63	65	
2.0	20	129/78	131	37	51.7	0.77	0.73	5.6	1.05	7.37	26	126	35	72	23	45	22	63	67	0.65
2.5	30		140	41	57.4	0.82	0.77	5.5	1.06			126			24			66	70	
3.0	30		140	44	63.3	0.88	0.80	5.7	1.10			127			24			68	74	
3.5	40	135/78	145	43	63.6	0.89	0.79	5.4	1.13	7.35	24	127	35	74	23	45	22	67	76	0.67
	Recovery		149	48	63.0	0.89	0.80	5.4	1.11			129			22			66	74	
	Recovery		140	39	56.3	0.81	0.72	5.1	1.13			126			25			65	74	
	Recovery		140	36	50.5	0.80	0.79	5.6	1.01			122			26			59	60	
	Recovery		138	34	50.1	0.75	0.70	5.1	1.07			123			25			63	67	
	Recovery	114/69	133	39	52.5	0.77	0.74	5.6	1.04	7.33	24	122	35	70	28	45	18	64	66	0.66

TABLE 9.53.4. Oxygen Breathing

Time min	Work rate watts	BP mmHg	HR min⁻¹	f min⁻¹	$\dot{V}_E$ L/min BTPS	$\dot{V}_{CO_2}$ L/min STPD	$\dot{V}_{O_2}$ L/min STPD	$\dot{V}_{O_2}$/HP ml/beat	R	pH	HCO₃⁻ meq/L	ET	P_{O_2}, mmHg a	(A − a)	ET	P_{CO_2}, mmHg a	(a − ET)	$\dfrac{\dot{V}_E}{\dot{V}_{CO_2}}$	$\dfrac{\dot{V}_E}{\dot{V}_{O_2}}$	$\dfrac{V_D}{V_T}$
	Rest									7.34	25	519			47					
	Rest		67	21	20.6	0.29									24			65		
	Rest		63	21	16.0	0.24									27			59		
	Rest		58	19	17.2	0.23									25			68		
	Rest	111/69	59	18	16.7	0.24				7.36	24	585	84	25	44	19	63		0.63
	Rest		66	18	14.4	0.13									25			72		
	Rest		64	20	17.1	0.23									25			67		
	Unloaded		90	23	25.9	0.33									23			67		
	Unloaded		93	28	26.0	0.37									25			64		
	Unloaded		90	23	24.6	0.34									23			67		
	Unloaded		95	25	28.4	0.40									25			66		
	Unloaded		93	25	29.8	0.42									24			66		
	Unloaded	116/75	94	24	28.6	0.41				7.35	25	615	52	25	46	21	65		0.66
0.5	10		92	26	33.1	0.43									25			67		
1.0	10		100	27	30.9	0.44									27			65		
1.5	20		103	29	35.8	0.52									26			64		
2.0	20	120/78	108	27	38.1	0.56				7.33	25	620	44	26	49	23	64		0.68
2.5	30		110	31	38.6	0.56									26			64		
3.0	30		114	28	40.6	0.60									26			64		
3.5	40		123	35	50.6	0.73									26			65		
4.0	40	132/81	125	34	50.8	0.75				7.31	25	612	51	26	50	24	64		0.69
4.5	50		132	34	52.5	0.79									27			63		
5.0	50		140	43	62.8	0.87									24			68		
5.5	60		150	40	63.5	0.91									25			66		
6.0	60	141/87	150	47	69.6	0.96				7.28	24	605	57	23	51	28	68		0.71
	Recovery		133	40	57.6	0.83									25			65		
	Recovery		112	31	42.1	0.82									31			48		

Interpretation

Comments

Resting respiratory function studies showed mild to moderate restrictive and obstructive components in ventilatory mechanics, an extremely low D_LCO, and severe arterial hypoxemia.

Analysis

Referring to flow chart 1, both the peak $\dot{V}O_2$ and anaerobic threshold are severely reduced. Proceeding to flow chart 4 through branchpoint 4.1, the breathing reserve is normal, but the high $\dot{V}E/\dot{V}CO_2$ at the *AT* (branchpoint 4.3) and high VD/VT (branchpoint 4.2) direct us to the boxes with lung disease with impaired oxygenation and abnormal pulmonary circulation. The findings support these diagnoses with high dead space ventilation increas-ing the ventilatory requirements at rest and all work levels. With O_2 breathing, there is no evidence of a right to left shunt, but ventilatory drive is reduced and the patient is able to tolerate a considerably higher work rate.

Conclusion

This patient with sarcoidosis with some disturbance in ventilatory mechanics has severe gas exchange abnormality due to marked pulmonary vascular disease. He has severe hypoxemia at rest and during exercise without supplemental oxygen; his ability to perform work is increased with oxygen. From sequential exercise testing it became evident that this man's pulmonary microcirculation was disappearing (increasing VD/VT and $\dot{V}E/\dot{V}O_2$ and worsening hypoxemia) despite stable ventilatory mechanics. The patient was treated with unilateral lung transplantation.

Case 54 Interstitial Pneumonitis: Pre- and Post-corticosteroid Therapy

Clinical Findings

This 37-year-old housewife developed progressive shortness of breath. She was found to have the pattern of interstitial lung disease on chest x-ray studies and was referred for exercise testing.

Exercise Findings

The patient performed exercise on a cycle ergometer. She pedalled at 60 rpm without added load for 3 minutes. The work rate was then increased 15 W per minute to her symptom-limited maximum. Arterial blood was sampled every second minute, and intra-arterial blood pressure was recorded from a percutaneously placed brachial artery catheter. Her resting and exercise ECGs were normal. In the initial study she stopped exercise because of short-ness of breath. After the first exercise test she was treated with prednisone. Her exercise test was repeated 6 months later, at which time she was taking 30 mg prednisone daily. She was asymptomatic at the time of the second test.

TABLE 9.54.1. Selected Respiratory Function Data

Measurement	Predicted	Before Treatment	After Treatment
Age, yr		37	
Sex		Female	
Height, cm		168	
Weight, kg	66	57	
Hematocrit, %		42	
VC, L	3.76	1.71	3.85
IC, L	2.50	1.31	2.25
FEV_1, L	3.08	1.52	3.10
FEV_1/VC, %	82	89	81
MVV, L/min	120	66	130
$D_{L}CO$, ml/mm Hg/min	28.5	16.2	

TABLE 9.54.2. Selected Exercise Data

Measurement	Predicted	Before Treatment	After Treatment
Peak $\dot{V}O_2$, L/min	1.72	1.35	2.01
Maximum HR, beats/min	183	149	174
Maximum O_2 pulse, ml/beat	9.4	9.1	11.6
$\Delta\dot{V}O_2$/ΔWR, ml/min/W	10.3	9.5	9.8
AT, L/min	>0.79	0.80	1.0
Blood pressure, mmHg (rest, max)		119/68, 190/81	125/75, 181/88
Maximum $\dot{V}E$, L/min		58	86
Exercise breathing reserve, L/min	>15	8	44
PaO_2, mmHg (rest, max ex)		65, 51	117, 98
$P(A - a)O_2$, mmHg (rest, max ex)		43, 65	−1, 26
$P(a - ET)CO_2$, mmHg (rest, max ex)		3, 3	−3, −2
VD/VT (rest, heavy ex)		0.40, 0.32	0.22, 0.15
HCO_3^-, mEq/L (rest, 2-min recov)		25, 21	24, 15

FIGURE 9.54.1.   Before treatment.

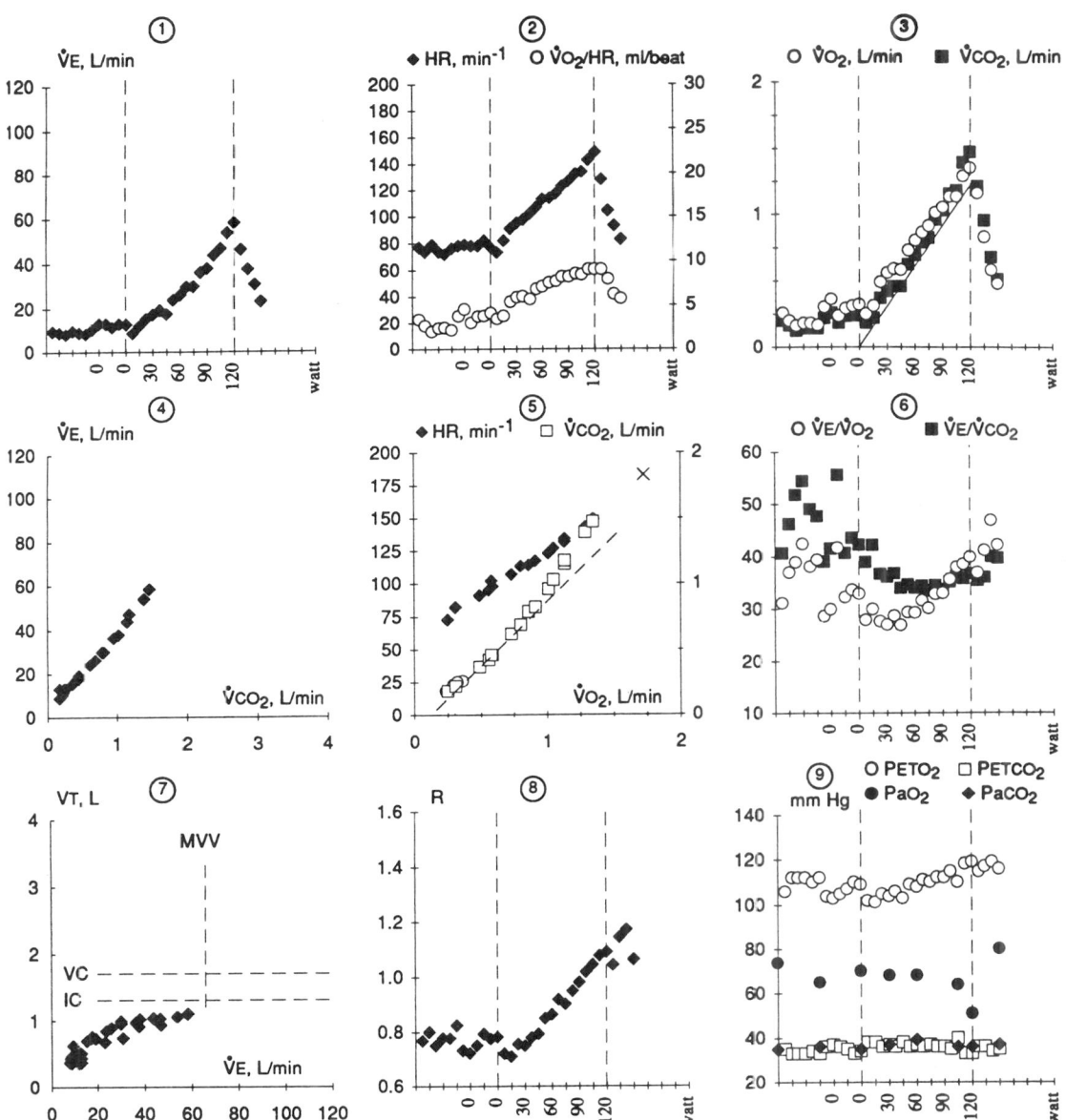

1. Vertical dashed lines in panels 1 to 3 and 6, 8, and 9 indicate the beginning and the end of increasing work period.

2. Unloaded cycling is performed for 3 minutes before the left vertical dashed line.

3. In panel 3, the diagonal line shows the increase of $\dot{V}O_2$ at a slope of 10 mL/min/w.

4. In panel 5, the diagonal dashed line has a slope of 1; the "x" in the upper right is the predicted maximum heart rate and $\dot{V}C_2$ for the subject.

TABLE 9.54.3. Before Treatment

Time min	Work rate watts	BP mmHg	HR min⁻¹	f min⁻¹	V̇E L/min BTPS	V̇CO₂ L/min STPD	V̇O₂ L/min STPD	V̇O₂/HR ml/beat	R	pH	HCO₃ meq/L	PO₂ mmHg ET	a	(A − a)	PCO₂ mmHg ET	a	(a − ET)	V̇E/V̇CO₂	V̇E/V̇O₂	VD/VT
	Rest									7.47	25		74			35				
	Rest		77	15	9.4	0.20	0.28	3.4	0.77			106			35			41	31	
	Rest		74	19	9.0	0.16	0.20	2.7	0.80			112			33			46	37	
	Rest		79	21	8.0	0.12	0.16	2.0	0.75			112			33			52	39	
	Rest		74	22	9.5	0.14	0.18	2.4	0.75			112			33			55	42	
	Rest		72	24	8.9	0.14	0.18	2.5	0.75			110			34			49	38	
	Rest	119/68	73	19	8.3	0.14	0.17	2.2	0.82	7.45	25	112	65	43	33	36	3	48	39	0.40
	Unloaded		73	20	10.3	0.22	0.30	3.8	0.73			104			36			39	29	
	Unloaded		79	25	12.9	0.26	0.36	4.6	0.72			103			37			41	30	
	Unloaded		73	34	12.9	0.18	0.24	3.1	0.75			105			36			56	42	
	Unloaded		73	23	11.3	0.23	0.29	3.7	0.73			107			35			41	32	
	Unloaded		82	29	12.9	0.24	0.31	3.8	0.77			110			33			43	34	
	Unloaded	125/68	77	24	12.6	0.25	0.32	4.2	0.73	7.44	23	109	70	37	34	35	1	42	33	0.35
0.5	15		73	20	8.7	0.18	0.25	3.4	0.72			102			38			39	28	
1.0	15		82	32	12.0	0.22	0.31	3.8	0.71			101			38			42	30	
1.5	30		91	22	15.4	0.37	0.49	5.4	0.73			105			36			37	28	
2.0	30	131/68	95	23	17.1	0.42	0.56	5.9	0.75	7.44	25	104	68	35	37	37	0	36	27	0.31
2.5	45		98	26	19.1	0.46	0.59	6.0	0.73			106			36			37	29	
3.0	45		102	23	17.6	0.46	0.58	5.7	0.79			103			38			34	27	
3.5	60		107	28	23.8	0.62	0.73	6.8	0.85			109			36			35	29	
4.0	60	146/75	113	29	25.9	0.69	0.80	7.1	0.83	7.43	25	108	63	38	37	39	2	34	29	0.32
4.5	75		114	31	29.8	0.79	0.86	7.5	0.92			111			36			34	32	
5.0	75		117	30	29.9	0.82	0.91	7.8	0.90			110			37			33	30	
5.5	90		123	37	36.2	0.96	1.01	8.2	0.95			112			36			34	33	
6.0	90		127	37	37.8	1.03	1.05	8.3	0.98			112			36			34	33	
6.5	105		132	42	43.8	1.15	1.13	8.6	1.02			115			35			35	36	
7.0	105	190/78	134	50	47.0	1.18	1.13	8.4	1.04	7.42	23	110	64	51	40	36	−4	36	38	0.31
7.5	120		143	51	54.0	1.39	1.29	9.0	1.08			118			33			36	39	
8.0	120	190/81	149	53	58.4	1.47	1.35	9.1	1.09	7.41	22	119	51	65	33	36	3	37	40	0.32
	Recovery		128	45	46.6	1.21	1.16	9.1	1.04			115			36			35	37	
	Recovery		104	41	37.6	0.95	0.83	8.0	1.14			117			36			36	41	
	Recovery		93	41	30.7	0.68	0.58	6.2	1.17			119			34			40	47	
	Recovery	190/81	83	34	23.1	0.51	0.48	5.8	1.06	7.36	21	116	80	35	35	37	2	40	42	0.36

Interpretation

Comments

The resting respiratory function studies indicate that this patient had severe restrictive lung disease before therapy, which improved markedly after therapy (Table 9.54.1). The resting ECG is normal. The "after-treatment" exercise test was performed 6 months after the first test.

Analysis

Referring to flowchart 1, the peak V̇O₂ and the anaerobic threshold are abnormal (Table 9.54.2). See flow chart 4: The patient's breathing reserve is low (branchpoint 4.1). VD/VT is high (branchpoint 4.2). This leads to the diagnosis of lung disease with an O₂ flow problem. Characteristically, this is a restrictive lung disease. Confirming restrictive lung disease as the major pathophysiologic disorder are a high

FIGURE 9.54.2.   After treatment.

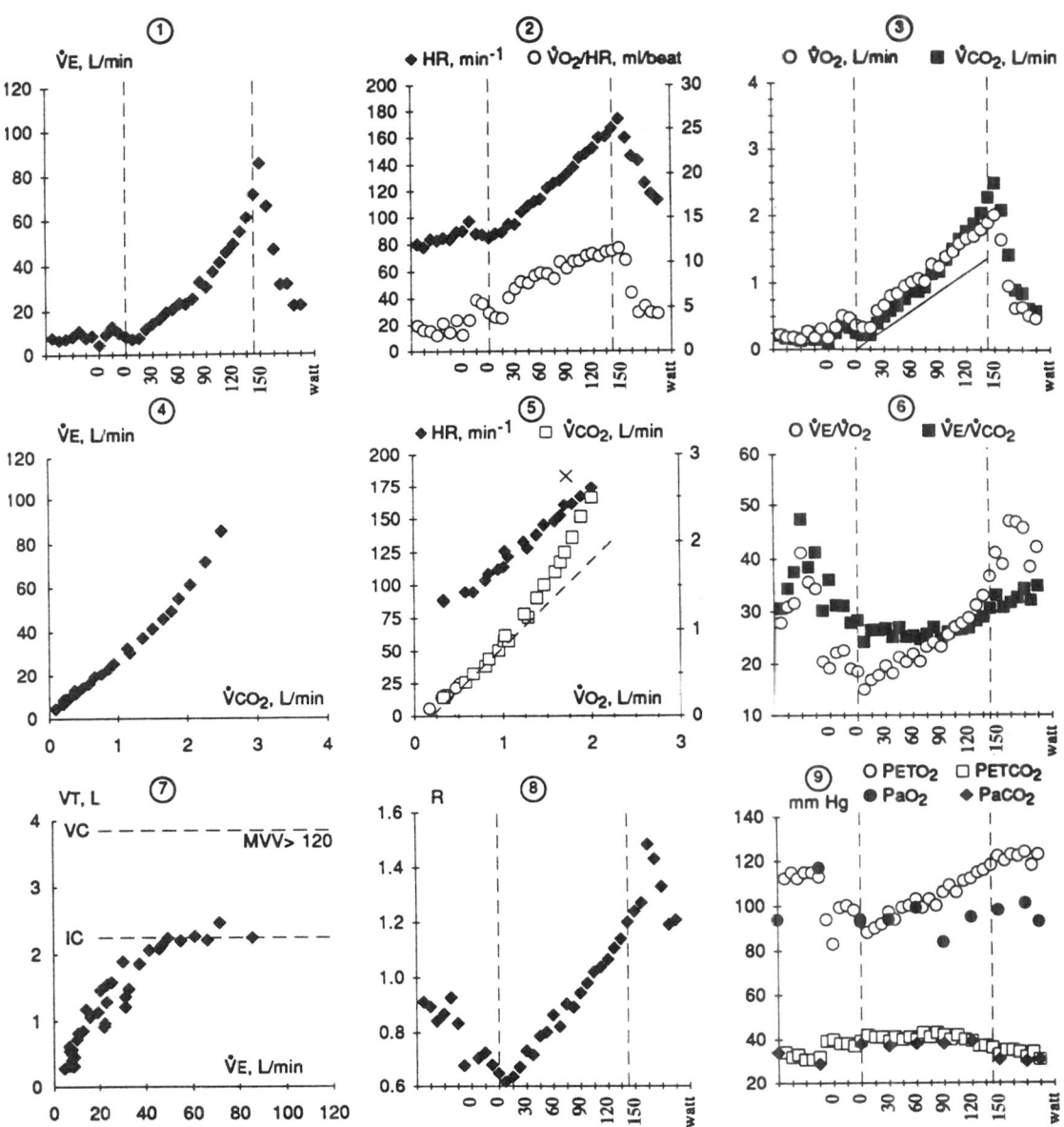

1. Vertical dashed lines in panels 1 to 3 and 6, 8, and 9 indicate the beginning and the end of increasing work period.

2. Unloaded cycling is performed for 3 minutes before the left vertical dashed line.

3. In panel 3, the diagonal line shows the increase of $\dot{V}O_2$ at a slope of 10 ml/min/w.

4. In panel 5, the diagonal dashed line has a slope of 1; the "x" in the upper right is the predicted maximum heart rate and $\dot{V}O_2$ for the subject.

TABLE 9.54.4. After Treatment

Time min	Work rate watts	BP mmHg	HR min⁻¹	f min⁻¹	V̇E L/min BTPS	V̇CO₂ L/min STPD	V̇O₂ L/min STPD	V̇O₂/HR ml/beat	R	pH	HCO₃ meq/L	PO₂ ET	PO₂ a	PO₂ (A−a)	PCO₂ ET	PCO₂ a	PCO₂ (a−ET)	V̇E/V̇CO₂	V̇E/V̇O₂	VD/VT
	Rest	125/75								7.45	23		94			94				
	Rest		80	15	7.7	0.21	0.23	2.9	0.91				112			34			31	28
	Rest		78	11	6.8	0.17	0.19	2.4	0.89				115			32			35	31
	Rest		84	13	7.1	0.16	0.19	2.3	0.84				112			33			37	32
	Rest		83	24	8.2	0.13	0.15	1.8	0.87				115			31			47	41
	Rest		85	13	10.7	0.25	0.27	3.2	0.93				115			31			38	36
	Rest	119/75	84	19	7.8	0.15	0.18	2.1	0.83	7.50	22	113	117	−1	32	29	−3	41	34	0.22
	Unloaded		89	28	8.7	0.21	0.31	3.5	0.68				94			39			30	20
	Unloaded		90	16	4.6	0.09	0.17	1.9	0.53				93			40			36	19
	Unloaded		97	20	9.2	0.24	0.34	3.5	0.71				99			38			31	22
	Unloaded		88	15	12.8	0.37	0.51	5.8	0.73				100			38			31	23
	Unloaded		87	14	10.1	0.32	0.47	5.4	0.68				98			37			28	19
	Unloaded	125/75	85	14	8.0	0.24	0.37	4.4	0.65	7.43	25	94	93	3	39	38	−1	28	18	0.17
0.5	15		88	21	6.9	0.27	0.34	3.9	0.62				88			42			24	15
1.0	15		89	23	7.5	0.27	0.33	3.7	0.64				90			41			26	17
1.5	30		95	14	11.5	0.39	0.58	6.1	0.67				92			41			26	18
2.0	30	125/69	95	12	14.1	0.49	0.67	7.1	0.73	7.44	25	97	94	8	39	37	−2	27	20	0.12
2.5	45		104	15	15.9	0.58	0.81	7.8	0.72				94			41			25	18
3.0	45		109	17	19.2	0.66	0.84	7.7	0.79				99			40			27	21
3.5	60		112	14	20.4	0.76	0.95	8.5	0.80				100			41			25	20
4.0	60	144/75	114	15	23.3	0.87	1.01	8.9	0.86	7.43	25	103	99	8	40	38	−2	25	22	0.10
4.5	75		122	18	23.1	0.87	1.06	8.7	0.82				99			43			25	20
5.0	75		126	16	25.3	0.93	1.03	8.2	0.90				103			41			26	23
5.5	90		128	22	32.6	1.14	1.28	10.0	0.89				100			43			27	24
6.0	90	156/75	133	16	30.3	1.17	1.24	9.3	0.94	7.42	24	106	84	26	42	38	−4	25	23	0.08
6.5	105		138	20	37.2	1.36	1.39	10.1	0.98				109			40			26	26
7.0	105		145	20	41.4	1.50	1.47	10.1	1.02				105			42			26	27
7.5	120		148	22	45.8	1.65	1.59	10.7	1.04				111			40			27	28
8.0	120	181/81	152	22	49.4	1.77	1.66	10.9	1.07	7.40	24	112	95	18	39	39	0	27	29	0.17
8.5	135		130	25	55.0	1.88	1.70	10.6	1.11				115			37			28	31
9.0	135		131	27	61.2	2.04	1.79	11.1	1.14				116			37			29	33
9.5	130		137	29	71.7	2.27	1.89	11.3	1.20				118			36			31	37
10.0	130	181/88	174	38	85.6	2.49	2.01	11.6	1.24	7.40	19	122	98	26	33	31	−2	33	41	0.15
	Recovery		160	30	66.5	2.08	1.64	10.3	1.27				120			35			31	39
	Recovery		146	22	46.9	1.42	0.96	6.6	1.48				123			35			32	47
	Recovery		143	23	31.3	0.90	0.63	4.4	1.43				122			34			33	47
	Recovery	181/81	126	26	31.4	0.85	0.64	5.1	1.33	7.36	17	124	101	25	32	30	−2	34	46	0.15
	Recovery	118	24	22.0	0.62	0.52	4.4	1.19					118			34			32	38	
	Recovery	175/75	113	23	22.2	0.58	0.48	4.2	1.21	7.36	17	123	93	30	31	31	0	35	42	0.18

VT/IC ratio (panel 7, Figure 9.54.1), breathing frequency exceeding 50 breaths per minute at the patient's maximum work rate (Table 9.54.3), P(A − a)O₂ increasing and PaO₂ decreasing systematically with work rate, and increased values of P(a − ET)CO₂ and VD/VT (Table 9.54.3).

After treatment, the peak V̇O₂ improved significantly and exceeded the predicted value. Arterial hypoxemia with exercise is no longer present and P(a − ET)CO₂ and VD/VT are normal, suggesting that the ventilation-perfusion abnormality observed before treatment was corrected. Moreover, the restrictive breathing pattern observed during pretreatment exercise resolved after treatment (compare panels 7 of Figs. 9.54.1 and 9.54.2).

Conclusion

Reduced exercise capacity due to restrictive lung disease, reversed after 6 months of therapy.

Case 55 Interstitial Pulmonary Fibrosis: Air and Oxygen Breathing

Clinical Findings

This 47-year-old man had developed dyspnea 12 years previously. A histologic diagnosis of pulmonary alveolar proteinosis was then made by open lung biopsy. Following whole lung lavage he became asymptomatic until 10 months prior to evaluation when progressive dyspnea first became evident when he was skiing at high altitudes. Although previously active in sports, he was unable to walk more than 30 yards on flat ground at a normal pace. He coughed with exercise and sometimes produced clear sputum. He denied smoking, wheezing, or edema. The results of his examination were normal except for digital clubbing and infrequent fine inspiratory rales at the lung bases. Chest x-ray showed increased interstitial markings with honeycombing.

Exercise Findings

The patient performed exercise on a cycle ergometer breathing room air, and, after a 30 minute rest, breathing 100% oxygen. He pedalled at 60 rpm without added load for 3 minutes. The work rate was increased 15 W every minute to his symptom-limited maximum. Arterial blood was sampled every second minute, and intra-arterial blood pressure was recorded from a percutaneously placed brachial artery catheter. When breathing room air, he stopped exercise because of fatigue and lightheadedness. When breathing oxygen he stopped because of leg pain and general fatigue. Resting and exercise ECGs were normal.

TABLE 9.55.1. Selected Respiratory Function Data

Measurement	Predicted	Measured
Age, yr		47
Sex		Male
Height, cm		174
Weight, kg	77	85
Hematocrit, %		41
VC, L	4.49	2.20
IC, L	2.99	1.14
TLC, L	6.48	3.17
FEV_1, L	3.58	2.01
FEV_1/VC, %	80	91
MVV, L/min, direct	151	112
MVV, L/min, indirect	143	80
$D_{L}CO$, ml/mm Hg/min	30.7	13.9

TABLE 9.55.2. Selected Exercise Data

Measurement	Predicted	Room Air	Oxygen
Peak $\dot{V}O_2$, L/min	2.60	1.23	
Maximum HR, beats/min	173	150	154
Maximum O_2 pulse, ml/beat	15.0	8.2	
$\Delta\dot{V}O_2/\Delta WR$, ml/min/W	10.3	8.6	
AT, L/min	>1.12	0.85	
Blood pressure, mmHg (rest, max)		120/75, 175/84*	138/87, 195/90*
Maximum $\dot{V}E$, L/min		72	56
Exercise breathing reserve, L/min	>15	8	32
PaO_2, mmHg (rest, max ex)		62, 37	568, 284
$P(A - a)O_2$, mmHg (rest, max ex)		30, 73	102, 365
$P(a - ET)CO_2$, mmHg (rest, max ex)		3, 10	4, 12
VD/VT (rest, heavy ex)		0.54, 0.54	0.51, 0.56
HCO_3^-, mEq/L (rest, 2-min recov)		23, 20	26, 22

*Systolic pulsus paradoxus of 70 mmHg.

FIGURE 9.55.1.   Air breathing.

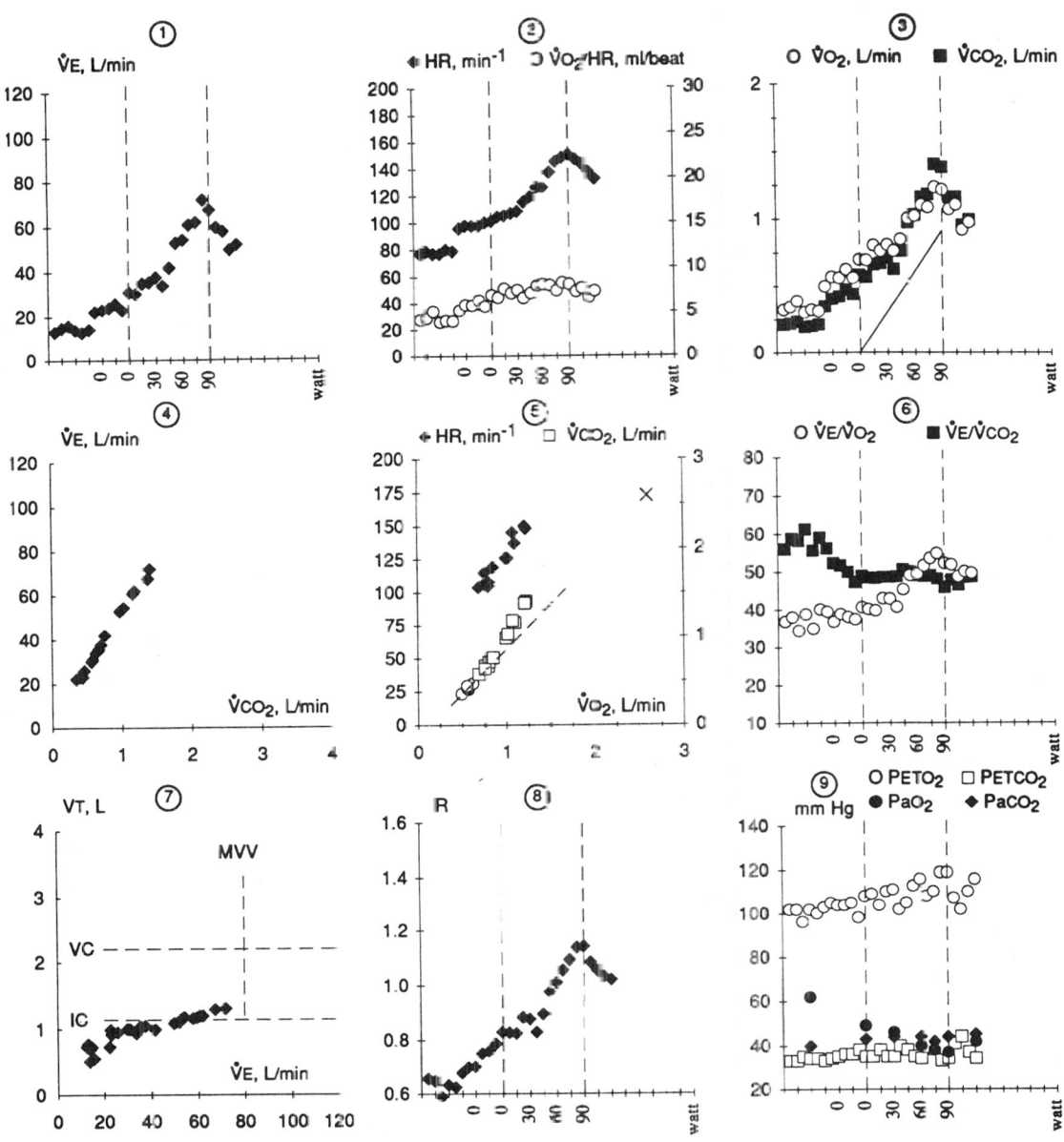

1. Vertical dashed lines in panels 1 to 3 and 6, 8, and 9 indicate the beginning and the end of increasing work period.
2. Unloaded cycling is performed for 3 minutes before the left vertical dashed line.
3. In panel 3, the diagonal line shows the increase of $\dot{V}O_2$ at a slope of 10 ml/min/w.
4. In panel 5, the diagonal dashed line has a slope of 1; the "×" in the upper right is the predicted maximum heart rate and $\dot{V}O_2$ for the subject.

TABLE 9.55.3. Air Breathing

Time min	Work rate watts	BP mmHg	HR min⁻¹	f min⁻¹	V̇E L/min BTPS	V̇CO2 L/min STPD	V̇O2 L/min STPD	V̇O2/HR ml/beat	R	pH	HCO3⁻ meq/L	PO2, mmHg ET	a	(A − a)	PCO2, mmHg ET	a	(a − ET)	V̇E/V̇CO2	V̇E/V̇O2	VD/VT
	Rest		77	17	13.2	0.21	0.32	4.2	0.66			102			33			56	37	
	Rest		79	20	14.6	0.22	0.34	4.3	0.65			102			33			59	38	
	Rest		77	28	15.8	0.23	0.39	5.1	0.59			96			35			58	34	
	Rest	120/75	77	27	13.9	0.19	0.30	3.9	0.63	7.37	23	102	62	30	34	40	6	61	39	0.54
	Rest		80	17	12.6	0.20	0.32	4.0	0.63			100			34			56	35	
	Rest		79	20	14.1	0.21	0.31	3.9	0.68			103			33			59	40	
	Unloaded		96	30	22.2	0.35	0.50	5.2	0.70			105			34			56	39	
	Unloaded		98	25	23.0	0.40	0.57	5.8	0.70			104			35			52	37	
	Unloaded		98	25	23.8	0.42	0.56	5.7	0.75			104			36			52	39	
	Unloaded		98	27	25.8	0.47	0.62	6.3	0.76			105			36			50	38	
	Unloaded		100	23	22.8	0.44	0.56	5.6	0.79			98			38			47	37	
	Unloaded	153/81	101	31	31.0	0.58	0.70	6.9	0.83	7.35	23	108	49	51	35	43	8	49	41	0.54
0.5	15		104	30	30.1	0.57	0.69	6.6	0.83			109			35			48	40	
1.0	15		105	35	34.8	0.66	0.80	7.6	0.83			104			38			48	40	
1.5	30		107	34	35.5	0.67	0.76	7.1	0.88			110			35			49	43	
2.0	30	159/75	108	36	37.6	0.71	0.81	7.5	0.88	7.34	23	111	46	55	35	44	9	49	43	0.55
2.5	45		115	36	33.8	0.63	0.76	6.6	0.83			102			40			49	40	
3.0	45		119	42	41.9	0.76	0.85	7.1	0.89			105			38			50	45	
3.5	60		126	46	52.8	0.98	1.00	7.9	0.98			113			35			50	49	
4.0	60	177/90	126	46	54.3	1.03	1.02	8.1	1.01	7.33	23	116	40	66	34	44	10	49	49	0.56
4.5	75		137	51	60.9	1.16	1.10	8.0	1.05			108			39			49	51	
5.0	75	186/90	145	52	62.1	1.18	1.08	7.4	1.09	7.33	22	110	38	73	38	42	4	49	53	0.54
5.5	90		148	55	72.0	1.40	1.23	8.3	1.14			119			33			48	55	
6.0	90	186/93	150	52	67.5	1.38	1.21	8.1	1.14	7.31	22	119	37	73	34	44	10	46	52	0.53
	Recovery		147	51	59.7	1.16	1.07	7.3	1.08			107			41			48	52	
	Recovery		144	50	57.9	1.16	1.10	7.6	1.05			102			44			46	49	
	Recovery		138	46	49.9	0.95	0.92	6.7	1.03			110			37			48	50	
	Recovery	174/90	132	47	52.1	0.99	0.97	7.3	1.02	7.27	20	116	42	64	34	45	11	49	50	0.56

Interpretation

Comments

This case of severe interstitial lung disease is presented to illustrate two major points: (1) The impaired peripheral oxygenation that may be caused by pulmonary fibrosis; and (2) the presence of a major increasing contribution of the carotid bodies to breathing, in association with arterial hypoxemia.

The results of the resting respiratory function studies indicate that this patient has a severe restrictive disorder, with no evidence of airflow obstruction (Table 9.55.1). The resting ECG is normal.

Analysis

Referring to flow chart 1, the peak V̇O2 and anaerobic threshold are reduced (Table 9.55.2). See flow chart 4: The breathing reserve is reduced (branchpoint 4.1). Following the low breathing reserve branch of

branchpoint 4.1, we consider branchpoint 4.2 and the high VD/VT. From this, we conclude that this patient has restrictive lung disease with an O₂ flow problem. Findings confirming this diagnosis are: (1) the high VT/IC ratio (panel 7, Fig. 9.55.1), (2) the low and progressively decreasing PaO₂ as work rate is increased (panel 9, Fig. 9.55.1), (3) a breathing frequency greater than 50 at the peak V̇O2 (Table 9.55.3), (4) an increased P(a − ET)CO₂ (panel 9, Fig. 9.55.1), (5) a steep heart rate response to the increasing oxygen uptake (panel 5, Fig. 9.55.1), (6) a low O₂ pulse with a flat contour as the work rate is increased (panel 2, Fig. 9.55.1), (7) a reduced ΔV̇O2/ΔWR (Table 9.55.2 and panel 3, Fig. 9.55.1), and (8) P(A − a)O₂ increasing with increasing work rate (Table 9.55.3). Note that all these confirmatory findings are characteristic of restrictive lung disease.

O₂ breathing allows the patient to increase his maximum work rate from 90 to 135 W (Table 9.55.4 and Fig. 9.55.2). This was accomplished primarily

FIGURE 9.55.2.   Oxygen breathing.

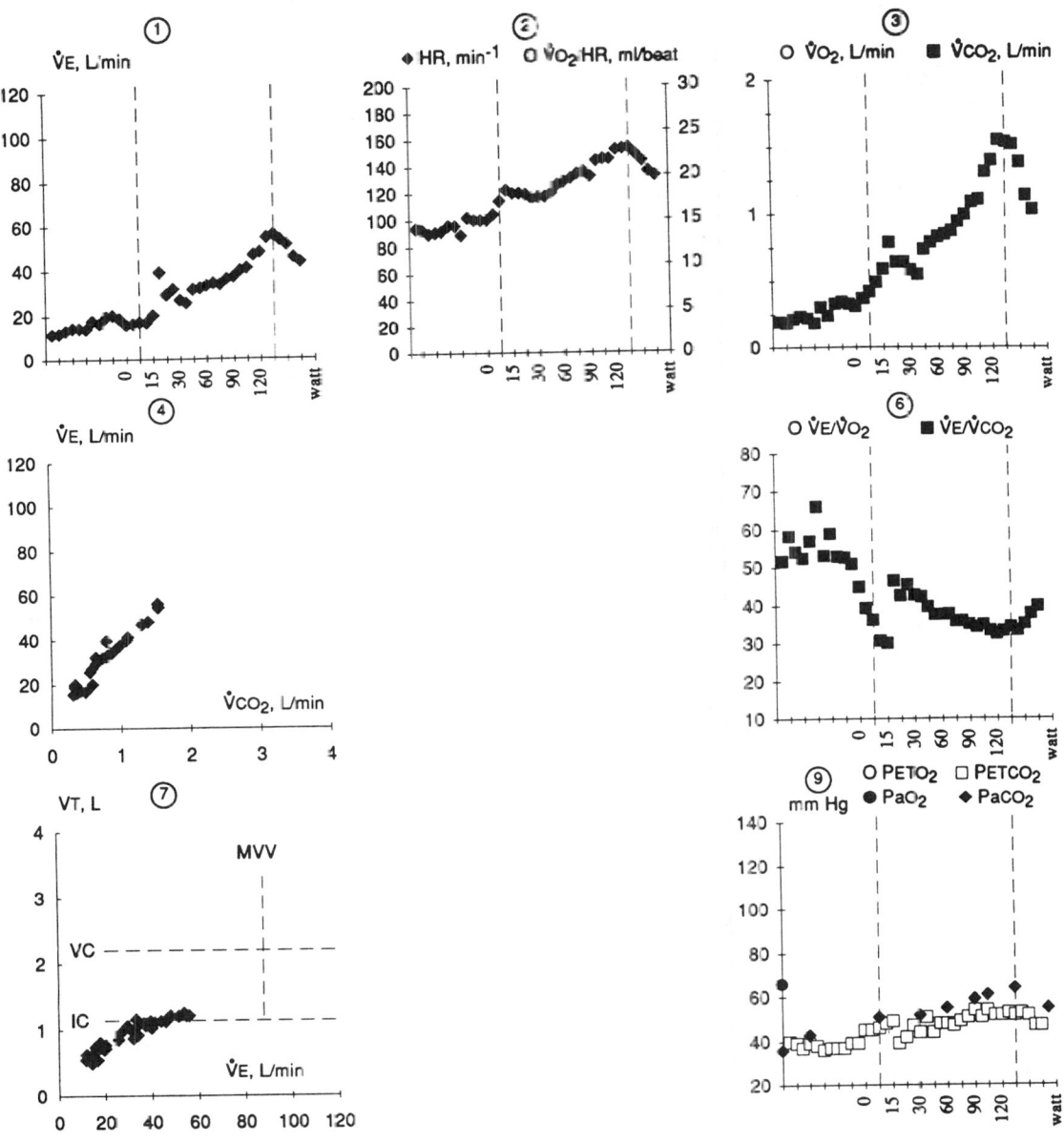

1. Vertical dashed lines in panels 1 to 3 and 6 and 9 indicate the beginning and the end of increasing work period.
2. Unloaded cycling is performed for 3 minutes before the left vertical dashed line.

TABLE 9.55.4. Oxygen Breathing

Time min	Work rate watts	BP mmHg	HR min⁻¹	f min⁻¹	$\dot{V}_E$ L/min BTPS	$\dot{V}_{CO_2}$ L/min STPD	$\dot{V}_{O_2}$ L/min STPD	$\dot{V}_{O_2}/HR$ ml/beat	R	pH	HCO_3^- meq/L	P_{O_2}, mmHg ET	a	(A−a)	P_{CO_2}, mmHg ET	a	(a−ET)	$\dot{V}_E/\dot{V}_{CO_2}$	$\dot{V}_E/\dot{V}_{O_2}$	V_D/V_T
	Rest	132/84								7.44	24	66			40				36	
	Rest		94	21	11.6	0.19									40				52	
	Rest		93	19	12.1	0.18									39				58	
	Rest		90	23	13.3	0.21									37				54	
	Rest	138/87	91	29	14.5	0.23				7.39	26	568	102		39	43	4		52	0.51
	Rest		92	23	14.5	0.22									38				57	
	Rest		96	25	14.0	0.18									36				66	
	Rest		96	22	17.8	0.30									37				53	
	Rest		89	30	16.7	0.24									37				59	
	Unloaded		102	28	19.8	0.33									37				53	
	Unloaded		100	26	20.1	0.34									39				53	
	Unloaded		100	25	18.9	0.33									39				51	
	Unloaded		100	21	15.7	0.31									45				45	
	Unloaded		104	22	16.4	0.37									45				39	
	Unloaded	192/108	114	24	17.2	0.42				7.33	26	540	122		46	51	5		36	0.47
0.5	15		122	22	16.9	0.49									48				31	
1.0	15		120	28	20.1	0.59									49				30	
1.5	15		120	35	39.6	0.79									39				46	
2.0	15		119	28	29.5	0.64									42				42	
2.5	30		116	37	32.2	0.64									47				45	
3.0	30	186/96	117	28	27.1	0.58				7.31	26	505	156		44	52	8		43	0.56
3.5	45		117	30	25.7	0.55									51				42	
4.0	45		120	32	32.0	0.74									44				40	
4.5	60		126	34	32.4	0.79									48				37	
5.0	60	192/99	128	29	33.5	0.83				7.28	25	467	191		48	55	7		37	0.54
5.5	75		131	32	34.6	0.85									47				38	
6.0	75		134	37	34.2	0.87									49				36	
6.5	90		136	33	36.5	0.94									51				36	
7.0	90	196/102	132	35	37.5	0.99				7.25	25	409	245		54	59	5		35	0.53
7.5	105		144	39	40.1	1.08									51				34	
8.0	105	207/102	145	37	41.3	1.10				7.23	25	350	302		54	61	7		35	0.55
8.5	120		145	40	47.0	1.31									52				33	
9.0	120		152	40	48.3	1.39									52				32	
9.5	135		153	45	54.7	1.54									53				33	
10.0	135	210/102	154	46	56.1	1.53				7.20	25	284	365		52	64	12		34	0.56
	Recovery		149	43	53.9	1.51									53				33	
	Recovery		144	43	51.7	1.38									52				35	
	Recovery		136	41	46.1	1.13									47				38	
	Recovery		133	39	44.1	1.03									47				40	
		192/102								7.22	22	475			55					

by decreasing ventilatory drive. In contrast to regulating arterial P_{CO_2} around 40 as the patient did when breathing air, 100% O_2 breathing attenuated ventilatory drive (carotid body inhibition) causing Pa_{CO_2} to increase to 64 at the maximum work rate achieved. At each work rate during O_2 breathing, the breathing frequency (f) is decreased (compare Table 9.55.3 with Table 9.55.4). O_2 breathing allows the patient to breathe less and to be less breathless. The breathing frequency is only 35 ($\dot{V}_E = 37.5$) at 90 W when breathing O_2 as compared to 52 ($\dot{V}_E = 67.5$) during air breathing, at the same work rate.

The heart rate is considerably more rapid during air breathing (150) than during O_2 breathing (132) at 90 W.

Conclusion

The patient has severe interstitial lung disease, with an important O_2 flow problem probably created by a combination of arterial hypoxemia and pulmonary vascular disease. O_2 breathing attenuates ventilatory drive and provides relief of dyspnea.

Case 56 Pulmonary Alveolar Proteinosis: Air and Oxygen Breathing

Clinical Findings

This 19-year-old man was hospitalized because of increasing shortness of breath, productive cough, and fatigue of 6 weeks' duration. He denied fever, sweats, chest pain, or exposure to infectious or toxic agents other than automobile paint fumes, tobacco, and occasional marijuana. He was thin, afebrile, tachycardia, and tachypneic with diffuse coarse rales bilaterally. Chest roentgenograms revealed a diffuse alveolar infiltrate, and blood gases showed hypoxemia and hypercapnia. An open lung biopsy showed pulmonary alveolar proteinosis. Exercise tests were performed while the patient was breathing room air and then 100% O_2 prior to bilateral lung lavage.

Exercise Findings

The patient performed exercise on a cycle ergometer twice in the same morning with a 40-minute rest period between tests. On both occasions, arterial blood was sampled every second minute, and intra-arterial pressure was recorded from a percutaneously placed brachial artery catheter. He pedalled at 60 rpm without an added load for 3 minutes. The work rate was then increased 15 W per minute to tolerance. The patient was well motivated and cooperative and stopped exercise on both occasions because of dyspnea and chest tightness. No ECG abnormalities were noted.

TABLE 9.56.1. Selected Respiratory Function Data

Measurement	Predicted	Measured
Age, yr		19
Sex		Male
Height, cm		180
Weight, kg	32	68
Hematocrit, %		49
VC, L	4.46	2.46
IC, L	2.98	1.50
TLC, L	6.7	3.40
FEV_1, L	3.79	2.20
FEV_1/VC, %	85	89
MVV, L/min		
Direct	134	101
Indirect	152	88
D_LCO, ml/mm Hg/min	36.5	8.4

TABLE 9.56.2. Selected Exercise Data

Measurement	Predicted	Room Air	Oxygen
Peak $\dot{V}O_2$, L/min	3.25	1.42	
Maximum HR, beats/min	201	150	150
Maximum O_2 pulse, ml/beat	16.2	9.5	
$\Delta\dot{V}O_2/\Delta WR$, ml/min/W	10.3	11.9	
AT, L/min	>1.31	1.4	
Work rate, max, W		75	120
Blood pressure, mmHg (rest, max ex)		120/57, 144/72	114/62, 132/72
Maximum $\dot{V}E$, L/min		84	73
Exercise breathing reserve, L/min			
Using direct MVV	>15	17	28
Using indirect MVV	>15	4	15
FaO_2, mmHg (rest, max ex)		52, 33	306, 164
P(A − a)O_2, mmHg (rest, max ex)		57, 76	371, 506
P(a − ET)CO_2, mmHg (rest, max ex)		−1, 5	1, 5
VD/VT (rest, max ex)		0.42, 0.59	0.49, 0.48
HCO_3^-, mEq/L (rest, recov)		23, 21	23, 20

FIGURE 9.56.1.   Air breathing.

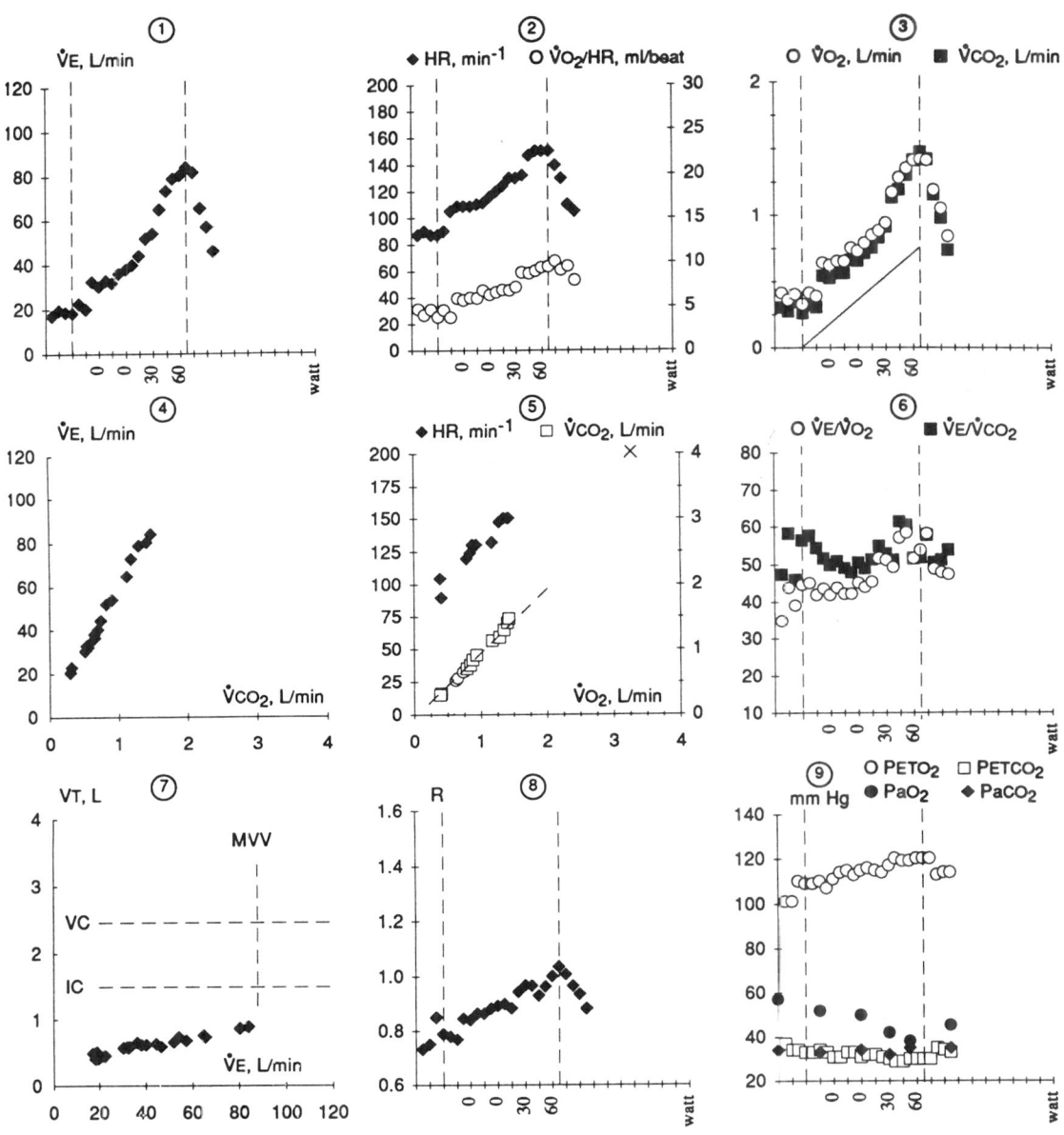

1. Vertical dashed lines in panels 1 to 3 and 6, 8, and 9 indicate the beginning and the end of increasing work period.
2. Unloaded cycling is performed for 3 minutes before the left vertical dashed line.
3. In panel 3, the diagonal line shows the increase of $\dot{V}O_2$ at a slope of 10 ml/min/w.
4. In panel 5, the diagonal dashed line has a slope of 1; the "x" in the upper right is the predicted maximum heart rate and $\dot{V}O_2$ for the subject.

TABLE 9.56.3. Air Breathing

Time min	Work rate watts	BP mmHg	HR min⁻¹	f min⁻¹	$\dot{V}E$ L/min BTPS	$\dot{V}CO_2$ L/min STPD	$\dot{V}O_2$ L/min STPD	$\dfrac{\dot{V}O_2}{HR}$ ml/beat	P	pH	HCO₃ meq/L	PO₂, mmHg ET	a	(A − a)	PCO₂, mmHg ET	a	(a − ET)	$\dfrac{\dot{V}E}{\dot{V}CO_2}$	$\dfrac{\dot{V}E}{\dot{V}O_2}$	$\dfrac{VD}{VT}$
	Rest	102/57								7.45	23	57			34					
	Rest		37	35	17.2	0.30	0.41	4.7	0.73			101			37			47	35	
	Rest		90	48	19.8	0.27	0.36	4.0	0.75			101			34			58	44	
	Rest		87	37	18.8	0.34	0.40	4.6	0.85			110			34			46	39	
	Rest		87	45	18.5	0.26	0.33	3.8	0.79			109			33			56	44	
0.5			90	50	22.7	0.32	0.41	4.6	0.78			109			33			58	45	
1.0		99/60	105	47	20.3	0.30	0.39	3.7	0.77	7.45	23	110	52	57	34	33	−1	54	42	0.42
1.5	Unloaded		109	57	32.7	0.54	0.64	5.9	0.84			107			33			52	44	
2.0	Unloaded		109	53	30.4	0.52	0.62	5.7	0.84			111			31			50	42	
2.5	Unloaded		109	57	33.3	0.56	0.65	6.0	0.86			114			31			51	44	
3.0	Unloaded		110	55	32.1	0.56	0.65	5.9	0.86			115			33			49	42	
3.5	Unloaded		111	56	36.4	0.66	0.75	6.8	0.88			113			33			48	42	
4.0	Unloaded	123/69	116	62	38.1	0.65	0.73	6.3	0.89	7.45	23	115	50	63	31	34	3	51	45	0.43
4.5	15		120	65	40.2	0.71	0.79	6.6	0.90			116			32			49	44	
5.0	15		124	70	44.4	0.75	0.85	6.9	0.88			115			32			51	45	
5.5	30		130	79	52.1	0.83	0.88	6.8	0.94			114			31			55	52	
6.0	30	126/72	130	73	54.2	0.91	0.94	7.2	0.97	7.46	22	117	42	75	30	32	2	53	51	0.43
6.5	45		132	85	64.9	1.13	1.17	8.9	0.97			120			29			51	49	
7.0	45		147	85	73.2	1.19	1.28	8.7	0.93			119			29			61	57	
7.5	60	144/72	150	93	78.8	1.30	1.35	9.0	0.96	7.43	23	119	38	76	30	35	5	60	58	0.59
8.0	60		150	93	80.4	1.41	1.41	9.4	1.00			120			30			51	51	
8.5	75		150	94	84.2	1.47	1.42	9.8	1.04			120			30			52	54	
	Recovery		140	92	81.8	1.42	1.41	10.1	1.01			120			30			57	58	
	Recovery		130	89	65.6	1.15	1.19	9.2	0.97			113			35			50	49	
	Recovery		110	84	57.3	0.98	1.05	9.5	0.93			114			34			51	48	
	Recovery	144/72	105	79	46.5	0.74	0.84	8.0	0.88	7.39	21	114	45	66	33	35	2	54	47	0.46

Interpretation

Comments

This case is presented to show the effects of O_2 breathing on work capacity in a patient with hypoxemia and restrictive lung disease and the differences between direct and indirect MVV measures in such patients. Resting respiratory function studies showed severe restrictive disease with low $D_{L}CO$, indicating loss of effective alveolar capillary bed, moderate hypoxemia, and mild hypocapnia

Analysis

Referring to flow chart 1, in the room air study the peak $\dot{V}O_2$ was low, but the anaerobic threshold was within normal limits (Table 9.56.2). This leads us to flow chart 3 and the category of lung disease through branchpoint 3.1 because of the borderline breathing reserve using the direct MVV. If we had used the indirect MVV, the breathing reserve would have been clearly low (abnormal). Confirmatory findings are high VD/VT, positive $P(a − ET)CO_2$, and wide $P(A − a)O_2$. Restrictive lung disease is further confirmed by the high breathing frequency of over 90 per minute (branchpoint 3.2). In the O_2 study, the patient exercised to a considerably higher work rate with a lower maximum $\dot{V}E$, confirming that the patient did indeed have ventilatory limitation during the room air study. The low O_2 pulse while the patient was breathing room air was due to the low arterial O_2 content (SaO_2 approximated 75% during late exercise) predominantly. This contributed to a reduced maximal arterio-venous O_2 content difference at maximal exercise. The patient developed a

FIGURE 9.56.2.   Oxygen breathing.

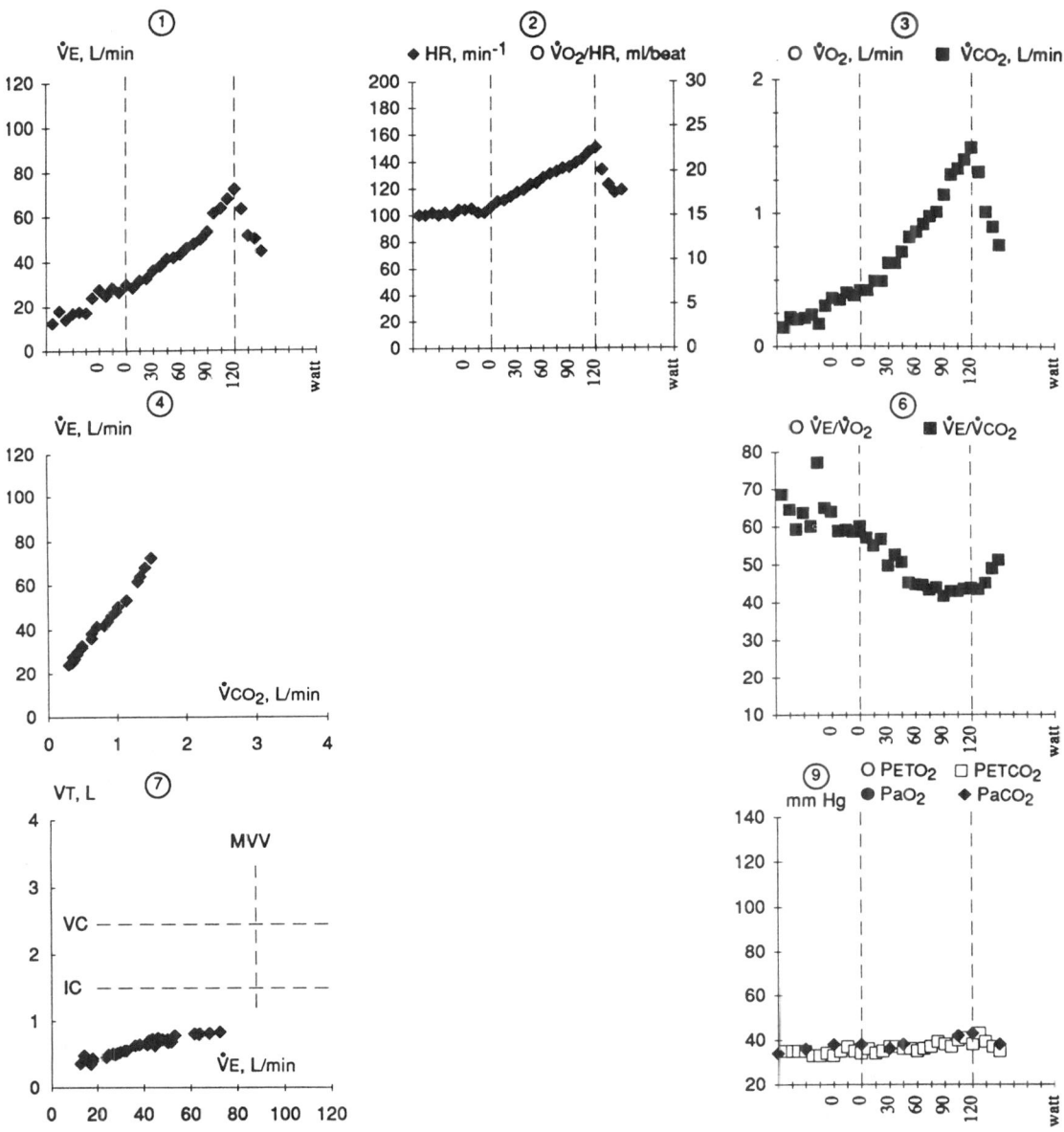

1. Vertical dashed lines in panels 1 to 3 and 6 and 9 indicate the beginning and the end of increasing work period.
2. Unloaded cycling is performed for 3 minutes before the left vertical dashed line.

TABLE 9.56.4.   Oxygen Breathing

Time min	Work rate watts	BP mmHg	HR min⁻¹	f min⁻¹	$\dot{V}_E$ L/min BTPS	$\dot{V}_{CO_2}$ L/min STPD	$\dot{V}_{O_2}$ L/min STPD	$\dot{V}_{O_2}$/HR ml/beat	R	pH	HCO_3^- meq/L	P_{O_2} ET	P_{O_2} a	P_{O_2} (A−a)	P_{CO_2} ET	P_{CO_2} a	P_{CO_2} (a−ET)	$\dot{V}_E/\dot{V}_{CO_2}$	$\dot{V}_E/\dot{V}_{O_2}$	V_D/V_T
	Rest	114/62								7.44	23	359				34				
	Rest		100	34	12.5	0.14									35				69	
	Rest		100	44	17.9	0.22									35				64	
	Rest		102	29	14.3	0.20									35				59	
	Rest	99/63	100	43	17.0	0.21				7.41	22	306	371		35	36	1		64	0.49
	Rest		102	40	17.8	0.24									33				60	
	Rest		100	48	17.2	0.17									33				77	
	Unloaded		104	52	23.9	0.30									34				65	
	Unloaded	102/63	104	56	27.7	0.36				7.40	23	221	454		33	38	5		64	0.53
	Unloaded		105	50	24.8	0.35									35				59	
	Unloaded		102	55	28.3	0.40									37				59	
	Unloaded		102	51	26.6	0.38									35				59	
	Unloaded	102/69	106	56	29.9	0.42				7.40	23	227	448		34	38	4		60	0.52
0.5	15		110	54	28.6	0.42									36				57	
1.0	15		111	56	31.7	0.49									34				55	
1.5	30		114	58	32.7	0.49									35				57	
2.0	30	102/60	117	57	36.1	0.63				7.39	21	189	488		37	36	−1		50	0.45
2.5	45		119	59	38.2	0.63									37				53	
3.0	45	108/60	123	64	41.4	0.71				7.39	23	183	512		36	38	2		51	0.48
3.5	60		124	59	42.0	0.82									36				45	
4.0	60		128	60	43.5	0.83									35				45	
4.5	75		131	62	46.2	0.92									36				44	
5.0	75		133	66	48.0	0.93									37				43	
5.5	90		135	69	50.1	1.01									39				44	
6.0	90		136	68	53.3	1.14									38				42	
6.5	105		139	76	61.8	1.29									37				43	
7.0	105	126/66	142	79	63.9	1.33				7.34	22	157	514		40	42	2		43	0.47
7.5	120		147	83	68.1	1.40									41				44	
8.0	120	132/72	150	87	72.5	1.49				7.32	22	164	506		38	43	5		44	0.49
	Recovery		134	80	63.6	1.31									43				43	
	Recovery		123	75	51.8	1.01									39				45	
	Recovery		117	74	50.3	0.90									37				49	
	Recovery	117/60	119	70	44.8	0.76				7.33	20	185	490		35	38	3		51	0.48

mild metabolic acidosis in both studies and some respiratory acidosis during O_2 breathing. The latter study demonstrates a large right to left shunt-like effect typical of this disorder (1).

Conclusion

This is a typical case of pulmonary alveolar proteinosis with restriction and severe gas exchange abnormalities. The patient was limited both by his ventilatory ability and by hypoxemia. Young patients with interstitial lung disease often develop strong ventilatory muscles that allow them to exercise at a higher rate than might otherwise be expected. The directly measured MVV, performed at a high breathing frequency, was 101 L/min, whereas the indirect MVV, calculated as 40 times the FEV_1 was 88 L/min. Bilateral lung lavage performed after this study was helpful in improving the patient's exercise tolerance.

Reference

1. Selecky PA, Wasserman K, Benfield JR, et al. The clinical and physiological effect of whole-lung lavage in pulmonary alveolar proteinosis: a ten-year experience. Ann Thorac Surg 1977;24:451-461.

Case 57 Alveolar Proteinosis: Pre- and Post-whole Lung Lavage

Clinical Findings

This 25-year-old graduate student was found to have alveolar proteinosis, proved by transbronchial lung biopsy, several years previously. He had had whole lung lavage twice previously, at yearly intervals, with improvement on both occasions. Despite the dyspnea associated with this illness, he was very physically active, running an average of 70 miles per week. He returned because of increasing dyspnea. Examination revealed a thin, muscular man who was not cyanotic. Chest roentgenograms showed bilateral infiltrates typical of alveolar proteinosis.

Exercise Findings

The patient performed exercise on a cycle ergometer with similar protocols before and shortly after separate lavages of the right and left lungs. He pedalled at 60 rpm without added load for 3 minutes. The work rate was then increased 25 or 30 W per minute to his symptom-limited maximum. Arterial blood was sampled every second minute, and intra-arterial blood pressure was recorded from a percutaneously placed brachial artery catheter. Resting 12-lead and exercise single-lead ECG were normal. On both tests, the patient stopped exercise because of leg fatigue.

TABLE 9.57.1. Selected Respiratory Function Data

Measurement	Predicted	Pre-lavage	Post-lavage
Age, yr		25	
Sex		Male	
Height, cm		165	
Weight, kg	70	52	
Hematocrit, %		48	47
VC, L	4.46	2.06	2.98
IC, L	2.98	1.36	1.60
TLC, L	5.93	3.28	4.10
FEV_1, L	3.63	1.67	2.44
FEV_1/VC, %	81	81	82
MVV, L/min	163	97	121
$D_{L}CO$, ml/mm Hg/min	29.5	20.0	28.7

TABLE 9.57.2. Selected Exercise Data

Measurement	Predicted	Pre-lavage	Post-lavage
Peak $\dot{V}O_2$, L/min	2.52	2.70	3.07
Maximum HR, beats/min	195	165	175
Maximum O_2 pulse, ml/beat	12.9	16.4	17.5
$\Delta\dot{V}O_2$/ΔWR, ml/min/W	10.3	9.2	9.1
AT, L/min	>1.02	2.1	2.1
Maximum $\dot{V}E$, L/min		125	133
Exercise breathing reserve, L/min	>15	−28	−12
PaO_2, mmHg (rest, max ex)		82, 53	93, 64
P(A − a)O_2, mmHg (rest, max ex)		16, 64	12, 55
P(a − ET)CO_2, mmHg (rest, max ex)		−1, 6	−1, −5
VD/VT (rest, heavy ex)		0.20, 0.36	0.25, 0.21
HCO_3^-, mEq/L (rest, heavy ex)		26, 21	24, 15

FIGURE 9.57.1.   Pre-whole lung lavage.

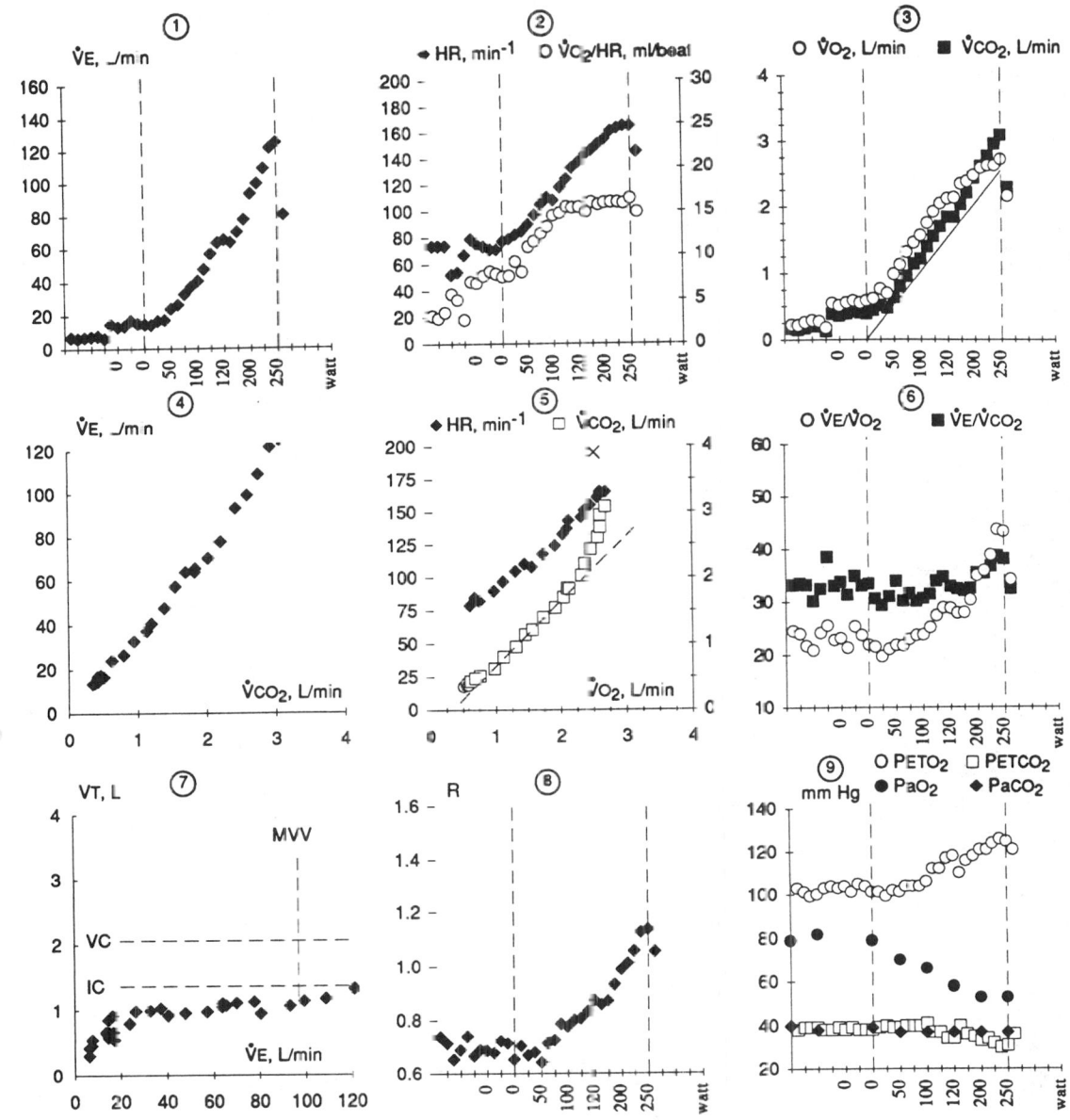

1. Vertical dashed lines in panels 1 to 3 and 6, 8, and 9 indicate the beginning and the end of increasing work period.
2. Unloaded cycling is performed for 3 minutes before the left vertical dashed line.
3. In panel 3, the diagonal line shows the increase of $\dot{V}O_2$ at a slope of 10 ml/min/w.
4. In panel 5, the diagonal dashed line has a slope of 1: the "x" in the upper right is the predicted maximum heart rate and $\dot{V}O_2$ for the subject.

TABLE 9.57.3. Pre-whole Lung Lavage

Time min	Work rate watts	BP mmHg	HR min⁻¹	f min⁻¹	V̇E L/min BTPS	V̇CO₂ L/min STPD	V̇O₂ L/min STPD	V̇O₂/HR ml/beat	R	pH	HCO₃⁻ meq/L	PO₂ mmHg ET	a	(A−a)	PCO₂ mmHg ET	a	(a−ET)	V̇E/V̇CO₂	V̇E/V̇O₂	VD/VT
	Rest									7.43	26	79			40					
	Rest		74	16	7.0	0.17	0.23	3.1	0.74			103			38			33	25	
	Rest		74	15	6.3	0.15	0.21	2.8	0.71			101			39			34	24	
	Rest		74	16	7.0	0.17	0.26	3.5	0.65			99			39			33	22	
	Rest		52	16	7.4	0.20	0.29	5.6	0.69	7.44	25	100	82	16	39	38	−1	30	21	0.20
	Rest		54	14	7.7	0.20	0.27	5.0	0.74			103			38			33	24	
	Rest		67	21	6.4	0.12	0.18	2.7	0.67			104			38			38	26	
	Unloaded		79	25	14.7	0.38	0.55	7.0	0.69			103			39			33	23	
	Unloaded		75	20	13.5	0.35	0.51	6.8	0.69			104			38			34	23	
	Unloaded		73	21	13.7	0.38	0.56	7.7	0.68			101			39			31	21	
	Unloaded		71	25	16.8	0.42	0.58	8.2	0.72			105			38			35	25	
	Unloaded		71	23	15.2	0.40	0.56	7.9	0.71			104			38			33	24	
	Unloaded		77	24	14.7	0.38	0.58	7.5	0.66	7.43	25	101	79	16	38	39	1	33	22	0.29
0.5	25		79	17	14.6	0.43	0.61	7.7	0.70			101			39			31	22	
1.0	25		82	18	16.5	0.51	0.76	9.3	0.67			99			40			29	20	
1.5	50		85	31	17.2	0.47	0.69	8.1	0.68			102			39			31	21	
2.0	50		90	30	23.9	0.63	0.98	10.9	0.64	7.43	24	101	70	27	39	37	−2	34	22	0.28
2.5	75		97	27	25.5	0.80	1.12	11.5	0.71			104			40			30	22	
3.0	75		105	33	32.8	0.95	1.31	12.5	0.73			104			40			32	23	
3.5	100		110	36	37.3	1.14	1.45	13.2	0.79			104			40			30	24	
4.0	100		108	44	40.7	1.21	1.56	14.4	0.78	7.44	25	106	66	39	41	37	−4	31	24	0.21
4.5	125		118	50	47.8	1.39	1.74	14.7	0.80			112			37			31	25	
5.0	125		124	59	57.4	1.55	1.92	15.5	0.81			112			37			34	27	
5.5	120		133	61	63.9	1.70	2.04	15.3	0.83			117			34			35	29	
6.0	120		137	61	65.6	1.84	2.11	15.4	0.87	7.43	24	118	58	51	34	37	3	33	29	0.27
6.5	175		143	58	64.1	1.83	2.13	14.9	0.86			110			40			32	28	
7.0	175		146	63	70.2	2.03	2.33	16.0	0.87			116			36			32	28	
7.5	200		151	69	77.8	2.21	2.37	15.7	0.93			118			35			33	30	
8.0	200		155	87	93.3	2.43	2.46	15.9	0.99	7.41	23	121	53	60	33	37	4	35	35	0.31
8.5	225		161	87	99.4	2.60	2.57	16.0	1.01			121			34			35	36	
9.0	225		163	93	108.9	2.76	2.61	16.0	1.06			124			32			37	39	
9.5	250		165	92	121.4	2.94	2.61	15.8	1.13			126			30			39	44	
10.0	250		165	96	124.9	3.07	2.70	16.4	1.14	7.36	21	125	53	64	31	37	6	38	43	0.36
	Recovery	145	85		80.6	2.27	2.15	14.8	1.06			121			36			32	34	

Interpretation
Comments

Respiratory function studies indicate moderately severe restrictive lung disease that improves after lung lavage (Table 9.57.1). The resting ECG is normal. The post-lavage exercise study was done 7 days after completion of whole lung lavage and 11 days after the pre-lavage study.

Analysis

Referring to flow chart 1, because this patient is so exceptionally well trained, his peak V̇O₂ and anaerobic threshold are substantially greater than predicted. Nevertheless, the rate of rise in V̇O₂ decreases above the anaerobic threshold before lavage (panel 3, Fig. 9.57.1). The peak V̇O₂, even before lavage, is significantly above predicted (Table 9.57.2). See flow chart 2: The O₂ pulse is supra-normal and his ECG is normal at peak V̇O₂. His blood gases, however, while normal at rest, become abnormal during exercise, with PaO₂ progressively decreasing and P(A − a)O₂ progressively increasing with work rate (Table 9.57.3) (branchpoint 2.1). The VD/VT is abnormal (branchpoint 2.3). At the maximum work rate performed, the patient has a marked tachypnea (Table 9.57.3). The tidal volume remains constant at the level of the inspiratory capacity from a relatively light work rate to the maximum (panel 7, Fig. 9.57.1), with the increase in minute ventilation achieved, almost solely, by increasing breathing frequency. This exercise response is consistent with

FIGURE 9.57.2.   Post-whole lung lavage.

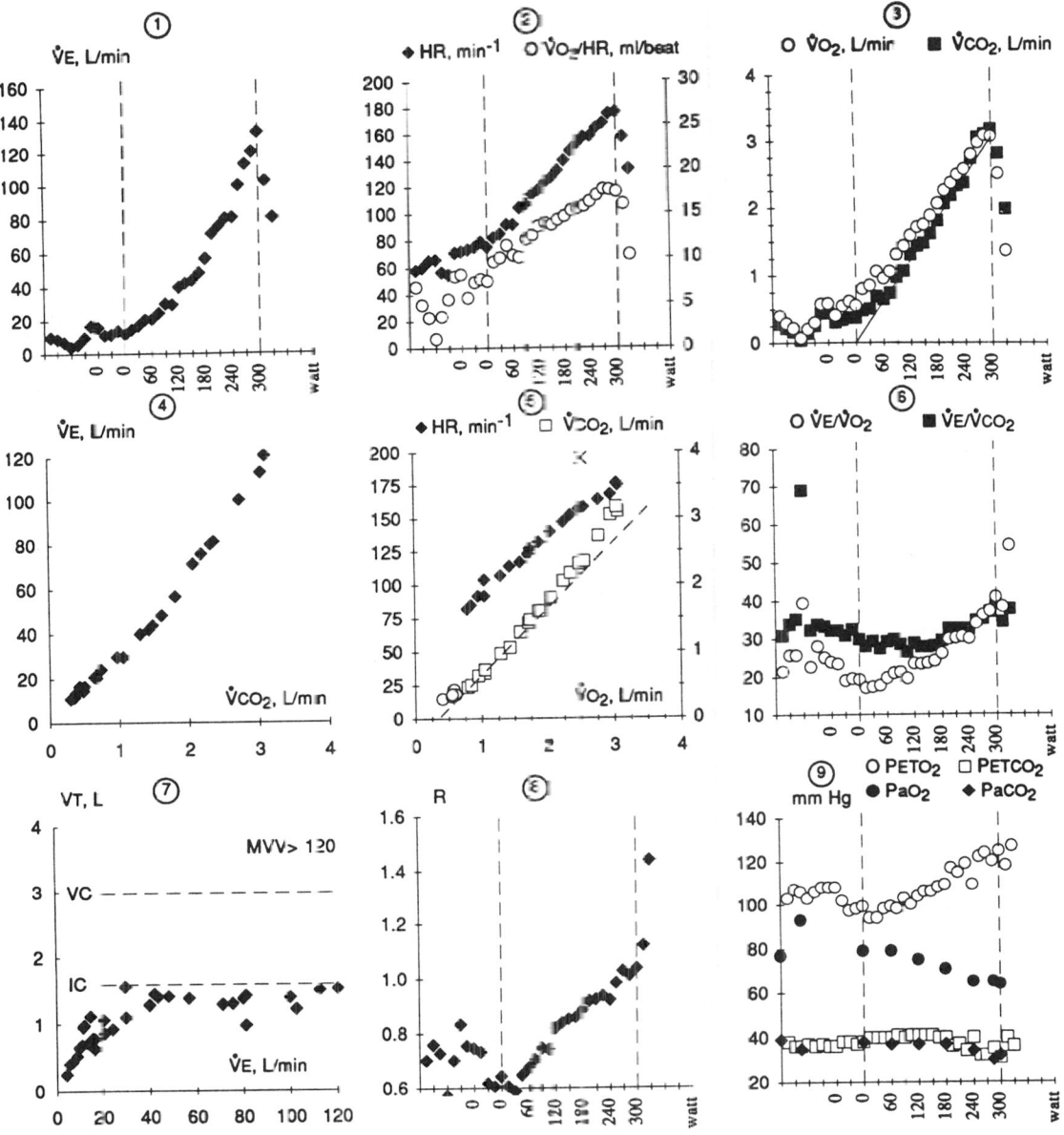

1. Vertical dashed lines in panes 1 to 3 and 6, 8, and 9 indicate the beginning and the end of increasing work period.
2. Unloaded cycling is performed for 3 minutes before the left vertical dashed line.
3. In panel 3, the diagonal line shows the increase of $\dot{V}O_2$ at a slope of 10 ml/min/w.
4. In panel 5, the diagonal dashed line has a slope of 1; the "x" in the upper right is the predicted maximum heart rate and $\dot{V}O_2$ for the subject.

TABLE 9.57.4. Post-whole Lung Lavage

Time min	Work rate watts	BP mmHg	HR min⁻¹	f min⁻¹	$\dot{V}E$ L/min BTPS	$\dot{V}CO_2$ L/min STPD	$\dot{V}O_2$ L/min STPD	$\dot{V}O_2$/HR ml/beat	R	pH	HCO₃⁻ meq/L	PO₂, mmHg ET	a	(A−a)	PCO₂, mmHg ET	a	(a−ET)	$\dot{V}E$/$\dot{V}CO_2$	$\dot{V}E$/$\dot{V}O_2$	VD/VT
	Rest									7.40	24		77			39				
	Rest		58	15	9.9	0.28	0.40	6.9	0.70			103			38			31	22	
	Rest		60	17	8.9	0.22	0.29	4.8	0.76			107			36			34	26	
	Rest		65	16	7.0	0.16	0.22	3.4	0.73	7.43	23	106	93	12	36	35	−1	35	26	0.24
	Rest		66	17	4.2	0.04	0.07	1.1	0.57			103			37			69	39	
	Rest		57	14	5.7	0.14	0.20	3.5	0.70			106			36			32	23	
	Rest		55	15	9.7	0.25	0.30	5.5	0.83			108			37			34	28	
	Unloaded		71	26	16.5	0.43	0.57	8.0	0.75			108			36			33	25	
	Unloaded		72	20	15.8	0.44	0.59	8.2	0.75			108			36			32	24	
	Unloaded		73	16	11.0	0.30	0.41	5.6	0.73			102			38			32	24	
	Unloaded		75	12	11.5	0.34	0.55	7.3	0.62			97			38			31	19	
	Unloaded		79	19	13.6	0.37	0.61	7.7	0.61			98			37			32	20	
	Unloaded		75	12	11.8	0.36	0.56	7.5	0.64	7.41	24	99	79	16	38	38	0	30	19	0.22
0.5	30		82	13	14.6	0.48	0.79	9.6	0.61			94			40			28	17	
1.0	30		85	21	16.5	0.50	0.85	10.0	0.59			94			40			29	17	
1.5	60		92	19	20.3	0.68	1.05	11.4	0.65			98			40			27	18	
2.0	60		92	24	20.8	0.64	0.95	10.3	0.67	7.41	23	99	79	20	40	37	−3	29	20	0.18
2.5	90		104	26	24.2	0.74	1.05	10.1	0.70			98			41			30	21	
3.0	90		107	27	29.8	0.97	1.30	12.1	0.75			103			40			28	21	
3.5	120		114	19	29.7	1.06	1.43	12.5	0.74			100			41			26	20	
4.0	120		117	31	40.0	1.30	1.59	13.6	0.82	7.40	23	104	75	31	41	37	−4	29	24	0.18
4.5	150		123	29	42.1	1.43	1.71	13.9	0.84			106			41			28	23	
5.0	150		127	31	43.7	1.48	1.74	13.7	0.85			106			41			28	24	
5.5	180		132	34	48.2	1.61	1.88	14.2	0.86			108			40			28	24	
6.0	180		140	41	56.8	1.81	2.05	14.6	0.88	7.40	23	109	71	38	40	37	−3	29	26	0.20
6.5	210		147	55	71.4	2.06	2.25	15.3	0.92			117			36			32	30	
7.0	210		152	58	75.8	2.18	2.36	15.5	0.92			115			37			33	30	
7.5	240		157	58	80.2	2.32	2.48	15.8	0.94			119			34			32	30	
8.0	240		158	57	81.3	2.36	2.56	16.2	0.92	7.40	21	109	65	49	40	34	−6	32	30	0.20
8.5	270		164	72	100.3	2.73	2.78	17.0	0.98			122			32			34	34	
9.0	270		168	75	113.0	3.04	2.96	17.6	1.03			124			32			35	36	
9.5	300		175	79	120.7	3.10	3.07	17.5	1.01	7.35	16	120	65	55	35	30	−5	37	37	0.21
10.0	300		176	96	132.8	3.17	3.06	17.4	1.04	7.30	15	125	64	55	31	32	1	39	41	0.29
	Recovery		157	84	102.9	2.80	2.50	15.9	1.12			118			40			34	38	
	Recovery		133	83	81.2	1.97	1.37	10.3	1.44			127			36			38	54	

restrictive lung disease, despite a supra-normal peak $\dot{V}O_2$.

Although the patient exceeds the predicted peak $\dot{V}O_2$ for sedentary males of his size, he clearly has physiologic abnormalities that limit his exercise performance, as evidenced by his improved exercise performance following bilateral whole lung lavage (Table 9.57.2, and contrasting data in Tables 9.57.3 and 9.57.4). Because of the mechanical limitation to lung expansion imposed by the alveolar filling disorder, and perhaps some pulmonary fibrosis, the patient must increase minute ventilation during exercise primarily by increasing breathing rate. The minute ventilation at maximum exercise exceeds his MVV (negative breathing reserve), reflecting his

high motivation and possibly some exercise bronchodilatation. In the second study the ventilatory pattern of restrictive disease persists but is more mild. The degree of arterial hypoxemia and the increase in P(A − a)O₂ are also considerably reduced following whole lung lavage (compare Table 9.57.3 with Table 9.57.4), whereas the upper portion of the $\dot{V}CO_2$ versus $\dot{V}O_2$ plot is shallower and O₂ pulse is increased at higher work rates (compare panels 5 and 2 of Figs. 9.57.1 and 9.57.2).

Conclusion

The patient has restrictive lung disease that improved following therapy.

Case 58 Pulmonary Microlithiasis: Air and Oxygen Breathing

Clinical Findings

This 63-year-old Iranian man had previously been diagnosed by lung biopsy as having pulmonary microlithiasis. He had never smoked. He had had slowly progressive dyspnea over 30 years until he was limited to walking a few steps. He occasionally had hemoptysis. He had been treated with corticosteroids and bronchodilators without apparent benefit. Exercise testing was requested to obtain optimal assessment of his cardiorespiratory function prior to possible therapeutic intervention. Resting ECG showed nonspecific ST-T wave changes.

Exercise Findings

Exercise tests recorded while the patient was breathing room air and then 100% O_2 were performed on the same day on a cycle ergometer with an intermediate rest period. On both occasions, arterial blood was sampled every second minute, and intra-arterial pressure was recorded from a percutaneously placed brachial artery catheter. The patient pedalled at 60 rpm without an added load for 3 minutes. The work rate was then increased 5 W per minute to tolerance. The patient was well motivated and cooperative and stopped exercise on both occasions because of dyspnea. No further ECG abnormalities were noted during or after exercise.

TABLE 9.58.1.   Selected Respiratory Function Data

Measurement	Predicted	Measured
Age, yr		63
Sex		Male
Height, cm		164
Weight, kg	69	55
Hematocrit, %		51
VC, L	3.36	1.37
IC, L	2.24	0.73
TLC, L	5.28	2.70
FEV_1, L	2.61	1.31
FEV_1/VC, %	78	92
MVV, L/min		
Direct	117	62
Indirect	104	52
$D_{L}CO$, ml/mm Hg/min	23.9	6.0

TABLE 9.58.2.   Selected Exercise Data

Measurement	Predicted	Room air	Oxygen
Peak $\dot{V}O_2$, L/min	1.69	0.60	
Maximum HR, beats/min	151	110	138
Maximum O_2 pulse, ml/beat	11.2	5.6	
$\Delta\dot{V}O_2/\Delta WR$, ml/min/W	10.3	10.3	
AT, L/min	>0.75	<0.55	
Work rate, max, W		15	40
Blood pressure, mmHg (rest, max ex)		147/84, 136/87	135/81, 153/99
Maximum $\dot{V}E$, L/min		63	54
Exercise breathing reserve, L/min			
Using direct MVV	>15	−1	8
Using indirect MVV	>15	−11	−2
PaO_2, mmHg (rest, max ex)		40, 34	364, 344
$P(A − a)O_2$ mmHg (rest, max ex)		48, 88	292, 304
$P(a − ET)CO_2$, mmHg (rest, max ex)		16, 17	21, 22
VD/VT (rest, max ex)		0.65, 0.64	0.68, 0.71
HCO_3^-, mEq/L (rest, recov)		31, 27	29, 28

FIGURE 9.58.1.   Air breathing.

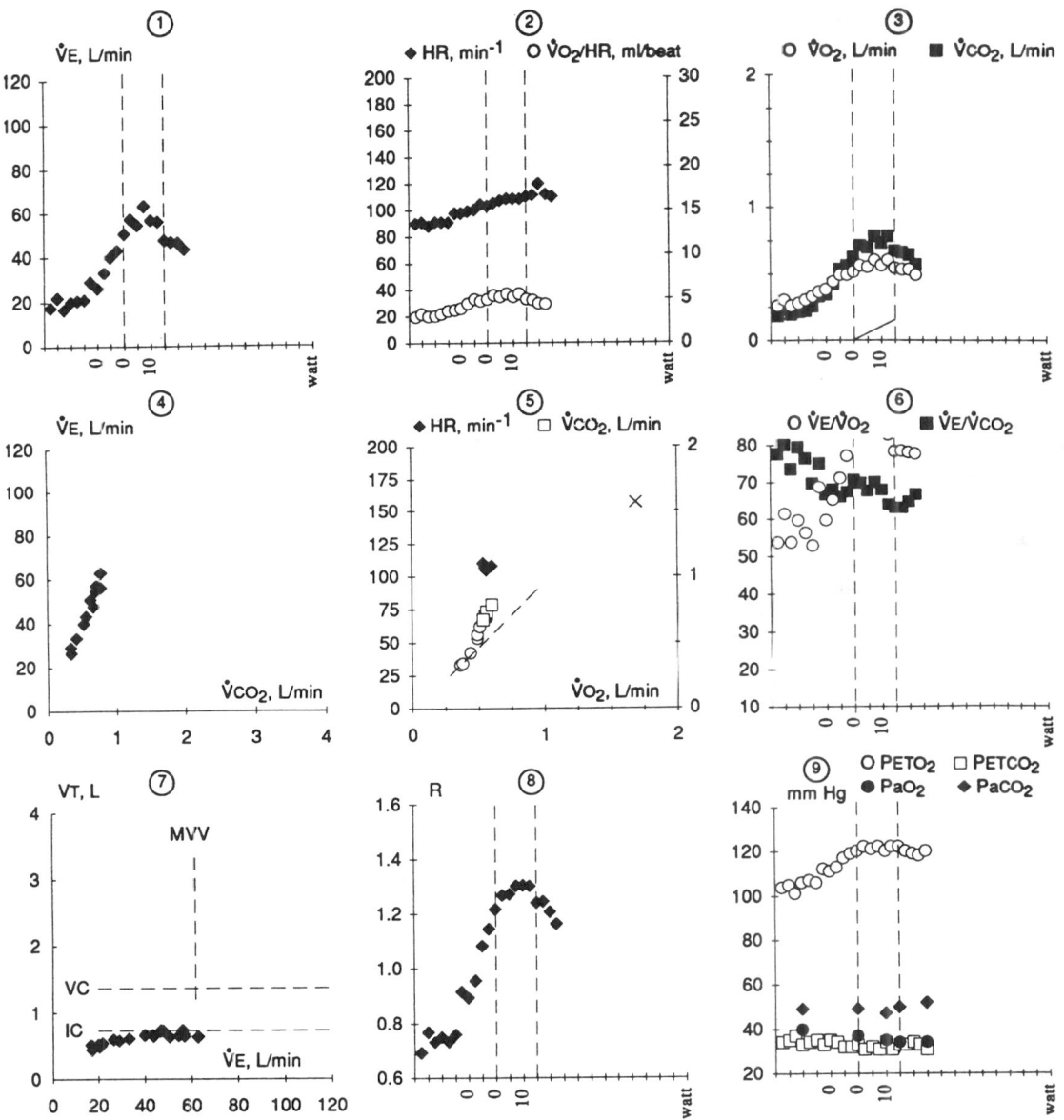

1. Vertical dashed lines in panels 1 to 3 and 6, 8, and 9 indicate the beginning and the end of increasing work period.
2. Unloaded cycling is performed for 3 minutes before the left vertical dashed line.
3. In panel 3, the diagonal line shows the increase of $\dot{V}O_2$ at a slope of 10 ml/min/w.
4. In panel 5, the diagonal dashed line has a slope of 1; the "x" in the upper right is the predicted maximum heart rate and $\dot{V}O_2$ for the subject.

TABLE 9.58.3. Air Breathing

Time min	Work rate watts	BP mmHg	HR min⁻¹	f min⁻¹	V̇E L/min BTPS	V̇CO₂ L/min STPD	V̇O₂ L/min STPD	V̇O₂/HR ml/beat	R	pH	HCO₃⁻ meq/L	PO₂, mmHg ET	a	(A − a)	PCO₂, mmHg ET	a	(a − ET)	V̇E/V̇CO₂	V̇E/V̇O₂	VD/VT
	Rest	147/84	90	39	17.3	0.15	0.26	2.9	0.69			104			34			78	54	
	Rest		91	40	21.8	0.25	0.30	3.3	0.77			105			35			80	61	
	Rest		88	32	16.7	0.15	0.26	3.0	0.73			101			37			74	54	
	Rest	147/84	91	33	19.9	0.21	0.28	3.1	0.75	7.41	31	106	40	48	33	49	16	79	60	0.65
	Rest		91	42	20.4	0.22	0.30	3.3	0.73			107			34			77	56	
	Rest		91	42	21.0	0.25	0.33	3.6	0.76			106			35			70	53	
	Unloaded		98	50	29.0	0.33	0.36	3.7	0.92			112			33			75	69	
	Unloaded		98	44	26.4	0.34	0.38	3.9	0.89			111			35			67	60	
	Unloaded		99	55	33.3	0.42	0.44	4.4	0.95			113			34			68	65	
	Unloaded		100	61	40.1	0.53	0.49	4.9	1.08			117			32			66	71	
	Unloaded		104	65	43.3	0.56	0.49	4.7	1.14			119			32			67	77	
	Unloaded	174/84	103	80	50.6	0.62	0.51	5.0	1.22	7.40	30	120	37	71	33	49	16	71	86	0.65
0.5	5		105	89	57.1	0.71	0.56	5.3	1.27			122			31			70	88	
1.0	5		107	84	54.5	0.70	0.55	5.1	1.27			121			32			68	86	
1.5	10		108	99	63.0	0.78	0.60	5.6	1.30			122			31			70	91	
2.0	10	186/90	108	83	56.7	0.73	0.56	5.2	1.30	7.39	28	120	35	77	34	47	13	68	89	0.64
2.5	15		108	77	56.2	0.78	0.60	5.6	1.30			122			31			64	83	
3.0	15	186/87	110	66	47.8	0.67	0.54	4.9	1.24	7.36	28	122	34	74	33	50	17	63	78	0.64
	Recovery		111	64	47.0	0.66	0.53	4.8	1.25			120			33			63	78	
	Recovery		120	65	46.8	0.64	0.53	4.4	1.21			119			34			64	78	
	Recovery		112	68	43.8	0.57	0.49	4.4	1.16			118			33			67	78	
	Recovery		110								7.33	27	120	34		31	52	21			

Interpretation

Comments

This case shows the effects of oxygen breathing on exercise capacity and blood gases in a patient severely disabled with interstitial lung disease. Resting respiratory function studies showed severe restrictive disease with low $D_{L}CO$, severe hypoxemia, and moderate hypercapnia.

Analysis

Referring to flow chart 1, in the room air study the peak V̇O₂ and the anaerobic threshold were reduced (Table 9.58.2). This leads us through branchpoints 1.1, 1.2, and 1.3 to flow chart 4. We arrive at the diagnosis of "lung disease with impaired peripheral oxygenation" through branchpoint 4.1 (low breathing reserve) and branchpoint 4.2 (high VD/VT). The patient filled all the requirements in both this box and the "abnormal pulmonary circulation" box. With O₂ breathing, a large shunt was not found. The high breathing frequency, negative value for breathing reserve, and high tidal volume to inspira-

tory capacity ratio all indicate severe ventilatory limitation. The gas exchange abnormalities (hypoxemia, positive P(a − ET)CO₂, and high VD/VT) were striking and reflect lung units with abnormally high and abnormally low ventilation-perfusion ratios. With O₂ breathing, exercise capacity was significantly increased, as arterial O₂ saturation and content increased. As a consequence of carotid body suppression with O₂, the ventilatory response was decreased compared to air breathing, and a more severe respiratory acidosis developed. In addition, note the extremely low O₂ pulse while the patient was breathing air. Arterial O₂ capacity was 21.3 ml/100 ml, and air breathing O₂ content was approximately 15 ml/100 ml. Thus, a major part of the reduction in O₂ pulse is due to arterial hypoxemia, with some reduction likely due to a low stroke volume.

Conclusion

This patient demonstrates the gas exchange and ventilatory defects of severe interstitial lung disease and demonstrates the improvement in exercise tolerance from O₂ supplementation.

FIGURE 9.58.2.   Oxygen breathing.

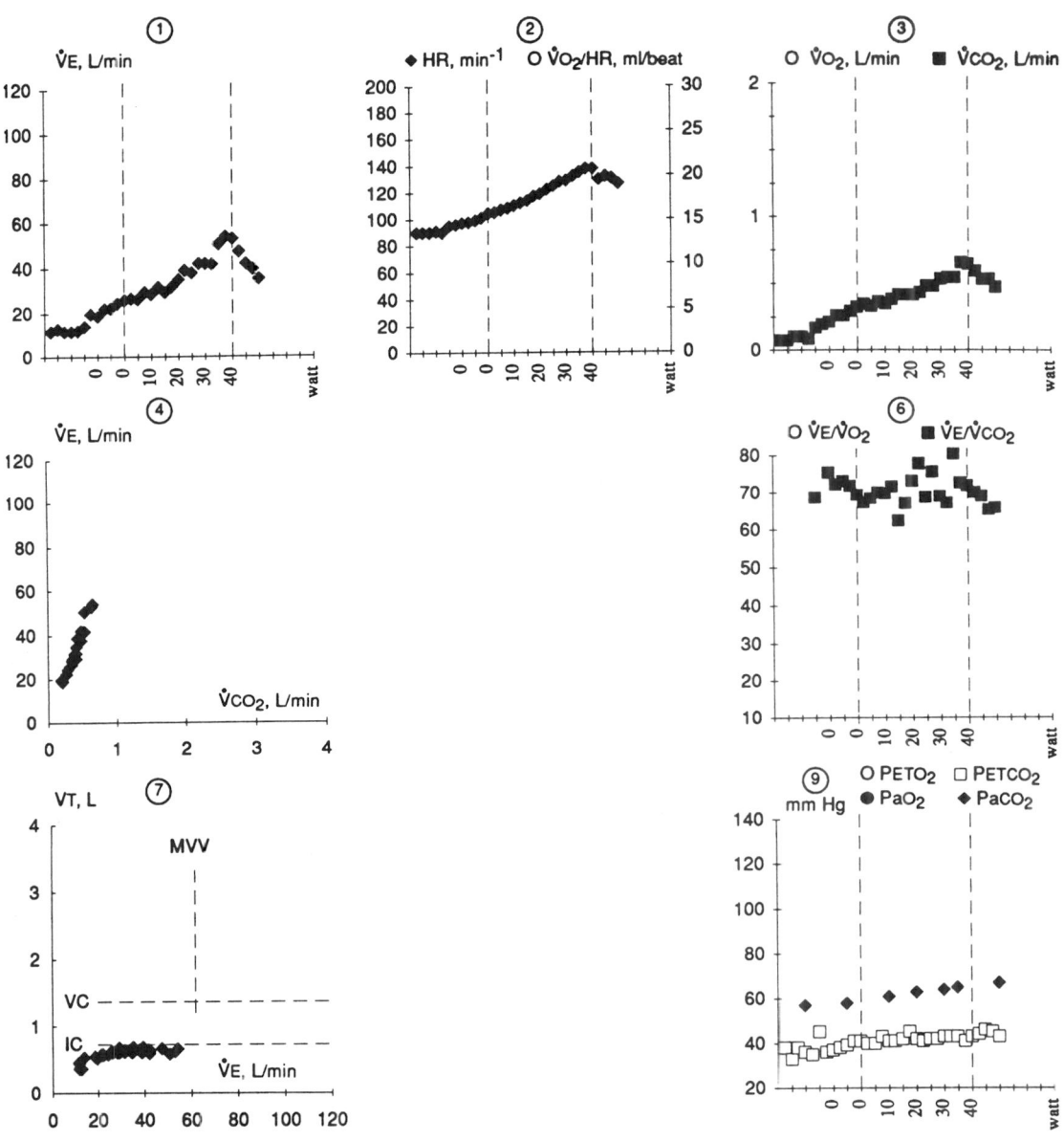

1. Vertical dashed lines in panels 1 to 3 and 6 and 9 indicate the beginning and the end of increasing work period.
2. Unloaded cycling is performed for 3 minutes before the left vertical dashed line.

TABLE 9.58.4. Oxygen Breathing

Time min	Work rate watts	BP mmHg	HR min⁻¹	f min⁻¹	$\dot{V}_E$ L/min BTPS	$\dot{V}_{CO_2}$ L/min STPD	$\dot{V}_{O_2}$ L/min STPD	$\dfrac{\dot{V}_{O_2}}{HR}$ ml/beat	R	pH	HCO₃ meq/L	P_{O_2}, mmHg ET	a	(A − a)	F_{CO_2}, mmHg ET	a	(a − ET)	$\dfrac{\dot{V}_E}{\dot{V}_{CO_2}}$	$\dfrac{\dot{V}_E}{\dot{V}_{O_2}}$	$\dfrac{V_D}{V_T}$
	Rest	120/78	90	31	11.6	0.07									38			128		
	Rest		90	35	12.8	0.07									33			140		
	Rest		90	25	11.5	0.10									38			94		
	Rest	135/81	91	26	11.6	0.10				7.32	29		364	292	36	57	21	94		0.68
	Rest		90	31	12.1	0.08									35			118		
	Rest		95	26	13.9	0.17									45			69		
	Unloaded		96	37	19.6	0.19									36			87		
	Unloaded		97	34	18.7	0.21									37			75		
	Unloaded		98	37	21.9	0.26									38			72		
	Unloaded	147/90	99	39	22.3	0.26				7.32	29		437	218	39	58	19	73		0.68
	Unloaded		101	42	24.4	0.29									41			72		
	Unloaded		104	41	25.7	0.32									41			69		
0.5	5		105	43	26.5	0.34									40			67		
1.0	5		107	43	26.2	0.33									40			68		
1.5	10		108	48	29.3	0.36									43			70		
2.0	10	147/90	110	47	28.4	0.35				7.29	29		423	229	41	61	20	70		0.68
2.5	15		112	51	31.5	0.38									41			71		
3.0	15		114	43	29.2	0.41									42			62		
3.5	20		117	49	31.6	0.41									45			67		
4.0	20	141/84	119	57	34.8	0.41				7.28	29		337	263	42	63	21	73		0.70
4.5	25		122	64	38.9	0.43									41			78		
5.0	25		125	58	37.9	0.48									42			69		
5.5	30		128	70	42.2	0.48									42			76		
6.0	30	153/99	129	66	42.1	0.53				7.26	28		361	288	43	64	21	69		0.70
6.5	35		132	64	41.7	0.54									43			67		
7.0	35		135	86	50.7	0.54				7.25	28		344	304	43	65	22	80		0.71
7.5	40		138	81	54.1	0.65									41			73		
8.0	40		138	84	53.1	0.64									43			72		
	Recovery		130	70	47.3	0.59									44			70		
	Recovery		132	65	42.0	0.53									46			69		
	Recovery		131	57	39.4	0.53									45			65		
	Recovery	151/102	127	51	35.2	0.47				7.23	28		380	266	43	67	24	66		0.70

Case 59 Pulmonary Vascular Disease, Thromboembolic

Clinical Findings

This 50-year-old shipyard worker had felt well until one year prior to evaluation when he noted the insidious but progressive development of dyspnea and easy fatigability. Six months later, he had had the abrupt onset of severe substernal chest pain and dyspnea, which resulted in hospitalization and treatment for a suspected myocardial infarction. Following discharge from the hospital, he had lost 25 to 30 pounds by watching his diet but remained somewhat dyspneic. There was no personal or family history of hypertension or diabetes mellitus. He had smoked 3 to 4 cigarettes daily until 2 years earlier. Physical examination was normal. Chest roentgenograms showed minimal pleural thickening bilaterally. Resting ECG showed normal QRS complexes and negative T waves in V1 to V3, suggesting right ventricular strain.

Exercise Findings

The patient performed exercise on a cycle ergometer. He pedalled at 60 rpm without added load for 3 minutes. The work rate was then increased 15 W per minute. Arterial blood was sampled every second minute, and intra-arterial blood pressure was recorded from a percutaneously placed brachial artery catheter. At 105 W work rate the pedal came off the cycle ergometer. After 30 minutes rest, the study was restarted with an increase of 20 W every minute. The patient stopped exercise because of overall fatigue and exhaustion; he denied having chest pain or dyspnea. There was a 0.5-mm ST segment depression in leads II, V5, and V6 that disappeared at 3 minutes of recovery.

TABLE 9.59.1. Selected Respiratory Function Data

Measurement	Predicted	Measured
Age, yr		50
Sex		Male
Height, cm		185
Weight, kg	86	92
Hematocrit, %		46
VC, L	5.10	4.68
IC, L	3.40	2.94
TLC, L	7.45	5.94
FEV_1, L	4.06	3.62
FEV_1/VC, %	80	77
MVV, L/min	161	152
$D_{L}CO$, ml/mm Hg/min	32.3	21.2

TABLE 9.59.2. Selected Exercise Data

Measurement	Predicted	Measured
Peak $\dot{V}O_2$, L/min	2.78	1.92
Maximum HR, beats/min	170	164
Maximum O_2 pulse, ml/beat	16.4	11.7
$\Delta\dot{V}O_2$/ΔWR, ml/min/W	10.3	8.9
AT, L/min	>1.25	1.25
Blood pressure, mmHg (rest, max)		125/80, 161/92
Maximum $\dot{V}E$, L/min		104
Exercise breathing reserve, L/min	>15	48
PaO_2, mmHg (rest, max ex)		83, 56
$P(A - a)O_2$, mmHg (rest, max ex)		26, 63
$P(a - ET)CO_2$, mmHg (rest, max ex)		5, 9
VD/VT (rest, heavy ex)		0.40, 0.45
HCO_3^-, mEq/L (rest, 2-min recov)		22, 19

FIGURE 9.59.1.

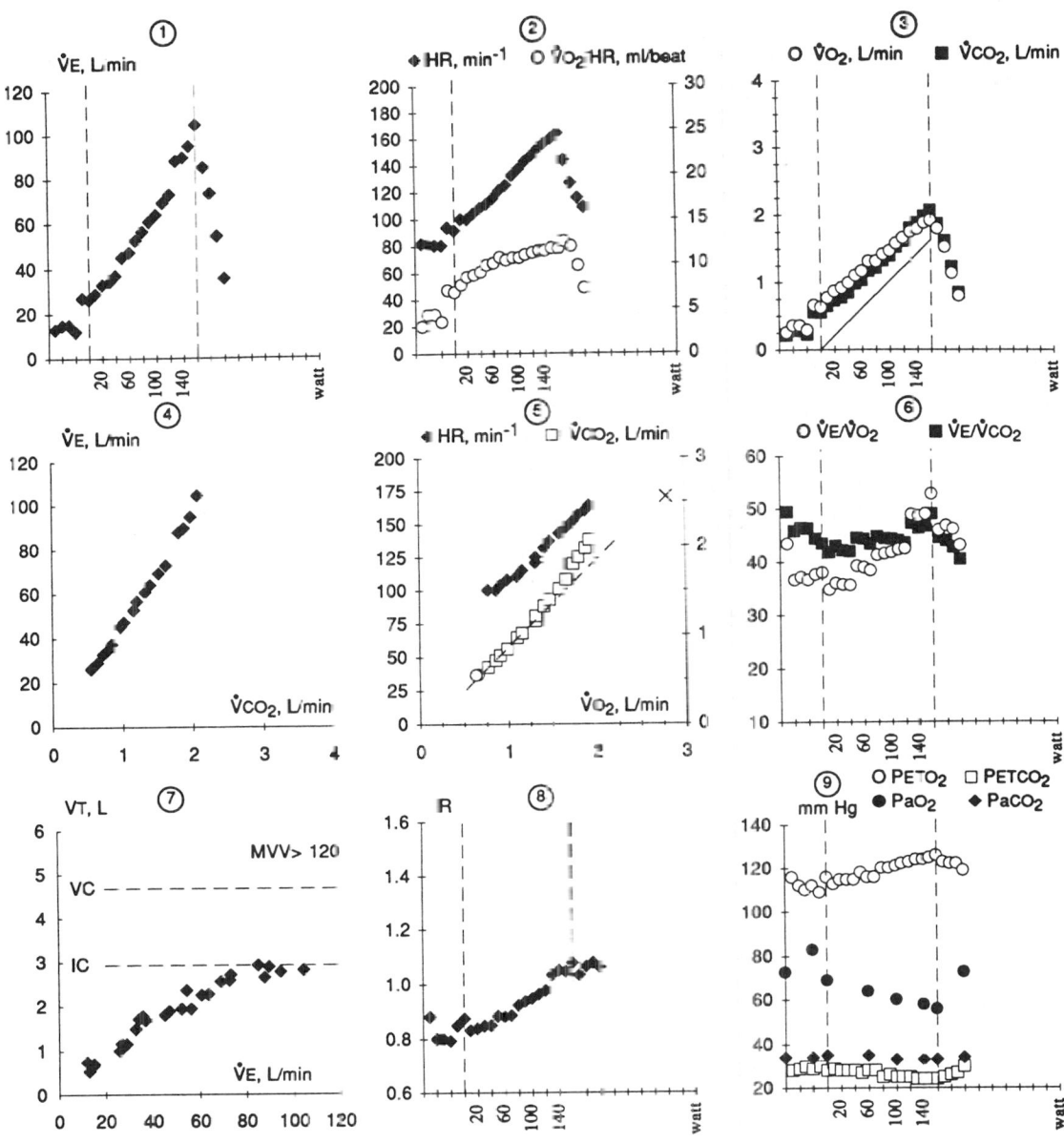

1. Vertical dashed lines in panels 1 to 3 and 6, 8, and 9 indicate the beginning and the end of increasing work period.
2. Unloaded cycling is performed for 3 minutes before the left vertical dashed line.
3. In panel 3, the diagonal line shows the increase of $\dot{V}_{O_2}$ at a slope of 10 ml/min/w.
4. In panel 5, the diagonal dashed line has a slope of 1; the "×" in the upper right is the predicted maximum heart rate and $\dot{V}_{O_2}$ for the subject.

Interpretation

Comments

This case is presented because it illustrates the use of exercise testing for detecting significant pulmonary vascular disease and correcting an erroneous diagnosis. The patient's physician assumed that symptoms of chest pain, dyspnea, and easy fatigability had been due to a myocardial infarction. That diagnosis could not be supported by myocardial enzyme concentrations or specific ECG changes. Radionuclide ventilation-perfusion scans, ordered because of the exercise study, confirmed the presence of

TABLE 9.59.3. Air Breathing

Time min	Work rate watts	BP mmHg	HR min⁻¹	f min⁻¹	$\dot{V}_E$ L/min BTPS	$\dot{V}_{CO_2}$ L/min STPD	$\dot{V}_{O_2}$ L/min STPD	$\dot{V}_{O_2}$/HR ml/beat	R	pH	HCO₃⁻ meq/L	Po₂, mmHg ET	a	(A − a)	Pco₂, mmHg ET	a	(a − ET)	$\dot{V}_E$/$\dot{V}_{CO_2}$	$\dot{V}_E$/$\dot{V}_{O_2}$	VD/VT
	Rest	125/80								7.41	21	116	73		28	34				
	Rest		82	24	12.9	0.22	0.25	3.0	0.88			116			28			49	43	
	Rest		82	22	14.7	0.28	0.35	4.3	0.80			112			29			46	37	
	Rest		81	21	14.8	0.28	0.35	4.3	0.80			110			30			46	37	
	Rest	119/83	81	16	12.0	0.23	0.29	3.6	0.79	7.42	22	112	83	26	29	34	5	46	37	0.40
	Unloaded		94	23	26.8	0.56	0.66	7.0	0.85			109			30			44	38	
	Unloaded	140/86	92	26	26.1	0.55	0.63	6.8	0.87	7.42	22	116	69	42	28	35	7	43	38	0.40
0.5	20		100	25	28.9	0.64	0.77	7.7	0.83			113			29			42	35	
1.0	20		100	22	32.8	0.72	0.86	8.6	0.84			115			28			43	36	
1.5	40		104	20	34.2	0.77	0.91	8.8	0.85			115			28			42	36	
2.0	40		108	22	37.1	0.84	0.99	9.2	0.85			115			28			42	36	
2.5	60		111	25	45.2	0.97	1.10	9.9	0.88			118			27			44	39	
3.0	60	146/86	115	25	47.2	1.02	1.16	10.1	0.88	7.42	22	116	64	47	28	35	7	44	39	0.42
3.5	80		121	27	52.5	1.16	1.31	10.8	0.89			116			28			43	38	
4.0	80		125	29	56.5	1.21	1.31	10.5	0.92			120			25			45	41	
4.5	100		132	27	60.8	1.32	1.41	10.7	0.94			120			26			44	41	
5.0	100	155/89	137	28	63.9	1.39	1.47	10.7	0.95	7.43	22	121	60	55	25	33	8	44	42	0.39
5.5	120		143	27	69.1	1.52	1.58	11.0	0.96			122			25			44	42	
6.0	120		147	28	72.8	1.62	1.66	11.3	0.98			123			25			43	42	
6.5	140		152	33	87.8	1.80	1.74	11.4	1.03			124			24			47	49	
7.0	140	161/92	156	31	89.7	1.88	1.79	11.5	1.05	7.40	20	124	58	60	24	33	9	46	49	0.42
7.5	160		160	34	94.8	1.97	1.88	11.8	1.05			125			24			47	49	
8.0	160	155/86	164	37	104.5	2.07	1.92	11.7	1.08	7.40	20	126	56	63	24	33	9	49	53	0.45
	Recovery		144	29	85.2	1.86	1.80	12.5	1.03			123			25			44	46	
	Recovery		127	27	73.4	1.62	1.52	12.0	1.07			122			26			44	47	
	Recovery		116	23	54.5	1.23	1.14	9.8	1.08			122			27			43	46	
	Recovery	152/86	109	20	35.7	0.84	0.79	7.2	1.06	7.37	19	119	73	45	30	34	4	40	43	0.36

many perfusion without ventilation defects, characteristic of pulmonary thromboembolic disease.

The results of the resting respiratory function studies indicate that this patient had normal lung mechanics. He had a significant reduction in diffusing capacity, however (Table 59.1). The ECG was suggestive of right ventricular strain.

Analysis

Referring to flow chart 1, the peak $\dot{V}_{O_2}$ is reduced while the anaerobic threshold is borderline low (Table 9.59.2). See flow chart 4: The breathing reserve is normal, which directs us to branchpoint 4.3. $\dot{V}_E/\dot{V}_{CO_2}$ at the *AT* is abnormally high (panel 6, Fig. 9.59.1) leading us to the diagnosis of abnormal pulmonary circulation. The vital capacity is normal (branchpoint 4.5) differentiating the abnormal pulmonary circulatory physiology diagnosis further to pulmonary vascular disease. We confirm this diagnosis with the abnormally high VD/VT, P(A − a)O₂, P(a − ET)CO₂, steep heart rate - $\dot{V}_{O_2}$ relationship and low relatively non-changing O₂ pulse. The patient was not tested with 100% O₂, but the lack of an abrupt decrease in PaO₂ during exercise suggests that a right to left shunt through a potentially patent foramen ovale does not exist.

Conclusion

This patient had pulmonary vascular disease, previously unrecognized, probably of thromboembolic origin. The patient eventually died of thromboembolic disease.

Case 60 Pulmonary Vasculitis: Air and Oxygen Breathing

Clinical Findings

This 54-year-old executive had apparently been in good health until 11 years previously, when he had had a documented acute myocardial infarction. Coronary arteriogram had been normal 1 year later. Five years ago he had developed fatigue, jaundice, Raynaud's phenomenon, renal failure, and peripheral neuropathy with a histologic diagnosis of membranoproliferative glomerulonephritis secondary to vasculitis. Diffuse cerebritis with panhypopituitarism had followed; this had responded well to corticosteroids, cyclophosphamide, and endocrine replacement therapy. Three years ago, progressive exertional dyspnea had begun without cough, pleurisy, or wheezing. A pulmonary nodule had developed and was biopsied. Histologic examination showed an organizing exudate, hemorrhage, and severe arteriolar wall thickening. The patient never smoked or abused drugs or alcohol. Physical examination revealed acrocyanosis without clubbing, clear lungs, and normal heart sounds. Exercise testing was performed to evaluate the possible efficacy of supplemental oxygen.

Exercise Findings

The patient performed exercise tests on the cycle ergometer. On both occasions he pedalled at 60 rpm without added load for 3 minutes. The work rate was then increased 15 W every minute.

The first test was done during air breathing, and the second was done while breathing 100% oxygen. Arterial blood was sampled every second minute, and intra-arterial blood pressure recorded from a percutaneously inserted brachial artery catheter.

During air breathing, the patient stopped because of leg fatigue and complained of shortness of breath. While breathing 100% O_2, the patient complained of leg fatigue only. Resting ECG showed a rightward axis, poor R wave progression in the precordial leads and T wave inversion in V4. There was no ectopy or abnormality of ST segments, although the T wave inversion increased during exercise.

TABLE 9.60.1. Selected Respiratory Function Data

Measurement	Predicted	Measured
Age, yr		54
Sex		Male
Height, cm		170
Weight, kg	74	64
Hematocrit, %		38
VC, L	4.03	4.07
IC, L	2.68	3.16
FEV_1, L	3.18	3.38
FEV_1/VC, %	79	83
MVV, L/min	137	143
D_Lco, ml/mmHg/min	26.5	8.0

TABLE 9.60.2. Selected Exercise Data

Measurement	Predicted	Room Air	Oxygen
Maximum work rate, W	160	90	90
Peak $\dot{V}O_2$, L/min	2.11	0.96	
Maximum HR, beats/min	166	132	131
Maximum O_2 pulse, ml/beat	12.7	7.3	
$\Delta\dot{V}O_2/\Delta$WR, ml/min/W	10.3	8.8	
AT, L/min	>0.97	<0.75	
Blood pressure, mm Hg (rest, max)		129/69, 204/84	126/75, 201/87
Maximum $\dot{V}E$, L/min		117	89
Exercise breathing reserve, L/min	>15	26	54
PaO_2, mm Hg (rest, max ex)		114, 90	692, 678
$P(A - a)O_2$, mm Hg (rest, max ex)		10, 41	−8, 4
$P(a - ET)CO_2$, mm Hg (rest, max ex)		7, 9	10, 12
VD/VT (rest, heavy ex)		0.44, 0.52	0.52, 0.57
HCO_3^-, mEq/L (rest, 2-min recov)		18, 12	18, 15

FIGURE 9.60.1. Air breathing.

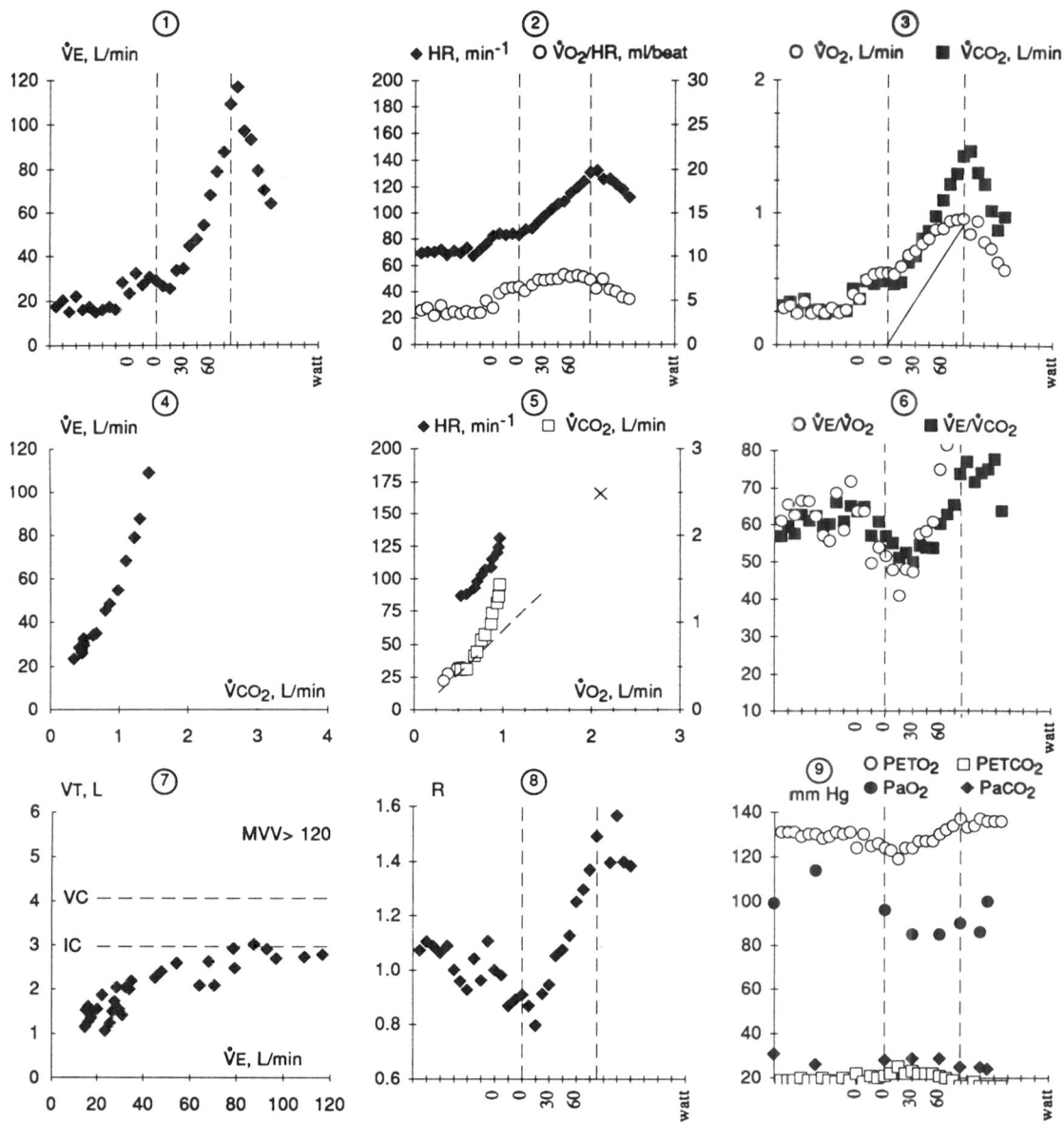

1. Vertical dashed lines in panels 1 to 3 and 6, 8, and 9 indicate the beginning and the end of increasing work period.
2. Unloaded cycling is performed for 3 minutes before the left vertical dashed line.
3. In panel 3, the diagonal line shows the increase of $\dot{V}O_2$ at a slope of 10 ml/min/w.
4. In panel 5, the diagonal dashed line has a slope of 1; the "x" in the upper right is the predicted maximum heart rate and $\dot{V}O_2$ for the subject.

TABLE 9.60.3. Air Breathing

Time min	Work rate watts	BP mmHg	HR min⁻¹	f min⁻¹	$\dot{V}_E$ L/min BTPS	$\dot{V}_{CO_2}$ L/min STPD	$\dot{V}_{O_2}$ L/min STPD	$\dot{V}_{O_2}$/HR ml/beat	R	pH	HCO₃ meq/L	PO₂ ET	PO₂ a	PO₂ (A−a)	PCO₂ ET	PCO₂ a	PCO₂ (a−ET)	$\dot{V}_E/\dot{V}_{CO_2}$	$\dot{V}_E/\dot{V}_{O_2}$	VD/VT
	Rest	129/69								7.38	18	99			31					
	Rest		69	12	17.5	0.29	0.27	3.9	1.07			131			19			57	61	
	Rest		70	13	20.1	0.32	0.29	4.1	1.10			131			19			59	66	
	Rest		70	10	15.2	0.25	0.23	3.3	1.09			131			19			57	62	
	Rest		72	12	22.3	0.34	0.32	4.4	1.06			129			20			63	67	
	Rest		68	10	16.1	0.25	0.23	3.4	1.09			130			19			61	66	
	Rest	126/69	71	13	17.3	0.26	0.26	3.7	1.00	7.44	17	130	114	10	19	26	7	62	62	0.44
	Rest		69	13	14.8	0.23	0.24	3.5	0.96			128			20			60	57	
	Rest		73	13	16.1	0.25	0.27	3.7	0.93			129			19			60	56	
	Rest		67	13	17.6	0.25	0.24	3.3	1.04			131			18			66	69	
	Rest		72	13	16.3	0.25	0.26	3.3	0.96			130			20			61	58	
	Unloaded		76	14	28.52	0.42	0.38	5.0	1.11			131			19			65	72	
	Unloaded		82	22	23.5	0.34	0.34	4.1	1.00			124			22			64	64	
	Unloaded		84	16	32.5	0.48	0.49	5.3	0.98			130			18			65	64	
	Unloaded		83	16	27.6	0.46	0.53	6.4	0.87			125			21			57	50	
	Unloaded		84	22	31.0	0.48	0.54	6.4	0.89			126			20			61	54	
	Unloaded	147/75	83	19	29.4	0.49	0.54	6.5	0.91	7.41	17	124	96	24	21	28	7	57	51	0.43
0.5	15		87	18	26.8	0.46	0.53	6.1	0.87			123			22			55	48	
1.0	15		88	21	25.8	0.47	0.59	6.7	0.80			119			25			51	41	
1.5	30		93	17	34.0	0.62	0.68	7.3	0.91			124			22			53	48	
2.0	30	156/78	98	16	34.9	0.67	0.71	7.2	0.94	7.39	17	124	85	35	23	29	6	50	47	0.39
2.5	45		103	20	45.2	0.80	0.76	7.4	1.05			127			22			54	57	
3.0	45		107	20	48.1	0.86	0.80	7.5	1.03			127			22			54	58	
3.5	60		109	21	54.5	0.98	0.87	8.0	1.13			127			22			54	61	
4.0	60	183/84	115	26	68.3	1.10	0.88	7.7	1.25	7.38	17	130	85	41	21	29	8	60	75	0.49
4.5	75		120	27	78.9	1.22	0.94	7.8	1.30			132			20			63	81	
5.0	75		124	29	87.6	1.30	0.95	7.7	1.37			134			19			65	90	
5.5	90	204/84	131	40	109.1	1.43	0.96	7.3	1.49	7.38	15	137	90	41	16	25	9	74	110	0.52
	Recovery		132	42	116.9	1.47	0.84	6.4	1.75			133			16			77	135	
	Recovery		126	36	97.1	1.31	0.94	7.5	1.39			134			18			72	100	
	Recovery	198/87	126	32	93.1	1.22	0.78	6.2	1.56	7.37	14	137	36	46	16	25	9	74	116	0.52
	Recovery	192/78	122	32	79.4	1.02	0.73	6.0	1.40	7.33	12	136	100	31	16	24	8	75	105	0.50
	Recovery		118	34	70.6	0.87	0.63	5.3	1.38			136			16			78	107	
	Recovery		112	31	64.4	0.97	0.57	5.1	1.70			136			16			64	108	

Interpretation

Comments

Except for the very low diffusing capacity, the results of this patient's respiratory function studies are normal (Table 9.60.1).

Analysis

Referring to flow chart 1, during air breathing, the peak $\dot{V}_{O_2}$ and the anaerobic threshold are significantly reduced (Table 9.60.2). See flow chart 4. The breathing reserve is normal (branchpoint 4.1). The $\dot{V}_E/\dot{V}_{CO_2}$ at the AT is significantly increased (Fig. 9.60.1, Table 9.60.3) (branchpoint 4.3) leading us to abnormal pulmonary circulation. The vital capacity is normal (branchpoint 4.5) leading us to a diagnosis of pulmonary vascular disease as opposed to moder-

ate to severe left ventricular failure. Confirmatory measurements are high VD/VT, P(a − ET)CO₂ and P(A − a)O₂ at the maximum work rate, steep heart rate − $\dot{V}_{O_2}$ relationship, low non-changing O₂ pulse and decreasing $\Delta \dot{V}_{O_2}/\Delta WR$ with increasing work rate.

PaO₂ decreases during exercise but remains within the normal range (panel 9, Fig. 9.60.1). The high PaO₂ measured during exercise with the patient breathing 100% O₂ confirms the absence of the development of a right to left shunt (usually through the foramen ovale) (branchpoint 4.7). This might be contrasted with Case 61, a patient with pulmonary vascular disease in whom a right to left shunt through the foramen ovale did develop during exercise.

100% O₂ breathing had little effect on this patient's exercise performance. This suggests that this

FIGURE 9.60.2.   Oxygen breathing.

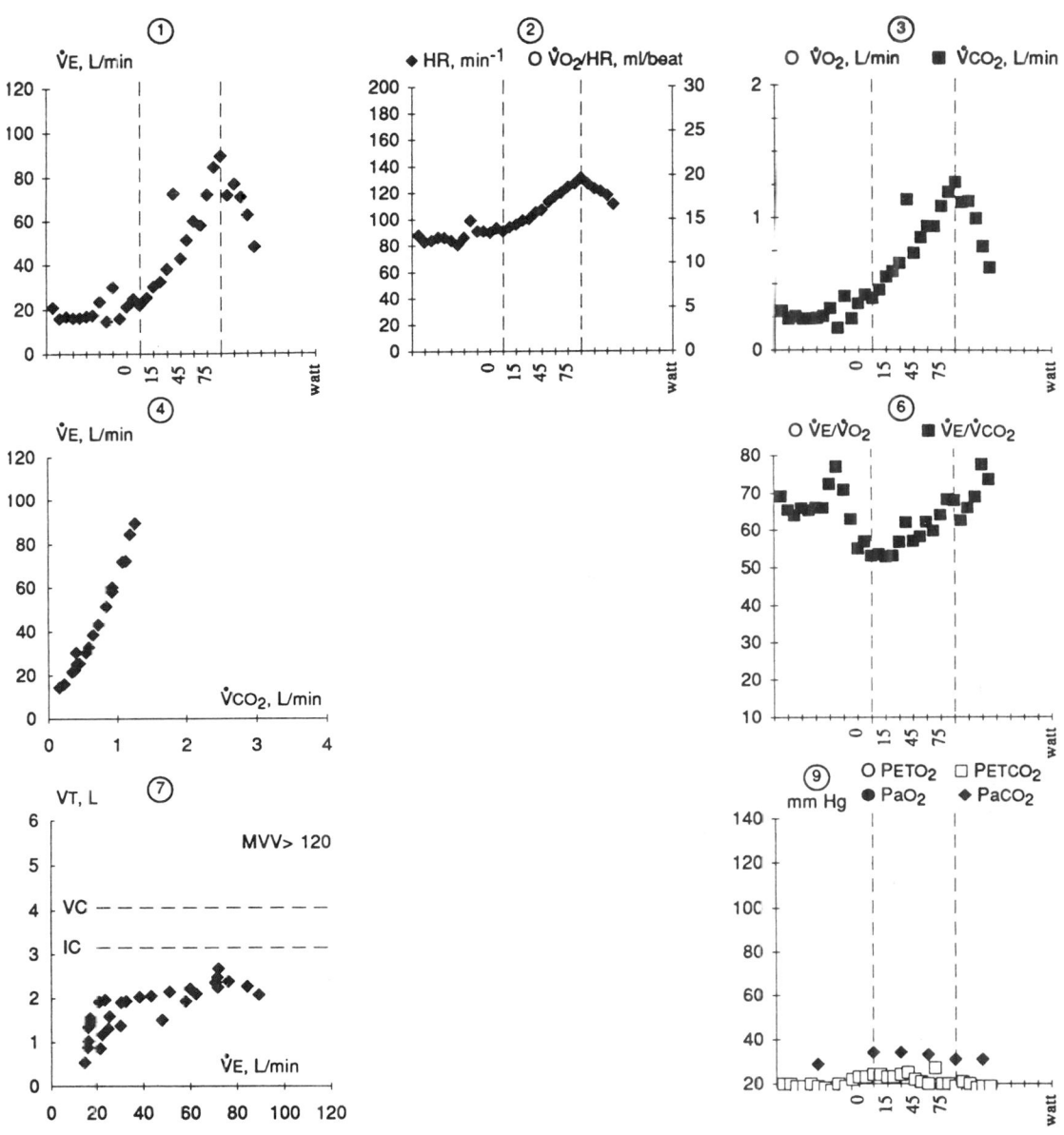

1. Vertical dashed lines in panels 1 to 3 and 6 and 9 indicate the beginning and the end of increasing work period.
2. Unloaded cycling is performed for 3 minutes before the left vertical dashed line.

TABLE 9.60.4. Oxygen Breathing

Time min	Work rate watts	BP mmHg	HR min⁻¹	f min⁻¹	$\dot{V}_E$ L/min BTPS	$\dot{V}_{CO_2}$ L/min STPD	$\dot{V}_{O_2}$ L/min STPD	$\frac{\dot{V}_{O_2}}{HR}$ ml/beat	R	pH	HCO₃⁻ meq/L	Po₂, mmHg ET	a	(A − a)	Pco₂, mmHg ET	a	(a − ET)	$\frac{\dot{V}_E}{\dot{V}_{CO_2}}$	$\frac{\dot{V}_E}{\dot{V}_{O_2}}$	$\frac{V_D}{V_T}$
	Rest		88	11	21.0	0.29									20			69		
	Rest		83	12	16.1	0.23									20			66		
	Rest		84	11	16.9	0.25									19			64		
	Rest		86	12	16.2	0.23									19			66		
	Rest		86	16	16.4	0.23									20			65		
	Rest	120/72	84	12	16.9	0.24				7.40	18		692	−8	19	29	10	66		0.52
	Rest		81	12	17.5	0.25									18			66		
	Rest		86	12	23.5	0.31									17			73		
	Unloaded		99	27	14.6	0.16									20			77		
	Unloaded		91	22	30.2	0.40									19			71		
	Unloaded		91	18	16.0	0.23									22			63		
	Unloaded		90	25	21.4	0.35									23			55		
	Unloaded		93	19	24.9	0.41									23			57		
	Unloaded	132/72	91	19	22.3	0.39				7.36	19		678	1	24	34	10	53		0.48
0.5	15		94	16	25.4	0.45									24			53		
1.0	15		96	16	30.4	0.55									23			53		
1.5	30		99	17	32.7	0.59									23			53		
2.0	30	156/75	100	19	38.4	0.65				7.35	18		645	34	24	34	10	57		0.53
2.5	45		105	27	72.3	1.13									25			62		
3.0	45		107	21	43.3	0.73									22			57		
3.5	60		113	24	51.4	0.85									21			58		
4.0	60	189/81	117	27	60.1	0.93				7.35	18		683	−3	20	33	13	62		0.56
4.5	75		120	30	58.1	0.93									27			60		
5.0	75		124	32	72.0	1.08									20			64		
5.5	90		127	37	84.3	1.19									20			68		
6.0	90	201/87	131	43	89.4	1.26				7.34	16		678	4	19	31	12	68		0.57
	Recovery		127	29	71.7	1.11									21			62		
	Recovery		123	32	76.5	1.12									20			66		
	Recovery		121	30	70.8	0.99									18			69		
	Recovery	186/78	118	30	62.9	0.78				7.31	15		682	0	19	31	12	77		0.61
	Recovery		111	32	48.3	0.62									19			74		

patient has little pulmonary vasodilatation in response to high O_2 breathing. Ventilation, however, is considerably reduced with O_2 breathing demonstrating a suppression of ventilatory drive during exercise. Despite this reduction in ventilation and dyspnea, there was no improvement in exercise performance. This suggests that the patient is not ventilatory limited.

Resting arterial bicarbonate is low, demonstrating a compensated metabolic acidosis at rest. The metabolic acidosis worsens with exercise (Table 9.60.2).

Conclusion

Severe pulmonary vascular disease has limited exercise performance.

Case 61 Pulmonary Hypertension with Patent Foramen Ovale

Clinical Findings

This 61-year-old woman had first noted mild exertional dyspnea 3 years prior to evaluation. Four months prior to evaluation she had "caught the flu" and soon thereafter developed recurring episodes of depression and confusion. Medical evaluation revealed hypoxemia. With oxygen therapy her mental status returned to normal. She also admitted to squeezing substernal chest pain, usually associated with exercise, but this symptom was not prominent. There was no history of cigarette smoking, exposure to environmental toxins, pulmonary emboli, or thrombophlebitis. She was given alprazolam for her mental symptoms and propranolol for systemic hypertension. On referral, examination revealed mild obesity, hypertension, and a prominent S4. Chest roentgenogram showed enlarged pulmonary arteries. Resting ECG revealed right axis deviation, an R much greater than S in V1, and negative T waves in leads V1 to V4.

Exercise Findings

The patient performed exercise on a cycle ergometer. She pedalled at 60 rpm without added load for 3 minutes. The work rate was then increased 5 W per minute to her symptom-limited maximum. Arterial blood was sampled every second minute, and intra-arterial blood pressure was recorded from a percutaneously placed brachial artery catheter. She stopped exercise because of shortness of breath. There were no arrhythmias, ST segment, or T wave changes with exercise. Following a rest period of 30 minutes, the exercise study was repeated while the patient was breathing 100% oxygen.

TABLE 9.61.1. Selected Respiratory Function Data

Measurement	Predicted	Measured
Age, yr		61
Sex		Female
Height, cm		147
Weight, kg	53	61
Hematocrit, %		37
VC, L	2.33	2.31
IC, L	1.56	1.59
TLC, L	3.66	4.53
FEV$_1$, L	1.90	1.59
FEV$_1$/VC, %	81	69
MVV, L/min	73	59
D$_{LCO}$, ml/mm Hg/min	17.6	17.3

TABLE 9.61.2. Selected Exercise Data

Measurement	Predicted	Room Air	Oxygen
Maximum work rate, W		20	25
Peak V̇O$_2$, L/min	1.23	0.62	
Maximum HR, beats/min	159	87	85
Maximum O$_2$ pulse, ml/beat	7.8	7.1	
AT, L/min	>0.61	Indeterminate	
Blood pressure, mmHg (rest, max)		186/90, 204/90	172/84, 210/102
Maximum V̇E, L/min		38	42
Exercise breathing reserve, L/min	>15	21	17
PaO$_2$, mmHg (rest, max ex)		71, 40	550, 70
P(A − a)O$_2$, mmHg (rest, max ex)		42, 79	138, 612
P(a − ET)CO$_2$, mmHg (rest, max ex)		5, 12	4, 9
VD/VT (rest, heavy ex)		0.31, 0.47	0.34, 0.47
HCO$_3^-$, mEq/L (rest, 2-min recov)		22, 20	22, 18

FIGURE 9.61.1.   Air breathing.

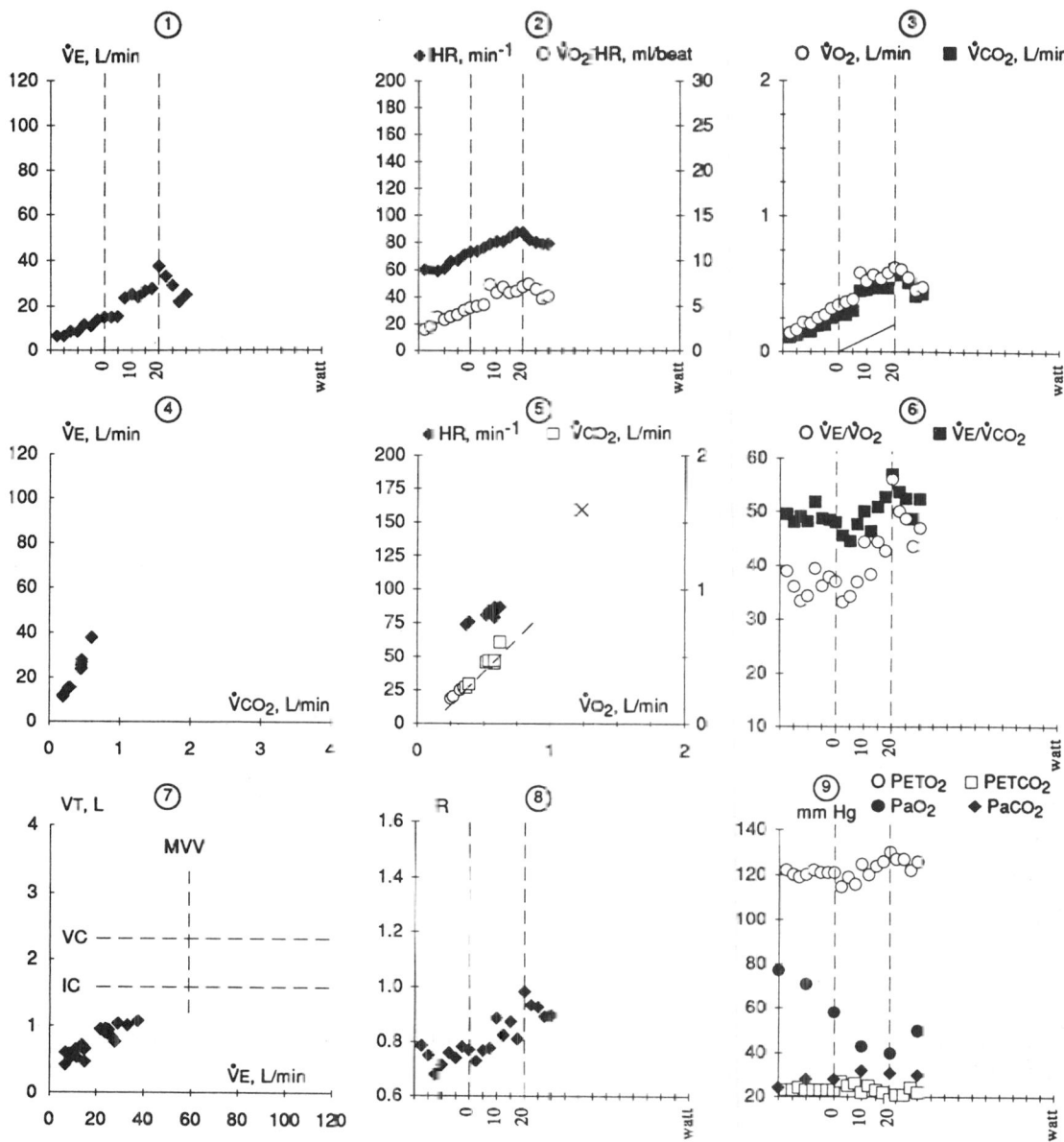

1. Vertical dashed lines in panels 1 to 3 and 6, 8, and 9 indicate the beginning and the end of increasing work period.
2. Unloaded cycling is performed for 3 minutes before the left vertical dashed line.
3. In panel 3, the diagonal line shows the increase of $\dot{V}O_2$ at a slope of 10 ml/min/w.
4. In panel 5, the diagonal dashed line has a slope of 1; the ′x″ in the upper right is the predicted maximum heart rate and $\dot{V}O_2$ for the subject.

FIGURE 9.61.2.   Oxygen breathing.

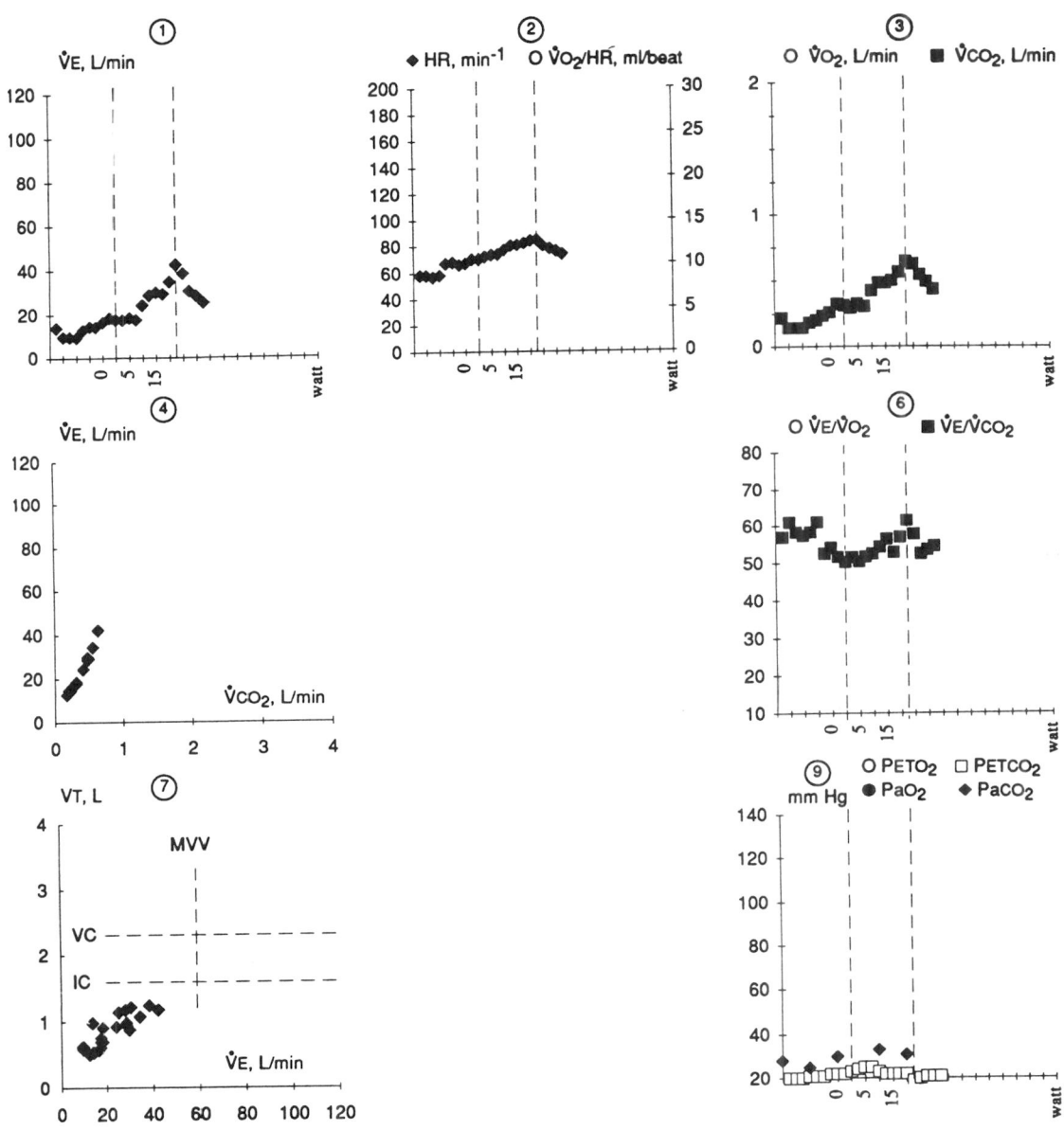

1. Vertical dashed lines in panels 1 to 3 and 6 and 9 indicate the beginning and the end of increasing work period.
2. Unloaded cycling is performed for 3 minutes before the left vertical dashed line.

TABLE 9.61.3. Air Breathing

Time min	Work rate watts	BP mmHg	HR min⁻¹	f min⁻¹	V̇E L/min BTPS	V̇CO₂ L/min STPD	V̇O₂ L/min STPD	V̇O₂/HR ml/beat	R	pH	HCO₃⁻ meq/L	PO₂ ET	PO₂ a	PO₂ (A−a)	PCO₂ ET	PCO₂ a	PCO₂ (a−ET)	V̇E/V̇CO₂	V̇E/V̇O₂	VD/VT
	Rest	186/90								7.56	21		77			24				
	Rest		60	16	6.8	0.11	0.14	2.3	0.73			122			23			49	39	
	Rest		60	11	6.7	0.12	0.16	2.7	0.75			120			23			48	36	
	Rest		59	17	8.8	0.15	0.22	3.7	0.68			119			24			49	33	
	Rest	206/114	61	14	8.4	0.15	0.21	3.4	0.71	7.52	22	120	71	42	23	28	5	48	34	0.31
	Unloaded		66	22	11.7	0.19	0.25	3.8	0.73			122			23			52	39	
	Unloaded		67	17	11.2	0.20	0.27	4.0	0.74			121			23			49	36	
	Unloaded		71	19	13.7	0.25	0.32	4.5	0.73			121			23			48	38	
	Unloaded	191/94	73	23	14.9	0.27	0.35	4.8	0.77	7.50	21	121	58	57	23	28	5	48	37	0.31
0.5	5		74	32	15.0	0.27	0.37	5.0	0.73			115			27			45	33	
1.0	5		76	23	15.3	0.30	0.39	5.1	0.77			119			25			44	34	
1.5	10		79	26	23.6	0.45	0.58	7.3	0.78			116			26			48	37	
2.0	10	202/96	81	27	25.3	0.46	0.52	6.4	0.88	7.47	23	125	43	72	22	32	10	50	44	0.42
2.5	15		81	25	23.9	0.47	0.57	7.0	0.82			120			25			46	38	
3.0	15		84	32	26.6	0.47	0.54	6.4	0.87			124			23			51	44	
3.5	20		87	36	27.8	0.47	0.58	6.7	0.81			126			22			53	43	
4.0	20	204/90	87	35	37.7	0.61	0.62	7.1	0.98	7.43	21	130	40	79	19	31	12	57	56	0.47
	Recovery		82	33	33.3	0.57	0.61	7.4	0.93			127			21			54	50	
	Recovery		80	28	29.1	0.51	0.55	6.9	0.93			127			21			52	49	
	Recovery		79	23	21.9	0.41	0.46	5.8	0.89			122			24			49	43	
	Recovery	198/87	79	27	24.8	0.43	0.48	6.1	0.90	7.45	20	126	50	67	22	30	8	52	47	0.41

TABLE 9.61.4. Oxygen Breathing

Time min	Work rate watts	BP mmHg	HR min⁻¹	f min⁻¹	V̇E L/min BTPS	V̇CO₂ L/min STPD	V̇O₂ L/min STPD	V̇O₂/HR ml/beat	R	pH	HCO₃⁻ meq/L	PO₂ ET	PO₂ a	PO₂ (A−a)	PCO₂ ET	PCO₂ a	PCO₂ (a−ET)	V̇E/V̇CO₂	V̇E/V̇O₂	VD/VT
	Rest	171/78								7.50	21		67			28				
	Rest		58	14	13.7	0.22									20			57		
	Rest		58	16	9.9	0.14									20			61		
	Rest		57	16	9.5	0.14									20			58		
	Rest	172/84	58	15	9.3	0.14				7.53	21	550	138		21	25	4	57		0.34
	Unloaded		67	25	12.6	0.18									21			58		
	Unloaded		68	27	14.5	0.20									21			61		
	Unloaded		66	26	14.3	0.23									22			53		
	Unloaded	180/87	67	29	16.5	0.26				7.48	22	386	297		22	30	8	54		0.40
	Unloaded		70	20	18.2	0.32									22			52		
	Unloaded		70	23	17.5	0.31									23			50		
0.5	5		72	28	17.3	0.29									24			51		
1.0	5		73	26	18.3	0.32									25			50		
1.5	10		74	25	17.6	0.30									25			52		
2.0	10	180/84	77	26	24.2	0.42				7.44	22	100	530		23	33	10	52		0.45
2.5	15		80	29	28.5	0.48									22			54		
3.0	15		81	34	29.9	0.48									22			56		
3.5	20		82	31	29.0	0.50									22			53		
4.0	20	210/102	84	32	34.5	0.56				7.45	21	70	612		22	31	9	57		0.47
4.5	25		85	36	42.3	0.64									19			61		
	Recovery		80	31	38.4	0.62									20			58		
	Recovery		78	25	30.5	0.54									21			53		
	Recovery		76	24	28.2	0.49									21			53		
	Recovery	198/92	74	22	25.2	0.43									21			54		

Interpretation

Comments

The results of this patient's resting respiratory function tests show mild airway obstruction (Table 9.61.1). The ECG is compatible with right ventricular hypertrophy. The exercise test was repeated with the subject breathing 100% oxygen to evaluate the possible development of a right to left shunt through a foramen ovale when exercise-induced right atrial pressure exceeds left atrial pressure—a possible cause of activity-induced hypoxemia, which might contribute to this patient's symptoms.

Analysis

Referring to flow chart 1, the peak oxygen uptake is reduced while the anaerobic threshold is indeterminate, but probably low (Table 9.61.2). See flow chart 4: The breathing reserve is normal (branchpoint 4.1). The $\dot{V}_E/\dot{V}_{CO_2}$ during exercise is high (branchpoint 4.3) supporting the diagnosis of abnormal pulmonary circulation. The patient is hyperventilating, however, and the arterial P_{CO_2} must be taken into account so that true V_D/V_T is calculated. The latter is increased. Branchpoint 4.5 further distinguishes between abnormal pulmonary circulation due to moderate to severe left ventricular failure and that due to pulmonary vascular disease, in that the vital capacity is normal. All confirmatory abnormalities are present supporting the diagnosis of pulmonary vascular disease.

At the lowest work rate, Pa_{O_2} abruptly decreases and continues to decrease as the work rate is increased. Moreover, $P(a - ET)_{CO_2}$ continues to increase as work rate is increased and the V_D/V_T become progressively more abnormal as work rate is increased (Tables 9.61.3 and 9.61.4). The changes in Pa_{O_2}, Pa_{CO_2} and V_D/V_T suggest the development of a right to left shunt during exercise. Clearly, the patient is also oxygen-flow limited in that $\dot{V}_{O_2}$ and oxygen pulse fail to increase with increasing work rate (panels 3 and 2, respectively, Fig. 9.61.1).

To document that a right to left shunt develops with exercise, Pa_{C_2} was measured at rest and during exercise while the patient was breathing 100% oxygen. At rest, Pa_{O_2} is at the lower limits of normal (550 mmHg); with mild exercise, it drops to 70 mmHg. This can only be explained by the development of a right to left shunt with exercise (contrast with Case 60).

Subsequently, the patient had right heart catheterization. Pulmonary artery pressures were confirmed to be at systemic pressure levels; the catheter slipped easily through a foramen ovale into the left atrium.

Conclusion

After diagnosis of "pulmonary vascular occlusive disease with exercise-induced right to left shunt through a patent foramen ovale" was made by the physicians who did the exercise studies, the patient had right heart catheterization. She was then diagnosed by cardiologist who did the catheterization study as "primary pulmonary hypertension with patent foramen ovale through which the catheter easily passed from right to left atrium."

Case 62 Left Ventricular Failure with Accompanying Lung Function Changes

Clinical Findings

This 66-year-old shipyard worker stated that he was in excellent health. Two weeks prior to evaluation he had had an episode of severe shortness of breath, awakening him from his sleep at a Colorado camp site at 11,000 feet of altitude. He had driven there from Los Angeles in the previous 24 hours. He had had no relief until he was driven down to an altitude of 7000 feet. He had a 40 pack year history of cigarette smoking with a nonproductive cough. He denied other symptoms. The physical examination was normal except for mild obesity. Chest roentgenograms revealed moderate nodular pleural plaques with evidence of minimal pulmonary fibrosis. Resting ECG showed left anterior superior hemiblock.

Exercise Findings

The patient performed exercise on a cycle ergometer. He pedalled at 60 rpm without added load for 3 minutes. The work rate was then increased 20 W per minute to his symptom-limited maximum. Arterial blood was sampled every second minute, and intra-arterial blood pressure was recorded from a percutaneously placed brachial artery catheter. The patient stopped exercising because of leg fatigue and shortness of breath. Exercise ECGs were normal except for the appearance of infrequent premature ventricular contractions during the last two work rates.

TABLE 9.62.1. Selected Respiratory Function Data

Measurement	Predicted	Measured
Age, yr		66
Sex		Male
Height, cm		178
Weight, kg	80	84
Hematocrit, %		41
VC, L	4.18	3.48
IC, _	2.79	2.96
TLC, L	6.56	5.95
FEV_1, L	3.26	2.76
FEV_1/VC, %	78	79
MVV, L/min	132	93
D_Lco, ml/mm Hg/min	25.6	22.7

TABLE 9.62.2. Selected Exercise Data

Measurement	Predicted	Measured
Peak $\dot{V}O_2$, L/min	2.12	1.58
Maximum HR, beats/min	154	141
Maximum O_2 pulse, ml/beat	13.7	11.6
$\Delta\dot{V}O_2/\Delta WR$, ml/min/W	10.3	7.7
AT, L/min	>0.95	1.1
Blood pressure, mmHg (rest, max)		167/86, 241/104
Maximum $\dot{V}E$, L/min		70
Exercise breathing reserve, L/min	>15	23
Pa_{O_2} mmHg (rest, max ex)		87, 90
P(a − a)O_2, mm Hg (rest, max ex)		19, 23
P(a − ET)CO_2, mmHg (rest, max ex)		−2, 3
V_D/V_T (rest, heavy ex)		0.38, 0.33
HCO_3, mEq/L (rest, 2-min recov)		24, 17

FIGURE 9.62.1.

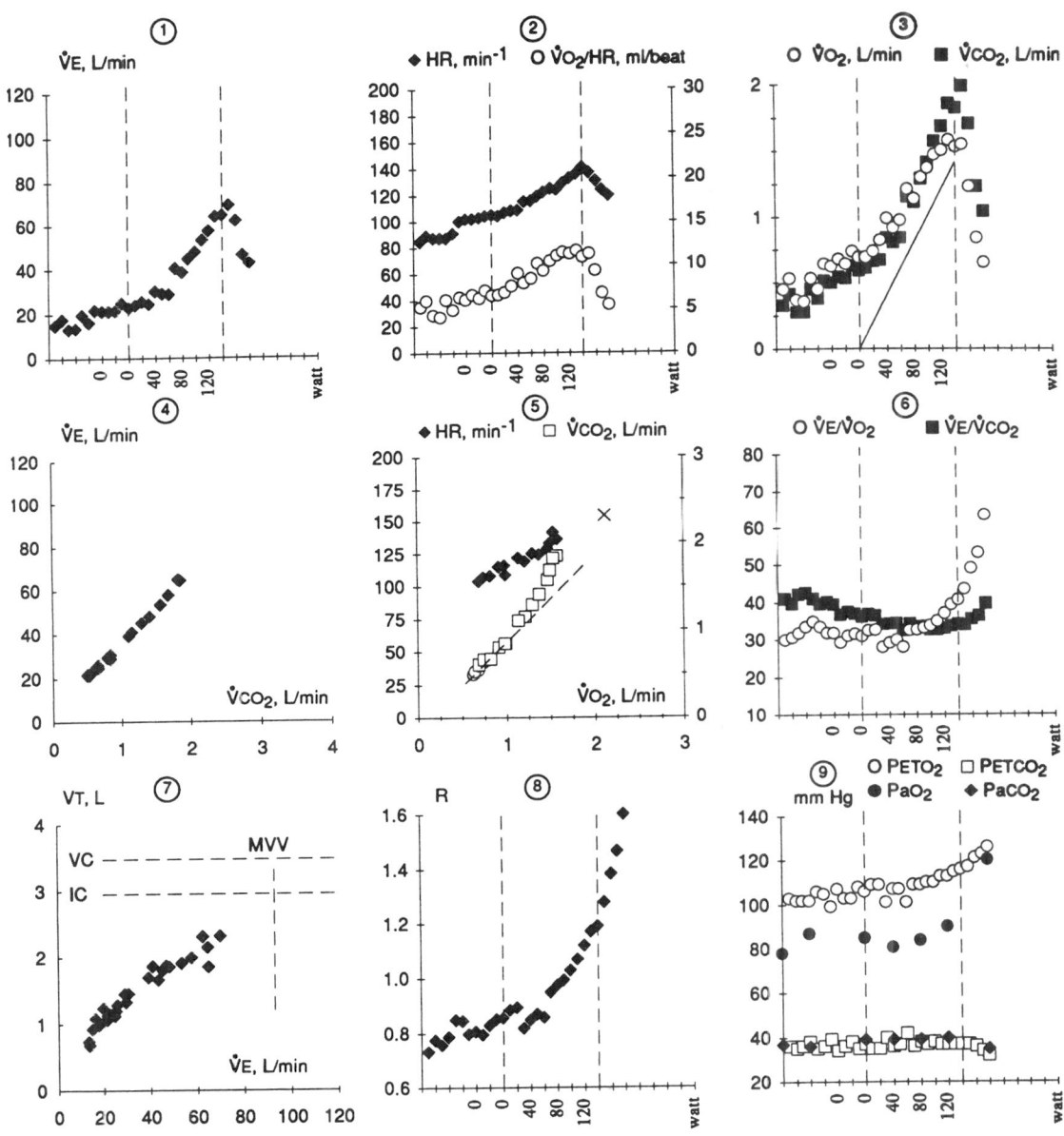

1. Vertical dashed lines in panels 1 to 3 and 6, 8, and 9 indicate the beginning and the end of increasing work period.

2. Unloaded cycling is performed for 3 minutes before the left vertical dashed line.

3. In panel 3, the diagonal line shows the increase of $\dot{V}O_2$ at a slope of 10 ml/min/w.

4. In panel 5, the diagonal dashed line has a slope of 1; the "x" in the upper right is the predicted maximum heart rate and $\dot{V}O_2$ for the subject.

Interpretation

Comments

Results of the resting respiratory function studies show the vital capacity to be at the low end of the normal range (Table 9.62.1). The resting ECG is abnormal, as noted in "Clinical Findings."

Analysis

Referring to flow chart 1, the peak $\dot{V}O_2$ is reduced and the anaerobic threshold is normal (Table 9.62.2). See flow chart 3. The breathing reserve is normal (branchpoint 3.1), and infrequent ventricular premature contractions appear during late exercise (branchpoint 3.3). This gives preference to the

TABLE 9.62.3. Air Breathing

Time min	Work rate watts	BP mmHg	HR min^{-1}	f min^{-1}	V̇E L/min BTPS	V̇CO2 L/min STPD	V̇C2 L/min STPD	V̇O2/HR ml/beat	R	pH	HCO3 meq/L	FO2, mmHg ET	a	(A−a)	PCO2, mmHg ET	a	(a−ET)	V̇E/V̇CO2	V̇E/V̇O2	VD/VT
	Rest	167/86								7.42	24		78			37				
	Rest		35	16	14.9	0.33	0.45	5.3	0.73			103			36			41	30	
	Rest		39	18	17.8	0.41	0.53	6.0	0.77			102			35			40	31	
	Rest		37	18	13.3	0.28	0.37	4.3	0.76			102			36			42	32	
	Rest	161/89	37	20	13.6	0.28	0.36	4.1	0.79	7.41	22	102	87	19	38	36	−2	43	33	0.38
	Rest		37	16	19.8	0.45	0.53	6.1	0.85			106			35			41	35	
	Rest		91	15	16.3	0.38	0.45	4.9	0.84			105			36			40	33	
	Unloaded		100	19	22.0	0.51	0.64	6.4	0.80			99			39			40	32	
	Unloaded		102	20	21.4	0.50	0.62	6.1	0.81			107			34			39	32	
	Unloaded		102	19	21.4	0.54	0.68	6.7	0.79			103			36			37	29	
	Unloaded		103	20	21.5	0.53	0.64	6.2	0.83			103			38			37	31	
	Unloaded		104	21	25.1	0.63	0.74	7.1	0.85			108			35			37	32	
	Unloaded	191/95	105	20	23.0	0.59	0.69	6.6	0.86	7.39	23	106	85	21	37	39	2	36	31	0.36
0.5	20		104	21	24.2	0.61	0.69	6.6	0.88			109			35			37	32	
1.0	20		107	20	25.8	0.66	0.74	6.9	0.89			109			35			37	33	
1.5	40		108	22	24.7	0.67	0.82	7.6	0.82			101			40			34	28	
2.0	40	194/92	109	21	30.5	0.84	0.99	9.1	0.85	7.39	23	107	31	24	36	39	3	34	29	0.33
2.5	60		115	22	29.4	0.80	0.92	8.0	0.87			107			37			34	30	
3.0	60		116	20	29.0	0.84	0.98	8.4	0.86			101			42			33	28	
3.5	80		119	22	41.1	1.15	1.21	10.2	0.95			109			36			34	32	
4.0	80	218/98	122	23	39.1	1.11	1.14	9.3	0.97	7.37	22	109	34	26	38	39	1	33	33	0.32
4.5	100		125	25	45.2	1.29	1.30	10.4	0.99			110			37			33	33	
5.0	100		124	26	48.3	1.41	1.37	11.0	1.03			110			38			33	34	
5.5	120		129	28	53.6	1.57	1.47	11.4	1.07			113			37			33	35	
6.0	120	239/98	133	29	57.8	1.38	1.50	11.3	1.12	7.34	21	113	90	23	37	40	3	33	37	0.33
6.5	140		136	30	64.5	1.35	1.58	11.6	1.17			115			37			33	39	
7.0	140	241/104	141	35	65.0	1.32	1.53	10.9	1.19			116			37			34	41	
	Recovery		137	30	69.7	1.98	1.55	11.3	1.28			117			37			34	43	
	Recovery		131	27	62.4	1.70	1.23	9.4	1.38			121			36			35	49	
	Recovery		124	25	46.8	1.23	0.84	6.8	1.46			123			34			36	53	
	Recovery	200/80	120	26	43.3	1.04	0.65	5.4	1.60	7.29	17	126	120	5	32	35	3	40	63	0.36

diagnostic box of "myocardial ischemia," rather than "poor effort," especially because the reduced ΔV̇O2/ΔWR strongly suggests a circulatory limitation. Because the low ΔV̇O2/ΔWR is somewhat incompatible with a normal AT, perhaps this analysis should be through flow chart 4. Because the breathing reserve is normal (branchpoint 4.1) and the V̇E/V̇CO2 at the AT and VD/VT are high (branchpoint 4.3), there is an abnormal pulmonary circulation. If we interpret the borderline reduced vital capacity as being low (branchpoint 4.5), this leads us to moderate to severe left ventricular failure. This is supported by the increase in P(a − ET)CO2 while P(A − a)O2 remains normal at the maximum work rate, a flattening of the O2 pulse and V̇O2 as the maximum work rate is approached, and a reduced

maximal O2 pulse. The abnormalities in gas exchange at the lung are most compatible with those found with left ventricular failure with disturbances in the pulmonary circulation which commonly accompany this disorder when it is moderate to severe. The ECG changes are compatible with this diagnosis. Systemic arterial hypertension could be contributory to the cardiac failure or a response to it.

Conclusion

This patient has left ventricular failure with the abnormal changes in the pulmonary circulation that accompany this disease when it becomes moderate to severe, and systemic arterial hypertension.

Case 63 Pulmonary Vascular Disease, Secondary to Interstitial and Obstructive Lung Disease

Clinical Findings

This 70-year-old retired shipyard worker complained of shortness of breath after climbing a flight of stairs. He had a 50 pack year smoking history but had stopped 3 months prior to the evaluation. He took triamterene, hydrochlorothiazide, and methyldopa for hypertension but denied any history of heart or lung disease. The physical examination was not remarkable. Resting ECG showed left axis deviation, left atrial enlargement, and left ventricular hypertrophy. Chest roentgenograms showed moderate pleural thickening with some calcification plus moderate interstitial fibrosis.

Exercise Findings

The patient performed exercise on a cycle ergometer. He pedalled at 60 rpm without added load for 3 minutes. The work rate was then increased 15 W per minute to his symptom-limited maximum. Arterial blood was sampled every second minute, and intra-arterial blood pressure was recorded from a percutaneously placed brachial artery catheter. Except for an increase in rate, the ECG pattern remained unchanged during exercise. The patient stopped exercise because of shortness of breath and a dry mouth.

TABLE 9.63.1. Selected Respiratory Function Data

Measurement	Predicted	Measured
Age, yr		70
Sex		Male
Height, cm		187
Weight, kg	87	76
Hematocrit, %		47
VC, L	4.69	3.64
IC, L	3.13	2.28
TLC, L	7.39	6.02
FEV_1, L	3.65	2.19
FEV_1/VC, %	78	60
MVV, L/min	140	90
$D_{L}CO$, ml/mm Hg/min	29.4	10.8

TABLE 9.63.2. Selected Exercise Data

Measurement	Predicted	Measured
Peak $\dot{V}O_2$, L/min	2.01	1.32
Maximum HR, beats/min	150	152
		8.7
Maximum O_2 pulse, ml/beat	13.4	
$\Delta\dot{V}O_2/\Delta WR$, ml/min/W	10.3	7.4
AT, L/min	>0.91	0.95
Blood pressure, mmHg (rest, max)		176/86, 227/89
Maximum $\dot{V}E$, L/min		88
Exercise breathing reserve, L/min	>15	2
PaO_2, mmHg (rest, max ex)		64, 52
$P(A-a)O_2$, mmHg (rest, max ex)		43, 68
$P(a-ET)CO_2$, mmHg (rest, max ex)		6, 4
VD/VT (rest, heavy ex)		0.45, 0.48
HCO_3^-, mEq/L (rest, 2-min recov)		27, 19

FIGURE 9.63.1.

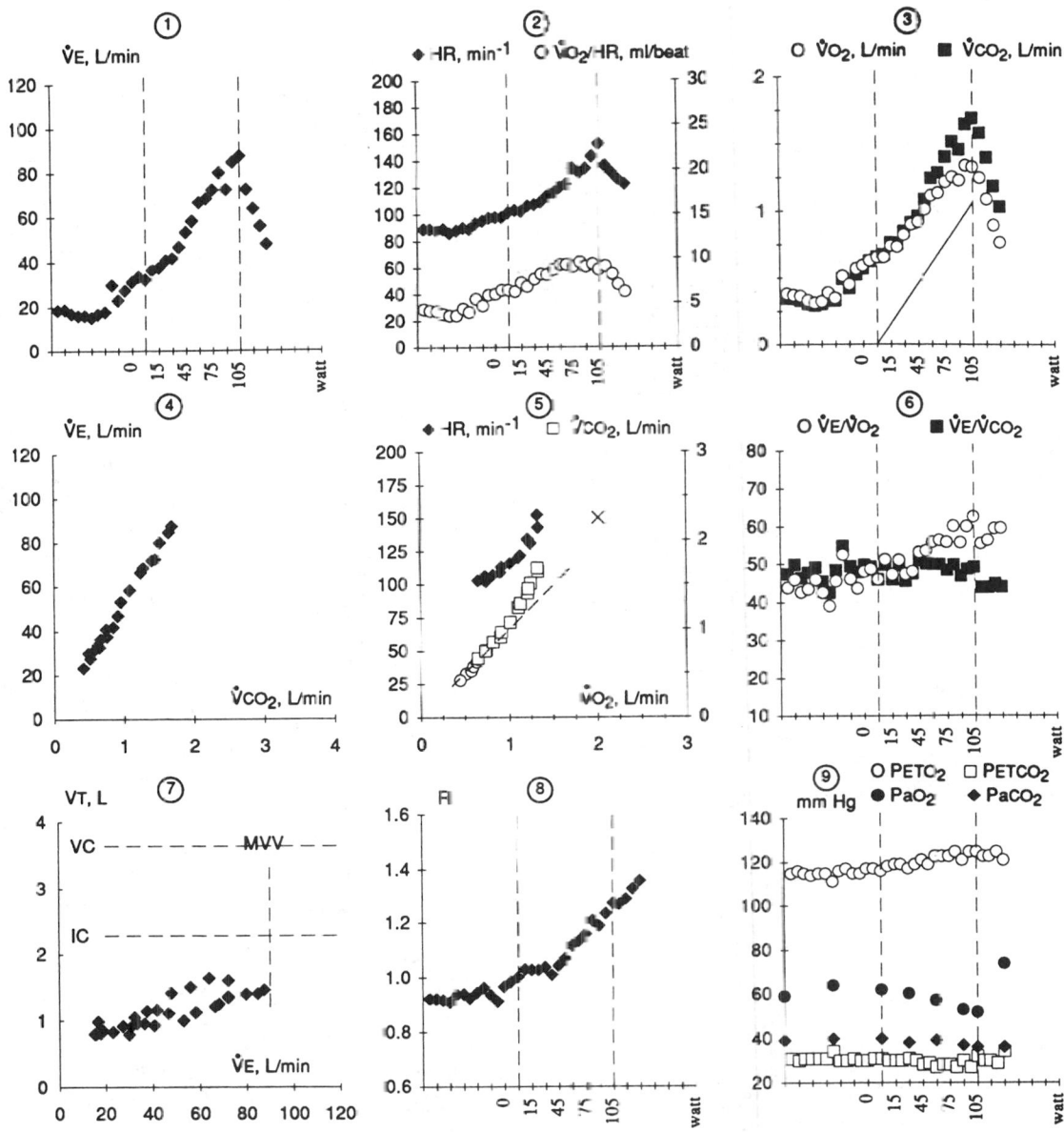

1. Vertical dashed lines in panels 1 to 3 and 6, 8, and 9 indicate the beginning and the end of increasing work period.

2. Unloaded cycling is performed for 3 minutes before the left vertical dashed line.

3. In panel 3, the diagonal line shows the increase of $\dot{V}O_2$ at a slope of 10 ml/min/w.

4. In panel 5, the diagonal dashed line has a slope of 1; the "×" in the upper right is the predicted maximum heart rate and $\dot{V}O_2$ for the subject.

Interpretation

Comments

This case is presented because of its mixed pathophysiologic features. Despite the patient's denial of a history of lung disease, the results of his respiratory function studies indicate that he has mild to moderate obstructive as well as mild restrictive lung disease as evidenced by the reduced FEV_1/VC, total lung capacity, and vital capacity. Accompanying these changes is a marked reduction in diffusing capacity (Table 9.63.1). The resting ECG reflects changes associated with long-standing systemic hypertension, for which he is being treated.

TABLE 9.63.3. Air Breathing

Time min	Work rate watts	BP mmHg	HR min⁻¹	f min⁻¹	V̇E L/min BTPS	V̇CO₂ L/min STPD	V̇O₂ L/min STPD	V̇O₂/HR ml/beat	R	pH	HCO₃⁻ meq/L	PO₂, mmHg ET	a	(A − a)	PCO₂, mmHg ET	a	(a − ET)	V̇E/V̇CO₂	V̇E/V̇O₂	VD/VT
	Rest									7.45	27		59			39				
	Rest	176/86	89	22	18.5	0.35	0.38	4.3	0.92			115			31			48	44	
	Rest		89	22	18.8	0.34	0.37	4.2	0.92			116			30			50	46	
	Rest		88	20	17.0	0.33	0.36	4.1	0.92			115			31			46	43	
	Rest		89	20	16.0	0.30	0.33	3.7	0.91			114			31			48	43	
	Rest		86	20	15.9	0.29	0.31	3.6	0.94			115			31			49	46	
	Rest		88	19	15.2	0.30	0.32	3.6	0.94			115			31			45	42	
	Rest	185/89	90	17	16.7	0.36	0.39	4.3	0.92	7.43	26	111	64	43	34	40	6	42	39	0.45
	Rest		89	22	17.8	0.33	0.35	3.9	0.94			116			30			48	46	
	Unloaded		93	38	30.0	0.49	0.51	5.5	0.96			117			30			55	52	
	Unloaded		95	28	23.1	0.42	0.45	4.7	0.93			115			31			49	46	
	Unloaded		97	30	27.4	0.52	0.57	5.9	0.91			115			30			48	44	
	Unloaded		98	34	31.2	0.57	0.59	6.0	0.97			117			30			50	48	
	Unloaded		98	35	33.5	0.62	0.63	6.4	0.98			117			31			49	48	
	Unloaded	197/89	101	31	32.4	0.65	0.65	6.4	1.00	7.43	26	116	62	48	31	40	9	46	46	0.49
0.5	15		103	38	36.5	0.67	0.65	6.3	1.03			118			30			50	51	
1.0	15		102	33	37.6	0.76	0.74	7.3	1.03			119			30			46	47	
1.5	30		106	44	40.9	0.75	0.73	6.9	1.03			119			30			50	51	
2.0	30	206/86	107	36	41.8	0.85	0.82	7.7	1.04	7.42	24	117	60	53	31	38	7	46	47	0.46
2.5	45		109	42	46.8	0.91	0.90	8.3	1.01			119			30			48	48	
3.0	45		113	53	53.3	0.96	0.92	8.1	1.04			121			28			51	53	
3.5	60		116	52	58.4	1.08	1.01	8.7	1.07			119			29			50	53	
4.0	60	209/86	120	55	66.6	1.24	1.11	9.3	1.12	7.42	25	123	57	57	27	39	12	50	56	0.52
4.5	75		122	55	68.4	1.28	1.13	9.3	1.13			123			28			50	56	
5.0	75		134	53	72.1	1.40	1.21	9.0	1.16			123			28			48	56	
5.5	90		131	57	79.9	1.51	1.25	9.5	1.21			125			27			50	60	
6.0	90	221/92	134	54	72.4	1.45	1.22	9.1	1.19	7.40	23	121	53	65	30	37	7	47	56	0.47
6.5	105		143	60	84.7	1.64	1.33	9.3	1.23			125			27			49	60	
7.0	105	227/89	152	60	87.5	1.68	1.32	8.7	1.27	7.38	21	125	52	68	32	36	4	49	62	0.48
	Recovery		136	45	72.4	1.57	1.24	9.1	1.27			123			30			44	55	
	Recovery		131	39	64.1	1.39	1.08	8.2	1.29			123			30			44	56	
	Recovery		126	37	56.0	1.18	0.89	7.1	1.33			125			29			45	59	
	Recovery	233/98	122	34	48.1	1.03	0.76	6.2	1.36	7.34	19	121	74	47	34	36	2	44	59	0.43

Analysis

Referring to flow chart 1, the peak V̇O₂ is reduced and the anaerobic threshold is borderline normal (Table 9.63.2). See flow chart 3. The breathing reserve is low (branchpoint 3.1), whereas the findings of a high VD/VT, P(a − ET)CO₂, and P(A − a)O₂ support the diagnosis of "lung disease." There is no heart rate reserve, however. The high breathing frequency during most of the exercise period (branchpoint 3.2) is more typical of restrictive than obstructive lung disease, although the patient manifests both disorders at rest. We must also consider the patient's other exercise findings. The plateau in V̇O₂ and O₂ pulse at low values as well as the low ΔV̇O₂/ΔWR, low heart rate reserve, and progressive hypoxemia are all characteristic of pulmonary vascular disease secondary to interstitial lung disease. See flow charts 4 (abnormal pulmonary circulation) and 5 (pulmonary vascular disease) for details.

Conclusion

Pulmonary vascular disease with reduced exercise performance, probably secondary to an interstitial lung disease.

Case 64 Pulmonary Arterio-venous Fistulae

Clinical Findings

This 26-year-old man with multiple pulmonary arterio-venous malformations and recurrent brain abscesses was referred for exercise testing to assess his pathophysiologic status before undergoing embolization therapy to his arterio-venous fistulae. He denied shortness of breath and, until recently, had worked as an aerobics instructor. The patient was well developed, muscular, and had no rales or murmurs on examination of the chest, but had marked finger clubbing and cyanosis. A recent study while the patient was at rest breathing oxygen showed a calculated right to left shunt of 53%.

Exercise Findings

The patient performed exercise on a cycle ergometer. He pedalled at 60 rpm without an added load for 3 minutes. The work rate was then increased continuously at a rate of 20 W per minute to tolerance. Blood was sampled every second minute, and intra-arterial pressure was recorded from a percutaneously placed brachial artery catheter. Heart rate and rhythm were continuously monitored; 12-lead ECGs were obtained during rest, exercise, and recovery. The patient appeared to give an excellent effort and stopped exercise because of general and leg fatigue, without dyspnea or chest pain. No arrhythmias or ischemic changes were noted on ECGs.

TABLE 9.64.1.   Selected Respiratory Function Data

Measurement	Predicted	Measured
Age, yr		26
Sex		Male
Height, cm		189
Weight, kg	87	64
Hemoglobin, g/100 ml		21.8
VC, L	5.55	4.18
IC, L	3.70	2.94
FEV₁, L	4.50	3.95
FEV₁/VC, %	81	94
MVV, L/min		
Direct	183	169
Indirect	180	158

TABLE 9.64.2.   Selected Exercise Data

Measurement	Predicted	Measured
Peak $\dot{V}O_2$, L/min	3.12	2.19
Maximum HR, beats/min	194	160
		13.7
Maximum O₂ pulse, ml/beat	16.1	
$\Delta\dot{V}O_2/\Delta WR$, ml/min/W	10.3	9.9
AT, L/min	>1.28	1.5
Blood pressure, mmHg (rest, max)		144/84, 180/90
Maximum $\dot{V}E$, L/min		123
Exercise breathing reserve, L/min	>15	35
SaO₂, % (rest, max ex)		76, 64
PaO₂, mmHg (rest, max ex)		39, 39
P(a − a)O₂, mmHg (rest, max ex)		74, 76
P(a − ET)CO₂, mmHg (rest, max ex)		9, 15
VE/VT (rest, max ex)		0.42, 0.52
HCO₃⁻, mEq/L (rest, 2-min recov)		22, 16

FIGURE 9.64.1.

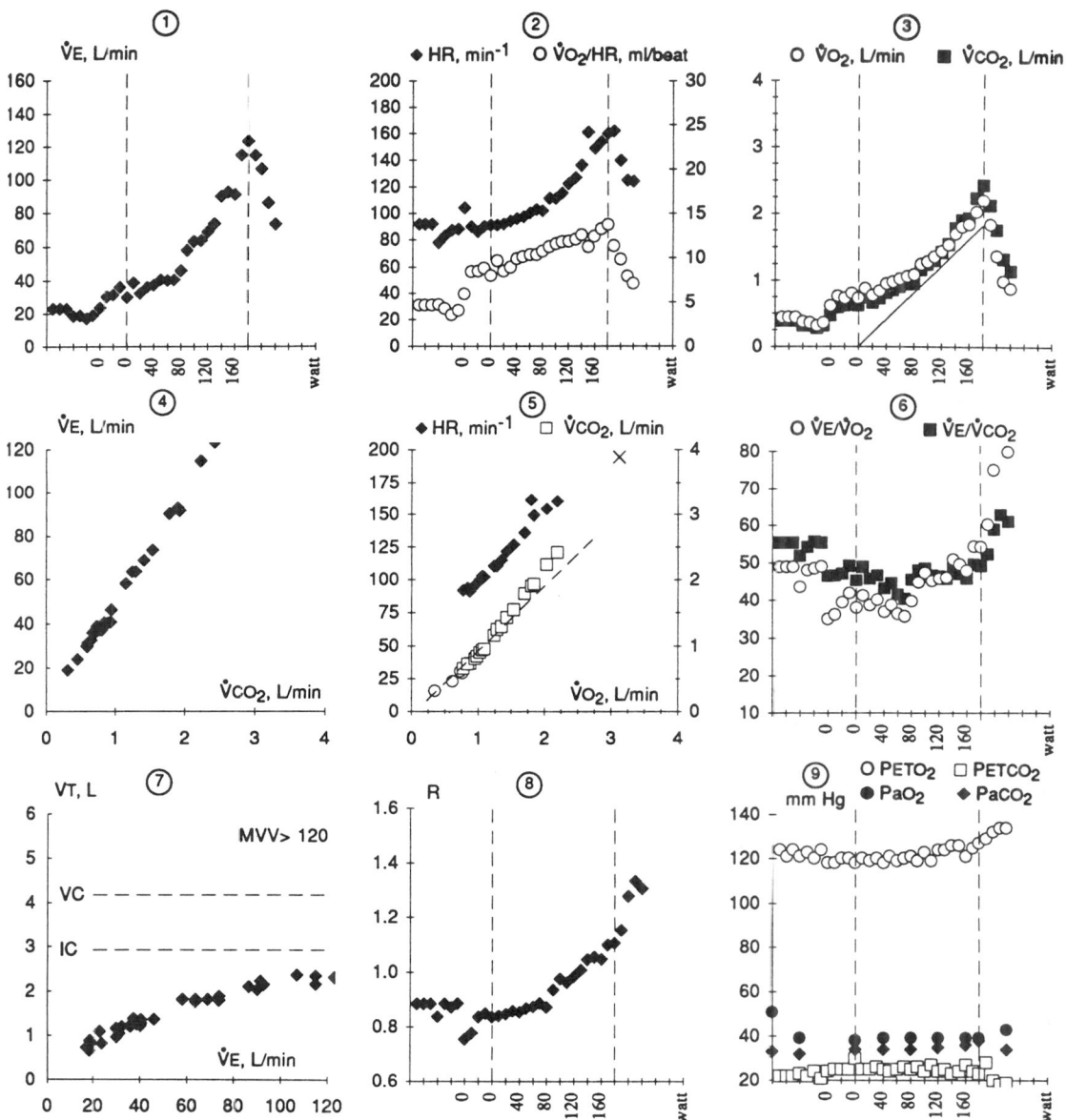

1. Vertical dashed lines in panels 1 to 3 and 6, 8, and 9 indicate the beginning and the end of increasing work period.

2. Unloaded cycling is performed for 3 minutes before the left vertical dashed line.

3. In panel 3, the diagonal line shows the increase of $\dot{V}O_2$ at a slope of 10 ml/min/w.

4. In panel 5, the diagonal dashed line has a slope of 1; the "x" in the upper right is the predicted maximum heart rate and $\dot{V}O_2$ for the subject.

TABLE 9.64.3. Air Breathing

Time min	Work rate watts	BP mmHg	HR min⁻¹	f min⁻¹	$\dot{V}_E$ L/min BTPS	$\dot{V}_{CO_2}$ L/min STPD	$\dot{V}_{O_2}$ L/min STPD	$\dot{V}_{O_2}$/HR ml/beat	R	pH	HCO₃ meq/L	P$_{O_2}$ ET	a	(A−a)	P$_{CO_2}$ ET	a	(a−ET)	$\dot{V}_E$/$\dot{V}_{CO_2}$	$\dot{V}_E$/$\dot{V}_{O_2}$	V_D/V_T
	Rest									7.43	22	51			33					
	Rest	92	21	22.3	0.38	0.43	4.7	0.88			24			22			55	49	
	Rest	92	21	22.3	0.38	0.43	4.7	0.88			21			22			55	49	
	Rest	92	21	22.3	0.38	0.43	4.7	0.88			24			22			55	49	
	Rest	78	28	18.5	0.31	0.37	4.7	0.54	7.45	22	21	39	74	23	32	9	52	44	0.42
	Rest	83	21	18.6	0.31	0.35	4.2	0.85			23			22			54	48	
	Rest	87	23	17.0	0.27	0.31	3.6	0.87			20			24			56	49	
	Unloaded		88	23	19.1	0.31	0.35	4.0	0.88			24			21			55	49	
	Unloaded		104	29	23.8	0.46	0.61	5.9	0.75			18			24			46	35	
	Unloaded		90	31	30.1	0.59	0.76	8.4	0.78			18			25			47	36	
	Unloaded		86	30	31.3	0.61	0.73	8.5	0.84			20			25			47	39	
	Unloaded		90	30	36.0	0.38	0.80	8.9	0.85			20			25			49	42	
	Unloaded	144/84	91	26	29.9	0.31	0.73	8.0	0.84	7.43	22	18	38	73	30	34	4	45	38	0.41
0.5	10		91	31	38.8	0.74	0.88	9.7	0.84			20			25			49	41	
1.0	20		92	27	32.4	0.36	0.78	8.5	0.85			19			25			46	39	
1.5	30		94	29	36.1	0.72	0.84	8.9	0.86			20			26			47	40	
2.0	40	150/90	96	27	37.2	0.31	0.95	9.9	0.86	7.42	22	18	39	72	25	34	9	43	37	0.39
2.5	50		97	30	40.4	0.35	0.98	10.1	0.87			21			24			45	39	
3.0	60		100	33	40.2	0.90	1.03	10.3	0.87			19			25			42	36	
3.5	70		103	32	40.6	0.94	1.06	10.3	0.89			20			26			40	36	
4.0	80	162/90	102	34	46.2	0.95	1.09	10.7	0.87	7.42	22	21	39	73	25	34	9	46	40	0.42
4.5	90		111	32	58.2	1.16	1.24	11.2	0.94			19			26			48	45	
5.0	100		111	36	63.6	1.25	1.28	11.5	0.98			23			24			48	47	
5.5	110		115	35	63.7	1.30	1.35	11.7	0.96			19			27			47	45	
6.0	120	174/96	122	38	69.0	1.42	1.44	11.8	0.99	7.33	20	24	39	76	24	35	11	46	46	0.45
6.5	130		127	39	73.7	1.54	1.53	12.0	1.01			24			25			46	46	
7.0	140		135	44	90.2	1.76	1.70	12.5	1.05			26			23			49	51	
7.5	150		161	43	92.9	1.90	1.80	11.2	1.06			26			24			47	50	
8.0	160	180/90	149	41	91.5	1.93	1.84	12.3	1.05	7.36	20	21	39	76	27	33	9	46	48	0.46
8.5	170		154	53	115.0	2.23	2.03	13.2	1.10			25			24			50	54	
9.0	180	180/96	160	53	123.3	2.42	2.19	13.7	1.11	7.31	19	27	39	76	23	33	15	49	54	0.52
	Recovery		162	49	115.0	2.12	1.84	11.4	1.15			29			28			52	60	
	Recovery		140	45	106.9	1.75	1.37	9.8	1.28			32			20			59	75	
	Recovery		125	41	86.4	1.32	0.99	7.9	1.33			34			18			63	84	
	Recovery	156/84	124	41	73.7	1.15	0.38	7.1	1.31	7.30	16	34	43	79	19	34	15	61	80	0.56

Interpretation

Comments

Resting respiratory function studies showed restrictive lung disease with good ventilatory ability. The patient was thin, cyanotic, and polycythemic. Resting arterial blood analysis showed hypoxemia and a chronic respiratory alkalosis.

Analysis

Referring to flow chart 1, the peak $\dot{V}_{O_2}$ is low, but the anaerobic threshold is normal (Table 9.64.2). Also striking are the severe hypoxemia, low $P_{ET}CO_2$, and high V_D/V_T. We are directed through branch-points 1.1, 1.2, and 1.3 to flow chart 3, which leads us through branchpoints 3.1 and 3.3 to "poor effort or musculo-skeletal disorder," which does not fit well with the patient's known findings. Using flow chart 4, the normal breathing reserve (branchpoint 4.1) and the high $\dot{V}_E/\dot{V}_{CO_2}$ at the AT (branchpoint 4.3), we are in the "abnormal pulmonary circulation pathophysiology" where the patient meets most of the criteria. If we had used flow chart 5, we would have arrived through branchpoints 5.1 and 5.3 at branchpoint 5.6 at "pulmonary vascular disease." The sustained reduction in arterial oxyhemoglobin saturation during exercise suggests a large right to left shunt.

The finding of a lower than predicted O_2 pulse in the presence of polycythemia is of interest, especially in view of the high oxyhemoglobin capacity of the blood (30.8 ml/100 ml versus the normal 21 ml/100 ml). Because of the low arterial oxyhemoglobin saturation, arterial content is only approximately 20 ml/100 ml. Likely, mixed venous oxyhemoglobin saturation is normal, resulting in a higher than normal oxyhemoglobin content (because of the polycythemia). Thus, there is no evidence of a reduced stroke volume or cardiac output. Much of the right ventricular output bypasses the aerated alveoli. In order to compensate for the venous blood that bypasses the gas exchange vessels in the lungs, the blood that does go through the pulmonary capillaries must be exposed to alveoli with lower P_{CO_2} than that of the arterial blood. Because the Pa_{CO_2} setpoint is about 35 mmHg, the Pa_{CO_2} and $P_{ET_{CO_2}}$ values must be very low as shown in panel 9 of Figure 9.64.1 , and the V_D/V_T values are much increased as work rate increases (Table 9.64.3) despite probably no real parenchymal disease.

Conclusion

The patient has a large right to left shunt at rest and during exercise because of pulmonary arteriovenous malformations. The high V_D/V_T and positive $P(a - _{ET})_{CO_2}$ values indicate that ventilation is relatively ineffective in removing CO_2 from the blood, consistent with a high fraction of right ventricular output bypassing the alveolar capillaries. In this patient, the wide $P(_A - a)_{O_2}$, positive $P(a - _{ET})_{CO_2}$, and high V_D/V_T which increase with exercise, indicate a large right to left shunt rather than the ordinary maldistribution of ventilation found in lung diseases without a right to left shunt.

Case 65 Poor Effort

Clinical Findings

This 37-year-old male electrician was referred for evaluation because of his 5-year exposure to asbestos while working in a shipyard. He stated that he had had a daily productive cough for a year and that he could only climb 6 or 7 steps before he had to stop to catch his breath. He stated that he had smoked approximately half a package of cigarettes daily for the last 13 years. He denied other problems and took no medications. Physical and chest roentgenographic examinations were normal.

Exercise Findings

The patient performed exercise on a cycle ergometer. He pedalled at 60 rpm without an added load for 3 minutes. The work rate was then increased 25 W per minute to his symptom-limited maximum. Blood was sampled every second minute, and intra-arterial blood pressure was recorded from a percutaneously passed brachial artery catheter. The patient was apprehensive and was unhappy about having a test performed. He breathed rapidly and shallowly on the mouthpiece despite reassurance and encouragement. He slowed his pedalling frequency after 2 minutes of incremental work and stopped pedalling at a work rate of 100 W, complaining of generalized fatigue, tingling in the hands, and lightheadedness. These symptoms resolved within 5 minutes. After an hour of rest, explanation, and encouragement to breathe at a slower rate, the test was repeated using an increment of 20 W/min. This time, the patient began to hyperventilate as soon as exercise began. He stopped cycling at a work rate of 60 W with a heart rate of 99. Complete data from the first test and selected data from the second test are presented. Resting and exercise ECGs were normal.

TABLE 9.65.1.   Selected Respiratory Function Data

Measurement	Predicted	Measured
Age, yr		37
Sex		Male
Height, cm		170
Weight, kg	80	87
Hematocrit, %		46
VC, L	4.52	4.20
IC, L	3.01	3.07
TLC, L	6.29	5.29
FEV, L	3.64	3.66
FEV/VC, %	81	87
MVV, L/min	152	129
D_LCO, ml/mm Hg/min	29.9	24.7

TABLE 9.65.2.   Selected Exercise Data

Measurement	Predicted	Measured
Peak $\dot{V}O_2$, L/min	3.00	1.43
Maximum HR, beats/min	183	112
Maximum O_2 pulse, ml/beat	16.4	12.8
$\Delta\dot{V}O_2/\Delta WR$, ml/min/W	10.3	10.1
AT, L/min	>1.26	Indeterminate
Blood pressure, mmHg (rest, max ex)		146/93, 174/105
Maximum $\dot{V}E$, L/min		64
Exercise breathing reserve, L/min	>15	65 nn
PaO_2, mmHg (rest, max ex)		89, 117
$P(A - a)O_2$ mmHg (rest, max ex)		6, 7
$P(a - ET)CO_2$, mmHg (rest, max ex)		0, −3
VD/VT (rest, max ex)		0.37, 0.19
HCO_3, mEq/L (rest, recov)		23, 20
Carboxyhemoglobin, rest, %		6.5

TABLE 9.65.3. Air Breathing

Time min	Work rate watts	BP mmHg	HR min^{-1}	f min^{-1}	$\dot{V}_E$ L/min BTPS	$\dot{V}_{CO_2}$ L/min STPD	$\dot{V}_{O_2}$ L/min STPD	$\dfrac{\dot{V}_{O_2}}{HR}$ ml/beat	R	pH	HCO$_3^-$ meq/L	P_{O_2}, mmHg ET	a	(A − a)	P_{CO_2}, mmHg ET	a	(a − ET)	$\dfrac{\dot{V}_E}{\dot{V}_{CO_2}}$	$\dfrac{\dot{V}_E}{\dot{V}_{O_2}}$	$\dfrac{V_D}{V_T}$
	Rest	146/93								7.42	23		95			36				
	Rest		72	37	20.9	0.41	0.39	5.4	1.05			117			33			43	46	
	Rest		73	31	15.1	0.29	0.32	4.4	0.91			109			36			43	39	
	Rest		73	32	9.8	0.16	0.21	2.9	0.76			104			38			44	34	
	Rest	153/102	73	29	11.3	0.20	0.32	4.4	0.63	7.41	23	97	89	6	37	37	0	44	28	0.37
	Rest		74	26	12.8	0.27	0.40	5.4	0.68			95			38			39	26	
	Rest		77	31	15.8	0.33	0.46	6.0	0.72			96			38			40	29	
	Unloaded		82	33	30.3	0.72	0.69	8.4	1.04			115			32			38	40	
	Unloaded		88	42	33.3	0.71	0.61	6.9	1.16			122			30			42	49	
	Unloaded		90	49	45.5	0.90	0.68	7.6	1.32			127			28			46	61	
	Unloaded		85	50	45.7	0.88	0.67	7.9	1.31			127			27			47	62	
	Unloaded		85	57	39.6	0.68	0.51	6.0	1.33			129			25			51	68	
	Unloaded		85	50	33.0	0.58	0.49	5.8	1.18			126			25			50	59	
	Unloaded	168/105	85	53	38.7	0.66	0.54	6.4	1.22	7.52	21	128	122	6	24	26	2	52	63	0.32
	Unloaded		83	54	45.6	0.79	0.65	7.8	1.22			129			23			52	63	
0.5	25		88	54	47.2	0.79	0.65	7.4	1.22			128			23			54	66	
1.0	25		89	56	60.6	0.99	0.79	8.9	1.25			127			24			56	71	
1.5	50		94	59	62.8	1.06	0.92	9.8	1.15			130			21			55	63	
2.0	50	168/102	94	54	54.7	0.97	0.95	10.1	1.02	7.56	19	126	123	5	23	22	−1	52	53	0.22
2.5	75		103	51	61.9	1.13	1.09	10.6	1.04			123			25			51	53	
3.0	75		103	51	62.9	1.19	1.15	11.2	1.03			126			23			49	51	
3.5	100		110	46	53.2	1.13	1.21	11.0	0.93			114			30			44	41	
4.0	100	174/105	112	46	64.0	1.39	1.43	12.8	0.97	7.52	20	120	117	7	28	25	−3	43	42	0.19
	Recovery		96	47	52.5	1.13	1.20	12.5	0.94			119			28			43	40	
	Recovery		86	46	45.4	0.91	0.90	10.5	1.01			122			27			46	46	
	Recovery		79	52	46.6	0.77	0.61	7.7	1.26			130			22			55	69	
	Recovery	168/108	78	43	34.9	0.55	0.45	5.8	1.22	7.54	20	130	126	3	22	24	2	57	69	0.33

TABLE 9.65.4. Selected Measures Early in Second Study

Time (min)	Work Rate	f (/min)	$\dot{V}_E$ (L/min)	R	pH	Pa_{CO_2} (mmHg)	HCO$_3^-$ (mEq/L)
0					7.42	34	22
0.5	Rest	32	26.6	1.08			
1	Rest	29	16.6	1.00			
1.5	Rest	22	17.7	0.97			
2	Rest	22	12.2	0.77	7.45	29	20
2.5	Rest	23	12.3	0.71			
3	Rest	25	18.3	0.80			
3.5	Unloaded	35	30.9	0.93			
4	Unloaded	39	34.9	1.07			
4.5	Unloaded	37	32.6	0.95			
5	Unloaded	46	44.5	1.08			
5.5	Unloaded	51	55.7	1.18			
6	Unloaded	49	51.0	1.14	7.57	21	19

Figure 9.65.1.

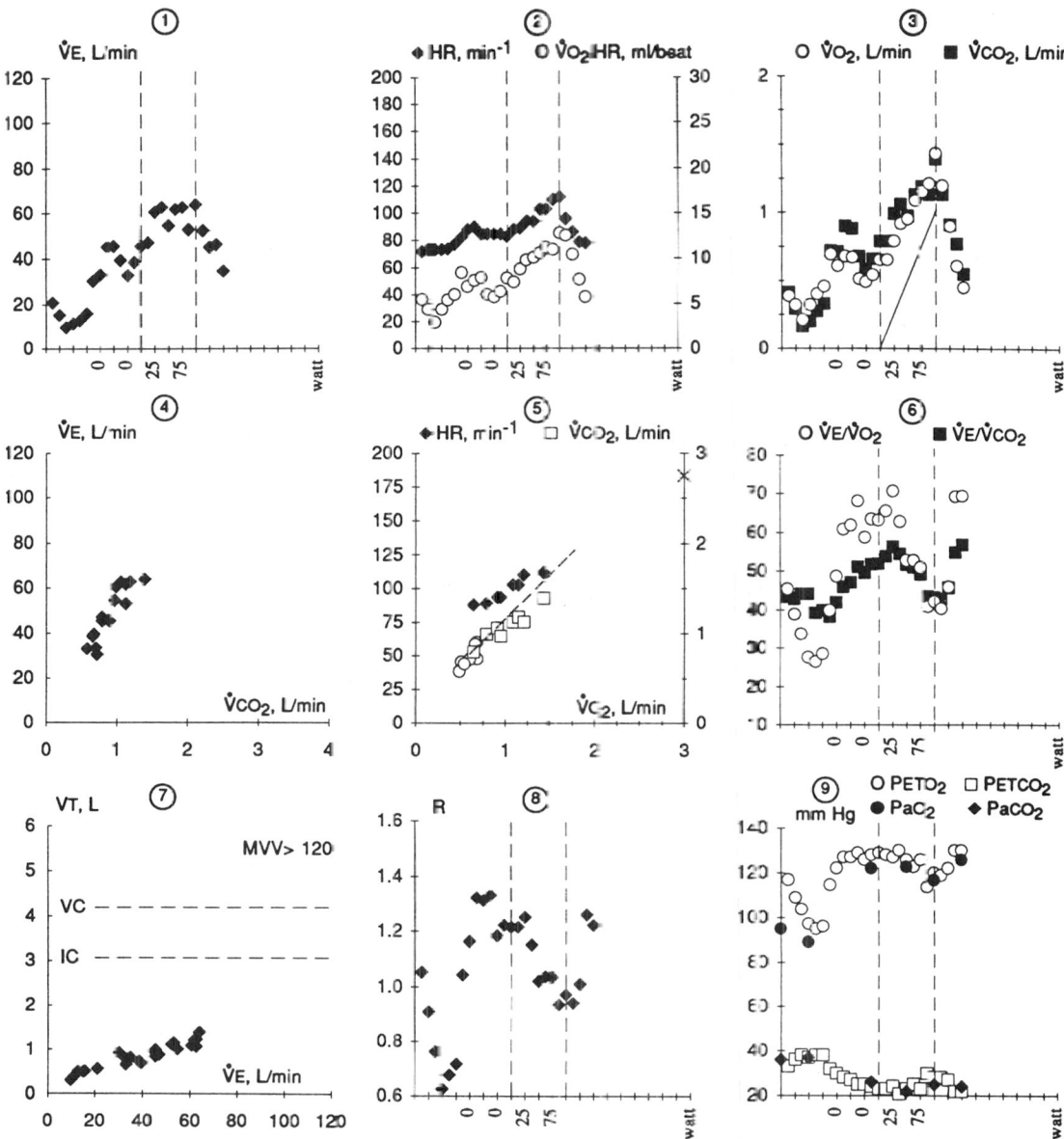

1. Vertical dashed lines in panels 1 to 3 and 6, 8, and 9 indicate the beginning and the end of increasing work period.

2. Unloaded cycling is performed for 3 minutes before the left vertical dashed line.

3. In panel 3, the diagonal line shows the increase of $\dot{V}O_2$ at a slope of 10 ml/min/w.

4. In panel 5, the diagonal dashed line has a slope of 1; the "x" in the upper right is the predicted maximum heart rate and $\dot{V}O_2$ for the subject.

Interpretation

Comments

Resting respiratory function was normal.

Analysis

Referring to flow chart 1, the peak $\dot{V}O_2$ was low, and the anaerobic threshold was indeterminate (Table 9.65.2). This leads us to flow chart 5. The indices of ventilation-perfusion matching at maximum work rate are normal (branchpoint 5.1). The heart rate reserve is high (branchpoint 5.2), and $\Delta\dot{V}O_2/\Delta WR$ is normal (branchpoint 5.5). This leads to the diagnosis of poor effort. The normal ECG, high breathing reserve, minimal decline in HCO_3^-, and R < 1.0 at exercise cessation, all signify the absence of organic cardiovascular or lung disease. We can also conclude that the patient gave a poor effort since he did not develop the metabolic acidosis that should be expected with a reasonable exercise effort.

We were unable to encourage him to improve his performance when tested an hour later. The abrupt hyperventilation and respiratory alkalosis early in the two studies ($Paco_2$ decreased from 37 to 22 in first study and 34 to 21 in second study, Tables 9.65.3 and 9.65.4) are typical of patients with anxiety or voluntary hyperventilation. An irregular breathing pattern reflected in the wild swings in gas exchange ratio shown in panel 8 of Figure 9.65.1 is more consistent with volitional lack of cooperation.

Conclusion

This case study shows poor effort on the part of the patient. There is no evidence of abnormal gas exchange, ventilatory limitation, metabolic acidosis or cardiovascular limitation. The symptoms and findings are typical of acute respiratory alkalosis of variable degree. Because of the high ventilatory equivalents that might suggest a gas exchange abnormality, blood gas analyses are helpful in excluding ventilation-perfusion mismatching.

Case 66 Poor Effort

Clinical Findings

This 59-year-old shipyard worker had been made aware of an abnormality in his chest x-ray 1 year prior to this evaluation. Retrospectively, he felt that he had had some shortness of breath for 2 years when jogging or climbing stairs. He had smoked cigarettes for 20 years, until age 35. Results of physical, laboratory, and roentgenographic examinations were normal except for prostatic enlargement and extensive pleural calcification.

Exercise Findings

The patient performed exercise on a cycle ergometer. He pedalled at 60 rpm without added load for 3 minutes. The work rate was then increased 20 W per minute to his symptom-limited maximum. Arterial blood was sampled every second minute, and intra-arterial blood pressure was recorded from a percutaneously placed brachial artery catheter. The patient pedalled irregularly during the test. He stopped pedalling, complaining of shortness of breath and leg fatigue, and stated he could go no further. Resting and exercise ECG were normal.

TABLE 9.66.1.   Selected Respiratory Function Data

Measurement	Predicted	Measured
Age, yr		59
Sex		Male
Height, cm		173
Weight, kg	73	72
Hematocrit, %		44
VC, L	3.65	3.05
IC, L	2.44	2.44
TLC, L	5.57	4.93
FEV$_1$, L	2.87	2.49
FEV$_1$/VC, %	79	82
MVV, L/min	121	110
D$_{LCO}$, ml/mm Hg/min	22.6	24.6

TABLE 9.66.2.   Selected Exercise Data

Measurement	Predicted	Measured
Maximum $\dot{V}O_2$, L/min	2.13	1.08
Maximum HR, beats/min	161	110
Maximum O_2 pulse, ml/beat	13.2	9.8
AT, L/min	>0.94	indeterminate
Blood pressure, mmHg (rest, max)		135/78, 144/78
Maximum $\dot{V}E$, L/min		30
Exercise breathing reserve, L/min	>15	80
PaCO_2, mmHg (rest, max ex)		98, 96
P(A − a)O_2, mmHg (rest, max ex)		0, 10
P(a − ET)CO_2, mmHg (rest, max ex)		0, −3
$\dot{V}D/VT$ (rest, heavy ex)		0.35, 0.36
HCO$_3^-$, mEq/L (rest, 2-min recov)		25, 24

FIGURE 9.66.1.

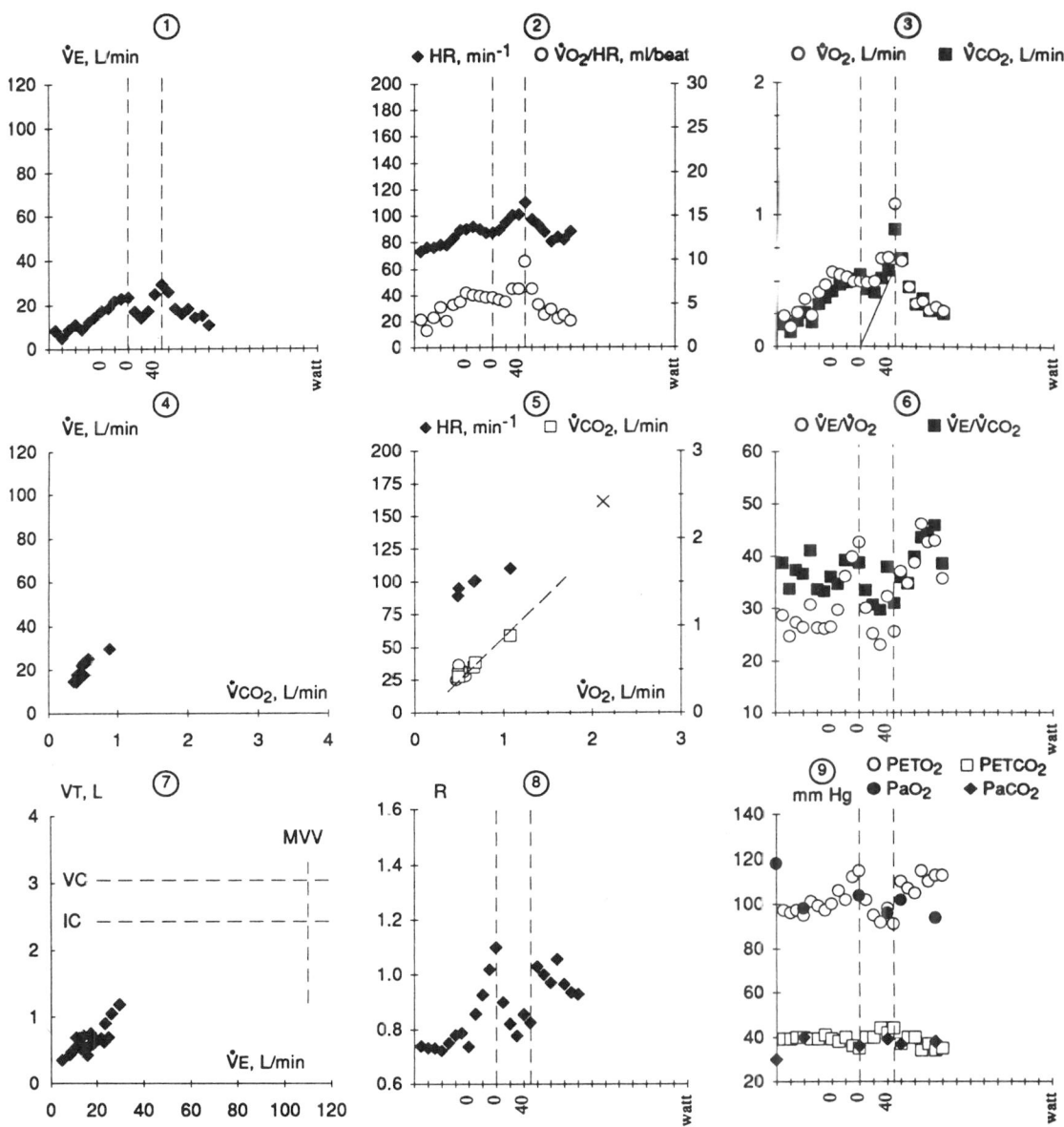

1. Vertical dashed lines in panels 1 to 3 and 6, 8, and 9 indicate the beginning and the end of increasing work period.

2. Unloaded cycling is performed for 3 minutes before the left vertical dashed line.

3. In panel 3, the diagonal line shows the increase of $\dot{V}O_2$ at a slope of 10 ml/min/w.

4. In panel 5, the diagonal dashed line has a slope of 1; the "x" in the upper right is the predicted maximum heart rate and $\dot{V}O_2$ for the subject.

TABLE 9.66.3. Air Breathing

Time min	Work rate watts	BP mmHg	HR min^{-1}	f min^{-1}	$\dot{V}_E$ L/min BTPS	$\dot{V}_{CO_2}$ L/min STPD	$\dot{V}_{O_2}$ L/min STPD	$\dot{V}_{O_2}$/HR ml/beat	R	pH	HCO$_3^-$ meq/L	P$_{O_2}$ mmHg ET	a	(A − a)	P$_{CO_2}$ mmHg ET	a	(a − ET)	$\dot{V}_E$/$\dot{V}_{CO_2}$	$\dot{V}_E$/$\dot{V}_{O_2}$	V$_D$/V$_T$
	Rest	135/78								7.51	24		118			30				
	Rest		73	19	8.2	0.17	0.23	3.2	0.74			97			39			39	29	
	Rest		76	14	4.9	0.11	0.15	2.0	0.73			96			39			34	25	
	Rest		73	19	8.7	0.19	0.26	3.4	0.73			97			40			37	27	
	Rest	132/78	73	20	11.2	0.26	0.36	4.6	0.72	7.41	25	95	98	0	40	40	0	37	26	0.35
	Rest		73	19	9.0	0.18	0.24	3.1	0.75			101			39			41	31	
	Rest		83	18	12.3	0.32	0.41	4.9	0.73			99			39			34	26	
	Unloaded		89	26	14.5	0.37	0.47	5.3	0.79			97			41			33	26	
	Unloaded		90	29	17.6	0.42	0.57	6.3	0.74			100			39			36	27	
	Unloaded		92	27	18.6	0.47	0.55	6.0	0.85			106			38			35	30	
	Unloaded		90	32	21.9	0.49	0.53	5.9	0.92			102			40			39	36	
	Unloaded		87	37	23.1	0.51	0.50	5.7	1.02			112			36			39	40	
	Unloaded	144/78	87	26	23.5	0.55	0.50	5.7	1.10	7.43	23	115	104	13	35	36	1	39	43	0.34
0.5	20		89	29	17.2	0.44	0.49	5.5	0.90			102			40			33	30	
1.0	20		95	20	14.3	0.41	0.50	5.3	0.82			95			40			31	25	
1.5	40		100	23	17.4	0.52	0.67	6.7	0.78			92			44			30	23	
2.0	40	144/78	101	36	25.0	0.58	0.68	6.7	0.85	7.41	24	98	96	10	42	39	−3	38	32	0.36
2.5	60		110	25	29.7	0.89	1.08	9.8	0.82			91			44			31	26	
	Recovery	150/78	97	25	26.2	0.67	0.65	6.7	1.03	7.41	23	110	102	12	37	37	0	36	37	0.32
	Recovery		93	31	18.6	0.46	0.46	4.9	1.00			107			40			35	35	
	Recovery		88	38	16.0	0.32	0.33	3.8	0.97			105			40			40	39	
	Recovery		81	28	18.5	0.37	0.35	4.3	1.06			115			34			44	46	
	Recovery		84	30	14.5	0.27	0.28	3.3	0.96			110			37			44	43	
	Recovery	132/84	82	30	15.4	0.28	0.30	3.7	0.93	7.4	24	113	94	16	34	38	4	46	43	0.42
	Recovery		88	16	11.0	0.25	0.27	3.1	0.93			113			35			39	36	

Interpretation

Comments

Resting respiratory function (Table 9.66.1) is within normal limits.

Analysis

Referring to flow chart 1, the peak $\dot{V}_{O_2}$ is significantly reduced and the anaerobic threshold is indeterminate (Table 9.66.2). See flow chart 5. The resting V$_D$/V$_T$ is normal, but it does not decrease appropriately during exercise. Only light exercise was performed, however, and the lack of a decrease might be spurious owing to the low tidal volume, tachypnea, and low work rate performed (Table 9.66.3). Because P(a − ET)$_{CO_2}$ and P(A − a)$_{O_2}$ are normal (branchpoint 5.1), we conclude that the indices of ventilation relative to perfusion are normal. Heart rate reserve (branchpoint 5.2) is high and the $\Delta\dot{V}_{O_2}$/ΔWR (branchpoint 5.5) could not be determined because the subject performed increasing work rate exercise for only two minutes. However, the breathing reserve as well as the heart rate reserve are high (Table 9.66.2). These findings place the patient in the diagnostic category of poor effort. The following findings are consistent with this diagnosis: (1) the normal exercise ECG; (2) R of only 0.82 at the peak $\dot{V}_{O_2}$; (3) minimal decline in HCO$_3^-$ induced by the exercise (Table 9.66.3); and the previously mentioned high heart rate reserve, high breathing reserve, normal blood gases, and normal indices of ventilation-perfusion mismatching.

Conclusion

This patient made a poor effort.

Case 67 Acute Hyperventilation and Anxiety in a Moderately Obese Man

Clincial Findings

This 56-year-old shipyard worker complained of progressive dyspnea on exertion, evident when climbing two flights of stairs. He had also noted anterior chest pain with exertion, relieved by rest, associated with dyspnea and diaphoresis but not with palpitations, lightheadedness, syncope, or numbness. He had stopped smoking 20 years previously after 20 pack years. He took no medications but had been told that he had hypertension several years ago. Physical examination and resting ECG were normal. Chest x-ray showed mild pleural thickening bilaterally.

Exercise Findings

After percutaneous insertion of a brachial artery catheter, while being positioned on the cycle ergometer, the patient became lightheaded and syncopal. The patient was placed on a gurney in the reverse Trendelenburg position. Continuous monitoring revealed a transient sinus bradycardia as low as 25 with normal blood pressure. The bradycardia lasted only a few minutes. After 15 minutes he felt well and was able to exercise. He pedalled at 60 rpm without added load for 3 minutes. The work rate was then increased 15 W every minute. Arterial blood was sampled every second minute, and intra-arterial blood pressure was recorded from the brachial artery catheter. Mild chest pain began at 45 W; exercise was stopped at 90 W because of the patient's continuing and increasing chest pain, which was typical of his usual symptom. There were no ST abnormalities nor was there arrhythmia during or after exercise.

TABLE 9.67.1. Selected Respiratory Function Data

Measurement	Predicted	Measured
Age, yr		56
Sex		Male
Height, cm		172
Weight, kg	75	98
Hematocrit, %		46
VC, L	4.10	3.16
IC, L	2.74	2.55
TLC, L	6.17	4.77
FEV_1, L	3.23	2.78
FEV_1/VC, %	79	88
MVV, L/min	137	98
$D_{L}CO$, ml/mm Hg/min	26.3	20.9

TABLE 9.67.2. Selected Exercise Data

Measurement	Predicted	Measured
Peak $\dot{V}O_2$, L/min	2.38	1.51
Maximum HR, beats/min	164	130
Maximum O_2 pulse, ml/beat	14.5	11.6
$\Delta\dot{V}O_2/\Delta WR$, ml/min/W	10.3	9.3
AT, L/min	>1.05	1.4
Blood pressure, mmHg (rest, max)		168/96, 228/111
Maximum $\dot{V}E$, L/min		79
Exercise breathing reserve, L/min	>15	19
PaO_2, mmHg (rest, max ex)		112, 100
P(A − a)O_2, mmHg (rest, max ex)		21, 25
P(a − ET)CO_2, mmHg (rest, max ex)		2, 0
VD/VT (rest, heavy ex)		0.30, 0.24
HCO_3^-, mEq/L (rest, 2-min recov)		24, 20

FIGURE 9.67.1.

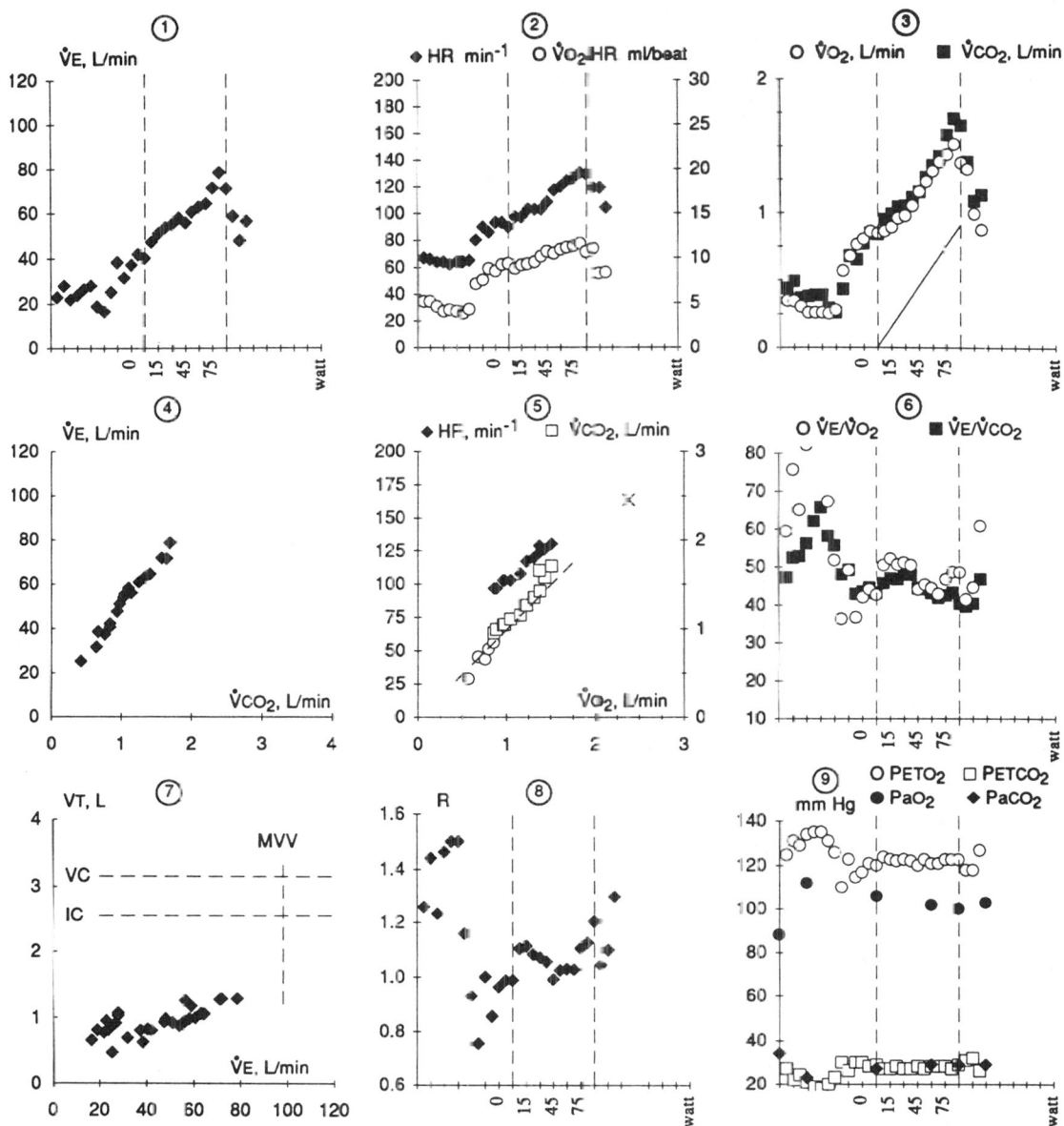

1. Vertical dashed lines in panels 1 to 3 and 6, 8, and 9 indicate the beginning and the end of increasing work period.

2. Unloaded cycling is performed for 3 minutes before the left vertical dashed line.

3. In panel 3, the diagonal line shows the increase of $\dot{V}O_2$ at a slope of 10 ml/min/W.

4. In panel 5, the diagonal dashed line has a slope of 1; the "x" in the upper right is the predicted maximum heart rate and $\dot{V}O_2$ for the subject.

Interpretation
Comments

Resting respiratory function studies reveal the patient to have a restrictive defect of the type generally seen with obesity (normal inspiratory capacity, but reduced expiratory reserve volume) (Table 9.67.1). The patient is, in fact, 23 kg overweight. Resting ECG is normal. As the patient was getting ready to cycle, he became lightheaded and hypotensive. His blood pressure decreased and he developed a marked bradycardia consistent with a vasovagal reaction. When placed in a supine position, the patient's pulse and blood pressure became normal and he resumed his position on the cycle ergometer for testing; however, he acutely hyperventilated at rest,

TABLE 9.67.3. Air Breathing

Time min	Work rate watts	BP mmHg	HR min⁻¹	f min⁻¹	V̇E L/min BTPS	V̇CO₂ L/min STPD	V̇O₂ L/min STPD	V̇O₂/HR ml/beat	R	pH	HCO₃⁻ meq/L	PO₂, mmHg ET	a	(A − a)	PCO₂, mmHg ET	a	(a − ET)	V̇E/V̇CO₂	V̇E/V̇O₂	VD/VT
	Rest	168/96								7.47	24		88			34				
	Rest		67	24	22.8	0.44	0.35	5.2	1.26			125			27			47	59	
	Rest		66	26	27.9	0.49	0.34	5.2	1.44			131			22			52	76	
	Rest		64	28	21.9	0.37	0.30	4.7	1.23			129			24			53	65	
	Rest	156/87	64	29	23.8	0.38	0.26	4.1	1.46	7.59	22	134	112	21	21	23	2	56	82	0.30
	Rest		62	29	26.7	0.39	0.26	4.2	1.50			135			19			62	93	
	Rest		64	27	27.9	0.39	0.26	4.1	1.50			135			18			66	98	
	Rest		64	23	18.8	0.29	0.25	3.9	1.16			131			20			58	67	
	Rest		65	25	16.6	0.26	0.28	4.3	0.93			126			23			56	52	
	Unloaded		80	53	25.2	0.43	0.57	7.1	0.75			110			30			48	36	
	Unloaded		90	61	38.6	0.68	0.68	7.6	1.00			123			26			49	49	
	Unloaded		86	45	31.7	0.65	0.76	8.8	0.86			115			30			43	37	
	Unloaded		93	46	37.5	0.77	0.80	8.6	0.96			117			30			44	42	
	Unloaded		93	52	42.2	0.85	0.86	9.2	0.99			121			28			44	44	
	Unloaded	207/108	90	49	40.4	0.84	0.85	9.4	0.99	7.52	22	120	106	17	29	27	−2	43	43	0.23
0.5	15		97	51	47.7	0.95	0.86	8.9	1.10			124			27			46	50	
1.0	15		97	55	51.1	0.99	0.89	9.2	1.11			123			27			47	52	
1.5	30		103	61	53.9	1.04	0.96	9.3	1.08			122			28			47	51	
2.0	30		103	61	55.4	1.05	0.98	9.5	1.07			123			27			48	51	
2.5	45		103	59	58.1	1.11	1.05	10.2	1.06			122			27			48	51	
3.0	45		108	59	56.0	1.15	1.16	10.7	0.99			120			28			44	44	
3.5	60		117	61	61.0	1.26	1.23	10.5	1.02			123			27			44	45	
4.0	60	216/108	120	59	63.2	1.35	1.31	10.9	1.03	7.49	22	121	102	20	28	29	1	43	44	0.28
4.5	75		124	61	64.5	1.42	1.38	11.1	1.03			121			28			42	43	
5.0	75		126	56	71.8	1.58	1.43	11.3	1.10			123			28			42	47	
5.5	90		130	61	78.7	1.70	1.51	11.6	1.13			123			27			43	49	
6.0	90	228/111	129	56	71.3	1.65	1.37	10.6	1.20	7.46	20	123	100	25	29	29	0	40	49	0.24
	Recovery		119	50	58.9	1.38	1.32	11.1	1.05			118			31			40	41	
	Recovery		119	49	48.2	1.09	0.99	8.3	1.10			118			32			40	44	
	Recovery		104	45	56.7	1.13	0.87	8.4	1.30			127			26			47	61	
										7.45	20		103			29				

demonstrating a marked respiratory alkalosis in his arterial blood (Table 9.67.3).

Analysis

In flow chart 1, the peak V̇O₂ is reduced while the anaerobic threshold is normal (Table 9.67.2), which directs us through branchpoints 1.1, 1.2, and 1.3 to flow chart 3. The breathing reserve (branchpoint 3.1) and ECG (branchpoint 3.3) are normal, directing us to "poor effort or musculoskeletal disorder." The VD/VT, P(A − a)O₂, and P(a − ET)CO₂ are normal and the heart rate reserve is high. The change in bicarbonate from rest to recovery is only 4 mEq/L, which is less than expected for a normal maximal exercise effort. These findings suggest that the patient's chest pain causing the physician to ask the patient to stop exercise was not supported by evidence of coronary artery disease, in that the ECG, ΔV̇O₂/ΔWR, heart rate-ΔV̇O₂ relationship and *AT* (Fig. 9.67.1, panel 5) were normal. On the other hand, the acute hyperventilation, demonstrated by the development of an abrupt alkalosis with an in-

crease in pH from 7.47 to 7.59 and PaCO₂ from 34 to 23 mmHg (Table 9.67.3), supports the diagnosis of an anxiety state. The high and irregular respiratory exchange ratio (R) at rest (Fig 9.67.1, panel 8) also supports this diagnosis. He does have significant obesity and hypertension however. Re-evaluation is in order when the patient is less anxious.

Conclusion

This study shows anxiety and acute resting hyperventilation with a non-physiological very irregular breathing pattern at rest and during exercise. The combination of high heart rate reserve and normal breathing reserve without objective evidence of either myocardial, pulmonary vascular, peripheral vascular, or underlying lung disease suggests that this patient's reduced maximum oxygen uptake, and perhaps symptom of dyspnea, is psychogenic. The pre-exercise vasovagal reaction and the acute hyperventilation in the anticipation of exercise are consistent with this interpretation.

Case 68 Skeletal Disease Limiting Exercise

Clinical Findings

This 60-year-old former shipyard worker had enjoyed apparent good health except for arthritis of the right hip of many years' duration and hypertension, which had not been treated. He had smoked cigarettes for a short period of time 3 decades previously. Chest roentgenograms showed fibrotic changes at both bases, but no rales were heard on physical examination.

Exercise Findings

The patient felt more comfortable walking on the treadmill than pedalling the cycle ergometer. After insertion of a brachial artery catheter he walked at 1.6 mph on the level followed by increments in grade of 2% per minute. He stopped exercise after 11 minutes because of pain in the right hip. He had no shortness of breath or palpitations. The ECG remained normal.

TABLE 9.68.1. Selected Respiratory Function Data

Measurement	Predicted	Measured
Age, yr		60
Sex		Male
Height, cm		175
Weight, kg	78	97
Hematocrit, %		44
VC, L	3.77	4.09
IC, L	2.52	3.01
TLC, L	5.77	5.72
FEV_1, L	2.96	3.21
FEV_1/VC, %	78	78
MVV, L/min	122	94
D_Lco, ml/min Hg/min	25.0	23.9

TABLE 9.68.2. Selected Exercise Data

Measurement	Predicted	Measured
Peak $\dot{V}o_2$, L/min	2.57	1.62
Maximum HR, beats/min	160	123
Maximum O_2 pulse, ml/beat	16.1	14.0
AT, L/min	>1.13	1.45
Blood pressure, mmHg (rest, max)		186/117, 213/123
Maximum $\dot{V}E$, L/min		52
Exercise breathing reserve, L/min	>15	42
Pao_2, mmHg (rest, max ex)		90, 80
$P(A - a)o_2$, mmHg (rest, max ex)		10, 32
$P(a - ET)co_2$, mmHg (rest, max ex)		1, -3
VD/VT (rest, heavy ex)		0.39, 0.25
HCO_3^-, mEq/L (rest, 2-min recov)		24, 23

FIGURE 9.68.1.

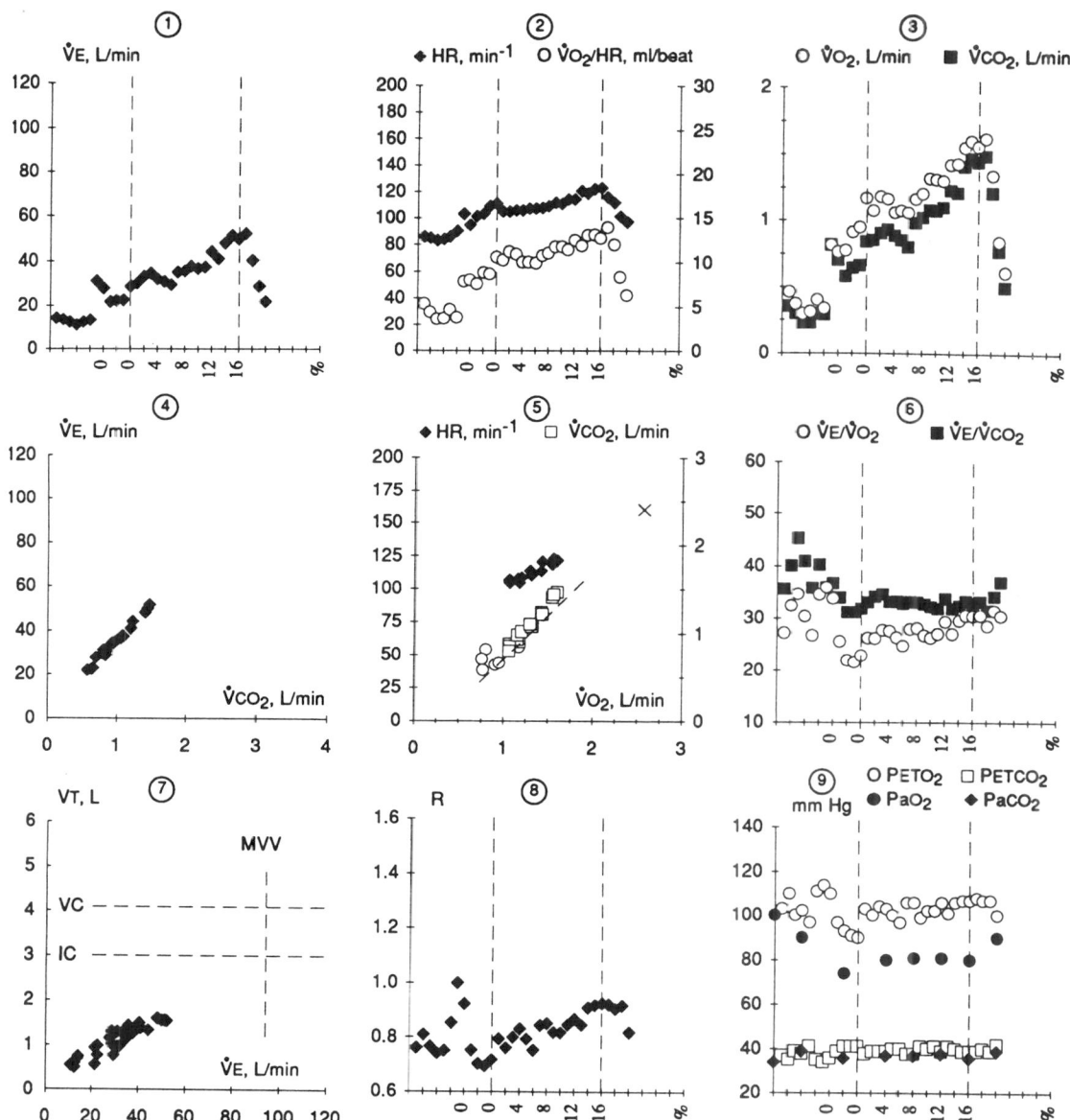

1. Vertical dashed lines in panels 1 to 3 and 6, 8, and 9 indicate the beginning and the end of increasing work period.

2. Zero grade walking is performed for 3 minutes before the left vertical dashed line.

3. In panel 5, the diagonal dashed line has a slope of 1; the "×" in the upper right is the predicted maximum heart rate and $\dot{V}O_2$ for the subject.

TABLE 9.68.3.   Air Breathing

Time min	Work rate watts	BP mmHg	HR min⁻¹	f min⁻¹	V̇E L/min BTPS	V̇CO₂ L/min STPD	V̇O₂ L/min STPD	V̇O₂/HR ml/beat	R	pH	HCO₃⁻ meq/L	PO₂, mmHg ET	a	(A − a)	FCO₂, mmHg ET	a	(a − ET)	V̇E/V̇CO₂	V̇E/V̇O₂	VD/VT
	Rest	186/117								7.44	23	100			34					
	Rest		86	19	14.1	0.35	0.46	5.3	0.76			103			37			36	27	
	Rest		85	20	13.7	0.30	0.37	4.4	0.81			110			35			40	32	
	Rest		83	25	12.5	0.23	0.30	3.6	0.77			100			39			45	35	
	Rest	192/126	84	20	11.1	0.23	0.31	3.7	0.74	7.41	24	102	90	10	38	39	1	41	30	0.39
	Rest		86	21	12.5	0.30	0.40	4.7	0.75			97			41			36	27	
	Rest		90	20	13.4	0.29	0.34	3.8	0.85			111			35			40	34	
	0		103	24	31.1	0.81	0.81	7.9	1.00			114			34			36	36	
	0		95	24	27.7	0.70	0.76	8.0	0.92			110			36			37	34	
	0		101	23	21.6	0.58	0.77	7.6	0.75			97			39			34	26	
	0	216/129	103	29	22.4	0.64	0.91	8.8	0.70	7.41	22	93	74	28	41	36	−5	31	22	0.21
	0		109	23	22.5	0.66	0.95	8.7	0.69			91			41			31	22	
	0		111	22	28.6	0.84	1.17	10.5	0.72			90			41			32	23	
0.5	2		105	24	30.1	0.85	1.07	10.2	0.79			103			38			33	26	
1.0	2		105	26	33.0	0.90	1.18	11.2	0.76			100			39			34	26	
1.5	4		106	28	34.6	0.93	1.16	10.9	0.80			104			39			35	28	
2.0	4	216/126	106	33	31.9	0.88	1.06	10.0	0.83	7.41	23	103	80	27	39	37	−2	33	27	0.27
2.5	6		107	32	30.9	0.85	1.07	10.0	0.79			100			40			33	26	
3.0	6		107	38	29.4	0.80	1.06	9.9	0.75			97			40			33	25	
3.5	8		108	31	35.0	0.98	1.16	10.7	0.84			106			38			33	28	
4.0	8	210/123	109	25	35.8	1.02	1.20	11.0	0.85	7.41	23	106	81	27	38	37	−1	33	28	0.28
4.5	10		112	30	37.8	1.08	1.32	11.8	0.82			99			41			33	27	
5.0	10		111	28	36.8	1.07	1.31	11.8	0.82			102			40			32	26	
5.5	12		114	28	37.4	1.10	1.30	11.4	0.85			102			41			32	27	
6.0	12	216/123	114	33	44.3	1.23	1.42	12.5	0.87	7.40	23	106	81	26	39	38	−1	34	29	0.31
6.5	14		121	30	44.1	1.21	1.43	11.8	0.85			107			41			32	27	
7.0	14		119	30	48.3	1.41	1.55	13.0	0.91			106			40			32	30	
7.5	16		122	33	51.5	1.47	1.60	13.1	0.92			107			39			33	30	
8.0	16	213/123	123	32	49.9	1.44	1.56	12.7	0.92	7.40	22	107	80	32	39	36	−3	33	30	0.25
	Recovery		116	34	52.2	1.49	1.62	14.0	0.92			108			39			33	30	
	Recovery		112	27	40.4	1.21	1.34	12.0	0.90			107			40			31	28	
	Recovery		101	28	28.7	0.77	0.84	8.3	0.92			107			39			34	31	
	Recovery	192/126	97	38	21.7	0.50	0.61	6.3	0.82	7.39	23	100	90	14	42	39	−3	37	30	0.34

Interpretation

Comments

The results of the respiratory function studies are within normal limits (Table 9.68.1). The patient had significant systemic hypertension at the time of the study (Table 9.68.3). Because of arthritis of the right hip, treadmill walking was used for exercise testing. The rate of walking was slow (1.6 mph) to avoid discomfort to the patient and also so the arterial pressure could be closely monitored.

Analysis

In flow chart 1, the peak V̇O₂ is significantly reduced but the anaerobic threshold is normal (Table 9.68.2). See flow chart 3. The breathing reserve at maximum exercise is high (branchpoint 3.1). The ECG is normal (branchpoint 3.3). The diagnosis at this point reveals either poor effort or that the patient has a musculoskeletal disorder. The normal VD/VT, borderline P(A − a)O₂, normal P(a − ET)CO₂, high heart rate reserve, and only 1 mEq/L decrease in bicarbonate 2 minutes after the start of recovery support either of these diagnoses. However, his history, normal ventilatory pattern, and minimal acid-base changes are most consistent with a musculoskeletal disorder limiting exercise at the measured peak V̇O₂.

Conclusion

Musculoskeletal disorder has limited exercise performance.

Case 69 Ankylosing Spondylitis

Clinical Findings

This 51-year-old airline employee had first developed symptoms of ankylosing spondylitis, primarily involving the neck and thoracic spine, approximately 6 years prior to evaluation. He had received some relief of pain with indomethacin. He had stopped smoking over 10 years previously. On the basis of pleural changes at the apices, he had been treated for tuberculosis several years ago although the tuberculin skin test was negative. To maintain fitness, he had begun running approximately 3 miles a day. In recent months he had felt as if he "could not get enough air into his lungs" and found himself taking gasping breaths. Physical examination revealed reduced neck movement and thoracic expansion. Chest roentgenograms revealed apical pleural thickening. ECG was normal.

Exercise Findings

The patient performed exercise on a cycle ergometer. He pedalled at 60 rpm without added load for 3 minutes. The work rate was then increased 20 W per minute to his symptom-limited maximum. He stopped exercise because of shortness of breath. Exercise ECGs were normal except for a single interpolated ventricular premature contraction.

TABLE 9.69.1. Selected Respiratory Function Data

Measurement	Predicted	Measured
Age, yr		51
Sex		Male
Height, cm		178
Weight, kg	80	79
Hematocrit, %		39
VC, L	4.62	3.61
IC, L	3.08	2.60
FEV$_1$, L	3.67	2.76
FEV$_1$/VC, %	79	76
MVV, L/min, direct	151	132 at f = 80/min
MVV, L/min, indirect	147	110

TABLE 9.69.2. Selected Exercise Data

Measurement	Predicted	Measured
Peak $\dot{V}O_2$, L/min	2.52	2.54
Maximum HR, beats/min	169	170
Maximum O$_2$ pulse, ml/beat	14.9	14.9
$\Delta\dot{V}O_2/\Delta WR$, ml/min/W	10.3	9.4
AT, L/min	>1.08	1.4
Blood pressure, mmHg (rest, max)		126/86, 206/84
Maximum $\dot{V}E$, L/min		108
Exercise breathing reserve, L/min	>15	2

FIGURE 9.69.1.

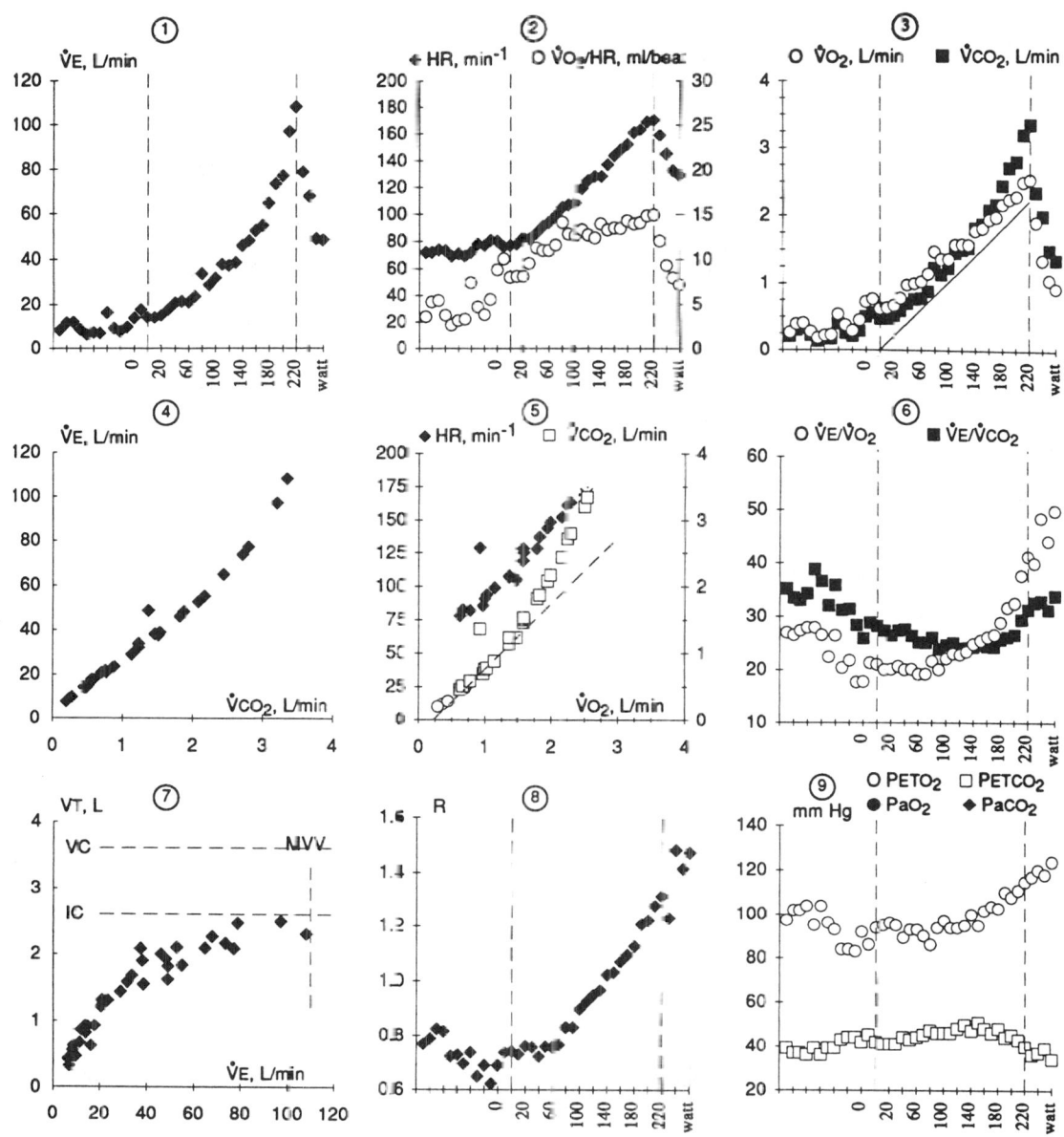

1. Vertical dashed lines in panels 1 to 3 and 6, 8, and 9 indicate the beginning and the end of increasing work period.
2. Unloaded cycling is performed for 3 minutes before the left vertical dashed line.
3. In panel 3, the diagonal line shows the increase of V̇O₂ at a slope of 10 ml/min/W.
4. In panel 5, the diagonal dashed line has a slope of 1 the "x" in the upper right is the predicted maximum heart rate and V̇O₂ for the subject.

Interpretation

Comments

The results of spirometry and total lung capacity measurement suggest that the patient has mild restrictive disease (Table 9.69.1) consequent to his ankylosing spondylitis. This is reflected in part by a reduction in the inspiratory capacity (loss of his ability to expand his chest wall). The resting ECG is normal.

TABLE 9.69.3. Air Breathing

Time min	Work rate watts	BP mmHg	HR min⁻¹	f min⁻¹	V̇E L/min BTPS	V̇CO₂ L/min STPD	V̇O₂ L/min STPD	V̇O₂/HR ml/beat	R	pH	HCO₃⁻ meq/L	PO₂, mmHg ET	e	(A−a)	PCO₂, mmHg ET	a	(a−ET)	V̇E/V̇CO₂	V̇E/V̇O₂	VD/VT
	Rest		72	15	8.3	0.20	0.26	3.6	0.77			97			39			35	27	
	Rest		72	17	11.5	0.30	0.38	5.3	0.79			102			37			34	26	
	Rest		74	14	12.1	0.33	0.40	5.4	0.83			102			37			33	27	
	Rest		73	14	8.7	0.22	0.27	3.7	0.81			104			36			34	28	
	Rest		69	15	6.3	0.13	0.18	2.6	0.72			95			39			39	28	
	Rest	126/86	71	16	7.2	0.16	0.22	3.1	0.73			104			36			37	27	
	Rest		69	22	7.0	0.16	0.23	3.3	0.70			96			39			32	22	
	Rest		72	26	16.2	0.39	0.53	7.4	0.74			93			39			36	26	
	Unloaded		78	19	9.1	0.24	0.37	4.7	0.65			84			43			31	20	
	Unloaded		77	18	7.8	0.20	0.29	3.8	0.69			84			44			31	22	
	Unloaded		81	21	9.7	0.28	0.45	5.6	0.62			83			44			28	18	
	Unloaded		80	15	13.9	0.49	0.71	8.9	0.69			92			42			26	18	
	Unloaded		76	19	17.7	0.56	0.76	10.0	0.74			86			45			29	21	
	Unloaded		77	16	14.3	0.46	0.62	8.1	0.74			94			42			28	21	
0.5	20		78	17	14.0	0.46	0.63	8.1	0.73			95			41			27	20	
1.0	20	158/86	83	16	14.3	0.51	0.67	8.1	0.76			96			41			26	20	
1.5	40		82	19	17.7	0.59	0.78	9.5	0.76			95			41			27	21	
2.0	40	174/84	86	17	20.7	0.70	0.97	11.3	0.72			89			44			28	20	
2.5	60		91	17	21.4	0.76	1.00	11.0	0.76			93			43			26	20	
3.0	60		94	16	21.0	0.78	1.03	11.0	0.76			93			44			25	19	
3.5	80		99	18	23.5	0.88	1.15	11.6	0.77			90			45			25	19	
4.0	80	178/78	105	20	33.6	1.23	1.48	14.1	0.83			86			47			26	22	
4.5	100		107	20	28.9	1.14	1.37	12.8	0.83			94			46			24	20	
5.0	100		108	20	31.8	1.23	1.37	12.7	0.90			97			46			24	22	
5.5	120		119	20	38.0	1.46	1.58	13.3	0.92			94			46			25	23	
6.0	120	190/86	125	18	37.5	1.51	1.59	12.7	0.95			94			48			24	23	
6.5	140		128	25	38.8	1.53	1.58	12.3	0.97			95			50			24	23	
7.0	140		128	23	46.1	1.82	1.78	13.9	1.02			100			47			24	25	
7.5	160		137	25	48.3	1.88	1.82	13.3	1.03			95			51			25	25	
8.0	160	206/84	144	25	52.7	2.08	1.94	13.5	1.07			102			48			24	26	
8.5	180		148	30	55.1	2.17	1.98	13.4	1.10			104			46			24	27	
9.0	180		152	31	64.8	2.44	2.16	14.2	1.13			103			48			25	29	
9.5	200		161	34	73.6	2.71	2.24	13.9	1.21			110			44			26	32	
10.0	200		163	37	77.2	2.80	2.29	14.0	1.22			108			45			26	32	
10.5	220		169	39	97.2	3.20	2.50	14.8	1.28			111			43			29	38	
11.0	220		170	47	108.3	3.34	2.54	14.9	1.31			115			40			31	41	
	Recovery		159	32	78.9	2.35	1.91	12.0	1.23			117			36			32	40	
	Recovery		145	30	67.9	2.00	1.35	9.3	1.48			120			37			33	48	
	Recovery	160/78	133	27	49.1	1.50	1.06	8.0	1.42			118			39			31	44	
	Recovery		129	30	48.8	1.37	0.93	7.2	1.47			124			34			34	50	

Analysis

In flow chart 1, the peak V̇O₂ and the anaerobic threshold are normal (Table 9.69.2). See flow chart 2. The ECG and O₂ pulse at peak V̇O₂ are normal (branchpoint 2.1). The subject is not obese (branchpoint 2.2). The normal ventilatory equivalent for CO₂ at the anaerobic threshold suggests that ventilation-perfusion matching is normal. The observation that tidal volume reaches the inspiratory capacity (panel 7, Fig. 9.69.1) reflects the changes that would be expected from restrictive pulmonary or chest wall disease. Note that the indirect MVV is close to the maximum exercise ventilation resulting in virtually no breathing reserve. This is further evidence of ventilatory limitation.

Conclusion

Exertional dyspnea secondary to restrictive changes in the chest wall consequent to ankylosing spondylitis.

Case 70 Myasthenia Gravis

Clinical Findings

This 62-year-old retired shipyard worker had been found to have myasthenia gravis 21 years earlier. He had taken 30 mg of pyridostigmine bromide with benefit for many years. He had a 20 pack history of smoking cigarettes but had stopped 21 years ago. He had a daily minimally productive cough. He took digoxin for an arrhythmia and reserpine for hypertension. He complained of gradually increasing shortness of breath in the last 3 years, evident when walking 2 to 3 blocks slowly or climbing a flight stairs. There was no evidence of pulmonary or cardiovascular disease on physical examination. Chest roentgenogram was normal except for old granulomatous disease. Resting ECG showed sinus bradycardia and ST segment depression in V5 or V6 consistent with digitalis effect.

Exercise Findings

The patient performed exercise on a cycle ergometer. He pedalled at 60 rpm without added load for 3 minutes. The work rate was then increased 15 W per minute to his symptom-limited maximum. Arterial blood was sampled every second minute, and intra-arterial blood pressure was recorded from a percutaneously placed brachial artery catheter. He stopped exercise complaining of leg pain and generalized fatigue. A single premature ventricular contraction occurred at 60W.

TABLE 9.70.1. Selected Respiratory Function Data

Measurement	Predicted	Measured
Age, yr		62
Sex		Male
Height, cm		178
Weight, kg	80	80
Hematocrit, %		39
VC, L	3.87	2.96
IC, L	2.58	2.08
TLC, L	5.95	4.64
FEV_1, L	3.03	2.42
FEV_1/VC, %	78	82
MVV, L/min	123	56
D_{CO}, ml/min Hg/min	24.7	25.6

TABLE 9.70.2. Selected Exercise Data

Measurement	Predicted	Measured
Peak $\dot{V}O_2$, L/min	2.21	1.09
Maximum HR, beats/min	158	102
Maximum O_2 pulse, ml/beat	14.0	10.8
$\Delta\dot{V}O_2/\Delta WR$, ml/min/W	10.3	10.5
AT, L/min	>0.97	>1.1
Blood pressure, mmHg (rest, max)		153/84, 210/84
Maximum $\dot{V}E$, L/min		37
Exercise breathing reserve, L/min	>15	19
Pa_{O_2}, mmHg (rest, max ex)		95, 86
$P(A - a)_{O_2}$, mmHg (rest, max ex)		8, 21
$P(a - ET)_{CO_2}$, mmHg (rest, max ex)		3, 1
V_D/V_T (rest, heavy ex)		0.39, 0.31
HCO_3^-, mEq/L (rest, 2-min recov)		25, 23

FIGURE 9.70.1.

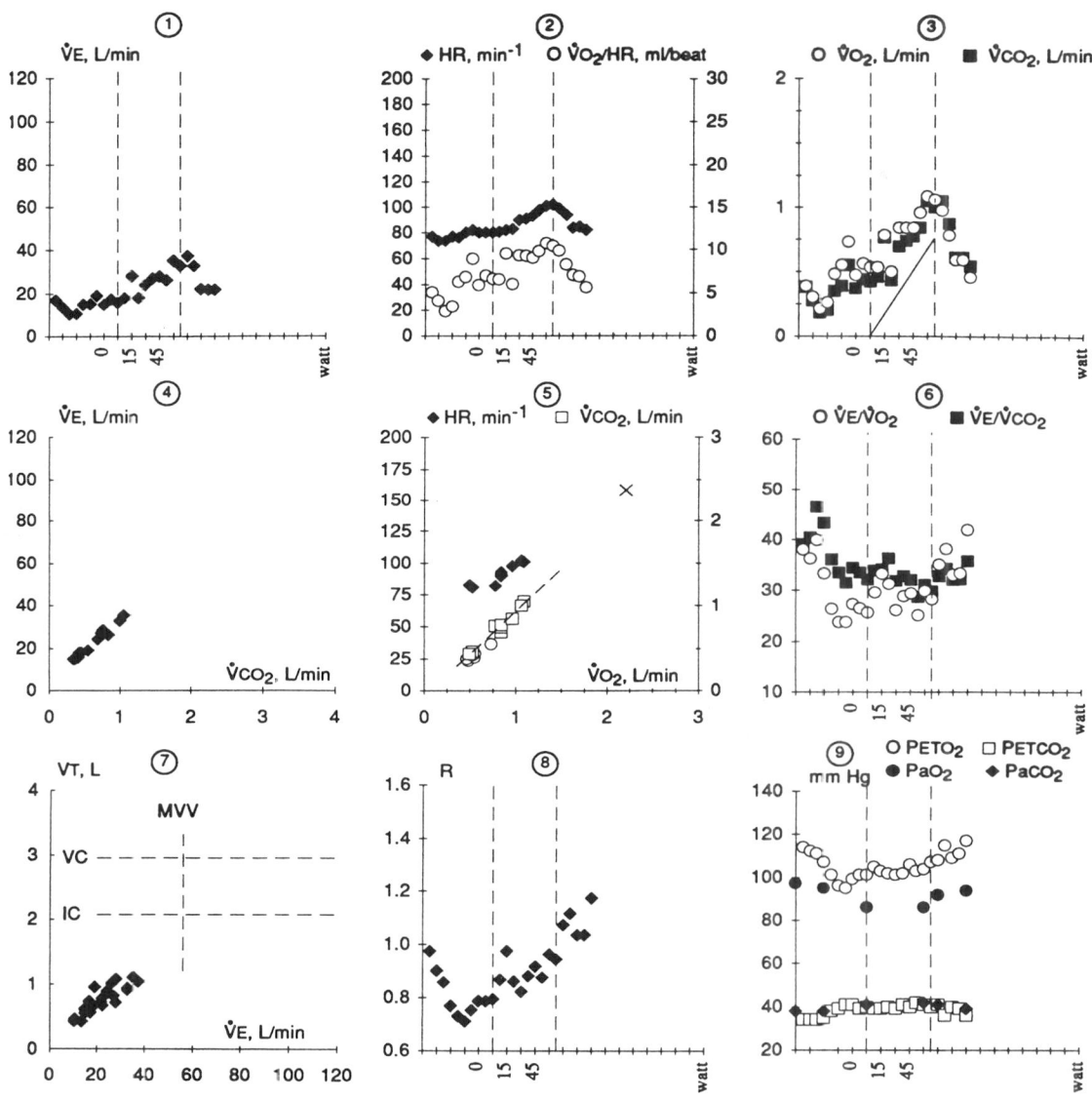

1. Vertical dashed lines in panels 1 to 3 and 6, 8, and 9 indicate the beginning and the end of increasing work period.

2. Unloaded cycling is performed for 3 minutes before the left vertical dashed line.

3. In panel 3, the diagonal line shows the increase of $\dot{V}O_2$ at a slope of 10 ml/min/W.

4. In panel 5, the diagonal dashed line has a slope of 1; the "x" in the upper right is the predicted maximum heart rate and $\dot{V}O_2$ for the subject.

TABLE 9.70.3. Air Breathing

Time min	Work rate watts	BP mmHg	HR min⁻¹	f min⁻¹	$\dot{V}E$ L/min BTPS	$\dot{V}CO_2$ L/min STPD	$\dot{V}O_2$ L/min STPD	$\dot{V}O_2$/HR ml/beat	R	pH	HCO_3^- meq/L	P_{O_2}, mmHg ET	a	(A − a)	P_{CO_2}, mmHg ET	a	(a − ET)	$\dot{V}E/\dot{V}CO_2$	$\dot{V}E/\dot{V}O_2$	VD/VT
	Rest	153/84								7.42	24		97			38				
	Rest		77	23	16.8	0.38	0.39	5.1	0.97			114			34			39	38	
	Rest		74	32	13.6	0.27	0.30	4.1	0.90			112			34			40	36	
	Rest		74	24	10.4	0.18	0.21	2.8	0.86			111			34			46	40	
	Rest	138/78	77	23	10.6	0.20	0.26	3.4	0.77	7.43	25	107	95	8	35	38	3	43	33	0.39
	Unloaded		76	27	14.9	0.35	0.48	6.3	0.73			107			38			36	26	
	Unloaded		80	25	15.2	0.39	0.55	6.9	0.71			96			39			34	24	
	Unloaded		82	20	19.0	0.55	0.73	8.9	0.75			95			41			31	24	
	Unloaded		80	24	14.8	0.37	0.47	5.9	0.79			99			41			34	27	
	Unloaded		80	31	17.4	0.44	0.56	7.0	0.79			101			39			34	26	
	Unloaded	165/81	80	27	15.8	0.42	0.55	6.6	0.79	7.41	26	101	86	15	40	41	1	32	25	0.30
0.5	15		81	27	17.9	0.46	0.55	6.5	0.87			105			39			34	29	
1.0	15		82	26	28.1	0.76	0.78	9.5	0.97			105			39			34	33	
1.5	30		83	28	18.0	0.43	0.50	6.0	0.86			105			40			36	31	
2.0	30	162/78	90	27	24.2	0.69	0.84	9.3	0.82			101			39			32	26	
2.5	45		91	33	27.0	0.74	0.84	9.2	0.88			105			41			33	29	
3.0	45		93	39	28.0	0.77	0.84	9.0	0.92			103			40			32	29	
3.5	60		98	26	26.2	0.84	0.96	9.8	0.88			103			42			29	25	
4.0	60	192/81	101	32	35.3	1.05	1.09	10.8	0.96	7.38	24	104	86	21	41	42	1	31	30	0.31
4.5	75		102	35	32.8	1.00	1.06	10.4	0.94			107			40			30	28	
	Recovery		99	36	37.4	1.05	0.98	9.9	1.07	7.38	24	108	92	19	41	41	0	33	35	0.33
	Recovery		94	36	32.8	0.87	0.78	8.3	1.12			115			36			34	38	
	Recovery		84	33	22.3	0.61	0.59	7.0	1.03			109			40			32	33	
	Recovery		85	28	22.0	0.61	0.59	6.9	1.03			111			39			32	33	
	Recovery	174/84	82	30	21.8	0.54	0.46	5.6	1.17	7.38	23	117	94	22	36	39	3	36	42	0.33

Interpretation

Comments

This patient appears to have mild restrictive lung or chest wall disease (Table 9.70.1). Because the diffusing capacity is within normal limits and the MVV is significantly reduced, the latter is more likely. The resting ECG is normal except for the digitalis effect.

Analysis

In flow chart 1, the peak oxygen uptake is reduced but the anaerobic threshold is normal (Table 9.70.2). See flow chart 3. The breathing reserve at the maximum work rate is normal (branchpoint 3.1). The ECG remained normal except for the digitalis effect (branchpoint 3.3). This suggests that the patient either made poor effort or had a musculoskeletal disorder. The indices of ventilation-perfusion mismatching are normal, supporting the concept that this patient does not have significant pulmonary disease. (VD/VT of 0.31 to 0.33 is considered to be normal in view of the low level of exercise performed.) The high heart rate reserve and small decrease in bicarbonate support the observation that the cardiovascular system was only minimally stressed. The reduced peak $\dot{V}O_2$, with the strikingly reduced MVV, suggests that this patient is limited by a chest wall defect.

Conclusion

Exercise limitation without cardiovascular or ventilatory impairment. Limitation is most likely secondary to myasthenia gravis.

Case 71 Aortic and Mitral Stenosis and Obstructive Airway Disease

Clinical Findings

This 43-year-old man developed dyspnea and precordial pain at rest and on exertion 3 weeks prior to study. He had a history of "passing out" with or without prior feelings of lightheadedness. He also noted cough and sputum production with exertion. He was a welder and an extremely heavy smoker, but he stated that he had reduced his smoking to several cigarettes daily. Evaluation, including cardiac catheterization, revealed severe aortic stenosis (1.4 cm^2 valvular area), normal coronary arteries, and an elevated pulmonary artery pressure of 50/25 mmHg and wedge pressure of 16 mmHg. Medications included an oral β-adrenergic blocker, theophylline, and a α-agonist inhaler. Physical examination was consistent with aortic stenosis and mitral valve disease, but the patient had no rales or wheezes.

Exercise Findings

The patient performed exercise on a cycle ergometer. He pedalled at 60 rpm without an added load for 3 minutes. The work rate was then increased 15 W per minute to tolerance. Blood was sampled every second minute, and intra-arterial blood pressure was recorded from a percutaneously placed brachial artery catheter. The resting ECG was normal except for an intraventricular conduction defect. The patient had neither chest pain nor ectopy during exercise, but he had expiratory wheezes and frequent premature atrial and ventricular contractions early in recovery. The arterial pressure tracing showed a delayed upstroke (200 milliseconds to peak pressure).

TABLE 9.71.1. Selected Respiratory Function Data

Measurement	Predicted	Before Bronchodilator	After Bronchodilator
Age, yr		43	
Sex		Male	
Height, cm		171	
Weight, kg	74	89	
Hemoglobin, g/100 ml		15.4	
VC, L	4.47	3.03	3.14
IC, L	2.98	2.03	2.23
TLC, L	6.32	6.54	
FEV$_1$, L	3.58	1.65	1.84
FEV$_1$/VC, %	80	54	
MVV, L/min	154	62	73
D$_L$CO, ml/mm Hg/min	27.2	19.8	

TABLE 9.71.2. Selected Exercise Data

Measurement	Predicted	Measured
Peak V̇O$_2$, L/min	2.70	1.48
Maximum HR, beats/min	177	140
Maximum O$_2$ pulse, ml/beat	15.3	10.6
ΔV̇O$_2$/ΔWR, ml/min/W	10.3	8.5
AT, L/min	>1.13	>1.0
Blood pressure, mmHg (rest, max ex)		96/69, 132/69
Maximum V̇E, L/min		59
Exercise breathing reserve, L/min	>15	14
PaO$_2$, mmHg (rest, mod ex)		84, 95
P(A − a)O$_2$, mmHg (rest, mod ex)		16, 14
P(a − ET)CO$_2$, mmHg (rest, mod ex)		3, 3
VD/VT (rest, max ex)		0.33, 0.32
HCO$_3^-$, mEq/L (rest, 2-min recov)		25, 24
Carboxyhemoglobin, %		4.3

FIGURE 9.71.1.

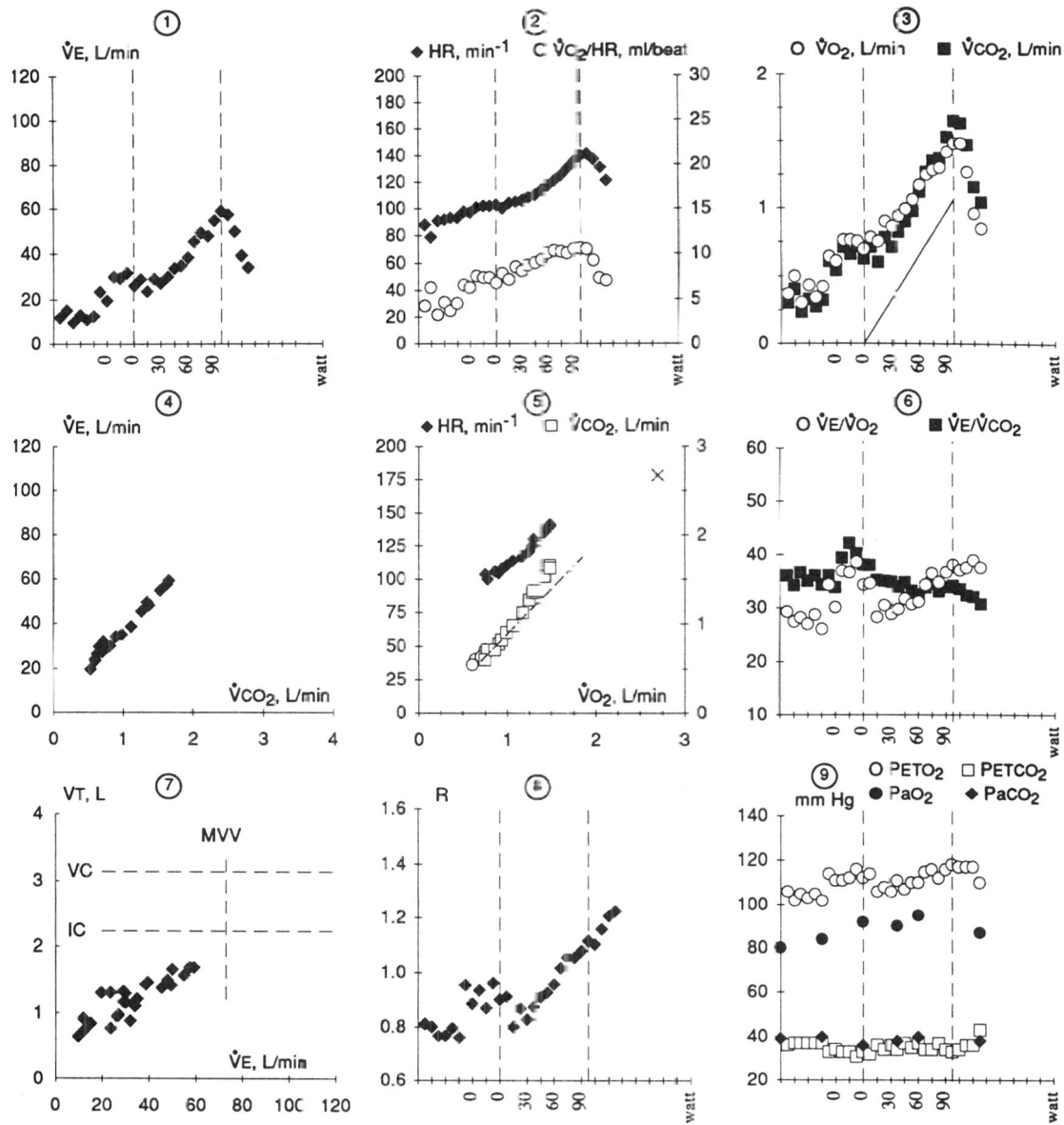

1. Vertical dashed lines in panels 1 to 3 and 6, 8, and 9 indicate the beginning and the end of increasing work period.
2. Unloaded cycling is performed for 3 minutes before the left vertical dashed line.
3. In panel 3, the diagonal line shows the increase of $\dot{V}O_2$ at a slope of 10 ml/min/W.
4. In panel 5, the diagonal dashed line has a slope of 1; the "x" in the upper right is the predicted maximum heart rate and $\dot{V}O_2$ for the subject.

Interpretation

Comments

Resting respiratory function tests reveal moderately severe obstructive lung disease with some response to inhaled albuterol and with a decreased D_LCO for the subject. Wheezing was noted during recovery from exercise. The carboxyhemoglobin level is increased. The patient has known significant valvular heart disease. The systemic blood pressure tracing showed a delayed upstroke (200 milliseconds to peak pressure), pulse pressure was low at rest, and

TABLE 9.71.3. Air Breathing

Time min	Work rate watts	BP mmHg	HR min⁻¹	f min⁻¹	$\dot{V}_E$ L/min BTPS	$\dot{V}_{CO_2}$ L/min STPD	$\dot{V}_{O_2}$ L/min STPD	$\dot{V}_{O_2}$/HR ml/beat	R	pH	HCO₃⁻ meq/L	PO₂, mmHg ET	a	(A−a)	PCO₂, mmHg ET	a	(a−ET)	$\dot{V}_E$/$\dot{V}_{CO_2}$	$\dot{V}_E$/$\dot{V}_{O_2}$	VD/VT
	Rest	93/63								7.42	25		80			39				
	Rest		88	13	11.9	0.30	0.37	4.2	0.81			106			36			36	29	
	Rest		79	18	15.2	0.40	0.50	6.3	0.80			102			37			34	27	
	Rest		91	15	9.7	0.23	0.30	3.3	0.77			105			37			37	28	
	Rest		92	17	13.0	0.33	0.43	4.7	0.77			103			37			35	27	
	Rest		93	16	11.1	0.27	0.34	3.7	0.79			105			37			36	29	
	Rest	96/69	93	17	12.4	0.32	0.42	4.5	0.76	7.41	25	102	84	16	37	40	3	34	26	0.33
	Unloaded		98	18	23.5	0.61	0.64	6.5	0.95			114			33			36	34	
	Unloaded		97	15	19.6	0.54	0.61	6.3	0.89			111			34			34	30	
	Unloaded		101	26	30.2	0.71	0.76	7.5	0.93			111			33			39	37	
	Unloaded		102	23	29.8	0.66	0.76	7.5	0.87			112			33			42	37	
	Unloaded		102	36	32.0	0.72	0.75	7.4	0.96			116			31			40	39	
	Unloaded	114/75	103	28	26.4	0.63	0.70	6.8	0.90	7.46	25	112	92	19	33	36	3	38	34	0.34
0.5	15		100	25	29.1	0.71	0.78	7.8	0.91			114			32			38	35	
1.0	15		104	31	23.8	0.60	0.75	7.2	0.80			106			36			35	28	
1.5	30		105	22	29.2	0.78	0.90	8.6	0.87			108			34			35	30	
2.0	30		106	28	27.2	0.71	0.86	8.1	0.83			106			36			35	29	
2.5	45	117/78	108	26	30.1	0.82	0.94	8.7	0.87	7.43	25	111	90	18	34	38	4	34	30	0.31
3.0	45		110	31	34.0	0.90	0.99	9.0	0.91			107			37			35	32	
3.5	60		114	29	35.0	0.98	1.06	9.3	0.92			110			35			33	31	
4.0	60	114/69	117	27	38.7	1.12	1.17	10.0	0.96	7.35	22	110	95	14	37	40	3	33	31	0.32
4.5	75		121	33	45.6	1.27	1.25	10.3	1.02			115			34			34	34	
5.0	75		125	35	49.6	1.35	1.28	10.2	1.05			116			34			35	36	
5.5	90		130	32	48.0	1.37	1.30	10.0	1.05			112			37			33	35	
6.0	90	132/69	135	35	54.9	1.53	1.42	10.5	1.08			116			34			34	37	
6.5	105		140	35	59.2	1.65	1.48	10.6	1.11			118			33			34	38	
7.0			141	34	57.6	1.63	1.48	10.5	1.10			117			34			34	37	
	Recovery		137	30	50.0	1.47	1.27	9.3	1.16			117			36			32	37	
	Recovery		131	27	39.5	1.16	0.96	7.3	1.21			117			36			32	39	
	Recovery	114/72	121	29	34.3	1.04	0.85	7.0	1.22	7.42	24	110	87	30	43	38	−5	31	37	0.24

systolic pressure did not increase normally during exercise.

Analysis

In flow chart 1, peak $\dot{V}_{O_2}$ and the anaerobic threshold are decreased. Proceeding to flow chart 4, the low breathing reserve (branchpoint 4.1) and high exercise VD/VT, (branchpoint 4.2) lead us to the diagnosis of lung disease with impaired peripheral oxygenation. This is an acceptable, but an incomplete, diagnosis because the impaired peripheral oxygenation was not due primarily to the increase in pulmonary vascular resistance, but rather to left-sided failure from valvular heart disease. The low anaerobic threshold, low $\Delta\dot{V}_{O_2}/\Delta WR$, and low, nearly flat O_2 pulse despite β-adrenergic blockade are all evidence of a low maximal cardiac output. Could the low cardiac output be exclusively on the basis of pulmonary vascular disease secondary to heart failure or emphysema? This is possible, but it seems unlikely, considering the symptoms of recurrent lightheadedness and the findings of severe aortic valve disease confirmed by cardiac catheterization and the slow upstroke in the arterial pressure tracing with exercise.

Conclusion

Exercise intolerance is due to the inability to increase cardiac output appropriately with exertion, primarily related to aortic valvular disease.

Case 72 Left Ventricular Failure and Mild Obstructive Airway Disease: Cycle and Treadmill

Clinical Findings

This 64-year-old shipyard worker was referred for evaluation. He stated that he was not limited in any of his activities; he had no shortness of breath walking on the level and only mild dyspnea after climbing 25 steps. He had smoked a half a pack of cigarettes daily until 1 year prior to this evaluation. Physical examination revealed no abnormality of the cardiovascular or respiratory systems except for a resting blood pressure of 160/84. Questionable pleural thickening was noted on chest x-ray studies. There was a small but consistent improvement in expiratory flow rates and MVV following inhalation of aerosolized isoproterenol.

Exercise Findings

The patient performed exercise on a cycle ergometer and, 1 month later, on a treadmill. He first pedalled at 60 rpm, without added load, for 3 minutes. The work rate was then increased 20 W per minute to his symptom-limited maximum. Arterial blood was sampled every second minute, and intra-arterial blood pressure was recorded from a percutaneously placed brachial artery catheter. The resting ECG was normal. He stopped exercising because of leg fatigue. Near the end of cycle exercise, 1 mm horizontal ST depression was noted in leads 2, 3, and AVF. On repeating testing 1 month later on the treadmill, the patient stopped exercising because he "could not get a good deep breath" and felt tired. There were no abnormal ECG findings on that test.

TABLE 9.72.1. Selected Respiratory Function Data

Measurement	Predicted	Measured
Age, yr		64
Sex		Male
Height, cm		182
Weight, kg	83	80
Hematocrit, %		47
VC, L	4.49	4.25
IC, L	2.99	3.95
TLC, L	6.94	7.61
FEV_1, L	3.51	2.96
FEV_1/VC, %	78	70
MVV, L/min	140	121
$D_{L}CO$, ml/mm Hg/min	28.8	28.1

TABLE 9.72.2. Selected Exercise Data

Measurement	Predicted		Measured	
	Cycle	Treadmill	Cycle	Treadmill
Peak $\dot{V}O_2$, L/min	2.19	2.43	1.56	1.65
Maximum HR, beats/min	156	156	143	157
Maximum O_2 pulse, ml/beat	14.1	15.6	10.9	10.5
$\Delta\dot{V}O_2/\Delta WR$, ml/min/W	10.3		9.7	
AT, L/min	>0.97	>1.08	1.0	1.1
Blood pressure, mmHg (rest, max)			194/98, 230/98	
Maximum $\dot{V}E$, L/min			68	77
Exercise breathing reserve, L/min			53	44
PaO_2, mmHg (rest, max ex)			98, 104	
$P(A - a)O_2$, mmHg (rest, max ex)			22, 18	
$P(a - ET)CO_2$, mmHg (rest, max ex)			2, −3	
VD/VT (rest, heavy ex)			0.30, 0.24	
HCO_3^-, mEq/L (rest, 2-min recov)			24, 17	

FIGURE 9.72.1.   Cycle ergometry.

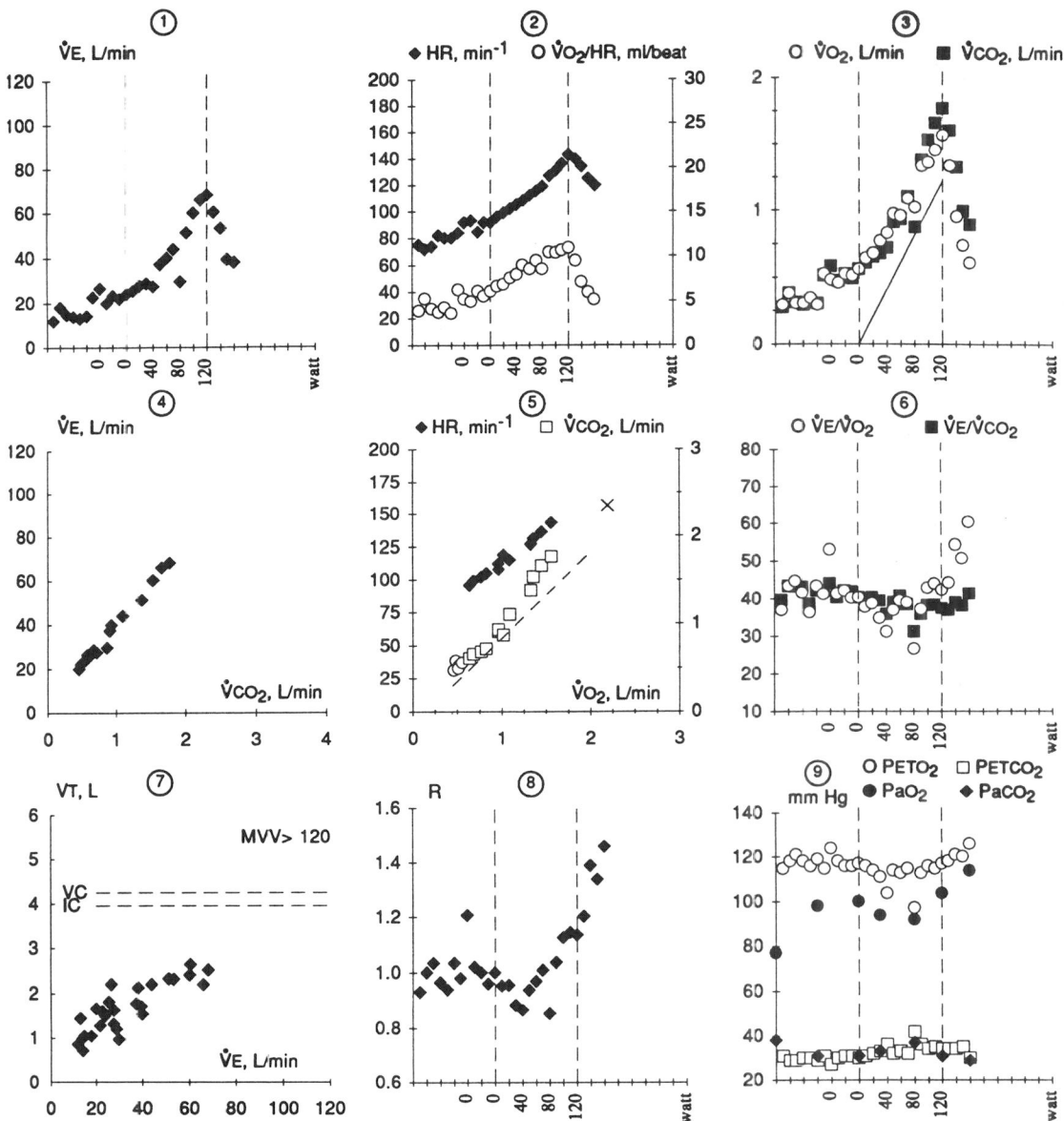

1. Vertical dashed lines in panels 1 to 3 and 6, 8, and 9 indicate the beginning and the end of increasing work period.

2. Unloaded cycling is performed for 3 minutes before the left vertical dashed line.

3. In panel 3, the diagonal line shows the increase of $\dot{V}O_2$ at a slope of 10 ml/min/W.

4. In panel 5, the diagonal dashed line has a slope of 1; the "x" in the upper right is the predicted maximum heart rate and $\dot{V}O_2$ for the subject.

TABLE 9.72.3. Cycle Ergometry

Time min	Work rate watts	BP mmHg	HR min⁻¹	f min⁻¹	$\dot{V}_E$ L/min BTPS	$\dot{V}_{CO_2}$ L/min STPD	$\dot{V}_{O_2}$ L/min STPD	$\dot{V}_{O_2}$/HR ml/beat	R	pH	HCO₃⁻ meq/L	PO₂ mmHg ET	a	(A−a)	PCO₂ mmHg ET	a	(a−ET)	$\dot{V}_E$/$\dot{V}_{CO_2}$	$\dot{V}_E$/$\dot{V}_{O_2}$	VD/VT
	Rest	194/98								7.42	24		77			38				
	Rest		75	14	11.9	0.27	0.29	3.9	0.93			115			31			40	37	
	Rest		72	17	17.9	0.38	0.38	5.3	1.00			118			29			43	43	
	Rest		74	14	14.6	0.31	0.30	4.1	1.03			121			29			43	45	
	Rest	176/95	82	14	13.7	0.29	0.30	3.7	0.97			118			30			43	42	
	Rest		80	9	13.1	0.32	0.34	4.3	0.94			116			30			39	36	
	Rest		80	20	14.3	0.30	0.29	3.6	1.03	7.48	23	119	98	22	29	31	2	42	43	0.30
	Unloaded		84	14	22.6	0.51	0.52	6.2	0.98			115			31			42	41	
	Unloaded		92	12	26.5	0.58	0.43	5.2	1.21			124			27			44	53	
	Unloaded		93	12	20.0	0.47	0.46	4.9	1.02			118			30			40	41	
	Unloaded	194/95	85	15	23.2	0.52	0.52	6.1	1.00			116			31			42	42	
	Unloaded		92	17	21.9	0.49	0.51	5.5	0.96			116			31			42	40	
	Unloaded		92	16	24.0	0.56	0.56	6.1	1.00	7.47	22	117	100	19	30	31	1	40	40	0.29
0.5	20		96	14	25.4	0.61	0.64	6.7	0.95			116			31			40	38	
1.0	20	209/92	99	17	27.7	0.65	0.68	6.9	0.96			114			32			40	39	
1.5	40		102	24	28.8	0.68	0.77	7.5	0.88	7.44	22	111	94	20	33	33	0	39	35	0.31
2.0	40		105	21	27.6	0.72	0.83	7.9	0.87			104			36			36	31	
2.5	60		108	21	37.4	0.91	0.97	9.0	0.94			114			32			39	37	
3.0	60	212/92	112	26	40.0	0.93	0.96	8.6	0.97			113			33			41	39	
3.5	80		115	20	44.0	1.10	1.09	9.5	1.01			115			32			38	39	
4.0	80		119	31	29.8	0.87	1.02	8.6	0.35	7.40	23	97	92	16	42	37	−5	31	27	0.23
4.5	100		127	22	51.3	1.38	1.33	10.5	1.04			113			36			36	37	
5.0	100	230/98	131	25	60.3	1.53	1.36	10.4	1.13			116			34			38	43	
5.5	120		136	30	66.1	1.66	1.45	10.7	1.14			115			35			38	44	
6.0	120		143	27	68.2	1.77	1.56	10.9	1.13	7.40	19	117	104	18	34	31	−3	37	42	0.24
	Recovery		140	23	60.7	1.60	1.33	9.5	1.20			118			34			37	44	
	Recovery	221/95	134	23	53.4	1.32	0.95	7.1	1.39			121			34			39	54	
	Recovery		125	23	39.5	0.99	0.74	5.9	1.54			120			35			38	51	
	Recovery		120	18	38.2	0.89	0.61	5.1	1.46	7.38	17	126	114	14	30	29	−1	41	60	0.27

Interpretation

Comments

This case is presented to contrast cycle with treadmill incremental exercise testing. Respiratory function measurements at rest suggest that this patient has mild obstructive lung disease (Table 9.72.1). Moreover, note that the patient hyperventilated at rest (Paco₂ and R values in Table 9.72.3) when first starting to breathe on the mouthpiece.

Analysis

The peak $\dot{V}_{O_2}$ is reduced in both the cycle and treadmill exercise studies while the anaerobic threshold is low normal (Table 9.72.2). Using flow chart 3, the breathing reserve is high (branchpoint 3.1), whereas the exercise ECGs (branchpoint 3.3) are equivocally abnormal. The patient did not have chest pain and the $\Delta\dot{V}_{O_2}/\Delta$WR is normal, but the O₂ pulse is abnormally low, indicating a circulatory abnormality—whether pulmonary vascular, peripheral arterial or

FIGURE 9.72.2.   Treadmill ergometry.

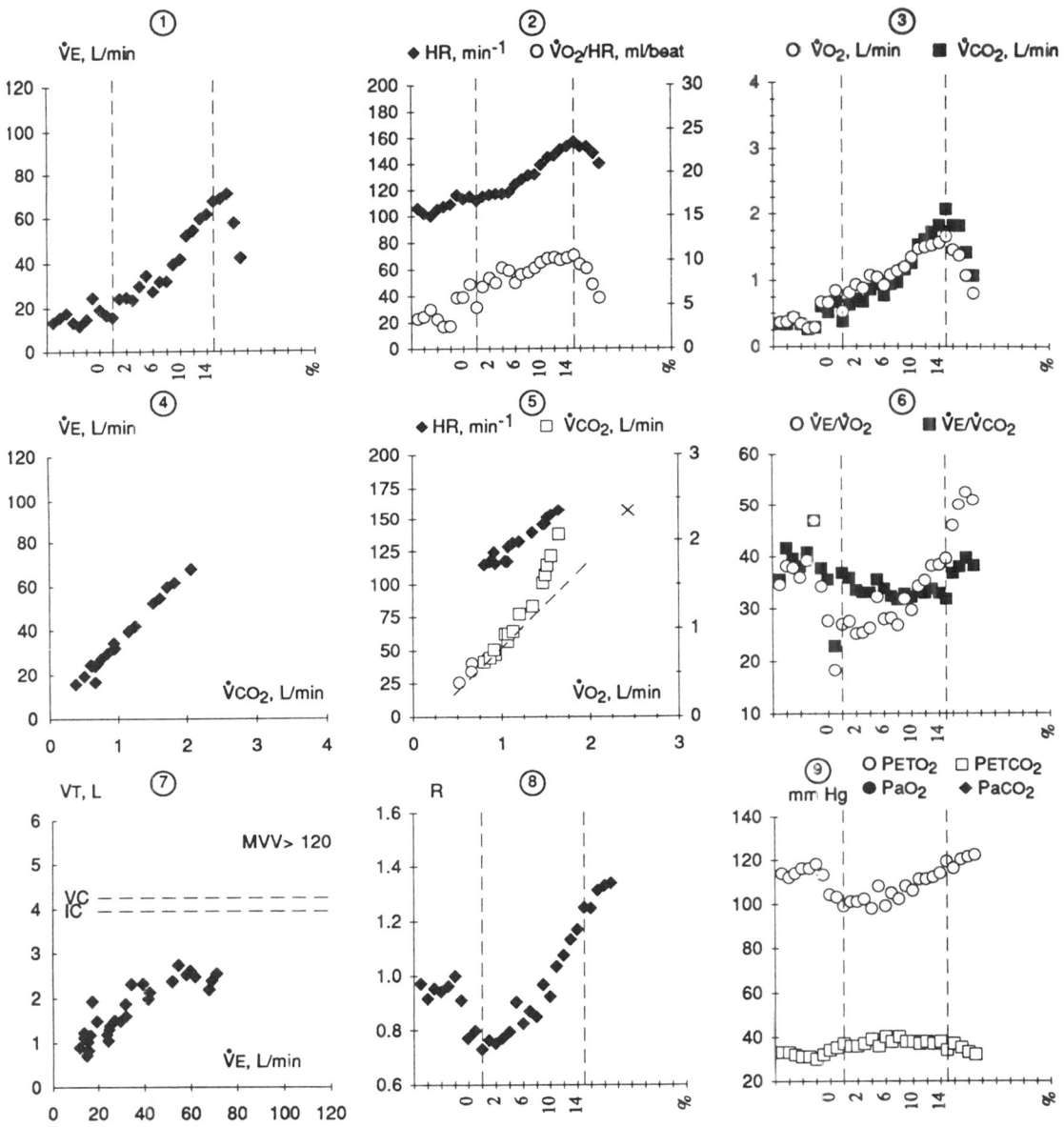

1. Vertical dashed lines in panels 1 to 3 and 6, 8, and 9 indicate the beginning and the end of increasing work period.

2. Zero grade walking is performed for 2 minutes before the left vertical dashed line.

3. In panel 5, the diagonal dashed line has a slope of 1; the "x" in the upper right is the predicted maximum heart rate and $\dot{V}O_2$ for the subject.

TABLE 9.72.4.   Treadmill Ergometry

Time min	Work rate watts	BP mmHg	HR min⁻¹	f min⁻¹	$\dot{V}_E$ L/min BTPS	$\dot{V}_{CO_2}$ L/min STPD	$\dot{V}_{O_2}$ L/min STPD	$\dot{V}_{O_2}$/HR ml/beat	R	pH	HCO₃ meq/L	Po₂, mmHg ET	a	(A−a)	Pco₂, mmHg ET	a	(a−ET)	$\dot{V}_E$ / $\dot{V}_{CO_2}$	$\dot{V}_E$ / $\dot{V}_{O_2}$	VD VT
	Rest		106	12	13.5	0.35	0.36	3.4	0.97			114			33			36	35	
	Rest		102	15	15.4	0.34	0.37	3.6	0.92			112			33			42	38	
	Rest		100	9	17.4	0.42	0.44	4.4	0.95			114			32			40	38	
	Rest		105	11	13.5	0.33	0.35	3.3	0.94			116			31			38	36	
	Rest		107	13	11.7	0.26	0.27	2.5	0.96			116			31			41	39	
	Rest		109	21	14.9	0.28	0.28	2.6	1.00			118			30			47	47	
	0		116	19	24.6	0.61	0.67	5.8	0.91			113			32			38	34	
	0		113	13	19.3	0.51	0.66	5.8	0.77			104			34			36	28	
	0		115	14	16.5	0.67	0.84	7.3	0.80			103			35			23	18	
	0		112	19	15.6	0.38	0.52	4.6	0.73			99			37			37	27	
0.5	2		115	23	24.2	0.62	0.81	7.0	0.77			101			36			36	27	
1.0	2		116	18	24.9	0.70	0.93	8.0	0.75			101			36			33	25	
1.5	4		117	20	23.8	0.67	0.87	7.4	0.77			102			37			33	25	
2.0	4		117	20	29.7	0.85	1.07	9.1	0.79			98			39			33	26	
2.5	6		118	15	34.6	0.94	1.04	8.8	0.90			108			36			35	32	
3.0	6		124	18	27.2	0.76	0.92	7.4	0.83			99			40			34	28	
3.5	8		128	17	31.8	0.94	1.08	8.4	0.87			105			38			32	28	
4.0	8		131	20	32.0	0.96	1.13	8.6	0.85			102			40			32	27	
4.5	10		132	17	39.5	1.16	1.20	9.1	0.97			108			38			33	32	
5.0	10		139	21	41.8	1.25	1.35	9.7	0.93			106			38			32	30	
5.5	12		145	22	52.3	1.52	1.47	10.1	1.03			111			37			33	34	
6.0	12		146	20	54.7	1.61	1.50	10.3	1.07			111			38			33	35	
6.5	14		151	23	59.9	1.72	1.52	10.1	1.13			112			37			34	38	
7.0	14		153	25	61.9	1.82	1.56	10.2	1.17			114			38			33	38	
7.5	16		157	31	67.8	2.06	1.65	10.5	1.25			119			34			32	39	
	Recovery		153	29	69.2	1.82	1.46	9.5	1.25			116			37			37	46	
	Recovery		153	28	71.2	1.81	1.38	9.0	1.31			120			35			38	50	
	Recovery		148	23	58.1	1.42	1.07	7.2	1.33			121			33			40	52	
	Recovery		140	20	42.4	1.07	0.80	5.7	1.34			122			32			38	51	

cardiac. The patient hyperventilates at rest but has no evidence of ventilation-perfusion mismatching or pulmonary vascular disease. The significant resting systemic hypertension does not increase inordinately during exercise and $\Delta \dot{V}_{O_2}/\Delta WR$ is normal, implying that peripheral arterial disease is not the primary disorder. The ECG findings, steep heart rate-$\dot{V}_{O_2}$ relationship in both forms of ergometry, (panel 5 in Figs. 9.72.1 and 9.72.2) constant and reduced O₂ pulse, and elevated ventilatory equivalents all suggest that the primary diagnosis is left ventricular failure presumably due to cardiac disease.

Conclusion

Left ventricular failure limiting exercise performance. This is confirmed by the absence of a cardiac reserve at the reduced maximum work rate, failure for $\dot{V}_{O_2}$ to rise normally with increasing work rate (treadmill exercise study), and the reduced maximum O₂ pulse in both forms of ergometry.

Case 73 β-adrenergic Blockade, Systemic Hypertension, Pulmonary Vascular Disease, and Mild Chronic Bronchitis

Clinical Findings

A 55-year-old former shipyard worker had first noted exertional dyspnea and a morning cough with small amounts of sputum approximately 5 years earlier. He retired 3 years previously because of an injury to the left foot. The patient had a 60 pack year smoking history but had stopped 1 year ago. Hypertension, diagnosed 1 year previously, was being treated with hydrochlorothiazide and propranolol. There is no history of angina or congestive heart failure. Examination revealed normal breath sounds, cardiovascular examination, and peripheral pulses. Chest roentgenograms showed minimal pleural plaques without evidence of parenchymal lung disease.

Exercise Findings

The patient performed exercise on a cycle ergometer. He pedalled at 60 rpm without added load for 3 minutes. The work rate was then increased 20 W per minute to his symptom-limited maximum. Arterial blood was sampled every second minute, and intra-arterial blood pressure was recorded from a percutaneously placed brachial artery catheter. Resting and exercise ECGs were normal except for relative bradycardia. The patient stopped exercise complaining of general fatigue and shortness of breath.

TABLE 9.73.1. Selected Respiratory Function Data

Measurement	Predicted	Measured
Age, yr		55
Sex		Male
Height, cm		173
Weight, kg	76	85
Hematocrit, %		48
VC, L	4.20	4.54
IC, L	2.80	3.66
TLC, L	6.26	6.88
FEV_1, L	3.32	3.16
FEV_1/VC, %	79	70
MVV, L/min	140	121
$D_{L}CO$, ml/mm Hg/min	28.1	16.6

TABLE 9.73.2. Selected Exercise Data

Measurement	Predicted	Measured
Peak $\dot{V}O_2$, L/min	2.35	1.59
Maximum HR, beats/min	165	113
Maximum O_2 pulse, ml/beat	14.3	14.4
$\Delta\dot{V}O_2/\Delta WR$, ml/min/W	10.3	9.8
AT, L/min	>1.01	0.95
Blood pressure, mmHg (rest, max)		181/107, 206/113
Maximum $\dot{V}E$, L/min		72
Exercise breathing reserve, L/min	>15	49
PaO_2, mmHg (rest, max ex)		73, 71
$P(A - a)O_2$, mmHg (rest, max ex)		31, 46
$P(a - ET)CO_2$, mmHg (rest, max ex)		3, 4
VD/VT (rest, heavy ex)		0.33, 0.35
HCO_3^-, mEq/L (rest, 2-min reccv)		24, 18

FIGURE 9.73.1.

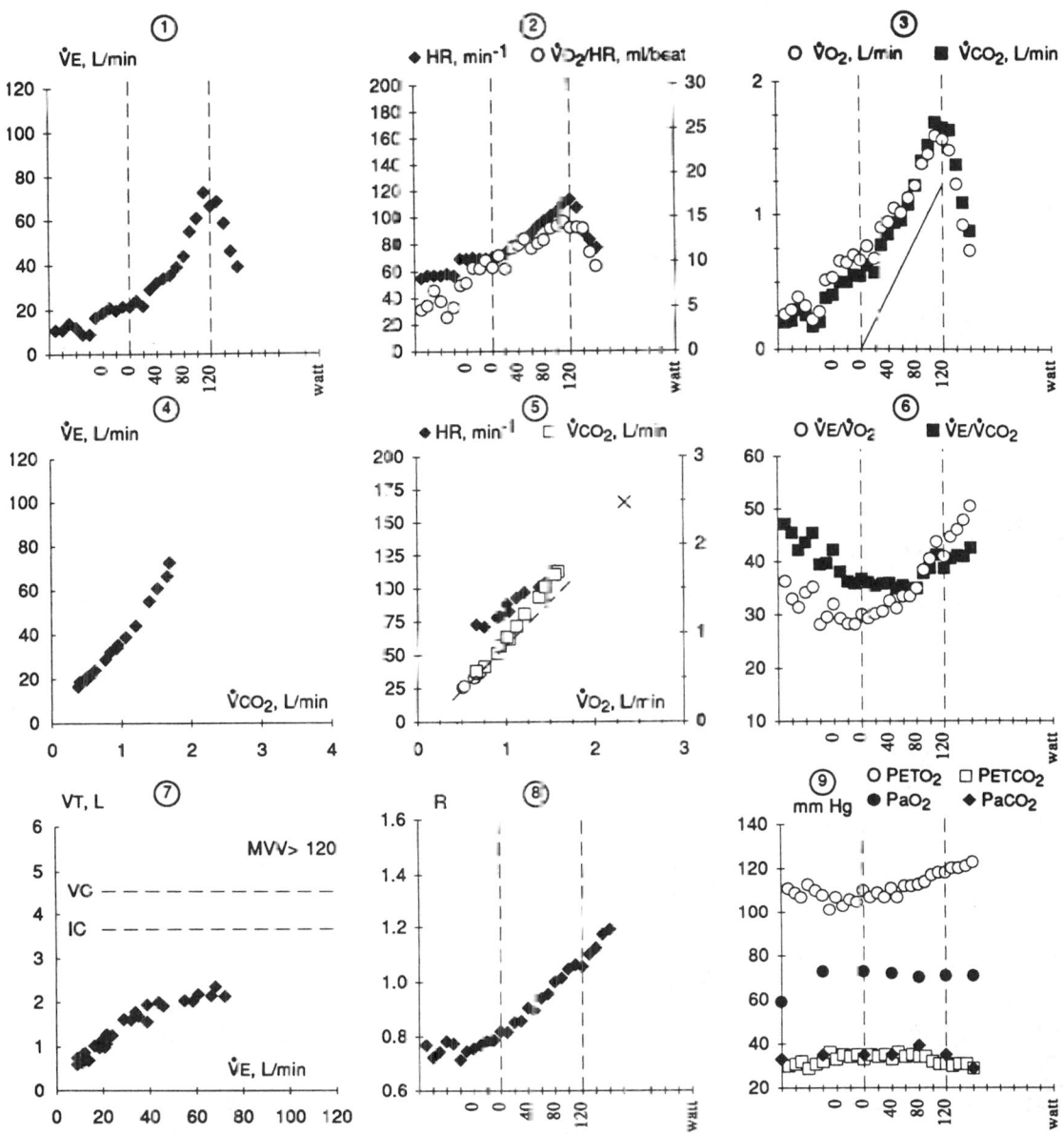

1. Vertical dashed lines in panels 1 to 3 and 6, 8, and 9 indicate the beginning and the end of increasing work period.
2. Unloaded cycling is performed for 3 minutes before the left vertical dashed line.
3. In panel 3, the diagonal line shows the increase of $\dot{V}O_2$ at a slope of 10 ml/min/W.
4. In panel 5, the diagonal dashed line has a slope of 1; the "x" in the upper right is the predicted maximum heart rate and $\dot{V}O_2$ for the subject.

TABLE 9.73.3. Air Breathing

Time min	Work rate watts	BP mmHg	HR min⁻¹	f min⁻¹	V̇E L/min BTPS	V̇CO₂ L/min STPD	V̇O₂ L/min STPD	V̇O₂/HR ml/beat	R	pH	HCO₃⁻ meq/L	Po₂ mmHg ET	a	(A − a)	Pco₂, mmHg ET	a	(a − ET)	V̇E/V̇CO₂	V̇E/V̇O₂	VD/VT
	Rest									7.47	24		59			33				
	Rest		55	15	10.7	0.20	0.26	4.7	0.77			111			30			47	36	
	Rest		57	17	11.0	0.21	0.29	5.1	0.72			109			31			46	33	
	Rest		57	20	13.9	0.29	0.39	6.8	0.74			107			32			42	31	
	Rest	182/107	57	14	12.1	0.25	0.32	5.6	0.78			113			29			44	34	
	Rest		58	15	9.0	0.17	0.22	3.8	0.77			110			31			45	35	
	Rest		57	12	8.9	0.20	0.28	4.9	0.71	7.44	23	108	73	31	32	35	3	39	28	0.33
	Unloaded		69	16	16.4	0.38	0.51	7.4	0.75			101			36			40	29	
	Unloaded	193/107	69	19	18.5	0.40	0.53	7.7	0.75			107			33			42	32	
	Unloaded		70	21	20.8	0.50	0.65	9.3	0.77			103			35			38	29	
	Unloaded		69	17	19.5	0.50	0.64	9.3	0.78			106			34			36	28	
	Unloaded		69	20	21.4	0.55	0.70	10.1	0.79			105			35			36	28	
	Unloaded		70	19	21.4	0.54	0.66	9.4	0.82	7.44	23	110	73	36	33	35	2	37	30	0.30
0.5	20		71	19	23.9	0.62	0.76	10.7	0.82			107			35			36	29	
1.0	20	194/107	73	17	21.6	0.57	0.67	9.2	0.85			109			34			35	30	
1.5	40		78	18	29.0	0.77	0.90	11.5	0.86			107			35			36	31	
2.0	40		79	20	32.2	0.85	0.94	11.9	0.90	7.44	23	111	72	40	33	35	2	36	32	0.30
2.5	60		83	19	33.9	0.93	1.04	12.5	0.89			107			36			35	31	
3.0	60	197/110	88	21	35.4	0.95	1.01	11.5	0.94			112			34			35	33	
3.5	80		93	20	39.0	1.07	1.12	12.0	0.96			112			35			35	33	
4.0	80		97	22	44.0	1.21	1.21	12.5	1.00	7.42	25	113	70	41	34	39	5	35	35	0.35
4.5	100		101	27	55.0	1.40	1.38	13.7	1.01			114			34			38	38	
5.0	100	206/113	104	28	61.0	1.52	1.45	13.9	1.05			117			32			39	40	
5.5	120		110	34	72.4	1.69	1.59	14.5	1.06			118			31			41	44	
6.0	120		113	31	66.4	1.65	1.56	13.8	1.06	7.42	22	118	71	46	31	35	4	39	41	0.35
	Recovery		107	29	68.4	1.63	1.48	13.8	1.10			120			30			40	45	
	Recovery	213/107	89	29	58.6	1.37	1.22	13.7	1.12			120			31			41	46	
	Recovery		83	24	46.0	1.08	0.92	11.1	1.17			121			31			41	48	
	Recovery		77	25	39.0	0.87	0.73	9.5	1.19	7.40	18	123	71	54	29	29	0	42	51	0.28

Interpretation

Comments

The mechanics of breathing are normal, but the diffusing capacity is significantly reduced (Table 9.73.1). The resting ECG is normal.

Analysis

In flow chart 1, peak V̇O₂ and the anaerobic threshold are reduced (Table 9.73.2). See flow chart 4. The breathing reserve is high (branchpoint 4.1). The ventilatory equivalent for CO_2 at the anaerobic threshold is high (branchpoint 4.3). This suggests that the patient has an abnormal pulmonary circulation. Confirmation of this is demonstrated by high VD/VT, P(A − a)O₂, and P(a − ET)CO₂ values (indices of ventilation-perfusion mismatching). Because there is no associated disturbance in respiratory mechanics, we must conclude that these findings are on the basis of primary pulmonary vascular disease. The significant reduction in diffusing capacity (D$_L$CO) is compatible with this conclusion. There is no abrupt decrease in PaO₂ or O₂ saturation at the start of exercise (branchpoint 4.5), indicating that a right to left shunt does not accompany the pulmonary vascular disease. Because the patient is being treated with propranolol, the heart rate response is unusually low for this kind of abnormality. Thus, the low heart rate and the systemic hypertension likely contribute to the low peak V̇O₂ and anaerobic threshold.

Conclusion

Exercise limitation is caused by pulmonary vascular disease, systemic hypertension, and impaired heart rate response secondary to β-adrenergic blockade.

Case 74 β-adrenergic Blockade, Obesity, and Asbestosis

Clinical Findings

This 61-year-old man was referred for follow-up cardiopulmonary exercise testing because of his 30-year work exposure to asbestos. He had stopped smoking 13 years before but had a 100 pack year history of cigarette smoking. He had noted dyspnea in the past 2 years (associated with an 11 kg weight gain) but denied cough, chest pain, claudication, or ankle edema. He had hypertension; his only medications were atenolol and nifedipine. Examination revealed rare crackles at the right lung base, normal heart sounds, and peripheral pulses. Resting ECG showed a prolonged PR interval, J-point elevations in leads V2 and V3, and nonspecific T wave abnormalities in the lateral chest leads. Chest roentgenograms revealed some diaphragmatic calcification, pleural thickening, and parenchymal scarring.

Exercise Findings

The patient performed exercise on a cycle ergometer. He pedalled at 60 rpm without an added load for 3 minutes. The work rate was then increased 15 W per minute to tolerance. Heart rate and rhythm were continuously monitored; 12-lead ECGs were obtained during rest, exercise, and recovery. Blood pressure was measured with a sphygmomanometer and oxygen saturation with an ear oximeter. The patient appeared to give a good effort and stopped exercise because of general fatigue; he denied chest pain or dyspnea during or after the study. The patient had no ectopy or abnormal ECG changes during or after exercise. Ear oximetry studies were normal.

TABLE 9.74.1. **Selected Respiratory Function Data**

Measurement	Predicted	Measured
Age, yr		61
Sex		Male
Height, cm		179
Weight, kg	81	120
Hematocrit, %		42
VC, L	4.41	2.97
IC, L	2.94	2.67
TLC, L	6.75	5.04
FEV_1, L	3.46	2.34
FEV_1/VC, %	78	78
MVV, L/min	140	92
D_LCO, ml/mm Hg/min	27.2	26.6

TABLE 9.74.2. **Selected Exercise Data**

Measurement	Predicted	Measured
Peak $\dot{V}O_2$, L/min	2.50	1.92
Maximum HR, beats/min	159	105
Maximum O_2 pulse, ml/beat	15.7	18.8
$\Delta\dot{V}O_2$/ΔWR, ml/min/W	10.3	9.6
AT, L/min	>1.10	1.3
Blood pressure, mmHg (rest, max ex)		140/90, 160/80
Maximum $\dot{V}E$, L/min		69
Exercise breathing reserve, L/min	>15	23

FIGURE 9.74.1.

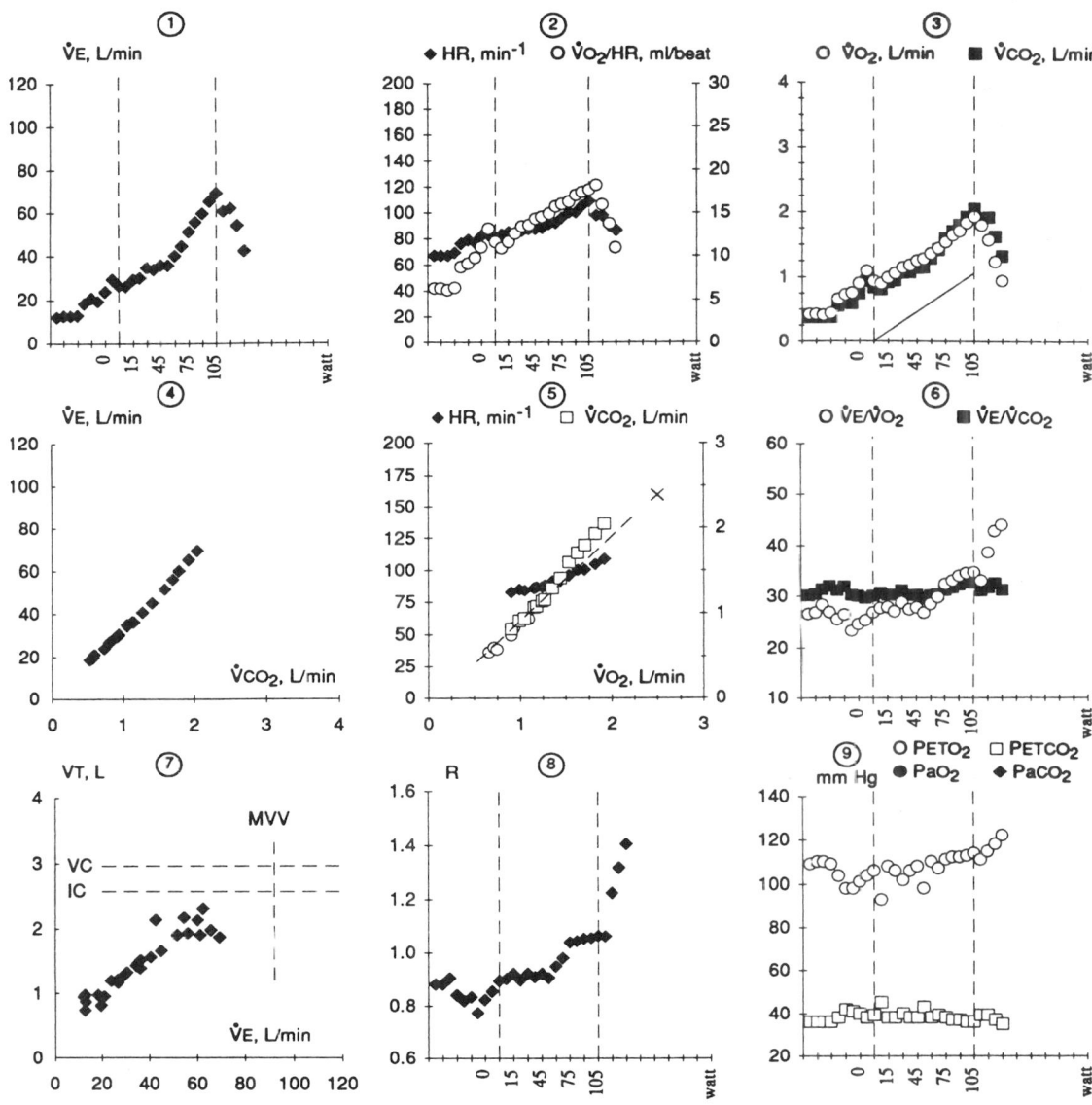

1. Vertical dashed lines in panels 1 to 3 and 6, 8, and 9 indicate the beginning and the end of increasing work period.

2. Unloaded cycling is performed for 3 minutes before the left vertical dashed line.

3. In panel 3, the diagonal line shows the increase of $\dot{V}O_2$ at a slope of 10 ml/min/W.

4. In panel 5, the diagonal dashed line has a slope of 1; the "x" in the upper right is the predicted maximum heart rate and $\dot{V}O_2$ for the subject.

TABLE 9.74.3. Air Breathing

Time min	Work rate watts	BP mmHg	HR min⁻¹	f min⁻¹	V̇E L/min BTPS	V̇CO2 L/min STPD	V̇O2 L/min STPD	V̇O2/HR ml/beat	R	pH	HCO3 meq/L	PO2 ET	PO2 a	PO2 (A−a)	PCO2 ET	PCO2 a	PCO2 (a−ET)	V̇E/V̇CO2	V̇E/V̇O2	VD/VT
	Rest	140/90																		
	Rest		67	13	12.3	0.37	0.42	6.3	0.83			109			36			30	27	
	Rest		67	17	12.7	0.37	0.42	6.3	0.83			110			36			30	27	
	Rest		67	13	12.7	0.37	0.41	6.1	0.90			110			36			31	28	
	Rest	130/80	69	15	13.1	0.37	0.44	6.4	0.84			109			36			32	27	
	Unloaded		76	19	18.5	0.54	0.66	8.7	0.82			104			38			31	26	
	Unloaded		79	22	21.0	0.60	0.72	9.1	0.83			98			42			32	27	
	Unloaded		77	24	19.6	0.58	0.75	9.7	0.77			98			41			30	23	
	Unloaded	130/80	82	20	23.9	0.74	0.90	11.0	0.82			101			40			30	25	
	Unloaded		83	23	29.6	0.93	1.09	13.1	0.85			104			38			30	25	
	Unloaded		80	23	26.9	0.83	0.93	11.6	0.89			106			39			30	27	
0.5	15		83	22	26.7	0.81	0.90	10.8	0.90			93			45			31	28	
1.0	15	145/80	85	23	29.5	0.91	0.99	11.6	0.92			108			38			30	28	
1.5	30		84	23	30.4	0.94	1.05	12.5	0.90			106			38			30	27	
2.0	30		86	24	35.0	1.06	1.15	13.4	0.92			102			40			31	29	
2.5	45		87	24	34.4	1.07	1.18	13.3	0.91			106			38			30	27	
3.0	45	140/80	87	24	36.4	1.14	1.24	14.3	0.92			108			38			30	28	
3.5	60		88	26	36.1	1.15	1.27	14.4	0.91			98			43			29	27	
4.0	60		91	26	40.6	1.23	1.35	14.8	0.95			110			38			30	28	
4.5	75		92	27	45.0	1.41	1.44	15.7	0.98			107			39			30	30	
5.0	75	150/90	96	27	51.6	1.59	1.53	15.9	1.04			111			38			31	32	
5.5	90		100	29	56.1	1.70	1.63	16.3	1.04			112			37			32	33	
6.0	90		100	28	60.0	1.79	1.70	17.0	1.05			112			37			32	34	
6.5	105		105	33	65.5	1.92	1.82	17.3	1.05			113			36			33	34	
7.0	105	160/80	109	37	69.4	2.04	1.92	17.6	1.06			114			36			32	35	
	Recovery		98	32	61.2	1.89	1.78	18.2	1.06			111			39			31	33	
	Recovery		98	27	62.4	1.91	1.56	15.9	1.22			115			39			31	39	
	Recovery		90	25	54.5	1.62	1.23	13.7	1.32			118			37			32	43	
	Recovery		86	20	42.8	1.32	0.94	10.9	1.40			122			35			31	44	

Interpretation

Comments

The reduced lung volumes are compatible with mild restrictive disease due to obesity (reduced ERV) and asbestosis. The nearly normal IC suggests that the restriction is primarily caused by obesity.

Analysis

In flow chart 1, peak V̇O2 is reduced (branchpoint 1.1), but the anaerobic threshold is normal (branchpoints 1.2 and 1.3), despite the patient's inability to raise his exercise heart rate above 105 beats/min. Going next to flow chart 3, the normal breathing reserve (branchpoint 3.1) and probably normal ECG (branchpoint 3.2) lead one to the diagnosis of poor effort or musculoskeletal disorder. There are no measures of VD/VT or arterial-alveolar pressure differences, but the normal ventilatory equivalents and normal ear oximetry are evidence against any major gas exchange abnormality during exercise. The high

heart rate reserve might lead one to consider poor effort, but the high recovery R of 1.40 (indicating a significant metabolic acidosis) is evidence against this diagnosis. The low maximum heart rate and accompanying high maximum O2 pulse are best explained by a high degree of β blockade from atenolol, which gives more time than usual for filling of the ventricles. The high V̇O2 at unloaded pedalling (nearly 1.0 L/min) is typical of obesity.

Conclusion

β-adrenergic blockade therapy of hypertension can cause significant reduction in maximum heart rate, peak V̇O2, and maximum work rate. Usually, as in this patient, the increase in O2 pulse is an important factor in overcoming the effect of reduction in maximum heart rate and minimizing the effect on maximum V̇O2. Obesity and the limited ability to increase heart rate can lead to the symptom of fatigue, however, as found in this case.

Case 75 Pulmonary Vascular Disease, Chronic Bronchitis, Asbestosis, and Myocardial Ischemia

Clinical Findings

This 51-year-old shipyard worker had noted increased dyspnea on exertion for 2 years, until he was unable to finish cleaning his one bedroom apartment. For several years he had a morning cough productive of small amounts of yellow sputum. He had over 40 pack years of cigarette smoking and continued to smoke. He denied chest pain, tightness, or pressure. Chest x-ray studies showed a streaky infiltrate in the lower lung fields with nodular scarring in the upper lung zones. Physical examination of the chest was normal. There was equivocal clubbing of the digits. Peripheral pulses were normal. ECG showed left axis deviation.

Exercise Findings

The patient performed exercise on a cycle ergometer. He first pedalled at 60 rpm, without added load, for 3 minutes. The work rate was then increased 15 W per minute to his symptom-limited maximum. Arterial blood was sampled every second minute, and intra-arterial blood pressure was recorded from a percutaneously placed brachial artery catheter. The patient stopped exercising because of severe knee cramps. During incremental exercise he developed premature atrial and ventricular contractions, and 3 to 4 mm ST segment depression in leads V4 and V5. He denied any chest pain or discomfort, dizziness or lightheadedness. The ST segments returned to normal within 1 minute of recovery.

TABLE 9.75.1. Selected Respiratory Function Data

Measurement	Predicted	Measured
Age, yr		51
Sex		Male
Height, cm		166
Weight, kg	70	55
Hematocrit, %		49
VC, L	3.88	3.83
IC, L	2.59	2.37
TLC, L	5.71	6.81
FEV_1, L	3.07	2.41
FEV_1/VC, %	79	63
MVV, L/min, direct	136	120
MVV, L/min, indirect	123	96
$D_{L}CO$, ml/mm Hg/min	26.9	21.5

TABLE 9.75.2. Selected Exercise Data

Measurement	Predicted	Measured
Peak $\dot{V}O_2$, L/min	1.99	1.77
Maximum HR, beats/min	169	150
Maximum O_2 pulse, ml/beat	11.8	11.8
$\Delta\dot{V}O_2/\Delta WR$, ml/min/W	10.3	9.7
AT, L/min	>0.86	1.2
Blood pressure, mmHg (rest, max)		132/72, 189/99
Maximum $\dot{V}E$, L/min		79
Exercise breathing reserve, L/min	>15	17
PaO_2, mmHg (rest, max ex)		69, 63
$P(A - a)O_2$, mmHg (rest, max ex)		30, 44
$P(a - ET)CO_2$, mmHg (rest, max ex)		10, 6
VD/VT (rest, heavy ex)		0.53, 0.47
HCO_3^-, mEq/L (rest, 2-min recov)		25, 17

FIGURE 9.75.1.

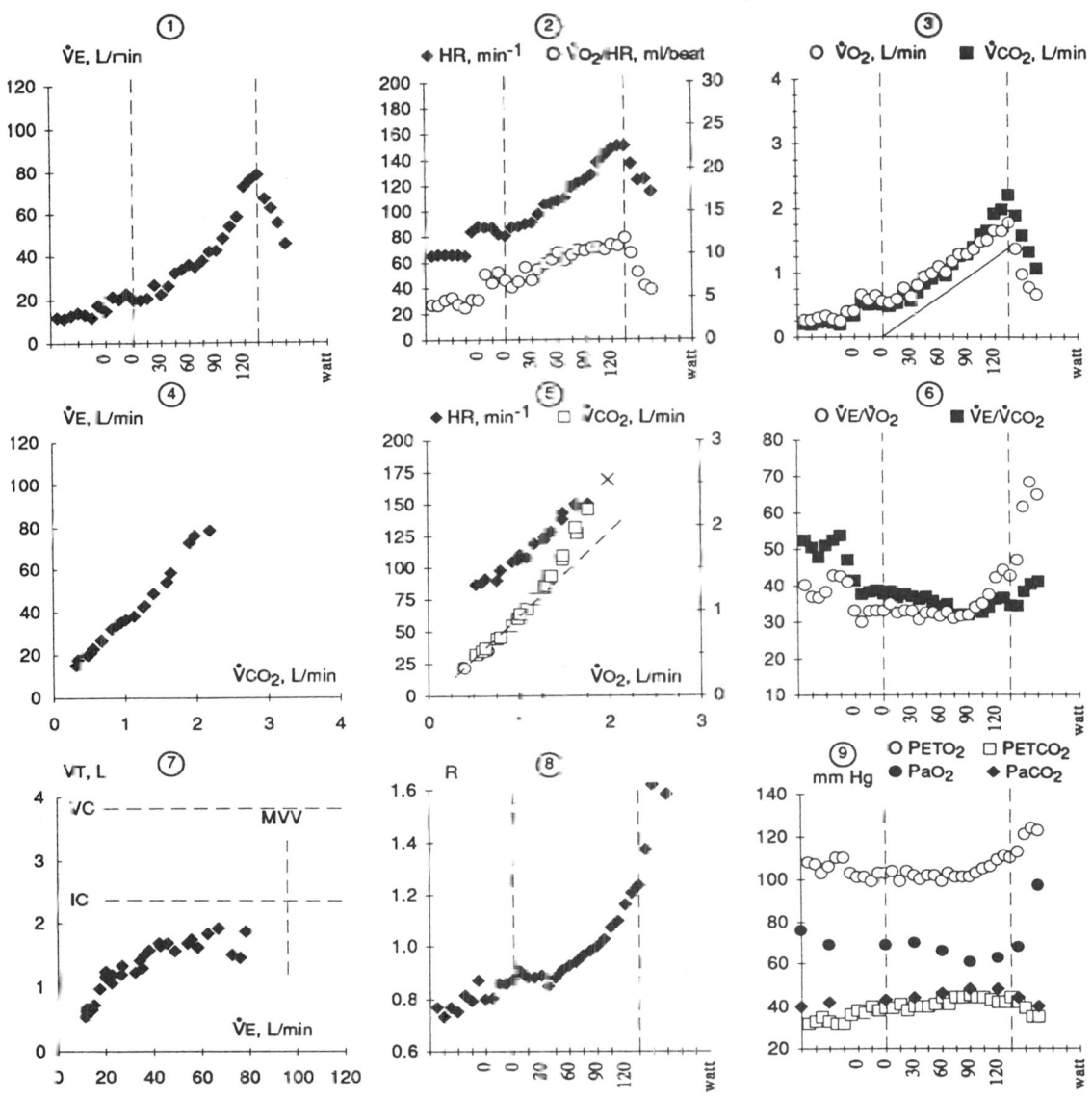

1 Vertical dashed lines in panels 1 to 3 and 5, 8, and 9 indicate the beginning and the end of increasing work period.

2. Unloaded cycling is performed for 3 minutes before the left vertical dashed line.

3. In panel 3, the diagonal line shows the increase of $\dot{V}O_2$ at a slope of 10 ml/min/W.

4. In panel 5, the diagonal dashed line has a slope of 1; the "x" in the upper right is the predicted maximum heart rate and $\dot{V}O_2$ for the subject.

Interpretation

Comments

Resting respiratory function tests are compatible with mild airflow obstruction (Table 9.75.1). The diffusing capacity is at the lower limits of normal. The resting ECG is essentially normal.

Analysis

In flow chart 1, the peak $\dot{V}O_2$ and the anaerobic threshold are normal (Table 9.75.2). See flow chart 2. The ECG at maximum exercise is abnormal suggesting ischemic changes. The arterial blood gases are also significantly abnormal during exer-

TABLE 9.75.3. Air Breathing

Time min	Work rate watts	BP mmHg	HR min⁻¹	f min⁻¹	$\dot{V}_E$ L/min BTPS	$\dot{V}_{CO_2}$ L/min STPD	$\dot{V}_{O_2}$ L/min STPD	$\dot{V}_{O_2}$/HR ml/beat	R	pH	HCO₃⁻ meq/L	P_{O_2} mmHg ET	a	(A−a)	P_{CO_2} mmHg ET	a	(a−ET)	$\dot{V}_E/\dot{V}_{CO_2}$	$\dot{V}_E/\dot{V}_{O_2}$	VD/VT
	Rest	132/72								7.42	25		76			40		52	40	
	Rest		65	18	12.0	0.20	0.26	4.0	0.77			108			32			52	40	
	Rest		66	21	11.4	0.19	0.26	3.9	0.73			107			33			51	37	
	Rest		66	19	12.6	0.23	0.30	4.5	0.77			103			35			48	37	
	Rest	159/81	66	22	14.1	0.24	0.32	4.8	0.75	7.39	25	106	69	28	33	42	9	51	38	0.52
	Rest		66	21	13.3	0.22	0.27	4.1	0.81			110			32			52	43	
	Rest		65	19	11.8	0.19	0.24	3.7	0.79			110			32			54	42	
	Unloaded		84	18	17.5	0.34	0.39	4.6	0.87			103			36			47	41	
	Unloaded		88	21	15.0	0.32	0.40	4.5	0.80			101			38			41	33	
	Unloaded		87	18	21.4	0.53	0.66	7.6	0.80			101			37			37	30	
	Unloaded	165/90	87	16	20.1	0.49	0.57	6.6	0.86			99			40			38	33	
	Unloaded		82	19	22.8	0.55	0.64	7.8	0.86			103			38			39	33	
	Unloaded		81	16	19.9	0.49	0.56	6.9	0.88	7.38	25	103	69	33	39	43	4	38	33	0.44
0.5	15		87	17	19.9	0.48	0.53	6.1	0.91			104			39			38	35	
1.0	15	180/93	88	18	20.6	0.52	0.59	6.7	0.88			99			41			37	32	
1.5	30		90	20	26.9	0.67	0.76	8.4	0.88			104			38			38	33	
2.0	30		91	21	22.5	0.56	0.63	6.9	0.89	7.37	25	102	70	32	40	44	4	37	33	0.43
2.5	45		98	22	26.4	0.68	0.80	8.2	0.85			100			40			36	31	
3.0	45	186/93	105	26	32.3	0.82	0.93	8.9	0.88			102			40			37	32	
3.5	60		106	24	34.2	0.90	0.99	9.3	0.91			102			41			36	32	
4.0	60		108	24	36.4	1.01	1.09	10.1	0.93	7.35	25	99	66	35	44	46	2	34	32	0.42
4.5	75		110	27	35.3	0.95	1.01	9.2	0.94			103			41			35	33	
5.0	75	189/93	119	24	38.1	1.13	1.17	9.8	0.97			101			44			32	31	
5.5	90		122	25	42.4	1.26	1.28	10.5	0.98			101			44			32	31	
6.0	90		124	26	43.0	1.28	1.28	10.3	1.00	7.31	24	101	61	41	45	48	3	32	32	0.41
6.5	105		128	31	48.8	1.40	1.36	10.6	1.03			103			44			33	34	
7.0	105	191/99	138	32	54.2	1.59	1.48	10.7	1.07			105			44			32	35	
7.5	120		143	36	58.6	1.64	1.49	10.4	1.10			106			43			34	37	
8.0	120		148	48	72.8	1.91	1.64	11.1	1.16	7.28	22	109	63	44	42	48	6	36	42	0.47
8.5	135		150	52	76.2	1.97	1.63	10.9	1.21			111			42			36	44	
9.0	135	189/99	150	42	78.7	2.19	1.77	11.8	1.24			110			44			34	42	
	Recovery		137	35	67.2	1.88	1.37	10.0	1.37	7.25	19	113	68	47	42	44	2	34	47	0.41
	Recovery	184/84	124	34	62.6	1.57	0.97	7.8	1.62			121			39			38	62	
	Recovery		125	32	55.9	1.32	0.78	6.2	1.69			124			35			40	68	
	Recovery		115	27	45.8	1.06	0.67	5.8	1.58	7.24	17	123	97	25	35	40	5	41	65	0.45

cise (branchpoint 2.1). The indices of ventilation-perfusion matching (VD/VT, $P(a - ET)CO_2$, and $P(A - a)O_2$) (branchpoint 2.3) are clearly abnormal, suggesting that this patient has lung disease and/or pulmonary vascular disease. Because the results of the resting respiratory function tests are not consistent with a diagnosis of restrictive lung disease and suggest that the patient's airflow obstruction is only mild, it is likely that the major abnormalities in ventilation-perfusion mismatching observed in this patient are attributable to pulmonary vascular disease. The ECG abnormalities that this patient developed as he approached his maximum work rate, despite the absence of chest pain, suggest that the patient also develops myocardial ischemia under exercise stress.

Conclusion

This study shows normal maximum exercise capacity in a patient with pulmonary vascular disease and myocardial ischemia. There is clear evidence of significant ventilation-perfusion mismatching of the type seen with pulmonary vascular disease; however, his pulmonary mechanics are only mildly abnormal. Presumably, this is an instance of changes in the pulmonary circulation disproportionate to airway or parenchymal disease. Additionally, the exercise induced ST segment depression and arrhythmia, typical of myocardial ischemia, suggest coronary artery disease. The pulmonary vascular disease and exercise hypoxemia possibly contribute to this cardiac abnormality.

Case 76 "Asthma," Obesity, and Anemia

Clinical Findings

This 50-year-old meatcutter and former smoker had severe exertional dyspnea and had been hospitalized on several occasions for what had been considered to be congestive heart failure with wheezing, leg edema, and orthopnea. He was referred for exercise testing to aid in distinguishing between cardiac and respiratory disease. He was anemic from unknown cause. Breath sounds were distant.

Exercise Findings

The patient performed exercise on a cycle ergometer. He pedalled at 60 rpm without an added load for 3 minutes. The work rate was then increased 15 W per minute to tolerance. Arterial blood was sampled every second minute, and intra-arterial pressure was recorded from a percutaneously placed brachial artery catheter. Heart rate and rhythm were continuously monitored; 12-lead ECGs were obtained during rest, exercise, and recovery. The patient appeared to give an excellent effort and stopped exercise because of severe dyspnea and exhaustion. He denied chest pain during or after the study. No arrhythmias or ischemic changes were noted on ECG.

TABLE 9.76.1. Selected Respiratory Function Data

Measurement	Predicted	Measured
Age, yr		50
Sex		Male
Height, cm		174
Weight, kg	77	91
Hemoglobin, g/100 ml		10.3
VC, L	4.40	3.11
IC, L	2.94	2.15
TLC, L	6.44	9.78
FEV$_1$, L	3.49	1.14
FEV$_1$/VC, %	79	37
MVV, L/min	147	45
D$_L$CO, ml/mm Hg/min	24.4	28.8

TABLE 9.76.2. Selected Exercise Data

Measurement	Predicted	Measured
Peak $\dot{V}O_2$, L/min	2.55	1.20
Maximum HR, beats/min	170	147
Maximum O$_2$ pulse, ml/beat	14.3	8.4
$\Delta\dot{V}O_2/\Delta WR$, ml/min/W	10.3	7.6
AT, L/min	>1.10	0.95
Blood pressure, mmHg (rest, max)		135/90, 180/84
Maximum $\dot{V}E$, L/min		41
Exercise breathing reserve, L/min	>15	4
PaO_2, mmHg (rest, max ex)		84, 76
P(A − a)O_2, mmHg (rest, max ex)		19, 21
P(a − ET)CO_2, mmHg (rest, max ex)		5, 5
VD/VT (rest, heavy ex)		0.43, 0.46
HCO$_3^-$, mEq/L (rest, 2-min recov)		31, 29

FIGURE 9.76.1.

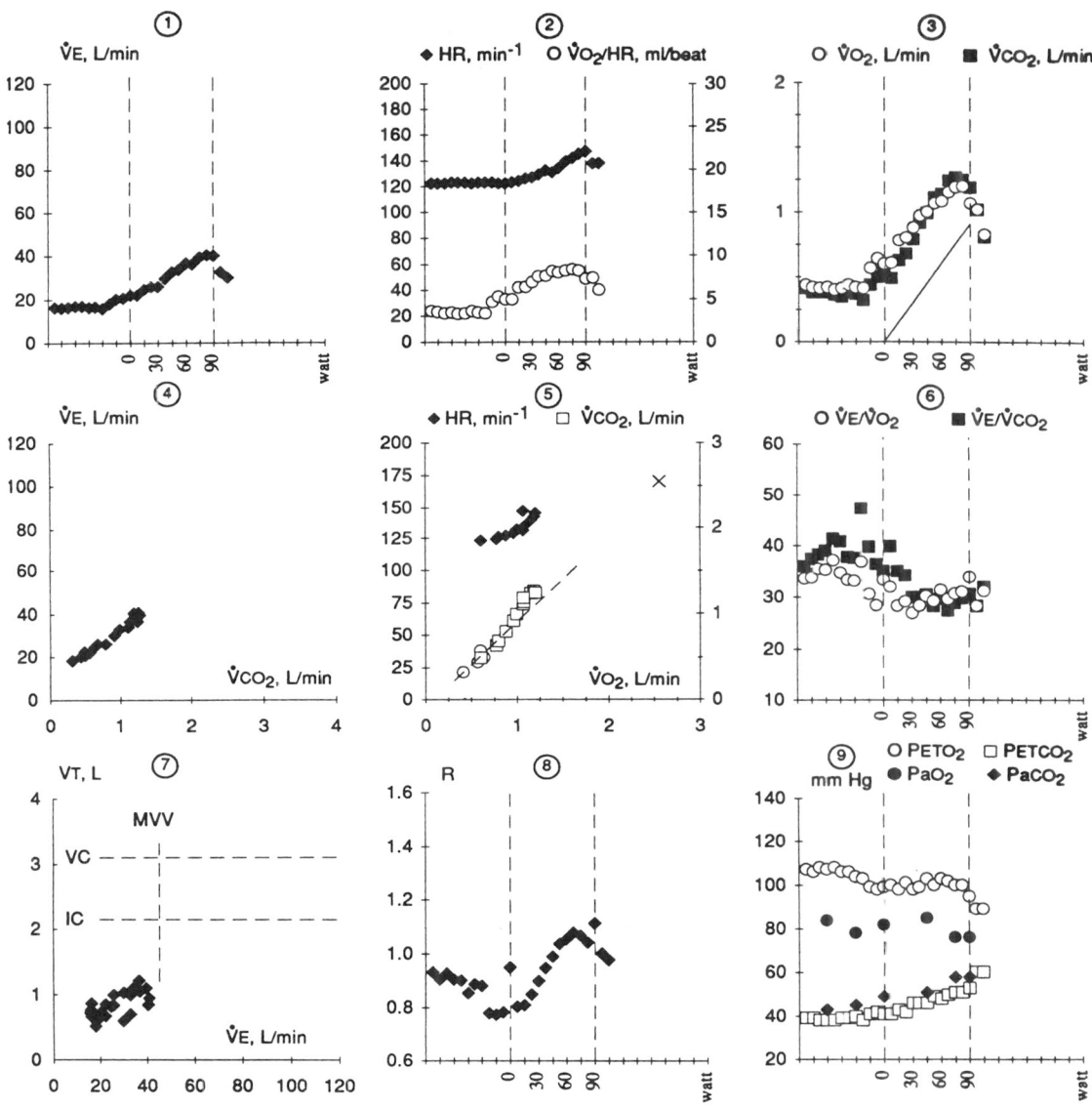

1. Vertical dashed lines in panels 1 to 3 and 6, 8, and 9 indicate the beginning and the end of increasing work period.

2. Unloaded cycling is performed for 2 minutes before the left vertical dashed line.

3. In panel 3, the diagonal line shows the increase of $\dot{V}O_2$ at a slope of 10 ml/min/W.

4. In panel 5, the diagonal dashed line has a slope of 1; the "x" in the upper right is the predicted maximum heart rate and $\dot{V}O_2$ for the subject.

TABLE 9.76.3. Air Breathing

Time min	Work rate watts	BP mmHg	HR min⁻¹	f min⁻¹	V̇E L/min BTPS	V̇CO₂ L/min STPD	V̇O₂ L/min STPD	V̇O₂/HR ml/beat	R	pH	HCO₃ meq/L	PO₂ ET	PO₂ a	PO₂ (A−a)	PCO₂ ET	PCO₂ a	PCO₂ (a−ET)	V̇E/V̇CO₂	V̇E/V̇O₂	VD/VT
	Rest		122	19	16.4	0.41	0.44	3.6	0.93			107			39			36	34	
	Rest		122	21	16.0	0.38	0.42	3.4	0.90			108			39			37	34	
	Rest		122	22	16.4	0.38	0.41	3.4	0.93			108			38			38	35	
	Rest	135/90	123	23	16.8	0.38	0.42	3.4	0.90	7.48	31	107	84	19	38	43	5	39	35	0.43
	Rest		123	25	17.0	0.36	0.40	3.3	0.90			108			38			41	37	
	Rest		123	25	16.4	0.35	0.41	3.3	0.85			106			39			41	35	
	Rest		122	22	16.6	0.39	0.44	3.6	0.83			106			39			38	33	
	Rest	123/84	123	22	15.8	0.37	0.42	3.4	0.83	7.46	31	104	78	22	40	45	5	38	33	0.43
	Unloaded		123	35	18.1	0.32	0.41	3.3	0.78			103			38			47	37	
	Unloaded		123	31	20.1	0.44	0.57	4.6	0.77			99			41			40	31	
	Unloaded		122	28	20.6	0.50	0.64	5.2	0.78			98			42			36	28	
	Unloaded	138/90	122	26	22.2	0.57	0.60	4.9	0.95	7.42	31	99	82	17	41	49	8	35	33	0.45
0.5	15		123	33	22.3	0.49	0.61	5.0	0.80			100			41			40	32	
1.0	15		124	30	24.6	0.63	0.78	6.3	0.81			98			43			35	28	
1.5	30		126	31	25.9	0.68	0.80	6.3	0.85			101			42			34	29	
2.0	30		127	26	25.9	0.79	0.88	6.9	0.90			98			46			30	27	
2.5	45		129	29	30.0	0.92	0.97	7.5	0.95			99			46			30	28	
3.0	45	140/78	132	33	32.9	0.99	1.00	7.6	0.99	7.38	30	103	85	14	46	51	5	30	30	0.41
3.5	60		131	31	33.9	1.11	1.07	8.2	1.04			100			49			28	29	
4.0	60		134	35	36.8	1.14	1.08	8.1	1.06			103			48			30	31	
4.5	75		139	30	36.6	1.24	1.15	8.3	1.08			102			50			27	30	
5.0	75	132/84	142	36	39.6	1.27	1.19	8.4	1.07	7.32	29	100	76	19	51	58	7	29	31	0.45
5.5	90		145	43	40.8	1.26	1.20	8.3	1.04			100			51			30	31	
6.0	90	180/84	147	48	40.4	1.19	1.07	7.3	1.11	7.32	29	95	76	21	53	58	5	31	34	0.46
	Recovery		138	47	32.8	1.02	1.02	7.4	1.00			89			60			28	28	
	Recovery		138	50	30.1	0.81	0.83	6.0	0.98			89			60			32	31	

Interpretation

Comments

Resting respiratory function studies showed severe obstructive lung disease with hyperinflation, no improvement in flow rates following inhaled albuterol, and an above predicted D$_L$CO. The predicted value for D$_L$CO was adjusted for the patient's anemia. The patient was also overweight, with arterial blood gases and pH suggesting a chronic compensated respiratory acidosis and an acute respiratory alkalosis. The respiratory acidosis increases with exercise.

Analysis

Referring to flow chart 1, the peak V̇O₂ and anaerobic threshold were both decreased (Table 9.76.2) Most striking is the ventilatory limitation accompanied by increasing respiratory acidosis and a low O₂ pulse. We are directed through branchpoints 1.1, 1.2, and 1.3 to flow chart 4. The low breathing reserve (branchpoint 4.1) and the high VD/VT (branchpoint 4.2) lead us to "lung disease with im-

paired peripheral oxygenation." The patient's data do not fit the conditions listed under this diagnosis perfectly, but he does have a low arterial O₂ content (anemia and slightly decreased arterial O₂ saturation) and many of the factors listed in the pulmonary vascular disease category. If we had used flow chart we might have arrived through branchpoints 5.1, 5.3, and 5.7 to the diagnosis of "obstructive lung disease." This is satisfactory, especially because of the severe respiratory acidosis that developed during exercise, but it accounts poorly for his low ΔV̇O₂/ΔWR and flat O₂ pulse, which indicate an O₂ flow problem. These latter abnormalities can be accounted for by his anemia.

Conclusion

As noted in Chapter 7, the flow charts cannot, and should not, always come to a single diagnosis. This is because the patient may have pathophysiologic features involving more than one organ system. In this patient, the primary problem appears to be severe obstructive lung disease with secondary pulmonary vascular disease, complicated by anemia.

Case 77 Mild Obstructive Airway Disease Complicated by Pulmonary Vascular Disease, with a Patent Foramen Ovale and Systemic Hypertension

Clinical Findings

This 64-year-old retired shipyard worker was evaluated because of increasing shortness of breath that had begun 7 years previously and had increased to become evident with walking two blocks or climbing a flight of stairs. He had smoked half a pack of cigarettes daily from age 40 to 60. He had been treated with isoniazid and ethambutol for pulmonary tuberculosis for 4 years, 2 decades before. Prostatic carcinoma had been diagnosed 8 months previously while he was having a transurethral prostatectomy. He took triamterene, hydrochlorothiazide, and methyldopa for the treatment of hypertension. Pulse was irregular without other evidence of cardiovascular disease. The chest x-ray studies revealed a single small pleural plaque on the left, evidence of old granulomatous disease in the right apex, and a flat diaphragm. Respiratory function tests done several days prior to exercise showed airway obstruction.

Exercise Findings

The patient performed exercise on a cycle ergometer. He pedalled at 60 rpm without added load for 3 minutes. The work rate was then increased 15 W per minute this symptom-limited maximum. Arterial blood was sampled every second minute, and intra-arterial blood pressure was recorded from a percutaneously placed brachial artery catheter. Resting ECG showed some premature atrial and premature ventricular contractions, poor R wave progression from leads V1 through V3, and left atrial enlargement. At 90 W there were occasional pairs of premature ventricular contractions and two epi-

sodes of ventricular bigeminy. The patient stopped exercising because of shortness of breath. Under questioning, he also conceded that he had felt some substernal tightness at the highest work rate.

TABLE 9.77.1. Selected Respiratory Function Data

Measurement	Predicted	Measured	
Age, yr		64	
Sex		Male	
Height, cm		178	
Weight, kg	80	82	
Hematocrit, %		47	

	Predicted	Before Bronchodilator	After Bronchodilator
VC, L	3.82	4.52	4.75
IC, L	2.55	3.25	
TLC, L	5.93	8.66	
FEV_1, L	2.98	2.69	2.78
FEV_1/VC, %	78	60	58
MVV, L/min	121	90	112
D_LCO, ml/mm Hg/min	24.8	14.0	

TABLE 9.77.2. Selected Exercise Data

Measurement	Predicted	Measured
Peak $\dot{V}O_2$, L/min	2.16	1.42
Maximum HR, beats/min	156	159
Maximum O_2 pulse, ml/beat	13.9	8.9
$\Delta\dot{V}O_2/\Delta WR$, ml/min/W	10.3	8.1
AT, L/min	>0.95	0.7
Blood pressure, mmHg (rest, max)		186/116, 263/128
Maximum $\dot{V}E$, L/min		91
Exercise breathing reserve, L/min	>15	91
PaO_2, mmHg (rest, max ex)		79, 57
$P(A - a)O_2$, mmHg (rest, max ex)		38, 65
$P(a - ET)CO_2$, mmHg (rest, max ex)		4, 9
V_D/V_T (rest, heavy ex)		0.38, 0.47
HCO_3^-, mEq/L (rest, 2-min recov)		24, 17

FIGURE 9.77.1.

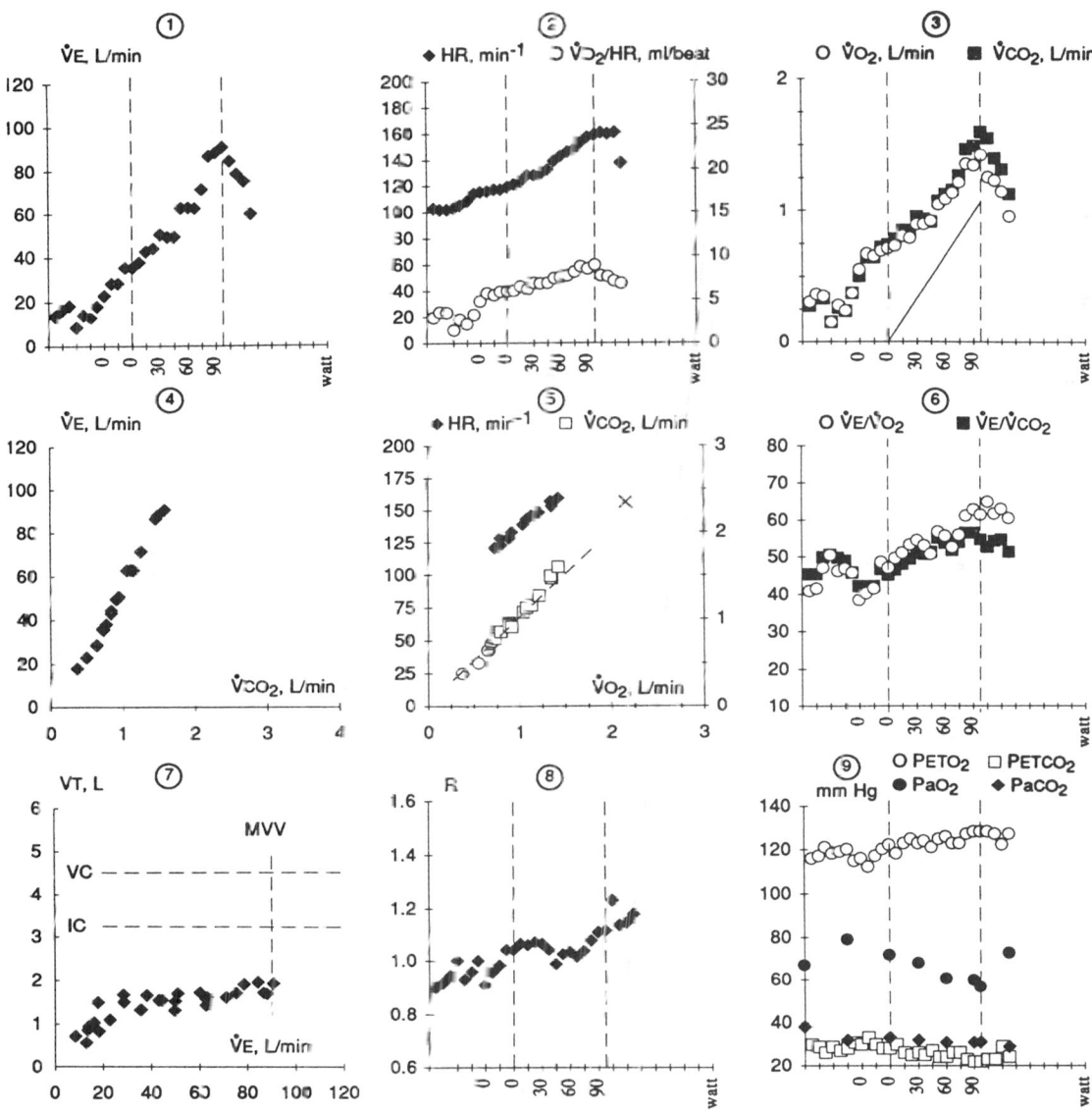

1. Vertical dashed lines in panels 1 to 3 and 6, 8, and 9 indicate the beginning and the end of increasing work period.

2. Unloaded cycling is performed for 3 minutes before the left vertical dashed line.

3. In panel 3, the diagonal line shows the increase of $\dot{V}O_2$ at a slope of 10 ml/min/W.

4. In panel 5, the diagonal dashed line has a slope of 1; the "x" in the upper right is the predicted maximum heart rate and $\dot{V}O_2$ for the subject.

TABLE 9.77.3. Air Breathing

Time min	Work rate watts	BP mmHg	HR min⁻¹	f min⁻¹	$\dot{V}_E$ L/min BTPS	$\dot{V}_{CO_2}$ L/min STPD	$\dot{V}_{O_2}$ L/min STPD	$\dot{V}_{O_2}$/HR ml/beat	R	pH	HCO_3^- meq/L	P_{O_2} ET	P_{O_2} a	P_{O_2} (A−a)	P_{CO_2} ET	P_{CO_2} a	P_{CO_2} (a−ET)	$\dot{V}_E/\dot{V}_{CO_2}$	$\dot{V}_E/\dot{V}_{O_2}$	V_D/V_T
	Rest	185/116								7.42	24	116	67		30	38				
	Rest		103	16	13.6	0.27	0.30	2.9	0.90			116			30			45	41	
	Rest		102	16	16.3	0.33	0.36	3.5	0.92			117			29			45	42	
	Rest		102	22	18.3	0.33	0.35	3.4	0.94			121			26			50	47	
	Rest		103	12	8.6	0.15	0.15	1.5	1.00			118			29			51	51	
	Rest		105	15	14.2	0.26	0.28	2.7	0.93			119			27			50	46	
	Rest	185/116	108	23	13.2	0.23	0.24	2.2	0.96	7.46	22	120	79	38	28	32	4	49	47	0.38
	Unloaded		114	12	17.9	0.37	0.37	3.2	1.00			115			31			46	46	
	Unloaded		115	21	22.9	0.50	0.55	4.8	0.91			116			30			42	38	
	Unloaded		116	17	28.4	0.64	0.67	5.8	0.96			112			33			42	40	
	Unloaded		117	19	28.5	0.64	0.65	5.6	0.98			117			30			42	41	
	Unloaded		117	27	35.8	0.72	0.69	5.9	1.04			120			28			47	49	
	Unloaded	236/126	119	27	35.6	0.74	0.71	6.0	1.04	7.43	22	122	72	46	28	33	5	45	47	0.39
0.5	15		121	23	38.1	0.78	0.73	6.0	1.07			118			30			46	50	
1.0	15		123	28	43.1	0.85	0.80	6.5	1.06			123			26			48	51	
1.5	30		128	29	44.5	0.85	0.79	6.2	1.08			125			25			49	53	
2.0	30	236/128	128	30	50.9	0.95	0.89	7.0	1.07	7.44	21	123	68	52	26	32	6	51	54	0.45
2.5	45		129	33	49.9	0.93	0.89	6.9	1.04			124			25			51	53	
3.0	45		133	38	49.8	0.91	0.92	6.9	0.99			121			27			51	51	
3.5	60		139	44	62.7	1.07	1.04	7.5	1.03			125			24			55	57	
4.0	60		143	39	63.2	1.12	1.08	7.6	1.04	7.44	21	126	61	59	24	31	7	53	55	0.45
4.5	75		146	40	62.7	1.15	1.13	7.7	1.02			123			26			52	52	
5.0	75		148	44	71.3	1.26	1.21	8.2	1.04			123			26			54	56	
5.5	90		153	50	86.6	1.46	1.35	8.8	1.08			127			23			56	61	
6.0	90		157	52	88.2	1.49	1.34	8.5	1.11	7.42	20	128	60	61	22	31	9	56	63	0.48
6.5	105	263/128	159	47	90.8	1.59	1.42	8.9	1.12	7.41	19	128	57	65	22	31	9	55	61	0.47
	Recovery		161	43	84.4	1.54	1.25	7.8	1.23			128			23			52	65	
	Recovery		160	41	78.6	1.39	1.22	7.6	1.14			127			23			54	62	
	Recovery		161	44	75.2	1.31	1.14	7.1	1.15			122			29			55	63	
	Recovery	233/139	138	35	60.3	1.12	0.95	6.9	1.18	7.39	17	127	73	51	24	29	5	51	60	0.40

Interpretation

Comments

This case is presented to illustrate the considerable amount of gas exchange abnormality that can occur during exercise, even with only mild abnormalities in spirometry, if there is considerable pulmonary vascular disease.

The results of the resting respiratory function studies indicate that this patient has mild airflow obstruction, hyperinflation, and a moderately severe abnormality in diffusing capacity (Table 9.77.1). The resting ECG is abnormal, as evidenced by premature atrial and ventricular contractions and poor R wave progression from V1 to V3. The arterial blood pressure is elevated. In such instances, one might have considered deferring the exercise test until blood pressure was under better control. The cuff-measured blood pressure is on the average 10 mmHg lower than the directly recorded blood pres-

sure, as described in Chapter 6. Because of the blood pressure elevation, the patient was exercised especially cautiously. The objective was to determine if this patient was primarily limited by his heart or lung disorder.

Analysis

Referring to flow chart 1, the peak $\dot{V}_{O_2}$ and AT are reduced (Table 9.77.2), which directs us through branchpoints 1.1, 1.2, and 1.3 to flow chart 4. The breathing reserve is low (branchpoint 4.1). The V_D/V_T is high (branchpoint 4.2) leading us to lung disease with impaired peripheral oxygenation. However the V_T/IC ratio is not high as in restrictive lung disease. Nor does a respiratory acidosis develop as in obstructive lung disease. The breathing reserve is zero despite the presence of only mild obstructive lung disease. The reason for the absence of a breathing reserve is the increasing ventilatory drive with exercise due to an increasing V_D/V_T and decreasing Pa_{O_2} (Table 9.77.3) as work rate is increased.

The lung disease with impaired peripheral oxygenation box asks that we confirm with abnormalities in the pulmonary circulation box. The presence of O_2 flow limitation due to pulmonary vascular disease is confirmed by an increasing V_D/V_T with work rate, a systematic increase in $P(A - a)_{O_2}$ with work rate, an increase in $P(a - ET)_{CO_2}$ with work rate, steep heart rate $-\Delta \dot{V}_{O_2}$ relationship with no heart rate reserve, low O_2 pulse, and low and decreasing $\Delta \dot{V}_{O_2}/\Delta WR$ with increasing work rate. These findings implicate the pulmonary circulation as the organ of major dysfunction. This abnormality is further complicated by changes in gas exchange accounted for by a right to left shunt presumably due to the opening of a foramen ovale during exercise (see the last item in the pulmonary vascular disease box). One hundred percent O_2 breathing during exercise might have confirmed the development of a right to left shunt.

Other gas exchange characteristics of a right to left shunt developing during exercise are an increasing rather than a decreasing $V_E/\dot{V}_{CO_2}$ ratio during exercise below the *AT* (lung getting less efficient as a gas exchanger), R becoming greater than 1 throughout exercise (panel 8, Fig. 9.77.1), $P_{ET_{CO_2}}$ decreasing with increasing work rate (panel 9, Fig. 9.77.1 and the calculated V_D/V_T and $P(a - ET)_{CO_2}$ not only remaining abnormal but becoming more abnormal as work rate increases (Table 9.77.3). These changes are explained by venous blood bypassing the lungs and mixing with arterial blood during exercise.

Conclusion

This patient has mild airflow obstruction but considerable pulmonary vascular disease, possibly secondary to emphysema. The probable opening of a foramen oval during exercise can account for this patient's increasing V_D/V_T, exercise induced hypoxemia and high ventilatory drive reflected in an increasing rather than a decreasing $V_E/\dot{V}_{CO_2}$ from the onset of exercise.

Case 78 Pulmonary Vascular Disease, Obstructive Airway Disease, and Talc Pneumoconiosis

Clinical Findings

This 63-year-old man had complained of progressive dyspnea for 10 years, but denied cough, sputum, wheezing, chest pain, or ankle edema. He had hypertension of 5 years' duration and was being treated with clonidine and dyazide. For several months he had noted epigastric burning pain, occasionally relieved by meals. He had been exposed to talc for over 40 years in his work and was an ex-smoker with a 40 pack year history of cigarette smoking. He had no heart murmurs. The chest roentgenogram showed pulmonary fibrosis. Resting ECG showed left anterior hemi-block and T-wave abnormalities in the anteroseptal region suggestive of ischemia. The patient was tested to evaluate the pathophysiology of his exertional dyspnea.

Exercise Findings

The patient performed exercise on a cycle ergometer. He pedalled at 60 rpm without an added load for 3 minutes. The work rate was then increased 20 W per minute to tolerance. Arterial blood was sampled every second minute, and intra-arterial pressure was recorded from a percutaneously placed brachial artery catheter. The patient stopped exercise because of shortness of breath. He had no chest pain and no further ECG abnormalities.

TABLE 9.78.1. Selected Respiratory Function Data

Measurement	Predicted	Measured
Age, yr		63
Sex		Male
Height, cm		163
Weight, kg	68	67
Hematocrit, %		53
VC, L	3.28	3.56
IC, L	2.19	2.28
TLC, L	5.17	6.00
FEV_1, L	2.55	2.20
FEV_1/VC, %	78	62
MVV, L/min	115	96
D_LCO, ml/mm Hg/min	23.9	10.7

TABLE 9.78.2. Selected Exercise Data

Measurement	Predicted	Measured
Peak $\dot{V}O_2$, L/min	1.84	1.02
Maximum HR, beats/min	157	161
Maximum O_2 pulse, ml/beat	11.7	6.7
$\Delta\dot{V}O_2/\Delta WR$, ml/min/W	10.3	5.2
AT, L/min	>0.81	0.8
Blood pressure, mmHg (rest, max)		162/84, 249/145
Maximum $\dot{V}E$, L/min		66
Exercise breathing reserve, L/min	>15	30
PaO_2, mmHg (rest, max ex)		79, 57
$P(A - a)O_2$ mmHg (rest, max ex)		33, 64
$P(a - ET)CO_2$ (rest, max ex)		4, 6
VD/VT (rest, max ex)		0.42, 0.44
HCO_3^-, mEq/L (rest, 2-min recov)		22, 17

FIGURE 9.78.1.

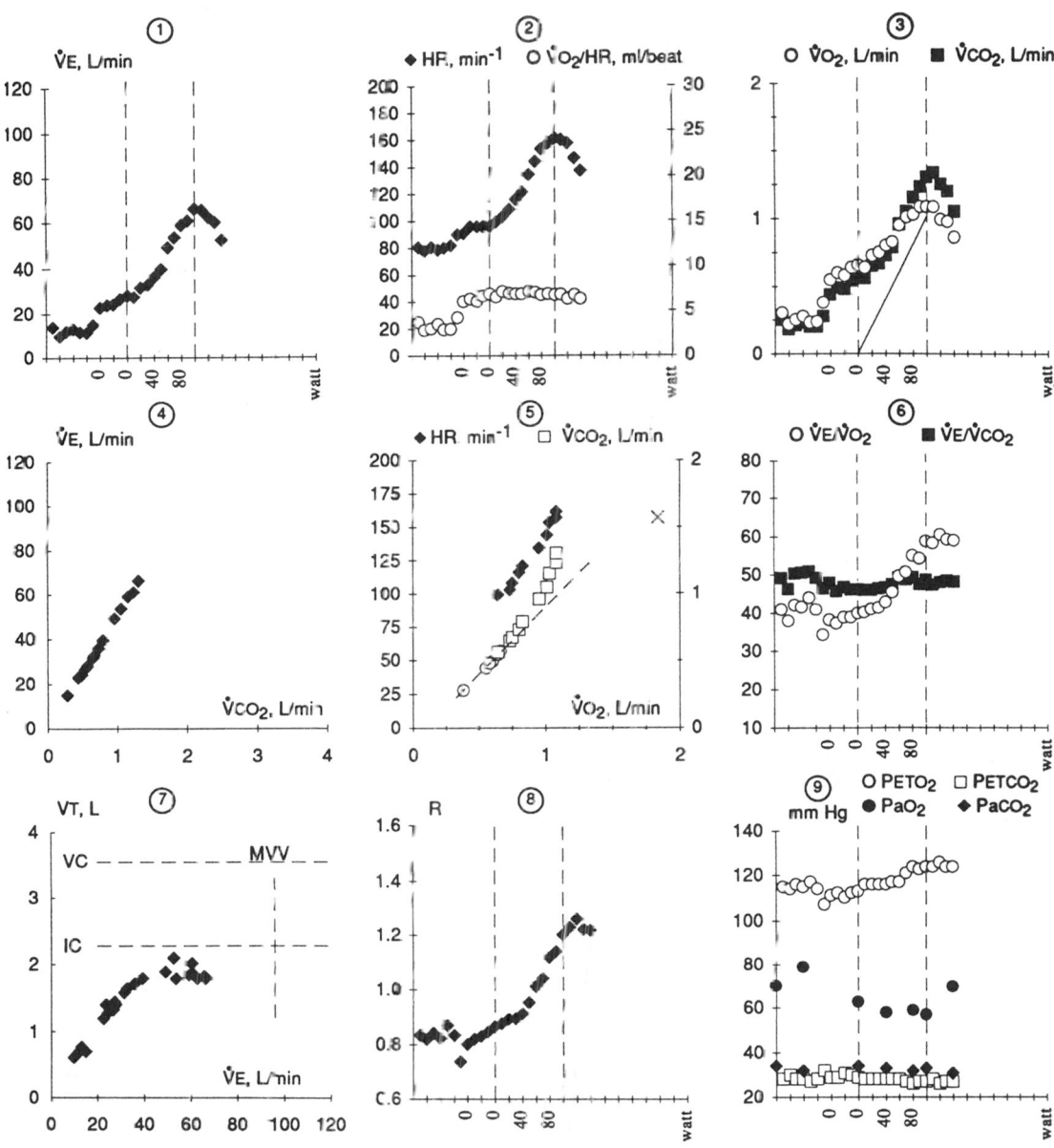

1. Vertical dashed lines in panels 1 to 3 and 6, 8, and 9 indicate the beginning and the end of increasing work period.
2. Unloaded cycling is performed for 3 minutes before the left vertical dashed line.
3. In panel 3, the diagonal line shows the increase of $\dot{V}_{C_2}$ at a slope of 10 ml/min/W.
4. In panel 5, the diagonal dashed line has a slope of 1; the "x" in the upper right is the predicted maximum heart rate and $\dot{V}_{C_2}$ for the subject.

TABLE 9.78.3. Air Breathing

Time min	Work rate watts	BP mmHg	HR min^{-1}	f min^{-1}	$\dot{V}_E$ L/min BTPS	$\dot{V}_{CO_2}$ L/min STPD	$\dot{V}_{O_2}$ L/min STPD	$\dot{V}_{O_2}$/HR ml/beat	R	pH	HCO$_3^-$ meq/L	PO$_2$, mmHg ET	a	(A − a)	PCO$_2$, mmHg ET	a	(a − ET)	$\dot{V}_E$/$\dot{V}_{CO_2}$	$\dot{V}_E$/$\dot{V}_{O_2}$	VD/VT
	Rest	162/84								7.43	22	70			34					
	Rest		81	19	13.9	0.25	0.30	3.7	0.83			115			28			49	41	
	Rest		78	16	9.7	0.18	0.22	2.8	0.82			114			30			46	38	
	Rest		81	17	12.0	0.21	0.25	3.1	0.84			116			28			50	42	
	Rest		79	17	13.1	0.23	0.28	3.5	0.82	7.46	22	115	79	33	28	32	4	51	42	0.42
	Rest		80	17	11.6	0.20	0.23	2.9	0.87			117			27			51	44	
	Rest	192/96	82	17	11.3	0.20	0.24	2.9	0.83			114			28			49	41	
	Unloaded	240/117	90	21	14.8	0.28	0.38	4.2	0.74			107			32			46	34	
	Unloaded		91	19	22.7	0.44	0.55	6.0	0.80			111			29			48	38	
	Unloaded		96	17	23.8	0.49	0.60	6.3	0.82			112			29			46	37	
	Unloaded		96	19	24.1	0.48	0.58	6.0	0.83			110			31			47	39	
	Unloaded		96	20	26.6	0.54	0.64	6.7	0.84			112			30			46	39	
	Unloaded	237/111	96	20	28.0	0.57	0.66	6.9	0.86	7.44	23	113	63	49	29	34	5	46	40	0.42
0.5	20		99	19	27.4	0.56	0.64	6.5	0.88			116			28			46	40	
1.0	20		103	20	31.6	0.65	0.73	7.1	0.89			116			28			46	41	
1.5	40		108	20	32.7	0.67	0.75	6.9	0.89			116			28			46	41	
2.0	40	240/114	116	21	35.9	0.73	0.80	6.9	0.91	7.45	23	116	58	56	28	33	5	47	43	0.42
2.5	60		121	22	39.4	0.79	0.83	6.9	0.95			117			28			48	45	
3.0	60		134	26	49.3	0.96	0.95	7.1	1.01			117			28			49	50	
3.5	80		144	30	53.7	1.05	1.01	7.0	1.04			121			27			49	51	
4.0	80	246/123	153	32	59.2	1.15	1.03	6.7	1.12	7.44	21	124	59	62	26	32	6	49	55	0.43
4.5	100		157	33	61.2	1.23	1.08	6.9	1.14			123			27			47	54	
5.0	100	249/145	161	37	66.4	1.30	1.08	6.7	1.20	7.40	20	124	57	64	27	33	6	49	59	0.44
	Recovery		160	36	65.8	1.33	1.08	6.8	1.23			124			28			47	58	
	Recovery		157	35	62.8	1.25	0.99	6.3	1.26			126			26			48	60	
	Recovery		146	30	60.5	1.20	0.98	6.7	1.22			124			27			48	59	
	Recovery	234/108	137	25	52.6	1.05	0.86	6.3	1.22	7.35	17	124	70	53	27	31	4	48	59	0.40

Interpretations

Comments

Resting studies showed a mild obstructive ventilatory defect with a severely reduced D$_L$CO. The patient had systemic hypertension at rest with a mildly abnormal ECG.

Analysis

Referring to flow chart 1, peak $\dot{V}_{O_2}$ is decreased. The anaerobic threshold is borderline abnormal. If one goes next to flow chart 3, the high breathing reserve and mildly abnormal ECG lead to the diagnosis of myocardial ischemia, but this is unsatisfactory because it does not take into account the severe gas exchange disturbances elicited. Flow charts 4 or 5 are preferable. Referring to flow chart 5, at branchpoint 5.1 we note abnormal VD/VT, P(a − ET)CO$_2$, and P(A − a)O$_2$, The breathing reserve is normal (branchpoint 5.3), and the PaO$_2$ progressively decreases (branchpoint 5.6), leading to the diagnosis of pulmonary vascular disease, with all the confirmatory findings described in the diagnostic box. The patient does have mild obstructive lung disease, but this is physiologically less important than the pulmonary vascular disease, as evidenced by the low and decreasing $\Delta\dot{V}_{O_2}/\Delta$WR (panel 3, Fig. 9.78.1), very steep heart rate—$\dot{V}_{O_2}$ relationship (panel 5, Fig. 9.78.1), high VD/VT, increased P(A − a)O$_2$, positive P(a − ET)CO$_2$, high ventilatory equivalents, and low and unchanging O$_2$ pulse, despite polycythemia. The systemic hypertension could also be contributing to a high afterload and low cardiac output state.

Conclusion

This patient has pulmonary vascular disease that is more severe than can be explained by uncomplicated obstructive lung disease, as well as coexistent exercise arterial hypertension. A subsequent lung biopsy demonstrated talc pneumoconiosis.

Case 79 Systemic Sclerosis and Primary Lung Cancer: Preoperative Evaluation

Clinical Findings

This 59-year-old woman with progressive systemic sclerosis was found to have a potentially operable squamous cell carcinoma of the lung by fiberoptic bronchoscopy. She had a 26 pack year history of cigarette smoking, complained of dyspnea after walking one block, and denied having a productive cough or hemoptysis. She had no history or overt signs or symptoms of heart disease. Her only medications were thyroid supplements and estrogens A cardiopulmonary exercise test was done to evaluate cardiac and lung function reserves in response to stress.

Exercise Findings

The patient performed exercise on a cycle ergometer. She pedalled at 60 rpm without an added load for 3 minutes. The work rate was then increased 5 W per minute to her symptom-limited maximum. Arterial blood was sampled every second minute, and intra-arterial blood pressure was recorded from a percutaneously passed brachial artery catheter. Resting and exercise ECGs were normal. The patient stopped exercise complaining of tired thighs.

TABLE 9.79.1. Selected Respiratory Function Data

Measurement	Predicted	Measured
Age, yr		59
Sex		Female
Height, cm		165
Weight, kg	62	75
Hematocrit, %		43
VC, L	2.73	2.26
IC, L	1.82	1.36
TLC, L	4.57	3.34
FEV_1, L	2.18	1.58
FEV_1/VC, %	80	70
MVV, L/min	82	73
$D_{L}CO$, ml/mm Hg/min	18.0	8.4

TABLE 9.79.2. Selected Exercise Data

Measurement	Predicted	Measured
Peak $\dot{V}O_2$, L/min	1.43	0.86
Maximum HR, beats/min	161	135
Maximum O_2 pulse, ml/beat	8.9	6.4
$\Delta\dot{V}O_2/\Delta WR$, ml/min/W	10.3	9.1
AT, L/min	>0.7	0.7
Blood pressure, mmHg (rest, max ex)		135/69, 180/81
Maximum $\dot{V}E$, L/min		38
Exercise breathing reserve, L/min	>15	35
PaO_2, mmHg (rest, max ex)		66, 55
$P(A - a)O_2$, mmHg (rest, max ex)		24, 51
$P(a - ET)CO_2$, mmHg (rest, max ex)		7, 13
V_D/V_T (rest, max ex)		0.40, 0.47
HCO_3^-, mEq/L (rest, recov)		25, 23

FIGURE 9.79.1.

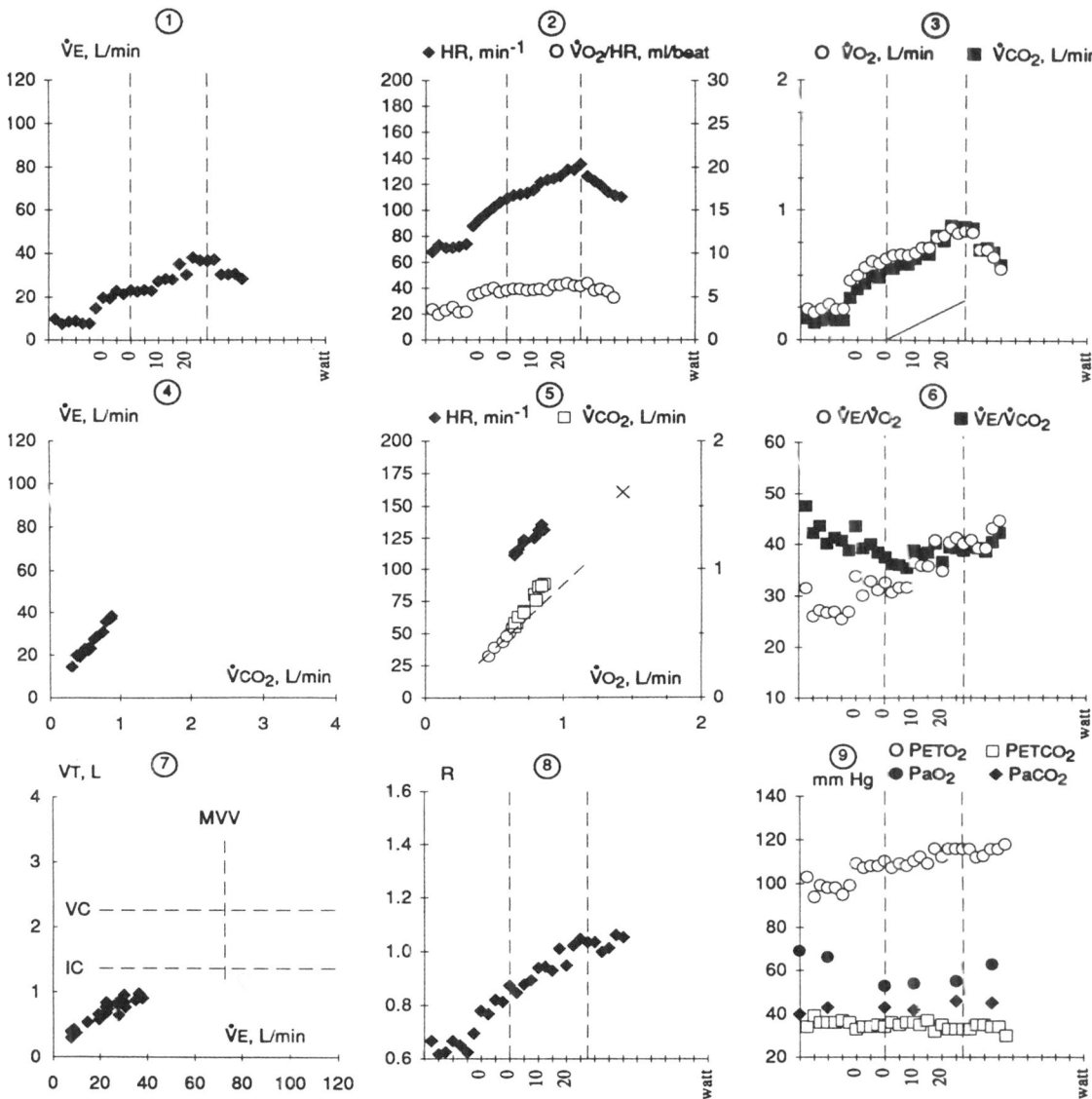

1. Vertical dashed lines in panels 1 to 3 and 6, 8, and 9 indicate the beginning and the end of increasing work period.

2. Unloaded cycling is performed for 3 minutes before the left vertical dashed line.

3. In panel 3, the diagonal line shows the increase of $\dot{V}O_2$ at a slope of 10 ml/min/W.

4. In panel 5, the diagonal dashed line has a slope of 1; the "x" in the upper right is the predicted maximum heart rate and $\dot{V}O_2$ for the subject.

TABLE 9.79.3.   Air Breathing

Time min	Work rate watts	BP mmHg	HR min⁻¹	f min⁻¹	V̇E L/min BTPS	V̇CO2 L/min STPD	V̇O2 L/min STPD	V̇O2/HR ml/beat	R	pH	HCO3 meq/L	PO2 ET	PO2 a	PO2 (A−a)	PCO2 ET	PCO2 a	PCO2 (a−ET)	V̇E/V̇CO2	V̇E/V̇O2	VD/VT
	Rest	132/69								7.40	24	69			40					
	Rest		68	26	9.8	0.16	0.24	3.5	0.67			103			34			47	32	
	Rest		73	25	7.6	0.13	0.21	2.9	0.62			94			39			42	26	
	Rest		71	22	8.4	0.15	0.24	3.4	0.63			99			36			44	27	
	Rest	135/69	71	21	9.0	0.18	0.27	3.8	0.67	7.38	25	93	66	24	36	43	7	40	27	0.40
	Rest		72	19	7.8	0.15	0.23	3.2	0.65			98			36			41	27	
	Rest		74	20	7.8	0.15	0.24	3.2	0.63			95			37			41	25	
	Unloaded		88	27	14.7	0.32	0.46	5.2	0.70			99			36			39	27	
	Unloaded		93	34	19.8	0.39	0.50	5.4	0.78			109			33			43	34	
	Unloaded		98	29	19.3	0.43	0.56	5.7	0.77			107			34			39	30	
	Unloaded		102	33	22.8	0.50	0.61	6.0	0.82			108			34			40	33	
	Unloaded		106	33	21.2	0.48	0.59	5.6	0.81			108			35			38	31	
	Unloaded	171/81	109	31	23.2	0.55	0.63	5.8	0.87	7.37	24	110	53	49	34	43	9	37	33	0.41
0.5	5		111	29	22.4	0.55	0.65	5.9	0.85			107			36			36	31	
1.0	5		112	28	23.2	0.58	0.66	5.9	0.88			109			35			36	32	
1.5	10		113	27	22.8	0.58	0.65	5.8	0.89			108			36			35	32	
2.0	10	174/78	115	33	27.2	0.63	0.67	5.8	0.94	7.35	23	110	54	52	36	42	6	39	36	0.42
2.5	15		121	34	26.3	0.67	0.71	5.9	0.94			112			35			38	36	
3.0	15		123	33	28.1	0.66	0.71	5.8	0.93			109			37			38	36	
3.5	20		124	40	35.5	0.80	0.79	6.1	1.01			116			32			40	41	
4.0	20		126	32	30.5	0.76	0.80	6.3	0.95			112			35			37	35	
4.5	25		131	42	38.3	0.88	0.86	6.6	1.02			116			33			39	40	
5.0	25	180/81	131	39	37.0	0.86	0.82	6.3	1.05	7.35	25	116	55	51	33	46	13	39	41	0.47
5.5	30		135	38	36.9	0.87	0.84	6.2	1.04			116			33			39	40	
	Recovery		126	39	37.2	0.86	0.83	3.6	1.04			116			33			39	41	
	Recovery		122	36	30.5	0.70	0.70	5.7	1.00			112			35			39	39	
	Recovery		119	36	30.5	0.71	0.70	5.9	1.01			113			35			39	39	
	Recovery	162/69	114	40	30.9	0.63	0.64	5.6	1.06	7.32	23	116	63	44	34	45	11	40	43	0.47
	Recovery		111	43	28.1	0.58	0.55	5.0	1.05			116			34			42	44	
	Recovery		110									118			30					

Interpretation

Comments

The resting respiratory function studies show mild restriction and mild obstruction, severe loss of available pulmonary capillary bed, and mild hypoxemia. She had no known cardiac disease.

Analysis

Referring to flow chart 1, the patient had a low peak V̇O2 and borderline anaerobic threshold (Table 9.79.2). If we use flow chart 3, we proceed through branchpoint 3.1 (normal breathing reserve) and through branchpoint 3.3 (normal ECG) to poor effort or musculo-skeletal disorder. This impression does not fit our patient well because she has unequivocal evidence of gas exchange abnormalities. If her anaerobic threshold were low, we would work through flow chart 4.

Because her breathing reserve is normal (branchpoint 4.1), we are directed to the right branch. Because the V̇E/V̇CO2 is high at the AT (branchpoint 4.3), we are given the diagnosis of "abnormal pulmonary circulation." The patient has all the physiologic abnormalities that define this disorder. While the VC is reduced (probably from systemic sclerosis), the increasing P(A − a)O2 with increasing work rate suggests that the abnormal pulmonary circulation is due to pulmonary vascular disease rather than left ventricular failure (branchpoint 4.5).

Conclusion

This patient has mild restrictive and obstructive lung disease but does not have ventilatory limitation during exercise. Rather she demonstrates significant gas exchange abnormalities characteristic of pulmonary vascular disease. This may be part of her systemic sclerosis and associated interstitial lung disease. Her peak V̇O2 of 11.5 ml/min/kg places her in a high risk category for pulmonary resection.

Case 80 Primary Pulmonary Hypertension

Clinical Findings

This 34-year-old female was referred for cardiopulmonary exercise testing because of exertional dyspnea known to be secondary to primary pulmonary hypertension. She is being treated with continuous intravenous prostacyclin and being followed closely. Her physician thought that she had not been doing too well, possibly due to repeated infections of her catheter or worsening of her underlying disease. Thus there was uncertainty as to whether she should be moved on to the lung transplantation list. This cardiopulmonary exercise test was done to obtain objective information on the state of her pulmonary circulation as compared to 3 years previously.

Exercise Findings

The patient performed exercise on a cycle ergometer while breathing through a mouthpiece with a nose clip in place for breath-by-breath measurements of gas exchange. Heart rate and rhythm were continuously monitored. The protocol consisted of 3 minutes of rest, 3 minutes of 0 load pedalling at 60 rpm, followed by a progressive increase in work rate of 10 watts per minute until she became too short of breath to continue. She also felt a little light headed and slight chest discomfort. 12 lead EKG recordings were obtained during rest, every minute of exercise, and recovery. The patient performed the exercise

test with good effort. Her exercise electrocardiograms were unchanged from rest except for rate increase.

TABLE 9.80.1. Selected Respiratory Function Data

Measurement	Predicted	Measured
Age, yr		34
Sex		Female
Height, cm		159
Weight, kg	61	62
Hematocrit, %		41
VC, L	2.99	2.47
IC, L	2.00	2.36
FEV$_1$, L	2.52	2.11
FEV$_1$/VC, %	84	85
MVV, L/min	98	88

TABLE 9.80.2. Selected Exercise Data

Measurement	Predicted	Measured
Peak $\dot{V}O_2$, L/min	1.77	0.85
Maximum HR, beats/min	186	153
Maximum O$_2$ pulse, ml/beat	9.5	5.0
$\Delta\dot{V}O_2/\Delta WR$, ml/min/W	10.3	6.0
AT, L/min	>0.78	0.6
Blood pressure, mmHg (rest, max)		118/74, 191/67
Maximum $\dot{V}E$, L/min		58
Exercise breathing reserve, L/min	>15	30
O$_2$ saturation, oximeter (rest, max)		94, <80

FIGURE 9.80.1.

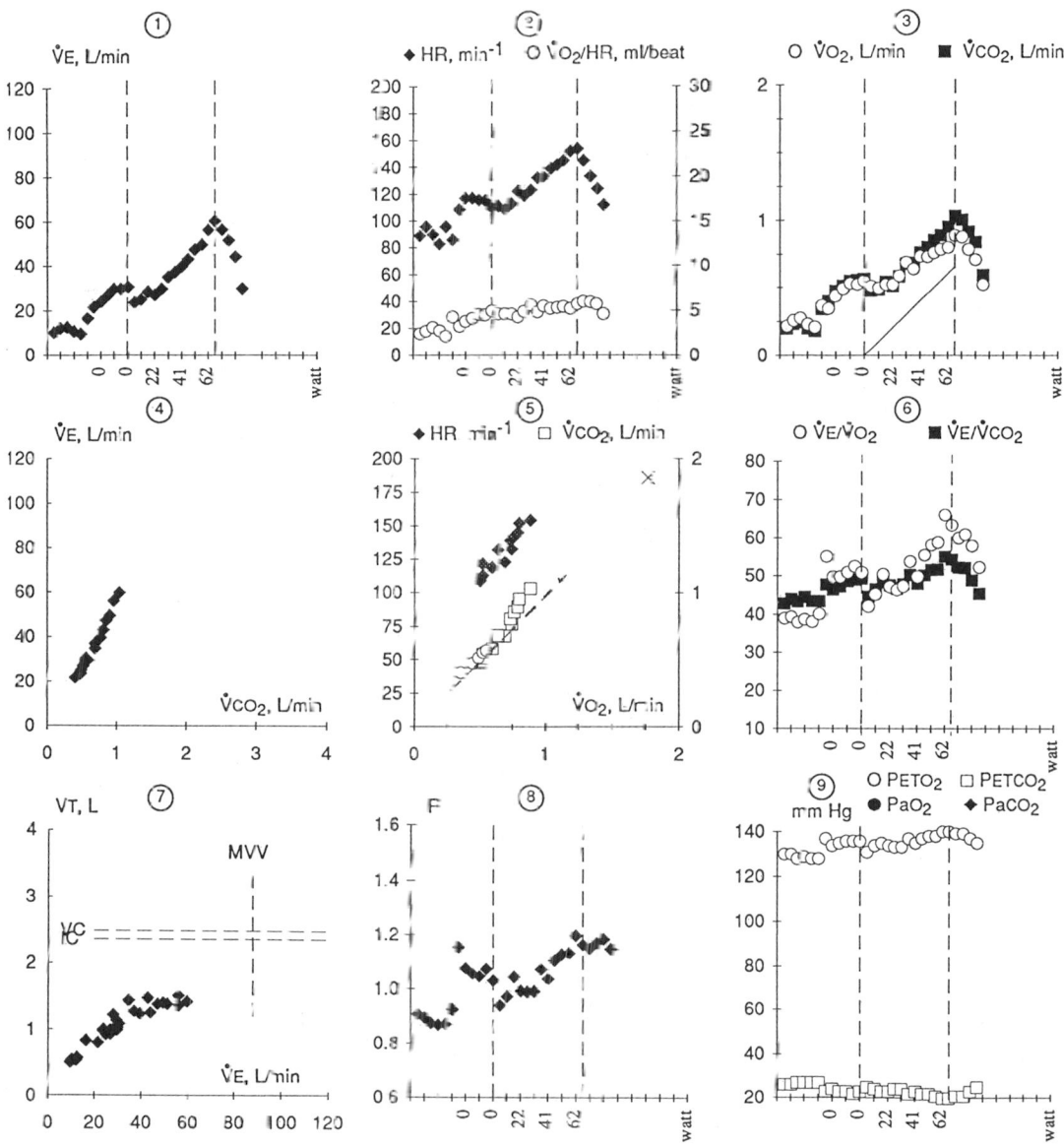

1. Vertical dashed lines in panels 1 to 3 and 6, 8, and 9 indicate the beginning and the end of increasing work period.

2. Unloaded cycling is performed for 3 minutes before the left vertical dashed line.

3. In panel 3, the diagonal line shows the increase of $\dot{V}O_2$ at a slope of 10 ml/min/W.

4. In panel 5, the diagonal dashed line has a slope of 1; the "x" in the upper right is the predicted maximum heart rate and $\dot{V}O_2$ for the subject.

TABLE 9.80.3. Air Breathing

Time (min)	Work rate (watts)	BP (mmHg)	HR (min⁻¹)	f (min⁻¹)	V̇E L/min BTPS	V̇CO₂ L/min STPD	V̇O₂ L/min STPD	V̇O₂/HR (ml/beat)	R	pH	HCO₃⁻ meq/L	PO₂, mmHg ET	a	(A − a)	PCO₂, mmHg ET	a	(a − ET)	V̇E/V̇CO₂	V̇E/V̇O₂	VD/VT
	Rest																			
	Rest	89	19	10.2	0.20	0.22	2.5	0.91				130			26			43	39	
	Rest	96	23	12.2	0.23	0.26	2.7	0.90				130			26			44	39	
	Rest	90	22	12.5	0.25	0.28	3.1	0.88				128			27			43	38	
	Rest	83	20	10.6	0.20	0.23	2.8	0.87				129			27			45	39	
	Rest	96	19	9.6	0.18	0.21	2.2	0.87				128			27			44	38	
	Rest	86	20	16.6	0.34	0.37	4.3	0.92				128			27			44	40	
	Unloaded	109	27	21.6	0.40	0.35	3.2	1.15				137			23			48	55	
	Unloaded	117	24	24.0	0.47	0.44	3.8	1.08				134			24			46	50	
	Unloaded	117	29	26.9	0.52	0.49	4.2	1.06				135			23			47	50	
	Unloaded	116	28	29.4	0.56	0.53	4.6	1.05				136			23			49	51	
	Unloaded	115	29	29.8	0.56	0.52	4.5	1.07				136			22			49	53	
	Unloaded	110	28	30.4	0.57	0.55	5.0	1.03				136			23			49	51	
0.5	4	111	24	23.5	0.48	0.51	4.6	0.94				131			25			45	42	
1.0	6	109	27	24.9	0.49	0.50	4.6	0.97				134			24			47	45	
1.5	17	113	23	28.2	0.54	0.52	4.6	1.04				135			23			48	50	
2.0	22	122	27	26.8	0.52	0.52	4.3	0.99				134			23			48	47	
2.5	25	119	26	29.5	0.58	0.59	5.0	0.99				133			24			47	46	
3.0	31	123	24	34.7	0.68	0.69	5.6	0.99				133			24			48	47	
3.5	36	132	29	37.0	0.69	0.64	4.8	1.07				137			22			50	54	
4.0	41	133	32	39.6	0.77	0.74	5.6	1.04				135			23			48	50	
4.5	47	139	29	43.0	0.81	0.73	5.3	1.11				137			22			50	56	
5.0	53	142	34	47.2	0.86	0.76	5.4	1.13				138			22			52	58	
5.5	56	145	35	49.4	0.90	0.79	5.4	1.13				138			21			52	59	
6.0	62	152	37	56.1	0.96	0.80	5.3	1.20				140			20			55	66	
6.5	65	154	42	59.9	1.04	0.89	5.8	1.16				140			20			54	63	
	Recovery	145	41	56.3	1.01	0.88	6.1	1.15				139			21			52	60	
	Recovery	133	37	51.3	0.92	0.79	5.9	1.17				139			21			52	61	
	Recovery	124	35	44.1	0.84	0.71	5.7	1.18				137			23			49	58	
	Recovery	112	30	29.7	0.60	0.52	4.6	1.15				135			25			45	52	

Interpretation

Comments

Resting spirometry was normal. Her electrocardiogram showed right ventricular hypertrophy and strain pattern.

Analysis

Referring to Table 9.80.2 and flow chart 1, her peak V̇O₂ and AT are low bringing us through branchpoints 1.1, 1.2, and 1.3 to flow chart 4. The breathing reserve is normal (branchpoint 4.1) and the ventilatory equivalent for V̇CO₂ at the AT (branchpoint 4.3) are high bringing us to abnormal pulmonary circulation. The vital capacity is normal (branchpoint 4.5) bringing us to the diagnosis of pulmonary vascular disease in contrast to the alternate diagnosis of left ventricular failure. She did not have arterial blood gas measurements therefore we can not use items 1–3 in the confirmatory box to support the diagnosis. But items 4–6 (non-invasive measurements) support the diagnosis.

Compared to the study of three years earlier, the peak V̇O₂ was unchanged. Also the ventilatory equivalents for CO_2 and O_2 were unchanged. However, the AT and O_2 pulse decreased slightly since the previous study.

Conclusion

This 34-year-old lady with primary pulmonary hypertension had significant O_2 transport problem causing her to be exercise limited. Gas exchange efficiency is poor as is characteristic of this disease. This study demonstrates the use of cardiopulmonary exercise testing to obtain quantitative information regarding the clinical status (progression) of a patient's underlying disease.

Case 81 Cardiomyopathy Due to Diastolic Dysfunction
Clinical Findings

This 29-year-old male executive has had exercise intolerance due to fatigue and dyspnea for about a year. He had been evaluated by a pulmonologist, allergist and a cardiologist, none of whom felt that they had an understanding of the cause of his symptoms. He had a history of asthma, but his physical signs and pulmonary function tests were not compatible with his symptoms. He was referred for cardiopulmonary exercise testing in order to get some help in the understanding of his symptoms and pathophysiology. He had three exercise tests, the one being presented here being the third. The first two were very similar to the one presented here and showed that the peak $\dot{V}O_2$ and AT were significantly reduced with high CO_2 output reflecting a low work rate metabolic acidosis, confirmed by arterial blood gases and lactate measurements on test 2 and 3. Also the O_2 pulse was significantly reduced and did not increase normally. The arterial blood gases and VD/VT were normal. Therefore, we knew that the low peak $\dot{V}O_2$ and AT were not due to lung or primary pulmonary vascular disease. Also, they were not due to peripheral arterial disease because the pattern of increase in $\dot{V}O_2$ and $\dot{V}CO_2$ was not compatible with this diagnosis (see chapter 8). In the absence of a murmur, ECG changes of myocardial ischemia, or history of congenital heart disease, he was diagnosed as either having a cardiomyopathy with diastolic dysfunction, or, less likely, a skeletal muscle myopathy in which the patient's muscles could not consume O_2 normally. Assuming that he did not have a skeletal muscle myopathy, the low O_2 pulse at peak $\dot{V}O_2$ indicate that his maximal stroke volume was about 65 ml. Because the patient's cardiologist did not believe that the patient had heart disease, the cardiopulmonary exercise test was repeated for a third time with systemic and pulmonary arterial and femoral venous catheters with blood gas and pH measurements, and direct arterial blood pressure tracings in search of a possible diagnosis of hypertrophic cardiomyopathy, other cardiomyopathy with diastolic dysfunction, or peripheral skeletal muscle myopathy.

Exercise Findings

Catheters were placed in the patient's right femoral vein, pulmonary artery and brachial artery, for the purpose of measuring blood gases, lactate and direct measurement of arterial pressures and wave form. The patient performed exercise on a cycle ergometer while breathing through a mouthpiece with a nose clip in place for breath-by-breath measurements of gas exchange. Heart rate and rhythm were continuously monitored. The protocol consisted of 3 minutes of rest, 3 minutes of 0 load pedalling at 60 rpm, followed by a progressive increase in work rate of 20 watts per minute until the patient became too symptomatic to continue. Blood was sampled for blood gases, pH and lactate at rest, at the end of 3 minutes of unloaded cycling, every minute during the incremental exercise period and at six minutes of recovery from the three sites. 12 lead EKG recordings were obtained during rest, every minute of exercise, and recovery. The patient performed the exercise test with good effort. His resting and exercise electrocardiograms were normal. No ectopic beats were noted.

TABLE 9.81.1. Selected Respiratory Function Data

Measurement	Predicted	Measured
Age, yr		29
Sex		Male
Height, cm		180
Weight, kg	81	86
Hematocrit, %		47
VC, L	4.95	4.29
IC, L	3.30	2.94
FEV$_1$, L	4.13	2.74
FEV$_1$/VC, %	83	64
MVV L/min	163	110

TABLE 9.81.2. Selected Exercise Data

Measurement	Predicted	Measured
Peak $\dot{V}O_2$, L/min	3.28	1.69
Maximum HR, beats/min	192	176
Maximum O_2 pulse, ml/beat	17.2	9.8
$\Delta\dot{V}O_2/\Delta WR$, ml/min/W	10.3	7.9
AT, L/min	>1.41	0.90
Blood pressure, mmHg (rest, max ex)		155/85, 160/90
Maximum $\dot{V}E$, L/min		90
Exercise breathing reserve, L/min	>15	20
PaO$_2$, mmHg (rest, max ex)		86, 105
P(A − a)O$_2$, mmHg (rest, max ex)		11, 17
P(a − ET)CO$_2$, mmHg (rest, max ex)		4, 7
VD/VT (rest, max ex)		0.47, 0.41
HCO$_3^-$, mEq/L (rest, recov)		26, 17
Lactate, mEq/L (recovery)		13.7

TABLE 9.81.3. Air Breathing

Time (min)	Work rate (watts)	BP (mmHg)	HR (min⁻¹)	f (min⁻¹)	V̇E L/min BTPS	V̇CO₂ L/min STPD	V̇O₂ L/min STPD	V̇O₂/HR ml/beat	R	pH	HCO₃⁻ meq/L	PO₂ mmHg ET	a	(A − a)	PCO₂ mmHg ET	a	(a − ET)	V̇E/V̇CO₂	V̇E/V̇O₂	VD/VT
	Rest																		30	
	Rest		74	17	12.0	0.26	0.34	4.6	0.76			105			36			39	30	
	Rest		72	15	9.7	0.20	0.27	3.8	0.74			104			37			41	36	
	Rest		70	16	9.2	0.16	0.21	3.0	0.76			106			37			47	34	
	Rest		71	15	9.0	0.17	0.22	3.1	0.77			105			37			44	39	
	Rest	155/85	69	15	8.9	0.15	0.19	2.8	0.79	7.40	25	107	86	14	37	41	4	49	35	0.47
	Rest		71	16	10.9	0.21	0.26	3.7	0.81			107			37			44		
	Unloaded		82	16	13.3	0.31	0.37	4.5	0.84			106			37			37	31	
	Unloaded		85	19	16.7	0.40	0.49	5.8	0.82			107			37			37	30	
	Unloaded		87	17	17.1	0.42	0.51	5.9	0.82			106			37			36	30	
	Unloaded		88	19	17.8	0.44	0.54	6.1	0.81			105			37			36	29	
	Unloaded		85	20	18.2	0.43	0.52	6.1	0.83			108			36			37	31	
	Unloaded	145/85	83	22	19.4	0.45	0.55	6.6	0.82	7.41	25	107	90	13	36	40	4	38	31	0.38
0.5	4		84	20	18.1	0.43	0.52	6.2	0.83			107			37			37	31	
1.0	14		87	23	21.4	0.52	0.63	7.2	0.83			108			36			37	30	
1.5	24		82	21	20.3	0.48	0.58	7.1	0.83			106			37			38	31	
2.0	34		89	21	23.1	0.59	0.69	7.8	0.86			107			37			35	30	
2.5	44	155/85	98	23	25.0	0.66	0.75	7.7	0.88	7.40	24	108	92	14	37	40	3	34	30	0.33
3.0	54		99	22	26.8	0.77	0.84	8.5	0.92			107			39			32	29	
3.5	64		103	27	30.5	0.84	0.86	8.3	0.98			110			38			33	32	
4.0	79		117	26	34.4	1.02	0.96	8.2	1.06			109			40			31	33	
4.5	85	175/90	124	28	39.2	1.14	1.05	8.5	1.09	7.38	24	111	95	17	39	41	2	32	35	0.31
5.0	94		130	30	46.2	1.30	1.13	8.7	1.15			115			37			33	38	
5.5	104		136	31	49.7	1.39	1.21	8.9	1.15			115			37			33	38	
6.0	114		144	29	51.7	1.49	1.31	9.1	1.14			114			38			33	37	
6.5	124	160/90	152	30	57.5	1.61	1.38	9.1	1.17	7.39	23	116	102	14	37	38	1	34	39	0.31
7.0	134		160	28	58.7	1.74	1.50	9.4	1.16			115			37			32	37	
7.5	144		166	31	64.7	1.87	1.62	9.8	1.15			115			37			33	38	
8.0	154		171	36	74.1	2.02	1.67	9.8	1.21			118			35			35	42	
8.5	164		178	48	89.3	2.11	1.69	9.5	1.25	7.35	21	123	106	12	31	38	7	40	50	0.41
9.0	152		178	54	90.2	2.08	1.64	9.2	1.27			124			31			41	52	
	Recovery		164	37	69.2	1.53	1.23	7.5	1.24	7.32	17	124	105	16	30	34	4	43	53	0.38
	Recovery		136	36	56.1	1.15	0.90	6.6	1.28			126			28			45	58	

The patient had a near syncopal event during the immediate recovery period as well as during spirometry. During these events he complained of dizziness and was diaphoretic. He admitted to these symptoms having occurred previously after exercise.

His blood pressure was noted to drop to 82/64 while his pulse remained in the 90 range. Lying him flat with his legs raised helped him recover from these two episodes. The typical cardiac slowing of a vasovagal event was not observed.

TABLE 9.81.4. Hemodynamic Responses to Exercise

Status	VO₂ (ml/min)	Heart rate (beats/min)	Systemic artery O₂ cont (ml/100 ml)	PO₂ (mmHg)	O₂ sat (%)	Pulmonary artery O₂ cont (ml/100 ml)	PO₂ (mmHg)	O₂ sat (%)	Femoral vein O₂ cont (ml/100 ml)	PO₂ (mmHg)	O₂ sat (%)	C(a − v̄)O₂ (ml/100 ml)	S.V. (ml)	C.O. (L/min)
Rest	250	71	20.0	86	97	12.1	33	60	6.0	20	32	7.9	44	3.1
C load	520	83	21.0	90	97	8.7	26	47	5.0	18	25	12.3	51	4.2
44 watts	720	98	21.0	92	97	8.6	26	44	4.9	18	25	12.4	59	5.8
85 watts	1000	124	21.0	95	97	8.2	25	39	5.8	21	29	12.8	63	7.8
124 watts	1340	152	21.5	102	97	7.9	25	37	7.4	26	35	13.6	65	9.8
164 watts	1680	176	22.0	106	97	6.1	23	29	6.7	25	31	15.9	60	10
(Max ex)	1640	164	22.0	105	97	4.8	20	22	5.1	23	24	17.2	58	9.5
6 min rec			21.0	99	97	14.5	45	69	17.0	55	80	6.5		

FIGURE 9.81.1.

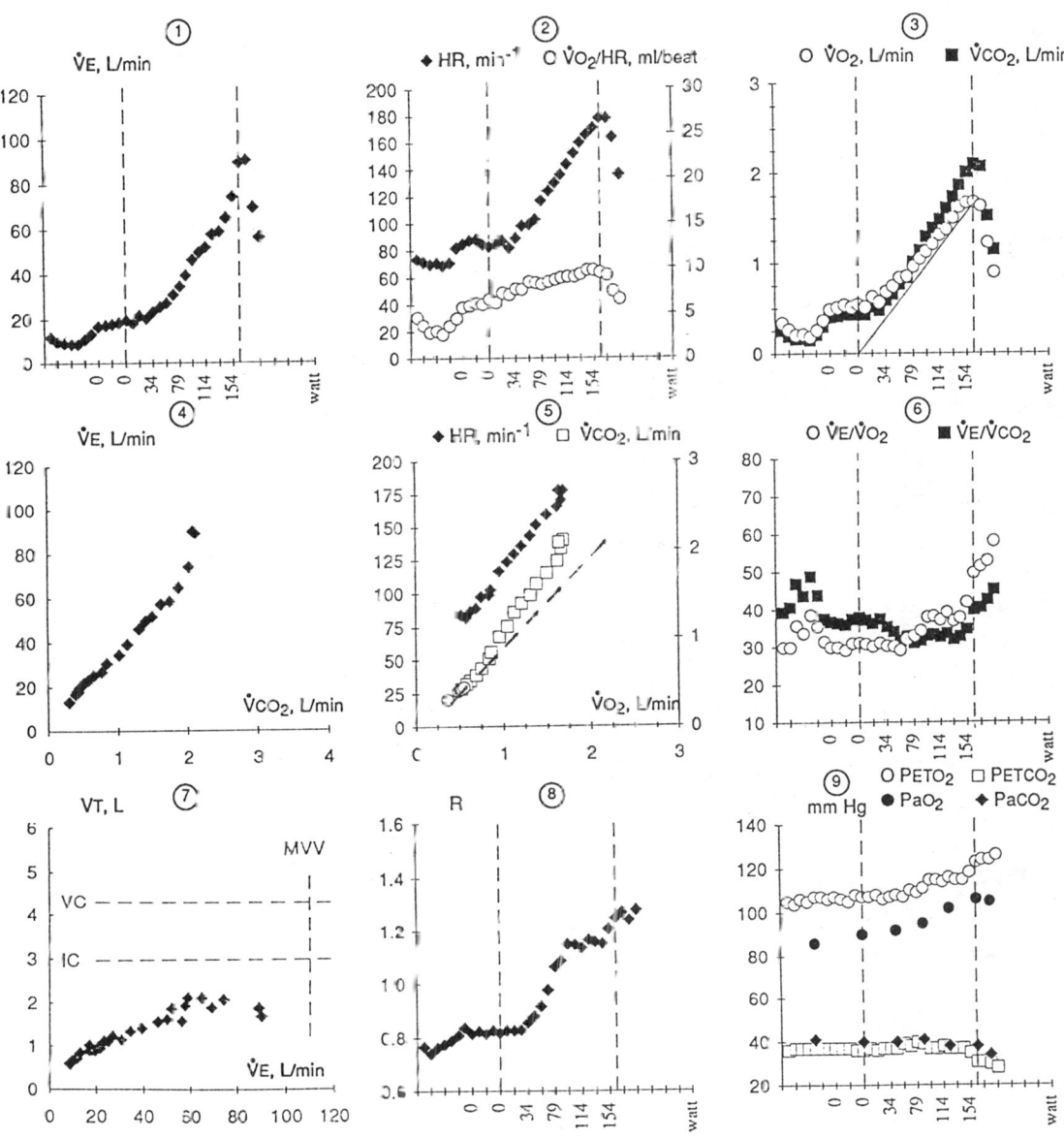

1. Vertical dashed lines in panels 1 to 3 and 6, 8, and 9 indicate the beginning and the end of increasing work period.
2. Unloaded cycling is performed for 3 minutes before the left vertical dashed line.
3. In panel 3, the diagonal line shows the increase of $\dot{V}O_2$ at a slope of 10 ml/min/W.
4. In panel 5, the diagonal dashed line has a slope of 1.

Interpretation

Comments

Respiratory function tests showed mild airflow obstruction.

Analysis

Referring to Table 9.81.2 and flow chart 1, his peak $\dot{V}O_2$ and *AT* are low bringing us through branchpoints 1.1, 1.2, and 1.3 to flow chart 4. The breathing reserve is normal (branchpoint 4.1) and the ventilatory equivalent for $\dot{V}CO_2$ at the anaerobic threshold (branchpoint 4.3) is borderline normal bringing us to the diagnosis of O_2 flow problem of non-pulmonary origin. The hematocrit is normal (branchpoint 4.4) and he has a low O_2 pulse which is non-changing as peak $\dot{V}O_2$ is approached. This brings us to heart disease. Although his electrocardiogram is normal, he has an abnormally steep heart rate increase relative to $\dot{V}O_2$ increase and a reduced $\Delta\dot{V}O_2/\Delta WR$ supporting the diagnosis of heart disease.

For the hemodynamic measurements, see Table 9.81.4 headed "Hemodynamic Responses to Exercise." The calculated stroke volume by direct Fick method was abnormally low at about 65 ml/beat on repeated measurements and explained the low peak $\dot{V}O_2$ and steep heart rate—$\dot{V}O_2$ relationship. The O_2 extraction across the leg is normal indicating that the patient does not have a skeletal muscle myopathy explaining his inability to extract O_2 normally. Note that his femoral vein PO_2 increased as work rate continued past the subjects anaerobic threshold. This paradoxical phenomenon has been previously observed in heart failure patients by Koike et al (1). O_2 extraction across the central circulation was normal, although the maximum O_2 extraction (75–80%) is reached at a lower $\dot{V}O_2$ than expected.

Conclusion

Twenty-nine-year-old man who developed a low cardiac output state judged to be due to diastolic cardiomyopathy. Pulmonary vascular disease, lung disease, peripheral arterial disease, skeletal muscle disease and other forms of heart disease were excluded.

Reference

1. Koike A, Wasserman F, Taniguchi K, et al. Critical capillary oxygen partial pressure and lactate threshold in patients with cardiovascular disease. J Am Coll Cardiol 1994; 23: 1644–1650.

Case 82 Transition from Normal to Left Ventricular Failure

Clinical Findings

This 71-year-old white collar worker was evaluated by cardiopulmonary exercise testing 4½ years earlier (age 66) and again at this time because of a recent worsening in exercise tolerance. The earlier studies showed that he had mild underlying lung or pulmonary vascular disease evidenced by a reduced diffusing capacity and slightly elevated ventilatory equivalent for CO_2 at the *AT* but normal lung mechanics. He tried to maintain a personalized exercise training program. He was doing well until about 9 months earlier when he developed painless hematuria. Work-up for this was complicated by a respiratory arrest. It was eventually revealed that the hematuria was due to a renal calculus. He now experiences dyspnea with exercise. His medications consist of a cholesterol lowering drug and inhaled bronchodilator medication.

Exercise Findings

For both evaluations, the patient performed exercise on a cycle ergometer while breathing through a mouthpiece with a nose clip in place for breath-by-breath measurements of gas exchange. Heart rate and rhythm were continuously monitored. The protocol consisted of 3 minutes of rest, 3 minutes of 0 load pedalling at 60 rpm, followed by a progressive increase in work rate of 15 watts per minute until he became too symptomatic to continue. He stopped exercise because of leg fatigue on both occasions; 12-lead EKG recordings were obtained during rest, every minute of exercise, and recovery. For the first test at age 66, he had a normal electrocardiogram.

For the test at age 71 he had a prolonged PR interval (0.21 sec) and some premature atrial contractions at rest which disappeared during exercise. There was no ectopy during exercise. The patient performed the exercise test with good effort.

TABLE 9.82.1.   Selected Respiratory Function Data

Measurement	Predicted	Measured
Age, yr		66
Sex		Male
Height, cm		164
Weight, kg	69	72
Hematocrit, %		43
VC, L	3.05	2.90
IC, L	2.03	2.00
FEV$_1$, L	2.48	2.30
FEV$_1$/VC, %	81	79
MVV, L/min	105	118
D$_{CO}$, ml/mm Hg/min	23	19

TABLE 9.82.2.   Selected Respiratory Function Data

Measurement	Predicted	Measured
Age, yr		71
Sex		Male
Height, cm		164
Weight, kg	69	74
Hematocrit, %		43
VC, L	2.96	3.01
IC, L	1.98	2.22
FEV$_1$, L	2.30	2.64
FEV$_1$/VC, %	78	88
MVV, L/min	93	110
D$_{CO}$, ml/mm Hg/min	23	12.3

TABLE 9.82.3.   Selected Exercise Data

Measurement	Predicted Age 66	Predicted Age 71	Measured Age 66	Measured Age 71
Peak V̇o$_2$, L/min	1.80	1.67	1.88	1.24
Maximum HR, beats/min	154	149	125	116
Maximum O$_2$ pulse, ml/beat	11.7	11.2	15.9	10.7
ΔV̇o$_2$/ΔWR, ml/min/W	10.3	10.3	14	7.2
AT, L/min	>0.85	>0.78	1.0	0.65
Maximum V̇E, L/min			90	63
Exercise breathing reserve, L/min	>15	>15	28	47

FIGURE 9.82.1.   Age 66.

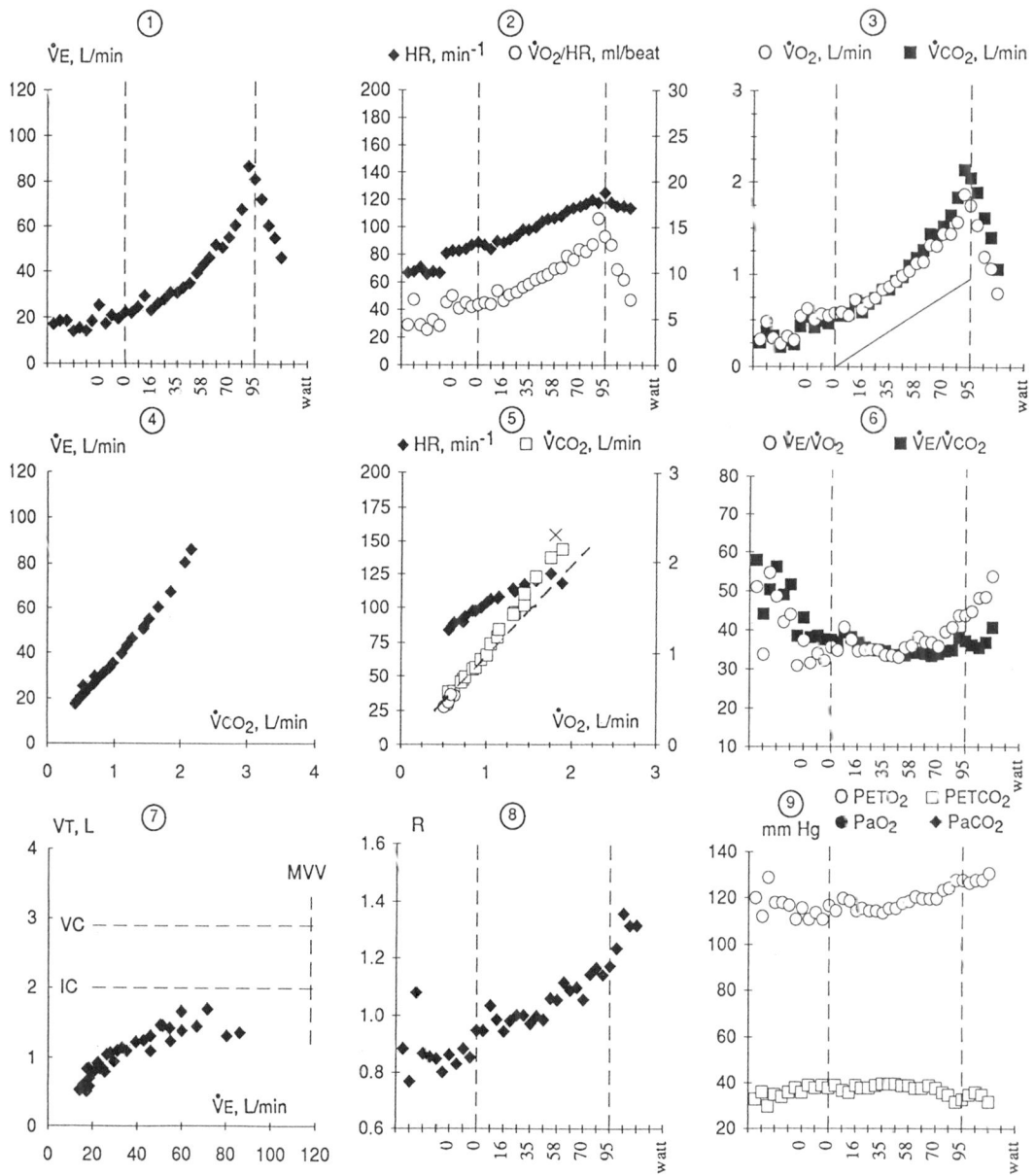

1. Vertical dashed lines in panels 1 to 3 and 6, 8, and 9 indicate the beginning and the end of increasing work period.

2. Unloaded cycling is performed for 3 minutes before the left vertical dashed line.

3. In panel 3, the diagonal line shows the increase of $\dot{V}O_2$ at a slope of 10 ml/min/W.

4. In panel 5, the diagonal dashed line has a slope of 1; the "x" in the upper right is the predicted maximum heart rate and $\dot{V}O_2$ for the subject.

TABLE 9.82.4. Age 66

Time (min)	Work rate (watts)	BP (mm Hg)	HR (min⁻¹)	f (min⁻¹)	V̇E L/min BTPS	V̇CO2 L/min STPD	V̇O2 L/min STPD	V̇O2/HR ml/beat	R	pH	HCO3⁻ mec/L	PO2 ET	a	(A−a)	PCO2 ET	a	(a−ET)	V̇E/V̇CO2	V̇E/V̇O2	VD/VT
	Rest																			
	Rest		67	34	17.2	0.26	0.29	4.4	0.88			120			33			58	51	
	Rest		68	32	18.6	0.37	0.49	7.2	0.77			112			36			44	34	
	Rest		71	27	18.7	0.34	0.31	4.4	1.08			129			30			51	55	
	Rest		66	27	14.2	0.22	0.26	3.9	0.87			118			35			56	49	
	Rest		68	26	15.6	0.28	0.33	4.9	0.85			118			34			49	42	
	Rest		67	27	14.4	0.24	0.29	4.3	0.85			117			36			52	44	
	Unloaded		81	22	18.5	0.44	0.55	6.8	0.80			111			38			39	31	
	Unloaded		83	32	25.4	0.54	0.63	7.5	0.86			116			36			43	37	
	Unloaded		83	21	17.5	0.42	0.51	6.1	0.83			111			39			38	32	
	Unloaded		84	26	21.0	0.50	0.57	6.8	0.88			114			38			39	34	
	Unloaded		87	25	19.5	0.47	0.56	6.4	0.85			111			39			38	32	
	Unloaded		89	24	22.4	0.56	0.59	6.6	0.95			117			38			38	36	
0.5	2		87	24	22.1	0.56	0.59	6.8	0.95			115			39			37	35	
1.0	7		84	29	24.6	0.58	0.55	6.6	1.03			120			37			39	41	
1.5	11		90	31	29.4	0.72	0.79	8.1	0.98			119			36			38	38	
2.0	16		89	28	23.4	0.59	0.62	7.0	0.94			115			39			37	35	
2.5	23		91	25	26.2	0.69	0.70	7.7	0.98			116			38			36	35	
3.0	26		94	26	28.0	0.75	0.75	7.9	1.00			115			38			35	35	
3.5	32		98	28	31.0	0.84	0.84	8.5	1.00			115			39			35	35	
4.0	35		98	28	31.1	0.85	0.87	8.9	0.97			114			40			35	34	
4.5	42		100	29	32.3	0.93	0.94	9.4	1.00			116			40			34	34	
5.0	44		104	32	35.3	0.98	1.00	9.6	0.99			116			40			34	33	
5.5	50		106	32	39.5	1.11	1.05	9.9	1.06			118			39			34	36	
6.0	58		107	34	43.0	1.19	1.13	10.5	1.05			119			39			34	36	
6.5	59		108	35	46.1	1.27	1.14	10.6	1.11			121			38			34	38	
7.0	70		112	35	51.6	1.45	1.33	11.9	1.09			120			38			34	37	
7.5	72		114	34	50.5	1.44	1.31	11.5	1.10			120			39			34	37	
8.0	70		115	44	54.9	1.53	1.45	12.6	1.06			120			38			34	36	
8.5	82		117	43	60.2	1.65	1.45	12.4	1.14			124			36			35	40	
9.0	87		120	46	67.2	1.84	1.58	13.1	1.17			125			35			35	41	
9.5	94		118	63	86.4	2.15	1.88	15.9	1.14			128			32			38	44	
10.0	95		125	61	80.5	2.06	1.75	14.0	1.17			123			33			37	44	
	Recovery		118	42	71.8	1.90	1.54	13.1	1.24			127			35			36	45	
	Recovery		115	38	60.1	1.69	1.20	10.4	1.35			128			36			36	48	
	Recovery		115	38	54.7	1.41	1.07	9.3	1.31			128			35			37	49	
	Recovery		114	42	46.2	1.06	0.81	7.1	1.32			131			32			41	54	

Interpretation

Comments

Resting pulmonary function tests were normal.

Analysis

Age 66: Referring to Table 9.82.3 and flow chart 1, his peak V̇O2 and AT are normal bringing us through branchpoint 1.1 to flow chart 2. At branchpoint 2.2 we find that he is not obese and would conclude that he would benefit from reassurance to continue his exercise program. The somewhat elevated V̇E/V̇CO2, while suggesting some uneven ventilation-perfusion relationships, was accompanied by a good breathing reserve.

Age 71: Referring to Table 9.82.3 and flow chart 1, his peak V̇O2 and AT are now reduced. We are directed through branchpoints 1.2 and 1.3 to flow chart 4. The breathing reserve is normal (branchpoint 4.1) and the ventilatory equivalent for V̇CO2 at the AT (branchpoint 4.3) is high bringing us to abnormal pulmonary circulation. The vital capacity is normal (branchpoint 4.5) suggesting a diagnosis of pulmonary vascular disease rather than left ventricular failure. He did not have arterial blood gas measurements therefore we can not use items 1–3 in the confirmatory box to support the diagnosis. Referring to items 4–6 (non-invasive measurements), he does not have a steep heart rate response to exercise. In fact he has a low maximum heart rate. His oxygen saturation by pulse oximetry was normal. Thus we conclude that a better choice

FIGURE 9.82.2.   Age 71.

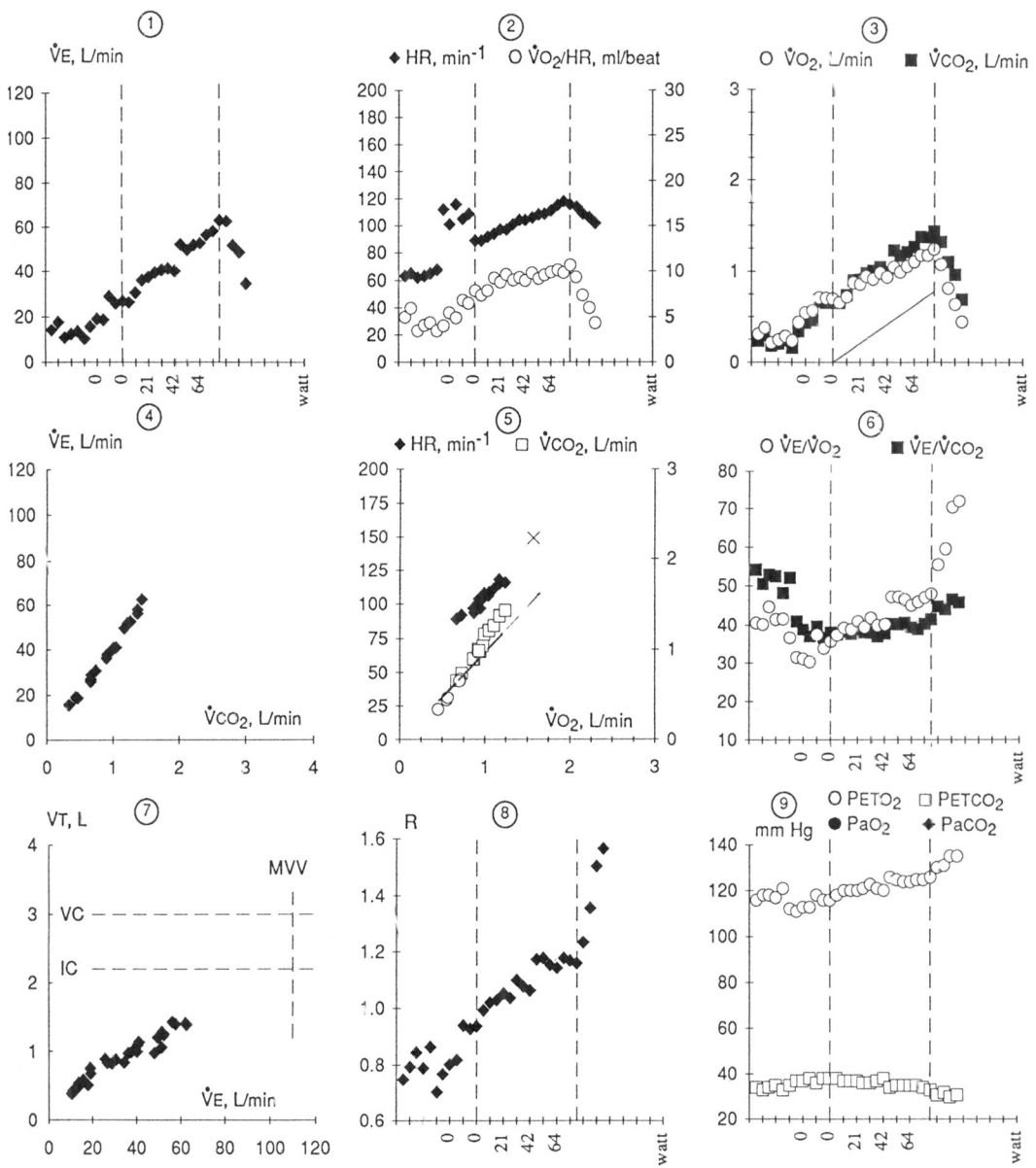

1. Vertical dashed lines in panels 1 to 3 and 6, 8, and 9 indicate the beginning and the end of increasing work period.

2. Unloaded cycling is performed for 3 minutes before the left vertical dashed line.

3. In panel 3, the diagonal line shows the increase of $\dot{V}O_2$ at a slope of 10 ml/min/W.

4. In panel 5, the diagonal dashed line has a slope of 1; the "x" in the upper right is the predicted maximum heart rate and $\dot{V}O_2$ for the subject.

TABLE 9.82.5. Age 71

Time (min)	Work rate (watts)	BP (mmHg)	HR (min⁻¹)	f (min⁻¹)	$\dot{V}_E$ /min BTPS	$\dot{V}_{CO_2}$ L/min STPD	$\dot{V}_{O_2}$ L/min STPD	$\dot{V}_{O_2}$/HR ml/beat	R	pH	HCO₃ meq/L	Po₂, mmHg ET	a	(A − a)	Pco₂, mmHg ET	a	(a − ET)	$\dot{V}_E$/$\dot{V}_{CO_2}$	$\dot{V}_E$/$\dot{V}_{O_2}$	VD/VT
	Rest																			
	Rest		63	28	14.5	0.23	0.31	5.0	0.75			116			34			54	41	
	Rest		65	35	17.8	0.31	0.39	5.9	0.79			118			33			51	40	
	Rest		62	26	11.2	0.18	0.21	3.4	0.85			118			34			53	45	
	Rest		63	28	12.4	0.20	0.26	4.0	0.79			117			35			53	41	
	Rest		65	25	13.5	0.25	0.29	4.4	0.86			121			33			48	42	
	Rest		68	27	10.4	0.17	0.24	3.5	0.70			112			35			52	37	
	Unloaded		112	27	15.8	0.34	0.45	4.0	0.77			111			37			41	31	
	Unloaded		101	28	19.0	0.44	0.55	5.5	0.80			113			37			39	31	
	Unloaded		116	25	13.9	0.47	0.57	4.9	0.82			113			38			37	30	
	Unloaded		105	35	29.0	0.67	0.72	3.8	0.94			118			36			40	37	
	Unloaded		109	29	25.9	0.66	0.71	6.5	0.93			116			38			37	34	
	Unloaded		89	32	27.0	0.66	0.70	7.9	0.94			116			38			38	36	
0.5	8		89	32	26.7	0.66	0.66	7.4	0.99			118			38			37	37	
1.0	11		92	35	30.7	0.74	0.72	7.9	1.02			120			37			38	39	
1.5	16		94	37	36.2	0.90	0.87	9.2	1.03			120			37			38	39	
2.0	21		97	38	37.7	0.90	0.86	8.8	1.05			120			37			39	41	
2.5	25		97	38	39.3	0.98	0.94	9.7	1.04			121			36			38	39	
3.0	32		101	37	40.6	1.01	0.91	9.0	1.10			123			36			38	42	
3.5	35		104	36	41.1	1.05	0.97	9.4	1.08			121			37			37	40	
4.0	42		104	40	40.2	0.99	0.93	9.0	1.06			120			38			38	40	
4.5	45		106	41	52.0	1.22	1.04	9.8	1.17			126			34			40	47	
5.0	52		108	41	49.6	1.17	0.99	9.2	1.18			125			35			40	47	
5.5	57		109	40	51.7	1.21	1.05	9.7	1.15			124			35			40	47	
6.0	64		111	42	52.5	1.26	1.11	10.0	1.14			124			35			39	45	
6.5	67		115	39	56.2	1.38	1.17	10.2	1.18			125			35			39	46	
7.0	70		118	41	57.8	1.37	1.17	9.9	1.17			125			34			40	47	
7.5	77		116	45	62.6	1.44	1.24	10.7	1.16			126			33			42	48	
	Recovery		111	44	62.2	1.32	1.07	9.4	1.24			130			31			45	55	
	Recovery		109	48	51.3	1.10	0.81	7.4	1.36			131			32			44	60	
	Recovery		106	49	48.2	0.96	0.64	6.0	1.50			135			30			47	70	
	Recovery		102	41	34.5	0.70	0.44	4.4	1.57			135			31			46	72	

would have been heart disease with left ventricular failure. This is an example in which the flow charts get you close to the diagnosis. However when the confirming data do not fit, another selection with similar pathophysiology should be considered.

This case was selected because of the sequential measurements at a 4½ year interval and a telephonic follow-up to the second study. The predicted peak $\dot{V}_{O_2}$ decreased 0.13 L/min but his actual peak $\dot{V}_{O_2}$ decreased 0.64 L/min over the 4½ year interval. Further his maximum O_2 pulse decreased from 15.9 to 10.7 at similar maximum heart rates. In a telephone call follow-up initiated by the patient, despite the absence of ECG changes to support myocardial

ischemia, he stated that his cardiologist, seeing the results of cardiopulmonary exercise testing, decided to do a coronary angiogram on him. Several major coronary vessels had high grade stenoses which were treated with angioplasty. The patient called back to inform us that since angioplasty, he had improved exercise tolerance, felt better and would return for follow-up study at a later date.

Conclusion

This 71-year-old man developed chronic heart failure over a 4½ year interval, probably due to myocardial ischemia.

Case 83 Psychogenic Dyspnea
Clinical Findings

This 73-year-old woman was referred for cardiopulmonary exercise testing because of exertional dyspnea which has been a progressive problem over the past year and had been worked up by internal medicine, cardiology and pulmonary specialists without reaching a diagnosis. A number of therapeutic options were tried without relief of symptoms. She had no problem at rest and had experienced no orthopnea or nocturnal dyspnea. She admitted to mild ankle edema toward evening. She did not experience typical angina type pain but did report pressure in the xiphoid area at times which was not related to breathing and which might also take place at rest. She had no history of gastroesophageal reflux. She had no breathing noises, although her daughter does say that she can hear her inhale at times (?sigh, not stridor). She had no difficulty in getting air out of her chest. She had right heart catheterization and left heart catheterization and selective right and left coronary angiography. The only abnormality reported was a somewhat elevated pulmonary artery pressure. She had an ejection fraction of 0.76. Her chest X-ray and CT scans of her chest and abdomen were normal. Ventilation and perfusion scans and echocardiogram were reported as normal. Her medications are metaprolol, procardia, premarin, zoloft, synthroid and magnesium.

Exercise Findings

An arterial catheter was inserted percutaneously in the left brachial artery under xylocaine anesthesia. The patient performed exercise on a cycle ergometer while breathing through a mouthpiece with a nose clip in place for breath-by-breath measurements of gas exchange. Heart rate and rhythm were continuously monitored. The protocol consisted of 3 minutes of rest, 3 minutes of 0 load pedalling at 60 rpm, followed by a progressive increase in work rate of 10 watts per minute until she became too symptomatic to continue. 12 lead EKG recordings were obtained during rest, every minute of exercise, and recovery. Blood pressure was monitored from the arterial catheter and recorded on a strip chart recorder. Arterial blood samples were taken at rest,

at the end of 3 minutes of unloaded cycling, and at one minute intervals (every 10 W) to maximum and at 2 minutes of recovery. A pulse oximeter was used for monitoring arterial O_2 saturation during the test.

The patient made good effort. She started hyperventilating at rest and increased her breathing rate to 50/minute as soon as she started to exercise. She started pedalling very rapidly so that unloaded cycling was equivalent to 10 W. She stated that she stopped exercise because she found it difficult to continue to pedal and because of shortness of breath. There were no ectopic beats or evidence of myocardial ischemia on the electrocardiogram.

TABLE 9.83.1. Selected Respiratory Function Data

Measurement	Predicted	Measured
Age, yr		73
Sex		Female
Height, cm		163
Weight, kg	63	76
Hematocrit, %		45
VC, L	2.79	2.35
IC, L	1.86	2.23
FEV$_1$, L	2.19	1.80
FEV$_1$/VC, %	78	77
MVV, L/min	84	67
D$_L$CO, ml/mm Hg/min	20.1	17.1

TABLE 9.83.2. Selected Exercise Data

Measurement	Predicted	Measured
Peak $\dot{V}O_2$, L/min	1.18	1.00
Maximum HR, beats/min	147	104
Maximum O_2 pulse, ml/beat	8.0	9.6
$\Delta \dot{V}O_2/\Delta WR$, ml/min/W	10.3	7.0
AT, L/min	>0.64	0.8
Blood pressure, mmHg (rest, max ex)		150/75, 175/95
Maximum $\dot{V}E$, L/min		53
Exercise breathing reserve, L/min	>15	14
PaO_2, mmHg (rest, max ex)		105, 122
P(A − a)O_2, mmHg (rest, max ex)		21, 6
P(a − ET)CO_2, mmHg (rest, max ex)		0, −1.4
VD/VT (rest, max ex)		0.28, 0.17
HCO$_3^-$, mEq/L (rest, recov)		19, 14
Lactate, mEq/L (rest, recov)		1.7, 9.7

FIGURE 9.83.1.

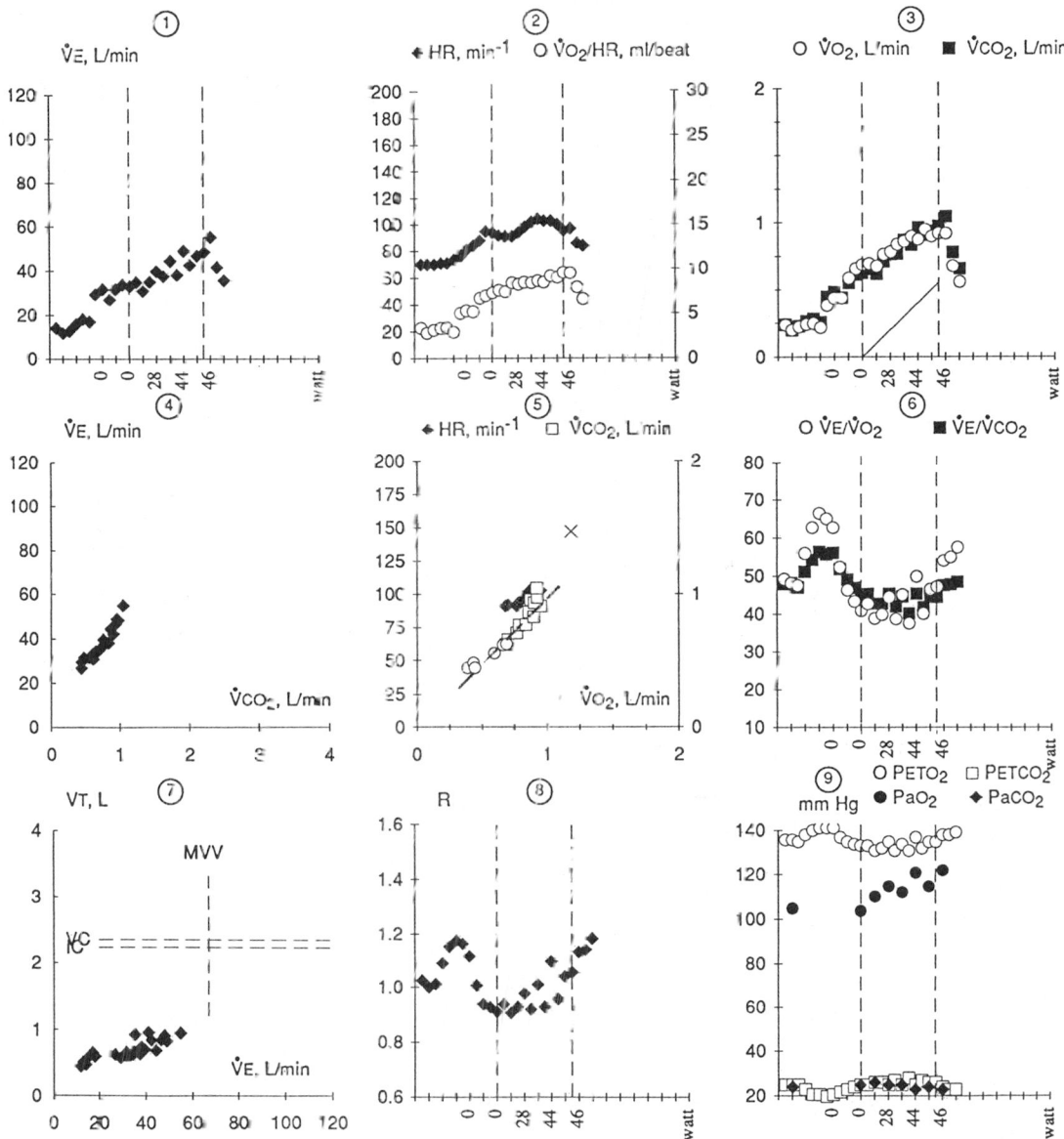

1. Vertical dashed lines in panels 1 to 3 and 6, 8, and 9 indicate the beginning and the end of increasing work period.
2. Unloaded cycling is performed for 3 minutes before the left vertical dashed line.
3. In panel 3, the diagonal line shows the increase of $\dot{V}CO_2$ at a slope of 10 ml/min/W.
4. In panel 5, the diagonal dashed line has a slope of 1; the "x" in the upper right is the predicted maximum heart rate and $\dot{V}CO_2$ for the subject.

TABLE 9.83.3. Air Breathing

Time (min)	Work rate (watts)	BP (mmHg)	HR (min⁻¹)	f (min⁻¹)	V̇E L/min BTPS	V̇CO₂ L/min STPD	V̇O₂ L/min STPD	V̇O₂/HR ml/beat	R	pH	HCO₃⁻ meq/L	PO₂, mmHg ET	a	(A − a)	PCO₂, mmHg ET	a	(a − ET)	V̇E/V̇CO₂	V̇E/V̇O₂	VD/VT
	Rest																			
	Rest		70	30	14.2	0.24	0.24	3.4	1.03			136		21	25			48	49	
	Rest	150/75	70	26	11.8	0.20	0.20	2.8	1.00	7.50	18	136	105		25	24	−1	48	48	0.21
	Rest		70	25	12.8	0.23	0.22	3.2	1.01			135			25			47	48	
	Rest		71	26	15.7	0.26	0.24	3.4	1.09			138			23			51	56	
	Rest		71	30	18.0	0.28	0.25	3.5	1.15			140			21			54	63	
	Rest		74	26	16.9	0.26	0.22	3.0	1.18			141			21			57	66	
	Unloaded		76	51	29.3	0.45	0.38	5.1	1.16			141			20			56	65	
	Unloaded		81	52	31.5	0.48	0.43	5.3	1.12			141			21			56	63	
	Unloaded		84	43	26.8	0.45	0.44	5.3	1.01			137			22			52	52	
	Unloaded		88	48	31.5	0.56	0.59	6.7	0.94			135			23			49	46	
	Unloaded		95	54	33.4	0.61	0.66	7.0	0.93			134			24			47	44	
	Unloaded	155/85	94	54	32.8	0.63	0.69	7.3	0.91	7.50	19	133	104	19	25	25	0	45	41	0.20
0.5	10		92	55	34.5	0.66	0.70	7.6	0.94			133			25			45	43	
1.0	7	165/90	91	50	30.8	0.62	0.68	7.5	0.91	7.47	19	131	110	12	26	26	0	43	39	0.20
1.5	16		91	52	34.9	0.71	0.76	8.4	0.93			132			26			43	40	
2.0	28	175/100	94	56	39.6	0.77	0.78	8.3	0.98	7.48	18	135	115	10	25	25	0	46	45	0.21
2.5	25		98	59	37.4	0.77	0.84	8.5	0.92			131			27			42	39	
3.0	31	190/100	102	64	44.3	0.87	0.86	8.4	1.01	7.47	18	134	112	13	25	25	0	45	45	0.20
3.5	31		104	51	38.0	0.83	0.90	8.6	0.93			131			28			40	38	
4.0	44	185/95	103	59	48.8	0.96	0.87	8.5	1.10	7.47	16	137	121	8	25	23	−2	46	50	0.16
4.5	47		103	50	42.3	0.91	0.95	9.2	0.96			132			27			42	40	
5.0	50	175/95	100	55	46.6	0.94	0.90	9.0	1.04	7.45	16	135	115	12	26	24	−2	45	47	0.17
5.5	55		96	53	48.1	0.98	0.92	9.6	1.06			135			26			45	47	
6.0	46	150/65	97	58	54.8	1.05	0.92	9.5	1.14	7.43	15	138	122	7	24	23	−1	48	54	0.19
	Recovery		86	43	41.1	0.78	0.68	7.9	1.15			138			23			48	55	
	Recovery		84	38	35.4	0.66	0.56	6.7	1.18			139			23			49	58	

Interpretation

Comments

Resting spirometry was normal.

Analysis

Referring to Table 9.83.2 and flow chart 1, her peak V̇O₂ is low normal and the AT is normal bringing us through branchpoints 1.1, to flow chart 2. Her ECG, arterial blood gases and O₂ pulse at peak V̇O₂ are normal (branchpoint 2.1) and she is overweight (branchpoint 2.2) but not excessively so. Her major problems with respect to her symptoms are twofold. First and primary is that she starts to hyperventilate with a very small tidal volume (almost panting) as evident from panel 7 and the non-physiological changes in the gas exchange ratio and the arterial blood gas measurements (panels 8 and 9) showing acute hyperventilation. The pattern of breathing is also abnormal in that she maintains a breathing rate of 50 to 60 from shortly after the start of unloaded cycling with a low tidal volume relative to her inspiratory capacity. Second, her heart rate response to exercise is impaired (low and very shallow slope of heart rate versus V̇O₂), presumably due to being on a β-adrenergic blocking drug in a dose which limits ability of heart rate and therefore cardiac output to increase normally (heart rate at maximum exercise = 104). Thus there are psychogenic and iatrogenic causes for this patient's symptoms.

Conclusion

Psychogenic dyspnea in a 73-year-old lady, complicated by heavy β-adrenergic blockade.

APPENDIX A

Symbols and Abbreviations

Dash (⁻) above any symbol indicates a *mean* value
Dot (·) above any symbol indicates a *time derivative*

GASES

	PRIMARY SYMBOLS		EXAMPLES
V	gas volume	V_A	volume of alveolar gas
$\dot{V}$	gas volume/unit time	$\dot{V}_{O_2}$	O_2 uptake/minute
P	gas pressure	P_{AO_2}	alveolar O_2 pressure
$\bar{P}$	mean gas pressure	$\bar{P}_{C_{O_2}}$	mean capillary O_2 pressure
F	fractional concentration of a particular gas	F_{IO_2}	fractional concentration of O_2 in inspired gas
f	respiratory frequency		
D	diffusing capacity	D_{CO}	diffusing capacity for CO
R	respiratory exchange ratio		
RQ	respiratory quotient		
Q	gas quantity		
$\dot{Q}$	gas quantity/unit time (gas flow)	$\dot{Q}_{O_2}$	O_2 consumed/minute
STPD	standard temperature and pressure (0°C, 760 mmHg), dry		
BTPS	body temperature and pressure, saturated with water vapor		

	SECONDARY SYMBOLS (small capitals)		EXAMPLES
I	inspired gas	F_{IO_2}	fractional concentration of O_2 in inspired gas
E	expired gas	V_E	volume of expired gas
A	alveolar gas	$\dot{V}_A$	alveolar ventilation/minute
ET	end tidal	P_{ETCO_2}	end-tidal CO_2 tension
T	tidal gas	V_T	tidal volume
D	dead space gas	V_D	physiological dead space volume
B	barometric	P_B	barometric pressure

BLOOD

PRIMARY SYMBOLS		EXAMPLES	
$\dot{Q}$	volume flow of blood/ unit time	$\dot{Q}c$	blood flow through pulmonary capillaries/ minute
C	concentration of gas in blood phase	Cao_2	content of O_2 in arterial blood
S	% saturation of Hb with O_2	$S\bar{v}o_2$	saturation of Hb with O_2 in mixed venous blood

SECONDARY SYMBOLS		EXAMPLES	
a	arterial blood	$Paco_2$	partial pressure of CO_2 in arterial blood
v	venous blood	$P\bar{v}o_2$	partial pressure of O_2 in mixed venous blood
c	capillary blood	Pc_{o_2}	partial pressure of O_2 in pulmonary capillary blood

LUNG VOLUMES AND FLOWS

V_T	tidal volume = volume of air inhaled or exhaled with each breath
VC	vital capacity = maximal volume that can be expired after maximal inspiration
IC	inspiratory capacity = maximal volume that can be inspired from the resting end-expiratory level
ERV	expiratory reserve volume = maximal volume that can be expired from the resting end-expiratory level
FRC	functional residual capacity = volume of gas in lungs at end-expiration
RV	residual volume = volume of gas in lungs after maximal expiration
TLC	total lung capacity = volume of gas in lungs after maximal inspiration
FEV_x	forced expired volume in x seconds, e.g., FEV_1 (one second)
MVV	maximal voluntary ventilation

VARIABLES AND PARAMETERS

$\dot{V}o_2$	oxygen uptake
$\dot{V}o_2$ max	maximal aerobic power
$\dot{V}co_2$	carbon dioxide output
$\dot{Q}o_2$	O_2 consumption
$\dot{Q}co_2$	CO_2 production
AT	anaerobic threshold
LT	lactate threshold
LAT	lactic acidosis threshold
R	gas exchange ratio
RQ	respiratory quotient
$\dot{V}E/\dot{V}o_2$	ventilatory equivalent for O_2
$\dot{V}E/\dot{V}co_2$	ventilatory equivalent for CO_2
VD/VT	physiological dead space/tidal volume ratio
VD	physiological dead space
BR	breathing reserve
HR	heart rate
HRR	heart rate reserve
WR	work rate
$\Delta\dot{V}o_2/\Delta WR$	change in $\dot{V}o_2$/change in WR

Glossary

Aerobic: Having molecular oxygen present; describes a metabolic process utilizing oxygen.

Alveolar to arterial P_{O_2} difference ($P(A - a)_{O_2}$): The difference between the ideal alveolar P_{O_2} and the mean arterial P_{O_2}. This difference is considered to be an index of the lungs' inefficiency with respect to oxygen exchange.

Alveolar ventilation ($\dot{V}_A$): Conceptually, this is the volume of inspired gas that reaches the alveoli per minute, or the volume of gas that is evolved from the alveoli per minute. In practice, it is computed as the theoretic alveolar ventilation necessary to produce the arterial CO_2 tension (Pa_{CO_2}) at the current CO_2 output level.

Anaerobic: Lacking or inadequate molecular oxygen; describes any metabolic process that does not use molecular oxygen.

Anaerobic threshold (AT): The exercise $\dot{V}_{O_2}$ above which anaerobic high-energy P_{O_4} production supplements aerobic high-energy P_{O_4} production, with consequential lowering of the cellular redox state, increase in lactate/pyruvate (L/P) ratio, and net increase in lactate production at the site of anaerobiosis. Exercise above the AT is reflected in the muscle effluent and central blood by an increase in lactate concentration and L/P ratio, and a metabolic acidosis. Gas exchange is also affected by characteristic slowing of $\dot{V}_{O_2}$ kinetics and an increase in CO_2 output over that produced from aerobic metabolism, resulting from HCO_3^- buffering of lactic acid.

Analog to digital converter: A device for transforming continuously changing information into discrete units over some small time frame within which the value is considered to be relatively constant. This transforms continuous data signals to a form that can be analyzed by a digital computer.

Arterial–end-tidal P_{CO_2} difference ($P(a - ET)_{CO_2}$): The difference between the mean arterial P_{CO_2} and the end-tidal P_{CO_2}. This is positive when the arterial P_{CO_2} is higher than the end-tidal P_{CO_2}.

Under certain conditions during exercise, the difference reflects the degree of lung inefficiency of ventilation.

Arterial–mixed venous O_2 content difference $(C(a - \bar{v})O_2)$: The difference in the O_2 content of the arterial and venous blood, usually expressed in milliliters of O_2 per deciliter or liter of blood.

ATPS: Used to express the conditions under which a gas volume is measured. Under ATPS conditions, gas volume is at ambient (e.g., room) temperature and pressure, and saturated with water vapor at ambient temperature.

Breath-by-breath: The expression of a particular physiologic value averaged over one entire respiratory cycle. These are usually expressed as the value that physiologic variable would have if maintained over an entire minute (e.g., ventilation expressed as L/min). Breath-by-breath is also used to describe a method for measurement of respiratory gas exchange in which the product of respired gas volume and simultaneously measured expired gas concentration are integrated.

Breathing reserve (BR): The difference between the maximum voluntary ventilation and the maximum exercise ventilation. Hence, this represents the body's residual potential for further increasing ventilation at maximum exercise.

BTPS: Used to express the conditions under which a gas volume is measured. Under BTPS conditions, gas volume is at body temperature and the ambient atmospheric pressure and fully saturated with water vapor at the subject's body temperature.

Carbon dioxide output ($\dot{V}CO_2$): The amount of CO_2 exhaled from the body into the atmosphere per unit time, expressed in milliliters or liters per minute, STPD. This may differ from CO_2 production rate under conditions in which additional CO_2 may be evolved from the body's stores or CO_2 is added to the body's stores. In the steady-state, CO_2 output equals CO_2 production rate. In rare circumstances, appreciable quantities of CO_2 can be eliminated from the body as bicarbonate via the gastrointestinal tract or by hemodialysis.

Carbon dioxide production ($\dot{Q}CO_2$): The amount of carbon dioxide produced by the body's metabolic processes and in some circumstances released by buffering reactions within the body, expressed in milliliters or liters per minute, STPD.

Cardiac output ($\dot{Q}$): The flow of blood from the heart in a particular period of time, usually expressed as liters per minute. It is the product of the average stroke volume per beat and the heart rate.

Constant work rate test: An exercise test in which a constant power output is required of the subject.

Dead space or physiologic dead space (V_D): This is the theoretic volume of gas taken into the lung that is not involved in CO_2 exchange, assuming that the CO_2 tension in the alveolar volume equilibrates with that of the pulmonary capillary blood as it leaves the lung. The physiologic dead space is made up of the anatomic dead space (the volume of the upper airways, trachea, and bronchi) and the alveolar dead space (the volume of alveoli that is ventilated but unperfused and a certain portion of those alveoli that are underperfused).

Dead space/tidal volume ratio (V_D/V_T): The proportion of the tidal volume that is made up of the physiologic dead space. This is an index of the relative inefficiency for pulmonary gas exchange to eliminate CO_2.

Diffusing capacity: This is a measure of the rate of uptake of a particular gas across the alveolar-capillary bed for a specified driving pressure for that gas. It is measured, therefore, as the volume of gas per unit time per pressure difference (e.g., ml/min/mmHg). It is also referred to as the pulmonary gas transfer index (a term that more properly reflects the measurement). It is most practical to use carbon monoxide as the test gas for measurement of diffusing capacity of the lungs, in which case it is referred to as $D_{L}CO$.

Diffusion defect: A defect in the lungs' ability for gas diffusion. This is typically caused either by an abnormally increased diffusion path length or by conditions in which the transit time of the red cell through the pulmonary capillary bed is so fast that insufficient time is available for complete equilibrium between the concentration of gas in the alveolus and the same gas in the alveolar capillary.

Disability: A legal term that considers the effect of a functional impairment on the patient's ability to perform a specific work task and other factors such as age, sex, education, social environment, job availability, and the energy requirements of the occupation.

End-tidal PCO_2 ($PETCO_2$): The PCO_2 of the respired gas determined at the end of an exhalation. This is commonly the highest PCO_2 measured during the alveolar phase of the exhalation.

End-tidal P_{O_2} ($P_{ET_{O_2}}$):   The P_{O_2} determined in the respired gas at the end of an exhalation. This is typically the lowest P_{O_2} determined during the alveolar portion of the exhalation.

Exponential: A process in which the instantaneous rate of change of a variable is proportional to the "distance" from a steady-state or required level; hence, the rate of change of the function under consideration is rapid when it is far from its steady-state value and slows progressively as the function approaches its steady-state. If the process is known to be, or may be reasonably estimated to be, exponential, the time to reach 63% of the final value, i.e., to approach within 37% of the final value, is termed the time constant (τ) of the response. If the process is exponential, this time constant is related to the half time (the time to reach 50% of the final value) by the equation $t1/2 = 0.693 \, \tau$.

Fick method for cardiac output: A means of estimating cardiac output from the uptake of O_2 by the lungs and the arterial–mixed venous O_2 content difference. $\dot{Q} = \dot{V}_{O_2}/C(a - \bar{v})_{O_2}$. When the same principle is used to measure cardiac output with CO_2 as the test gas, the CO_2 output is divided by the $C(\bar{v} - a)_{CO_2}$.

Frequency response: This reflects the fidelity with which a device can track rapidly changing physiologic information. The frequency response of the device is usually determined by applying rapidly changing signals of a particular amplitude that span a range of frequencies, and then establishing the range over which the device accurately tracks the signal.

Gas exchange ratio (R):   The ratio of the carbon dioxide output to the oxygen uptake per unit time. This gas exchange ratio reflects not only tissue metabolic exchange of the gases, but also the influence of transient changes in gas storage of O_2 and, especially, CO_2. For example, the gas exchange ratio exceeds the respiratory quotient during hyperventilation as additional CO_2 is evolved from the body's stores, whereas the gas exchange ratio is less than the respiratory quotient during transient hypoventilation when CO_2 is retained in the body's stores. See also Respiratory Quotient.

Half time (t 1/2):   Unlike the time constant, which requires evidence that the process approximates an exponential function for its determination, the half time of a response is a simple description of the time to reach half of the change to the final value, regardless of the function. The half time

is generally representative of the speed by which a process approaches the steady-state.

Heart rate reserve (HRR):   The difference between the predicted highest heart rate attainable during maximum exercise and the actual highest heart rate. It is usually determined during exercise testing involving large muscle masses, such as during cycle or treadmill ergometry.

Ideal alveolar P_{O_2}:   A term that describes the alveolar P_{O_2} that would be obtained if the lung were an ideal gas exchanger, i.e., with ventilation uniformly matched to perfusion.

Impairment: A medical term reflecting an abnormality of or decrease in physiologic function that persists after treatment. For exercise, it could represent any defect in the ventilatory-circulatory-metabolic coupling of external to internal respiration.

Incremental exercise test: An exercise test designed to provide gradational stress to the subject. The work rate is usually increased over uniform periods of time, for example, every 4 minutes, every minute, every 15 seconds, or even continuously (e.g., ramp pattern increment).

Lactate: The anion of lactic acid.

Lactate threshold (*LT*):   The exercise $\dot{V}_{O_2}$ above which a net increase in lactate production results in a sustained increase in central blood lactate concentration.

Lactic acid: A three-carbon carboxylic acid ($CH_3CHOHCOOH$) that is an end-product of anaerobic metabolism of glucose or glycogen. Another major product is pyruvic acid ($CH_3CO COOH$), which can undergo conversion to acetyl coenzyme A and can thereby be further oxidized. The relative amounts of lactic acid and pyruvic acid are determined by the cytosolic redox state; a low redox state, reflected by a high ratio of $NADH+H^+/NAD^+$, favors the generation of lactate from pyruvate. The conversion of pyruvate into lactate maintains the supply of NAD^+ necessary for glycolysis to continue. The presence of lactic acid is a marker of anaerobic metabolism.

Lactic acidosis threshold (*LAT*):   The exercise $\dot{V}_{O_2}$ above which arterial standard HCO_3^- decreases because of a net increase in lactate production. This can be detected by an increase in CO_2 output (from dissociation of H_2CO_3 as HCO_3^- buffers lactic acid) above that which would be predicted from aerobic metabolism alone during a progressively increasing work rate exercise test.

Laminar flow: A condition in which the flow of a fluid (gas or liquid) through a conduit is characterized by the uniform direction of flow of any plane sheet of the fluid, each of which flows parallel to any other in the direction of flow. Under conditions of laminar flow, the pressure difference between an upstream point and a downstream point is directly proportional to flow. The proportionality constant is the resistance of the conduit.

Mass spectrometer: A device that separates and measures molecules of gas of a particular type, in a mixed gas stream, on the basis of their mass. Two types are commonly used. The fixed collector uses a magnetic means of separating the gases; these are then counted at different specific sensors. Alternatively, a quadrapole mass spectrometer utilizes shifts in an electromagnetic field to separate the gases such that only one gas arrives at the counter at a particular time.

Maximal oxygen uptake ($\dot{V}O_2$ max): The maximal oxygen uptake ($\dot{V}O_2$ max) is the highest possible oxygen uptake that a given subject can achieve for a given form of ergometry. It may be different than the peak oxygen uptake. Maximal oxygen uptake may be determined by repeated studies at higher and higher work rates to determine the highest possible value, or the $\dot{V}O_2$ max can be accepted when $\dot{V}O_2$ reaches a plateau during a single maximum work rate test. See peak oxygen uptake.

Maximum exercise heart rate: The highest obtainable heart rate during a maximum effort test.

Maximum exercise ventilation: The highest minute ventilation achieved during a maximum work rate test. This is usually determined by tests that tax large muscle masses, such as cycle or treadmill ergometry.

Maximum voluntary ventilation (MVV): The upper limit of the body's ability to ventilate the lungs. This is conventionally measured at rest from maximal volitional effort for short periods of time, e.g., 12 seconds, and expressed in units of liters per minute, BTPS.

Mets: Oxygen uptake required for a given task divided by resting oxygen uptake.

Minute ventilation ($\dot{V}I$ or $\dot{V}E$): The volume of air taken into or exhaled from the body in one minute. This is conventionally expressed at body temperature, saturated with water at atmospheric pressure (BTPS).

Mixed venous blood: A sample of blood representative of the flow-weighted venous blood returning from all the organs of the body. Usually, blood obtained from the pulmonary artery is considered to be mixed venous blood.

Mixed venous O_2 or CO_2: The average partial pressure, or gas content, of the blood returning from all the tissues of the body and, having been fully mixed in the right heart, is normally represented by the concentration or partial pressure of that gas in the pulmonary arterial blood.

Mixing chamber: A device that mixes the dead space and alveolar gas to produce a gas that is representative of the mixed expired gas. This is typically achieved by exhaling into a baffled chamber that mixes several breaths. The mixed expired concentration of a gas can be measured downstream from the chamber.

O_2 content (CO_2): The volume of O_2 (STPD) in a given volume (L, dl, or ml) of blood. This includes the major component that is bound to hemoglobin and that amount physically dissolved in the blood.

O_2 debt: The additional oxygen utilized in excess of the baseline needs of the body following a bout of exercise.

O_2 deficit: The oxygen equivalent of the total energy utilized to perform work that did not derive from reactions utilizing atmospheric oxygen taken into the body after the start of the exercise. For moderate intensity exercise, the O_2 deficit represents the energy equivalent of the depletion of the high-energy phosphate stores and oxygen stored in the body at the start of the work. For heavy or severe exercise, the oxygen deficit includes, in addition, the energy equivalent of anaerobic processes used to produce energy.

O_2 delivery: The amount of oxygen delivered to a tissue per unit time. It is, therefore, the product of the oxygen content of arterial blood and the blood flow to that tissue.

O_2 difference: The difference between the O_2 uptake predicted for a work rate during an incremental exercise test and the highest O_2 uptake attained.

O_2 flow: The amount of oxygen actually flowing per unit time, either from the heart or into a region of interest, such as a muscle or a muscle fiber. This, therefore, is a product of the oxygen content of the arterial blood and the total or regional blood flow.

O_2 pulse: The oxygen uptake divided by the heart rate. Hence, it represents the amount of oxygen extracted by the tissues of the body from the O_2 carried in each stroke volume.

Oximeter: A device that uses transmission techniques to estimate the saturation of hemoglobin with oxygen. Direct oximetry is done on blood samples. For indirect oximetry, a site for measurement, such as the earlobe or finger, is selected because blood comes close to the skin, traverses the capillary bed with little loss of oxygen, and hence, the mean capillary value will reflect arterial values. See pulse oximeter.

Oxygen consumption ($\dot{Q}_{O_2}$): The amount of oxygen utilized by the body's metabolic processes in a given time, expressed in milliliters or liters per minute, STPD.

Oxygen uptake ($\dot{V}_{O_2}$): The amount of oxygen extracted from the inspired gas in a given period of time, expressed in milliliters or liters per minute, STPD. This can differ from oxygen consumption under conditions in which oxygen is flowing into or being utilized from the body's stores. In the steady-state, oxygen uptake equals oxygen consumption.

Peak oxygen uptake (Peak $\dot{V}_{O_2}$): The highest oxygen uptake achieved during a maximum work rate test. The peak oxygen uptake may differ from the maximal oxygen uptake ($\dot{V}_{O_2}$ max) because the latter is sometimes determined by repeated studies at increasing work rates to obtain the $\dot{V}_{O_2}$ that cannot be exceeded by the subject. The $\dot{V}_{O_2}$ max is used to describe the $\dot{V}_{O_2}$ when it reaches a plateau value during a single maximum work rate test. See maximal oxygen uptake.

Phase I: The period of time following the onset of exercise that is required for the products of exercise metabolism to reach the lungs. Phase I is a result of the transit delay from the site of increased metabolism. Normally, this period is 15 to 20 seconds.

Phase II: The period of time following the onset of exercise when the mixed venous blood gas concentrations and blood flow continue to change in the exercising muscles. Phase II reflects the "kinetic phase" of gas exchange that begins at the end of Phase I and continues until a steady-state is obtained.

Phase III: The steady-state phase of gas exchange during moderate exercise or the period of exercise after 3 minutes for heavy exercise. For moderate exercise, it reflects the period in which the mixed venous gas concentrations and blood flow have become constant. This generally occurs by 3 minutes in healthy subjects. For heavy exercise, $\dot{V}_{O_2}$ is observed to increase slowly during this phase. This is likely related to lactate metabolism and

may result from changing work efficiency, the effect of the increasing acidemia on muscle blood flow and on rightward shift in the oxyhemoglobin dissociation curve.

Physiologic dead space: See dead space.

Pneumotachograph: A device used to measure gas flow. It is typically composed of a screen across which the pressure drop stemming from the flow of gas may be measured. This determines the instantaneous gas flow. Flow may be integrated over time to yield the volume of air respired.

Power: See work rate.

Pulse oximeter: A noninvasive device for estimating arterial blood oxygen saturation using a combination of spectrophotometry and pulse plethysmography. The pulse oximeter probe is designed to be placed on the earlobe or finger tip.

Pulse pressure: The difference between the systolic and the diastolic blood pressure.

Pump calibrator: A device that simulates the airflow and gas concentration waveforms encountered during respiration. Because the "metabolic rate" of such a device can be precisely calculated, it is useful for calibration of an exercise gas exchange measurement system.

R: See gas exchange ratio.

RQ (respiratory quotient): The ratio of the rate of carbon dioxide production to oxygen consumption. This ratio reflects the metabolic exchange of the gases in the body's tissues and is dictated by substrate utilization. See gas exchange ratio.

Ramp exercise test: See incremental exercise test. An exercise testing protocol in which the work rate is continuously increased at a constant rate, e.g., 10 W/min.

Response time: A means of characterizing the rate at which a device or system responds to a given signal. For example, in response to a sudden application of a constant level of input, how long does the output take to become constant? This can be characterized by the time constant, half time, or the time to reach 90% of the final value.

Set-point: This is a term used in control system theory that reflects the particular value of a regulated variable that the output of the system regulates. For example, a CO_2 set point is considered to be the operating level of arterial P_{CO_2}, which is maintained at its relatively constant (i.e., set-point) value by changes in ventilation at a given level of CO_2 output.

Steady-state: This is a characteristic of a physiologic system in which its functional demands are being met such that its output per unit time becomes constant. The time to achieve a steady-state commonly differs for different physiologic systems. For example, following the onset of constant load exercise, oxygen uptake rises to reach its steady-state appreciably faster than CO_2 output or ventilation. A constant value attained by the system is not sufficient, however, to determine that the system is in a steady-state. If the system reaches the limit of its output, and, as a result, its output becomes constant, as in the case of oxygen uptake reaching its maximum value, a steady-state does not prevail. The system in this instance is in a limited state, not a steady-state.

STPD: Used to express the conditions under which a gas volume is measured. Under STPD conditions, gas volume is at standard conditions of temperature and pressure and free of water vapor. The standard conditions are 0°C, 760 mmHg, and dry gas.

Stroke volume: The volume of blood ejected from either ventricle of the heart in a single beat.

Sustainable work rate: This is a relative term that reflects the extent to which a particular work rate may be sustained for sufficient time for the successful completion of a particular occupational, recreational, or laboratory-induced work rate. Therefore, at a sustainable work rate, the subject does not fatigue within the time constraints of the requirements of the test.

Thermodilution blood flow measurement: A technique in which a measured bolus of physiologic fluid of known temperature, usually at 0°C, is injected into a vascular stream, such as in the right atrium, and the temperature of the blood is measured at a mixed downstream point, such as in the pulmonary artery. The addition of the cold bolus of fluid decreases the blood temperature at the downstream point; the amount of cooling is a function of the blood flow. Thermodilution cardiac output measurements are usually performed using a thermistor-tipped pulmonary artery catheter (Swan-Ganz type).

Tidal volume to inspiratory capacity ratio (V_T/ IC): The ratio of the volume of air actually breathed during a breath (V_T) to the volume potentially available for that breath, the latter estimated from the end-expiratory lung volume to the maximum inspiratory volume at rest (IC). Hence, it reflects the proportion of the potential inspiratory volume excursion that is actually utilized for a particular breath.

Transducer: A device that transforms energy from one form to another. For example, a pressure transducer is a device that changes fluid pressure into an electrical signal that can be analyzed and used for display or recording.

Turbulent flow: A condition in which the fluid (gas or liquid) flow has characteristic eddies, whorls, and diverse directional currents, such that additional energy needs to be applied to create a given fluid flow. Under conditions of turbulent flow, the relationship between flow and pressure is nonlinear. See laminar flow.

V-slope method: A technique that allows detection of the onset of lactic acidosis during an incremental exercise test when one notes an accelerated rate of CO_2 output compared to oxygen uptake.

$\Delta\dot{V}O_2(6 - 3)$: The difference in oxygen uptake between the sixth and the third minute of a constant load exercise test. Normal subjects typically attain a steady-state for constant load exercise within 3 minutes during moderate exercise; hence, the $\Delta\dot{V}O_2(6 - 3)$ is zero. A positive value for this index reflects a degree of continuing non-steady-state for the work and usually signals fatiguing exercise.

$\dot{V}O_2$ max: See maximal oxygen uptake and peak oxygen uptake.

$\Delta\dot{V}O_2/\Delta$work rate (WR): The increase in oxygen uptake in response to a simultaneous increase in work rate. Under appropriate conditions (e.g., steady-state aerobic work), this may be used to estimate the efficiency for muscular work.

Wasted ventilation ($\dot{V}D$): The difference between the computed alveolar ventilation and the measured minute ventilation. Also known as the physiologic dead space ventilation, this term is meant to reflect the volume of the respired air that did not participate in alveolar capillary gas exchange, and it is equal to $V_D \times f$.

Work: A physical quantification of the force operating on a mass that causes it to change its location. Under conditions where force is applied and no movement results (e.g., during an isometric contraction), no work is performed, despite increased metabolic energy expenditure. The unit of work is the joule $= kg\ m^2/sec^2$.

Work rate or power: This reflects the rate at which work is performed, i.e., work per unit time. Work rate is usually measured in watts (kg m^2/ sec^3 or joule/sec) or alternatively in kilopond meters per minute (kpm/min); 1 W is equivalent to 6.12 kpm/min.

Calculations, Formulae, and Examples

This appendix presents the most essential formulae for calculating gas exchange and other related variables during exercise. An example accompanies the formula for each variable, using typical data acquired during exercise testing. Calculation of these variables uses well-defined and tested formulae, but several areas deserve particularly close attention. Thus, we address the specific problems of water vapor in the calculation of $\dot{V}O_2$, the problem of making corrections for the dead space of the breathing valve, and aspects of data collection for breath-by-breath gas exchange analysis.

FORMULAE AND EXAMPLE OF GAS EXCHANGE CALCULATION

The formula for calculating each variable takes into account the condition under which each measurement is made and certain conventions. For the example calculation, we assume that expired gas is collected for 2 minutes into a meteorologic balloon or a Douglas bag. Volume is measured in a large spirometer; fractional concentrations of O_2 and CO_2 are measured to within 0.04% using gas analyzers or a mass spectrometer. The gas concentrations are fractions of total gas volume excluding water vapor. An arterial blood sample is obtained during the collection of expired gas.

The measurements used for the example calculation are given in Table C.1.

Minute Ventilation ($\dot{V}E$)

The volume of gas exhaled divided by the time of collection in minutes determines minute ventilation ($\dot{V}E$). By convention, $\dot{V}E$ is reported at body temperature saturated with water vapor at ambient pressure (BTPS), as in formula 1. It may be necessary during calculation to obtain $\dot{V}E$ (STPD) using formula 2, or from the appropriate tables (see Appendix E).

TABLE C.1. Measurements Used for Example of Calculation of Gas Exchange

Measured volume: 54.2 L (ATPS)
Collection time: 2 min
Number of breaths: 41 in 2 min
Heart rate (HR) = 120/min
Body temperature = 37°C
F_{IO_2} = 0.2093 (20.93%)
F_{ICO_2} = 0.0004 (0.04%)
F_{EO_2} = 0.162 (16.2%)
F_{ECO_2} = 0.041 (4.1%)
(Fractions of dry gas volume)

Hemoglobin — 15 g/100 mL
Valve dead space = 64 ml
Ambient temperature (T) = 22°C
Barometric pressure (P_B) = 760 mmHg
Partial pressure of water, saturated at 22°C (P_{H_2O}) = 19 mmHg
Pa_{O_2} = 91 mmHg
Pa_{CO_2} = 36 mmHg
pH = 7.44
Sa_{O_2} = 95%
P_{ETCO_2} = 38 mmHg
$P\bar{v}_{O_2}$ = 27 mmHg
$S\bar{v}_{O_2}$ = 50%

A. Most commonly, ventilation is measured at ambient temperature and gas is fully saturated with water vapor at that temperature (ATPS). Formula 1 is used to convert volume from ATPS to BTPS. The temperature and water vapor correction factors can also be found in Appendix E.

$$\dot{V}_E(L/min, BTPS) = \dot{V}_E(L/min, ATPS) \times \frac{(273 + 37)}{273 + T}$$
$$\times \frac{P_B - P_{H_2O} \text{ (at T)}}{P_B - 47} \quad (1)$$

where T is ambient temperature (°C), body temperature is 37°C, P_{H_2O} at 37°C is 47 mm Hg, and P_B is barometric pressure.

B. From $\dot{V}_E$ (BTPS), $\dot{V}_E$ (STPD) can be obtained using formula 2. This converts $\dot{V}_E$ (BTPS) to STPD (273 °K, barometric pressure = 760 mm Hg, and no water vapor present) for $\dot{V}_{CO_2}$ and $\dot{V}_{O_2}$ calculations.

$\dot{V}_E$ (L/min, STPD)

$$= \dot{V}_E (L/min, BTPS) \times \frac{273}{(273 + 37)} \times \frac{(P_B - 47)}{760}$$

which becomes,

$$\dot{V}_E (L/min, STPD) = \dot{V}_E (L/min, BTPS) \times 0.826, \quad (2)$$

if P_B = 760 mm Hg.

Example:

$$\dot{V}_E (L/min, ATPS) = \frac{\text{Total Volume (ATPS)}}{\text{Total Collection Time}}$$

$$= \frac{54.2}{2 \text{ min}} = 27.1$$

then, from formula 1

$$\dot{V}_E (L/min, BTPS) = 27.1 \times \frac{310}{(273 + 22)} \times \frac{(760 - 19)}{(760 - 47)}$$

$$= 29.6$$

and, from formula 2,

$$\dot{V}_E (L/min, STPD) = 29.6 \times 0.826 = 24.3$$

Respiratory Frequency (f)

$$f (min^{-1}) = \frac{\text{number of complete breaths}}{\text{total time for complete breaths}} \quad (3)$$

Example:

$$f (min^{-1}) = \frac{41 \text{ breaths}}{2 \text{ min}} = 20.5$$

Tidal Volume (V_T)

$$V_T (L, BTPS) = \frac{\dot{V}_E (L/min, BTPS)}{f} \quad (4)$$

Example:

$$V_T (L, BTPS) = \frac{29.6}{20.5} = 1.44$$

CO$_2$ Output ($\dot{V}_{CO_2}$)

The CO$_2$ output and O$_2$ uptake are reported under STPD conditions. If $\dot{V}_E$ and $\dot{V}_I$ are measured at or converted to STPD conditions, F_{ECO_2} is the fraction of dry gas volume, and F_{ICO_2} is zero or negligible:

$$\dot{V}_{CO_2} (L/min, STPD) = \dot{V}_E (L/min, STPD) \times F_{ECO_2} \quad (5)$$

or, for P_B = 760 mm Hg,

$$\dot{V}_{CO_2} (L/min, STPD) = \dot{V}_E (L/min, BTPS)$$
$$\times 0.826 \times F_{ECO_2} \quad (6)$$

Example: Substituting $\dot{V}_E$ and F_{ECO_2} (Table C.1) into formula 5,

$$\dot{V}_{CO_2} (L/min, STPD) = 24.3 \times 0.041 = 0.997$$

O_2 Uptake ($\dot{V}O_2$)

For the derivation of the formula for $\dot{V}O_2$ and consideration of water vapor, see Appendix C, Special Considerations. Formula 7 should be used only after determining the dry expired gas fraction.

If $\dot{V}E$ is measured at or converted to STPD, F_{IO_2} is 0.2093 (dry room air), F_{ECO_2} and F_{EO_2} are fractions of CO_2 and O_2 in dry gas respectively, and $F_{ICO_2} = 0$, then:

$$\dot{V}O_2 \text{ (L/min, STPD)} = \dot{V}E \text{ (L/min, STPD)} \times (\Delta F_{O_2})\text{true, dry} \qquad (7)$$

where (ΔF_{O_2}) true, dry $= 0.265 - 1.265 \times F_{EO_2} - 0.265 \times F_{ECO_2}$ for a person breathing room air. The (ΔF_{O_2}) true, dry can also be obtained from the nomogram in Appendix E.

Example: Substituting from Table C.1 into formula 7:

(ΔF_{O_2})true, dry $= 0.265 - 0.205 - 0.0108 = 0.049$
$\dot{V}O_2$ (L/min, STPD) $= 24.3 \times 0.049 = 1.19$

Gas Exchange Ratio (R)

$$R = \frac{\dot{V}CO_2 \text{ (L/min, STPD)}}{\dot{V}O_2 \text{ (L/min, STPD)}} \qquad (8)$$

Example:

$$R = \frac{0.997}{1.19} = 0.84$$

Ventilatory Equivalents for CO_2 and O_2 ($\dot{V}E/\dot{V}CO_2$, $\dot{V}E/\dot{V}O_2$)

The ventilatory equivalents for CO_2 and O_2 are measurements of the ventilatory requirement for that metabolic rate. By convention they are expressed as $\dot{V}E$ (L/min, BTPS) divided by $\dot{V}CO_2$ or $\dot{V}O_2$ (L/min, STPD). Because the portion of the ventilation wasted in clearing the breathing valve deadspace is disregarded in determining the ventilatory requirement, the product of valve deadspace (V_{DM}) × respiratory frequency (f) is subtracted from the total $\dot{V}E$:

$$\dot{V}E/\dot{V}CO_2 = \frac{\dot{V}E \text{ (L/min, BTPS)} - [f \text{ min}^{-1} \times V_{DM}(L)]}{\dot{V}CO_2 \text{ (L/min, STPD)}} \qquad (9)$$

$$\dot{V}E/\dot{V}O_2 = \frac{\dot{V}E \text{ (L/min, BTPS)} - [f \text{ min}^{-1} \times V_{DM}(L)]}{\dot{V}O_2 \text{ (L/min, STPD)}} \qquad (10)$$

Example:

$$\dot{V}E/\dot{V}CO_2 = \frac{29.6 - [20.5 \times 0.064]}{0.997} = 28.4$$

$$\dot{V}E/\dot{V}O_2 = \frac{29.6 - [20.5 \times 0.064]}{1.19} = 23.8$$

Oxygen Pulse ($\dot{V}O_2$/HR)

$\dot{V}O_2$/HR (ml, STPD/beat)

$$= \frac{\dot{V}O_2 \text{ (L/min, STPD)} \times 1000 \text{ ml/L}}{HR \text{ (beats/min)}} \qquad (11)$$

Example:

$$\dot{V}O_2\text{/HR (ml, STPD/beat)} = \frac{1.19 \times 1000}{120} = 9.9$$

Alveolar PO_2 (P_{AO_2})

P_{AO_2} (mm Hg)

$$= F_{IO_2} \times (P_B - 47) - \frac{P_{ACO_2}}{R}(1 - F_{IO_2}(1 - R)) \qquad (12)$$

where P_B is barometric pressure in mm Hg, P_{ACO_2} is ideal alveolar P_{CO_2} in mm Hg, R is the gas exchange ratio, and F_{IO_2} is the fraction of inspired O_2, dry. Usually, the assumption that $P_{ACO_2} = P_{aCO_2}$ is used and the term $F_{IO_2} \times (1 - R)$ may be dropped because it is so small that it has an insignificant effect on the calculated P_{AO_2}, especially during air breathing. This simplifies the formula to:

$$P_{AO_2} \text{ (mm Hg)} = F_{IO_2} \times (P_B - 47) - \frac{P_{aCO_2}}{R} \qquad (13)$$

Whereas R is often assumed to be 0.8 at rest, R should always be calculated during exercise because it will range from 0.7 to 1.4 and have an appreciable effect on alveolar PO_2 calculation.

Example: Substituting into formula 13,

$$P_{AO_2} \text{ (mm Hg)} = (0.2093 \times 713) - \frac{36}{0.84} = 106$$

Alveolar-Arterial PO_2 Difference ($P[A - a]O_2$)

$$P(A - a)O_2 \text{ (mm Hg)} = P_{AO_2} - P_{aO_2} \qquad (14)$$

where P_{AO_2} is determined as above and P_{aO_2} is arterial PO_2.

Example:

$$P(A - a)O_2 \text{ (mm Hg)} = 106 - 91 = 15$$

Arterial End-Tidal P_{CO_2} Difference ($P[a - ET]CO_2$)

$$P(a - ET)CO_2 = Pa_{CO_2} - P_{ETCO_2} \qquad (15)$$

where Pa_{CO_2} is arterial P_{CO_2} and P_{ETCO_2} is end-tidal P_{CO_2}.

Example:

$$P(a - ET)CO_2 = 36 - 38 = -2 \text{ mm Hg}$$

Physiologic Dead Space (V_D)

$$V_D \text{ (L)} = V_T \text{ (L)} \times \frac{(Pa_{CO_2} - P\bar{E}_{CO_2})}{Pa_{CO_2}} - V_{Dm} \text{ (L)} \quad (16)$$

where V_T is tidal volume, Pa_{CO_2} is arterial P_{CO_2}, $P\bar{E}_{CO_2}$ is mixed expired P_{CO_2}, and V_{Dm} is breathing valve dead space. Mixed expired P_{CO_2} can be calculated from:

$$P\bar{E}_{CO_2} = \frac{\dot{V}_{CO_2} \text{ (L/min, STPD)}}{\dot{V}_E \text{ (L/min, STPD)}} \times (P_B - 47 \text{ mmHg})$$

Example:

$$P\bar{E}_{CO_2} = \frac{0.997}{24.3} \times 713 = 29$$

$$V_D \text{ (L)} = 1.44 \times \frac{36 - 29}{36} - 0.064 = 0.22$$

Physiologic Dead Space/Tidal Volume Ratio (V_D/V_T)

$$\frac{V_D}{V_T} = \frac{(Pa_{CO_2} - P\bar{E}_{CO_2})}{Pa_{CO_2}} - \frac{V_{Dm} \text{ (L)}}{(V_T \text{ (L)} - V_{Dm} \text{ (L)})} \quad (17)$$

Example:

$$\frac{V_D}{V_T} = \frac{36 - 29}{36} - \frac{0.064}{1.44} = 0.15$$

The V_D/V_T must be calculated using the arterial P_{CO_2}. There has been an unfortunate trend of calculating V_D/V_T "noninvasively" during exercise by substituting P_{ETCO_2} for Pa_{CO_2} in the foregoing formulas, or by calculating Pa_{CO_2} from P_{ETCO_2} using a regression formula derived from normal subjects. As shown in Chapter 3, P_{ETCO_2} and Pa_{CO_2} are nearly equal only in normal subjects at rest. During exercise, the $P(a - ET)CO_2$ becomes negative and larger in magnitude in normal subjects, whereas it becomes larger and more positive in patients with lung disease who have increased V_D/V_T. Therefore, the relationship between Pa_{CO_2} and P_{ETCO_2} during exercise is unpredictable (1). Furthermore, small errors in Pa_{CO_2} may result in clinically important differences in the calculated V_D/V_T.

Cardiac Output

The cardiac output ($\dot{Q}$) can be determined by thermal indicator dilution or by the Fick method using $\dot{V}_{O_2}$ and arterial-mixed venous O_2 content difference:

$$\dot{Q}\text{(L/min)} = \frac{\dot{V}_{O_2} \text{ (ml/min, STPD)}}{(Ca_{O_2} - C\bar{v}_{O_2}) \text{ ml } O_2/\text{L blood}} \quad (18)$$

where Ca_{O_2} is O_2 content in arterial and $C\bar{v}_{O_2}$ is O_2 content in mixed venous blood. These can be calculated from:

$$\begin{aligned} C_{O_2} &\text{ (ml } O_2/100 \text{ ml)} \\ &= (S_{O_2} \times 0.01 \times 1.34 \text{ ml } O_2/\text{g Hb} \times [\text{Hb}]) \\ &\quad + (0.003 \text{ ml } O_2/\text{mm Hg}/100 \text{ ml} \times P_{O_2}) \quad (19) \end{aligned}$$

where [Hb] is hemoglobin concentration in g/100 ml blood and S_{O_2} is the oxyhemoglobin saturation in per cent. Note that this calculation gives O_2 content in ml O_2/100 of blood and is converted to ml O_2/L blood by multiplying by 10.

Example:

$$\begin{aligned} Ca_{O_2}&\text{(ml } O_2/100 \text{ ml)} \\ &= (95\% \times 0.01 \times 1.34 \times 15) + (0.003 \times 91) = 19.4 \\ C\bar{v}_{O_2}&\text{(ml } O_2/100 \text{ ml)} \\ &= (50\% \times 0.01 \times 1.34 \times 15) + (0.003 \times 27) = 10.1 \\ (Ca_{O_2} &- C\bar{v}_{O_2}) \\ &= 19.4 - 10.1 = 9.3 \text{ ml } O_2/100 \text{ ml} = 93 \text{ ml } O_2/\text{L} \end{aligned}$$

$$\dot{Q}\text{(L/min)} = \frac{1190 \text{ (ml/min, STPD)}}{93 \text{ ml } O_2/\text{L blood}} = 12.8$$

The foregoing method of cardiac output measurement requires a sample of mixed venous blood. A noninvasive determination of cardiac output can be made, however, using an analogous formula for CO_2 and an estimate of mixed venous CO_2 content (indirect Fick). The mixed venous P_{CO_2} can be approximated by several techniques, for example, single-exhalation (2) and rebreathing (3). With the rebreathing method, a mixture of CO_2 and high inspired O_2 is rebreathed, and the P_{CO_2} of the rebreathed gas rapidly approaches that of mixed venous blood. The mixed venous content of CO_2 ($C\bar{v}_{CO_2}$) can then be estimated using hemoglobin concentration and the CO_2 dissociation curve adjusted for estimated oxygen saturation (4). The arterial P_{CO_2} is used to determine arterial CO_2 content (Ca_{CO_2}) and, using $\dot{V}_{CO_2}$, cardiac output is:

$$\dot{Q}(L/min) = \frac{\dot{V}_{CC_2}\ (ml/min,\ STPD)}{(C\bar{v}_{CO_2} - Ca_{CO_2})\ ml\ CO_2/L\ blood} \quad (20)$$

The arterial P_{CO_2} must be used in this calculation rather than the end-tidal P_{CO_2}. This is because the CO_2 content versus P_{CO_2} curve (CO_2 dissociation curve) is steep, and a small error in P_{CO_2} results in a large error in CO_2 content. In addition, the P_{ETCO_2} is higher than Pa_{CO_2} in normal subjects but usually lower than Pa_{CO_2} in patients with a substantial alveolar dead space during exercise. The accuracy of the cardiac output also depends on an extremely accurate blood gas analysis for both arterial and mixed venous P_{CO_2} values. In addition, the oxygen content of the blood greatly affects the relationship between P_{CO_2} and CO_2 content (Haldane effect), and the mixed venous oxygen is not known using these estimates. Additionally, above the AT, the CO_2 dissociation curve is displaced downward. This results in a reduced mixed venous CO_2 content for a given $P\bar{v}_{CO_2}$. Because of these reasons, cardiac output measurements by this indirect, noninvasive method should be considered approximate.

CALCULATIONS AT MAXIMUM EXERCISE
Breathing Reserve (BR)

BR (L/min) = MVV (L/min)
$$\qquad - \dot{V}_E\ (L/min)\ at\ maximum\ exercise \quad (21)$$

BR (%)
$$= \frac{MVV\ (L\ min) - \dot{V}_E\ (L/min)\ at\ maximum\ exercise}{MVV\ (L/min)}$$
$$\times 100 \quad (22)$$

where MVV is maximum voluntary ventilation at rest.

Example: If MVV is 82 L/min and $\dot{V}_E$ at maximum exercise is 65 L/min, then:

$$BR\ (L/min) = 82 - 65 = 17\ L/min$$

$$BR\ (\%) = \frac{82 - 65}{82} \times 100 = 21\%$$

Heart Rate Reserve (HRR)

HRR (beats/min) = Predicted maximum HR
$$\qquad - HR\ at\ maximum\ exercise \quad (23)$$

HRR (%)
$$= \frac{Predicted\ maximum\ HR - HR\ at\ maximum\ exercise}{Predicted\ maximum\ HR}$$
$$\times 100 \quad (24)$$

where predicted maximum HR (adults) = 220 − age (years). Example: For a 60-year-old man, predicted maximum HR = 220 − 60 = 160 beats/min. If HR at maximum exercise is 145 beats/min, then:

$$HRR\ (beats/min) = 160 - 145 = 15$$

$$HRR\ (\%) = \frac{160 - 145}{160} \times 100 = 9\%$$

SPECIAL CONSIDERATIONS FOR CALCULATION OF GAS EXCHANGE VARIABLES
Water Vapor and Oxygen Uptake ($\dot{V}_{O_2}$)

Oxygen uptake ($\dot{V}_{O_2}$) is determined by collection and analysis of expired gas. The usual calculation method determines $\dot{V}_{O_2}$ from expired ventilation, expired CO_2 fraction, and expired O_2 fraction, and is based on the assumption that the inspired and expired volume of nitrogen (and other inert gases) does not differ during the collection period. During rest and exercise, this method has been found to be satisfactory (5, 6). Nevertheless, errors may be introduced if careful attention to methods and calculations is not taken. This is especially true of how water vapor is handled because this variable can greatly affect the result.

If the Scholander or Haldane method of gas analysis or a mass spectrometer is used, or water vapor is removed by drying the gas prior to measurement, then measured gas concentration is relative to total gas minus the volume of water vapor. Thus, the dilution of the concentration of each gas caused by water vapor can be ignored and calculations are relatively simple:

$$\dot{V}_{O_2} \text{ (L/min, STPD)} = (F_{IO_2} \times \dot{V}_I \text{ [L/min, STPD])}$$
$$- (F_{EO_2} \times \dot{V}_E \text{ [L/min, STPD])}$$

where F_{IO_2} and F_{EO_2} are the O_2 fractions of dry gas volumes. If, over the period of collection, the volumes of inspired and expired nitrogen (and other inert gases) are equal during breathing, then:

$$\dot{V}_I \times F_{IN_2} = \dot{V}_E \times F_{EN_2},$$

and

$$\dot{V}_I = (F_{EN_2}/F_{IN_2}) \times \dot{V}_E$$

where F_{IN_2} and F_{EN_2} are the fractional concentrations of nitrogen and other inert gases.

Because $(F_{IN_2} + F_{IO_2} + F_{ICO_2}) = 1$ and $(F_{EN_2} + F_{EO_2} + F_{ECO_2}) = 1$, then:

$$\dot{V}_I = \frac{(1 - F_{EO_2} - F_{ECO_2})}{(1 - F_{IO_2} - F_{ICO_2})} \times \dot{V}_E$$

and

$$\dot{V}_{O_2} \text{ (L/min, STPD)} = \left[\frac{F_{IO_2} \times (1 - F_{EO_2} - F_{ECO_2})}{(1 - F_{IO_2} - F_{ICO_2})} - F_{EO_2} \right]$$
$$\times \dot{V}_E \text{ (L/min, STPD)}$$

The quantity in brackets is called the true O_2 difference, (ΔF_{O_2}) true.

If we assume that $F_{ICO_2} = 0$, or is negligible, then:

$$(\Delta F_{O_2}) \text{ true} = \frac{(F_{IO_2} - F_{EO_2} - F_{IO_2} \times F_{ECO_2})}{(1 - F_{IO_2})}$$

and

$$\dot{V}_{O_2} \text{ (L/min, STPD)} = \dot{V}_E \text{ (L/min, STPD)} \times (\Delta F_{O_2}) \text{ true}$$

For room air inspired gas, F_{IO_2} (dry) = 0.2093, and:

$$\dot{V}_{O_2} \text{ (L/min, STPD)} = \dot{V}_E \text{ (L/min, STPD)}$$
$$\times (0.265 - 1.265 \times F_{EO_2} - 0.265 \times F_{ECO_2}) \quad (25)$$

If water vapor is not removed from the gas and the method of gas analysis measures gas fraction of the total gas volume including water vapor, as is the case for most discrete O_2 analyzers, then the water vapor will reduce each dry gas fraction by the factor:

$$\frac{(P_B - P_{H_2O})}{P_B} \text{ or } (1 - F_{H_2O})$$

In this case, the determination of $\dot{V}_{O_2}$ is affected by water vapor as follows. First, $\dot{V}_{O_2}$ can be expressed using $\dot{V}_I$ and $\dot{V}_E$ measured under the conditions of measurement, i.e., at temperature T and containing some water vapor:

$$\dot{V}_{O_2} \text{ (L/min, STPD)} = \frac{273}{273 + T} \times \frac{P_B}{760}$$
$$\times (\dot{V}_I \times F_{IO_2} - \dot{V}_E \times F_{EO_2}) \quad (26)$$

where $\dot{V}_I$ and $\dot{V}_E$ are L/min at temperature T, and F_{IO_2} and F_{EO_2} are fractions of $\dot{V}_I$ and $\dot{V}_E$ respectively, including the volume of water vapor.

Because $\dot{V}_I = (F_{EN_2}/F_{IN_2}) \times \dot{V}_E$, and $(F_{EN_2} + F_{EO_2} + F_{ECO_2} + F_{EH_2O}) = 1$ and $(F_{IN_2} + F_{IO_2} + F_{ICO_2} + F_{IH_2O}) = 1$, then substituting into equation 26 gives:

$$\dot{V}_{O_2} \text{ (L/min, STPD)} = \dot{V}_E \text{ (L/min at T)}$$
$$\times k(T, P_{H_2O}) \times (\Delta F_{O_2}) \text{ true} \quad (27)$$

where

$$k(T, P_{H_2O}) = \frac{273}{273 + T} \times \frac{P_B}{760}$$

and

$$(\Delta F_{O_2}) \text{true}$$
$$= \frac{F_{IO_2} \times (1 - F_{ECO_2} - F_{EH_2O}) - F_{EO_2} \times (1 - F_{IH_2O})}{(1 - F_{IO_2} - F_{IH_2O})}$$

The calculation of $\dot{V}_{O_2}$ is simpler if the expired gas is dried prior to analysis for O_2 and CO_2. Beaver (8) provides a nomogram for calculation of oxygen uptake in the presence of water vapor, however, that can be used to determine $\dot{V}_{O_2}$ and R from a sample of mixed expired gas assumed to be fully saturated with water vapor at a known temperature (see Appendix E). The subject is assumed to be breathing room air and the O_2 and CO_2 analyzers display the fractions of total expired gas including water vapor. Substantial errors would result if water vapor were not taken into account. Again, the correction is not needed when gas fractions are measured as fractions of dry gas.

Breath-by-breath measurement systems must deal with the effect of water vapor on calculation of $\dot{V}_{O_2}$. Rapidly responding gas analyzers or a respiratory mass spectrometer are used. A mass spectrometer may be adjusted to "ignore" water vapor if the sum of ion voltages is made up of only those measuring N_2, O_2, CO_2, and argon, with water vapor ignored in both inspired and expired gases. If this method is used, then the volume to be multiplied by true O_2 fraction should be adjusted to the dry volume.

Rapidly responding O_2 analyzers and infrared CO_2 analyzers used without drying the analyzed gas read fractions of total gas volume and therefore read lower concentrations than if the same gas were measured after being dried. As shown in equation 27, the values can be used in a breath-by-breath system if F_{EH_2O} and F_{IH_2O} are known (8). The assumption that expired gas is fully saturated at some known temperature is the starting point for several approaches to dealing with this in breath-by-breath systems.

First, the expired gas sample can be kept warm to prevent condensation. If gas is fully saturated at a known temperature, F_{EH_2O} can be estimated. A heated sampling tube is necessary and the temperature must be accurately known. For example, assuming a value of 37°C when actual expired gas temperature is 32°C can result in a 7 to 8% error in $\dot{V}O_2$. During exercise, expired gas rapidly cools in the mouthpiece and breathing valve to as low as 32°C. Because gas for analysis is most often sampled at this location in breath-by-breath systems, then even if the gas is rewarmed, there will have been some unknown loss of water vapor to condensation.

A second approach is to allow the sampled gas to cool to a known temperature. This avoids the problem of indeterminate loss of water vapor from cooling followed by rewarming. Auchincloss et al. (9) described a water bath that cooled expired gas to 15°C prior to rewarming and analysis. If a small-diameter sampling tube and low flow rate can be used, then gas may be allowed to cool to ambient temperature. This latter method is convenient and simple, but care should be taken that water droplets do not alter resistance and flow characteristics of the sampler and do not affect the linearity and response of the analyzer.

Deno and Kamon described a dryer for use in on-line breath-by-breath systems (10). Removing water vapor by passing gas through a tube containing calcium sulfate is generally unsuitable for breath-by-breath methods because it introduces unacceptable delay times, may distort the gas concentration profile, and cannot meet the challenge of large gas sample flows. Deno and Kamon used a copper condenser tube and separator immersed in an ice bath at 1°C. Even at flow rates of saturated 38° air up to 1 L/min, P_{H_2O} was constantly 5 mmHg.

Response times were comparable with those reported for breath-by-breath systems, albeit at moderately high sample flow rates (1 L/min).

Another approach used by many modern exercise systems employs special conducting tubing that allows water vapor to pass out of the gas being conveyed to the gas analyzer until water vapor equilibrium is reached with the atmosphere. Thus, water vapor partial pressure in the gas analyzers is equal to the ambient P_{H_2O} rather than saturated at some imprecisely known emperature. This method avoids the need to know the precise temperature and temperature changes of the respired gas and does not adversely affect the response time.

Oxygen Uptake ($\dot{V}O_2$) and Oxygen Breathing

The foregoing calculation of $\dot{V}O_2$ is intended for measurement during room air breathing. The use of the same equations during breathing of oxygen-enriched inspired gas mixtures has several potential problems. The relationship of $\dot{V}I$ to $\dot{V}E$ is subject to large differences for small measurement errors when F_{IO_2} and F_{EO_2} are high and F_{IN_2} and F_{EN_2} are low. In addition, the assumption that $\dot{V}I \times F_{IN_2} = \dot{V}E \times F_{EN_2}$ is not valid for a transient wash-out period during which hyperoxic gas is inspired and more nitrogen is removed during expiration than is added during inspiration. Lastly, if the subject is breathing 100% oxygen, the equations given previously cannot be used at all because there is no inspired or expired nitrogen.

Although calculation of $\dot{V}O_2$ during enriched oxygen breathing is theoretically possible, the accuracy of $\dot{V}O_2$ using conventional equations and measurements is almost certainly less than when the subject is breathing room air. $\dot{V}O_2$ calculated with $F_{IO_2} > 0.21$ should be interpreted with caution.

An alternative approach to testing subjects during oxygen breathing is to ignore or not make measurements of $\dot{V}O_2$. Often, a reason for exercise testing is to determine the need for supplemental oxygen in a particular patient. This question can usually be answered by comparison of maximum work rate, heart rate, respiratory frequency, minute ventilation, $\dot{V}E/\dot{V}CO_2$, and exercise endurance between a maximum exercise test on room air with a similar test during oxygen breathing. An objective improvement in exercise capacity and decreased $\dot{V}E$ and $\dot{V}E/\dot{V}CO_2$ are encouraging signs of a beneficial effect of supplemental O_2.

Valve Dead Space and Physiologic Dead Space

The physiologic dead space consists of the anatomic dead space and the alveolar dead space. During measurement, the volume of the breathing valve and mouthpiece apparatus is considered to be in series with the anatomic dead space. This apparatus dead space is usually subtracted from the V_D calculated by the Engoff modification of the Bohr equation:

$$V_D = V_T\,(L) \times \frac{Pa_{CO_2} - P\bar{E}_{CO_2}}{Pa_{CO_2}} - V_{Dm}\,(L)$$

where V_D is subject dead space, V_T is tidal volume, and V_{Dm} is the volume of the apparatus (or valve dead space).

Bradley and Younes (11), Suwa and Bendixen (12), and Singleton et al. (13) reported that the effective dead space of the valve (the correction term [V_{Dm}]) may be different from the measured mechanical dead space. The reader is referred to their thorough analyses of the proper correction value under various conditions.

In practice, most reports of V_D during exercise have corrected for apparatus dead space by subtracting the entire mechanical dead space. Any potential error can be minimized if the valve dead space is small and the subject's tidal volume is relatively large compared to V_{Dm}. Valves with large dead spaces may be necessary, however, because they usually offer smaller breathing resistances at high inspiratory and expiratory flows. These high flows would be encountered when studying healthy normal subjects with large tidal volumes during exercise. On the other hand, patients with small tidal volumes will usually not generate high flows during exercise and the small dead space valves are recommended.

Calculations for Breath-by-Breath Analysis

Breath-by-breath methods use the same formulae as for mixed expired gas collections. Conceptually, the expired volume is divided into small sequential samples. The volume of each is determined and, when multiplied by the gas concentrations appropriate for that sample adjusted for the time difference between the flow and gas concentration signals, gives the volume of CO_2 eliminated or O_2 taken up for that sample. The results are summed mathematically and then reported either per breath or per unit time. Thus, the term "breath-by-breath" applies to the method of expired gas analysis and data reduction and does not necessarily mean that each breath is individually reported.

If V_E is the sum of all volume exhaled between time 0 and time T then:

$$V_E = \sum_{t=0}^{T} Vexp(t + \Delta t)$$

where $Vexp(t + \Delta t)$ is the volume expired between time t and $t + \Delta t$, Δt is a time interval, and T is the total time of expiration for single or multiple breaths.

This is satisfactory if volume is directly measured over small time intervals. If expired flow rather than volume is measured, then:

$$V_E = \int_0^T \dot{V}exp(t)dt$$

where $\dot{V}exp(t)$ is the expired flow over the infinitesimally small time interval dt at time t. The volume exhaled over that time is the product $\dot{V}exp(t) \times dt$. In practice, a small constant Δt is substituted for dt and the mean flow during the time interval ($t + \Delta t$) is used as $\dot{V}exp(t)$:

$$V_E = \sum_{t=0}^{T} \dot{V}exp(t + \Delta t) \times \Delta t$$

where $\dot{V}exp(t + \Delta t)$ is the mean flow rate during the time interval $t + \Delta t$. The minute ventilation ($\dot{V}_E$) is the volume per unit time.

In a breath-by-breath system, the $\dot{V}_{CO_2}$ is calculated by multiplying the nearly instantaneous F_{ECO_2} for each small time interval by the simultaneous expired volume during that interval. These products are then integrated:

$$V_{CO_2} = \int_{t=0}^{T} \dot{V}exp(t)dt \times F_{ECO_2}(t)$$

where $\dot{V}exp(t)dt$ is the instantaneous expired volume and $F_{ECO_2}(t)$ is the instantaneous expired CO_2 concentration at time t, adjusted for the delay between when the gas is sampled and when the analyzer reads the appropriate concentration. In practice, the small time interval Δt is substituted for dt:

$$V_{CO_2} = \sum_{t=0}^{T} \dot{V}exp(t + \Delta t) \times \Delta t \times F_{ECO_2}(t)$$

where $\dot{V}exp(t + \Delta t)$ is the mean flow for the time period t to $t + \Delta t$, $F_{ECO_2}(t)$ is the mean expired CO_2 during this time period, and Δt is a small time interval. For the volume of O_2 taken up, the true O_2 difference [(ΔF_{O_2}) true] is substituted for $F_{E_{CO_2}}$ in this equation. The $\dot{V}_{CO_2}$ and $\dot{V}_{O_2}$ are equal to the volume of CO_2 or O_2 divided by the time during exhalation, whether expressed per breath or per minute or other time unit.

An analog integrator or analog-to-digital converter and digital computer can perform the necessary multiplication and summation. The respired gas is not, strictly speaking, measured and analyzed continuously, but instead data are rapidly sampled, e.g., every 20 milliseconds. The resultant expired flow versus time curve is, therefore, made up of sequential points sampled at intervals Δt or at a frequency $f = 1/\Delta t$. The rate of sampling is important because rapid and large changes in expired flow (or gas concentration) may occur during exercise and could be missed if the data are sampled at too slow a rate. Bernard (14), using generalized simulated curves of expired flow and expired CO_2, found that a sample rate of 30 Hz was adequate during exercise, and that rates of 40, 50, and 100 Hz achieved little improvement in fidelity. Beaver et al. (15), in their analysis, suggested that a sampling frequency equal to twice the highest frequency occurring in the signal to be measured should be used. They suggested that for human exercise testing a frequency of 50 Hz is satisfactory to record flow and mass spectrometer signals.

A minor consideration is the method of summation or numeric integration. Bernard (14) suggested that the trapezoidal rule was adequate for integration of respiratory signals. This assumes, as previously, that the mean expired flow and gas concentrations during the time period between t and $t + \Delta t$ is equal to the average of the values measured at the beginning and end of the time period.

A serious potential problem deals with time alignment of the appropriate expired flow (or volume) and expired gas concentration because of the appreciable time required for gas transport and measurement by most gas analyzers. For breath-by-breath analysis, it is essential that the appropriate instantaneous flow rate be multiplied by the proper time-matched expired gas concentration. Flow rates can be determined accurately and nearly instantaneously; flow at the mouth will reach the transducer with a delay determined by the speed of sound (approximately 100 ft/s) and the distance to the transducer. However, gas analyzer measurements cannot with current technology be made without some delay and distortion inherent to the transport of gas to the analyzer and the intrinsic characteristics

of the analyzer. The accuracy of a breath-by-breath system is dependent on the ability of the system to match flow rate and appropriate gas concentration prior to integration. Thus, each flow sampled must be stored until the appropriate expired gas concentration value has been determined. This matching process is usually performed as part of the computer program for on-line exercise systems.

Bernard (14) used simulated curves of expired CO_2 and expired flow to estimate potential error caused by the time delay between measurements of these two variables. Using perfectly time-matched hypothetic curves as standard, less than a 5% difference in calculated $\dot{V}_{CO_2}$ was found if the time misalignment was less than or equal to 25 milliseconds. Of importance is that the theoretic sampling rate was 100 Hz, the signals were given random noise, and the product of flow and CO_2 was integrated using the trapezoid rule.

Two factors contribute to the time alignment problem. Most systems use a capillary tube with a pump to draw a continuous expired gas sample into the analyzer. The gas transport time is dependent on the dimensions of the tube and the pump flow rate; transport time is typically on the order of 200 to 400 milliseconds. Second, the gas analyzer output itself has an intrinsic response time that further adds to the delay. For infrared CO_2 analyzers, electrochemical O_2 analyzers, and respiratory mass spectrometers, the time constants for response are in the range of 50 to 100 milliseconds. The net result is that an instantaneous change in gas concentration at the sampling end of the tubing can be accurately measured, but only after introducing corrections to account for these delays. The mixing and diffusion of gas within the sampling tubing may further distort the result. These must also be accounted for in these corrections.

In most solutions to this problem, an instantaneous or step change in gas concentration is introduced at the sampling inlet and the time course of the gas analyzer output is observed. Attempts are then made to determine optimal methods of compensating for the gas transport delay and gas analyzer response characteristics.

Although the gas analyzer response time component is certainly important, matching of flow and gas concentration signals for gas transport delay, i.e., the time simply to reach the analyzer, alone considerably improves results. Using this method, Bates et al. (16) found a 10-fold reduction in error from the uncorrected value and suggested that this simple adjustment might be sufficient.

To account for the gas analyzer response time, an additional correction function is usually used. This function is derived from analysis of the total response of the gas analyzer system. Beaver et al. (15) indicated that the most significant wave shape distortion is removed by a total delay correction equal to transport delay plus one time constant and analyzed the magnitude of potential errors. Investigators have used various functions to describe the response characteristics of their gas analyzers or mass spectrometers (16–19). We (20) found that an equal area method for analyzer delay time adds a one time constant delay if the analyzer response curve is exponential and an empirically determined longer delay time if the curve is sigmoid. Factors that affect selection of an optimal method included the level of noise in the measured signal, the sampling rate, and the type of calculation desired.

The importance of matching flow rate and appropriate gas concentration cannot be overly stressed for a breath-by-breath system. Although not all investigators agree on the optimal way of dealing with gas analyzer response time, a satisfactory balance among degree of accuracy, speed, and reproducibility can be reached.

References

1. Lewis D, Sietsema KE, Casaburi R, Sue DY. Inaccuracy of noninvasive estimates of V_D/V_T in clinical exercise testing. Chest 1994;106:1476–1480.
2. Kim TS, Rahn H, Farhi LE. Estimation of the true venous and arterial P_{CO_2} by gas analysis of a single-breath. J Appl Physiol 1996;21:1338–1344.
3. Jones NL, Campbell EJM, McHardy GJR, et al. The estimation of carbon dioxide pressure of mixed venous blood during exercise. Clin Sci 1967;32:311–327.
4. McHardy GJR. The relationship between the differences in pressure and content of carbon dioxide in arterial and venous blood. Clin Sci 1967;32:299–309.
5. Wagner JA, Horvath SM, Dahms TE, Reed S. Validation of open-circuit for the determination of oxygen consumption. J Appl Physiol 1973;34:859–863.
6. Wilmore JH, Costill DL. Adequacy of the Haldane transformation in the computation of exercise V_{O_2} in man. J Appl Physiol 1973;35:85–89.
7. Beaver WL, Wasserman K, Whipp BJ. On-line computer analysis and breath-by-breath graphical display of exercise function tests. J Appl Physiol 1973;34:128–132.
8. Beaver WL. Water vapor corrections in oxygen consumption calculations. J Appl Physiol 1973;35:928–931.
9. Auchincloss JH, Gilbert R, Baule GH. Control of water vapor during rapid analysis of respiratory gases in expired air. J Appl Physiol 1970;28:245–247.
10. Deno NS, Kamon E. A dryer for rapid response on-line expired gas measurements. J Appl Physiol 1979;46:1196–1199.
11. Bradley PW, Younes M. Relation between respiratory valve dead space and tidal volume. J Appl Physiol 1980;49:528–532.
12. Suwa K, Bendixen HH. Change in P_{aCO_2} with mechanical dead space during artificial ventilation. J Appl Physiol 1968;24:556–563.
13. Singleton GJ, Olsen CR, Smith RL. Correction for mechanical dead space in the calculation of physiological dead space. J Clin Invest 1972;51:2768–2772.
14. Bernard TE. Aspects of on-line digital integration of pulmonary gas transfer. J Appl Physiol 1977;43:375–378.
15. Beaver WL, Lamarra N, Wasserman K. Breath-by-breath measurement of true alveolar gas exchange. J Appl Physiol 1981;51:1662–1675.
16. Bates JHT, Priak GK, Tanner TE, McKinnon AE. Correcting for the dynamic response of a respiratory mass spectrometer. J Appl Physiol 1983;55:1015–1022.
17. Noguchi H, Ogushi Y, Yoshiya I, Itakura N, Yambayashi H. Breath-by-breath V_{CO_2} and V_{O_2} require compensation for transport delay and dynamic response. J Appl Physiol 1982;52:79–84.
18. Mitchell RR. Incorporating the gas analyzer response time in gas exchange computations. J Appl Physiol 1979;47:1118–1122.
19. Arieli R, Van Liew HD. Corrections for the response time and delay of mass spectrometers. J Appl Physiol 1981;51:1417–1422.
20. Sue DY, Hansen JE, Blais M, Wasserman K. Measurement and analysis of gas exchange during exercise using a programmable calculator. J Appl Physiol 1980;49:456–461.

Placement of a Brachial Artery Catheter

EQUIPMENT

1. Appropriate catheter.
2. Cournand-type needle with sharp, hollow stylus.
3. A 2-ml syringe with a 26-gauge needle for local anesthesia.
4. Sterile saline suitable for intravascular injection.
5. Heparinized saline, 50 ml, for catheter flushing.

SELECTION OF CATHETER

Because we most often insert the catheter into a brachial artery, we use a polyethylene catheter that is 25 cm long and has a diameter of 1.37 mm. The tip is tapered to fit a guidewire (50 cm × 0.63 mm) that fits through a 19-gauge thin-walled Cournand-style needle. The catheter is long enough so the end used for collection can be brought around the back of the arm and sampling can be done without the subject's altering the position of his or her arm or being aware of when blood is sampled. For radial artery catherization, any number of small, short polyethylene catheters designed for insertion into the radial artery can be used.

ARTERY SELECTION

The brachial or radial artery is generally used. Complications such as thrombosis are exceedingly rare when appropriate precautions are taken. We find the brachial artery to be preferable, however, because it is larger and the catheter has less effect on compromising its lumen. Moreover, the patient's arm need not be secured to a board, and sliding of the catheter in and out of the artery when the patient moves is not a problem. The radial pulse should be palpated to check for continued patency. If the radial artery is used for the arterial catheterization, do an Allen test to verify that there is blood flow through the ulnar artery to the hand.

POSITIONING THE ARM FOR BRACHIAL ARTERY CATHERIZATION

Positioning the arm is extremely important:

1. Extend the arm; place a rolled towel or cushion under the elbow for maximum extension.
2. Pronate the hand.
3. Palpate the brachial artery on the medial side of the antecubital fossa.

LOCAL ANESTHESIA

If the patient is not allergic to the local anesthetic agent, anesthetize the skin and area around the artery. If time allows (approximately 1 hour before placing the catheter), a topical local anesthetic ointment (e.g., lidocaine + privacaine) can be used to anesthetize the skin surface. For injection, we use 1 or 2% lidocaine without epinephrine. After positioning the arm, inject the local anesthetic 1) intradermally above the artery; 2) subcutaneously just above the artery; and 3) subcutaneously on either side of the artery. The total amount should be about 1 to 2 ml, as excessive amounts of anesthetic can make palpation of the brachial pulse more difficult.

ARTERIAL PUNCTURE AND CATHETER INSERTION

1. Locate the artery between the fingers in the area of anesthesia.
2. Use a 19-gauge Cournand-style needle with the sharp, hollow stylus inserted.
3. Holding the needle by its shield, while keeping the stylus in the needle with one's thumb (be sure not to cover the hole in the stylus), penetrate the skin over the artery. Position the tip of the needle above the artery. Then abruptly insert the stylus and the needle tip into the artery.
4. When the tip of the stylus enters the artery, blood will flow out of the proximal hole in the stylus.
5. Advance the needle 1 mm to be sure that the tip of needle is in the artery (the stylus protrudes a little beyond the tip of the needle).
6. Remove the stylus. At this point, blood should shoot out of the needle with arterial pressure, indicating that the needle tip is well within the lumen of the artery. If blood does not flow readily, withdraw the needle slightly (it might have gone into the posterior wall of artery). Once a strong stream of arterial blood is evident,

it is safe to advance the needle further into the lumen of the artery using the continuous stream of blood to document the needle's position. The needle advance may be facilitated by depressing the hub slightly to reduce the possibility of impaling the posterior wall of the artery with the needle tip. Do not advance the needle without the stylus in place if there is no flow of blood. It may damage the artery.

7. If there is no blood flow, slowly withdraw the needle without the stylus because the needle tip may have passed through the inner wall of the artery. If there is still no blood flow, withdraw the tip of the needle to the skin. Clear the needle and stylus of any blood or clot, then try again.
8. With the needle tip in the lumen of the artery, documented by freely flowing blood, thread the guidewire for the catheter through the needle and slide it about 3 inches into the lumen of the artery. If the guidewire does not slip easily past the needle tip, the needle lumen is not centered in the lumen of the artery, and the needle must be repositioned. Do not try to advance the guidewire if any resistance is encountered.
9. Remove the needle, leaving the guidewire in place. To avoid a hematoma at the site, compress over the site at which the needle was inserted because the guidewire is narrow relative to the withdrawn needle.
10. Now slide the smoothly tapered end of the catheter over the wire. When the catheter reaches the skin, slide it through the skin and arterial wall using a gently rotating motion while holding the skin back so that it does not move with the catheter.
11. When the catheter position is well established several inches into the artery, remove the guidewire. Blood should readily flow out of the end of the catheter.
12. Attach a Luer-lock stopcock to the end of the catheter and flush the system immediately with heparinized saline.
13. Cover the site of insertion with sterile gauze and fix the catheter with tape.

DIFFICULT PUNCTURES

Limit yourself to 15 minutes of effort. If you are not successful by then, stop trying and ask someone with more experience to help or rely only on noninvasive measurements. The latter will provide a considerable amount of information.

APPENDIX E

Tables and Nomogram

TABLE E.1 Partial Pressure of Water of Saturated Gas at Centigrade Temperature T

T	P_{H_2O}	T	P_{H_2O}	T	P_{H_2O}
10	9.20	20	17.53	30	31.83
11	9.84	21	18.65	31	33.70
12	10.51	22	19.82	32	35.67
13	11.23	23	21.07	33	37.73
14	11.98	24	22.38	34	39.90
15	12.78	25	23.76	35	42.18
16	13.63	26	25.21	36	44.57
17	14.53	27	26.74	37	47.08
18	15.47	28	28.35	38	49.70
19	16.47	29	30.04	39	52.45
20	17.53	30	31.83	40	55.34

TABLE E.2. Factors for Conversion from ATPS to BTPS (37°C)

	T°C	16	17	18	19	20	21	22	23	24	25	26	27	28	29	30
	600	1.138	1.132	1.126	1.120	1.115	1.109	1.103	1.097	1.090	1.084	1.078	1.071	1.065	1.058	1.051
	610	1.136	1.131	1.125	1.119	1.114	1.108	1.102	1.096	1.090	1.083	1.077	1.071	1.064	1.058	1.051
	620	1.135	1.130	1.124	1.118	1.113	1.107	1.101	1.095	1.089	1.083	1.076	1.070	1.064	1.057	1.050
	630	1.134	1.129	1.123	1.117	1.112	1.106	1.100	1.094	1.083	1.082	1.076	1.069	1.063	1.056	1.050
	640	1.133	1.128	1.122	1.116	1.111	1.105	1.099	1.093	1.087	1.081	1.075	1.069	1.062	1.056	1.049
	650	1.132	1.127	1.121	1.116	1.110	1.104	1.098	1.092	1.087	1.081	1.074	1.068	1.062	1.056	1.049
	660	1.131	1.126	1.120	1.115	1.109	1.103	1.098	1.092	1.086	1.080	1.074	1.068	1.061	1.055	1.049
	670	1.130	1.125	1.119	1.114	1.108	1.103	1.097	1.091	1.085	1.079	1.073	1.067	1.061	1.055	1.048
	680	1.129	1.124	1.118	1.113	1.107	1.102	1.096	1.090	1.085	1.079	1.073	1.067	1.060	1.054	1.048
P_B	690	1.128	1.123	1.118	1.112	1.107	1.101	1.095	1.090	1.084	1.078	1.072	1.066	1.060	1.054	1.047
	700	1.128	1.122	1.117	1.111	1.106	1.100	1.095	1.089	1.083	1.077	1.072	1.066	1.059	1.053	1.047
	710	1.127	1.121	1.116	1.111	1.105	1.100	1.094	1.088	1.083	1.077	1.071	1.065	1.059	1.053	1.047
	720	1.126	1.121	1.115	1.110	1.104	1.099	1.093	1.088	1.082	1.076	1.070	1.065	1.059	1.052	1.046
	730	1.125	1.120	1.115	1.109	1.104	1.098	1.093	1.087	1.082	1.076	1.070	1.064	1.058	1.052	1.046
	740	1.124	1.119	1.114	1.109	1.103	1.098	1.092	1.087	1.081	1.075	1.070	1.064	1.058	1.052	1.046
	750	1.124	1.118	1.113	1.108	1.102	1.097	1.092	1.086	1.080	1.075	1.069	1.063	1.057	1.051	1.045
	760	1.123	1.118	1.113	1.107	1.102	1.096	1.091	1.086	1.080	1.074	1.069	1.063	1.057	1.051	1.045
	770	1.122	1.117	1.112	1.107	1.101	1.096	1.090	1.085	1.079	1.074	1.068	1.062	1.057	1.051	1.045
	780	1.122	1.116	1.111	1.106	1.101	1.095	1.090	1.084	1.079	1.073	1.068	1.062	1.056	1.050	1.044

T°C is ambient temperature in degrees centigrade; P_B is barometric pressure.

TABLE E.3. Factors for Conversion from ATPS to STPD

T°C	16	17	18	19	20	21	22	23	24	25	26	27	28	29	30
600	0.729	0.725	0.722	0.718	0.714	0.710	0.706	0.703	0.699	0.695	0.691	0.686	0.682	0.678	0.674
610	0.741	0.738	0.734	0.730	0.726	0.723	0.719	0.715	0.711	0.707	0.703	0.698	0.694	0.690	0.685
620	0.754	0.750	0.746	0.742	0.739	0.735	0.731	0.727	0.723	0.719	0.715	0.710	0.706	0.702	0.697
630	0.766	0.762	0.759	0.755	0.751	0.747	0.743	0.739	0.735	0.731	0.727	0.722	0.718	0.714	0.709
640	0.779	0.775	0.771	0.767	0.763	0.759	0.755	0.751	0.747	0.743	0.739	0.734	0.730	0.726	0.721
650	0.791	0.787	0.783	0.779	0.775	0.771	0.767	0.763	0.759	0.755	0.751	0.746	0.742	0.737	0.733
660	0.803	0.800	0.796	0.792	0.788	0.784	0.780	0.775	0.771	0.767	0.763	0.758	0.754	0.749	0.745
670	0.816	0.812	0.808	0.804	0.800	0.796	0.792	0.788	0.783	0.779	0.775	0.770	0.766	0.761	0.757
680	0.828	0.824	0.820	0.816	0.812	0.808	0.804	0.800	0.795	0.791	0.787	0.782	0.778	0.773	0.768
PB 690	0.841	0.837	0.833	0.829	0.824	0.820	0.816	0.812	0.807	0.803	0.799	0.794	0.790	0.785	0.780
700	0.853	0.849	0.845	0.841	0.837	0.832	0.828	0.824	0.820	0.815	0.811	0.806	0.802	0.797	0.792
710	0.866	0.861	0.857	0.853	0.849	0.845	0.840	0.836	0.832	0.827	0.823	0.818	0.813	0.809	0.804
720	0.878	0.874	0.870	0.865	0.861	0.857	0.853	0.848	0.844	0.839	0.835	0.830	0.825	0.821	0.816
730	0.890	0.886	0.882	0.878	0.873	0.869	0.865	0.860	0.856	0.851	0.847	0.842	0.837	0.833	0.828
740	0.903	0.899	0.894	0.890	0.886	0.881	0.877	0.872	0.868	0.863	0.859	0.854	0.849	0.844	0.840
750	0.915	0.911	0.907	0.902	0.898	0.894	0.889	0.885	0.880	0.875	0.871	0.866	0.861	0.856	0.851
760	0.928	0.923	0.919	0.915	0.910	0.906	0.901	0.897	0.892	0.887	0.883	0.878	0.873	0.868	0.863
770	0.940	0.936	0.931	0.927	0.923	0.918	0.913	0.909	0.904	0.900	0.895	0.890	0.885	0.880	0.875
780	0.953	0.948	0.944	0.939	0.935	0.930	0.926	0.921	0.916	0.912	0.907	0.902	0.897	0.892	0.887

T°C is ambient temperature in degrees centigrade; PB is barometric pressure.

TABLE E.4. Estimated $\dot{V}O_2$ for Various Activities

Activity	Estimated $\dot{V}O_2$ (ml/kg/min)	Activity	Estimated $\dot{V}O_2$ (ml/kg/min)
Basic postures		Hitching trailers, operating jacks or heavy levers	12.25
Sitting only (desk work, writing, calculating)	4.25	Masonry, painting, paperhanging	14.0
Standing only (bartending)	8.75		
Walking 3.0 mph	10.5	**Walking: moderate work**	
3.5 mph	14.0	Carrying trays, dishes	14.70
		Gas station mechanical work (changing tires, etc.)	15.75
Sitting: light or moderate work			
Driving a car	4.25	**Heavy arm work**	
Driving a truck	5.30	Lifting and carrying	
Hand tools, light assembly	5.30	(a) 20–44 lbs	15.75
Working heavy levers	7.0	(b) 45–64 lbs	21.0
Riding mower	8.75	(c) 65–84 lbs	26.25
Crane operator	8.75	(d) 85–100 lbs	29.75
Driving heavy truck (including frequent on and off with some arm work)	10.5		
		Heavy tools	
		Jackhammers, pneumatic drills	21.0
Standing: moderate work		Shovel, pick	28.0
Light assembly at slow pace	8.75		
Gas station operator	9.45	**Carpentry**	
Scrubbing, waxing, polishing (floors, walls)	9.45	Light interior repair (tile laying)	14.0
Heavy assembly (farm machinery, plumbing)	10.5	Building and finishing interior	15.75
Light welding	10.5	Putting in sidewalk	17.5
Stocking shelves (light objects)	10.5	Exterior remodeling (hammering, sawing)	21.0
Janitorial work	10.5		
Assembly line with light or medium parts at moderate pace	12.25	**Miscellaneous**	
		Pushing objects of 75 lb or more (desks, file cabinets)	28.0
Assembly line with brief lifting every 5 minutes (45 lbs or less)	12.25	Laying railroad track	24.5
Same as above (parts > 45 lbs)	14.0	Cutting trees—chopping wood	
		Hand saw	19.25
		Automatic	10.5

(From Tennessee Heart Association: Physician's Handbook for Evaluation of Cardiovascular and Physical Fitness. Nashville, Tennessee Heart Association, 1972; reprinted with permission.)

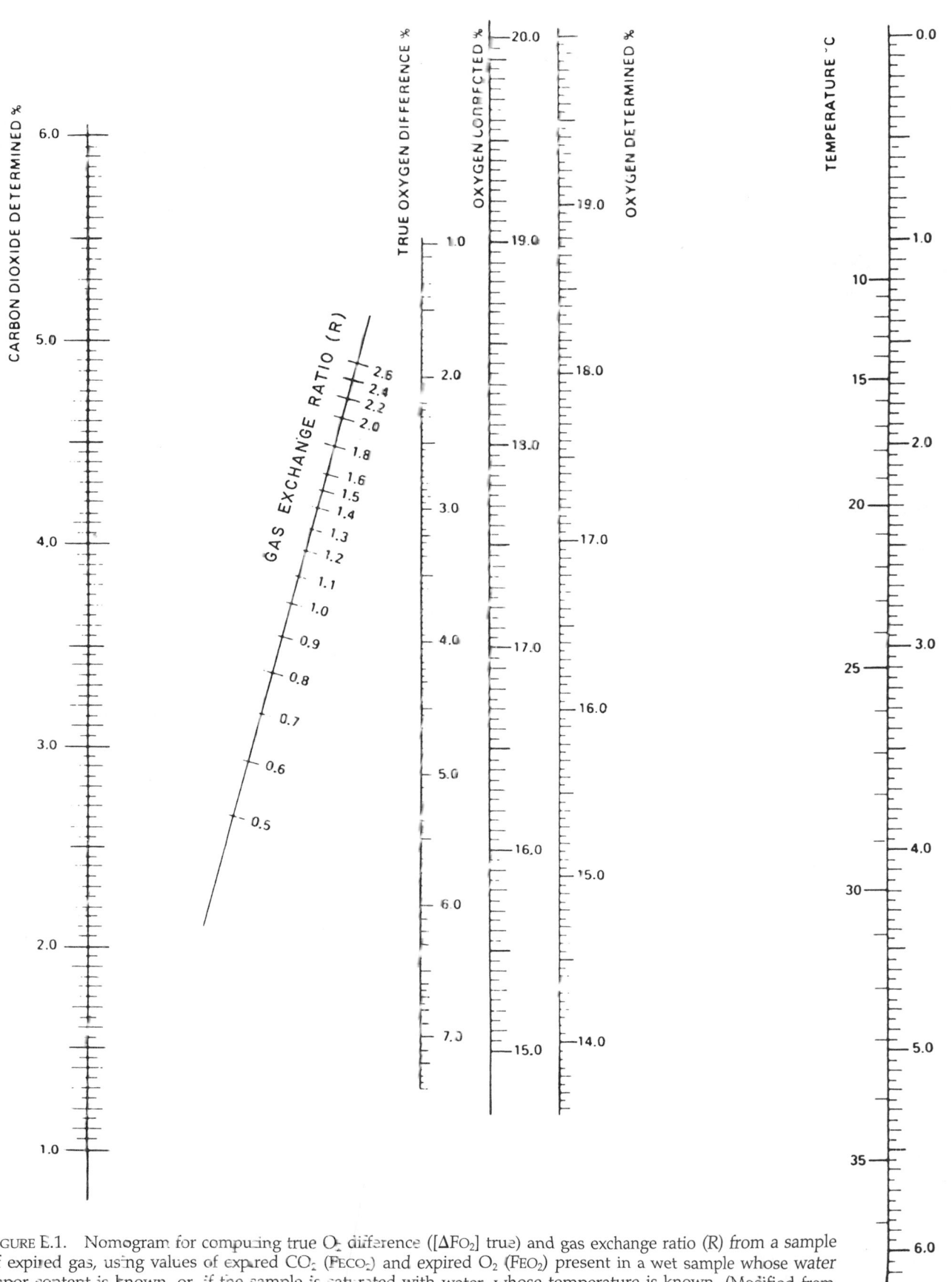

FIGURE E.1.   Nomogram for computing true O_2 difference ($[\Delta F_{O_2}]$ true) and gas exchange ratio (R) from a sample of expired gas, using values of expired CO_2 (F_{ECO_2}) and expired O_2 (F_{EO_2}) present in a wet sample whose water vapor content is known, or, if the sample is saturated with water, whose temperature is known. (Modified from Beaver WL. Water vapor corrections in oxygen consumption calculations. J Appl Physiol, 1973, 35:928–931.)

Index

Page numbers in *italic* indicate figures. Page numbers followed by "t" indicate tables.

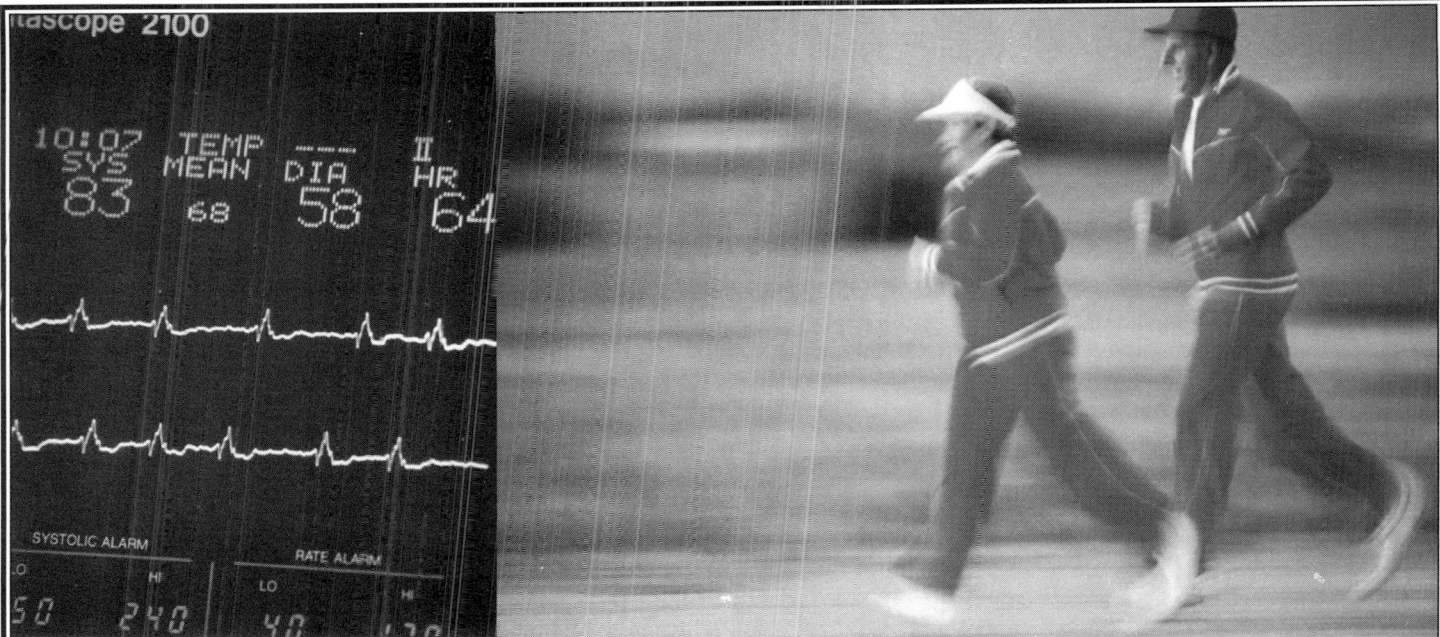
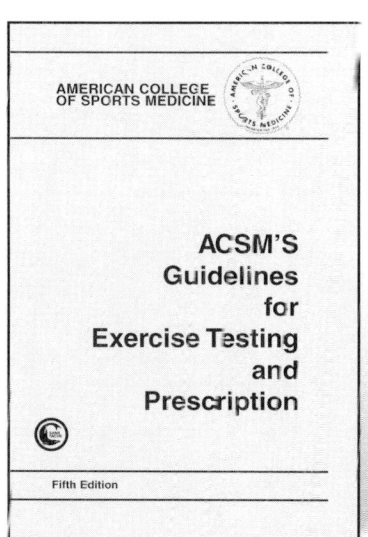
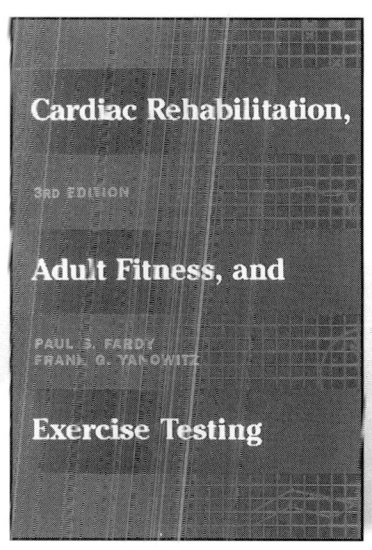
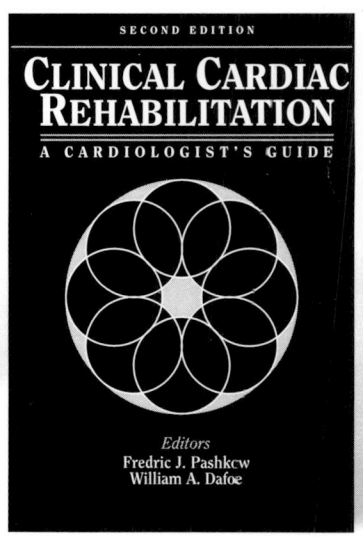
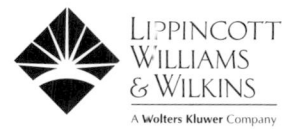